Medical
Problems in
Dentistry

Commissioning Editor: Alison Taylor
Development Editor: Clive Hewat
Project Manager: Hemamalini Rajendrababu/Bryan Potter
Designer: Charles Gray
Illustration Manager: Merlyn Harvey
Illustrator: Antbits

Medical Problems in Dentistry

6th EDITION

Professor Crispian Scully CBE

MD, PhD, MDS, MRCS, FDSRCS, FDSRCPS, FFDRCSI, FDSRCSE, FRCPath, FMedSci, FHEA, FUCL, DSc, DChD, DMed (HC), Dr HC

Professor of Special Care Dentistry, UCL – Eastman Dental Institute, London, UK
Professor of Oral Medicine, Pathology and Microbiology, University of London, UK
Visiting Professor at Universities of Edinburgh, Granada, Helsinki, Middlesex and West of England;
Honorary Consultant at University College Hospitals, London, UK; Great Ormond Street Hospital, London;
St. Savvas Hospital, Athens, Greece, and European Institute for Oncology, Milan, Italy

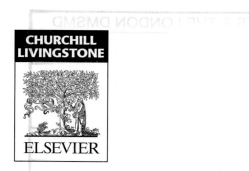

CHURCHILL LIVINGSTONE

ELSEVIER

EDINBURGH   LONDON   NEW YORK   OXFORD   PHILADELPHIA   ST LOUIS   SYDNEY   TORONTO 2010

CHURCHILL
LIVINGSTONE
ELSEVIER

Sixth Edition © 2010, Elsevier Limited. All rights reserved.

ISBN 9780702030574

British Library Cataloguing in Publication Data
A catalogue record for this book is available from the British Library

Library of Congress Cataloging in Publication Data
A catalog record for this book is available from the Library of Congress

Notice

Knowledge and best practice in this field are constantly changing. As new research and experience broaden our knowledge, changes in practice, treatment and drug therapy may become necessary or appropriate. Readers are advised to check the most current information provided (i) on procedures featured or (ii) by the manufacturer of each product to be administered, to verify the recommended dose or formula, the method and duration of administration, and contraindications. It is the responsibility of the practitioner, relying on their own experience and knowledge of the patient, to make diagnoses, to determine dosages and the best treatment for each individual patient, and to take all appropriate safety precautions. To the fullest extent of the law, neither the Publisher nor the Author assumes any liability for any injury and/or damage to persons or property arising out of or related to any use of the material contained in this book.

The Publisher

ELSEVIER your source for books, journals and multimedia in the health sciences

www.elsevierhealth.com

Working together to grow libraries in developing countries

www.elsevier.com | www.bookaid.org | www.sabre.org

ELSEVIER BOOK AID International Sabre Foundation

The Publisher's policy is to use **paper manufactured from sustainable forests**

Printed in China

PREFACE

The aim of this book is to provide a basis for the understanding of how general medical and surgical conditions influence oral health and oral healthcare. It is particularly relevant to dental professionals and other persons working in the oral healthcare sciences. The reader should thus be able to understand relevant illness identified from the history, physical examination, and investigations; be able to present a succinct and, where appropriate, unified list of all problems that could influence oral healthcare; and formulate a diagnosis/treatment plan for each problem (appropriate to the level of training). The reader should also be able to communicate appropriately with other healthcare providers; to retrieve medical information using the recommended further reading sections and computer, in a manner that reflects understanding of medical language, terminology, and the relationship among medical terms and concepts; to refine search strategies to improve relevance and completeness of retrieved items; and to identify and acquire full-text electronic documents available from the internet sites quoted.

Though dentistry remains largely a technical subject, there are a number of reasons why dental professionals should have this basis to their education and training. Dentistry is a profession and not a trade; medical problems can influence oral health and healthcare, whilst oral health and healthcare can influence general health and healthcare; dental professionals need to understand patients and their attitudes to healthcare; they need to communicate at a reasonable level with other health professionals and with patients and sometimes the media; dental professionals may need to act as advocates for patients; and, finally, dental professionals themselves can find themselves in need of healthcare. Since the first edition of this book, the importance of medicine in dentistry, interactions between medicine and dentistry, and the need for medical knowledge by the whole dental team have all radically increased – as has the whole of medicine.

The knowledge base of medicine has been extended and effective new technologies, techniques and drugs have been developed, many of which have resulted in complications relevant to oral healthcare. Many patients who would in earlier times have succumbed, are alive and live to much greater ages, thanks to advances such as public health improvements, transplants, pacemakers, radiotherapy and/or potent drugs – and they need good oral health and may well need oral healthcare. A wider range of medical problems has thus become relevant to oral healthcare sciences. The world has changed further and the relevance of the book has grown even more, with an increasing number of persons who require special care, and with increasing travel, not least by dental staff and trainees to developing countries. An ever increasing number of medical conditions also appear to be influenced by dental health and healthcare: the range of conditions possibly linked to periodontal disease (pre-eclampsia; pre-term and low birthweight babies; endometriosis; ischaemic heart disease; cerebrovascular disease; aspiration pneumonia; diabetes mellitus; metabolic syndrome; chronic kidney disease; osteoporosis; Alzheimer disease; pancreatic cancer; and even oral cancer) is a prime example.

In general terms, dental professionals need to develop strategies to identify patients at risk of medical problems, to assess the severity of those risks and, where necessary, recognize the need for help and be able to seek advice from a colleague with special competence in the relevant fields. This text has become one of the most widely used sources of information for all dental staff who need to contend with the increasing variety of medical problems, particularly as they are aware that they face a growing risk of litigation if they do not keep themselves familiar with current knowledge, in line with the increasing acceptance of the need for continuing professional education and development.

The management of patients with these various diseases should take into consideration the severity of the condition; the type of operative procedure envisioned, and in particular the amount of trauma, likely distress and time taken; other risk factors; and the healthcare setting (skills/facilities) available. Issues of access and informed consent, and the desirability of preventive oral healthcare and avoidance of harm, apply to virtually all situations. The comments and recommendations herein should be used as guidelines to care, not commandments. Unfortunately, there are very few randomized controlled trials available to provide evidence for the various practices, and so many of the recommendations have to be based on consensus. Since the fifth edition, my co-author for 25 years, Professor Rod Cawson, has sadly passed away. Nevertheless, the fact that this text had become a best-seller and prize-winner, and has provided probably the most comprehensive coverage available worldwide, stimulated me into renewed efforts to keep it abreast of the understanding of diseases and developments in medical and surgical care relevant to the oral healthcare sciences.

I have updated and re-organized the whole text. Key points have been added in relation to the most important medical conditions, and the focus on dentally relevant and changing areas has been increased. Much of the material is presented alphabetically in order to enhance access. This edition is, therefore, essentially a complete re-write and the opportunity has been used to remove the arrows inserted in the previous editions.

This edition now also includes, for the first time, a number of disorders not previously included, plus alternative and complementary medicine, health promotion, men's issues and occupational issues. Included in a number of new areas are autoinflammatory disorders, biological response modifiers, cosmetic procedures, craniofacial transplantation, drug reactions, drug-resistant microbial infections (nosocomial infections, tuberculosis and HIV), IgG$_4$-related plasmacytic disease, osteomyelitis, osteonecrosis, immune reconstitution syndrome and transgender issues. New illustrations have also been added, as well as selected recent references and up-to-date Internet websites. Eponymous conditions appear in a separate chapter. National and even international guidelines that have been beginning to appear have been included where considered relevant. In an effort to keep the size manageable, and the publisher happy, I have removed some of the less relevant material.

One of the major differences between most textbooks and original articles is that the latter are peer-reviewed. In an effort to try to enhance the quality of this edition, I have therefore sought peer review from an Advisory Board constituted from a group of specialist colleagues from the UK, who have scrutinized the material relevant to their particular areas of interest, to try to ensure that only accurate and contemporary material has been included, that there are no obvious deficits and that the latest advances have been incorporated. Nevertheless, any errors that might remain are mine, and readers should always check the most recent guidelines, drug doses, and potential reactions and interactions before use, discuss management issues with the patient, and never proceed with any intervention without the clear formal informed consent of the patient and consultation with their healthcare advisers.

This book has never purported to be a comprehensive textbook, particularly of oral physiology or oral medicine and pathology, though a considerable amount of relevant material is discussed herein. The content provided is for information and educational purposes only: in no way should it be considered as a substitute for medical consultation with a qualified professional. A physician should always be consulted for any health problem or medical condition. Commonly used acronyms such as BP (blood pressure), ECG (electrocardiogram), ESR (erythrocyte sedimentation rate); FBP (full blood picture), LA (local anaesthesia), GA (general anaesthesia), IHD (ischaemic heart disease), NSAIDS (non-steroidal anti-inflammatory drugs), CNS (central nervous system), CT (computed tomography), MRI (magnetic resonance imaging) and TMJ (temporomandibular joint) are not given full explanation on each occasion they appear. Clinicians are advised always to consult the latest guidelines from bodies such as the National Institute for Health and Clinical Excellence (NICE), the Royal Colleges of Surgeons, the Royal Colleges of Physicians, the British Dental Association (BDA), the General Dental Council (GDC), the Resuscitation Council and those of the various specialist medical and dental societies or associations. The increasing spectre of litigation increasingly influences decisions and, although in some instances guidelines may have not led to clarity, clinicians may find their decisions difficult to defend if they fail to record very good reason for not adhering to the guidelines. Further information can be found on the Internet (all sites were verified 1 August 2009 and many have been used to source material), or in recent texts, such as:

- http://health.nih.gov/
- http://www.nlm.nih.gov/medlineplus/medlineplus.html
- http://www.mayoclinic.com/health/diseases/index
- http://www.cochrane.org
- http://emedicine.medscape.com
- http://www.rcseng.ac.uk/fds
- http://en.wikipedia.org/wiki/
- http://www.dh.gov.uk/
- http://www.cancerbackup.org.uk/Home
- http://www.sign.ac.uk/index.html
- http://www.library.nhs.uk/default.aspx
- Oral and Maxillofacial Diseases (Scully C, Flint SF, Porter SR, Moos K, 2010. Dunitz, Taylor & Francis, London)

I am especially grateful to the Editorial Advisory Board for their advice on this edition, and to Dr Athanasios Kalantzis for his helpful suggestions on the previous edition. Drs Oslei Paes de Almeida, Jose Vicente Bagan, Pedro diz Dios, and Andy Wolff have, through various discussions, been helpful. I am also grateful to Dr David Croser, Dr Francesco D'Aiuto, Mrs Lesley Derry, Dr Janice Fiske, Professor Stephen Flint, Professor Mark Griffiths, Dr Anne Hegarty, Dr Stephen Henderson, Dr Kevin Johnston, Mr David Koppel, Dr Samintharaj Kumar, Professor Kursheed Moos, Professor Jonathan Sandy and Dr Rosie Shotts for other helpful comments, and to John Evans for assistance. I am, as always, grateful to Dental Protection for guidance.

I am grateful to Professor Peter Simpson (Royal College of Anaesthetists) and the late Professor John Lowry (Standing Dental Advisory Committee) for their permission to reproduce the SDAC Executive Summary on Conscious Sedation; to the Health and Safety Executive for permission to use material from their website on latex allergy; to Dr Christine Randall for material on endocarditis prophylaxis; and to C Kurt-Gabel, L Taylor & Dr C Howard, Directors of A to E Training & Solutions Ltd, for their help and advice on the management of medical emergencies (the treatment algorithms, reproduced with their permission, were developed as part of the A to E Medical Emergencies in Dental Practice course [info@ atoetraininigandsolutions.co.uk]). Dr Mike Rubens, Ms Lesley Garlick, Professor Rodney Grahame, Dr Navdeep Kumar, Dr Mohamed El-Maaytah, Professor Stephen Flint, Professor Stephen Porter, Professor John Langdon and Professor Jonathan Shepherd have kindly helped with some of the illustrations.

Any comments or criticisms from readers will of course be gratefully received, though I hope that the further significant improvements in this edition, together with the dearth of criticism of previous editions, means that I have fulfilled the aims as best I can. As Rod Cawson said in the preface to one of his other books: "Some people will criticize this for being too brief, some for being too long but, sad as it may be, this is the best I can do".

Crispian Scully
London
2010

CONTENTS

EDITORIAL ADVISORY BOARD

SECTION

GENERAL

MEDICAL EMERGENCIES

The knowledge base of medicine has been extended, and effective new technologies, techniques and drugs have been developed. This has allowed patients, who in earlier times would have succumbed, to remain alive and live to much greater ages; such patients may be prone to medical emergencies.

Collapse or other emergencies in the dental surgery are a cause for anxiety for all involved Atherton et al., 1999a (Box 1.1).

This chapter is limited to the main diagnostic and management issues in emergency management for easy reference; fuller discussion of these conditions can be found in the relevant chapters. In general terms, dental professionals need to develop strategies to identify patients at risk of such medical emergencies, to assess the severity of those risks and, where necessary, recognize the need for help and be able to seek advice from a colleague with special competence in the relevant fields. All dental staff need to contend with the increasing variety of medical problems, particularly as they are aware that they face a growing risk of litigation if they do not keep themselves familiar with current knowledge, in line with the increasing acceptance of the need for continuing professional education and development.

The comments and recommendations herein should be used as guidelines to care, not commandments. Unfortunately, there are very few randomized controlled trials available to provide evidence for the various practices, and so many of the recommendations have to be based on consensus.

Annual theoretical and practical training of all clinical staff is required to manage these rare events effectively. Clinical dental staff have an obligation to be conversant with the current Resuscitation Council (UK) guidelines (2006 revised 2008) (see Further reading). The UK General Dental Council (GDC), in *Standards for dental professionals* and associated supplementary guidance (2005; see Useful websites), states that all dental professionals are responsible for putting patients' interests first, and acting to protect them. Central to this responsibility is the need to ensure that they are able to deal with medical emergencies that may arise. All members of the dental team need to know their roles in the event of an emergency. GDC guidance *Principles of dental team working* states that dental staff who employ, manage or lead a team should make sure that:

- there are arrangements for at least two people to be available to deal with medical emergencies when treatment is planned to take place
- all members of staff, not just the registered team members, know their role if a patient collapses or there is another kind of medical emergency
- all members of staff who might be involved in dealing with a medical emergency are trained and prepared to deal with such an emergency at any time, and regularly practise simulated emergencies together.

The GDC has stipulated that 10 hours of training and retraining in emergency management is a mandatory requirement of continuing professional development in every 5-year period.

The most common medical emergencies apart from the simple faint are fitting in an epileptic patient, angina pectoris (ischaemic chest pain), hypoglycaemia in a diabetic patient and haemorrhage. Myocardial infarction and cardiopulmonary arrest are more immediately dangerous, but fortunately less common (Box 1.2).

Emergencies are rare, occurring at rates of 0.7 cases per dentist per year (Girdler and Smith, 1999) or once every 3–4 years (Atherton et al., 1999b). A medical emergency occurring in dental practice is most likely to be the result of an acute deterioration of a known medical condition. It may pose an immediate threat to an individual's life and needs rapid intervention. It is best prevented!

PREVENTION

Emergency management algorithms are of paramount importance and dentists are ultimately responsible for the performance of their staff in delivery.

Confidence and satisfactory management of emergencies can be improved by the following.

- Repeatedly assessing the patient whilst undertaking treatment, noting any changes in appearance or behaviour.
- Never practising dentistry without another competent adult in the room.

Box 1.1 Common emergencies

- Collapse
- Chest pain
- Shortness of breath
- Mental disturbances
- Reactions to drugs or sedation
- Bleeding

Box 1.2 Likely causes of sudden loss of consciousness and collapse

- Simple faint
- Diabetic collapse secondary to hypoglycaemia
- Epileptic seizure
- Anaphylaxis
- Cardiac arrest
- Stroke
- Adrenal crisis

- Always having accessible the telephone numbers for the emergency services and nearest hospital accident and emergency department. The patient's general medical practitioner details should be recorded in the notes.
- Training staff in emergency service contact protocols and emergency procedures: this should be repeated annually. All dental clinics should have a defined protocol for how the emergency services are to be alerted. The protocol should include clear directions for the emergency services to locate and access the clinic and, in a large building, a member of the team should meet the paramedics at the main entrance.
- Having a readily accessible emergency drugs box and equipment checked on a weekly basis (Table 1.1 and Figs 1.1–1.3).
- Taking a careful medical history, assessment of disease severity, careful treatment scheduling and planning and, in some cases, administration of medication prior to treatment.

- Using the simple intervention of laying the patient supine prior to giving local analgesia (LA) will prevent virtually all simple faints – the commonest emergency.
- Ensuring diabetic patients have had their normal meals, appropriately administered medication, and are treated early in the morning session or immediately after lunch is likely to prevent hypoglycaemic collapse.

All this is particularly important when sedation is used, when there are invasive or painful procedures, or when medically complex individuals are being treated. 'Forewarned is forearmed', and dental practitioners must ensure that medical and drug histories are updated at each visit prior to initiating treatment. It is suggested disease severity should be assessed using a risk stratification system, for example the American Society of Anesthesiologists (ASA) classification (see Chs. 2 and 3). This may help identify high-risk individuals.

Few emergencies can be treated definitively in the dental surgery, and the role of the dental team is one of support

Table 1.1 Suggested minimal equipment and drugs for emergency use in dentistry (after Resuscitation Council, 2006).

Equipment	General comments	Detail
Oxygen (O$_2$) delivery	Portable apparatus for administering oxygen Oxygen face (non-rebreathe type) mask with tube Basic set of oropharyngeal airways (sizes 1, 2, 3 and 4) Pocket mask with oxygen port Self-inflating bag valve mask (BVM; 1-L size bag), where staff have been appropriately trained Variety of well-fitting adult and child face masks for attaching to self-inflating bag	Two portable oxygen cylinders (D size) with pressure reduction valves and flow meters. Cylinders should be of sufficient size to be easily portable but also allow for adequate flow rates (e.g. 10L/min, until the arrival of an ambulance or the patient fully recovers. A full 'D' size cylinder contains 340L of oxygen and should allow a flow rate of 10L/min for up to 30 minutes. Two such cylinders may be necessary to ensure the oxygen supply does not fail
Portable suction	Portable suction with appropriate suction catheters and tubing (e.g. the Yankauer sucker)	
Spacer device for inhalation of bronchodilators		
Automated external defibrillator (AED)	All clinical areas should have immediate access to an AED (Collapse to shock time less than 3 minutes)	
Automated blood glucose measuring device		
Equipment for administering drugs intramuscularly	Single-use sterile syringes (2-ml and 10-ml sizes) and needles (19 and 21 sizes)	Drugs as below
Emergency	**Drugs required**	**Dosages for adults**
Anaphylaxis	Adrenaline (epinephrine) injection 1:1000, 1 mg/ml	Intramuscular adrenaline (0.5 ml of 1 in 1000 solution) Repeat at 5 minutes if needed
Hypoglycaemia	Oral glucose solution/tablets/gel/powder [e.g. 'GlucoGel®' formerly known as 'Hypostop®' gel (40% dextrose)] Glucagon injection 1 mg (e.g. GlucaGen HypoKit)	Proprietary non-diet drink or 5 g glucose powder in water Intramuscular glucagon 1 mg
Acute exacerbation of asthma	(Beta-2 agonist) Salbutamol aerosol inhaler 100 mcg/activation	Salbutamol aerosol Activations directly or up to six into a spacer
Status epilepticus	Buccal or intranasal midazolam 10 mg/ml	Midazolam 10 mg
Angina	Glyceryl trinitrate[a] spray 400 mcg/metered activation	Glyceryl trinitrate, two sprays
Myocardial infarct	Dispersible aspirin 300 mg	Dispersible aspirin 300 mg (chewed)

No corticosteroid is included.
[a]Do not use nitrates to relieve an angina attack if the patient has recently taken sildenafil as there may be a precipitous fall in blood pressure; analgesics should be used. Where possible, all emergency equipment should be single use and latex free. The kit does not include any intravenous injections

and considered intervention using algorithms that can 'do no harm'. Previously it has been suggested that 20 or more drugs should be available to the dental surgeon for the management of emergencies but this is impractical, may be a source of confusion and, if incorrectly administered, life threatening. The Resuscitation Council (2006) recommendations for equipment and drugs are detailed in Table 1.1.

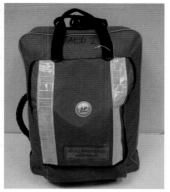

Fig. 1.1 Emergency kit

30 chest compressions 2 breaths

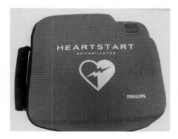

Fig. 1.2 Automatic defibrillator

Other agents (e.g. flumazenil) and equipment (e.g. a pulse oximeter) are needed if conscious sedation is administered. General anaesthesia (GA) must only be undertaken by anaesthetists and where advanced life support (ALS) is available.

MANAGING EMERGENCIES

For all medical emergencies, a structured approach to assessment and reassessment prevents any symptoms and signs being missed and any incorrect diagnoses being made. The sequence is best remembered as 'ABCDE' (Box 1.3).

Dental staff should be trained in basic cardiopulmonary resuscitation (CPR) so that, in the event of cardiac arrest, they should be able to:

- recognize cardiac arrest
- summon immediate help (dial for the emergency services)
- initiate CPR according to current resuscitation guidelines (evidence suggests that chest compressions can be effectively performed in a dental chair)
- ventilate with high-concentration oxygen via a bag and mask
- apply an automated external defibrillator (AED) as soon as possible after collapse. Follow the machine prompts and administer a shock if indicated with a maximum collapse to shock time of 3 minutes.

EMERGENCY PROCEDURE

- Call for local assistance.
- Assess patient – ABCDE (as Box 1.3) – and give oxygen if appropriate.

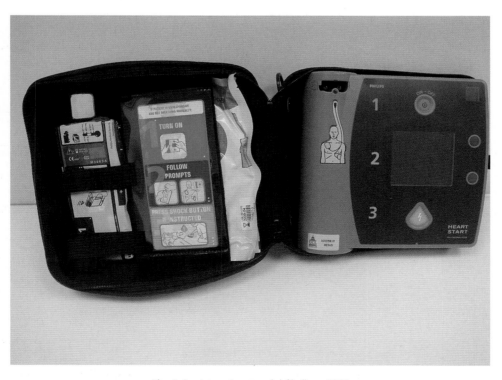

Fig. 1.3 Automatic external defibrillator (AED)

- Use acronym MOVE:

  Monitor – reassess ABCDE regularly, attach AED if appropriate

  Oxygen – 15 L/min through non-rebreathe mask

  Verify emergency services are coming

  Emergency action – correct positioning and drug administration.

Intramuscular (i.m.) injection is nowadays used for giving emergency drugs. The most accessible site in a clothed patient sitting in a dental chair is the lateral aspect of the thigh. The vastus lateralis is a large muscle with no large nerves or arteries running through it. In an emergency, the injection can be administered through clothing. The mid point between the pelvis and the knee is the preferred site.

The Advanced Medical Priority Dispatch System (AMPDS) is a medically approved, unified system used to despatch appropriate aid to medical emergencies including systematized caller interrogation and pre-arrival instructions. AMPDS gives a main response category:

- A (immediately life-threatening)
- B (urgent call)
- C (routine call).

This may well be linked to a performance targeting system where calls must be responded to within a given time period. For example, in the UK, calls rated as 'A' on AMPDS are targeted with getting a responder on scene within 8 minutes.

COLLAPSE (Table 1.2)

The cause of sudden loss of consciousness may be suggested by the medical history:

- collapse at the sight of a needle or during an injection is likely to be a simple faint
- following some minutes after an injection of penicillin, collapse is more likely to be due to anaphylaxis
- collapse of a diabetic at lunchtime, for example, is likely to be caused by hypoglycaemia
- collapse of a patient with angina or previous myocardial infarction may be caused by a new or further myocardial infarction.

The clinical features of the episode may also aid diagnosis; for example, severe chest pain suggests a cardiac cause. A structured and systematic assessment regardless of perceived causative factors is required to mitigate management errors.

Box 1.3 Assessment in emergencies

Airway	Identify foreign body obstruction and stridor
Breathing	Document respiratory rate, use of accessory muscles, presence of wheeze or cyanosis
Circulation	Assess skin colour and temperature, estimate capillary refill time (normally, this is 2 seconds with hand above heart), assess rate of pulse (normal is 70 beats/min)
Disability	Assess conscious level by acronym **60-100**: • **A**lert • responds to **V**oice • responds to **P**ainful stimulus • Blood glucose **U**nresponsive
Exposure	Respecting the patient's dignity, try to elicit the cause of acute deterioration (e.g. rash, or signs of recreational drug use)

Table 1.2 Common emergencies

Emergency	1. Call for assistance	2. Give oxygen	3. Other main actions	4. Alert emergency services
Anaphylaxis	Yes	Yes	Adrenaline i.m. (0.5 ml of 1 in 1000 adrenaline) Legs up position	Yes
Angina	Yes	Yes	Glyceryl trinitrate sublingually	Only if no spontaneous recovery after action (3)
Asthma exacerbation	Yes	Yes	Sit patient up and forwards, salbutamol inhaled via spacer	Only if no spontaneous recovery after action (3)
Cardiac arrest	Yes	Yes	CPR	Yes
Choking	Yes	Yes	Back slap five times, then abdominal thrust five times	Only if no spontaneous recovery after action (3)
Epileptic fit	Yes	Yes	Protect patient from harm Consider midazolam i.m. or sublingually/buccal mucosa	Only if no spontaneous recovery after 5 minutes, persistent altered conscious state or the fit characteristics are different to those previously described
Faint	Yes	No*	Lay patient flat	Only if no spontaneous recovery after action (3)
Hypoglycaemia	Yes	Yes	Glucose If unconscious, glucagon i.m.	Only if no spontaneous recovery after action (3)
Myocardial infarction	Yes	Yes	Aspirin chewed	Yes

CPR, cardiopulmonary resuscitation; i.m., intramuscular.
*But oxygen will do harm

The principles of the *chain of survival*, which applies to emergencies where the patient is not breathing and has no pulse, involve four stages:

- early recognition and call for help
- early CPR
- early defibrillation; and
- early advanced life support.

Simple faint

Fainting (syncope) is the most common cause of sudden loss of consciousness. It is associated with a loss of postural tone, with spontaneous recovery. Up to 2% of patients may faint before or during dental treatment. Young, fit, adult males in particular are prone to faint, especially before, during and after injections.

Vasovagal (vasodepressor) attack (or pressure on the vagus) is the usual cause of a simple faint. The diagnosis rests on the history, upright posture, an emotional or painful stimulus, gradual not sudden fading of consciousness, sweating, nausea, pallor, other manifestations of autonomic activity, and rapid recovery on lying down. Simple faints tend to occur, and recur, in young people.

Other causes of sudden loss of consciousness include:

- Situational syncope provoked by coughing, micturition or postural change.
- Sudden cardiac syncope due to arrhythmia or circulatory obstruction – typically in older people.
- Orthostatic hypotension.
- Neurological disorders.

which should be considered in the differential diagnosis.

Predisposing factors for vasovagal attack include:

- anxiety
- pain
- fatigue
- fasting (rarely)
- high temperature and relative humidity.

Signs and symptoms of a simple faint include:

- premonitory dizziness, weakness or nausea
- pallor
- cold clammy skin
- dilated pupils
- pulse is initially slow and weak, then rapid and full
- loss of consciousness.

The simple precaution of laying patients flat *before* giving injections will prevent fainting. Very rarely patients, can suffer *malignant vasovagal syncope* with recurrent, severe and otherwise unexplained syncope, and their clinical history is intermediate between that of vasovagal and cardiac syncope and diagnosis confirmed by tilt test.

Management

- Lie individuals flat, ideally with their legs raised.
- Leave them in this position until fully recovered.
- Slowly return the chair to the upright position.

- Record that the event occurred and identify the likely cause.
- Aim to prevent further episodes.

Anaphylaxis

- Always detail known allergies and the severity of any previous type 1 hypersensitivity reactions.
- Avoid possible allergens and, when this is not possible, refer for specialist assessment.
- Life-threatening anaphylaxis may occur despite no previous history of allergen exposure.
- Anaphylaxis is the most severe allergic response and manifests with acute hypotension, bronchospasm, urticaria rash and angioedema (Fig. 1.4).
- The causal agents include:
  penicillins – the most common cause, but also other antimicrobials (cephalosporins, sulfonamides, tetracyclines, vancomycin)
  latex
  muscle relaxants
  non-steroidal anti-inflammatory drugs (NSAIDs)
  opiates
  radiographic contrast media
  others – vaccines, immunoglobulins, various foods and insect bites.
- Strict avoidance of the causal agent is essential.
- Where there is a previous history of anaphylaxis, the patient should carry a self-administered i.m. injection device, for example EpiPen® (ALK-Abelló, Hungerford, Berkshire, UK) or Twinject® (Verus Pharmaceuticals, San Diego, California, USA) (or less commonly epinephrine aerosol, such as MedihalerEpi). The standard dosage of epinephrine supplied by an EpiPen for adults is 0.3 ml of 1 in 1000 (0.3 mg). Child-sized dosages (0.15 mg) are available as the EpiPen JR.
- Diagnosis is as follows:
  facial flushing, itching, paraesthesiae, oedema or sometimes urticaria, or peripheral cold clammy skin
  stridor or wheeze
  abdominal pain, nausea
  loss of consciousness
  pallor going on to cyanosis
  rapid, weak or impalpable pulse.

Cardiac arrest

- Cardiac arrest can occur in a patient with no previous history of cardiac problems, but is more likely in those with a history of ischaemic heart disease, diabetics and older people.
- Previous angina or myocardial infarction predisposes to cardiac arrest.
- Ventricular fibrillation accounts for most sudden cardiac arrests. Causes are myocardial infarction, hypoxia, drug overdose, anaphylaxis or severe hypotension.
- After airway and breathing assessment, basic life support (BLS) needs to be initiated immediately to maintain adequate cerebral perfusion until the underlying cause is reversed (Fig. 1.5).

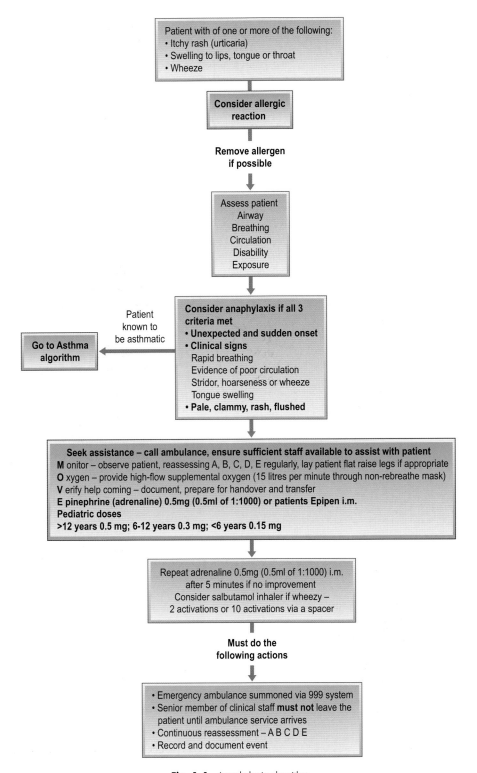

Fig. 1.4 Anaphylaxis algorithm

- Basic life support comprises:
  initial assessment
  airway maintenance
  chest compression
  ventilation.

Management

See Figs 1.5 and 1.6.

Diabetic collapse: hypoglycaemia

- Hypoglycaemia is the most dangerous complication of diabetes mellitus because the brain becomes starved of glucose.
- Diabetics treated with insulin, those with poor blood glucose control or poor awareness of their hypoglycaemic episodes have a greater chance of losing consciousness.
- Remember a collapse in a diabetic may be caused by other emergencies, for example a faint or myocardial infarction.

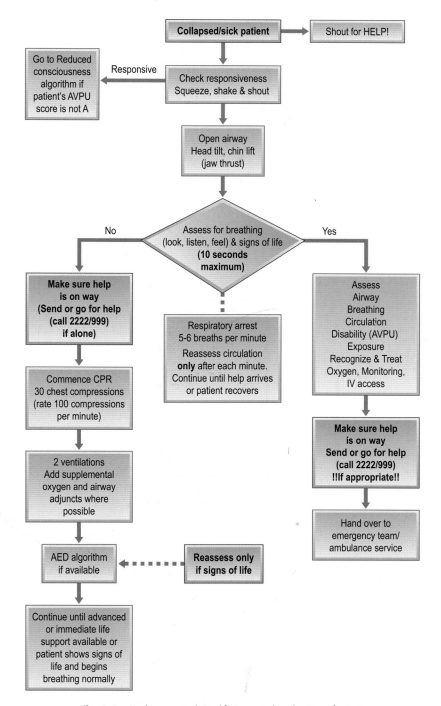

Fig. 1.5 Cardiac arrest – basic life support algorithm (*see fig 1.6)

Ischaemic heart disease is common in long-standing diabetes.

- Hypoglycaemia may present as a deepening drowsiness, disorientation, excitability or aggressiveness, especially if it is known that a meal has been missed.
- A management algorithm is provided in Fig. 1.7.

Fitting

- Fits are usually seen in known epileptics.
- Various factors may precipitate a fit including not eating, cessation of anticonvulsant therapy, menstruation

and some drugs, such as alcohol, flumazenil or tricyclic antidepressants.

- Fits may also affect people with no history of epilepsy, especially following hypoxia from loss of consciousness for other reasons, or in hypoglycaemia.
- Diagnosis of a tonic-clonic (Grand/mal) seizure:
  loss of consciousness with rigid, extended body, which is sometimes preceded by a brief cry
  widespread jerking movements
  possible incontinence of urine and/or faeces
  slow recovery with the patient sometimes remaining dazed (post-ictal).

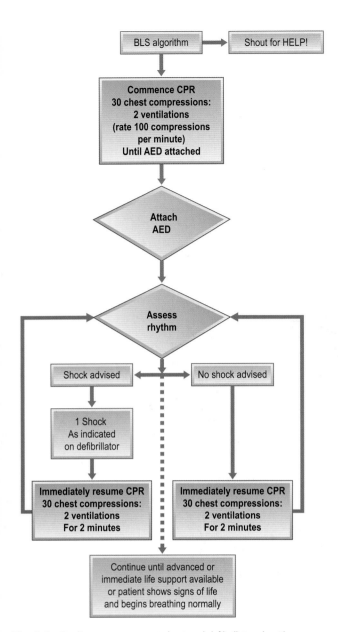

Fig. 1.6 Cardiac arrest – automated external defibrillator algorithm

- A management algorithm for the fitting patient is shown in Fig. 1.8.

Chest pain

- Acute severe chest pain is usually caused by angina or, less commonly, myocardial infarction.
- Patients with 'unstable' angina and those with a recent history of hospital admission for ischaemic chest pain have the highest risk, and should not be considered for routine dental treatment in primary care.
- Diagnostic features include:
  severe crushing retrosternal pain radiating down the left arm
  breathlessness but may be described as 'heartburn'
  vomiting and loss of consciousness if there is an infarct
  pulse may be weak or irregular if there is an infarct.
- Management is detailed in Fig. 1.9.

Shortness of breath

Acute severe asthma

- Anxiety, infection, or exposure to an allergen or drugs may precipitate asthma.
- High-risk asthmatics include those individuals:
  taking oral medication in addition to inhaled β_2 agonists and corticosteroids
  who regularly use a nebulizer at home
  who have required oral steroids for their asthma within the last year
  who have been admitted to hospital with asthma within the last year.
- Diagnostic features are:
  breathlessness
  expiratory wheeze
  use of accessory muscles – shrugging shoulders with each respiratory cycle with increased severity
  rapid pulse (usually over 110/min) with increasing severity but this may slow in life-threatening exacerbation.
- Management is detailed in Fig. 1.10

Foreign body respiratory obstruction

Causes of respiratory obstruction include laryngeal spasm and foreign body. Although these may occur in any individual, the sedated patient poses a significant risk. Prevention of foreign body inhalation, including teeth, crowns, filling materials or endodontic instruments is far better than the event occurring. At the least, such an event causes great embarrassment, at worst respiratory obstruction, lung abscess or death. Use a rubber dam.

Diagnosis is as follows:

- breathing is irregular with crowing or croaking on inspiration
- violent respiratory efforts using accessory muscles
- deepening cyanosis.

Management is as follows (see Fig. 1.11):

- Inspect and clear the airway by suction or a finger sweep.
- If the patient cannot cough out the object, use back slaps or an abdominal thrust (formerly termed the Heimlich manoeuvre) to clear the airway (Fig. 1.12)
- If the obstruction is not in the pharynx but lower in the respiratory tract, endoscopy or tracheostomy may be needed.
- Give oxygen.
- Reassure the patient.

LESS COMMON EMERGENCIES

Stroke

- Stroke may rarely occur in apparently healthy patients, but is more common in older and hypertensive individuals. A history of stroke predisposes to a further event.

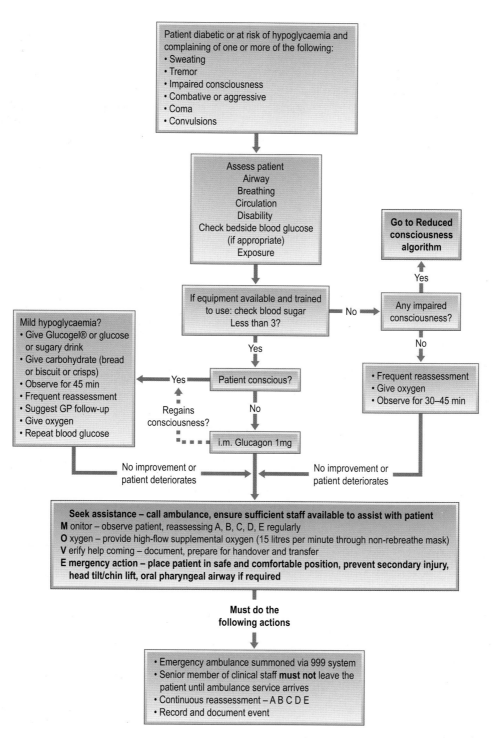

Fig. 1.7 Hypoglycaemia algorithm

- Diagnosis varies with the size and site of brain damage but typically includes:
  loss of consciousness
  unilateral weakness of the arm and leg
  facial palsy.
- Management details are shown in Box 1.4.

Adrenal crisis: collapse of a patient with a history of corticosteroid therapy

- Collapse in a patient with Addison disease or a history of systemic corticosteroid therapy may be caused by adrenal insufficiency,

triggered by general anaesthesia, trauma, infections or other stress, but has never been recorded in primary dental care.
- Prevention of this emergency is contentious and will be dealt with in Ch. 6.
- Diagnosis is as follows:
  pallor
  pulse – rapid, weak or impalpable
  loss of consciousness
  rapidly falling blood pressure.
- Management is detailed in Fig. 1.13.

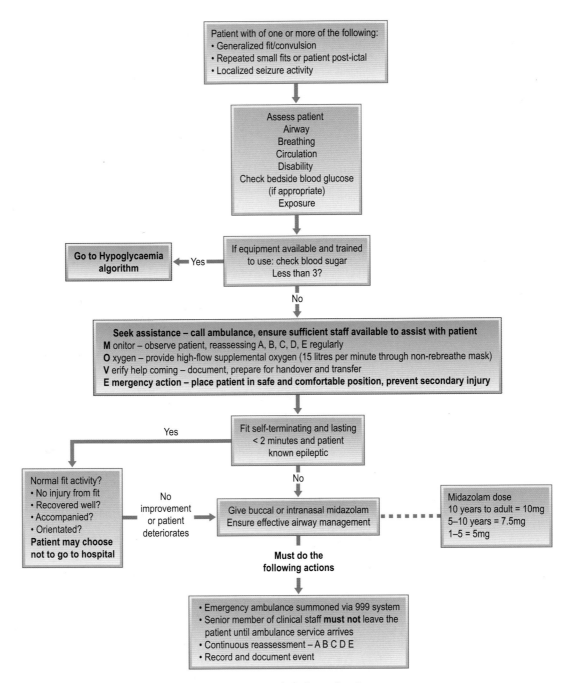

Fig. 1.8 Fitting/convulsions algorithm

REACTIONS TO DRUGS OR SEDATION

Intravascular injection of local anaesthetic agent

Diagnostic features may include:

- agitation
- confusion
- drowsiness
- fitting
- eventually loss of consciousness.

Management is detailed in Box 1.5.

Temporary facial palsy, diplopia or localized facial pallor

- These occur rarely as a result of the anaesthetic agent acting on the facial nerve or orbital contents and the transient effects resolve.
- If the individual is unable to blink, the eyelids should be taped closed until the anaesthetic abates.

Local anaesthetic allergy

Allergy to LA is managed as for anaphylaxis, but is very rare.

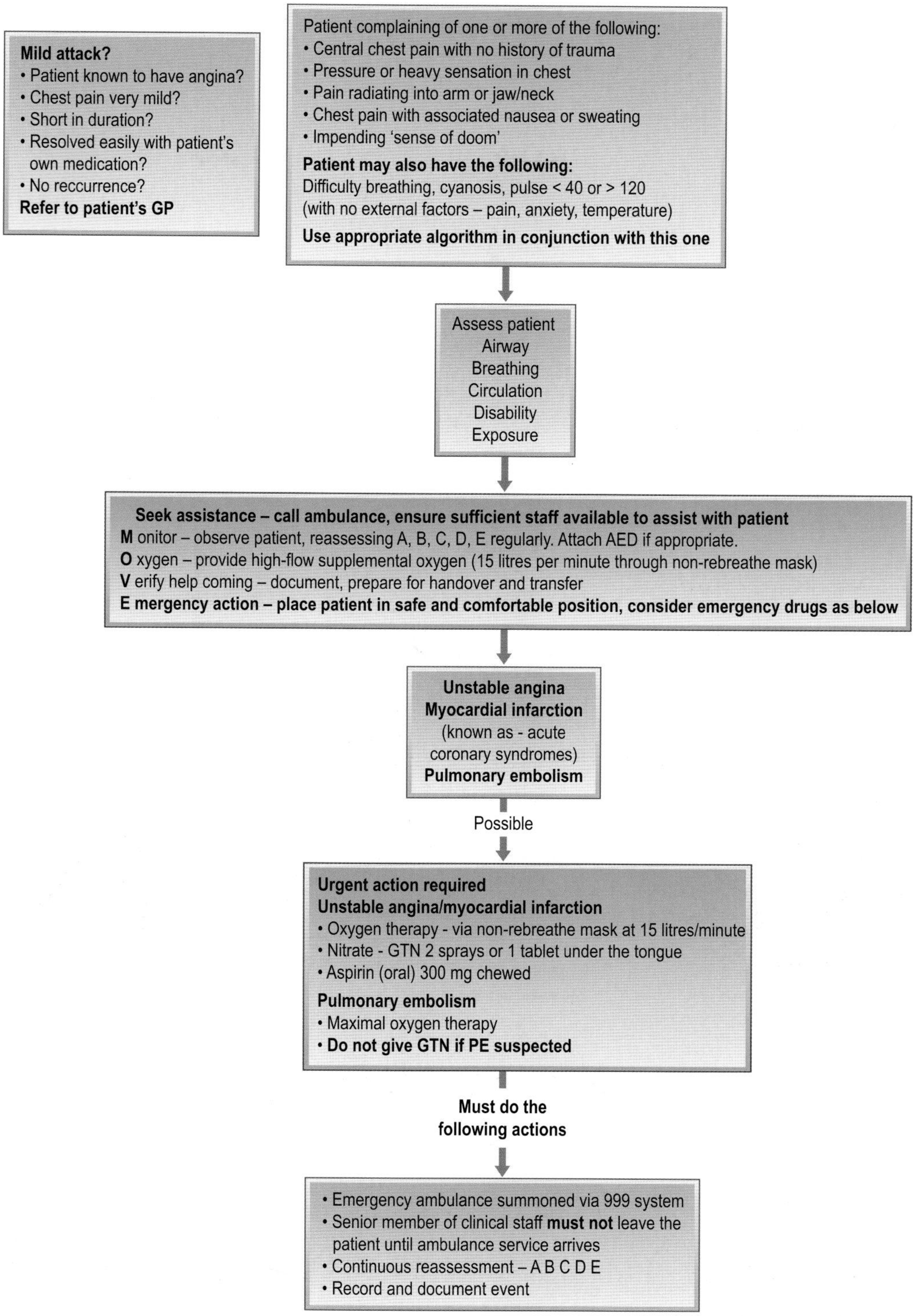

Mild attack?
• Patient known to have angina?
• Chest pain very mild?
• Short in duration?
• Resolved easily with patient's own medication?
• No reccurrence?
Refer to patient's GP

Patient complaining of one or more of the following:
• Central chest pain with no history of trauma
• Pressure or heavy sensation in chest
• Pain radiating into arm or jaw/neck
• Chest pain with associated nausea or sweating
• Impending 'sense of doom'
Patient may also have the following:
Difficulty breathing, cyanosis, pulse < 40 or > 120
(with no external factors – pain, anxiety, temperature)

Use appropriate algorithm in conjunction with this one

Assess patient
Airway
Breathing
Circulation
Disability
Exposure

Seek assistance – call ambulance, ensure sufficient staff available to assist with patient
M onitor – observe patient, reassessing A, B, C, D, E regularly. Attach AED if appropriate.
O xygen – provide high-flow supplemental oxygen (15 litres per minute through non-rebreathe mask)
V erify help coming – document, prepare for handover and transfer
E mergency action – place patient in safe and comfortable position, consider emergency drugs as below

Unstable angina
Myocardial infarction
(known as - acute
coronary syndromes)
Pulmonary embolism

Possible

Urgent action required
Unstable angina/myocardial infarction
• Oxygen therapy - via non-rebreathe mask at 15 litres/minute
• Nitrate - GTN 2 sprays or 1 tablet under the tongue
• Aspirin (oral) 300 mg chewed
Pulmonary embolism
• Maximal oxygen therapy
• **Do not give GTN if PE suspected**

Must do the
following actions

• Emergency ambulance summoned via 999 system
• Senior member of clinical staff **must not** leave the
  patient until ambulance service arrives
• Continuous reassessment – A B C D E
• Record and document event

Fig. 1.9 Chest pain algorithm

Cardiovascular reactions to local anaesthetic

• Usually only palpitations are experienced.
• The likely cause should be identified and the patient reassured.
• Await natural subsidence of symptoms.
• If chest pain occurs, treat as above.
• Where possible, defer further immediate dental treatment.

Hypotension resulting from interaction with antihypertensive drugs

• Assess and clear the airway.
• Assess breathing and administer oxygen.
• Assess circulation.
• Lay the patient flat.
• Reassure.

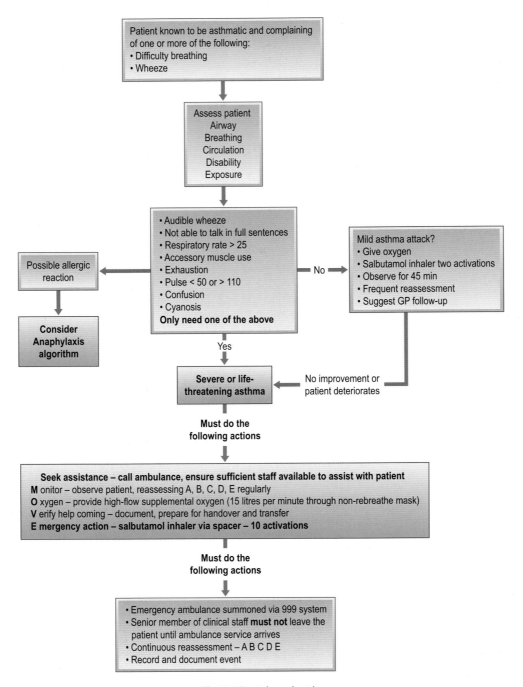

Fig. 1.10 Asthma algorithm

- Summon assistance.
- Where possible, defer further immediate dental treatment.

SEDATION EMERGENCIES

Respiratory failure

- Causes include drug overdose or hypoxia.
- Diagnosis is as follows:
  respiratory rate slows and then stops
  ashen cyanosis
  pulse initially rapid and weak; later irregular or impalpable
  cardiac arrest may follow.
- Management is as follows:

assess patient using ABCDE
call an ambulance
administer no further sedation
lay patient flat
commence ventilation with bag and mask containing high
  oxygen concentration
consider flumazenil administration
defer dental treatment.

Sedative drug overdose or drug interaction

- Accidental overdose or the combination of the sedative agent with another drug used by the patient may be responsible.

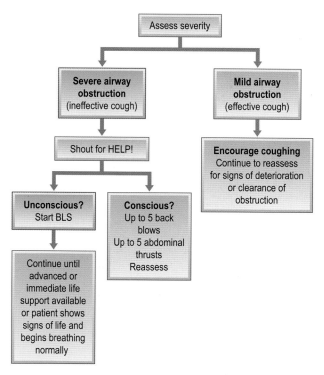

Fig. 1.11 Choking algorithm

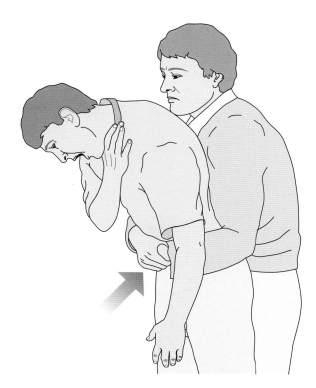

Fig. 1.12 Abdominal thrust

- Diagnosis is as follows:
  pallor
  decreased pulse rate
  hypotension
  respiratory depression.
- Management is as follows:
  stop drug
  give oxygen and ventilate artificially if required
  for midazolam overdose, give flumazenil
  if the patient progresses to cardiac arrest, commence cardiopulmonary resuscitation.
  call the emergency services
  defer dental treatment.

MENTAL DISTURBANCES

Hyperventilation syndrome

- Causes of hyperventilation include:
  anxiety or neurosis
  pain
  cardiovascular disease
  nervous system disease
  acidosis (either metabolic or drug-associated)
  poor respiratory exchange, but in this case it is a compensatory physiological response.
- The clinical features vary widely, but neurological and psychological features may include:
  anxiety
  weakness
  light-headedness
  dizziness
  disturbed consciousness

Box 1.4 Management of stroke

- Assess, clear airway and check breathing
- Check pulse and capillary refill
- Reassure the patient
- Give high-flow oxygen
- Call ambulance
- Defer dental treatment

---

  perioral and peripheral paraesthesiae
  tetany
  muscle pain or stiffness.
- The most common underlying diagnosis is psychological and is typically seen in a young woman overbreathing secondary to anxiety until carbon dioxide washout results in paraesthesia.
- Cardiovascular and respiratory features may include:
  palpitations
  chest pain
  breathlessness.
- Management is detailed in Box 1.6.

Disturbed or aggressive behaviour

- Disturbed or aggressive behaviour may be occasioned by:
  an underlying psychiatric disorder
  drugs: especially barbiturates, alcohol or other drugs of addiction or drug withdrawal, or corticosteroids
  pain or discomfort
  infections, particularly in the elderly
  hypoglycaemia or other endocrine disorders

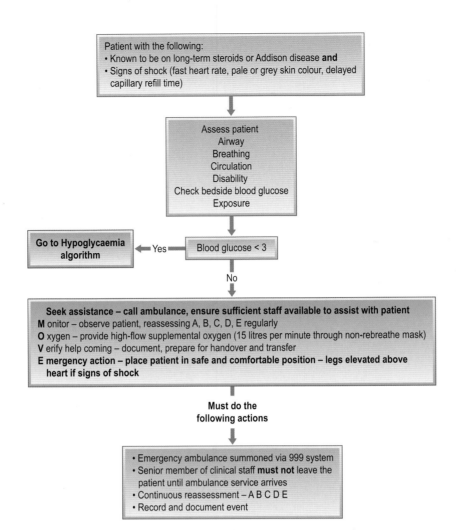

Fig. 1.13 Adrenal insufficiency algorithm

Box 1.5 Management of intravascular injection of local anaesthetic

- Stop the local anaesthetic administration
- Lay the patient flat
- Reassure the patient
- Assess and maintain the airway
- Check breathing and circulation
- Most patients recover spontaneously within half an hour
- Stabilize and defer further dental treatment until another day

Box 1.6 Management of hyperventilating patients

- Assess airway breathing and circulation; identify any disability
- Reassure patient
- Encourage patient to decrease respiratory rate slowly
- If there is obvious sympathetic overactivity, as shown particularly by tachycardia or arrhythmias, a cardiologist's opinion should be obtained, as treatment with a beta-blocker may be necessary
- Defer dental treatment until medical assessment has taken place

---

temporal lobe epilepsy
cerebral tumours.
- Management is detailed in Box 1.7.

Bleeding.
- Post-extraction bleeding causes are usually secondary to local trauma.
- Haemorrhagic disease, though uncommon, must always be considered (see Box 1.8 and Ch. 8).
- Management is detailed in Box 1.8.

COLLAPSE OF UNCERTAIN CAUSE (Table 1.2 and Fig 1.14)

USEFUL WEBSITES

http://www.resus.org.uk/pages/guide.htm
http://www.alsg.org
http://www.erc.edu
http://en.wikipedia.org/wiki/Medical_emergency
http://www.ncemi.org/cse/contents.htm
http://www.atoetrainingandsolutions.co.uk

Box 1.7 Management of disturbed and not to restrain or aggressive behaviour

- Reassure and try to calm the patient and not to restrain
- Do not sedate, as this may confuse the diagnosis and may occasionally be fatal. Midazolam or diazepam are likely also to worsen the excitement of a psychotic patient
- Call an ambulance
- If the patient is violent and uncontrollable, call the police
- Defer dental treatment

Box 1.8 Management of the bleeding patient

- Assess airway, breathing and circulation disability and exposure
- Reassure the patient. Post-extraction bleeding often worries the patient excessively because a little blood dissolved in saliva gives the impression of a major bleed
- Partners or relatives anxiety can prevent early resolution and should be asked to remain in the waiting room
- Gently clean the mouth
- Locate the source of the bleeding
- Suture the socket under local analgesia
- Enquire into the patient's history, especially family history of abnormal bleeding
- If the bleeding is persistent or severe and there has been an estimated loss of more than about 500 ml, or if the patient is already compromised secondary to severe anaemia, then the patient should be admitted to hospital
- Tranexamic acid mouthwash 5% may help in the interim to stabilize the clot
- If the bleeding is uncontrollable, call an ambulance

RESUSCITATION AND EMERGENCIES

The GDC does not have any guidelines on resuscitation but would refer registrants to the Resuscitation Council, which does have the relevant guidance. However, 5.3 and 5.4 of *Standards for dental professionals* (both page 9) expects the

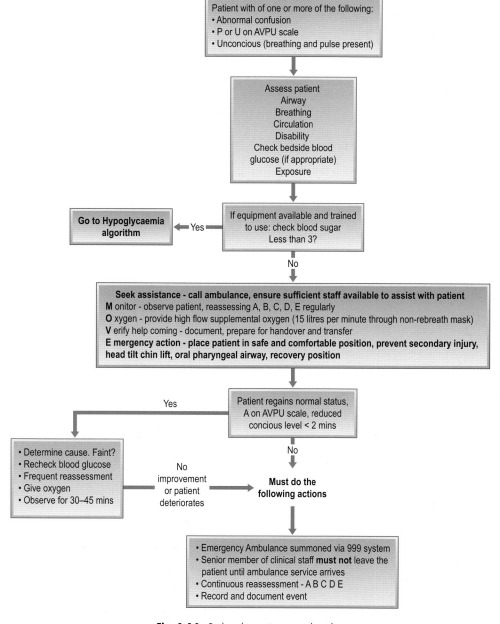

Fig. 1.14 Reduced consciousness algorithm

registrant to find out about current best practice, laws and regulations which affect their work. Full details are available at: http://www.gdc-uk.org/NR/rdonlyres/FFD61DA5-A09E-4B38-8FFB-BA342E9F0AF4/16687/147158_Standards_Profs.pdf

For emergencies, the GDC's *Principles of dental team working* standard 5.7 covers medical emergencies (page 11) and is available at the following link: http://www.gdc-uk.org/NR/rdonlyres/79B1032C-4B07-460E-A2BA-D7A388D7754E/31247/Dental_Working_Team.pdf

REFERENCES AND FURTHER READING

American Academy of Pediatric Dentistry; American Academy of Pediatric Dentistry Committee on Sedation and Anesthesia, 2005–2006. Guideline on the elective use of minimal, moderate, and deep sedation and general anesthesia for pediatric dental patients. Pediatr Dent 27 (Suppl 7), 110–118.

Atherton, G.J., McCaul, J.A., Williams, S.A., 1999a. Medical emergencies in general dental practice in Great Britain Part 3: perceptions of training and competence of GDPS in their management. Br Dent J 186(5): 234–7.

Atherton, G.J., McCaul, J.A., Williams, S.A., 1999b. Medical emergencies in general dental practice in Great Britain Part 1: their prevalence over a 10-year period. Br Dent J 186, 72–79.

Balmer, M.C., Longman, L.P., 2008. A practical skill one day medical emergencies course for dentists and DCPs. Br Dent J 204, 453–536.

Boyd, B.C., Fantuzzo, J.J., Votta, T., 2006. The role of automated external defibrillators in dental practice. N Y State Dent J 72, 20–23.

Cardiopulmonary resuscitation – guidelines for clinical practice and training, 2004. Resuscitation Council (UK), Royal College of Anaesthetists, Royal College of Physicians. Intensive Care Society, London.

Cardiopulmonary resuscitation – guidelines for clinical practice and training in primary care, 2002. Resuscitation Council (UK), London.

Chiu, C.Y., Lin, T.Y., Hsia, S.H., Lai, S.H., Wong, K.S., 2004. Systemic anaphylaxis following local lidocaine administration during a dental procedure. Pediatr Emerg Care 20, 178–180.

Conscious sedation for dentistry: the competent graduate, 2000. Dental Sedation Teachers Group.

Coulthard, P., 2006. Conscious sedation guidance, 2000 Evid Based Dent 7, 90–91.

Coulthard, P., Bridgman, C.M., Larkin, A., et al., 2000. Appropriateness of a Resuscitation Council (UK) Advanced Life Support Course for primary care dentists. Br Dent J 188, 507–512.

Dym, H., 2008. Preparing the dental office for medical emergencies. Dent Clin North Am 52, 605–608 x.

Fukayama, H., Yagiela, J.A., 2006. Monitoring of vital signs during dental care. Int Dent J 56, 102–108.

Girdler, N.M., Smith, D.G., 1999. Prevalence of emergency events in British dental practice and emergency management skills of British dentists. Resuscitation 41, 159–167.

Greenwood, M., 2000. Medical emergencies in the dental practice. Periodontol 2008 (46), 27–41.

Haas, D.A., 2002. Emergency drugs. Dent Clin North Am 46, 815–830.

Hodgson, T.A., Buchanan, J.A.G., Davies, R.C., 2003. Medical emergencies in dental practice: a practical approach. Fits and faints. Private Dent 8 (8), 33–36.

Hodgson, T.A., Buchanan, J.A.G., Davies, R.C., 2003. Medical emergencies in dental practice: a practical approach. Chest pain, asthma and inhaled foreign body. Private Dent 8 (9), 22–26.

Hodgson, T.A., Buchanan, J.A.G., Davies, R.C., 2003. Medical emergencies in dental practice: a practical approach. Anaphylaxis, adrenal and diabetic emergencies. Private Dent 8 (10), 28–33.

JOE Editorial Board, 2008. Medical emergencies and drugs: an online study guide. J Endod 34 (Suppl 5), e201–203.

Johnston, S.L., Unsworth, J., 2003. Adrenaline given outside the context of life threatening allergic reactions. BMJ 326, 589–590.

Joint Royal Colleges Ambulance Liaison Committee clinical practice guidelines 2006 for use in UK ambulance services (version 4.0). http://jrcalc.org.uk/guidelines.html.

Kaeppler, G., Daublander, M., Hinkelbein, R., Lipp, M., 1998. [Quality of cardiopulmonary resuscitation by dentists in dental emergency care]. Mund Kiefer Gesichtschir 2 (2), 71–77.

Koerner, K.R., Taylor, S.E., 2000. Emergencies associated with local anesthetics. Dent Today 19 (10), 72–79.

Lepere, A.J., Finn, J., Jacobs, I., 2003. Efficacy of cardiopulmonary resuscitation performed in a dental chair. Aust Dent J 48, 244–247.

Müller, M.P., Hänsel, M., Stehr, S.N., Weber, S., Koch, T., 2008. A state-wide survey of medical emergency management in dental practices: incidence of emergencies and training experience. Emerg Med J 25, 296–300.

Prescribing in dental practice. British National Formulary, 2005 British Medical Association and the Royal Pharmaceutical Society of Great Britain, London.

Principles of dental team working, 2005. General Dental Council, London.

Proceedings of the 2005 International Consensus on Cardiopulmonary Resuscitation and Emergency Cardiovascular Care Science with Treatment Recommendations, 2005. Resuscitation 67, 157–341.

Project Team of the Resuscitation Council (UK), 1999. Emergency medical treatment of anaphylactic reactions. J Accid Emerg Med 16, 243–247.

Resuscitation Council guidelines 2006. Medical emergencies and resuscitation: standards for clinical practice and training for dental practitioners and dental care professionals in general dental practice. Resuscitation Council (UK), London, 2006 (revised 2008).

Resuscitation guidelines 2005. Resuscitation Council (UK), London.

Robb, N.D., Leitch, J, 2006. Medical emergencies in dentistry. Oxford University Press, Oxford.

Roberts, J.R., 1998. Emergency medicine and surgery. WB Saunders, Philadelphia.

Rosenberg, M.B., 2004. Medical emergencies in the pediatric patient: airway management. J Mass Dent Soc 52 (4), 46–48.

Scully, C., 1997. The prevention and management of emergencies. Br Dent J Launchpad 4, 18–22.

Scully, C., Kalantzis, A., 2005. Oxford handbook of dental patient care. Oxford University Press, Oxford.

Sharma, P.R., Hargreaves, A.D., 2006. Malignant vasovagal syncope. Dent Update 33 (4), 246–248, 250.

Standards in conscious sedation for dentistry, 2000. Report of an Independent Expert Working Group funded by the Society for the Advancement of Anaesthesia in Dentistry, London.

Training in conscious sedation for dentistry. Dental Sedation Teachers Group, 2005. http://www.dstg.co.uk.

Health care aims to improve the health of patients but can itself carry risks. The first principle should be to do no harm (*primum non nocere*). Nevertheless, a recent report from the UK estimated that up to 18% of the population believe that they have suffered from a 'medical error', 10% of hospital admissions may result in something going wrong and 5% have had adverse effects from medical care.

Morbidity and mortality in the dental surgery has become rare. Operations are now associated with less morbidity and mortality than formerly, but there remains room for improvement. Deaths as a result of the use of general anaesthesia (GA) in the dental surgery in the past were few but nevertheless provoked widespread public concern and, as a result of legislation, it is no longer acceptable, in the UK, for a dentist to act as anaesthetist (this had been the case for some time in certain other countries) and GA must only be given in a hospital with critical care facilities – because of the need to have resuscitation equipment available. If working in hospital, however, dentists may be required to assess patients for GA, to ensure essential prerequisites are met before GA. Dentists can themselves provide conscious sedation and local anaesthesia (LA), and may need to manage GA patients post-operatively and therefore they must have an understanding of risk assessment and perioperative care.

As has been stated, the first principle should be to do no harm and, therefore, at the start of a patient's visit, it is essential:

1. to assess the patient's needs;
2. to obtain a careful medical, dental, family, social (and sometimes developmental) history, and make a risk assessment
3. to obtain the patient's consent to any investigations required
4. to obtain the patient's consent to an agreed treatment plan.

RISK ASSESSMENT

Dentistry should be very safe, provided that the patient is healthy and the procedure is not dramatically invasive; thus morbidity and mortality following dental procedures is even less excusable than when it follows more invasive interventions. Surgical procedures are generally the most hazardous. Drugs, particularly those acting on the neurological system (e.g. sedatives and anaesthetic agents), are also potentially dangerous and should be particular carefully administered. Risks come mainly, however, when dental staff are overambitious in terms of their skill or knowledge, the patient is not healthy and/or the procedure is invasive (tissues are disrupted).

Most oral care can be given under LA and then morbidity is minimal. By contrast, GA with intravenous or inhalational agents is only occasionally required for dental treatment and then only in a hospital setting: control of vital functions is impaired or lost to the anaesthetist. GA is only permitted in a hospital with appropriate resuscitation facilities and carried out by a qualified anaesthetist. Conscious sedation is considerably safer than GA, though not as safe as LA. Even so, it must be carried out in appropriate facilities, by adequately trained personnel and with due consideration of the possible risks.

Adequate risk assessment is essential and endeavours to anticipate and prevent trouble. The criteria of 'fitness' for a procedure are not absolute but depend on a number of factors as shown in Box 2.1.

A patient attending for dental treatment and apparently 'fit' may actually have serious systemic disease(s) and be taking drugs (including recreational drugs), either or both of which might influence the health care required. Many patients with life-threatening diseases now survive as a result of advances in surgical and medical care, and either or both can significantly affect the dental management or even the fate of the patient. Though this is most likely when treating hospital patients and other risk groups such as the older person, one study showed 30% of dental patients to have a relevant medical condition. The risk is greatest when surgery is needed, and when GA or sedation are given – and these problems may be compounded if close medical support is lacking.

No interventional procedure is entirely free from risk but care can be improved by making an adequate assessment based on history, clinical signs and, where appropriate, investigations, and minimizing trauma and stress to the patient (Table 2.1).

Although every care must be taken to identify the medically compromised patient, it must be appreciated that the means to do so in conventional dental settings are limited and by no means always successful. It is impossible to legislate for

Box 2.1 Factors influencing outcomes of health care procedures

- Health of the patient
- Type of procedure
- Duration of the procedure
- Degree of trauma and stress
- Degree of urgency of the procedure
- Skill and experience of the operator
- Skill and experience of the anaesthetist/sedationist

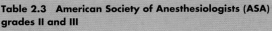

Table 2.1 Risk assessment and management

Risks increased by	Risks reduced by
Increasing age	Planned treatment
Medical treatments	Non-invasive procedures
Surgical treatments	Monitoring
Lengthy dental procedures	Reassurance
Drug use – medication or recreational	Competent operator

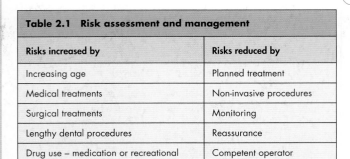

Table 2.2 American Society of Anesthesiologists (ASA) classification

ASA class	Definition
I	Normal, healthy patient
II	A patient with mild systemic disease (e.g. well-controlled diabetes, asthma, hypertension or epilepsy), pregnancy, anxiety
III	A patient with severe systemic disease limiting activity but not incapacitating (e.g. epilepsy with frequent seizures, uncontrolled hypertension, recent myocardial infarct, uncontrolled diabetes, severe asthma, stroke)
IV	A patient with incapacitating disease that is a constant threat to life (e.g. cancer, unstable angina or recent myocardial infarct, arrhythmia or recent cerebrovascular accident)
V	Moribund patient not expected to live more than 24 hours with or without treatment

Table 2.3 American Society of Anesthesiologists (ASA) grades II and III

	ASA II	ASA III
COPD	Cough or wheeze; well controlled	Breathless on minimal exertion
Angina	Occasional use of GTN	Regular use of GTN or unstable angina
Hypertension	Well controlled on single agent	Poorly controlled; multiple drugs
Asthma	Well controlled with inhalers	Poorly controlled; limiting lifestyle
Diabetes	Well controlled; no complications	Poorly controlled or complications

COPD, chronic obstructive pulmonary disease (see Ch. 15); GTN, glyceryl trinitrate.

Another assessment tool, which is virtually identical to the ASA scale but can be modified by factors such as those shown in Table 2.4, is the prognosis and assessment of risk scale (PARS), which categorizes patients into groups I–V. Other factors considered in PARS are shown in Table 2.5.

The Karnofsky scale, which has been adapted for use in many areas, including hospices, cancer clinics, etc., is a quick and easy way to indicate how a patient is feeling on a given day, without going through several multiple choice questions or symptom surveys (Table 2.6). The medical complexity classification is another tool (Table 2.7).

Often dental treatment in medically compromised patients may have to be delayed until expert advice has been sought. Patients undergoing procedures under GA must be pre-assessed by the anaesthetist. Good communication is therefore essential with both patient and other health professionals.

all possibilities and there have been many cases where apparently fit people have died suddenly within a short time of being declared healthy on medical examination.

The main aims are to ensure that procedures are carried out:

- promptly but safely
- on the correct patient and the correct site
- with minimal complications and the best possible outcome.

Assessment of the risks involved must include not only the health of the patient but also the severity of the procedure and the drugs/anaesthesia to be used.

Patients may be assessed using a risk-stratification scoring system such as the Physical Status Classification of the American Society of Anesthesiologists (ASA) classification (Table 2.2). ASA I and II patients can be treated in general dental practice or community services. ASA III patients are often best treated in a hospital-based clinic where expert medical support is available. ASA IV and V patients are usually hospitalized or bedridden, and are generally only seeking emergency dental treatment.

Dental treatment must be significantly modified if the patient has an ASA score of III or IV: a relatively high percentage of patients aged 65–74 years (23.9%) and 75 years or over (34.9%) do have an ASA score of III or IV. Controversies can arise in relation to scores of II and III; Table 2.3 summarizes these scores for some of the more common disorders.

CONSENT

The patient's autonomy must be respected at all times. Patients can determine what investigations and treatment they are or are not willing to receive. They must be given sufficient information about their condition, suggested treatment(s) (including alternative management if available), any associated risks of the proposed treatment and possible outcomes if nothing is done before they are asked to make a decision. They have the right to refuse treatment even if this could adversely affect the outcome or result in their death. Depending on the situation, time should be allowed for the patient to think about and discuss the proposed treatment with those close. Consent is not an isolated event, but involves a continuing dialogue between clinician and patient (and occasionally their relatives or partner). *Patients who undergo procedures performed without their valid consent may be entitled to claim damages in the civil courts by making a claim of negligence. The clinician is also vulnerable in the criminal courts to a charge of assault and battery following a complaint to the police by the person who received the treatment.*

Information about what investigations or treatment will involve, the benefits and risks (including side-effects and complications) and the alternatives to the particular procedure

Table 2.4 Dental care modifications and American Society of Anesthesiologists (ASA) and prognosis and assessment of risk scale (PARS) scales

ASA	Definition	PARS	Dental care modifications
I	Normal, healthy patient	I	None
II	A patient with mild systemic disease (e.g. well-controlled diabetes, asthma, hypertension or epilepsy), pregnancy, anxiety	II	Dental care should focus on elimination of acute infection before medical/surgical procedure (e.g. prosthetic cardiac valve)
III	A patient with severe systemic disease limiting activity but not incapacitating (e.g. epilepsy with frequent seizures, uncontrolled hypertension, recent myocardial infarct, uncontrolled diabetes, severe asthma, stroke)	III	Dental care should focus on elimination of acute infection and chronic disease before medical/surgical procedure (e.g. organ transplant patients)
IV	A patient with incapacitating disease that is a constant threat to life (e.g. cancer, unstable angina or recent myocardial infarct, arrhythmia or recent cerebrovascular accident)	IV	All potential dental problems should be corrected before medical/surgical procedure (e.g. prior to radiotherapy to head and neck)
V	Moribund patient not expected to live more than 24 hours with or without treatment	V	Control of acute dental pain and infection only

Table 2.5 Prognosis and assessment risk scale

	Comment
Medical status Physical status	Any complicating medical factors
Oral hygiene Psychological needs Functional ability	
Mental status	Level of understanding
Social environment Family environment	Support or significant events planned shortly after treatment
Access issues Financial issues	Access to dental building, etc.
Communication needs	Is an interpreter required?
Behaviour	Is behaviour management needed?
Consent	Is patient competent to give consent?

Table 2.6 Karnofsky scale

100	Able to work. Normal, no complaints, no evidence of disease
90	Able to work. Able to carry out normal activity, minor symptoms
80	Able to work. Normal activity with effort, some symptoms
70	Independent, not able to work. Cares for self, unable to carry out normal activity
60	Disabled, dependent. Requires occasional assistance, cares for most needs
50	Moderately disabled, dependent. Requires considerable assistance and frequent care
40	Severely disabled, dependent. Requires special care and assistance
30	Severely disabled. Hospitalized, death not imminent
20	Very sick. Active supportive treatment needed
10	Moribund. Fatal processes are rapidly progressing

Table 2.7 The medical complexity classification

	Medical condition	Status	Complications
MC-0	No significant medical problems	MC-0	No complications anticipated
MC-1	Controlled and stable condition/disease	MC-1A	No complications anticipated
		MC-1B	Minor complications anticipated
		MC-1C	Major complications anticipated
MC-2	Poorly controlled and/or unstable condition/disease	MC-2A	No complications anticipated
		MC-2B	Minor complications anticipated
		MC-2C	Major complications anticipated
MC-3	Cardiac or other conditions needing continuous monitoring		

proposed is crucial for patients when making up their minds. The courts have stated that patients should be told about 'significant risks which would affect the judgement of a reasonable patient'.

'Significant' has not been legally defined, but the General Medical Council (GMC) requires doctors to tell patients about 'serious or frequently occurring' risks. In addition, if patients make clear they have particular concerns about certain kinds of risk, ensure they are informed about these risks, even if they are very small or rare. Always answer questions honestly. Sometimes, patients may make it clear that they do not want to have any information about the options, but want the health professional to decide on their behalf. In such circumstances, ensure that the patient receives at least very basic information about what is proposed. Where information is refused, this should be documented in the patient's notes and/or on a consent form. The important thing is for the clinician to record sufficient details of the consent process in order to be able to reconstruct the discussions and the thinking that led to a particular course of treatment in the event of a challenge at a later stage – possibly years later.

The patient's open agreement to proceed with the investigation or treatment proposed after full discussion and the patient's receipt of sufficient information is sometimes called 'informed consent'.

When obtaining consent, patients should be informed of:

- details of diagnosis and prognosis with and without treatment
- uncertainties about the diagnosis
- options available for treatment
- the purpose of all aspects of a proposed investigation or treatment
- the likely benefits and probability of success
- any possible adverse effects, the risks of the procedure proposed
- the likelihood of one or more of the risks coming to pass
- likely outcomes if a procedure is not carried out
- the need for drains, catheters, tracheostomy, etc.
- a reminder that patients can change their mind at any stage
- a reminder that patients have the right to a second opinion.

Other issues that should be discussed at this stage include:

- time of appointment or admission
- starving instructions
- management of usual medication
- specific pre-operative preparation that may be required
- transport to where the procedure will be performed
- specific anaesthetic issues
- anticipated duration of procedure
- likely recovery period
- likely discharge date
- specific post-operative care
- follow-up requirements
- anticipated date of return to full activity.

'Informed' consent means that the patient must be fully aware of the procedure, its intended benefits, its possible risks and the level of these. In particular, patients must be warned:

- about pre-operative preparation
- of possible adverse effects

- about post-operative sequelae (e.g. pain)
- where they will be during their recovery
- of the possibility of intravenous infusions, catheters, naso-gastric tubes, any deformity, swelling, bruising, pain, etc.

All questions should be answered honestly. Information should not be withheld that might influence the decision-making process. Patients should never be coerced. Finally, for consent to be valid, the person who obtains it must have sufficient knowledge of the proposed treatment and its risks, and should be the person who is undertaking the procedure.

At any time the information on the form can be augmented by making an additional record in the patient's notes of conversations/discussions/warnings.

Consent may be:

- implied (a patient lying in the dental chair with their mouth open is consenting to a dental examination), or
- expressed
  verbal (a patient who gives you permission to take a blood test or perform simple dental procedures after you have explained the reasons these are necessary)
- written.

Although rarely a legal requirement (but frequently a contractual obligation), it is good practice to seek written consent; this is essential where the treatment is complex or involves significant risks or adverse effects. Written consent must be obtained from all patients having an operation. The possible benefits of the treatment must be weighed against the risks and always discussed by the person carrying out the procedure or, if for some reason this is not possible, a delegated person with the appropriate expertise to do so (i.e. a person who is competent to carry out the surgery proposed themselves as an independent practitioner in their own right). Written consent is also essential when provision of clinical care is not the primary purpose, the treatment is part of a project or research, or there are significant consequences for personal or social life. A signature on a consent form does not itself prove the consent is valid: the point of the form is to record the patient's decision and also increasingly the content of the discussions that have taken place. Your Trust or organization may have a policy setting out when you need to obtain written consent. A signed consent form is not a legal waiver; if, for example, patients do not receive enough information on which to base their decision, then the consent may not be valid, even though the form has been signed. A signed consent form will not protect the clinician if there is doubt as to whether consent was actually 'informed'. Ideally the form should be designed to serve as an *aide-memoire* to health professionals and patients, by providing a checklist of the kind of information patients should be offered, and by enabling the patient to have a written record of the main points discussed. However, the written information provided for the patient in no way should be regarded as a substitute for face-to-face discussions with the patient. Patients are also entitled to change their mind after signing the consent form, if they retain capacity to do so.

Consent in relation to dentistry is the expressed or implied agreement of the patient to undergo a dental examination, investigation or treatment. The law in relation to consent continues to evolve (as does most legislation) and there are significant variations between countries. However, the principles remain essentially the same, as follows.

- Before examining, treating or caring for competent adult patients, their consent must be obtained.
- Adults are assumed to be competent unless demonstrated otherwise. If there are doubts about their competence, the question to ask is: 'Can this patient understand, retain and then weigh up the information needed to make this decision?'
- Patients may be competent to make some health care decisions, even if they are not competent to make others.
- Giving and obtaining consent is usually a process, not a one-off event. *Patients can change their minds and withdraw consent at any time.*

For consent to be valid, patients must receive sufficient information about their condition and proposed treatment. It is the health care professional's responsibility to explain all the relevant facts to the patient, and to ascertain that they understand them. If patients are not offered as much information as they reasonably need to make their decision, and in a form they can understand, their consent may not be valid. For example, information for those with visual impairment should be provided in the form of audio tapes, Braille or large print.

Patients whose first language is not English may need the help of an interpreter. Most National Health Service (NHS) Trusts and organizations have access to experienced interpreters. It is preferable to rely on a neutral (i.e. not a family member) interpreter when examining and seeking consent from a patient for surgery or treatment.

Make sure to keep the patient, other staff and, where appropriate and in accordance with the patient's wishes, the patient's relatives and/or partner, fully informed. If there is any reason to believe that the consent may be disputed later, or if there are concerns about an individual's attitude or behaviour, meticulous documentation in the case notes is invaluable. Maintain good, clear, contemporaneous records of the nature of all discussions that take place, including the names of those involved. Good communication and documentation can prevent future dispute and litigation.

SPECIFIC PROBLEMS

- No one else can make a decision on behalf of a competent adult.
- In an emergency, a life-saving procedure can be performed without consent.
- All actions must, however, be justifiable to one's peers.
- No one can give or withhold consent on behalf of a mentally incapacitated patient; decisions lie primarily with the clinicians, who should act in the patient's best interest. Where there is doubt, ultimately a Court will decide on the best course of action, having taken expert advice.

The UK Department of Health's *Reference guide to consent for examination or treatment* (also available at www.doh.gov.uk/consent) offers a comprehensive summary of the law on consent. The Mental Capacity Act 2005 provides guidance for health care professionals who treat this group of patients.

Guidance has been published by the UK Department of Health (Mental Capacity Act 2005 Code of Practice: http://www.dca.gov.uk/legal-policy/mental-capacity/mca-cp.pdf).

Essentially, everyone aged 16 or more is presumed to be competent to give consent for themselves, unless the opposite is demonstrated.

Competent adults, namely persons aged 16 and over who have the capacity to make their own decisions about treatment, can consent to dental treatment and they are also entitled to refuse treatment, even where it would clearly benefit their health. If a patient is mentally competent to give consent but is physically unable to sign a form, you should complete this form as usual, and ask an independent witness to confirm that the patient has given consent orally or non-verbally.

If the patient is 18 or over and is not legally competent to give consent, you should use a form for adults who are unable to consent to investigation or treatment. Patients will not be legally competent to give consent if:

- they are unable to comprehend and retain information material to the decision; and/or
- they are unable to weigh and use this information in coming to a decision.

You should always take all reasonable steps (e.g. involving more specialist colleagues) to support a patient in making their own decision before concluding that they are unable to do so.

Relatives *cannot* be asked to sign this form on behalf of an adult who is not legally competent to consent for him or herself, unless the patient has appointed a friend or relative to act for them, creating a lasting power of attorney (LPA). This LPA must have been created when the patient was competent and the LPA must be lodged with the Court of Protection. An LPA may allow the relative or friend to take decisions about the health of the patient should the patient be found to be lacking capacity.

Children under the age of 16 years may also have capacity to consent if they have the ability to understand the nature, purpose and possible consequences of the proposed investigation or treatment, as well as the consequences of non-treatment. Children below 16 who have *Gillick* competence (understand fully what is involved in the proposed procedure) may therefore consent to treatment without their parents' authority or knowledge, although their parents will ideally be involved.

'Gillick competence' is a term used in medical law to decide whether a child (16 years or younger) is able to consent to medical treatment, without the need for parental permission or knowledge:

> As a matter of Law the parental right to determine whether or not their minor child below the age of sixteen will have medical treatment terminates if and when the child achieves sufficient understanding and intelligence to understand fully what is proposed.

The standard is based on a House of Lords' decision in the case *Gillick v West Norfolk and Wisbech Area Health Authority* [1985] 3 All ER 402 (HL). The case is binding in England, and has been approved in Australia, Canada and New Zealand. Similar provision is made in Scotland by The Age of Legal Capacity (Scotland) Act 1991. In Northern Ireland, although separate legislation applies, the then Department of Health and Social Services Northern Ireland stated that there was no reason to suppose that the House of Lords' decision would not be followed by the Northern Ireland Courts.

Where a child under 16 years old is not deemed competent to consent, a person with parental responsibility (e.g. their legal parent or guardian, or a person appointed by the Courts) has authority to consent for investigations or treatment, that are in the child's best interests.

There are several legal tests which have been described in relation to consent. The *Bolam* test states that a doctor who:

> acted in accordance with a practice accepted as proper by a responsible body of medical men skilled in that particular art is not negligent if he is acting in accordance with such a practice, merely because there is a body of opinion which takes a contrary view.

However, a judge may on certain rare occasions choose between two bodies of expert medical opinion, if one is to be regarded as 'logically indefensible' (*Bolitho* principle). The main alternative to the *Bolam* test is the *'prudent-patient test'* widely used in North America. According to this test, doctors should provide the amount of information that a 'prudent patient' would want.

Obtaining consent from adult patients without capacity

The more elective the procedure, the more care should be taken in ensuring that the patient/parent/guardian/carer have been consulted. In true emergency situations, a dentist may rely on the best intent principle in relation to the overall well-being of the patient, although, where there is any doubt, advice should be taken. Involve the patient as far as possible; some incapacitated patients may be quite capable of giving partial consent. Decide who else should be involved in any decision to proceed with the patient's treatment. The current position (in the UK) is that no adult can consent to the treatment of another adult (with the exception of cases under the Mental Capacity Act 2005). Before anyone can give valid consent to treatment, she or he must possess the requisite capacity. The law presumes that, in the absence of evidence to the contrary, patients over the age of 16 years are capable of giving (or withholding) consent to treatment. The broad test of capacity is that the person concerned should be able to understand the nature and purpose of the treatment and must be able to weigh the risks and benefits. They should be able to retain and weigh this information as well as communicate their decision.

Where there is doubt, a decision has to be made as to the capacity of the patient. This presents a problem for dentists providing care for patients with learning impairment. Where the patient lacks the capacity to consent, then the dentist would normally act in the patient's best interests and treatment should not be withheld simply because consent has not been obtained, or a charge of failure in duty of care could be made. If a person is incapable of giving or refusing consent, and has not validly refused such care in advance, treatment may still be given lawfully if it is deemed to be in the patient's best interests. However, this should happen only after full consideration of its potential benefits and unwanted effects, and in consultation with the carer(s), relatives and other people close to the patient. Where treatment involves taking irreversible decisions

or carrying greater risks, then the agreement of another dentist or doctor is appropriate. For those with learning difficulties, it is important to discuss with the parent, carer or, in their absence, two professionals who should sign their approval in the best interests of the patient. The discussions and agreement should be documented in the patient's record and, whilst this does not constitute consent, it represents good practice.

The Mental Health Act 1983 is primarily concerned with the care and treatment of people who are diagnosed as having a mental health problem which requires that they be detained or treated in the interests of their own health and safety or with a view to protecting other people. This act is now over 20 years old and new legislation has been passed through parliament in the form of the Mental Health Bill 2007.

The Mental Capacity Act 2005 (MCA) came into force in UK in 2007, and the law applies to everyone involved in care, treatment or support of people aged 16 years and over in England and Wales and who lack capacity to make all or some decisions for themselves. This applies to situations where a person may lack capacity to make a decision at a particular time due to illness, drugs or alcohol. Assessments of capacity should be time and decision specific.

A new criminal offence of ill-treatment or wilful neglect of people who lack capacity came into force in UK in April 2007. Within the law, 'helping with personal hygiene (that would include toothbrushing)' will attract protection from liability as long as the individual has complied with the MCA by assessing a person's capacity and acted in their best interests. 'Best interest' decisions made on behalf of people who lack capacity should be least restrictive of their basic rights and freedoms.

In Scotland, the position is complicated by the fact that the dentist has to comply with the *Adults with Incapacity Act 2000*. This requires that the patient's doctor issues a certificate before treatment. The document is a procedure-specific document and a new one will be required for each treatment plan or in the event of a change to the plan. Episodes requiring GA or sedation not included in the original treatment plan will need further certification. The interesting nuance is that the dentist can assess capacity, but it is the doctor who has to assess incapacity. This has created significant practical difficulties for many health care providers.

Obtaining consent for child patients

Social pattern changes have meant that the position relating to who is able to consent to treatment for a child has changed. Parental responsibility lies with the natural mother, natural father (if married to the mother at birth), adoptive parents and those who have temporary residence orders (where the child lives with them). The local authority may acquire responsibility. The natural father not married to the natural mother does *not* have parental responsibility. Parental responsibility can be granted by court order, by agreement with the mother or, on her death, if stated in her will. Step-parents can be granted parental responsibility by court order.

The information provided is an example of UK law. It is important to remember that the legal situation with regard to consent varies around the world and is subject to continued debate and development.

THE USE OF RESTRAINT

Occasionally, patients may need some assistance in order to be able to undergo or cooperate with investigations or treatment. The dividing line between this and trespass to the person can be fine. Three forms of trespass to the person exist:

- assault – the fear or threat of impending harm
- battery – the unlawful application of force or unwanted touching
- false imprisonment – the infliction of restraint.

These issues must be considered carefully where the patient lacks the necessary capacity to understand the procedure being carried out. Any physical intervention is subject to the rule of 'reasonableness'. Sometimes it is necessary to control movements during operative procedures or to support an arm, for example, for the injection of intravenous drugs to prevent patients injuring themselves. It is wise to involve the carer or relatives' assistance at such times and to ensure that this is documented. Learning disabilities teams may be able to assist and are likely to have developed protocols and procedures to deal with such problems.

MEDICAL HISTORY

The history (or anamnesis) is the information gained by a health care professional with the aim of formulating a diagnosis, providing medical care and identifying medical problems relevant to health care. The history is obtained from either the patient or people who know the patient and can provide the necessary information. History-taking also allows the health care professional to develop rapport with their patient, place the diagnosis in the context of the patient's life and identify relevant physical signs, and assess mental state and attitude towards health care. Age and cultural factors may also be important (Appendix 2.1).

It may occasionally be helpful formally to assess the patient's feeling about health care and, for this, tools such as the Corah anxiety scale are available (Box 2.2; see Ch. 10).

When taking a history, a structured guide such as that shown in Box 2.3 should be followed. Patients should also be given a form to supply all the information they can about their health and any medication they are receiving. Medical and drug history should be regularly updated at subsequent dental visits.

PERSONAL DETAILS

The personal details of the patient include their age, sex, educational status, religion, occupation, relationship status, address and contact details. This is necessary information for administrative purposes and, since the questions are largely non-threatening, this stage provides a gentle introduction into the meeting of patient and clinician, and provides a format for individual introduction suitable to the particular culture.

PRESENTING COMPLAINT

This should be recorded in the patient's own words (e.g. 'pain in my face').

Box 2.2 Corah dental anxiety scale

If you had to go to the dentist tomorrow, how would you feel about it?
- I would look forward to it as a reasonably enjoyable experience
- I wouldn't care one way or the other
- I would be a little uneasy about it
- I would be afraid that it would be unpleasant and painful
- So anxious, that I sometimes break out in a sweat or almost feel physically sick

When you are waiting in the dentist's office for your turn in the chair, how do you feel?
- Relaxed
- A little uneasy
- Tense
- Anxious
- So anxious, that I sometimes break out in a sweat or almost feel physically sick

When you are in the dentist's chair waiting while he gets his drill ready to begin work on your teeth, how do you feel?
- Relaxed
- A little uneasy
- Tense
- Anxious
- So anxious, that I sometimes break out in a sweat or almost feel physically sick

You are in the dentist's chair to have your teeth cleaned. While you are waiting and the dentist is getting out the instruments which he will use to scrape your teeth around the gums, how do you feel?
- Relaxed
- A little uneasy
- Tense
- Anxious
- So anxious, that I sometimes break out in a sweat or almost feel physically sick

---

Box 2.3 Essentials of history-taking

- Personal details
- Presenting complaint (PC)
- History of presenting complaint (HPC)
- Relevant medical history (RMH)
- Drug history
- Social history
- Family history

HISTORY OF PRESENTING COMPLAINT

The timing of the complaint and its evolution should be elicited. If the patient has pain, a useful mnemonic is 'SOCRATES': S – site, O – onset (gradual/sudden), C – character, R – radiation, A – associations (other symptoms), T – timing/duration, E – exacerbating and alleviating factors, S – severity (rate the pain on a visual analogue scale of 1–10).

RELEVANT MEDICAL HISTORY

This includes any past medical and surgical problems: patients should be asked if they carry a medical warning card or device. Careful note should be taken of it, particularly in respect of corticosteroid or warfarin use, a bleeding disorder or diabetes (see e.g. Medic-Alert and Talisman; Figs 2.1–2.3). The completion of such a form provides a useful basis for the dentist to enquire

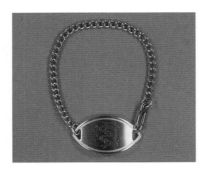

Fig. 2.1 Medic-Alert bracelet the patient's main diagnosis or drug treatment is engraved on the reverse, together with the telephone number of the company that holds details of the medical history

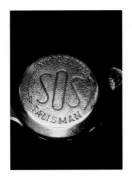

Fig. 2.3 Talisman warning emblem

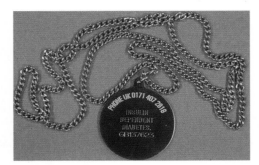

Fig. 2.2 Diabetes alert necklace

Box 2.4 Review of systems (see Table 2.8)

- Allergies
- Bleeding disorders
- Cardiorespiratory disorders
- Drug treatment
- Endocrine disorders
- Fits or faints
- Gastrointestinal disorders
- Hospital admissions and attendances
- Infections
- Jaundice and liver disorders
- Kidney disorders
- Likelihood of pregnancy
- Mental state
- Neurological problems

further and the following chapters describe in more detail the nature and relevance of any diseases that are mentioned. The completion of such a form and appropriate response to its contents is also useful evidence when faced with any medico-legal claims. The medical history is crucial but has limitations, not least since patients may be ill-informed.

Functional enquiry or review of systems (ROS) helps disclose undeclared medical problems. Patients should be asked specifically about conditions; Box 2.4 offers an alphabetical list that is easy to recall.

The relevance of the main points from the history is shown in Table 2.8 and it may also be necessary to enquire about constitutional symptoms (e.g. fever, weight loss, night sweats, fatigue/malaise/lethargy, sleeping pattern, appetite, fever, rash, lumps/bumps/masses), musculoskeletal conditions (pain, stiffness, swelling of the joints) and skin complaints (bruising; Fig. 2.4) rash, blistering, lumps (Fig. 2.5).

DRUG HISTORY

Ask if the patient has any allergies to medication or other substances. If they state they have an allergy, ask them to describe what reaction occurred.

Often, a medical problem is revealed only after a drug history has been elicited, but some patients may be unaware of the name of, or reason for taking, their medication. Ask the patient if they are taking any prescription-only medication (POM; this

may be tablets, injections, patches or inhalers) or any over-the-counter (OTC) medications, including herbal preparations. Multiple drug use is common in older people with complex medical histories (Fig. 2.6). Sometimes, the nature of the drug used may be suggested from the name (Table 2.9).

SOCIAL HISTORY

Find out tactfully about the occupation, marital status, partner's job and health, housing, dependents, mobility, lifestyle habits (alcohol, tobacco, betel etc and recreational drugs), culture and faith. Any social or religious engagements that are dependent on the patient being unimpeded following an elective treatment (wedding/examination/job interview) need discussion and possibly treatment should be rescheduled; see also Chs 25, 28 and 30.

FAMILY HISTORY

The medical history of blood relatives may be very informative. *The history may also radically change with time, so it is essential that the history be updated before each new course of treatment, every sedation session and especially before surgery or GA.* For example, patients not pregnant at one course of treatment could well be by the next. One study followed a small group of middle-aged and older dental patients, and found that nearly 20% developed significant medical disorders (mostly cardiovascular) over a period of 5 years.

Table 2.8   Relevance of medical history to dentistry

Condition	Main features	Other comments	Relevance in dentistry
Allergies	Range from urticaria to anaphylaxis	Rashes? Racial origins may be important, especially in the case of drug reactions. The risk of developing carbamazepine-induced Stevens–Johnson syndrome is strongly associated with the presence of HLA-B*1502 in individuals of Han Chinese, Hong Kong Chinese or Thai origin	Common allergies are to latex, iodine, Elastoplast and drugs (hence the acronym 'LIED'). Anaesthetics, analgesics (e.g. aspirin or codeine) and antibiotics (e.g. penicillin) are the main offending drugs
Bleeding disorders	Bleeding and/or bruising	Haematological/lymphatic: lymph node swelling? Bleeding or bruising? History of involvement of other members of the family or of admission to hospital for control of bleeding is particularly important	Significant hazard to surgery
Cardiorespiratory disorders	Wheezing, cough, dyspnoea, chest pain, swelling of ankles, palpitations, hypertension	Chest pain? Shortness of breath? Exercise tolerance? Orthopnoea? Oedema? Palpitations? Cough? Sputum? Wheeze? Haemoptysis? Patient's ability to climb 15–20 stairs without pain, dyspnoea or tiredness may indicate degree of fitness of the cardiorespiratory system	Often a contraindication to GA or conscious sedation
Drug treatment	Obtaining useful answers about drug treatment including over-the-counter medications will necessitate asking: 'Do you ever take any injections, drugs, pills, tablets or medicines or herbal preparations of *any* kind?'	Drug use may be the only indication of serious underlying disease. Corticosteroids, anti-hypertensives, anticonvulsants, anticoagulants, antibiotics, insulin and oral hypoglycaemics are all important in this respect	Most serious drug interactions are with GA agents (intravenous or inhalational), mono-amine oxidase inhibitors and antihypertensive drugs. Aspirin and other NSAIDs may be a hazard in anticoagulated, asthmatic, diabetic or pregnant patients, those with peptic ulcer, or children under 16 years. If the patient does not know the name of medicines, defer treatment until the drug is identified by the patient's doctor or the Drugs Information Unit or Pharmacy or by checking *Monthly Index of Medical Specialties* (MIMS), *Physicians' Desk Reference* (PDR) or *British National Formulary* (BNF)
Endocrine disorders	Diabetes mellitus may lead to collapse	*Diabetes:* irritability, aggression, lassitude, anorexia, weight loss *Hyperthyroid:* heat intolerance, emotional lability, sweating, diarrhoea, oligomenorrhoea, weight loss despite increased appetite, tremor, palpitations, visual disturbances *Hypothyroid:* dislike of cold weather, lethargy, tiredness, depression, dry skin and hair, hoarseness, menorrhagia, constipation *Hyperadrenocorticism:* weight gain and redistribution, moon face, hirsutism, skin striae, purpura *Hypoadrenalism:* weakness, weight loss, hypotension, pigmentation	Hypoglycaemia is the main problem
Fits or faints	History of fits or faints	Type? Frequency? Precipitating factors? Awareness may allow preventive measures to be instituted	Fainting, epilepsy and other causes of loss of consciousness can disrupt dental treatment and may result in injury to the patient
Gastrointestinal disorders	Abdominal pain, frequency and type of stool, bleeding and weight loss	Difficulty swallowing? Indigestion? Nausea/vomiting/haematemesis? Bowel habit? Faecal colour, consistency, blood (or melaena), smell, difficulty flushing away, tenesmus (feeling of incomplete evacuation) or urgency?	Crohn disease or coeliac disease may lead to oral complications, and gastric disorders may increase the risk of vomiting during GA
Hospital admissions and attendances	Hospital admissions may also indicate underlying disease, and past operations may suggest the possibility of future complications that can influence dental treatment		A history of operations may provide knowledge of possible reactions to GA and surgery. A patient who has had a tonsillectomy, for example, without complications is most unlikely to have a congenital bleeding disorder. Retinal operations, since they may use intraocular gases, may be a contraindication to GA or relative analgesia, which may cause rapid expansion of the ocular gas causing blindness

(Continued)

Table 2.8   Relevance of medical history to dentistry—cont'd

Condition	Main features	Other comments	Relevance in dentistry
Infections	Various possibly rashes and/or fever	Ever attended a clinic for STIs, or been admitted to hospital for an infection, or been accepted or refused for blood donation? Men who have sex with men, abusers of intravenous drugs and patients who have attended STI clinics are more likely to have a history of infection with HIV, hepatitis viruses, herpes simplex, syphilis, gonorrhoea and many other infections (see Chs 21)	The possibility of transmission of infections and their sequelae must be considered. Carriers of MRSA may be a hazard to others; carriers of *Neisseria meningitides* may be sources of meningitis outbreaks
Jaundice and liver disorders	A history of jaundice may imply carriage of hepatitis viruses, although jaundice is a clinical sign of other underlying liver diseases		Liver disease can lead to prolonged bleeding and impaired drug metabolism can result (Ch. 9). Jaundice after an operation may have resulted from halothane hepatitis and, if this is suspected, a different general anaesthetic, such as isoflurane, desflurane or sevoflurane, should be given
Kidney and genitourinary disorders	Manifestations of chronic kidney disease may include hypertension, pallor and bruising	Incontinence (stress or urge), dysuria (pain), haematuria, nocturia, frequency, polyuria, hesitancy, terminal dribbling? Vaginal discharge?	Can affect dental management, as excretion of some drugs is impaired. Tetracyclines should be given in lower doses. Complications of renal failure or transplants can produce oral signs
Likelihood of pregnancy		Menses (periods) – frequency, regularity, heavy or light, duration, painful? First day of last menstrual period (LMP)? Number of pregnancies and births? Menarche? Menopause? Any chance of pregnancy now? Which trimester?	Any essential procedures involving drugs (even aspirin), radiography or GA should be arranged during the middle trimester
Mental state	Behavioural changes	Appearance and behaviour; thought (speech) form, rate, quantity, pattern, flight of ideas, loosening of associations; mood (subjective); affect (observed); thought content, preoccupations, obsessions, overvalued ideas, ideas of reference, delusions; suicidality; abnormal experiences, hallucinations, passivity, thought interference; cognition; consciousness; attention/concentration; memory; orientation; intelligence; executive function; insight. It may sometimes be useful to assess the degree of patients' anxiety in a relatively objective way by using the Corah dental anxiety scale (see above)	Anxiety is inexorably associated with attending for dental treatment. Anxious patients may sometimes react aggressively and anxiety may limit extent of dental treatment that can be provided under LA
Neurological		Special senses – any changes in sight, smell, hearing and/or taste? Seizures, faints, fits, funny turns? Headache? Pins and needles (paraesthesiae) or numbness? Limb weakness, poor balance? Speech problems? Sphincter disturbance?	Movement disorders can significantly disrupt operative procedures. Access can be a barrier to care

GA, general anaesthesia; HIV, human immunodeficiency virus; LA, local analgesia; MRSA, meticillin-resistant *Staphylococcus aureus*; NSAID, non-steroidal anti-inflammatory drug; STI, sexually transmitted infection.

CLINICAL EXAMINATION

It is important for dental professionals not merely to inspect and examine the mouth and neck, but to look at the whole patient. Examination of a patient's appearance, behaviour and speech, body language, and inspection of the face, neck, arms and hands can reveal many significant conditions (Fig. 2.7). A search should be made for such readily visible signs such as anxiety, movements and tremors, and tiredness, and also for facial changes (e.g. expression, pallor, cyanosis or jaundice), dyspnoea or wheezing, or finger clubbing. However, it must be stressed that even very ill patients can look remarkably well.

Facial movement and sensation should be tested in the course of testing the cranial nerves (see Ch. 13). Eyes and ears should be observed and examined (Fig. 2.8). Maxillary, mandibular or zygomatic deformities or swellings may be more reliably confirmed by inspection from above (maxillae/zygomas) or behind (mandible). The degree and direction of opening of the mandible should be assessed; this can be disturbed in temporomandibular joint (TMJ) disease, and other conditions causing restricted mouth-opening (trismus) discussed in Ch. 4.

Inspection of the major salivary glands may reveal swelling of the parotid gland, which causes outward deflection of the lower part of the ear lobe, which is best observed by looking at the patient from behind (Fig. 2.9).

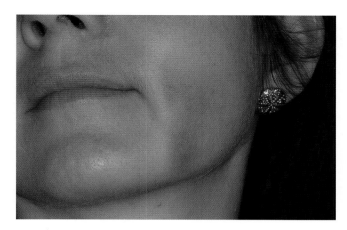

Fig. 2.4 Facial bruising

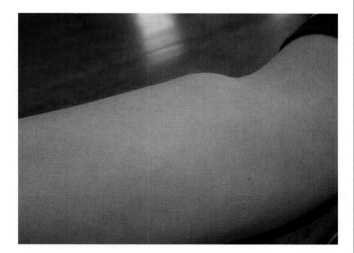

Fig. 2.5 Lipoma

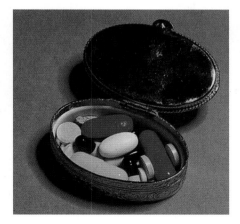

Fig. 2.6 Pill box presented by an outpatient who proved to be taking eight different medications, including a corticosteroid daily

Table 2.9 Drug names and possible identification

Drugs ending in…	Possible type of drug[a]
-am	Benzodiazepines
-ase	Fibrinolytics
-apine	Antipsychotics
-asone/one	Corticosteroids
-azine	Antipsychotics
-azole	Azole antifungals
-azosin	α-adrenoreceptor blockers
-cillin	Penicillins
-cin	Some antimicrobials
-coxib	Newer non-steroidal anti-inflammatory drugs
-cycline	Tetracyclines
-dopa	Antiparkinsonian agents
-dronate/dronic	Bisphosphonates
-erol	β_2 agonists (used for asthma)
-fibrate	Fibrates
-imab/umab	Monoclonal antibodies
-ipine	Calcium channel blockers
-lukast	Leukotriene receptor antagonists
-navir	Protease inhibitors
-nitrate	Nitrates
-olol	Beta-blockers
-ovir	Antivirals
-parin	Heparins
-prazole	Proton pump inhibitors
-pril	Angiotensin-converting enzyme inhibitors
-relin	Gonadorelin analogues
-salazine	Salicylate derivatives
-sartan	Angiotensin receptor antagonist
-setron	$5HT_3$ antagonists
-statin	Statins
-terol	β_2-adrenergic agonist
-tidine	H_2 receptor antagonists
-triptan	$5HT_1$ agonists
-tropium	Antimuscarinic bronchodilators
-vudine	Nucleoside reverse transcriptase inhibitors

[a]Always check in *British National Formulary* (BNF).

Examination of the neck is crucial. The patient should be observed from the front but also the neck should be palpated as swollen lymph nodes are sometimes a sign of disease (Fig. 2.10). One third of lymph nodes of the body are in the neck.

In-patients must always have a full physical examination before an operation, which may include inspection, palpation, percussion and auscultation, and includes examination of the lymph nodes and at least the following systems:

- cardiovascular – pulse, blood pressure, heart sounds
- respiratory – respiratory rate, lung expansion, tracheal position, lung sounds

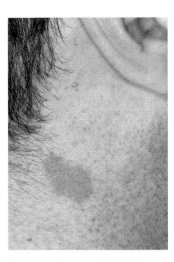

Fig. 2.7 Café-au-lait patch indicative of neurofibromatosis

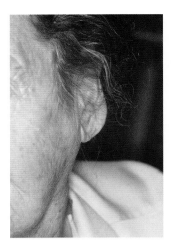

Fig. 2.9 Salivary gland swelling

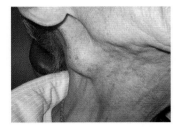

Fig. 2.10 Cervical lymphadenopathy

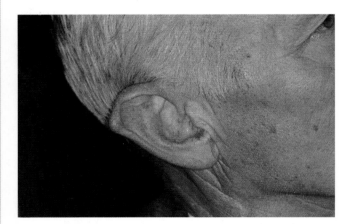

Fig. 2.8 Gouty tophi

- gastrointestinal – any swelling or restriction of movement or tenderness should be noted, together with palpation for masses and tenderness
- neurological – especially the cranial nerves.

Speech disturbances may suggest drug intoxication, xerostomia, learning disorder, neurological or muscle diseases. Loss of weight or emaciation can be features of anorexia, malignant disease, tuberculosis or human immunodeficiency virus (HIV) infection.

Hands can show a number of features. Deformities can be seen in arthritis (Fig. 2.11). Palmar erythema can be seen in liver disease and rheumatoid arthritis. Finger-clubbing may be congenital or seen in cardiorespiratory disease and liver cirrhosis. Koilonychia (spoon-shaped nails) is seen in iron deficiency; leukonychia (white nails) in liver cirrhosis; nail defects in lichen planus (Fig. 2.12), chronic candidosis and psoriasis; nail haemorrhages in infective endocarditis; and pigmentation in drug use (e.g. zidovudine; Fig. 2.13). Raynaud phenomenon can be a feature of connective tissue disorders. Finger-joint deformities can be features of rheumatoid arthritis. Dupuytren contracture may be

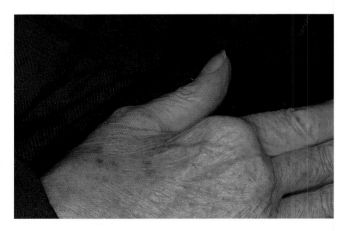

Fig. 2.11 Arthritis

seen in alcoholic cirrhosis and muscle contractures in cerebral palsy.

Hair changes can be features of several conditions. Alopecia may be autoimmune, or seen in lichen planus, or occur after radiation. Hirsutism is seen in adrenogenital syndrome, Cushing disease or due to ciclosporin, corticosteroids, minoxidil, phenytoin or androgenic steroids.

Eyes may show features of disease. Exophthalmos can be seen in hyperthyroidism, ptosis in myopathy and Horner syndrome. Blue sclerae can be features of infancy, and osteogenesis imperfecta. Conjunctival haemorrhage can indicate trauma, fractured zygoma or purpura. Jaundice can imply liver disease.

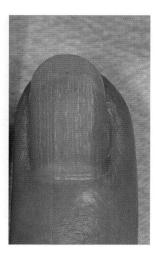

Fig. 2.12 Lichen planus nail

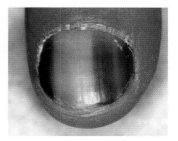

Fig. 2.13 Nail discolouration may be seen after trauma or in local disease, such as fungal infections, in drug use (as here) or in systemic disease

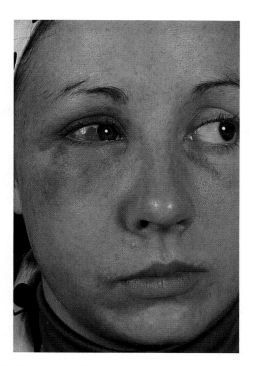

Fig. 2.14 Subconjunctival haemorrhage associated with zygomatic fracture

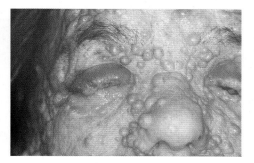

Fig. 2.15 Neurofibromatosis

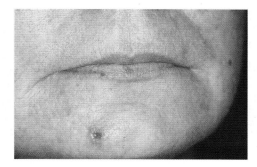

Fig. 2.16 Basal cell carcinoma

The face may be unusual in many syndromes, such as Down syndrome, mucopolysaccharidoses; may exhibit bruising from trauma (Fig. 2.14) or purpura; cushingoid facies in Cushing disease or due to corticosteroid treatment; masklike facies in scleroderma. Facial telangiectasia is seen in hereditary haemorrhagic telangiectasia, cirrhosis and CREST (calcinosis, Raynaud, oesophageal dysfunction, scleroderma, telangiectasia) syndrome. Facial palsy may indicate stroke or Bell palsy. Neurofibromatosis (Fig. 2.15), tumours (Fig. 2.16) and cysts (Fig. 2.17) may present as lumps. Infection may cause swelling (Fig. 2.18). Myxoedema may indicate hypothyroidism. 'Butterfly rash' over the face may indicate systemic lupus erythematosus, angiofibromas may underlie tuberous sclerosis (epiloia; Fig. 2.19). A malar flush can be seen in mitral valve stenosis; xanthelasmas in hyperlipidaemia; cyanosis in hypoxia – cardiac or respiratory disease. Pallor is seen in anaemia or an imminent faint; purpura in thrombocytopenia or trauma; hyperpigmentation can be racial, or due to suntan, Addison disease or chronic drug (e.g. phenothiazine) use; hypopigmentation can be due to vitiligo (Fig. 2.20).

Cervical lymph node enlargement is seen in HIV and other infections, malignancy, leukaemia. Salivary gland swellings can represent mumps, Sjögren syndrome, sialosis or tumour. The lips can show cheilitis (e.g. factitious; Fig. 2.21), lichen planus (Fig. 2.22) or erythema multiforme. Angular stomatitis can be associated with denture-related stomatitis, anaemia, haematinic deficiency, diabetes, HIV and other diseases (Fig. 2.23). Lip swelling may be seen in infections, Crohn disease, sarcoidosis or angioedema. Lip pigmentation may underlie Peutz–Jegher syndrome. 'Hanging jaw' is a feature of myasthenia gravis. Prognathism and thickened facies can

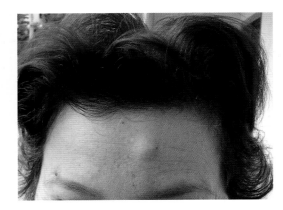

Fig. 2.17 Sebaceous cyst

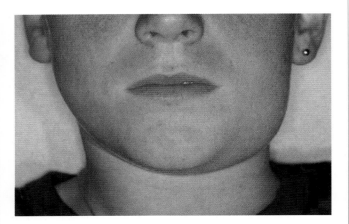

Fig. 2.18 Cat scratch disease

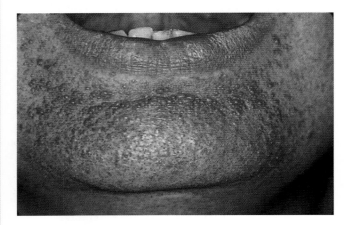

Fig. 2.19 Tuberous sclerosis showing adenoma sebaceum

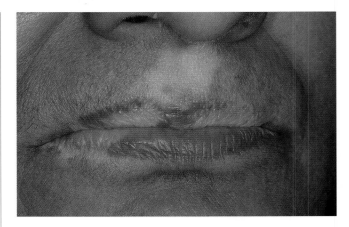

Fig. 2.20 Vitiligo

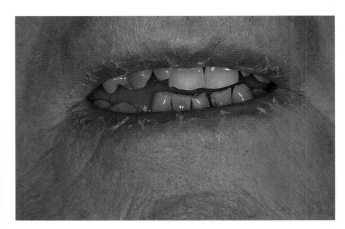

Fig. 2.21 Exfoliative cheilitis

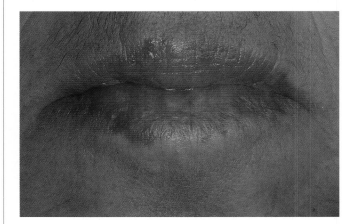

Fig. 2.22 Lichen planus on lips

be features of acromegaly. Lumps may indicate neoplasms (Fig. 2.24).

Most evidence shows that the history and physical examination often reveal most if not all of the clinically useful data. Before any investigations are initiated, the patient's consent must be obtained. Confidentiality must be respected: the history and examination and investigation findings should not be divulged except when there is expressed consent.

INVESTIGATIONS

Investigations are useful only when the appropriate tests are requested, and interpreted in the light of the history, clinical findings, knowledge and experience. It is useless and potentially dangerous to request investigations, the results of which will have no influence on the diagnosis or management.

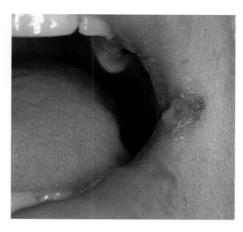

Fig. 2.23 Angular stomatitis

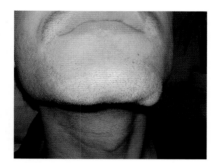

Fig. 2.24 Osteoma

Screening for latent medical problems is *sometimes* appropriate, mainly when effective action can be taken on the basis of the results. Several relevant treatable conditions, particularly hypertension and diabetes, are frequently unsuspected. For example, blood and urine glucose levels may be abnormal in 5% or more of dental patients. However, it is important not to undertake testing that may cause unnecessary anxiety, trauma, delay or expense.

Many studies have shown the *disadvantages* of 'routine' and 'screening' tests, even pre-operatively, carried out with little focus; too often, trivial or inexplicable findings are revealed and unnecessary anxiety and stress caused.

PRE-OPERATIVE TESTS

Pre-operative tests may provide information to reduce possible harm or increase benefit to the patient by altering surgical or sedation/anaesthetic management, and may help risk assessment and discussion with the patient relevant to informed consent. They may predict post-operative complications and establish a baseline measurement for later reference. However, it is important before requesting any investigation that there is a high enough likelihood of finding an abnormal result and that an abnormal result would genuinely change the patient's management. The National Institute for Health and Clinical Excellence (NICE) guidelines are generic and lack consensus; hospitals may have their own guidelines and individual clinicians remain ultimately responsible.

Table 2.10	Grades of surgery
Grade	**Examples of procedures**
1	Excision of lumps and bumps, incision of abscesses, tooth removal
2	Arthroscopy, herniorraphy, varicose veins
3	Hysterectomy, thyroidectomy
4	Major bowel, cardiac, head and neck, and joint surgery, and neurosurgery

For the purpose of pre-operative tests, NICE categorize surgical procedures on the basis of complexity and physiological insult into four grades (Table 2.10).

Chest radiograph (X-ray)

The likelihood of identifying undiagnosed cardiorespiratory disease and the desirability to re-evaluate patients with known conditions need to be balanced against the radiation exposure. In general, ASA I patients do not require pre-operative chest X-rays (CXRs) with the *possible* exception of smokers over the age of 60 undergoing grade 3 or 4 surgery. Certain types of surgery *may* warrant a CXR at some point in the patient's work-up (e.g. cardiothoracic, oesophageal and major head and neck surgery). ASA III patients with cardiovascular disease undergoing anything more than grade 1 surgery should probably have a CXR. This should not be repeated if one has been done within 6 months unless the patient has had a change in their symptoms or signs; in many cases, it could be argued that echocardiography provides more useful information and avoids radiation exposure. Respiratory disease that has changed in its nature or severity with time is a probable indication for CXR with the exception of patients between the ages of 16 and 40 undergoing grade 1 surgery.

Electrocardiogram

An electrocardiogram (ECG) may on occasions provide evidence of asymptomatic cardiovascular disease and, in those with known cardiac disease, is useful in estimating risks of GA and surgery. An ECG should be obtained for smokers, and patients with history or symptoms of cardiac, respiratory or renal disease undergoing grade 4 surgery, and all patients over the age of 60 regardless of the grade of surgery.

Full blood count (full blood picture)

Full blood count (FBC) may identify and quantify pre-existing anaemia and help assessment of the patient's likely tolerance of any blood loss. FBC is probably indicated in all patients undergoing grade 3 and 4 surgery, particularly in patients with cardiovascular or respiratory disease, for all patients with renal disease and for all patients over 60 undergoing grade 2 surgery. The white cell count (WCC) may be useful if infection is suspected, and the platelet count where there is suspicion or history of bleeding tendency.

Sickle test

A sickle test should be requested for all patients of African and West Indian origin, and probably also for those of Mediterranean and Indian origin.

Haemostasis tests

Haemostatic tests are platelet count, prothrombin time (PT), international normalized ratio (INR) and activated partial thromboplastin time (APTT). Indications for pre-operative tests of haemostasis are patients taking anticoagulants, or patients on haemodialysis, or where there is a past history or family history of abnormal bleeding, bruising, liver, kidney or vascular disease, or before surgery likely to cause a large blood loss so that the need for transfusion is likely, and before arterial reconstructive surgery or surgery for cancer especially where liver metastases may have resulted in a bleeding tendency. Investigations should be considered where regional anaesthesia is planned, particularly spinal and epidural techniques.

Renal function tests (urea and electrolytes)

Renal function should be assessed in all patients with known renal disease, diabetes, liver dysfunction, and those with an ileus, who are parenterally fed or who are likely to have intravenous fluid administration and perioperative fluid loss.

All adults and children should have urea and electrolyte tests (U&Es) before grade 4 surgery (U&Es are otherwise not generally required in children). These tests are needed in all adults of ASA III or undergoing grade 3 surgery. Older patients may have asymptomatic deteriorating renal function, so U&Es should be obtained for those aged 60 and over, and before grade 3 surgery. In patients with cardiovascular disease, U&Es are needed in those aged 60 and over undergoing grade 2 surgery.

IMAGING

X-RAYS (RADIOGRAPHY)

Radiography, fully discussed elsewhere, is particularly helpful diagnostically since it is inexpensive, rapidly achieved and widely available. Conventional radiography is useful for imaging: bone and joint disease, fractures and dislocations, antral and dental disease (see Table 2.11.) Plain X-rays have a relatively low radiation dose and special procedures can achieve soft-tissue imaging, albeit with a higher radiation dose.

Radiography requests are essential to enable the radiographic staff to give you the best or most appropriate radiographs for the region under investigation.

1. Fill in the request form as fully as possible with full, relevant, clinical findings.
2. Request the region required rather than specific views, except for dental panoramic tomography, when the term 'DPT' will suffice.

Table 2.11 Radiographs recommended for demonstrating various head and neck sites

Region required	Standard views	Additional views
Skull[a]	PA 20 Lateral Townes (1/2 axial view)	SMV Tangential
Facial bones	OM OM 30 Lateral	Zygoma Reduced exposure SMV
Paranasal sinuses	OM for maxillary antra	Upper occlusal or lateral SMV DPT, tomography
Orthodontics	DPT Cephalometric lateral skull	
Pre- and post-osteotomy	DPT Cephalometric lateral skull Cephalometric PA skull	
Nasal bones	OM 30 Lateral Soft tissue lateral	
Mandible	DPT	Lateral obliques PA mandible Mandibular occlusal
Temporomandibular joints	Transcranial lateral obliques or DPT (mouth open and closed)	Transpharyngeal Arthrography Reverse Townes Reverse DPT Consider CT scan/MRI

[a]CT scanning is valuable in craniofacial injuries.
CT, computed tomography; DPT, dental panoramic tomogram; MRI, magnetic resonance imaging; OM, occipitomental; PA, posteroanterior; SMV, submentovertex.

COMPUTED AXIAL TOMOGRAPHY

A computed tomography (CT) or computed axial tomography (CAT) scan is a type of repeated special radiograph taken across 'slices' of the body to build up a complex image, using several beams simultaneously from a number of different angles (Fig. 2.25).

Advantages

- It provides good anatomical representation of hard tissues (bone and cartilage).
- It is generally better than magnetic resonance imaging (MRI) for examining lymph nodes.
- It provides good cross-sectional representation.
- Multiplanar reconstruction is possible from the raw data of the initial examination.
- Three-dimensional reconstruction is possible.
- It provides guidance for biopsies.
- Compared with MRI:
  it is more widely available

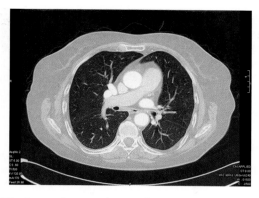

Fig. 2.25 Computed tomography scan of chest

imaging is more rapid (in seconds compared with MRI, which takes minutes)

it is affected less by motion artefact, since it is quicker

it can be used on patients for whom MRI is inappropriate (e.g. claustrophobics, or people with pacemakers, ferrous or paramagnetic aneurysm clips).

Disadvantages

- CT gives a significant radiation dose.
- It provides phasic imaging of vascular structures and tumours.
- CT is an expensive procedure.
- The whole CT procedure may take up to 1 h, but often takes less than 30 min.
- Some patients experience claustrophobia in the CT scanner.

Indications

Computed tomography allows visualization of 3–10-mm sections of the body in two dimensions with enough clear distinction between black, grey and white areas of the image to allow pathological diagnosis in many cases.

It is particularly useful in examining the chest or abdomen. CT using contrast media makes it possible to visualize abnormalities more clearly.

Contraindications

Contraindications include pregnancy and history of severe allergies; this may preclude the use of a contrast agent.

Procedure

1. Patients may be asked not to eat beforehand.
2. Patients may have to swallow or be injected intravenously with contrast material that will show up against the tissue on the final pictures.
3. The patient must lie on a couch, which will move through the scanner.

4. The radiographer can see, hear and communicate with the patient (by means of a two-way microphone and speaker system) at all times.
5. The scanner will take a series of pictures.
6. The patient must lie still while images are being taken in order to ensure that they are in focus, and may be asked to hold their breath so the scan is not blurred.

SCINTIGRAPHY/NUCLEAR MEDICINE

Radionuclide (radioisotope) scans can be particularly useful to detect abnormalities in bone, salivary glands, thyroid gland and lymph nodes. Common radionuclide agents used include technetium 99^m (Tc-99m)-labelled diphosphonates for bone scans, and gallium for imaging lymph nodes.

Radionuclide scanning involves administration of a radionuclide with an affinity for the organ or tissue of interest and recording of the distribution of radioactivity. A very small amount of a mildly radioactive liquid is injected into a vein, usually in the arm, and after the injection the patient will have to wait up to 3 h before the scan can be taken. The distribution of the radionuclide is detected in the tissue/organ under examination where the isotope is concentrated, by a gamma camera, which produces the images or scans after processing by a computer. Detectors record activity in retaining organs at time of acquisition. Time/activity curves can be plotted to provide functional analysis. The images can then be produced on film, coloured paper or as graphs or numerical data. The amount of radioactivity given to a patient is small, not dangerous to either the patient or to anyone nearby, and usually clears from the body within 24 h.

POSITRON EMISSION TOMOGRAPHY

Radioactive molecules made from radionuclides (radioactive isotopes) with short half-lives such as ^{11}C, ^{15}O or ^{13}N are injected intravenously. Depending on the type of molecule injected, positron emission tomography (PET) can provide information on different biochemical functions. For example, if glucose is used, the PET scan will show an image of glucose metabolism, or how much energy the body is using in a specific area (such as the brain or a tumour).

MAGNETIC RESONANCE IMAGING (NUCLEAR MAGNETIC RESONANCE)

Magnetic resonance imaging (MRI) is a safe, non-invasive procedure that allows three-dimensional images of internal organs to be created with radio waves and large powerful electromagnets to align hydrogen atoms (protons) within the body (Fig. 2.26).

Advantages

- There is no ionizing radiation.
- It provides new, rapidly developing, good multiplanar imaging.
- It provides good soft-tissue differentiation, which is better than that with CT.

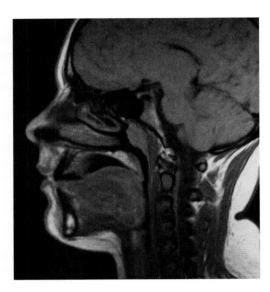

Fig. 2.26 Magnetic resonance image of head and neck

- It provides good imaging of bone marrow.
- It provides good imaging of perineural infiltration.
- Pictures can be taken from multiple angles.
- It can be performed through clothing and through dense tissue such as bone.
- There is less distortion from dental restorations than with CT.

Disadvantages

Magnetic resonance imaging is dangerous for people with pacemakers or defibrillators and inappropriate for those with ferrous or paramagnetic aneurysm clips. MRI is currently relatively expensive and time-consuming (it can take anything from 30 min to 1 h and 30 min, or even 2 h), rather noisy and some patients experience claustrophobia. It can also be affected by motion artefact, since it is slow.

Indications

Magnetic resonance imaging, like CT, can be used to produce cross-sectional views of the body or a body part, but MRI can also be used for other views such as sagittal. MRI allows a clear distinction between black, grey and white areas of the image to allow pathological diagnosis in many cases.

Again like CT, MRI can be used on any part of the body but is frequently used to examine the head and brain, since it is there that it produces clearer results than does CT. MRI is also useful in detecting abnormalities in soft tissues and in chest or abdominal examination.

Contraindications

These include:

- presence of a cardiac pacemaker, defibrillator or monitor
- vascular or surgical clips
- any type of orthopaedic prosthesis, rods or pins

- dentures or appliances of any type in the mouth, which must be removed before the scan (implants, fixed crowns or restorations are not a contraindication; see below)
- an intrauterine contraceptive device (IUD)
- pregnancy – any effects of MRI on pregnancy are unclear
- history of allergies – may preclude the use of contrast agent.

Procedure

1. Patients may be asked not to eat for 1 h before the scan; not to smoke for 2 h before; and not to drink tea, coffee, alcohol or soft drinks containing caffeine (cola, etc.) for 2 h before, as these can affect blood flow and so affect the scan. Iron interferes with the scan and thus iron-containing medications should not be taken.
2. As the MRI scan uses magnetism, metals may affect it. Persons with certain types of metal surgical clips, metal pins or plates, cardiac monitors or pacemakers cannot therefore have an MRI scan. The patient must remove everything metal, including watches, any jewellery including piercings, metal clothes closures, belts, metal-containing prostheses, hair clips, shoes, mobile phones, personal organizers, keys, purses and wallets containing magnetic strip credit cards. These must all be left outside the room.
3. MRI scans are noisy, so the patient wears ear plugs.
4. The patient must lie on a couch that can move backwards and forwards through the cylinder.
5. The patient must lie still while images are being taken in order to ensure that they are in focus, and may be asked to hold their breath so the scan is not blurred.
6. The radiographer can see, hear and communicate with the patient (by means of a two-way microphone and speaker system) at all times.
7. The MRI is in a special room to exclude radio waves as these interfere with the scan.

ULTRASOUND (ULTRASONOGRAPHY)

Ultrasound is the use of high-frequency sound waves (a frequency over 20 000 Hz; 20 kHz), which are reflected at interfaces between tissues. An ultrasound scan uses very high frequency sound waves not audible to the human ear, passed through the body using a transmitter or scanner that is normally placed on the skin surface. The pattern of the reflected sound waves or 'echoes' is used to create an outline of the organ in question, so ultrasonography is used for soft tissues rather than bony structures. It can measure size, detect structural abnormalities, determine whether a lump is solid or fluid-filled, or monitor growth of the fetus during pregnancy.

Advantages

- Ultrasound examination is completely painless and safe.
- It produces no ionizing radiation.
- It is inexpensive and provides a good screening test.
- The equipment is mobile.

- It provides good differentiation between cystic and solid soft-tissue masses.
- Advanced technique (Doppler) assesses flow characteristics in vessels.

Indications

- To diagnose disease in liver, gallbladder, pancreas, urinary bladder, prostate, kidney, thyroid gland, lymph nodes, salivary glands, ovaries or testicles, and breast.
- In obstetrics, to check that there are no fetal abnormalities, and to monitor fetal growth.
- For ophthalmic imaging.
- To examine blood flow.
- To diagnose aneurysms.
- For echocardiography.

Contraindications

None known.

Procedure

1. Ultrasound examination takes between 15 min and 1 h.
2. Usually, a lubricating silicone gel applied to the skin is used to help conduct the sound waves into the body.
3. Patients must lie still during the examination.
4. For some more specialized kinds of ultrasound examination, the probe is inserted into the body.
5. In abdominal ultrasound scanning, large amounts of gas in the intestine can interfere with the images. Therefore, in these instances, low-fibre foods should be taken for 24–36 h before the examination. Some examinations of the intestines, for example, require a preparatory enema and fasting for several hours before the appointment. Others, as used in obstetrics, may require a full bladder.

LABORATORY INVESTIGATIONS

HISTOPATHOLOGY

A biopsy of adequate size and representative of the lesion should be taken, placed in a fixative and sent to the pathology laboratory carefully labelled and with the appropriate form of request for histopathological examination.

- Specimens for *routine histological examination* should be fixed in 10% formol saline; at least ten times the volume of the specimen is needed for adequate fixation.
- Specimens for *immunofluorescent investigations* are not usually carried out on formol saline-fixed tissue, but should be sent in a suitable transport medium for immediate freezing at −70°C and direct immunofluorescence. Serum should also be sent for indirect immunofluorescence.

If tuberculosis or a systemic mycosis is suspected, a fresh tissue specimen should be sent for culture.

MICROBIOLOGY

Specimens should be collected before antimicrobials are started. If pus is present, a sample should be sent in a sterile container, in preference to a swab. Requests for culture and antibiotic sensitivity should indicate possible aetiology, present antimicrobial therapy and any drug allergies. If tuberculosis is suspected, this must be clearly indicated on the request form.

If the microbiological specimen cannot be dealt with within 2 h, the swab should be placed in transport medium and kept in the refrigerator at 4°C (not a freezer) until dealt with by the microbiology department.

Actinomycosis

Preferably send pus for culture but, in the absence of adequate pus, send a dressing that has been in contact with the wound for several hours.

Candidosis

Swabs from the lesions and from the fitting surface of the denture may be sent for Gram stain or culture.

Viral hepatitis or HIV infection

Many centres have defined protocols for the collection of specimens from patients with suspected hepatitis or HIV infection. Particular care must be taken to avoid needlestick injuries and contaminating the outside of the containers, and to indicate the hazard of the infection. Special coloured plastic bags (usually red) to indicate this hazard can be used for transporting the specimen. Consent is required when testing, particularly for HIV.

Other viral infections

Swabs must be sent in viral transport medium: dry swabs are no use. Acute and convalescent serum samples (10 ml blood in plain container) should be taken. The convalescent serum is collected 2–3 weeks after the acute illness.

Syphilis

Oral lesions should be cleaned with saline to remove oral treponemes before a smear is made for dark-ground examination: 10 ml of serum should be sent for VDRL (Venereal Disease Research Laboratory) testing (Ch. 21).

HAEMATOLOGY

Blood for film and red cell indices must be collected into a tube containing potassium EDTA (ethylenediamine tetra-acetic acid; 4 ml into an EDTA tube). EDTA inhibits clotting through its action on cation-dependent proteolytic enzymes critical to the clotting cascade. The blood must be gently mixed to ensure that the anticoagulant is well distributed; clotted samples are useless. Blood for assay of corrected whole blood folate levels is also collected in an EDTA tube. Most other necessary investigations are performed on serum (Appendix 2.2). Any venepuncture episode requires consent, both for the insertion of the needle and the investigations being carried out on the blood sample. See Table 2.12 for potential complications.

BIOCHEMISTRY

There is currently some variation as to whether serum or plasma is needed for certain biochemical tests depending on the laboratory involved. Special containers may be required for automated multichannel analysers, which give a full biochemical profile on a single blood specimen. However, most biochemical estimations can be carried out on serum (collect blood in a plain container), although plasma (collect in a lithium heparin tube) may be needed for estimation of electrolytes, cortisol and proteins. Blood glucose assays are carried out on a sample in a fluoride bottle. Urinalysis is also available (Appendix 2.3+2.4).

IMMUNOLOGY

Most tests of humoral immunity and complement components are carried out on serum (plain tube). Autoantibodies are detected in serum. In order to prevent the rapid decay of complement components, the serum should be separated as soon as possible and frozen at –20°C at least and preferably at –70°C. Serum for immune complexes and cryoglobulins may need special handling, details of which can be obtained from the relevant laboratory.

Tests of cell-mediated immunity are expensive and can often only be carried out once special preparations have been made (consult the laboratory; Appendix 2.5).

Table 2.12	Complications of venepuncture
Complication	**Remarks**
Failure in a young normal adult	Relax. Correct application of tourniquet. Warm the arm/hand. Check that the syringe and needle will aspirate. Try the other arm; use a sphygmomanometer cuff at just below diastolic pressure; make sure that you can palpate the vein before trying again
Difficult patients	
Fat arm: veins difficult to locate	Remember that the veins are there. Palpate the antecubital fossa over the usual vein site (see text) If unsuccessful, try the veins on the radial side of the wrist or on the back of the hand (painful)
Thin arm: veins move away from the needle	Most annoying! Insert the needle deliberately alongside the vein, preferably at a Y-junction and immobilize the vein with your other hand before penetrating vein from the side
Haematoma formation	Most annoying to the patient! Owing to poor technique, inadequate pressure to puncture site or removing needle before tourniquet removed. May cause venous thrombosis. Try not to penetrate through the other side of the vein. Keep firm pressure with swab on vein after venepuncture until haemostasis secured. In the elderly, maintain this pressure for several minutes

See below for direct immunofluorescence specimens.

The presence of autoantibodies does not always indicate disease and absence does not necessarily exclude it. The type of autoimmune disorder or disease that occurs and the amount of destruction depends on which systems or organs are targeted by the autoantibodies, and how strongly. Disorders caused by organ-specific autoantibodies, those that primarily target a single organ, such as the thyroid in Graves disease and Hashimoto thyroiditis, are often the easiest to diagnose as they frequently present with organ-related disease.

Once a diagnosis has been made and a treatment plan has been decided on, it must be explained to the patient and informed consent must be obtained.

USEFUL WEBSITES

For Department of Health key consent documents, see: www.dh.gov.uk
The GDC has produced a supporting guidance to its standards specifically on consent, Principles of patient consent, which can be found at the following link:
http://www.gdc-uk.org/NR/rdonlyres/FFD61DA5-A09E-4B38-8FFB-BA342E9F0AF4/16688/147163_Patient_Cons.pdf
http://www.nice.org.uk/nicemedia/pdf/Preop_Fullguideline.pdf

FURTHER READING

Abraham-Inpijn, L., Russell, G., Abraham, D.A., et al., 2008. A patient-administered medical risk related history questionnaire (EMRRH) for use in 10 European countries (multicenter trial). Oral Surg Oral Med Oral Pathol Oral Radiol Endod 105, 597–605.

Brown J. Scully C, 2004. Advances in oral health care imaging; part two Private Dentistry. 9;2, 67–71.

Brown J. Scully C, 2004. Advances in oral health care imaging; part three Private Dentistry. 9;3, 78–79.

Geist, S.M., Geist, J.R., 2008. Improvement in medical consultation responses with a structured request form. J Dent Educ 72, 553–561.

General Medical Council. Consent to investigation and treatment: www.gmc-uk.org.

Goodchild, J.H., Glick, M., 2003. A different approach to medical risk assessment. Endodont Topics 4, 1–8.

Hainsworth, J.M., Hill, K.B., Rice, A., Fairbrother, K.J., 2008. Psychosocial characteristics of adults who experience difficulties with retching. J Dent 36, 494–499.

Henwood, S., Wilson, M.A., Edwards, I., 2006. The role of competence and capacity in relation to consent for treatment in adult patients. Br Dent J 200, 18–21.

Leslie, D., Lipsky, P., Notkins, A.L., 2001. Autoantibodies as predictors of disease. J Clin Invest 108, 1417–1422.

Lockwood, A.J., Yang, Y.F., 2008. Nitrous oxide inhalation anaesthesia in the presence of intraocular gas can cause irreversible blindness. Br Dent J 204, 247–248.

Longmore, M., Wilkinson, I., Turmezei, T., Cheung, C.K., Smith, E., 2007. Oxford handbook of clinical medicine, 7th edn. Oxford University Press, Oxford.

Pyle, M.A., Lalumandier, J.A., Sawyer, D.R., 2000. Prevalence of elevated blood pressure in students attending a college oral health program. Spec Care Dentist 20, 234–239.

Royal College of Surgeons of England, 2002. Code of practice for the surgical management of Jehovah's witnesses. Royal College of Surgeons of England, London.

Thikkurissy, S., Smiley, M., Casamassimo, P.S., 2008. Concordance and contrast between community-based physicians' and dentist anesthesiologists' history and physicals in outpatient pediatric dental surgery. Anesth Prog 55, 35–39.

Appendix 2.1 Suggested medical questionnaire for patients to complete

Other useful formats are available such as that referenced in the Resuscitation Council UK document 2006 on Medical Emergencies for Dental Practitioners.

		YES	NO	DETAILS
1	Have you had an operation or anaesthetic before?			
2	Have you had any problems with anaesthetics?			
3	Have any of your relatives had any problems with anaesthetics?			
4	Are you taking any drugs or other medications (inhalers, Pill)?			
5	If female, are you or could you be pregnant?			
6	Have you had any steroid drugs in the past? If yes, when?			
7	Have you any allergies (drugs/plasters/antiseptics/foodstuffs)?			
8	Do you have heart disease or have you had a heart attack?			
9	Do you ever have to take antibiotics routinely prior to dental surgery?			
10	Do you get chest pains, indigestion, or tummy acid in the throat?			
11	Do you have an hiatus hernia?			
12	Do you have high blood pressure?			
13	Do you get breathless walking, climbing stairs or lying flat?			
14	Do you have asthma, bronchitis, or chest disease?			
15	Have you ever had a convulsion or a fit?			
16	Do you have arthritis or muscle disease?			
17	Do you have anaemia or other blood disorder?			
18	Do you know your sickle status (if relevant)?			
19	Have you ever had liver disease or been jaundiced?			
20	Have you ever had kidney disease?			
21	Do you have diabetes (sugar in your urine)?			
22	Do you smoke? If yes, how many a day (also last six months)?			
23	Do you drink alcohol? If yes, how many units per week?			
24	Do you have any crowns, loose or artificial teeth? Indicate:			
25	Do you wear contact lenses?			
26	Is there anything else you think the surgeon or anaesthetist should know?			

Appendix 2.2 Interpretation of haematological results

Blood	Normal range[a]	Level ↑	Level ↓
Haemoglobin	Male 13.0–18.0 g/dl Female 11.5–16.5 g/dl	Polycythaemia (rubra vera or physiological); myeloproliferative disease; dehydration	Anaemia
Haematocrit (packed cell volume or PCV)	Male 40–54% Female 37–47%	Polycythaemia; dehydration	Anaemia
Mean cell volume (MCV) MCV = PCV/RBC	78–99 fl	Macrocytosis in vitamin B_{12} or folate deficiency; liver disease; alcoholism; hypothyroidism; myelodysplasia; myeloproliferative disorders; aplastic anaemia; cytotoxic agent	Microcytosis in iron deficiency, thalassaemia, chronic disease
Mean cell haemoglobin (MCH) MCH = Hb/RBC	27–31 pg/cell	Pernicious anaemia	Iron deficiency; thalassaemia; sideroblastic anaemia
Mean cell haemoglobin concentration (MCHC) MCHC = Hb/PCV	32–36 g/dl		Iron deficiency; thalassaemia; sideroblastic anaemia; anaemia in chronic disease
Red cell count (RBC)	Male 4.2–6.1 × 10^{12}/L Female 4.2–5.4 × 10^{12}/L	Polycythaemia	Anaemia; fluid overload
White cell count (total)	4–10 × 10^{9}/L	Infection; inflammation; leukaemia; intense exercise; trauma; stress; pregnancy	Early leukaemia; some infections; bone marrow disease; drugs including corticosteroids and chemotherapy; idiopathic
Neutrophils	Average 3.3 × 10^{9}/L	Pregnancy; exercise; infection; bleeding; trauma; malignancy; leukaemia; corticosteroids	Some infections; drugs; endocrinopathies; bone marrow disease; idiopathic
Lymphocytes	Average 2.5 × 10^{9}/L	Physiological; some infections; leukaemia; lymphoma	Some infections; some immune defects (e.g. HIV, AIDS); lymphoma; corticosteroids; SLE
Eosinophils	Average 0.15 × 10^{9}/L	Allergic disease; parasitic infestations; skin disease; malignancy including lymphoma	Some immune defects
Platelets	150–400 × 10^{9}/L	Thrombocytosis in bleeding; myeloproliferative disease; chronic inflammatory states	Thrombocytopenia related to leukaemia; drugs; HIV; other infections; idiopathic; autoimmune; DIC
Reticulocytes	0.5–1.5% of RBC	Haemolytic states; during treatment of anaemia	Chemotherapy; bone marrow disease
Erythrocyte sedimentation rate (ESR)	0–15 mm/h	Pregnancy; infections; anaemia; inflammation; connective tissue disease; temporal arteritis; trauma; infarction; tumours	–
Plasma viscosity	1.4–1.8 cp	As ESR	

[a]Adults unless otherwise stated. Check values with your laboratory.

AIDS, acquired immune deficiency syndrome; DIC, disseminated intravascular coagulopathy; Hb, haemoglobin; HIV, human immunodeficiency virus; MCH, mean corpuscular haemoglobin; MCHC, mean corpuscular haemoglobin concentration; SLE, systemic lupus erythematosus.

Appendix 2.3 Interpretation of biochemical results[a]

Biochemistry[b]	Level[c] ↑	Level[c] ↓
Acid phosphatase	Prostatic malignancy; renal disease; acute myeloid leukaemia	–
Alanine transaminase (ALT)[d]	Liver disease; infectious mononucleosis	Hypothyroidism; hypophosphatasia; malnutrition
Alkaline phosphatase	Puberty; pregnancy; Paget disease; osteomalacia; fibrous dysplasia; malignancy in bone; liver disease; hyperparathyroidism (some); hyperphosphatasia	–
Alpha₁-antitrypsin	Liver cirrhosis	Congenital emphysema
Alpha-fetoprotein (AFP)	Pregnancy; gonadal tumour; liver disease	Fall in level in pregnancy indicates fetal distress
Amylase	Pancreatic disease; mumps; some other salivary diseases	–
Angiotensin-converting enzyme (ACE)	Sarcoidosis	–
Antistreptolysin O titre (ASOT)	Streptococcal infections; rheumatic fever; drugs[f]	–
Aspartate transaminase (AST)[e]	Liver disease; biliary disease; myocardial infarct; trauma; drugs[f]	–
Bilrubin (total)	Liver or biliary disease; haemolysis	–
Brain natriuretic peptide	Cardiac failure	–
Caeruloplasmin	Pregnancy; cirrhosis; hyperthyroidism; leukaemia	Wilson disease
Calcium	Primary hyperparathyroidism; malignancy in bone; renal tubular acidosis; sarcoidosis; thiazides; calcium supplements; excess vitamin D	Hypoparathyroidism; renal failure; rickets; nephrotic syndrome; chronic renal failure; lack of vitamin D; low magnesium levels; acute pancreatitis
Cholesterol	Hypercholesterolaemia; pregnancy; hypothyroidism; diabetes; nephrotic syndrome; liver or biliary disease	Malnutrition; hyperthyroidism
Complement (C3)	Trauma; surgery; infection	Liver disease; immune complex diseases (e.g. lupus erythematosus)
Complement (C4)	–	Liver disease; immune complex diseases; HANE (hereditary angioneurotic oedema)
Cortisol (see Steroids)	–	–
Creatine kinase (CK)	Myocardial infarct; trauma; muscle disease; rhabdomyolysis; statins	–
Creatinine	Renal failure; urinary obstruction	Pregnancy
C-reactive protein (CRP)	Inflammation; trauma; myocardial infarct; malignant disease	–
C1 esterase inhibitor	–	Hereditary angiodema
Erythrocyte sedimentation rate (ESR)	Inflammation; trauma; myocardial infarct; malignant disease	–
Ferritin	Liver disease; haemochromatosis; leukaemia; lymphoma; other malignancies; thalassaemia	Iron deficiency
Fibrinogen	Pregnancy; pulmonary embolism; nephritic syndrome; lymphoma	Disseminated intravascular coagulopathy (DIC)
Folic acid	Folic acid therapy	Alcoholism; dietary deficiency; haemolytic anaemias; malabsorption; myelodysplasia; phenytoin; metho-trexate; trimethoprim; pyrimethamine; sulfasalazine; cycloserine; oral contraceptives; pregnancy
Free thyroxine index (FTI; serum T4 and T3 uptake)	Hyperthyroidism	Hypothyroidism
Gamma-glutamyl transpeptidase (GGT)	Alcoholism; obesity; liver disease; myocardial infarct; pancreatitis; diabetes; renal diseases; tricyclics	–
Globulins (total; see also Protein)	Liver disease; multiple myeloma; autoimmune disease; chronic infections	Chronic lymphatic leukaemia; malnutrition; protein-losing states
Glucose	Diabetes mellitus; pancreatitis; hyperthyroidism; hyperpituitarism; Cushing disease; liver disease; post head injury	Hypoglycaemic drugs; Addison disease; hypopituitarism; hyperinsulinism; severe liver disease

(Continued)

Appendix 2.3 Interpretation of biochemical results[a]—cont'd

Biochemistry[b]	Level[c] ↑	Level[c] ↓
Hydroxybutyrate dehydrogenase (HBD) immunoglobulins	Myocardial infarct	–
Total immunoglobulins	Liver disease; infection; sarcoidosis; connective tissue disease	Immunodeficiency; nephrotic syndrome; enteropathy
IgG	Myelomatosis; connective tissue disorders	Immunodeficiency; nephrotic syndrome
IgA	Alcoholic cirrhosis; Berger disease	Immunodeficiency
IgM	Primary biliary cirrhosis; nephrotic syndrome; parasites; infections	Immunodeficiency
IgE	Allergies; parasites	–
Lactate dehydrogenase (LDH)	Myocardial infarct; trauma; liver disease; haemolytic anaemias; lymphoproliferative diseases	Radiotherapy
Lipase	Pancreatic disease	–
Lipids (triglycerides)	Hyperlipidaemia; diabetes mellitus; hypothyroidism; hyper-vitaminosis D	–
Magnesium	Renal failure	Cirrhosis; malabsorption; diuretics; Conn syndrome; renal tubular defects
Nucleotidase	Liver disease	–
Percent carbohydrate-deficient transferrin	Alcoholism	–
Phosphate	Renal failure; bone disease; hypoparathyroidism; hyper-vitaminosis D	Hyperparathyroidism; rickets; malabsorption syndrome; insulin
Potassium	Renal failure; Addison disease; ACE inhibitors; potassium supplements	Vomiting; diabetes; Conn syndrome; diuretics; Cushing disease; malabsorption; corticosteroids; salbutamol
Protein (total)	Liver disease; multiple myeloma; sarcoid; connective tissue diseases	Pregnancy; nephrotic syndrome; malnutrition; enteropathy; renal failure; lymphomas
Albumin	Dehydration	Liver disease; malnutrition; malabsorption; nephrotic syndrome; multiple myeloma; connective tissue disorders
Alpha$_1$-globulin	Oestrogens	Nephrotic syndrome
Alpha$_2$-globulin	Infections; trauma	Nephrotic syndrome
Beta-globulin	Hypercholesterolaemia; liver disease; pregnancy	Chronic disease
Gamma-globulin	(see Immunoglobulins)	Nephrotic syndrome; immunodeficiency
SGGT (see GGT)	–	–
SGOT (see AST)	–	–
SGPT (see ALT)	–	–
Sodium	Dehydration; Cushing disease	Cardiac failure; renal failure; SIADH (syndrome of inappropriate antidiuretic hormone); Addison disease; diuretics
Steroids (corticosteroids)	Cushing disease; some tumours	Addison disease; hypopituitarism
Thyroxine (T4)	Hyperthyroidism; pregnancy; oral contraceptive	Hypothyroidism; nephrotic syndrome; phenytoin
Troponin	Myocardial infarction	–
Urea	Renal failure; dehydration; gastrointestinal bleed	Liver disease; nephrotic syndrome; pregnancy; malnutrition
Uric acid	Gout; leukaemia; renal failure; multiple myeloma	Liver disease; probenecid; allopurinol; salicylates; other drugs
Vitamin B$_{12}$	Liver disease; leukaemia; polycythaemia rubra vera	Pernicious anaemia; gastrectomy; Crohn disease; ileal resection; vegans; metformin

[a]Absolute value ranges may differ from laboratory to laboratory. There are also many more causes of abnormal results than are outlined here.
[b]Serum or plasma.
[c]Adult levels; always consult your own laboratory.
[d]ALT = SGPT (serum glutamate–pyruvate transaminase).
[e]AST = SGOT (serum glutamate–oxaloacetic transaminase).
[f]Ampicillin, cefalothin, cloxacillin, erythromycin, indometacin, methotrexate, opioids.
SI values: 10^{-1}, deci (d); 10^{-2}, centi (c); 10^{-3}, milli (m); 10^{-6}, micro (μ); 10^{-9}, nano (n); 10^{-12}, pico (p); 10^{-15}, femto (f).

Appendix 2.4 Urinalysis: interpretation of results[a,e]

	Colour	Protein	Glucose[b]	Ketones	Bilrubin[c]	Urobilinogen[c]	Blood[d]
Comment	–	Tetrabromphenol blue dye binds to some proteins in urine – mainly albumin. Not all proteins are detected and the sensitivity is not high	–	–	–	–	Tests for intact red cells and free haemoglobin (Hb)
Health	Yellow	Usually no protein, but a trace can be normal in young people	Usually no glucose, but a trace can be normal in 'renal glycosuria' and pregnancy	Usually no ketones but ketonuria may occur in vomiting, fasting or starved patients	Usually no bilrubin	Usually present in normal healthy patients, particularly in concentrated urine	Usually no blood
False positives	Red: beet	Alkaline urine. Container contaminated with disinfectant (e.g. chlorhexidine). Blood or pus in urine. Polyvinyl pyrrolidone infusions	Cefamandole. Container contaminated with hypochlorite	Patients on L-dopa or any phthalein compound	Chlorpromazine and other phenothiazines	Infected urine. Patients taking ascorbic acid, sulfonamides or paraminosalicylate	Menstruation. Container contaminated with some detergents
Disease	Brown: homogentisic acid, bilrubin, urobilin, porphyrins Red: Hb Milky in chyluria	Renal diseases. Also cardiac failure, diabetes, endocarditis, myeloma, amyloid, some drugs, some chemicals	Diabetes mellitus. Also in pancreatitis, hyperthyroidism, Fanconi syndrome, sometimes after a head injury, other endocrinopathies	Diabetes mellitus. Also in febrile or traumatized or starved patients on low carbohydrate diets	Only where conjugated bilirubin is increased – hepatocellular and obstructive liver disease	Haemolytic or hepatic, hepatocellular or obstructive disease. Prolonged antibiotic therapy	Genitourinary diseases. Also in bleeding tendency, haemolysis, rhabdomyolysis, some infections where bacteria contain hydroperoxidase, some drugs, endocarditis

[a]Using test strips (e.g. Ames reagent strips, BM-Test-5L, Diastix or Diabur strips). Normal or non-fresh urine may be alkaline; normal urine may be acid.
[b]Dopa, ascorbate or salicylates may give false negatives.
[c]May be false negative if urine not fresh.
[d]Ascorbic acid may give false negative.
[e]Nitrites and leukocyte esterase positivity suggests a urinary tract infection.
Hb, haemoglobin

Appendix 2.5 Some important autoantibodies

Autoantibodies	Main associations
Anti-actin antibodies	Autoimmune hepatitis, coeliac disease
Anti-epithelial antibodies	
Basement membrane zone	Pemphigoid
Intercellular cement (desmoglein)	Pemphigus
Anti-ganglioside antibodies	
Anti-GD3	Guillain–Barré syndrome
Anti-GM1	Travellers' diarrhoea
Anti-GQ1b	Miller–Fisher syndrome (see Guillain–Barré syndrome)
Anti-gastric parietal cell antibody	Pernicious anaemia
Anti-glomerular basement membrane antibody (Anti-GBM antibody)	Goodpasture syndrome
Anti-Hu antibody	Neuroblastoma
Anti-intrinsic factor antibodies	Pernicious anaemia
Anti-islet cell antibodies*	Diabetes type 1

(Continued)

Appendix 2.5 Some important autoantibodies—cont'd

Autoantibodies	Main associations
Anti-Jo 1 antibody (GAD65)	Polymyositis, dermatomyositis
Anti-liver/kidney microsomal 1 antibody (anti-LKM 1 antibodies)	Chronic hepatitis C
Anti-Ku antibody	Polymyositis/scleroderma (PM/Scl) overlap syndrome
Anti-mitochondrial antibody	Primary biliary cirrhosis
Anti-neutrophil cytoplasmic antibodies (ANCA)	
pANCA (perinuclear; anti-myeloperoxidase)	Ulcerative colitis, polyarteritis nodosa
cANCA (cytoplasmic proteinase 3; anti-PR3)	Wegener granulomatosis
Antinuclear antibodies (ANA) Anti-extractable nuclear antigen antibodies (Anti-ENA antibodies):	
Anti-p62 antibodies	Primary biliary cirrhosis
Anti-sp100 antibodies	Primary biliary cirrhosis
Anti-glycoprotein210 antibodies	Primary biliary cirrhosis
Anti-ds (double-stranded) DNA antibody	Antibody with the highest specificity for systemic lupus erythematosus (SLE) and found in most patients
Anti-Ro (Robair) antibody	Sjögren syndrome
Anti-La (Lattimer) antibody	Sjögren syndrome
Anti-RNP antibody	Mixed connective tissue disease (MCTD)
Anti-Sm antibody	SLE
Anti-PM/Scl (anti-exosome) antibody	PM/Scl overlap syndrome
Anti-Scl 70 antibodies Anti-topoisomerase antibodies	Scleroderma
Anti-centromere antibodies	CREST syndrome
Anti-smooth muscle antibody	Autoimmune hepatitis
Anti-steroid 21-hydroxylase (21-OH) antibody	Addison disease
Anti-thyroid antibodies	
Thyroid peroxidase antibodies (TPOAb)	Hashimoto thyroiditis, Graves disease
TSH receptor antibodies (TRAb)	Graves disease
Thyroglobulin antibodies	Autoimmune thyroid disease
Anti-transglutaminase antibodies	
Anti-tTG (tissue transglutaminase)	Coeliac disease
Anti-eTG (epidermal transglutaminase)	Dermatitis herpetiformis
Rheumatoid factor (RF)	Rheumatoid arthritis (high rate of false positives in SLE and other conditions)
Lupus anticoagulant Anti-thrombin antibodies	SLE

TSH, thyroid-stimulating hormone.

*Anti-insulin; anti-glutamic acid decarboxylase; and 1CA512.

Assessment of the patient has been discussed in Ch. 2. Any form of surgery or invasion of bone or soft tissues causes an inflammatory response, with variable pain and swelling; therefore it is crucial that the benefits outweigh the risks. It is also important only to undertake a procedure or use a drug for which the clinician is aware of interactions and able to manage any potential complications (Table 3.1).

Finally, never alter a patient's medication personally, even aspirin given by another health professional, as this is considered at the least discourteous and, at worst, practising medicine without a licence. Always consult with the patient's health professional.

PAIN AND ITS MANAGEMENT

Pain is an unpleasant sensory and/or emotional experience associated with actual or potential tissue damage. Pain is a complicated process that involves an intricate interplay between important chemicals (neurotransmitters), which bind to neurotransmitter receptors (nociceptors) on the surface of cells. These function much like gates or ports and enable pain messages to pass through and on to neighbouring cells; normally, nociceptors only respond to strong, potentially harmful stimuli. However, when tissues become injured or inflamed, they release chemicals (Box 3.1) that make nociceptors more sensitive and cause them to transmit pain signals in response to lesser stimuli – even gentle stimuli such as a breeze or caress. This is referred to as *allodynia*, a state in which pain is produced by innocuous stimuli.

Pain is initiated with the activation of nociceptors at the free nerve endings of A-delta and C fibres, followed by transduction, whereby one form of energy (mechanical, thermal, chemical) is converted into another (electrical – nerve impulse). Lightly myelinated A-delta nerve fibres are responsible for sharp stabbing pain usually resulting from stimulation of mechanoreceptors (e.g. primary pain following acute injury). Stimulation of unmyelinated C-polymodal nerve fibres gives rise to pain described as dull, aching and poorly localized (e.g. infection, secondary pain following acute injury, visceral pain). Pain may be superficial or deep somatic, visceral or neuropathic, based on the site of action of the noxious stimulus. Following transduction, neural impulses are carried along the peripheral nerves, spinal cord and brainstem, which act as relay centres (where the pain signal can potentially be blocked, enhanced or otherwise modified). They continue through the thalamus (which also serves as the storage area for body images and plays a key role in relaying messages between the brain and various parts of the body) until they reach the cerebral cortex, the headquarters for complex thoughts, where pain perception takes place.

The main excitatory neurotransmitters for pain are substance P and glutamate. Inhibitory neurotransmitters include gamma-aminobutyric acid (GABA), serotonin, norepinephrine (noradrenaine) and opioid-like chemicals, such as endorphins and enkephalins (which block pain by locking on to opioid receptors and switching on pain-inhibiting pathways or circuits). Endorphins may also be responsible for the 'feel-good' effects experienced after vigorous exercise and the pleasurable effects of tobacco smoking.

It must be borne in mind that pain has emotional, sensory, behavioural and cognitive components, and can be influenced by temperament, context, previous experience, pain sensitivity,

Table 3.1 More common drug interactions of significance in oral health care. (NB There are many others; check text and Ch. 29)				
Drug group used in dentistry	Specific drugs used in dentistry	Interacting drug	Main uses of interacting drug	Possible outcomes (check text and Ch. 29)
Analgesics	Acetaminophen (paracetamol)	Alcohol (ethanol)	Abuse	Liver toxicity
	Aspirin	Alcohol	Alcoholism	Risk of gastrointestinal bleeding
		Corticosteroids	Immune suppression	Risk of gastrointestinal ulceration
		Hypoglycaemics	Diabetes	Enhanced hypoglycaemia
		Warfarin	Cardiac disease	Risk of gastrointestinal bleeding
	NSAIDs	Antihypertensives	Hypertension	Reduced antihypertensive effect
		Corticosteroids	Immune suppression	Risk of gastrointestinal ulceration
		Lithium	Manic depression	Lithium toxicity
		Methotrexate	Rheumatoid disease	Methotrexate toxicity
		Warfarin	Cardiac disease	Risk of gastrointestinal bleeding

(Continued)

Table 3.1 More common drug interactions of significance in oral health care. (NB There are many others; check text and Ch. 29)—cont'd

Drug group used in dentistry	Specific drugs used in dentistry	Interacting drug	Main uses of interacting drug	Possible outcomes (check text and Ch. 29)
Antibacterials	Ampicillin, amoxicillin	Beta-blockers	Hypertension	Antihypertensive levels lowered. Greater severity of anaphylactic reactions
	Any antibacterial	Oral contraceptives	Contraception	Failed contraception
	Erythromycin	Benzodiazepines	Anxiety states	High benzodiazepine levels
		Carbamazepine	Epilepsy, trigeminal neuralgia	Carbamazepine toxicity
		Ciclosporin	Immunosuppression	Ciclosporin toxicity
		Digoxin	Cardiac failure	Digitalis toxicity
		Statins	Hyperlipidaemia	Muscle damage
		Terfenadine	Allergies	Arrhythmias
		Theophylline	Asthma	Theophylline toxicity
		Warfarin	Anticoagulation	Bleeding tendency increased
	Metronidazole	Ethanol (alcohol)	Abuse	Disulfiram-type reaction
		Lithium	Manic depression	Lithium toxicity
		Warfarin	Anticoagulation	Bleeding tendency increased
	Tetracyclines	Antacids	Gastric disease	Reduced tetracycline absorption
		Digoxin	Cardiac failure	Digitalis toxicity
Antifungals	Fluconazole	Statins	Hyperlipidaemia	Muscle damage
		Warfarin	Anticoagulation	Bleeding tendency increased
	Miconazole	Statins	Hyperlipidaemia	Muscle damage
		Warfarin	Anticoagulation	Bleeding tendency increased
Epinephrine-containing LAs		Beta-blockers (non-selective)	Hypertension	Hypertension and bradycardia
		Cocaine	Abuse	Arrhythmias
		COMT inhibitors (tolcapone, entacapone)	Parkinsonism	Hypertension, tachycardias, arrhythmias
		Halothane	GA	Arrhythmias
		Tricyclics	Depression	Hypertension, tachycardias, arrhythmias
Benzodiazepine sedatives		Alcohol (ethanol)	Abuse	Benzodiazepine toxicity
		Cimetidine	Gastric disorders	Benzodiazepine toxicity
		Digoxin	Cardiac disease	Digitalis toxicity
		Fluoxetine	Depression	Benzodiazepine toxicity
		Isoniazid	Tuberculosis	Benzodiazepine toxicity
		Oral contraceptives	Contraception	Benzodiazepine toxicity
		Phenytoin	Epilepsy	Phenytoin toxicity
		Protease inhibitors	HIV/AIDS	Benzodiazepine toxicity
		Theophylline	Asthma	Theophylline toxicity

AIDS, acquired immune deficiency syndrome; COMT, catechol-O-methyltransferase; GA, general anaesthesia; HIV, human immunodeficiency virus; LA, local analgesia; NSAIDs, non-steroidal anti-inflammatory drugs.

coping skills and cognitive development, and biological, psychological and cultural factors.

PREVENTION AND TREATMENT OF PAIN

Prevention and treatment of pain and suffering is essential. Furthermore, inadequate pain control during a clinical procedure may also make management and pain control far more difficult for future health care procedures. Pre-emptive analgesia is the clinical concept of introducing analgesic management before the onset of noxious stimuli, which helps to prevent pain potentiation. Reassurance, explanation, a calm environment and gentle handling will help, but frequently need to be supplemented with analgesics, hypnosis, local anaesthesia (LA), conscious sedation (oral, inhalational or intravenous) or general anaesthesia (GA).

ANALGESICS

Analgesics may act at different levels of the pain transmission pathway: aspirin and other non-steroidal anti-inflammatory agents (NSAIDs), acetaminophen (paracetamol), corticosteroids and LA act peripherally, while opioids act on the central nervous system (CNS). Neurogenic pain, originating in damaged C fibres, may also respond to membrane-stabilizing drugs, such as anticonvulsants (e.g. carbamazepine). Tricyclic antidepressants (e.g. amitriptyline) also have a role in the modulation of pain pathways. Muscle relaxants and hypnosis may be indicated for pain related to muscle spasm.

Adjuncts to analgesia include transcutaneous electrical nerve stimulation (TENS), dorsal column stimulation (DCS), acupuncture, rubbing the skin locally, psychological techniques and neurosurgical procedures.

Analgesic drug use, contraindications and potential reactions and interactions are fully discussed in Ch. Table 3.1 summarizes the main problems relevant to de

CONTROL OF MILD PAIN

Non-opioids analgesics may be used (Table 3.2).

Acetaminophen (paracetamol; *N*-acetyl-para-aminophenol; APAP) has approximately the same analgesic activity as aspirin, and is a useful analgesic and antipyretic (reduces fever) but has no anti-inflammatory activity. Acetaminophen appears to act by reducing the oxidized form of the cyclo-oxygenase (COX) enzyme, preventing it from forming pro-inflammatory cytokines, and it also modulates the endogenous cannabinoid system. Acetaminophen is metabolized by the liver and by P450 enzymes, responsible for its toxic effects due to a minor alkylating metabolite (*N*-acetyl-*p*-benzoquinone imine, abbreviated as NAPQ1). Acetaminophen causes no gastric irritation and is remarkably safe but, in overdose, it can cause liver damage. Acetaminophen accounts for most drug overdoses in the USA, the UK and the Antipodes. Up to 4 g daily is the maximum dose for an adult, but acetaminophen toxicity is increased by starvation and by alcohol, anticonvulsants, barbiturates and possibly zidovudine. *Co-methiamol* is a combination tablet of paracetamol with methionine included to ensure that sufficient levels of glutathione in the liver are maintained in order to minimize the liver damage if an overdose is taken.

Box 3.1 Chemical mediators of pain

- Bradykinin
- Hydrogen ions
- Leukotrienes
- Potassium ions
- Prostaglandins
- Serotonin
- Substance P
- Thromboxane

Table 3.2   Non-opioid analgesics

Analgesic	Tablet contains	Route	Adult dose	Comments
Non-NSAIDs				
Acetaminophen (paracetamol)	500 mg	Oral	500–1000 mg up to six times a day (max. 4 mg daily)	Mild analgesic. Not anti-inflammatory. Hepatotoxic in overdose or prolonged use. Contraindicated in liver or renal disease, anorexia, or those on zidovudine. Available with methionine to prevent liver damage in overdose, as co-methiamol
Nefopam	30 mg	Oral or i.m.	30–60 mg up to three times daily	Moderate analgesic. Contraindicated in convulsive disorders. Caution in pregnancy, older patients, renal or liver disease. May cause nausea, dry mouth, sweating
NSAIDs[a]				
Aspirin	300 or 325 mg	Oral	300-600 mg up to six times a day after meals (use soluble or dispersible or enteric-coated aspirin) (max. 4 g daily)	Mild anti-inflammatory analgesic. Causes gastric irritation. Interferes with haemostasis. Contraindicated in bleeding disorders, children, asthma, late pregnancy, peptic ulcers, renal disease, aspirin allergy
Mefenamic acid	250–500 mg	Oral	250—500 mg up to three times a day	Mild anti-inflammatory analgesic. May be contraindicated in asthma, gastrointestinal, renal and liver disease, and pregnancy. May cause diarrhoea or haemolytic anaemia
Diflunisal	250 or 500 mg	Oral	250–500 mg twice a day	Anti-inflammatory analgesic for mild to moderate pain. Long action: twice-daily dose only. Effective against pain from bone and joint. Contraindicated in pregnancy, peptic ulcer, allergies, renal and liver disease
Ibuprofen	200 mg	Oral	200–400 mg up to four times a day	Mild analgesic. Fewer adverse effects than other NSAIDs. Causes gastric irritation. Interferes with haemostasis. Contraindicated in bleeding disorders, older people, asthma, late pregnancy, peptic ulcers, renal disease, aspirin allergy

[a]There are many other NSAIDs (see Table 3.3).
NSAIDs, non-steroidal anti-inflammatory drugs; i.m., intramuscular.

Table 3.3   Non-steroidal anti-inflammatory drugs

Group	Subgroup	Examples
Carboxylic acids	Carbo- and hetero-cyclic acids	Etodolac Indometacin Sulindac Tolmetin
	Fenamic acids	Flufenamic acid Meclofenamic acid Mefenamic acid
	Phenylacetic acids	Alcofenac Diclofenac Fenclofenac
	Proprionic acids	Fenbufen Fenoprofen Flurbiprofen Ibuprofen Ketoprofen Naproxen Oxaprozin Tiaprofenic acid
	Salicylic acids	Aspirin (acetyl salicylic acid) Diflunisal
Enolic acids	Oxicams	Isoxicam Piroxicam (restricted use because of gastrointestinal effects and rashes) Tenoxicam
	Pyrazolones	Butazones Propazones
Non-acidic compounds		Nabumetone

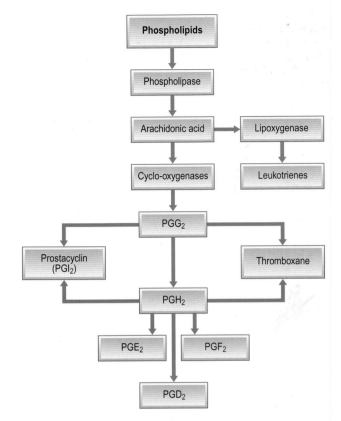

Fig. 3.1   Cyclo-oxygenase pathway

Box 3.2 Non-steroidal anti-inflammatory drugs: contraindications

- Allergy
- Asthma
- Bleeding tendency
- Cardiac failure
- Drug interactions (e.g. lithium)
- Peptic ulceration
- Pregnancy
- Renal disease
- Transplant patients

NSAIDs act peripherally to reduce pain and are equi-analgesic with centrally acting weak opioids such as codeine. A wide range of non-steroidal anti-inflammatory drugs (NSAIDs) is available (Table 3.3). NSAIDs act by blocking COX, which converts arachidonic acid to prostaglandins, some of which are involved in inflammation and pain. Other prostaglandins stimulate protective gastric mucus secretion, blood platelet formation and renal excretion. Most NSAIDs block cyclo-oxygenase 1 (COX-1) particularly, which is responsible for the prostaglandins affecting stomach, platelets and kidneys – and they can thus also damage the stomach and interfere with haemostasis and renal function (Fig. 3.1 and Box 3.2).

All NSAIDs can cause serious gastrointestinal effects: azapropozone is the highest risk and ibuprofen the lowest. They cause gastric irritation, ulceration and bleeding, especially in older patients and patients taking corticosteroids. Piroxicam use is limited now to treatment by specialists – of osteoarthritis, rheumatoid arthritis and ankylosing spondylitis. Ketoprofen and ketorolac also have high gastrointestinal adverse effects. NSAIDs should not be used in patients with current or past peptic ulcers, and not used in combinations. COX-2 inhibitors have much less effect on the stomach, platelets and kidneys but still some and, unfortunately, are also associated with a thrombotic risk (e.g. myocardial infarction and stroke), as are non-selective NSAIDs such as diclofenac and ibuprofen, especially when used at high doses and for long periods. NSAIDs can also

worsen asthma and are contraindicated in pregnancy, and in older patients. Misoprostol or H_2 antagonists or proton-pump inhibitors can help protect the stomach. NSAIDs inhibit platelet function and can interact with lithium to cause lithium toxicity. They also block renal prostaglandin synthesis and rarely cause acute renal failure, particularly in older patients with cardiac failure and those with renal damage, such as diabetic nephropathy. In these groups, renal function should be monitored.

Aspirin is a typical NSAID, which has the effects described above but also irreversibly inhibits platelet function and therefore causes a prolonged bleeding time for the life of the platelets (about 7–8 days minimum). Other NSAIDs also inhibit platelet function, but do so reversibly and therefore prolong the bleeding time only for the life of the drug (typically 48–72 h). COX-2 inhibitors, such as celecoxib and rofecoxib, are NSAIDs that spare the COX-1 enzyme and thus cause less gastric

Table 3.4 Opioids[a]

Analgesic	Tablet contains	Route	Adult dose	Comments
Codeine phosphate	15 mg	Oral	10–60 mg up to six times a day (or 30 mg i.m.)	Analgesic for moderate pain. Contraindicated in late pregnancy and liver disease. Avoid alcohol. May cause sedation and constipation. Weakens cough reflex
Dextropropoxyphene	65 mg	Oral	65 mg up to four times a day	Analgesic for moderate pain. Risk of respiratory depression in overdose, especially if taken with alcohol. Can cause dependence. Occasional hepatotoxicity. No more effective as an analgesic than paracetamol/acetaminophen or aspirin alone. Available with acetaminophen as co-proxamol
Dihydrocodeine tartrate	30 mg	Oral	30 mg up to four times a day (or 50 mg i.m.)	Analgesic for moderate pain. May cause nausea, drowsiness or constipation. Contraindicated in children, hypothyroidism, asthma and renal disease. Interacts with MAOI. May increase post-operative dental pain. Reduce dose for elderly. Available with paracetamol as co-drydamol
Pentazocine	25 mg	Oral	50 mg up to four times a day (or 30 mg i.m. or i.v.)	Analgesic for moderate pain. May produce dependence. May produce hallucinations. May provoke withdrawal symptoms in narcotic addicts. Contraindicated in pregnancy, children, hypertension, respiratory depression, head injuries or raised intracranial pressure. There is a low risk of dependence
Buprenorphine	0.2 mg	Sublingual	0.2–0.4 mg up to four times a day (or 0.3 mg i.m.)	Potent analgesic. More potent analgesic than pentazocine, longer action than morphine, no hallucinations, may cause salivation, sweating, dizziness and vomiting. Respiratory depression in overdose. Can cause dependence. Contraindicated in children, pregnancy, MAOI, liver disease and respiratory disease
Meptazinol	No tablet available	i.m. or i.v.	75–100 mg up to six times a day	Potent analgesic. Claimed to have a low incidence of respiratory depression. Side-effects as buprenorphine
Phenazocine	5 mg	Oral or sublingual	5 mg up to four times a day	Potent analgesic for severe pain. May causes nausea
Pethidine	No tablet available	s.c. or i.m.	25–100 mg up to four times a day	Potent analgesic. Less potent than morphine. Contraindicated with MAOI. Risk of dependence
Morphine	As required	s.c., i.m., oral or suppository	5–10 mg	Potent analgesic. Often causes nausea and vomiting. Reduces cough reflex, causes pupil constriction, risk of dependence
Diamorphine	10 mg	s.c., i.m. or oral	2–5 mg by injection, 5–10 mg orally	Potent analgesic. More potent than pethidine and morphine. Euphoria and dependence

i.m., intramuscular; i.v., intravenous; MAOI, monoamine oxidase inhibitor; s.c., subcutaneous.
[a]Not usually appropriate for dental pain.

damage; they do not affect platelets and are preferred for patients with peptic ulceration, but are contraindicated in cardiac disease and should not be used together with aspirin. Rofecoxib has been shown to increase the risk of myocardial infarction and has been withdrawn.

CONTROL OF MODERATE PAIN

If acetaminophen or NSAIDs fail to control the pain, an opioid may be indicated (Table 3.4). Weak oral opioids, such as codeine, provide useful analgesia by a central action. The analgesic efficacy of codeine (methylmorphine) is partly dependent on its O-demethylation to morphine via cytochrome P450, which exhibits genetic polymorphism and therefore the degree of pain relief, and the adverse effects may vary significantly between individuals. Despite this, codeine is widely used for post-operative pain relief at an adult dose of 30–60 mg often in combination with acetaminophen, though the NHS does not recommend it for dental pain.

Opioids activate the mu_1 receptor in the CNS that is responsible for analgesia. Activation of the mu_2 receptor by opioids can lead to the undesired effects of respiratory depression, sedation, constipation, nausea and vomiting. Opioids also depress the ventilation rate by depressing the response of the brain to carbon dioxide. Opioids may be contraindicated in patients who have acute or chronic respiratory disease and seizures.

Tramadol is another mild opioid that acts as an opioid receptor agonist and also inhibits spinal monoamine reuptake. It is an effective analgesic, but is contraindicated in epilepsy and porphyria, and patients on antidepressants or antipsychotics. Because its action is only partially opioid based, tramadol causes less sedation and respiratory depression than other opioids in equi-analgesic doses, but nausea and vomiting can be troublesome. Tramadol in combination with antidepressant drugs may precipitate the serotoninergic syndrome, and the use of 5-hydroxytryptamine 3 ($5HT_3$) antagonists to prevent its nausea and vomiting may reduce analgesic efficacy.

CONTROL OF SEVERE PAIN

Severe pain requires treatment with potent opioids (e.g. morphine, pethidine, oxycodone or fentanyl; Tables 3.4 and 3.5). The benefits of opioids must be weighed against their adverse effects. Choice of drug and route of administration depend on the particular clinical situation and care must be taken when converting from one form of drug or administration route to another as doses will vary.

Opioids can cause respiratory depression – supplemental oxygen may be indicated. Respiratory depression can be reversed with naloxone. Other effects include pinpoint pupils, sedation, nausea, constipation and pruritus. These symptoms must be anticipated and appropriately treated.

Post-operatively, morphine may be administered orally but, as some patients may need to be kept nil by mouth, or gastrointestinal absorption may be reduced or unpredictable, intramuscular or subcutaneous administration may be needed. Nevertheless, intramuscular injections are painful, absorption unpredictable and dangerous, and analgesia cannot be accurately titrated to clinical need. Intravenous morphine is the only way to establish a suitable degree of analgesia reliably, but issues about the timing of administration and who may safely administer it have led to the development of more demand-dependent systems of analgesic delivery.

Oxycodone and fentanyl are no more effective than morphine, but may cause fewer adverse effects.

Patient-controlled analgesia

The disadvantages of giving morphine as required (prn) are due to the peak effects, which may oversedate and cause nausea and vomiting while, during the trough, the patient may have inadequate analgesia. Patient-controlled analgesia (PCA), which consists of an infusion pump that delivers a small bolus whenever a demand button is pressed within the confines of a set 'lock-out' time, solves some of these problems.

CONTROL OF CHRONIC AND NEUROPATHIC PAIN

Sustained-release oral formulations of morphine or oxycodone or transdermal administration of fentanyl may help some patients with chronic pain. Antidepressants and anticonvulsants can also be useful. Psychological therapies as well as alternative techniques, such as TENS, may also help, as may one of several neurosurgical procedures.

Table 3.5 The analgesic ladder			
			Severe pain
			Acetaminophen + injected opioid (morphine)
		Moderate pain	
		Acetaminophen ± oral opioid (codeine, dihydrocodeine or NSAID)	
Mild pain			
Acetaminophen (paracetamol)			

NSAID, non-steroidal anti-inflammatory drug.

CHOICE OF ANAESTHETIC TECHNIQUE FOR DENTAL PROCEDURES

Dental professionals should ensure that due regard is given to all aspects of behavioural management and anxiety control before deciding to prescribe or proceed with treatment under LA, conscious sedation or GA. The choice of the appropriate method for any particular patient for a specific procedure depends on several factors, including the type of procedure or operation indicated, the physical and mental health of the patient (see Appendix 3.3), the effects of the agents used and the patient's wishes. Attempts have been made to grade patients as to physical fitness for operation (Ch. 2) and these may help the decision-making. The degree of cooperation must be taken into account; this may be lacking in some children and other people. Other factors that may influence the decision include social circumstances (e.g. is the patient able to be accompanied, and cared for at home?), urgency and facilities available at the time.

Hypnotics can be useful pre-operatively, to help the patient sleep (Table 3.6); all can impair decision-making and driving, and most, apart from antihistamines and chlormethiazole, act on receptors for gamma-aminobutyric acid.

Local anaesthesia should be used wherever possible for outpatient dentistry (Table 3.7), with conscious sedation if necessary. GA and so-called 'sedation with intravenous barbiturates' are significant causes of morbidity or even mortality, and should be given only in a hospital with critical care facilities.

Table 3.6 Hypnotics			
	Duration of action	**Examples**	**Comments**
Benzodiazepines	Long acting	Diazepam, flunitrazepam, flurazepam, nitrazepam	Residual effects on following day (hangover effect). Dependence can result
	Shorter acting	Loprazolam, lormetazepam, temazepam	–
Pyrazolopyrimidine	Very short action	Zaleplon	–
Cyclopyrrolone	Short	Zopiclon	Dependence is possible
Imidazopyridine	Short	Zolpidem	Dependence is possible
Chlormethiazole	Medium	Chlormethiazole	Pronounced hangover. Anticholinergic effects such as dry mouth
Antihistamines	Medium	Diphenhydramine, promethazine	–

LOCAL ANAESTHESIA (LOCAL ANALGESIA)

The first use of cocaine as LA in surgery is credited to an Austrian ophthalmologist, Koller, who, in 1884, used cocaine at the suggestion of Sigmund Freud, who had discovered its analgesic properties. Subsequently, dozens of LA compounds have been developed and used in solution to block nerve conduction temporarily.

Local anaesthetic molecules bind specifically to sodium channel proteins in axonal membranes of neurons near the injection site, with essentially no effects centrally unless given in overdose. LAs comprise:

- ester-type agents (e.g. procaine, benzocaine)
- amide-type agents (e.g. lidocaine, bupivacaine).

LAs used in dentistry are mostly amides (Box 3.3).

A vasoconstrictor is usually included to maintain the duration of anaesthesia. Adrenaline (epinephrine) is the commonly used vasoconstrictor; felypressin (Octapressin®) is an alternative used with prilocaine. Vasoconstrictor solutions may also contain antioxidants such as bisulfites, which can cause adverse reactions.

Adverse reactions to LAs may also include dose-related toxic responses (cardiovascular and CNS) in normal individuals, and idiosyncratic or allergic responses. It is questionable whether there have been many genuine (immunoglobulin E (IgE)-mediated) allergic reactions to lidocaine. However, there have been occasional reactions to other components, such as the preservative. Most adverse reactions to LA administration are unrelated to the drug and are caused by fainting, or due to inadvertent entry of the drug into the circulation. One study showed blood aspiration into the LA cartridge in nearly 3% of injections. LA injections should be given with an aspirating syringe to avoid intravascular injection of epinephrine in particular. It is also wise to use a safety syringe in order to reduce the risk of needlestick (sharps) injury. The LA should then be slowly injected. Reactions unrelated to the LA agents include psychomotor responses, sympathetic or other nerve stimulation. Arrhythmias and electrocardiogram (ECG) changes such as ST segment depression may be detectable during dental extractions or operations under LA, presumably due to trigeminal stimulation. Patients being treated with digoxin for atrial fibrillation or congestive heart failure are more prone to these arrhythmias.

Overdosage has caused deaths associated with LA, but otherwise mortality is very rare indeed. Over a 10-year period, there were only three deaths in persons receiving dental care under LA in Britain (1980–1989). *All* were related to the use of

---

Box 3.3 Amide local anaesthetic agents

- Lidocaine
- Prilocaine
- Mepivacaine
- Articaine (carticaine)
- Bupivacaine and etidocaine (sometimes used for their prolonged action)

---

prilocaine. This fact does not suggest that prilocaine is dangerous but serves to emphasize that it is not necessarily safer than lidocaine. *Amide LAs have been given to millions of patients, many of whom must have been medically compromised, for nearly half a century, with few serious untoward reactions.* It is difficult, therefore, to believe that, in moderated doses, they can cause significant toxic or allergic reactions.

Convincing reports of authenticated allergic reactions to other injected LA agents are rare. Amide LAs such as lidocaine also far more rarely cause contact dermatitis that the ester-type agents and few cases have been reported worldwide. The risk of hypersensitivity to all other amide LAs, such as prilocaine or mepivacaine, is equally low. The most sensitizing component of LA solutions has been the preservative. Initially, methylparabens was used for this purpose and, as a consequence of reactions, parabens are rarely used now. Allergies to components in LA solutions may possibly be due to sulfite antioxidants or latex in the LA cartridge diaphragm or bung. Ester LAs such as amethocaine can be potent sensitizers. They are mainly used in surface anaesthetics.

Attempts to confirm putative allergy to LAs by skin testing (prick tests or intracutaneous tests) are time-consuming, usually uninformative, can provoke anaphylaxis in the rare instances of true allergy, and are therefore rarely justified. Challenge tests are also typically negative. If a patient claims to be allergic to an LA, then either a non-cross-reacting agent should be used or, alternatively, a GA may be required. However, experienced clinicians have found that giving a challenge dose hardly ever has any adverse effect. Where there are multiple supposed allergies, it may be best first to administer sterile saline subcutaneously to demonstrate any non-allergic response, and then give rising concentrations of diluted LA at 30-min intervals (resuscitation facilities must be at hand). Clearly, it is of great importance to avoid labelling patients inappropriately as allergic to LAs in the first place. The common adverse reactions of inadvertent intravenous administration of LA should be appropriately recognized and explained to the patient.

The overall incidence of complications of all types from LA is reportedly around 4.5%, but most of these are of a trifling nature. Local adverse effects may include blanching of the facial skin (Fig. 3.2), transient facial palsy (LA misplaced and entering the parotid gland where it affects the facial nerve), visual disturbance (misplaced posterior superior alveolar nerve LA can produce diplopia, mydriasis, palpebral ptosis and abduction difficulties of the affected eye), persistent anaesthesia (prilocaine and articaine are mildly neurotoxic, and any LA injection can physically damage nerves), trismus (damage to nerve supply or medial pterygoid muscle, or bleeding into the area) or lip trauma (due to the patient biting an anaesthetized lip). None of these is common or permanent.

Drug interactions with LA solutions are rare, if at least theoretically, possible (see Table 3.1 and Ch. 29). Epinephrine was alleged to be potentiated in patients taking tricyclic antidepressants but this has been disproved. In patients on beta-blockers, interactions may be possible because of the unopposed beta-sympathomimetic activity of epinephrine, but this only happens when excessively large doses of an epinephrine-containing LA are given (unlikely in dentistry). Other interactions are exceedingly rare (see below).

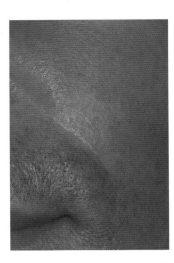

Fig. 3.2 Skin vasoconstriction after dental local anaesthetic injection

Local anaesthetic creams (e.g. Ametop; amethocaine (tetracaine), or EMLA; lidocaine plus prilocaine) effectively reduce the pain of needle pricks and are thus useful for skin injections in children. LA may also usefully be given by intraligamentary injection. Most LAs are metabolized in the liver.

LOCAL ANAESTHETIC AGENTS

Lidocaine

Lidocaine (lignocaine) is the most widely used LA in many countries. Because of its effectiveness and the paucity of significant adverse reactions to it after half a century of use, lidocaine with epinephrine is the standard against which other LAs are judged. It is an amide-type with a rapid onset of action, providing LA of intermediate to long duration. Less than 10% of lidocaine is excreted unchanged in the urine. Lidocaine is metabolized mainly by the liver with an elimination half-life of 1–2 h and rapidly undergoes first-pass metabolism. The main metabolites also have LA activity and contribute to the effects of lidocaine as they have longer half-lives. Lidocaine can cross the placenta and may enter breast milk.

Serious adverse effects of lidocaine are exceedingly rare and most adverse reactions are due to misplacing the needle, incompetent administration or overdose. There may not, however, be a linear relationship between the dose of lidocaine and the resultant blood level. In general, toxicity is more likely in children, older people and some acutely ill patients. Early features of overdose include tinnitus, circumoral paraesthesia, metallic taste, light-headedness, nausea, vomiting and double vision. At higher levels, nystagmus, slurred speech, auditory and visual hallucinations, localized muscle twitching and tremors of the hands and feet are possible. Convulsions followed by loss of consciousness, respiratory arrest and eventual cardiovascular collapse may also occur. Lidocaine may cause some degree of depression of atrial and atrioventricular nodal activity, intraventricular conductivity and ventricular contraction. *Excessive* doses of lidocaine have been followed by death.

Lidocaine should not be given in a dose exceeding 4.4 mg/kg body weight. The maximum dose of lidocaine for the average adult therefore is 300 mg. If lidocaine is used in combination

Table 3.7 Possible indications for and contraindications to local anaesthesia (LA)

LOCAL ANAESTHESIA	
May be contraindicated	**May be indicated**
In patients on beta-blockers if very large doses are given	After a recent meal
In patients with sensory loss in the trigeminal region	If there are inadequate facilities for general anaesthesia (GA)
In local infection	If there is no GA available
In LA 'allergy'	In poor-risk patient for GA
Doses should be reduced in liver disease	For minor surgery or procedure
Very young children	
Needle phobics	
Haemangioma in field	
Pseudocholinesterase deficiency	
Bleeding tendency	
Major surgery	
Uncooperative patient	
Sepsis in field	

with epinephrine, the safe dose is up to 7 mg/kg, increasing the maximum dose of lidocaine to 500 mg for an average adult. A dental LA cartridge of 2.2 ml containing lidocaine 2% with epinephrine contains 44 mg of lidocaine, and thus the maximum safe number of cartridges for a normal adult would be 11 cartridges (seven cartridges if used without epinephrine). Lidocaine solution with epinephrine contains sodium metabisulfite to prevent oxidation of epinephrine; it should not be given to patients allergic to sulfites. Lidocaine may be contraindicated (Table 3.8) in patients with some cardiac disorders (especially hypovolaemia, heart block or other conduction disturbances), porphyria and myasthenia gravis. Lidocaine should be used in lower doses in children and older patients, cardiac, hepatic or renal disease. Impaired lidocaine metabolism may be found in severe cardiac failure and liver disease. Factors that affect hepatic blood supply and/or enzyme function can also significantly influence lidocaine metabolism.

Epinephrine can cause unopposed alpha-adrenergic activity in patients taking beta-blockers but only if LAs are given in far larger doses than appropriate for dentistry. Beta-blockers may also reduce hepatic blood flow and inhibit hepatic microsomal enzymes. By contrast, phenytoin, benzodiazepines and barbiturates may induce hepatic enzymes, lowering levels of free lidocaine.

Prilocaine

Prilocaine is an amide-type LA of fast onset and intermediate duration of action. Prilocaine metabolism is similar to that of lidocaine, being rapidly metabolized by the liver and excreted in the urine as *o*-toluidine. The main adverse effect of prilocaine is a dose-dependent production of methaemoglobinaemia

Table 3.8 Indications for and contraindications to local anaesthesia (LA) with lidocaine

LA WITH LIDOCAINE	
May be contraindicated	May be indicated
In patients with porphyria	Lidocaine is the LA of choice in pregnancy
In patients on suxamethonium, since apnoea is prolonged	

Table 3.9 Indications for and contraindications to local anaesthesia (LA) with prilocaine

LA WITH PRILOCAINE	
May be contraindicated in patients	May be indicated
With G6PD deficiency; there is a greater risk of methaemoglobinaemia	In some patients with cardiovascular disease
With porphyria	
Taking antimalarials; there is a greater risk of methaemoglobinaemia	
Taking sufonamides; there is a greater risk of methaemoglobinaemia	

G6PD, glucose-6-phosphate dehydrogenase.

Table 3.10 Indications for and contraindications to local anaesthesia (LA) with articaine

LA WITH ARTICAINE	
May be contraindicated	May be indicated
In patients with porphyria	In patients on beta-blockers
Heart block	
Cholinesterase deficiency	
Narrow angle glaucoma	

Table 3.11 Indications for and contraindications to local anaesthesia (LA) with bupivacaine

LA USING BUPIVACAINE	
May be contraindicated	May be indicated
In pregnancy: may cause maternal cardiac effects and fetal hypoxia	When unusually prolonged analgesia is required
In cardiac disease	

resulting in impaired oxygen-carrying capacity. Cyanosis may occur 2–3 h following administration. The local and systemic adverse effects of prilocaine on the CNS and heart are similar to those of lidocaine. Prilocaine may occasionally cause local neurotoxicity. The maximum adult dose of prilocaine is 400 mg. Prilocaine is contraindicated in methaemoglobinaemia and possibly in porphyria or children (Table 3.9).

Articaine (carticaine)

Articaine is an amide-type LA that has an onset and duration of anaesthesia similar to other intermediate-acting amide LAs. The most significant benefit of articaine over lidocaine is that it may have somewhat faster onset and greater depth of action. It can also be used in patients taking beta-blockers.

Articaine is mildly neurotoxic and can cause prolonged anaesthesia but its other adverse effects, toxic reactions and drug interactions (solutions containing a vasoconstrictor) are the same as for other amide LAs (Table 3.10). The maximum recommended adult dose for articaine is 7 mg/kg. It is not for use in children under 4 years of age. It should possibly not be given in porphyria.

Bupivacaine

Bupivacaine is an amide-type LA with a slow onset but long duration of action. It is therefore useful intraoperatively for patients under GA, to reduce the trigeminal nerve stimulation that can cause arrhythmias, and to give prolonged pain control post-operatively. It binds to plasma proteins and has a plasma half-life of 1.5–5.5 h. Bupivacaine is largely metabolized in the liver. Maximum dose is 2.5 mg/kg.

Bupivacaine is the most cardiotoxic of the LAs (Table 3.11), the cardiotoxic effects being enhanced by hypoxia, hypercapnia, acidosis and hyperkalaemia. It inhibits cardiac conductivity and contractility, and may induce ventricular fibrillation. Bupivacaine therefore should not be used for patients with cardiac disease. Levobupivacaine, the L-isomer of bupivacaine, is of similar potency to bupivacaine but has the advantage of being significantly less cardiotoxic and neurotoxic than racemic bupivacaine.

Mepivacaine

Mepivacaine is an amide-type LA with a more rapid onset and shorter duration of action than lidocaine and is rapidly metabolized in the liver. It binds to plasma proteins and has a plasma half-life of 2–3 h. About 50% of the metabolites of mepivacaine are excreted in urine. Mepivacaine can cross the placenta.

VASOCONSTRICTORS

Epinephrine (adrenaline)

The addition of epinephrine to an LA improves haemostasis and anaesthesia: 1 in 80 000 to 1 in 100 000 epinephrine enhances pulpal anaesthesia ninefold, and soft-tissue anaesthesia fourfold. It also increases the duration of action of lidocaine and increases its safety margin. There is controversy about the possible systemic effects of epinephrine in an LA solution (Table 3.12). Epinephrine is a potent sympathomimetic having significant

Table 3.12 Indications for and contraindications to local anaesthesia (LA) containing epinephrine

LA CONTAINING EPINEPHRINE	
May be contraindicated in patients	**May be indicated**
After radiotherapy to the area	For maximally effective anaesthesia
With a liability to dry socket	
Who are asthmatic and who can be sensitive to sulfites	
On digoxin, as it may precipitate arrhythmias	
With cardiac bypass grafts, as it may precipitate arrhythmias	
On beta-blockers – hypertensive crises may result, but only in overdose	
Who are taking noradrenaline-uptake blockers, St John's wort, atomoxetine, antipsychotic drugs or other psychoactive agents	
Who have used drugs of abuse, especially cannabis, ephedrine, clenbuterol or cocaine in the previous 24 h. Additive sympathomimetic effects may develop	
Who are taking anti-emetics	
With untreated hyperthyroidism	
With phaeochromocytoma	

beta-adrenergic activity (beta-1 action raises cardiac rate and contraction force while beta-2 activity causes bronchodilation) and can thus cause a rise in blood pressure, and some alpha activity, which causes vasoconstriction of vessels of the skin and mucosae.

The cardiac effects of epinephrine-containing LA solutions are usually slight but can be significant. Even with the use of aspirating techniques, up to 20% of all LA injections made into the highly vascular head and neck region may result in a significant rapid, albeit transient, rise of peripheral blood levels of epinephrine. There is also a slow rise in peripheral blood levels of epinephrine as a consequence of the gradual release of LA solution from the site of injection into local blood vessels. Epinephrine in LAs can raise cardiac output or blood pressure. This is seen in healthy persons and others with cardiovascular disease. This does not happen when epinephrine is omitted. There is a very small rise in systolic blood pressure (BP; up to 8 mmHg) and a slight fall in diastolic pressure when lidocaine with 1:100 000 epinephrine is used, and up to a 14-mmHg rise with 1:25 000 epinephrine. By virtue of the enhanced anaesthesia, epinephrine may reduce the release of endogenous catecholamines. This is shown by data using tritiated epinephrine where the rise in peripheral blood catecholamine levels associated with intraoral injection of epinephrine-containing LA was mainly due to endogenous epinephrine. Patients with hypertension have greater elevation of systolic pressures after administration of LAs, but patients with ischaemic heart disease or prosthetic cardiac valves have changes similar to those of healthy persons. However, systolic and diastolic pressures and cardiac rate can be

raised even before the patient attends for dental treatment. The mere sight of a clinician can cause a slight rise in BP ('white-coat hypertension'). Immediately before the injection of LA there can be significant rises in cardiac rate, systolic pressure and, to a lesser extent, diastolic pressure. Cardiac rate may fall but systolic pressure may rise slightly during administration of the LA. Similar cardiovascular changes may be seen when saline is injected or even if a syringe is placed in the mouth but the needle does not touch the mucosa. Anxiety clearly underlies these changes.

The clinical significance, if any, of the above remains unclear, but some argue that epinephrine is best avoided in cardiac patients or persons on beta-blockers. However, this remains debatable. If a less effective LA is used, pain may not be completely abolished and this can cause significant adverse effects on the heart. Also, in the case of patients on beta-blockers, interactions have only resulted when excessively large doses of an epinephrine-containing LA have been given.

Epinephrine-containing LAs may cause a significant but transient fall in plasma potassium, an effect particularly noticeable in patients on non-potassium-sparing diuretics (e.g. thiazide and loop diuretics). This hypokalaemic action appears due to a beta-2 adrenergic action on membrane-bound ATPase. Epinephrine-containing LAs may also cause a transient rise in plasma glucose levels, due to alpha-2 adrenergic inhibition of insulin release, but these changes appears to have no clinical significance.

In the case of cocaine intoxication, epinephrine-containing LAs and other adrenergic vasoconstrictors are completely contraindicated. Epinephrine-containing LAs may also slightly delay wound healing after dental surgery and may increase the frequency of post-extraction alveolar osteitis ('dry socket').

Epinephrine is rapidly inactivated by the liver via both catechol-*O*-methyl transferases (COMTs) and monoamine oxidases (MAOs). The metabolites are excreted in urine, mainly as glucuronides or ethereal sulfate conjugates.

Felypressin

Felypressin is a synthetic analogue of vasopressin with little of its antidiuretic or oxytocin-like actions. Theoretically, it can cause coronary artery vasoconstriction and might affect the uterus in pregnancy, but these effects are unlikely with dental LA preparations. The administration of large amounts of felypressin to patients receiving GA with halothane may result in cyanosis and a slight rise in BP, but these changes are not serious.

Felypressin has little toxicity, even if given intravenously in amounts far in excess of those used for LA (Table 3.13). Over the years however, prilocaine with felypressin has *not* been shown to be safer than lidocaine with epinephrine, which generally provides deeper and more effective pain control.

OTHER METHODS OF LOCAL ANALGESIA

Intraligamentary (intraligamental) injections

Intraligamentary injections given after topical anaesthesia are recommended for restorative procedures in mandibular teeth in haemophiliac patients. The intraligamentary injection administered with a computer-controlled local anaesthetic delivery system (wand) is successful particularly when an inferior alveolar nerve block fails to provide profound pulpal anaesthesia in

Table 3.13 Possible indications for and contraindications to prilocaine with felypressin

LA CONTAINING FELYPRESSIN	
May be contraindicated	May be indicated
In cardiac patients	For better anaesthesia than with prilocaine alone
In patients with a liability to dry socket	
Theoretically in pregnant patients	

LA, local anaesthesia.

Table 3.14 Indications and contraindications for local anaesthesia (LA) by intraligamentary injection

LA BY INTRALIGAMENTARY INJECTION	
May be contraindicated	May be indicated
Possibly in patients predisposed to infective endocarditis	In bleeding tendencies

mandibular posterior teeth of patients presenting with irreversible pulpitis. Indications and contraindications are shown in Table 3.14.

Electronic dental analgesia

A number of dedicated electronic dental analgesia (EDA) systems are available. Some studies found that many patients (60%) preferred EDA to LA for restorative dentistry; however, others found that the levels of effectiveness of EDA were similar to those of topical anaesthesia, reducing the discomfort of LA injections in only 26% of cases. Indications and contraindications are shown in Table 3.15.

CONSCIOUS SEDATION

Changes in the provision of GA for UK dental services, and recommendations by repeated working groups that GA for dental treatment should only be used when there is no other method of pain and anxiety management appropriate for that patient, have led to the growing use of conscious sedation. This is defined as:

a technique in which the use of a drug or drugs produces a state of depression of the central nervous system enabling treatment to be carried out, but during which verbal contact with the patient is maintained throughout. No interventions are required to maintain a patent airway, spontaneous ventilation is adequate and cardiovascular function is maintained. The drugs and techniques used to provide conscious sedation for dental treatment should carry a margin of safety wide enough to render loss of consciousness unlikely.

Table 3.15 Indications for and contraindications to electronic dental analgesia

ELECTRONIC DENTAL ANALGESIA	
May be contraindicated	May be indicated
Demand-type pacemakers	–
Cerebrovascular disease	
Epilepsy	

Theoretcal and clinical training in conscious sedation is cricial before providing this service.

Only patients who are in ASA categories I and II are suitable for treatment under conscious sedation outside a hospital department. It can be helpful for treating patients with needle phobia or other fears, pronounced gag reflex or anxiety and for complex procedure such as endodontic and surgical work. Conscious sedation is normally used in conjunction with appropriate LA.

Most anxious patients can be treated with oral sedation (with benzodiazepines such as temazepam) or intravenous techniques with benzodiazepines (e.g. midazolam), or transmucosal sedation with benzodiazepines (usually nasal or sublingual midazolam) or inhalational sedation (with nitrous oxide and oxygen). Others may respond to a combination or alternative techniques, such as intravenous sedation with propofol or more than one drug.

Particular care is necessary in patients who are old, pregnant, very young or have cardiovascular, respiratory, liver, kidney or psychiatric disorders (Table 3.16). All patients should have thorough medical, dental and social histories taken and dental examinations recorded for each course of treatment. BP measurement (Fig. 3.3), colour, pulse and respiration are important as they determine patient selection and monitoring of the procedure. The ASA status should be determined.

Written informed consent must be obtained before each operation. Suitable consent forms are supplied by the medical defence societies. It is desirable, and there is increasing pressure, to provide patients with written information relevant to their treatment. Due consideration should be given to the patient's regular medication, if any (Table 3.17).

Sedated and anaesthetized patients may lose their cough reflex and not be able to protect their airway adequately. Material from the mouth or elsewhere can thus be aspirated into the larynx/lungs. Thus the airway must be protected by the anaesthetist/sedationist.

PRE-MEDICATION

Pre-medication may still be administered for the purposes of reducing anxiety, decreasing secretions, reducing pain and vomiting (Table 3.18).

CONDUCTING CONSCIOUS SEDATION

In conducting sedation in the UK, the requirements of the Code of Practice issued by the General Dental Council must be fulfilled (Box 3.4; see Appendix 00). Suitable resuscitative equipment, including a defibrillator, must always be available.

Table 3.16 Indications for and contraindications to conscious sedation

INTRAVENOUS SEDATION	
May be contraindicated	**May be indicated**
In psychotic personalities	In patients having involuntary movements (e.g. chorea, Parkinsonism)
In severe (disabling) heart disease	In uncooperative patients (e.g. learning impairment)
In respiratory infections	In patients who faint with local anaesthesia
In airways obstruction	In patients with a tendency to retch
In fascial space infections	Where stress may induce attacks of angina
In chronic obstructive pulmonary disease	Where stress may induce attacks of epilepsy
In the unescorted patient	Where stress may induce attacks of asthma
In pregnancy	Where stress may induce attacks of hypertension
In children	In patients too anxious to accept treatment under LA
In needle phobics	In many prolonged operations, such as removal of third molars or preparation for multiple implants for which GA would otherwise be needed
In liver disease	In upper airways obstruction
In myasthenia gravis	In claustrophobic patients
In glaucoma	
INHALATIONAL SEDATION	
May be contraindicated	**May be indicated**
In psychoses	In children
In pregnancy during the first trimester	In drug users
In claustrophobic patients (mask phobia)	In myasthenia gravis
In Respiratory infections	In asthma
After some eye surgery	In needle phobics
In patients with vitamin B12 deficiency, or an metho-frexale	In patients with tendency to retch
Where access to the nose is required	In epileptics

Table 3.17 Pre-operative modification of regularly used medications before operation under conscious sedation or general anaesthesia

Medication	Action (always discuss with the physician responsible for the patient)
ACE inhibitors	Continue
Alpha-blockers	Continue
Analgesics	Continue
Anticholinesterase eye drops	May theoretically prolong the effect of suxamethonium and mivacurium
Anticoagulants	Continue consult haematologist
Anticonvulsants	Continue
Antimicrobial	Continue
Anti-arrhythmics	Continue
Aspirin	Continue except for some surgery (e.g. urological and neurosurgery)
Beta-blockers	Continue
Calcium-channel blockers	Continue
Contraceptive pill	Continue
Corticosteroids	Continue, and raise dose (see Ch. 6)
Digoxin	Continue
Diuretics (potassium-sparing)	Omit on morning of operation
Diuretics (thiazides or loop)	Continue
Heparin	Last prophylactic dose must be 6 hours before operation
Insulin or antidiabetics	See Ch. 6. Consult diabetologist; usually change to a sliding scale
Lithium	Stop 1 day before major surgery
Monoamine oxidase inhibitors (MAOIs)	Dangerous hypertensive interaction with certain opioid drugs. Preferably stop a few weeks before surgery if opioids are to be used
Non-steroidal anti-inflammatory drugs (NSAIDs)	Continue
Oral hypoglycaemics	Last dose is administered the night before a morning operating list or morning of an afternoon list
Selective serotonin reup-take inhibitors (SSRIs)	May interact with other drugs that facilitate serotonin (e.g. tramadol and other antidepressants): possibility of serotonin syndrome (dangerous neuromuscular and autonomic overactivity)
Statins	Continue
Tricyclic antidepressants	Exaggerate the effects of catecholamines
Warfarin	Continue usually; consult haematologist

ACE, angiotensin-converting enzyme.

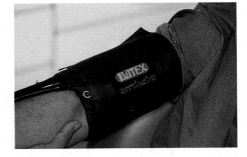

Fig. 3.3 Blood pressure measurement using sphygmomanometry

Table 3.18 Pre-medication

Aim	Drugs used
Reducing anxiety	Temazepam 10–30 mg po (adults); oral midazolam 0.5 mg/kg or alimemazine (trimeprazine) 2 mg/kg po (children)
Decreasing secretions	Glycopyrrolate
Analgesia	NSAIDs are commonly administered in adults; paracetamol in children
Antiemetics	Promethazine or alimemazine

NSAIDs, non-steroidal anti-inflammatory drugs; po, per os (orally).

Box 3.4 Requirements before using conscious sedation (see also www.doh.gov.uk/sdac)

- Written medical history
- Previous dental history
- Written instructions have been provided pre- and post-operatively
- The presence of an accompanying adult
- The patient has complied with pre-treatment instructions
- The medical history has been checked and acted on
- Records of drugs employed, dosages and times given including site and method of administration
- Previous conscious sedation/general anaesthesia history
- Pre-sedation assessment
- Any individual specific patient requirements
- Suitable supervision has been arranged
- There is written documentation of consent for sedation (consent form)
- Records of monitoring techniques
- Full details of dental treatment provided
- Post-sedation assessment

The dental surgery should be large enough to allow adequate access for the dental team all around the patient. The dental chair must be capable of being placed in the horizontal position. Dedicated purpose-designed relative analgesia (inhalational sedation; IS) machines for dentistry should be used. Such machines should be maintained according to manufacturers' guidance with regular documented servicing. Gas supply lines for IS machines must be connected by non-interchangeable colour-coded pipelines to the medical gas supply or a mobile four-cylinder stand. On installed pipelines there must be a low-pressure warning device and an audible alarm. Nitrous oxide and oxygen cylinders must be stored safely with regard to current regulations. Cylinders must be secured safely to prevent injury. There should be adequate scavenging of waste gases. Inadequate scavenging may result in unacceptable risks to health of the dental team. Scavenging of gases should not rely on window-opening or air-conditioning alone and it should confirm to current Control of Substances Hazardous to Health (Regulations 1988, UK; COSHH) standards. The long-term exposure limit (LTEL) represents a time-weighted average (TWA) over an 8-h reference period defined in COSHH Regulation EH40 as the procedure whereby the occupational exposures in any 24-h period are treated as equivalent to a single uniform exposure for 8 h – the TWA exposure; recommended

LTELs range from 25 to 100 ppm. Breathing systems should have separate inspiratory and expiratory limbs to allow proper scavenging. Active and passive systems are available for scavenging. Nasal masks should be close fitting to provide a good seal without air entrainment valves. All the appropriate equipment for the administration of sedation must be available in the surgery. This includes syringes, needles, cannulae, surgical wipes/tapes/dressings, tourniquets and labels. Purpose-designed, calibrated and appropriately maintained equipment is essential for all infusion techniques. It is mandatory to be able to administer supplementary oxygen or oxygen under intermittent positive pressure ventilation (IPPV) to the patient, should the need arise.

There must be at least one other person present at all times, suitably qualified and experienced to monitor the level of sedation and well-being of the patient. The levels of theoretical and practical training required by team members, regulations regarding standard and emergency equipment, monitoring, recovery facilities, consent, and instructions to patients and carers have been described in two UK Department of Health reports (see Further reading). An overview of the practical techniques only is provided here.

The clinical record for conscious sedation should include the reason for conscious sedation, evidence of the consent process and the following (Box 3.5). Instructions should be given in written form when sedation is proposed. Patients often fail to take in what they are told or quickly forget. The patient's name

Box 3.5 Inhalation sedation technique

1 Check that the IS (relative analgesia) machine and scavenging are functioning properly and that an alternative supply of oxygen (O_2) is available
2 Recline the patient with legs uncrossed and position the mask over the patient's nose
3 Close the air entrainment valve on the mask (if present) and start administering 100% O_2 at a flow rate to approximate the patient's minute volume. This has been achieved when the reservoir bag moves with each breath without collapsing or overinflating and the patient does not have to mouth-breathe. (Correct flow rates are typically 5–8 L/min for an adult. Paediatric minute volumes vary with age)
4 Turn the nitrous oxide (N_2O) inspired concentration to 10% and advise the patient that they may start to feel warm, light-headed or experience tingling of the extremities
5 After ensuring that the patient's speech (which may be slurred) is maintained for 1 min, increase the N_2O in increments of 5–10% at 1-min intervals until a relaxed state is reached. Inspired N_2O concentrations of 25–35% are typically used; concentrations exceeding 50% should be avoided
6 Supplement the inhalational sedation throughout with positive comments of reassurance and instructions
7 Delayed patient's verbal or motor responses, visual or auditory changes, warmth and paraesthesia are all signs of an adequately sedated patient. Inability to maintain mouth-opening, snoring (indicating some degree of airway compromise) or moving into a state of restlessness are signs of oversedation and the concentration of N_2O should thus be decreased
8 Protection of the airway with the use of a rubber dam or butterfly sponge is important in the sedated patient
9 Monitor clinical signs (e.g. pulse and respiratory rate, unobstructed breathing and lack of cyanosis) throughout the surgery. Pulse oximetry may help
10 Turn O_2 concentration to 100% at the end of the procedure

and the reason for having sedation must be confirmed. This apparently obvious precaution avoids embarrassing confusion between patients coming from a crowded waiting room. The operation site should be confirmed and, if appropriate, marked in ink by the operator. This must be done while the patient is conscious, and checked with the patient. One of the most effective methods of lessening anxiety is by reassurance and brief discussion of a patient's particular anxieties.

Appliances such as orthodontic removable appliances or dentures should be removed pre-operatively. The sedationist must be aware of the presence of crowned, fragile or loose teeth, bridges which could be damaged, contact lenses, hearing aids or colostomy bags. The bladder should be emptied pre-operatively.

It is essential that a dental professional does not administer sedation in the absence of a second trained person. The latter is required not merely to assist and help deal with any mishaps, but also to act as a chaperone. Fantasies of sexual assault may arise during benzodiazepine sedation. Further, the patient may become disinhibited and make advances to the dentist.

Monitoring for intravenous sedation must include constant monitoring of conscious state, colour, BP, respiration and pulse. Use should be made of a BP monitor and pulse oximeter (Fig. 3.4): this provides a measure of the degree of haemoglobin oxygen saturation by means of spectrophotometry. Pulse oximeters are usually accurate and are a valuable safety measure. They pass red light at 660 nm (absorbed by oxygenated haemoglobin) and infrared light at 920 nm (absorbed by deoxygenated haemoglobin) across the vascular bed (usually of a finger or ear lobe), which permits display of the percentage haemoglobin saturated with oxygen. This is safe when above 90%. A stethoscope and, ideally, also an ECG monitor (Fig. 3.5) should be used. However, this is rarely practicable in the absence of expert interpretation of the tracing, such as in a hospital, unless an automatic read-out of possible diagnoses is available. Disadvantages of using ECG are that it can generate anxiety in the patient and is disturbed by movements, so its use is often restricted to patients with serious cardiac disease being treated in a hospital.

PREPARATION AND CHOICE OF TECHNIQUE

Only patients of ASA class I and II are suitable for sedation as outpatients. ASA III patients should be referred to at least an appropriate secondary care unit and ASA IV patients to the hospital service, ideally with an anaesthetist present. Unlike sedation in the hospital operating-theatre setting, fasting is *not* required for conscious sedation in the dental practice where resorting to GA in the event of failure is not an option. There are few absolute contraindications, but special care should be taken with children and the elderly. Treatment during pregnancy should be avoided where possible, certainly avoiding the use of nitrous oxide and probably benzodiazepines in the first trimester.

'Standard' sedation techniques involve the use of *one only* of the options outlined below.

Oral sedative drug alone

This method is ideal where it is not possible to use one of the titratable techniques (e.g. needle-phobic patients for whom nitrous oxide is unlikely to provide sufficient relaxation). Oral sedation should only be used by those capable of intravenous cannulation. Benzodiazepines may cause paradoxical hyperexcitability in some children or oversedation in older people and the level of sedation cannot be altered.

Pre-medication before conscious sedation

Pre-medication may be desirable to lessen anxiety. However, this is not usually feasible in general dental practice as it delays recovery. Any premedication is typically given 30–35 min pre-operatively. If pre-medication has to be given, benzodiazepines are useful because of their anxiolytic and amnesic actions, their relative freedom from side-effects and wide safety margin. Diazepam, lorazepam and temazepam are increasingly widely used for pre-medication. Beta-blockers may also be used and may help to prevent arrhythmias induced by surgery. Opioids such as pethidine are traditional pre-medicants because of their sedative action. However, they frequently cause nausea, vomiting and respiratory depression. Promethazine or trimeprazine/alimemazine may be used for their sedative and antiemetic effect, for pre-medication of children, but they have a prolonged action and are often ineffective. They also raise blood sugar levels – a consideration when treating diabetics. Patients vary widely in their requirements for pre-medication and this may be discussed with the anaesthetist/sedationist.

Inhalational sedation with nitrous oxide and oxygen

This technique does not cause significant cardiorespiratory or respiratory depression in patients who are well enough to have outpatient treatment. Nitrous oxide diffuses into body cavities and thus is contraindicated after recent eye retinal surgery where

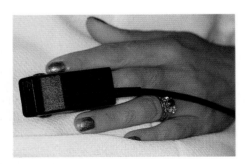

Fig. 3.4 Pulse oximetry to monitor blood oxygen saturation (nail varnish should be removed!)

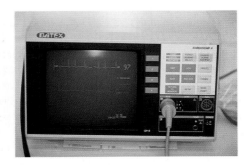

Fig. 3.5 Cardiac monitor

parfluoropropane sulphur hexafluoride has been used, and where there is bowel obstruction, cysts on pathological cavities. The gases persist in the eye for up to 3 month after surgery. Chronic exposure may interfere with vitamin B12. An 'IS machine' with built-in safety features is used to titrate nitrous oxide and non-hypoxic (30%+) flows of oxygen (Box 3.5). The oxygen concentration is set to 100% at the end of surgery to minimize diffusion hypoxia. Patients are monitored using clinical signs (i.e. responsiveness, adequate breathing, pulse and colour). Before being allowed to leave professional supervision, the patient should be able to walk unaided without stumbling or feeling unstable. Adults who have received inhalation sedation may leave unaccompanied.

Intravenous sedation with midazolam alone

Midazolam is currently the accepted benzodiazepine of 'standard' intravenous sedation, and has displaced diazepam (Box 3.6). Benzodiazepines may cause disinhibition in children and intravenous sedation for children under 12 is only appropriate for a minority of cases. Outpatient sedation is contraindicated for patients with cardiorespiratory disease of ASA grade IV, and in those with significant renal or hepatic dysfunction.

Patients must be accompanied post-operatively and receive advice similar to that issued after GA. Flumazenil is a specific antagonist at the benzodiazepine binding site on the GABA receptor and will reverse sedation in emergencies.

Advanced techniques

More experienced and suitably trained teams working in tightly controlled clinical settings with additional facilities as outlined by the Department of Health may use 'alternative techniques'

Box 3.6 Intravenous sedation technique

1 Establish reliable intravenous access
2 Inject 2–3 mg of midazolam over 30 s and assess the patient's response over the next 2–3 min
3 Administer further 0.5–1-mg increments of midazolam at 2-min intervals until adequate sedation is achieved, as indicated by a relaxed but cooperative patient with slight speech slurring (eyelid signs, as formerly used in diazepam sedation, are not reliable)
4 Careful titration is necessary because some patients may require more and some may require a lot less than the average dose requirement of 0.07 mg/kg (i.e. 5 mg for a 70 kg person)
5 Protection of the airway with the use of rubber dam or butterfly sponge is particularly important in the patient sedated with midazolam
6 Sedation will realistically be maintained for about 30 min of operating time. The patient must be monitored clinically as during inhalational sedation (see earlier) and also with pulse oximetry
7 Signs of oversedation are as with inhalation sedation (see earlier). In addition, if oxygen (O_2) saturation is seen to fall, the patient's airway and respiratory effort must be reassessed. Simply instructing the patient to take deeper breaths and administering supplemental nasal or face-mask O_2 may be all that is necessary for surgery to continue, provided verbal contact is also still maintained. However, in the presence of other signs of oversedation (see earlier), it may be advisable not to start surgery.
8 Only if this fails should flumazenil (200 μg bolus then 100 μg increments at 1-min intervals until improvement) be used and it should never be used solely to hasten post-operative recovery
9 Direct post-operative observation for 15 min and discharge with an escort after 1 h

---

such as: sedation for children under 12 other than with nitrous oxide; inhalational sedation using anything other than nitrous oxide (e.g. sevoflurane); intravenous sedation with propofol; the use of additional intravenous drugs, an opioid or ketamine; or combined inhalational and intravenous sedation (except use of nitrous oxide to site a cannula).

Where techniques involve the continuous intravenous administration of a drug, or where three or more drugs are used together regardless of their routes, a dedicated non-operator sedationist must be present. This may be a dentist or doctor, registered for 4 years with experience of at least 100 procedures who has undergone recognized training in conscious sedation in the context of the dental environment. It has been suggested that an anaesthetist with 2 years' experience would comply with *most* of these requirements.

DRUGS USED FOR CONSCIOUS SEDATION (TABLE 3.19)

Nitrous oxide

Nitrous oxide with oxygen is overall the safest agent for conscious sedation because of its rapid reversibility and lack of respiratory or cardiodepressant effects. Other agents are available but the administrator's experience and facilities, and the relative safety of the different agents, must be taken into consideration (Table 3.19). For needle phobics, children, epileptics, some drug users or those with asthma and myasthenia gravis, IS is preferable to intravenous sedation because it provides better control of the patient. For inhalation sedation, clinical monitoring of the patient is adequate. For claustrophobic patients, or those with upper airways obstruction, inhalation sedation may be contraindicated (see below).

Benzodiazepines

Benzodiazepines are potent sedative drugs. They act on the limbic system and block reuptake of GABA. They also have mild muscle-relaxant, taming and anticonvulsant activity. They also have a desirable amnesic effect. They can depress respiration, but do not affect the cardiovascular system. The depth of sedation necessary is established by the patient showing Eve's sign (the inability to touch accurately the end of the nose). Flumazenil reverses the effect of benzodiazepines. Benzodiazepines may be ineffective in children, in whom they may paradoxically cause hyperactivity, and may be ineffective in persons on long-term medication with psychoactive drugs. Be very careful about prescribing benzodiazepines in combination with an opioid as both are respiratory depressants.

Benzodiazepines are usually given intravenously, but some can be given orally, rectally or intranasally. Diazepam has been widely used for conscious sedation. It is a mild respiratory depressant with minimal risk to healthy persons, but potentially dangerous to those with cardiorespiratory disease and particularly chronic obstructive pulmonary disease. Diazepam is metabolized to products that have sedative actions (desmethyl diazepam, temazepam and oxazepam) and thus effects can persist, with a half-life of 20–72 h. Midazolam is now the most commonly used agent. Midazolam is considerably (two or three times) more potent than diazepam, amnesia is more profound

Table 3.19 Agents for conscious intravenous sedation[b]

Drug	Proprietary names	Adult dose	Comments
Diazepam	Valium	Up to 20 mg	Benzodiazepine: gives sedation with amnesia but no analgesia. Give slowly intravenously in 2.5-mg increments until ptosis begins (i.e. eyelids begin to droop; Verril's sign) – rapid injection may cause respiratory depression. Then give local analgesia Disadvantages: • may cause pain or thrombophlebitis • drowsiness returns transiently 4–6 h post-operatively due to metabolites desmethyl diazepam, triazolam and oxazepam, and enterohepatic recirculation • may cause mild hypotension and respiratory depression
	Diazemuls	Up to 20 mg	Preferred to Valium. It has most of the actions above but causes less thrombophlebitis and therefore can be given into veins on dorsum of hand. Expensive. Do not give intramuscularly
Midazolam	Hypnovel	0.07 mg/kg (up to 7.5 mg total dose)	Benzodiazepine. Compared to diazepam: • onset of action is quicker (30 s) • amnesia is more profound, starting 2–5 min after administration and lasting up to 40 min (with no retrograde amnesia) • recovery is more rapid. Midazolam is virtually completely eliminated within 5 h without the recurrence of drowsiness that may follow the use of diazepam • incidence of venous thrombosis is less than with diazepam • at least twice as potent • signs of sedation are less predictable – very slow injection required. Occasional deaths in elderly
Propofol	Propofol, Diprivan	2 mg/kg	Contraindicated in children under 18 years. May cause pain on injection. Contraindicated in patients taking anticonvulsants. Occasional fits or anaphylaxis

[b]Midazolam is the main agent used.

and recovery more rapid (Table 3.20). The maximal effect of midazolam on the brain appears to be about 10–15 min after intravenous administration. Intranasal midazolam has a faster onset of sedation than oral diazepam, with better sedation and faster recovery.

Propofol

Propofol, an agent mainly used for GA, is also useful as a sedative, especially in intensive care units (ICUs) (see below). Propofol appears to have the advantages of a rapid sedative response, with a quicker recovery and better effects on mood compared with midazolam. However, propofol may cause life-threatening adverse events, particularly when used to sedate critically ill children. This problem, first noted in 1992 when a report was published of five children with croup or bronchiolitis in an ICU who were sedated with propofol and subsequently died from metabolic acidosis and myocardial failure, possibly related to impaired fatty-acid oxidation at the level of the mitochondria. Subsequently termed 'propofol syndrome', sporadic cases and series have been described in the literature since then. The agent is therefore contraindicated for children under the age of 18 years, either during surgical or diagnostic procedures or in the ICU.

POST-OPERATIVE CARE

The immediate post-operative period is a particularly dangerous time and the patient must be closely supervised with pulse oximetry, until completely conscious, by the dental surgeon and then by the nurse or other responsible adult, until the patient

Table 3.20 Midazolam: possible adverse reactions and contraindications

Adverse reactions	Contraindications
Hiccough	Hypersensitivity to midazolam
Cough	Erythromycin use (potentiates midazolam)
Oversedation	Concomitant use of barbiturates, alcohol, narcotics or other central nervous system depressants, cimetidine, omeprazole, Kava or Valerian
Pain at the injection site	Glaucoma
Nausea and vomiting	Depressed vital signs, shock or coma
Headache	
Blurred vision	
Fluctuations in vital signs	
Hypotension	
Respiratory depression	
Respiratory arrest	

is alert and able to stand without dizziness or ataxia. A member of the dental team should supervise the patient during recovery. The first stage of recovery is normally in the dental chair. Once patients have recovered sufficiently to move to a resting area, they should be carefully guided and supported. During recovery, patients should be laid on their side in the semi-prone (tonsillar) position and the airway must be protected. Up to 20% of patients may become hypoxic after intravenous sedation and therefore supplemental oxygen should be given during recovery. Equipment and drugs for dealing with medical emergencies must be on hand. The sedationist must be constantly available to see the patient for any emergency.

The criteria for discharge are that the patient should be able to walk unaided without stumbling or feeling unstable. The decision to discharge a patient into the care of the responsible adult escort after any type of sedation must be the responsibility of the dentist or anaesthetist/sedationist (see also Appendices to this chapter). The patients must be accompanied home by a responsible adult. If this is not possible, sedation is contraindicated. Exceptions may be made occasionally in the case of inhalation sedation with nitrous oxide and oxygen when, at the discretion of the sedationist, the patient may leave unaccompanied if the patient is medically fit and responsible. Arrangements should be made for the patient to travel home by private car driven by the escort, or taxi rather than public transport. When this is not possible, the escort must be made aware of the added responsibilities of caring for the patient during the journey home. If either the patient or the escort appears to be unwilling or unable to comply with these requirements, sedation should not be given. It is desirable that the escort should look after the patient for the rest of the day. Alternatively, arrangements should be made for a reliable adult to undertake that care.

GENERAL ANAESTHESIA

It is inappropriate in this book to discuss anaesthetic agents or intraoperative care in detail, since GA is the remit of specialist anaesthetists and, in the UK, must be given only in a hospital (see *A conscious decision; a review of the use of general anaesthesia and conscious sedation in primary dental care,* Department of Health, 2003). However, dental surgeons working in hospital may have to care for such patients perioperatively. Indications for GA are shown in Table 3.21. Due consideration should be given to the patient's medication if any (Table 3.7), which should be discussed with the anaesthetist.

Table 3.21 Indications for and contraindications to general anaesthesia

GENERAL ANAESTHESIA	
May be contraindicated	**May be indicated**
In pregnancy	In refusal or allergy to local anaesthesia
In unescorted patients	For acute local infections (but not Ludwig angina)
In severe infections in the floor of the mouth	For injection phobia
In severe anaemia (especially sickle cell anaemia)	For learning impairment
In severe renal disease	For major surgery
In severe hepatic disease	For multiple extractions
In severe respiratory disease	
In severe cardiac disease	

PRE-OPERATIVE PREPARATION

It is the anaesthetist's responsibility to assess suitability for, and the best approach to, GA but a thorough clerking by the surgical team makes this process more efficient. Information about previous GA (tolerance and associated problems), induction or airway management (e.g. starvation, mouth-opening, dentition, heartburn and reflux) and history or family history of conditions important to GA (e.g. cholinesterase deficiency, malignant hyperpyrexia) are important.

PRE-OPERATIVE STARVATION GUIDELINES

If gastric contents are regurgitated there is the risk of aspiration of these into the lungs and asphyxiation or Mendelsohn syndrome. This risk has traditionally been reduced whenever possible, by minimizing intake of food and drink before GA. Many patients however are, in reality, starved for excessive times. Prolonged fast of fluid is illogical since, in fasting patients, the stomach can secrete up to 50 ml of gastric juice an hour. Further, ingested clear fluids rapidly leave the stomach of healthy people, with about half the volume disappearing in 10–20 min. Prolonged fluid deprivation has also been shown to increase the volume and decrease the pH of gastric juice, which increases the likelihood and consequences of gastric acid aspiration. Although patients who are likely to have delayed gastric emptying through underlying disease or drug treatment should not drink before GA, there is now overwhelming evidence in favour of allowing other patients with ASA grades I or II to drink clear fluids up to 2 h before the procedure. If medication needs to be administered pre-operatively, tablets and capsules can be swallowed with a small quantity of water at any time before GA.

The risks apply mainly (and rarely) to GA. Protective reflexes should remain largely intact in conscious sedation, and so the risks of aspiration should be less. Guidelines available are somewhat equivocal but there are no hard data to support starvation before conscious sedation.

If aspiration is likely, metoclopramide hastens gastric emptying and may contribute to risk reduction. Ranitidine or sodium citrate can neutralize the acidity of gastric secretions in those at risk of aspiration.

RAPID SEQUENCE INDUCTION

It may not be appropriate to wait for adequate starvation when emergency surgery is required. In such circumstances, a rapid sequence induction of GA is required. In addition, certain conditions may render starvation times less effective (Box 3.7).

Patients with significant reflux or gastro-oesophageal incompetence are also at risk of aspirating the contents of their stomachs whether filled with food or not and, in general, should

Box 3.7 Conditions rendering pre-operative starvation ineffective

- Trauma at less than the usual starvation time after eating
- Use of potent opioids pre-operatively
- Any acute abdominal condition (particularly bowel obstruction)
- Active labour

also be considered for a rapid sequence induction. In this, the patient breathes 100% oxygen for at least 3 min to extend the time during which the patient may remain well saturated while apnoeic if there are difficulties intubating (pre-oxygenation). A predetermined dose of induction agent is delivered as a bolus while an assistant applies backward pressure to the cricoid cartilage. The latter manoeuvre occludes the oesophagus and further reduces the likelihood of regurgitation. A fast-acting muscle relaxant (suxamethonium or rocuronium) is given, the patient intubated, and cricoid pressure only released when endotracheal tube position is confirmed and its cuff inflated.

INTRAVENOUS ANAESTHETICS (TABLE 3.22)

Most intravenous sedative and GA agents are modulators of the GABA$_A$ receptor, facilitating inhibitory neurotransmission at a site on the receptor away from that of GABA itself. Ketamine, however, is an N-methyl-D-aspartate (NMDA) receptor blocker and clonidine-like agents are α_2-receptor agonists.

Etomidate

Etomidate, an imidazole derivative, causes less cardiovascular depression than either propofol or thiopentone/thiopental, although its use, even in hypotensive patients, has declined owing to other undesirable effects such as nausea and vomiting, pain on injection and excitatory movements. It inhibits the enzymes 11β-hydroxylase and 17α-hydroxylase suppressing adrenal function, an effect which may occur even after a single dose.

Ketamine

Ketamine anaesthesia is dissociative, separating the electrical activity of the thalamocortical system from the limbic system. There is a delay preceding the onset of anaesthesia. Unlike other induction agents, ketamine stimulates the sympathetic nervous system, increasing heart rate and BP (but also cerebral blood flow, intracranial pressure, and both myocardial and cerebral oxygen demand). Ketamine should be avoided in patients with raised intracranial pressure and open eye injuries and used with caution in hypertension. It is a bronchodilator and useful in patients with severe bronchospasm refractory to other bronchodilators. Vivid and unpleasant dreams may follow its use.

Propofol

Propofol is the most commonly used intravenous induction agent (see above). It is a highly lipid-soluble, weak organic acid, formulated as a 1% or 2% lipid emulsion with soya bean oil and egg phosphatide. Patients with egg allergy are usually sensitive to egg *albumin* and therefore may still be given propofol.

Propofol suppresses upper airway reflexes, making coughing and laryngospasm rare, and it is therefore particularly suited to the use of the laryngeal mask airway (LMA). Propofol causes systemic vascular resistance to fall and is associated with less reflex tachycardia than other induction agents. BP invariably falls and propofol should be administered slowly and cautiously to older or haemodynamically compromised patients. Awakening is due largely to redistribution rather than metabolism. Pain on injection may be decreased by the addition of lidocaine or formulation in an alternative base.

Thiopentone/thiopental

Thiopentone/thiopental is a barbiturate that leaves airway reflexes relatively preserved, but airway manipulation without a muscle relaxant (i.e. the LMA) can cause laryngospasm. Thiopentone/thiopental was the agent originally described for rapid sequence induction and is often (by convention only) the agent of choice in these circumstances. Thiopentone/thiopental is contraindicated in patients with porphyria. Accidental extravascular injection causes pain and necrosis, and intra-arterial injection may result in gangrene.

Total intravenous anaesthesia

Anaesthesia may be maintained by repeated boluses or an infusion of intravenous agents – total intravenous anaesthesia (TIVA). Infusion pumps can deliver propofol by a continuous infusion that maintains a constant level in the plasma – target-controlled infusion (TCI).

AIRWAY MANAGEMENT

Effective GA abolishes pain and awareness during surgery, and also the tone of head and neck muscles that normally maintain the airway patency and the cough and gag reflexes

Table 3.22 Drugs for intravenous anaesthesia			
Drug	**Proprietary names (UK)**	**Adult dose**	**Comments**
Etomidate	Hypnomidate	0.2 mg/kg	Good for outpatient anaesthesia. Pain on injection: use large vein and give fentanyl 200 µg first. After operation give naloxone 0.1–0.2 mg and oxygen. Little cardiovascular effect. Often involuntary movements, cough and hiccough. Hepatic metabolism. Avoid in repeated doses on traumatized patient – may suppress adrenal steroid production
Ketamine	Ketalar	0.5–2 mg/kg	Rise in blood pressure, cardiac rate and intraocular pressure. Little respiratory depression. Often hallucinations. Contraindicated in hypertension, psychiatric, cerebrovascular or ocular disorders. Rarely used in dentistry
Propofol	Diprivan	2 mg/kg	May cause pain on injection. Occasional fits or anaphylaxis. Contraindicated in children under 18
Thiopentone/ thiopental	Intraval	2.5 mg/kg (2.5% solution)	Ultra short-acting barbiturate. No analgesia. Danger of laryngospasm. Rapid injection may cause apnoea. Irritant if injected into artery or extravascularly

crucial to protect the airway from aspiratable material. Some form of airway-opening technique is thus always required, with an additional need to protect the patient's respiratory tract from aspiratable material.

Airway manoeuvres with or without a face mask

The airway of an unconscious patient may be maintained patent using a head-tilt and chin-lift or jaw-thrust technique. Where GA is being administered, a face mask is usually necessary to deliver both oxygen and GA to keep the patient alive and asleep, respectively. An oropharyngeal and/or nasopharyngeal airway may be used to aid manual airway maintenance. Although a head-down lateral position with vigilant observation and suction may help minimize the risk of airway soiling from aspiratable material, more reliable means of airway protection are generally needed. Furthermore, the insertion of a more substantial airway-opening device means the anaesthetist is free to deliver an appropriate GA at the same time.

Laryngeal mask

The laryngeal mask airway is an inflatable 'mask' that acts as a face mask but is connected to a tube or stem so that it may be inserted into the oropharynx just at the laryngeal entrance. An airway seal is achieved by inflation of the 'mask' cuff, which also provides some degree of isolation from the oesophagus. The LMA requires less skill to insert than does an endotracheal tube and usually presents a smaller risk of trauma to tissues and teeth. Once inserted, it does not need to be held in place and it is possible to maintain an airway probably for as long as necessary. Although the classic LMA (cLMA) offers reasonable protection from material coming from the airway above, it does not however guarantee airway protection from gastric material; therefore, where there is a risk of regurgitation, endotracheal intubation is usually required. The ProSeal LMA™, which has a second lumen which 'sits' at the opening of the oesophagus creating a channel through which gastric contents may be vented away from the trachea or through which a nasogastric tube may be inserted, may reduce the risk of inadvertent aspiration. The intubating LMA (ILMA) is another variation of the cLMA that may be used to aid the intubation of the trachea either when this has proved difficult or where there is a need to avoid positioning the head and neck for intubation in the usual manner (e.g. cervical spine injury or rheumatoid arthritis). The cLMA, though a bulky device that limits surgical access to the mouth, has become an acceptable alternative to intubation for many dental, oral, maxillofacial and ear, nose and throat procedures.

Intubation

Use of a tracheal tube with an inflated cuff is the only way to *guarantee* protection of the respiratory tract from soiling. Indications for intubation are shown in Box 3.8.

A cuffed tracheal tube may be inserted orally, nasally or as a surgical airway (tracheostomy or crico-thyroidotomy). A muscle relaxant is usually used for intubation (see Box 3.9 for intubation technique).

Box 3.8 Indications for intubation

- Restricted access to airway or whole patient (ENT, neurosurgery, prone)
- Protection against contamination of airway from above
- Protection against contamination of airway from below
- Requirement for muscle relaxation where resulting airway pressure may exceed that suitable for a LMA

ENT, ear, nose and throat; LMA, laryngeal mask airway.

Box 3.9 Intubation technique

1 Check equipment and monitoring
2 Induce anaesthesia and manually ventilate the patient before a muscle relaxant is administered
3 Flex the patient's neck with the atlanto-occipital joint extended ('sniffing the morning air'), allowing direct visual alignment of the larynx with the open mouth at laryngoscopy
4 Hold the laryngoscope blade (in the left hand) and pass along the right side of the floor of the mouth displacing the tongue to the right
5 When the epiglottis is seen, advance the tip of the blade into the space between it and the base of tongue
6 Lift laryngoscope up and away, bringing the vocal cords into view, allowing the introduction of the endotracheal tube either directly or after first inserting a bougie and 'rail-roading' the endotracheal tube over it
7 Commence ventilation and inflate the tube cuff until the leak disappears. Confirm the tube position by auscultating both lung bases and apices, looking for chest movement and preferably demonstration of carbon dioxide in the exhaled gases with a capnograph. An endotracheal tube inserted too far will tend to go down the right bronchus, in which case partially deflate the cuff and withdraw the tube slightly. If in doubt, remove the tube, ensure the patient is well oxygenated and anaesthetized, and start again

---

Endotracheal intubation may be difficult in some instances and this difficulty may be suggested by a high Mallampati score (Table 3.23), and a number of other factors (Box 3.10).

Fibreoptic intubation

For patients who are known or at high risk of difficult intubation, an awake fibreoptic procedure allows intubation without the patient losing their protective airway reflexes and ability to breathe. Anaesthesia of the entire upper airway from nasopharynx to glottis is established using topical LA in a variety of concentrations with or without some carefully titrated sedation. A short narrow endoscope with endotracheal tube mounted is introduced via the nose or mouth into the trachea by direct visualization – and the tube rail-roaded over it. GA is subsequently induced in the normal way and the cuff inflated. Fibreoptic intubation is often performed in patients who are asleep (not at risk of aspiration and unlikely to be difficult to ventilate) for the purpose of avoiding a traumatic direct laryngoscopy where a nasal tube is required, to avoid neck manipulation in those with cervical spine pathology and to teach and develop the skill of fibreoptic intubation.

MUSCLE RELAXANTS

With the exception of the rapid sequence induction situation, an ability to ventilate the patient manually with a bag and face

Table 3.23 Mallampati scoring

Class	Definition
1	Full visibility of tonsils, uvula and soft palate
2	Visibility of hard and soft palate, upper portion of tonsils and uvula
3	Soft and hard palate and base of the uvula are visible
4	Only hard palate visible

Box 3.10 Observations that suggest difficulty in intubation

- Neck – reduced distance from thyroid cartilage to mandibular symphysis, short and/or fat, thyroid goitre, neck masses
- Retrognathic mandible with Class II malocclusion, particularly Class II division 1
- Trismus
- Ankylosing spondylitis
- Rheumatoid arthritis

mask should always be verified prior to the administration of a muscle relaxant. These are neuromuscular-blocking drugs. There are two main categories – non-depolarizing and depolarizing. Non-depolarizing agents (mivacurium, rocuronium, vecuronium and atracurium) act by blocking acetylcholine (ACh) receptors at the motor end plate. Depolarizing agents (suxamethonium) are ACh agonists that, after an initial stimulation, desensitize muscle fibres to further ACh stimulation, preventing nearby Na^+ channels repolarizing and producing a neuromuscular block.

Suxamethonium

Suxamethonium is the only depolarizing muscle relaxant in use. The usefulness is in its rapid action and very brief effects. The rapid onset and short duration of action of suxamethonium make it useful for induction of GA. Suxamethonium may stimulate muscarinic receptors in the SA node causing bradycardia (atropine should be given before a repeat dose and considered in all infants). Because of the initial muscle spasm, it can result in hyperkalaemia post-operatively. The small rise in K^+ is usually of little significance but may be dangerous in patients with pre-existing electrolyte abnormalities, renal failure, burns, spinal injuries and progressive neuromuscular disorders. Muscle pains also occur post-operatively and intraocular pressure rises. Prolonged neuromuscular block (suxamethonium apnoea) occurs in 4% of patients owing to inherited deficiency in the enzyme plasma cholinesterase, apnoea ranging from 10 min to several hours. Suxamethonium may also precipitate malignant hyperpyrexia.

Atracurium

Atracurium is an antagonist at the neuromuscular junction nicotinic acetylcholine receptor. Histamine release can occasionally cause hypotension or bronchospasm. Atracurium is eliminated completely independently of hepatic and renal metabolism by ester hydrolysis and spontaneous breakdown. Cis-atracurium causes less histamine release but has a slower onset time.

Vecuronium

Vecuronium is an aminosteroidal muscle relaxant, which does not affect the cardiovascular system or release histamine. It is metabolized by hepatic de-acetylation and renal excretion.

Rocuronium

Rocuronium is an aminosteroidal muscle relaxant used as an alternative to suxamethonium for rapid sequence intubation.

Mivacurium

Mivacurium is a benzylisoquinolinium muscle relaxant, which has a shorter duration of action than the other non-depolarizing relaxants. It is metabolized by plasma cholinesterase and therefore patients prone to suxamethonium apnoea should also not receive mivacurium.

Reversal of neuromuscular blockade

Neostigmine is an anticholinesterase that reverses the competitive effects of non-depolarizing muscle relaxants. Neostigmine also acts at autonomic ganglia and is therefore given with either atropine or glycopyrrolate to prevent bradycardia.

Sugammadex is used for the reversal of rocuronium and vecuronium neuromuscular blockade.

ANAESTHETIC GASES

General anaesthesia acts via effects on proteins in cell membranes, probably ion channels. Several inhalational and intravenous anaesthetic agents appear similarly to facilitate the function of inhibitory ion-channels while attenuating the function of excitatory ion-channels, to produce a state of anaesthesia. Nitrous oxide has been used for many years for GA. Halothane was the main drug used for inhalational anaesthesia until the 1980s but the rare severe liver injury following repeated exposures to halothane in some patients (Ch. 9) led to the development of other volatile agents such as enflurane, isoflurane, desflurane and sevoflurane. Arrhythmias may accompany halothane use, especially if adrenaline is given. Cardiac rhythm is also more stable with the other agents, though they cause greater respiratory depression than halothane, and induction is less pleasant. Enflurane causes cardiorespiratory depression and can be epileptogenic. Immediate recovery is slower after isoflurane than halothane and there may be some coughing. Recovery after sevoflurane is rapid but it may agitate children. Desflurane may cause apnoea or breath-holding, and increased secretions, and is not for use in children (Table 3.24).

Following induction of GA and the establishment of airway control, anaesthesia is maintained by the continuous administration of either a volatile anaesthetic or intravenous agent, with or without nitrous oxide or another means of analgesia.

The potency of an inhalational agent is determined by its lipid solubility or oil:gas partition coefficient, whereas its speed of action is determined by its blood:gas partition coefficient. Historically, some volatile anaesthetic agents were inflammable or even explosive, but modern agents are not inflammable.

Table 3.24	Inhalational agents	
Drug	**Proprietary names (UK)**	**Comments**
Desflurane	Suprane	Less potent than isoflurane. May cause apnoea or coughing and is contraindicated in children
Enflurane	Ethrane/ Alyrane	Less potent anaesthetic than halothane. Non-explosive. Less likely to induce arrhythmias or affect liver than halothane. Induction and recovery are slower than with halothane
Halothane	Fluothane	Non-explosive. Anaesthetic but weak analgesic. Causes fall in blood pressure, cardiac arrhythmias and bradycardia. Hepatotoxic on repeated administration. Post-anaesthetic shivering is common, vomiting rare. Contraindicated for dental procedures in patients younger than 18 years unless treated in hospital
Isoflurane	Forane/ Aerrane	Isomer of enflurane. It causes less cardiac but more respiratory depression than halothane. Induction and recovery are slower than with halothane
Nitrous oxide	–	Analgesic but weak anaesthetic. Non-explosive. No cardiorespiratory effects. May cause eye damage from expansion of intravitreal gases
Sevoflurane	Sevoflurane	Rapid action and recovery. May cause agitation in children

The commonly used volatile agents are all bronchodilators but depress ventilation.

Nitrous oxide

Nitrous oxide has a very low blood:gas partition coefficient and thus a very rapid onset and offset, but it approaches anaesthetic potency only in a grossly hypoxic mixture. It has good analgesic properties (useful for inhalational pain relief with oxygen as Entonox). Nitrous oxide with its analgesic properties may also be used as a 'carrier' gas to complement the sleep-inducing properties of a volatile agent. In addition, nitrous oxide, which moves into blood faster than nitrogen moves out, has the ability to increase the alveolar concentration of a volatile agent and speed up its effects. Conversely, at the end of GA, nitrous oxide rapidly leaves the blood, reducing the concentration of available oxygen in the alveoli (diffusion hypoxia). Additional oxygen is thus usually administered to a patient recovering from nitrous oxide anaesthesia to counteract this. Nitrous oxide has additional undesirable properties in some circumstances. It contributes to post-operative nausea and vomiting, and expands enclosed gas spaces and may thus be detrimental to certain bowel, ocular, and middle ear procedures. Prolonged exposure to nitrous oxide affects vitamin B_{12} metabolism and can result in megaloblastic and neurological syndromes.

Isoflurane

Isoflurane is the longest established and cheapest of the three commonly used volatile anaesthetics (isoflurane, sevoflurane, desflurane). It is irritant and unpleasant to inhale, and is therefore rarely used for induction of anaesthesia but otherwise has properties that make it a good maintenance agent. It may reduce systemic vascular resistance and cause a reflex tachycardia.

Sevoflurane

Sevoflurane has a faster onset than isoflurane and is more pleasant to inhale like halothane it also causes a fall in systemic vascular resistance but, because it attenuates reflex changes in heart rate, the BP tends to fall further. Compared to isoflurane, a greater proportion of sevoflurane is metabolized to potentially toxic by-products and there are theoretical if controversial concerns regarding its suitability in renal failure. It is considerably more expensive than isoflurane.

Desflurane

Desflurane has a blood:gas partition coefficient lower than that of nitrous oxide, and thus the onset and offset of its effects are rapid. Like isoflurane, it is unsuitable for inhalation induction but its effects wear off rapidly, even after prolonged anaesthesia, and this can be an advantage for long surgical cases where prolonged administration of other agents may be associated with prolonged recovery. Desflurane's unusual physical properties necessitate an electrically heated vaporizer.

Halothane

The risk of cardiac arrhythmias and hepatotoxicity means halothane has been superseded by other volatile agents in most situations. Because of a relatively high blood:gas coefficient, halothane does not wear off as quickly as sevoflurane. Thus induction is slower but also anaesthesia will be deeper for longer when the mask is removed; this may be an advantage where airway manipulation with minimal risk of laryngospasm is necessary.

Enflurane

Enflurane is an isomer of isoflurane. Its cardiovascular side-effects fall between those of halothane and isoflurane, and it has been associated with epileptiform electroencephalogram (EEG) changes. Its use has therefore declined.

ANALGESIA

Opioids are commonly used at induction and act rapidly so that effective analgesia is established before surgery. Alfentanil, fentanyl, morphine and remifentanil are opioids that are frequently used.

COMPLICATIONS OF GENERAL ANAESTHESIA

Many patients have a relatively smooth post-operative recovery, especially after short procedures. Superficial vein thrombosis may follow intravenous injections that are irritant or cannulae that have entered the tissues. Analgesics usually suffice, though antibiotics are occasionally indicated.

Medical emergencies such as anaphylaxis, Addisonian crisis and acute severe asthma, among others, may occur perioperatively, as they may at any time.

Local complications after GA

Operative care carried out expeditiously, with careful handling of tissues, asepsis, wound toilet and careful closure of the wound, will minimize local complications, as will the appropriate use of analgesics and antimicrobials. Nevertheless, some pain is to be expected after surgical procedures, and bleeding or wound infection is not always totally avoidable.

Pain

Pain after surgery usually starts after anaesthetic drugs have worn off, and may result from unavoidable operative trauma. Alternatively, it may result from a complication such as infection. Post-operatively, analgesics should be given as necessary, but if a GA has been given, the anaesthetist should be consulted first. Immediately after oral surgery it may be necessary to use a long-acting local analgesic or a strong analgesic such as morphine. In some cases this is best controlled by the patient (PCA). However, after most dental procedures, a combination of ibuprofen, paracetamol and codeine (Tables 3.3 and 3.4) should be effective.

Wound infection

Wound infection is uncommon after oral and maxillofacial procedures unless there has been significant contamination, such as in a road traffic accident, or if foreign bodies are present, local vascularity is poor or the patient is immunocompromised. Infection may cause pain, discharge or sepsis and is best managed by drainage, wound toilet, antimicrobials and analgesics as indicated. The diagnosis must first be made, and treatment guided by the likely pathogen (Ch. 21). If streptococci are implicated, the first-choice therapy in the absence of allergy is amoxicillin ± clavulanate. If staphylococci are involved, flucloxacillin is appropriate. For anaerobic infections, metronidazole is the first choice. For Gram-negative infections (e.g. contamination of wound with bowel organisms, urinary tract infection, hospital-acquired and aspiration pneumonia), it is best to take advice from the microbiologist; useful antibiotics include amoxicillin, piperacillin plus tazobactam, and gentamicin.

Bleeding

Post-operative haemorrhage is usually due to a local cause (i.e. damaged soft tissues; see Ch. 8). It responds to local pressure, insertion of haemostatic agents or suturing of the soft tissues. Patients should be given written as well as verbal guidance on how to care for their wounds. If there is a contributing systemic cause (e.g. anticoagulated patients), appropriate pre- and post-operative measures must be taken.

Systemic complications after GA

Drowsiness, headache, sore throat, muscle pains and vomiting are seen in over 60% of patients after outpatient GA. Headache seems more common in women, especially if halothane has been used. Sore throat, if the patient was intubated, and muscle pains if suxamethonium has been given, are common. More important complications are shown in Box 3.11.

Box 3.11 Post-operative complications

- Collapse
- Respiratory complications
- Cardiac complications
- Delayed recovery of consciousness
- Nausea and vomiting
- Fever
- Jaundice
- Behavioural problems
- Low urine output
- Thrombosis
- Death

Collapse

There may be signs of weakness, sweating, rapid pulse and pallor, hypotension, shock or loss of consciousness. The causes can be difficult to find but may include haemorrhage, pulmonary embolism, cardiac arrest (usually myocardial infarction), sepsis, anaphylaxis, adrenal insufficiency and adverse reactions to GA agents. These are outlined in Ch. 1.

Post-operative nausea and vomiting (PONV)

Post-operative vomiting is both unpleasant for the patient and dangerous if protective laryngeal reflexes have not returned after GA or sedation, and may have serious sequelae (risk of aspiration with intermaxillary fixation, wound dehiscence, etc.). Risk factors include female sex, non-smokers, those with a previous history of PONV or travel sickness, and use of post-operative morphine. Volatile agents are thought to be responsible for most vomiting immediately after waking from GA. One possible explanation is that these agents potentiate the function of $5HT_3$ receptors in addition to their effect on the $GABA_A$ receptor. Optimum prevention or treatment is by combining drugs with different modes of action. In many cases, the cause of post-operative nausea is unclear, but some patients seem to be particularly susceptible. An antiemetic is usually effective (Tables 3.18 and 3.25).

Metoclopramide, and domperidone, however, are best avoided in the young and older people, as they can induce dystonic reactions. Parenteral administration may be needed if vomiting is severe.

Fever

A transient rise in temperature post-operatively is common within a few hours of GA and major operations and is regarded as 'physiological'. Persistent fever shortly post-operatively may

Table 3.25 Antiemetics

Class	Used mainly for nausea and vomiting related to	Main possible adverse effects
Antihistamines (e.g. cyclizine)	Many causes, including post-operative	May cause sedation
Dexamethasone	Post-operative nausea and vomiting or that associated with cancer chemotherapy	
Domperidone	Cancer chemotherapy	Few problems with sedation or dystonic reactions
Metoclopramide	Gastrointestinal disorders, including post-operative	May cause dystonic reactions
Nabilone	Cancer chemotherapy	A cannabinoid that may cause drowsiness
Phenothiazines	Neoplastic disease, radiation, general anaesthesia or drug use, including post-operative	May cause dystonic reactions
5HT$_3$ antagonists (granisetron, ondansetron, tropisetron)	Post-operative nausea and vomiting or that associated with cancer chemotherapy	May cause headaches or hypersensitivity reactions

5HT$_3$, 5-hydroxytryptamine 3 (serotonin).

indicate malignant hyperthermia (Ch. 23). Persistent fever for several days post-operatively, especially if spiking, may indicate haematoma, wound infection, deep vein thrombosis (DVT), UTI, infection of an intravenous line or more serious pulmonary infection. Persistent mild fever continuing or appearing several weeks post-operatively may indicate infective endocarditis (Ch. 5).

Jaundice

Post-operative jaundice after GA can result from many causes, including viral and drug-induced hepatitis. Halothane should be avoided if the patient has been exposed to it within the previous 6 months or has had a previous episode of halothane hepatitis. In a series of 300 patients who had been given halothane on more than one occasion within a month, and who subsequently developed hepatitis, no fewer than 46% died.

Alcoholic hepatitis can be a problem. GA for high-risk patients cannot be avoided for emergencies, such as maxillofacial injuries, and this group of patients includes an unduly high proportion of alcoholics.

Aggravation of pre-existing liver disease (including gallstones), hepatic necrosis secondary to circulatory failure, transfusion reactions and Gilbert syndrome are other causes.

Behavioural complications

Causes of confusion after GA or sedation may include: drugs (anaesthetic, analgesic, others), hypoglycaemia, alcohol or other drug withdrawal, pre-existing psychiatric states, hypoxia, infection (wound, lungs, urinary tract, abscess, septicaemia), urine retention or disturbed urea and electrolytes. Amnesia that persists for at least 5 h is common after sedation with diazepam or midazolam. As a result, patients are likely to forget post-sedation instructions, or worse, have an accident as a result of forgetting to take normal precautions when using power tools or other dangerous equipment. Bizarre behaviour has also been described even 24 h after sedation. It is also important to make sure that the patient is not anticipating going abroad immediately after the GA or sedation. Airports are difficult to navigate even by the fully alert, and complications might develop on board an aircraft or at a destination where medical care is limited.

Low urine output

Absolute anuria is usually caused by urine retention – a common post-operative complication, especially in the older male. The patient should be catheterized unless urine can be passed after a warm bath. If the patient is already catheterized, make sure the catheter is not blocked. Low urine output is a cardinal sign of dehydration, hypovolaemia and shock. The patient should be given fluids orally or intravenously. Start with a fluid challenge and continue according to the response. Care must be taken with patients in heart failure.

Deep vein thrombosis

Deep vein thrombosis is mainly seen after prolonged major operations under GA, and affects the leg veins. It may lead to pulmonary embolism (Ch. 5). Always suspect this in a patient whose haemoglobin saturation falls several days after major surgery or they develop hypotension, tachycardia, chest pain, etc. (see Ch. 5). Factor V Leiden deficiency and other causes of thrombophilia should be considered (Ch. 5).

Awareness

For patients, the possibility of being awake during GA is a cause of worry. Unfortunately, it is not unheard of, is an established cause of complaints against anaesthetists and is a precipitant of post-traumatic stress disorder. Awareness most often manifests as recollection of an auditory perception; sensations of pain are less likely. These experiences are more likely to occur when GA may become light, such as during airway manipulation and transfer of the patient into the operating room. Significant awareness is generally felt to be unlikely during surgery where a muscle relaxant has not been used, because movement in response to a noxious stimulus precedes awareness – and depth of anaesthesia may be adjusted accordingly. There is currently much interest in depth of anaesthesia monitoring, which utilizes various calculations from a simplified EEG recording (e.g. BIS), but whether or not these technologies are likely to reduce the incidence of awareness is unknown.

Delayed recovery of consciousness after GA

Important causes are overdose of GA agents or the use of long-acting opioids for pre-medication, suxamethonium sensitivity, diabetic coma or hypoglycaemia, cardiac complications as mentioned earlier or cerebrovascular accidents. The latter may be either in susceptible patients (elderly hypertensives) or as a result of emboli. Occasionally, neurotic patients may feign persistent unconsciousness.

Patients should not be discharged from recovery if they are at risk of laryngospasm or not fully conscious. Certain conditions resulting in an abnormally prolonged time to recovery of either consciousness or ventilation may, however, cause more subtle respiratory problems or post-operative confusion, as shown in Box 3.12.

Box 3.12 Causes of delayed recovery from GA

- Residual intravenous or gaseous agents, sedatives, opioids
- Residual muscle relaxation (use a nerve stimulator)
- Anticholinergic drugs
- Hypoxia, hypercapnia
- Hypothermia
- Hypothyroidism
- Electrolytes (Na+, Ca2+ particularly)
- Cerebrovascular accident or other pathology

Cardiac complications

Myocardial infarction, cardiac failure or severe arrhythmias can follow GA and are the main risks in those with pre-existing cardiac disease (Ch. 5). Pre-existing cardiac disease may be aggravated or myocardial infarction can follow at an unpredictable interval after the anaesthetic, especially in those with ischaemic heart disease (Ch. 5). Myocardial infarction is one of the chief causes of deaths associated with anaesthesia. There is no logical reason why GA *per se* should be expected to cause myocardial infarction or arrhythmias, and evidence is emerging that certain GA agents may have myocardial *protective* properties. Nevertheless, perioperative cardiac complications account for many of the deaths 'under GA', although these can probably be explained by gross haemodynamic abnormalities (blood loss, hypotension, hypertension, bradycardia, tachycardia) and/ or metabolic abnormalities (hypoxia, hypercapnia, electrolyte problems) in patients who can not compensate for them. Cardiac risk factors are notoriously difficult to apply generally though there have been many scoring systems over the years. Shock (circulatory failure leading to tissue and organ hypoperfusion) is more likely to be a complication of major surgery: contributory factors include pre-existing heart disease, dehydration, haemorrhage, sepsis or anaphylactic reactions.

Laryngospasm

Upper airway stimulation causes coughing in a fully awake patient and no reaction in one who is deeply anaesthetized.

Instead of a coordinated cough, the patient inbetween these states is at risk of their vocal cords closing and failing to open again (laryngospasm). This results in stridor when mild to moderate, but complete airway obstruction when severe. The cords often relax with positive airway pressure (and increasing the inspired volatile concentration when inducing anaesthesia) but occasionally it is necessary to re-administer a muscle relaxant.

Other respiratory complications

Airway obstruction is particularly important in dental surgery because of operating around the airway and the risk of inhaling foreign material. Facilities such as suction must always be immediately available for locating and clearing any blockage. *The recovery period is the most dangerous time and great care must be taken to keep the airway clear.*

Lung alveoli begin to collapse within minutes of GA, as respiratory muscle tone is lost (atelectasis). This occurs particularly in lower zones and with higher inspired oxygen concentrations when there is less nitrogen to 'splint' open the alveoli. If excessive, it may cause shunting to occur with a tendency to impaired post-operative gas exchange. This is extremely common but quickly compensated for in the healthy patient. At the other end of the spectrum, patients with poor pre-operative respiratory function or inadequate pain relief preventing coughing and clearance of secretions may develop pneumonia and respiratory failure. Immobility for any reason leaves patients at risk of thromboembolism and thus GA is a contributory factor. This is reflected in the markedly different risk associated with different types of surgery. After prolonged GA, especially in older people, there is high risk of atelectasis (Ch. 15); therefore, the patient should be strongly encouraged to undertake breathing exercises and to cough up any sputum. Accumulation of secretions is a frequent cause of lower airway obstruction and subsequent chest infection. This can be particularly severe in patients with chronic bronchitis (Ch. 15). A transient rise in temperature is common and is usually caused by atelectasis or localized pulmonary infection that may not be clinically detectable. Physiotherapy may be helpful. In dentistry, inhalation of a tooth or fragments of materials is another possible cause of atelectasis and subsequent lung abscess. Also, if an emergency operation has had to be carried out despite an acute upper respiratory tract infection, lower respiratory tract infection is more likely. Occasionally, bronchospasm can result from a hypersensitivity reaction to an intravenous anaesthetic or other drug used during the operation.

Respiratory weakness may be due to the action of muscle relaxants. Reversal of the action of neuromuscular blocking drugs depends on many factors but, if delayed, results in weak respiratory movements that cannot be made stronger by the patient's conscious efforts. Suxamethonium apnoea is discussed in Ch. 23. Impaired chest movements may be caused by damage to the chest, a common accompaniment of maxillofacial injuries, particularly when they result from road traffic accidents (Ch. 24). This may inhibit respiration and coughing.

Respiratory depression can result from the effects of the anaesthetic and ancillary drugs. Midazolam and pentazocine, for example, form a potent combination of respiratory depressants, which can be aggravated by hypoxia, often from a similar cause, and have caused occasional deaths.

Malignant hyperpyrexia

See Ch. 23.

PARTICULAR CONSIDERATIONS OF OUTPATIENT SEDATION OR GA IN DENTISTRY

Since the operation site is close to the airway, any inflammatory oedema, haemorrhage or foreign bodies can endanger respiration. Appropriate instruction must be given pre-operatively, recorded in the case notes and re-emphasized before discharge. Patients must be made aware that, after a GA, it is dangerous to drive a vehicle, ride a bicycle, pillion on a motorcycle, work with unguarded machinery or make important decisions. They should also be warned not to drink alcohol or take certain drugs, particularly sleeping tablets. Obviously, it is impossible to control the behaviour of irresponsible patients, but it is essential to point out the dangers in the clearest possible terms. Patients may also fail to take in or forget verbal instructions, particularly after benzodiazepine use. To protect both the patient and operator, the patient and escort should be given written instructions, and every other item should be checked (Fig. 3.6). In the case of sedation given in the dental surgery, it is important to use a questionnaire to make sure that nothing has been forgotten and, in the event of any mishap, to provide documentary evidence that this assessment has been carried out.

Mark each item with a tick or N/A for *every* sedation given | Patient label

STAFF CHECK   DATE:
Experienced qualified DSA present?
Another dentist/doctor/nurse/DSA is within easy call?
Operator and assistants know emergency procedures?

EQUIPMENT CHECK
Site of emergency equipment known?
Have the following been checked by the operator?
Oxygen
Suction — dental unit
Suction — mobile/back-up
Positive pressure ventilating bag
Sphygmomanometer
Pulse oximeter
Other automatic monitor (BP/ECG)
Emergency drugs (Flumazenil)
Sedation equipment
Have the following been checked?
Dental equipment
Dental unit

PATIENT CHECK
Patient, parent or guardian know what is planned?
Written consent has been obtained?
Written pre- + post-operative instruction issued?
Medical and dental history checked?
Routine medication taken?
Last meal or drink checked?
Fasting patient?
If Yes — has glucose been given?
Patient has consumed alcohol today?
If Yes — advise to postpone session?
Responsible escort present?
Weight recorded?
BP recorded?

OPERATOR'S NAME IN CAPITALS:

Fig. 3.6 Checklist for operators before giving sedation (courtesy of Miss AM Skelly)

DEATH IN PATIENTS RECEIVING GA FOR DENTAL TREATMENT

Although deaths are now uncommon during or immediately after GA for dental treatment, they are more frequent than with other pain and anxiety control methods. Every death is a tragedy for the individual and family. Investigation of deaths has too often highlighted factors that seemed potentially avoidable. In the UK, there has been a fall in the number of deaths associated with GA for dental treatment outside hospital since the 1960s, in line with the decline in the use of GA in dental practice. Tragically though, there were a number of deaths in children associated with GA for dental treatment outside hospital in the late 1990s. Investigations and inquiries into these deaths have been critical of the standard of care provided in fundamental areas such as pre-operative assessment, monitoring of electrical heart activity, blood pressure, oxygen and carbon dioxide levels, start of resuscitation and transfer to specialist critical care. GA for dental treatment is not permitted in the UK outside a hospital with critical care facilities (amendment in 'Maintaining Standards' published by the British General Dental Council, 2001). Dentists arranging or providing dental treatment under GA should also make sure they have explored and discussed with the patient all possible alternatives and enquired about possible contraindications. They must also take measures to avoid need for GA in the future.

USEFUL WEBSITES

http://www.aagbi.org
http://www.bma.org.uk
http://www.emedicine.com/perioperativecare/index.shtml
http://www.gdc-uk.org/Current+registrant/standards+fort+Dental+professionals
http://www.gdc-uk.org/NR/rdonlyres/FFD61DA5-A09E-4B38-8FFB-BA342E9F0AF4/16688/147163_Patient_Cons.pdf
http://www.surgical-tutor.org.uk/default-home.htm?principles/perioperative.htm~right

Conscious sedation and general anaesthesia

The statement by the General Dental Council (GDC) on both conscious sedation and general anaesthesia is found in an annex to the GDC's Standards for dental professionals. It supports the recommendations and guidance of the Department of Health. Full details are available at: http://www.gdc-uk.org/NR/rdonlyres/FFD61DA5-A09E-4B38-8FFB-BA342E-9F0AF4/16687/147158_Standards_Profs.pdf

A conscious decision – a review of the use of general anaesthesia and conscious sedation in primary dental care: http://www.dh.gov.uk/en/Publicationsandstatistics/Publications/PublicationsPolicyAndGuidance/DH_4074702

Conscious sedation in the provision of dental care: http://www.dh.gov.uk/en/Publicationsandstatistics/Publications/PublicationsPolicyAndGuidance/DH_4069257

Consent

The GDC has produced supporting guidance to its standards specifically on consent – *Principles of patient consent:*

http://www.gdc-uk.org/NR/rdonlyres/FFD61DA5-A09E-4B38-8FFB-BA342E9F0AF4/16688/147163_Patient_Cons.pdf

FURTHER READING

A conscious decision. Report of an expert group chaired by the Chief Medical and Dental Officer. Department of Health, London, 2000.

Ashford, R.U., Scollay, J., Harrington, P., 2002. Obtaining informed consent. Hosp Med 62, 374.

Astarita, C., Gargano, D., Romano, C., et al., 2001. Long term absence of sensitization to mepivacaine as assessed by a diagnostic protocol including patch test. Clin Exp Allergy 31, 1762–1770.

British Medical Association and Law Society. Assessment of mental capacity: guidance for doctors and lawyers. BMJ, London, 2004.

Cohn, S.L., Goldman, L., 2003. Preoperative risk evaluation and perioperative management of patients with coronary artery disease. Med Clin North Am 87, 111–136.

Conscious sedation in the provision of dental care. Report of an expert group on sedation for dentistry. Standing Dental Advisory Committee, 2003. http://www.advisorybodies.doh.gov.uk/sdac/conscious_sedation03.pdf.

Conscious sedation. A referral guide for dental practitioners. Society for the Advancement of Anaesthesia in Dentistry and Dental Sedation Teachers Group, 2001.

Crowe, S., 2002. Obtaining consent in the elderly patient. Hosp Med 63, 61.

Department of Constitutional Affairs. Mental Capacity Act 2005 – summary, p.1. http://www.dh.gov.uk/assetRoot/04/10/85/96/04108596.pdf.

Department of Health, 2001. General anaesthesia for dental treatment in a hospital setting with critical care facilities. www.doh.gov.uk/dental/consciousguidance2.htm

Department of Health, 2002. Guidelines for conscious sedation in the provision of dental care. Standing Dental Advisory Committee.

Doyle, R., 1999. Assessing and modifying the risk of postoperative pulmonary complications. Chest 115 (Suppl 5), S77–S81.

Flynn, P.J., Strunin, L., 2005. General anaesthesia for dentistry. Anaesth Intensive Care Med 6, 263–265.

Furness, P.M., 2003. Obtaining and using human tissues for research: ethical and practical dilemmas. Hosp Med 64, 198–199.

General anaesthesia, sedation and resuscitation in Dentistry. Report of an expert working party prepared for the Standing Dental Advisory Committee 1990. (AKA The Poswills Report).

Haas, D.A., 2002. An update on analgesics for the management of acute postoperative dental pain. J Can Dent Assoc 68, 476–482.

Hollenberg, S.M., 1999. Preoperative cardiac risk assessment. Chest 11 (Suppl 5), S51–S57.

Implementing and ensuring safe sedation practice for healthcare procedures in adults. Academy of Medical Royal Colleges, London.

Jolly, D.E., 2000. General health assessment. In: Nunn, J.H. (ed.), Disability and oral care, FDI World Dental Press, London.

Maintaining standards. General Dental Council, November 1997, revised November 2001.

Mental Capacity Act 2005, s2(1).

McKenna, G., Manton, S., 2008. Pre-operative fasting for intravenous conscious sedation used in dental treatment: are conclusions based on relative risk management or evidence? Br Dent J 205, 173–176.

Padfield, A., 2007. 'Just a little whiff of gas'; a partial history of UK dental chair anaesthesia. Anaesth News 243, 27–28.

Penarrocha-Diago, M., Sanchis-Bielsa, J.M., 2000. Ophthalmologic complications after intraoral local anesthesia with articaine. Oral Surg Oral Med Oral Pathol Oral Radiol Endod 90, 21–24.

Powell, C.A., Caplan, C.E., 2001. Pulmonary function tests in the preoperative pulmonary evaluation. Clin Chest Med 22, 703–714.

Reference guide to consent for examination or treatment. Department of Health, London, March 2001.

Resuscitation guidelines for use in the United Kingdom. Resuscitation Council (UK), London, 2000.

Sedation in dentistry. The competent graduate. Dental Sedation Teachers Group, 2000.

Sedgwick, E., 2001. Patients' right to refuse treatment. Hosp Med 63, 196–197.

Smetana, G.W., 2003. Preoperative pulmonary assessment of the older patient. Clin Geriatr Med 19, 35–55.

Smith, A.F., Pittaway, A.J., 2003. Premedication for anxiety in adult day surgery. Cochrane Database Syst Rev CD002192.

Standards for conscious sedation in dentistry: alternative techniques. Report of an expert group on sedation for dentistry. Standing Dental Advisory Committee, 2007. http://www.rcseng.ac.uk/fds/docs/SCSDAT%202007.pdf.

Standards for conscious sedation. Report of an independent expert working group convened by the Society for the Advancement of Anaesthesia in Dentistry, October 2000.

Wheeler, R., 2006. Consent in surgery. Ann R Coll Surg Engl 88, 261–264.

Appendix 3.1 General anaesthesia, sedation and resuscitation

Recommendations from the Poswillo Report (Department of Health, 1990)

- The use of general anaesthesia should be avoided wherever possible.
- The same general standards in respect of personnel, premises and equipment must apply irrespective of where the general anaesthetic is administered. (Para 3.8)
- Dental anaesthesia must be regarded as a postgraduate subject. (Para 3.11)
- All anaesthetics should be administered by accredited anaesthetists who must recognize their responsibility for providing dental anaesthetic services. (Para 3.13)
- Anaesthetic training should include specific experience in dental anaesthesia. (Para 3.14)
- Health authorities should review the provision of consultant dental anaesthetic sessions to ensure that they are sufficient to meet local needs. (Para 3.14)
- Doctors and dentists with knowledge, experience and competence sufficient to satisfy the College of Anaesthetists and the Faculty of Dental Surgery are to be under no detriment. (Para 3.16)
- The no detriment arrangements must have been implemented within 2 years of the publication of this report. (Para 3.17)
- The administration of general anaesthesia in dental surgeries and clinics equipped to the recommended standards of monitoring necessary for patient safety shall continue. (Para 3.17)
- An electrocardiogram, a pulse oximeter and a non-invasive blood pressure device are essential for the non-invasive monitoring of a patient under general anaesthesia. (Paras 3.16 and 3.19)
- A capnograph is to be used where tracheal anaesthesia is practised. (Para 3.20)
- A defibrillator must be available. (Para 3.21)
- Equipment conforming to recognized standards should be purchased and installed, regularly serviced and maintained in accordance with the manufacturer's instructions. (Para 3.21)
- Intravenous agents should be administered via an indwelling needle or cannula, which should not be moved until the patient has fully recovered. (Para 3.22)
- Appropriate training must be provided for those assisting the anaesthetist and dentist. (Paras 3.25 and 4.15)
- At no time should the recovering patient be left unattended. (Para 3.26)
- Adequate recovery facilities should be available. (Para 3.26)
- Good contemporaneous records of all treatments and procedures should be kept. (Para 3.26)
- Written consent should be obtained on each occasion prior to the administration of a general anaesthetic. (Para 3.30)
- Consideration should be given to developing a national general anaesthetic/sedation consent form for general dental practitioners. (Para 3.31)
- Patients should be provided with comprehensive pre- and post-treatment instructions and advice. (Para 3.31)

Appendix 3.2 Classification of operations and admissions

CLASSIFICATION OF OPERATIONS

EMERGENCY

Immediate life-saving operation, resuscitation simultaneous with surgical treatment (e.g. trauma, ruptured aortic aneurysm). Operation usually within 1 h.

URGENT

Operation as soon as possible after resuscitation (e.g. irreducible hernia, intussusception, oesophageal atresia, intestinal obstruction, major fractures). Operation within 24 h.

SCHEDULED

An early operation but not immediately life-saving (e.g. malignancy). Operation usually within 3 weeks.

ELECTIVE

Operation at a time to suit both patient and surgeon (e.g. cholecystectomy, joint replacement).

DAY CASE

A patient who is admitted for investigation or operation on a planned non-resident basis (i.e. no overnight stay).

CLASSIFICATION OF ADMISSIONS

ELECTIVE

At a time agreed between the patient and the surgical service.

URGENT

Within 48 h of referral/consultation.

EMERGENCY

Immediately following referral/consultation, when admission is unpredictable and at short notice because of the clinical need.

Appendix 3.3 Checks and instructions for patients

ROUTINE CHECKS BEFORE CONSCIOUS SEDATION FOR DENTAL TREATMENT

Always check the following.

1 Patient's name (and hospital number).
2 Nature, side and site of operation.
3 Medical history, particularly of cardiorespiratory disease or bleeding tendency.
4 That consent has been obtained in writing from patient or, in a person under 16 years of age, from parent or guardian, and that the patient adequately understands the nature of the operation and sequelae.
5 That necessary oral investigations (e.g. radiographs) are available.
6 What the patient has had by mouth, including drugs, over the previous 4 h.
7 That the patient has emptied his or her bladder.
8 That the patient's dentures have been removed and bridges, crowns and loose teeth have been noted by the anaesthetist.
9 That any pre-medication (and, where indicated, regular medication such as the contraceptive pill, anticonvulsants or antidepressants) has been given but not usually within the previous 4 h.
10 That the anaesthetic and suction apparatus are working satisfactorily and that emergency drugs are available and not date-expired.
11 That the patient is escorted by a responsible adult.
12 That the patient has been warned not to drive, operate unguarded machinery, drink alcohol or make important decisions for 24 h post-operatively.

INSTRUCTIONS TO PATIENTS BEFORE CONSCIOUS SEDATION (PREFERABLY IN WRITING)

1 You must be accompanied by a responsible adult, over the age of 18 years, who will undertake to escort you home and remain with you for 24 h after treatment. You must not be accompanied by children under 14 years of age.
2 Do not wear nail varnish or make-up.
3 After sedation, you must not on the same day:
   a drive a motor vehicle
   b ride a bicycle or motorcycle, even as a passenger
   c cook or use unguarded machinery
   d take alcohol
   e take sedative drugs without medical advice
   f make important decisions or sign any documents.
4 If you develop a cold before your appointment, please telephone the hospital or dental surgery for advice.

Patients who fail to comply with these simple safety precautions will not be given sedation.

INSTRUCTIONS TO PATIENTS AFTER TOOTH EXTRACTION (PREFERABLY IN WRITING)

After a tooth has been extracted, the socket will usually bleed for a short time. This bleeding stops because a healthy blood clot forms in the tooth socket. These clots are easily disturbed and if this happens bleeding will recur. To avoid disturbance of the clot, please follow these instructions.

1 After leaving the hospital or dental surgery do not rinse out your mouth for 24 h, unless you have been told otherwise by the dentist.
2 Do not disturb the clot in the socket with your tongue or fingers.
3 For the rest of the day, take only soft foods.
4 Try not to chew on the affected side for at least 3 days.
5 Avoid unnecessary talking, excitement or exercise for the rest of the day.
6 Do not take alcoholic or very hot drinks for the rest of the day.
7 If the tooth socket continues to bleed after you have left the surgery, do not be alarmed – much of the liquid that appears to be blood is actually saliva. If bleeding persists, make a small pad from a clean handkerchief or cotton wool, place over the socket and close the teeth firmly on it. Keep up the pressure for 15–30 min. If the bleeding still does not stop, seek dental or medical advice.

Appendix 3.4 Standing Dental Advisory Committee: Report of an Expert Group on Sedation for Dentistry

CONSCIOUS SEDATION IN THE PROVISION OF DENTAL CARE

EXECUTIVE SUMMARY

- Despite the publication of a number of authoritative documents on pain and anxiety control for dentistry, it has become evident that there remain areas of confusion and lack of consensus.
- This document is designed to lay down specific recommendations to all practitioners providing *conscious sedation* for the provision of dental care in general dental practice, community and hospital settings.
- The effective management of pain and anxiety is of paramount importance for patients requiring dental care and *conscious sedation* is a fundamental component of this.
- Competently provided *conscious sedation* is safe, valuable and effective.
- It is absolutely essential that a wide margin of safety be maintained between *conscious sedation* and the unconscious state of general anaesthesia. *Conscious sedation* must

under no circumstances be interpreted as light general anaesthesia.

- A high level of competence based on a solid foundation of theoretical and practical supervised training, progressive updating of skills and continuing experience is the key to safe practice.
- Education and training must ensure that *all* members of the dental team providing treatment under *conscious sedation* have received appropriate supervised theoretical, practical and clinical training.
- Training in the management of complications, in addition to regularly rehearsed proficiency in life-support techniques, is essential for all clinical staff. Retention and improvement of knowledge and skills relies upon regular updating.
- Operating chairs and patient trolleys must be capable of being placed in the head-down tilt position and equipment for resuscitation from respiratory and cardiac arrest must be readily available.
- Dedicated purpose-designed machines for inhalational sedation should be used.
- It is essential to ensure that hypoxic mixtures cannot be delivered.
- There should be adequate active scavenging of waste gases.
- All equipment for the administration of intravenous sedation including appropriate antagonist drugs must be available in the treatment area and appropriately maintained.
- Supplemental oxygen delivered under intermittent positive pressure, together with back-up, must be immediately available.
- It is important to ensure that each exposure to *conscious sedation* is justified. Careful and thorough assessment of the patient ensures that correct decisions are made regarding the planning of treatment.
- A thorough medical, dental and social history should be taken and recorded prior to each course of treatment for every patient.
- There are few absolute contraindications for *conscious sedation*, though special care is required in the assessment and treatment of children and elderly patients.
- Patients must receive careful instructions and written valid consent must be obtained.
- Fasting for *conscious sedation* is not normally required but some authorities recommend the same fasting requirements as for general anaesthesia.

- Recovery from sedation is a progressive step down from completion of treatment through to discharge. A member of the dental team must supervise and monitor the patient throughout this period.
- The decision to discharge a patient into the care of the escort following any type of sedation must be the responsibility of the sedationist.
- The patient and escort should be provided with details of potential complications, aftercare and adequate information regarding emergency contact.
- The three standard techniques of inhalation, oral and intravenous sedation employed in dentistry are effective and adequate for the vast majority of patients. The simplest technique to match the requirements should be used.
  - The only currently recommended technique for inhalation sedation is a titrated dose of nitrous oxide with oxygen and it is absolutely essential to ensure that a hypoxic mixture cannot be administered.
  - The standard technique for intravenous sedation is the use of a titrated dose of a *single* drug; for example the current use of a benzodiazepine.
  - Oral premedication with an effective low dose of a sedative agent may be prescribed.
  - No single technique will be successful for all patients.
- All drugs and all syringes in use in the treatment area must be clearly labelled and each drug should be given according to accepted recommendations.
- Stringent clinical monitoring during the procedure is of particular importance and all members of the clinical team must be capable of undertaking this.
- *Conscious sedation* for children must only be undertaken by teams which have adequate training and experience.
  - Nitrous oxide/oxygen should be the first choice for paediatric dental patients.
  - Intravenous sedation for children is only appropriate in a minority of cases.
- The management of any complication, including loss of consciousness, requires the *whole* dental team to be aware of the risks, appropriately trained and fully equipped. It is vitally important for the whole team to be prepared and regularly rehearsed.
- Attention must be given to risk awareness, risk control and risk containment.
- Evidence of active participation in continuing professional development (CPD) and personal clinic audit is an essential feature of clinical governance.

SIGNS AND SYMPTOMS

This chapter summarizes a range of the more important medical conditions, arranged alphabetically.

ABDOMINAL PAIN

Abdominal pain is common, and often trivial and due to gastroenteritis. Acute and severe pain may however be a symptom of serious intra-abdominal disease, from inflammatory bowel disease to various 'surgical problems'. Such a surgical emergency (an 'acute abdomen') includes appendicitis, intestinal obstruction, perforated peptic ulcer, perforated diverticulitis, ectopic pregnancy, twisted ovarian cyst, a leaking abdominal aneurysm, mesenteric embolism or thrombosis, biliary tract disease, pancreatitis or a kidney stone. Gangrene and intestinal perforation can follow as little as 6 h after interruption of the intestinal blood supply from appendicitis, a strangulating obstruction or an arterial embolus.

ALOPECIA

Alopecia (hair loss) may be *temporary* and caused for instance by radiotherapy; cytotoxic chemotherapy; other drugs (e.g. anticoagulants, retinoids, beta-blockers and oral contraceptives); or tinea capitis (ring worm). More permanent alopecia may be the following.

• *Involutional alopecia* – the gradual progressive permanent thinning of the hair which is normal with ageing in both sexes.
• *Androgenic alopecia* – a genetically predisposed condition that affects both sexes, earlier in men than women (as early as the teens or early 20s), with the hairline receding and hair from the crown gradually and permanently disappearing (male pattern baldness).
• *Alopecia areata* – patchy hair loss in children and young adults of uncertain cause, often sudden in onset and sometimes resulting in complete baldness. However, in 90% of cases, the hair regrows within a few years.
• *Alopecia universalis* – loss of all body hair of uncertain cause, with a low chance of regrowth, especially when in children.
• Autoimmune diseases, particularly lupus erythematosus, may cause hair loss.

AMENORRHOEA

Amenorrhoea – absence of menstruation (menses), except before puberty, during pregnancy or early lactation, and after the menopause – is pathological. It may be caused by anatomical abnormalities, endocrine dysfunction (hypothalamic, pituitary, adrenal, thyroid or other), cirrhosis, ovarian failure, or genetic defects. Amenorrhoea is either primary (menarche has not occurred by age 16) or secondary (menses have not occurred for 3 or more months in women who have had menses).

ANAEMIA

Anaemia is a reduction in the haemoglobin level for the age and sex. Anaemia may be normocytic, microcytic or macrocytic according to the cause (Ch. 08).

ANGINA PECTORIS (SEE CHEST PAIN)

ANOREXIA

Anorexia, or loss of appetite, is a non-specific symptom seen in many conditions, but notably in: malignant disease (Ch. 22); chronic infections and eating disorders (Ch. 27).

ANOSMIA

Anosmia (loss of sense of smell) is usually due to nasal occlusion from the common cold, rhinitis, hay fever or nasal polyps. Some loss of smell may be normal with ageing but medications may change or impair the ability to detect odours. It can also arise from damage to the olfactory nerves from head injury, radiotherapy or certain viral infections. Systemic causes include cerebrovascular accidents, Alzheimer dementia, tabes (syphilis), brain tumours, and many endocrine, nutritional, and nervous disorders.

ANXIETY

Anxiety may be normal, or part of a psychiatric disorder (Ch. 10), but it may also be caused by stress; stimulant drugs such as amphetamines, caffeine, cocaine, ecstasy and many others – or their withdrawal; neurological disorders (brain trauma, infections, inner ear disorders); cardiovascular disorders (heart failure, arrhythmias); endocrine diseases (adrenal or thyroid hyperfunction, hypoglycaemia, phaeochromocytoma); or respiratory diseases (asthma, chronic obstructive pulmonary disease).

APHASIA

Aphasia is a language disorder that impairs both the expression and understanding of language as well as reading and writing. Aphasia results from damage to the left cerebral hemisphere of the brain, often as the result of a stroke, head injury or brain tumour. Speech disorders such as dysarthria or apraxia of speech, which also result from brain damage, may be associated.

ARRHYTHMIAS (SEE CH. 5)

ASCITES

Ascites is the accumulation of fluid in the peritoneal cavity. It may be from peritoneal sources (bacterial, fungal or parasitic disease; cancer (malignant ascites); endometriosis or starch peritonitis) or from extraperitoneal sources (cirrhosis, congestive heart failure, hypoalbuminaemia, myxoedema or ovarian disease, e.g. Meig syndrome).

ATAXIA

Ataxia is incoordination or clumsiness of movement that is not the result of muscular weakness but of cerebellar, vestibular or sensory (proprioceptive) disorders. In ataxia, there is uncoordinated movement – defined as an abnormality of muscle control or an inability to coordinate movements finely. Causes of ataxia include: drugs (e.g. alcohol, aminoglutethimide, anticholinergics, phenytoin, carbamazepine, phenobarbital and tricyclic antidepressants), stroke or transient ischaemic attack (TIA), multiple sclerosis, head trauma, poisoning, hereditary (congenital cerebellar ataxia, Friedreich ataxia, ataxia telangiectasia) or post-infectious (typically following chickenpox or encephalitis).

Cerebellar ataxia is produced by lesions of the cerebellum or its afferent or efferent connections in the cerebellar peduncles, pons or red nucleus.

Vestibular ataxia is produced by lesions anywhere along the eighth nerve pathway from labyrinth to brainstem and in the vestibular nuclei. Labyrinthitis is a typical cause. Nystagmus is frequently present, typically unilateral, and most pronounced on gaze away from the side of vestibular involvement. Vestibular ataxia is also gravity-dependent – incoordination of limb movements cannot be demonstrated when the patient is examined lying down but only when the patient attempts to stand or walk.

Sensory ataxia can result from abnormalities anywhere along the afferent pathway from peripheral nerve to the parietal lobe cortex. Clinical findings include defective joint position and vibration sense in the leg and sometimes the arms, unstable stance with Romberg sign (sways with eyes shut), and a gait of slapping quality.

BACK PAIN

Back pain is a very common complaint; nearly four out of five people experience it at some time. Most cases do not have a definable cause but sedentary jobs and lifestyles may predispose, as can obesity, or strenuous sports such as football and gymnastics. Women who have been pregnant, smokers and workers who repetitively lift heavy objects are all at greater risk of back pain. At the other extreme, back pain can be a symptom of spinal metastasis and be virtually a death warrant. Back pain can develop from spinal causes (muscular disorders or strain, back overuse or injury, pressure on a nerve root or ruptured intervertebral vertebral disc ('slipped disc') or spinal arthritis, fractures or metastases. Non-spinal causes include menstruation or pre-menstrual syndrome (PMS), endometriosis, ovarian cysts or cancer.

BLEEDING TENDENCIES

Prolonged bleeding usually has a local cause such as excessive operative trauma.

Other causes include: haemorrhagic disease involving platelet activation and function, contact activation, the clotting protein factors, or antithrombin function; uncontrolled hypertension (rarely); or aspirin or other non-steroidal anti-inflammatory drugs (NSAIDs), that interfere with platelet function (but rarely severe).

BLINDNESS (SEE VISUAL IMPAIRMENT)

BRADYCARDIA

Bradycardia may have intrinsic or extrinsic causes.

Intrinsic causes include: myocardial infarction, ischaemia or idiopathic degeneration; infiltrative diseases (sarcoidosis, amyloidosis or haemochromatosis); collagen diseases; myotonic muscular dystrophy; surgical trauma; or endocarditis.

Extrinsic causes include: autonomically mediated syndromes (vomiting, coughing, micturition, defaecation, etc.); carotid-sinus hypersensitivity from vagal hypertonicity; drugs (beta-adrenergic blockers, calcium-channel blockers, clonidine, digoxin, antiarrhythmic agents); hypothyroidism; hypothermia; neurological disorders (affecting the autonomic nervous system); or electrolyte imbalances (hypokalaemia, hyperkalaemia).

CERVICAL LYMPH NODE ENLARGEMENT (SEE LYMPHADENOPATHY)

CHEST PAIN

Angina and myocardial infarction are the main causes of acute chest pain (Table 4.1).

Table 4.1   Main causes of acute chest pain

Cause of Pain	Features	Predisposing Factors
Myocardial infarction	Severe persistent crushing retrosternal pain possibly radiating to left arm. Unrelieved by glyceryl trinitrate. May be nausea or vomiting	Coronary heart disease. Hypertension
Angina pectoris	Retrosternal pain possibly radiating to left arm. Often previously experienced. Relieved in 3 min by glyceryl trinitrate	Coronary heart disease. Hypertension
Acute abdominal pain	Pain location is of particular importance. Depending on cause there may be concomitant symptoms such as gastro-oesophageal reflux, nausea, vomiting, diarrhoea, constipation, jaundice, melaena, haematuria, haematemesis, weight loss, and mucus or blood in the stool	Serious causes: ruptured abdominal aortic aneurysm, perforated viscus, mesenteric isch-aemia, ruptured ectopic pregnancy, intestinal obstruction, appendicitis, pancreatitis
Dissecting aneurysm	Sudden severe chest or upper back pain, often described as a tearing, ripping or shearing sensation, that radiates down the back, loss of consciousness, shortness of breath	Men between 40 and 70 years
Oesophagitis	Low retrosternal pain on lying down or stooping. Improved by antacids	Hiatus hernia
Anxiety (hyperventilation)	Anxious patients with precordial pain. Overbreathing, panic and precordial pain	Stress
Trauma	Obvious history	–
Lung infection or tumour	Pain on inspiration. May be accompanied by dyspnoea or cough	Pneumonia. Pleurisy. Bronchogenic carcinoma

Table 4.2   Causes of finger clubbing

Hereditary	Respiratory	Cardiovascular	Gastrointestinal	Metabolic
	Lung cancer Bronchiolitis Fibrosing alveolitis Asbestosis HIV, fungal and mycoplasmal infections Mesothelioma	Endocarditis Cyanotic congenital heart disease	Ulcerative colitis Crohn disease Coeliac disease Liver disease	Thyrotoxicosis Acromegaly

HIV, human immunodeficiency virus.

CLUBBING OF FINGERS

Finger-clubbing is enlargement of the end of the digit. The cause is uncertain but might be due to hypoxia and circulating hormones such as erythropoietin. Clubbing can be hereditary but is usually acquired (Table 4.2).

COMA

Level of consciousness is assessed by the Glasgow Coma Scale (Ch. 24). A coma is profound unconsciousness in which the person is alive but unable to react or respond to stimuli. Coma results from central nervous system (CNS) diseases and conditions that affect CNS function, especially brain trauma, stroke, tumour, epilepsy, infection (e.g. meningitis), metabolic abnormalities (diabetic coma, ketoacidosis or electrolyte abnormality – hypernatraemia, hypercalcaemia), intoxication (e.g. alcohol, drugs of abuse, analgesics, anticonvulsants, antihistamines, benzodiazepines, digoxin, heavy metals, hydrocarbons, barbiturates, insulin, lithium, organophosphates, phencyclidine, phenothiazines, salicylates, or tricyclic antidepressants), or shock, hypoxia or hypotension (arrhythmia, heart failure).

Persistent coma is termed the vegetative state.

CONFUSION

The confused patient has fluctuating consciousness, and impaired orientation and short-term memory. Delusions or hallucinations can cause severe agitation. Confusional states need to be differentiated from dementia, in which there are similar disturbances of orientation and memory, but consciousness is unimpaired. Patients are usually more confused at night. The confused patient should receive immediate medical attention since brain damage may result from many of the causes (see Coma).

CONSTIPATION

Constipation is the passage of small amounts of hard, dry faeces, usually fewer than three times a week. Some believe they are constipated, or irregular, if they do not have a bowel movement every day but there are no criteria for what can be regarded as 'normal'.

Constipation is the most common gastrointestinal complaint. Common causes include: lifestyle habits; inadequate dietary fibre, liquids or exercise; changes in life or routine, such as pregnancy, older age, and travel; abuse of laxatives, or ignoring the urge to have a bowel movement. Medications such as codeine, opioids, antacids that contain aluminium, antispasmodics, antidepressants, iron supplements, diuretics and anticonvulsants may be implicated. More important are colorectal disease (obstruction, scar tissue (adhesions), diverticulosis, tumours, strictures, irritable bowel syndrome, Hirschsprung disease) and systemic disease, such as neurological disorders (multiple sclerosis, Parkinson disease, chronic idiopathic intestinal pseudo-obstruction, stroke, spinal cord injuries), metabolic and endocrine conditions (diabetes, thyroid dysfunction, uraemia) or immunological disorders (amyloidosis, lupus, scleroderma).

COUGH

A cough is a sudden voluntary or involuntary explosive expiratory manoeuvre that tends, or intends, to clear material (sputum) from the airways. Transient cough may be simply a mechanism to expel mucus or an inhaled foreign body.

Cough is typical of respiratory, and sometimes of cardiac, disorders. Angiotensin-converting enzyme (ACE) inhibitors may produce a cough. A morning cough persisting until sputum is expectorated typifies chronic bronchitis. A cough that comes on exposure to cold air or during exercise may suggest asthma. One associated with rhinitis or wheezing or that is seasonal may be an allergic response. If induced by postural change, it may suggest chronic lung abscess, tuberculosis, bronchiectasis or a pedunculated tumour. If associated with eating, it suggests a disturbance of the swallowing mechanism, or possibly a pharyngeal pouch or a tracheo-oesophageal fistula.

CYANOSIS

Cyanosis is a bluish or purplish tinge to the skin due to very low oxygen saturation (SaO_2) and thus excess reduced haemoglobin. Approximately $5\,g/dl$ of reduced (deoxygenated) haemoglobin has to be present in the capillaries to generate the dark blue colour of cyanosis. For this reason, patients who are anaemic may be hypoxaemic without showing any cyanosis.

Peripheral cyanosis is a dusky or bluish tinge to the fingers and toes and, when unaccompanied by hypoxaemia, is caused by peripheral vasoconstriction as in the cold, and especially in Raynaud disease.

Central cyanosis (where the colour is also seen in the lips or within the mouth) is more serious and usually an indication of hypoxaemia, often because either of cardiac failure or of respiratory disease, or both together in cor pulmonale. Central cyanosis is an indication of gross hypoxia; such patients must not be given conscious sedation in the dental surgery, but should be treated in hospital.

Many factors, from natural skin pigment to room lighting, can affect detection of cyanosis and, if hypoxaemia is suspected, measurement of the oxygen level is necessary (arterial blood gas determination, pulse oximetry).

DEAFNESS

Deafness is common and, in over 30% of cases, is hereditary. Deafness may occasionally be associated with congenital malformations such as first arch syndromes. Deafness is caused by conductive hearing loss or sensorineural hearing loss.

Conductive hearing loss is due to disorders involving the middle or external ear – when sounds that should be carried from the tympanic membrane to the inner ear are blocked by, for example, ear wax, fluid or infection in the middle ear, or abnormal bone growth.

Sensorineural hearing loss is due to neural disorders such as defects of the cochlear nerve or its central connections, as in damage to the inner ear or auditory nerve (e.g. in birth defects, head injury, tumours, certain drugs, hypertension or stroke). Hearing can be lost by exposure to very loud noises, particularly over a long period of time (pop music, explosions, loud machinery, etc.). Age-related aural changes include especially *presbycusis* – the most common hearing problem in the elderly and linked to changes in the inner ear.

It is important when communicating with deaf people to face them, without wearing a face mask, and to speak clearly, in the absence of extraneous noise. The deaf alphabet helps enormously (Fig. 4.1).

DELIRIUM

Delirium is a state of mental confusion, caused by a disturbance in the normal functioning of the brain, which develops quickly and usually fluctuates in intensity. More common in older people, delirium affects at least one in ten hospitalized patients, and is common in many terminal illnesses.

The symptoms come on quickly, in hours or days, in contrast to those of dementia. The delirious patient has diminished awareness of, and responsiveness to, their environment, and the hallmark is a fluctuating level of consciousness. There may be limited awareness of the environment, confusion or disorientation (especially of time), memory impairment—especially of recent events, hallucinations, illusions and misinterpreted stimuli, mood disturbance, possibly including anxiety, euphoria or depression, and language or speech impairment.

There are many possible causes of delirium, including the following:

- Metabolic encephalopathy – hepatic or renal failure, diabetes, hyperthyroidism or hypothyroidism, vitamin deficiencies, fluid and electrolytes imbalance or severe dehydration.
- Drug intoxication – alcohol, anticholinergics (including atropine, scopolamine, chlorpromazine and diphenhydramine), sedatives (including barbiturates and benzodiazepines), antidepressants (including lithium, anticonvulsant drugs, corticosteroids), anticancer drugs (including methotrexate and procarbazine, cimetidine), street drugs, for example marijuana, LSD (lysergic acid diethylamide), amphetamines, cocaine, opioids, PCP (phenylcyclidine), inhalants.
- Poisons, for example carbon monoxide, heavy metals, insecticides (such as parathion and sevin), mushrooms

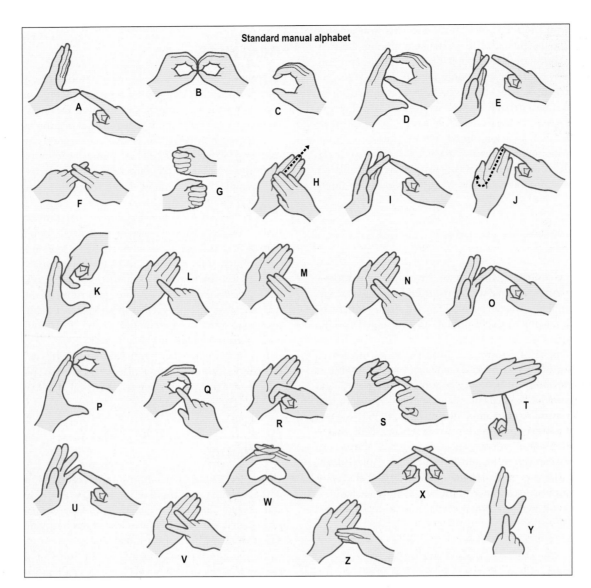

Fig. 4.1 Manual alphabet

(such as *Amanita* species), plants –such as jimsonweed (Datura) and morning glory (*Ipomoea* spp.).

- Fever, cerebral disorders (infection, head trauma, epilepsy, cerebrovascular accident, brain tumour), blood gas changes (hypoxaemia, hypercapnia) or post-surgical.

DEMENTIA

Dementia is a condition in which there is progressive loss of mental ability, including the ability to remember, think and reason (Ch. 10). The most common features include changes in memory, behaviour, mood and personality, and difficulty in communicating or understanding. Alzheimer disease is the most common form and responsible for about 50% of dementia. Vascular dementia is the second leading cause, a result of several TIAs, or small strokes. Other causes include Parkinson disease, Huntington disease, human immunodeficiency virus (HIV) infection and Creutzfeldt–Jakob disease. Dementia may occasionally be reversible if caused by brain diseases

or conditions such as brain tumours, depression or alcohol dependence.

DIARRHOEA

Diarrhoea is defined as loose, watery stools passed more than three times in a day. Diarrhoea may have a temporary cause, such as an infection; this is common and usually lasts a day or two and resolves spontaneously. Prolonged diarrhoea can be a sign of other disorders, particularly intestinal disease. Causes include infections: bacterial infections or toxins, such as pre-formed staphylococcal enterotoxin (from *S. aureus*) in contaminated food or water; viral; parasites; food intolerances (e.g. to lactose); reaction to drugs, such as antibiotics like clindamycin, and antacids containing magnesium; intestinal diseases (inflammatory bowel disease, coeliac disease or irritable bowel syndrome); or after surgery (e.g. after gastric surgery or cholecystectomy).

Where food hygiene is poor, diarrhoea can be life-threatening, especially if due to infections such as shigellosis (bacillary

Table 4.3 Causes of diplopia

Structure Involved	Site	Causes	Features that may be Associated
Extraocular muscles	Orbit	Trauma Exophthalmos Myasthenia gravis	Middle-third facial fracture Thyrotoxicosis Myopathy elsewhere
Cranial nerves III, IV and VI	Orbit	Trauma, tumour, sarcoid	Middle-third facial fracture
	Superior orbital fissure	Trauma, tumour, sarcoid	Often several muscles paralysed. Involvement of ophthalmic division of trigeminal. Pupil often normal
	Cavernous sinus	Aneurysms, infection, fistula, trauma	Similar to superior orbital fissure syndrome
	Skull base	Aneurysms. tumours, meningitis, fractures	May be involvement of single nerves; may be pupil dilatation
Cranial nerve nuclei	Brainstem	Vascular lesions, tumours, multiple sclerosis	May be involvement of trigeminal or facial nerves or complex neurological disorders

dysentery) or cholera. The passing of blood in the stools is typical of severe dysentery.

DIPLOPIA

Double vision (diplopia) is the simultaneous perception of two images of a single object. These images may be displaced horizontally, vertically or diagonally (i.e. both vertically and horizontally) in relation to each other. Diplopia is caused by misalignment of the eyes due to visual functional defects, mainly caused by eye muscle or neurological disorders; by a structural defect in the eye's optical system; or by drugs (e.g. alcohol, phenytoin, carbamazepine or lamotrigine). Diplopia may be an occasional transient complication of dental local anaesthetic injections, presumably because the anaesthetic tracks to the inferior orbital fissure, where it can block orbital nerves.

Diplopia is not uncommon after maxillofacial trauma (from trauma and/or alcohol or drugs) but usually resolves spontaneously within a few days. Persistent diplopia after trauma can be caused by blow-out fractures of the floor of the orbit, entrapment of (or damage to) the orbital muscles or damage to the suspensory ligament to the frontal process or the zygomatic bone. Later fibrous adhesions between the orbital periosteum and coverings of the eye may cause permanent limitation of movement, as may injury to cranial nerves III, IV and VI (Table 4.3). Paralytic strabismus is characterized by variable deviation of the ocular axes according to the position of gaze and is the usual type of strabismus that follows maxillofacial injuries.

DIZZINESS

Dizziness (vertigo) is a sensation of feeling unsteady or giddy, sometimes with a sensation of movement, spinning or floating. Dizziness is often due to disorders of the labyrinth – this interacts with other systems, such as the brain, eyes and musculoskeletal systems, to maintain the body's position. Movement of fluid in the semicircular canals signals the direction and speed of rotation of the head. Dizziness can be due to central vestibular disorders (a problem in the brain or its connecting nerves); peripheral vestibular disorder (labyrinthine disturbances); Ménière disease – an inner-ear fluid balance disorder

Box 4.1 Causes of dry mouth

Iatrogenic
- Drugs (antimuscarinics, sympathomimetics)
- Cancer therapy (irradiation of salivary glands, radioactive iodine, cytotoxic drugs)
- Graft-versus-host disease

Salivary gland disease
- Aplasia
- Sjögren syndrome
- Sarcoidosis
- HIV disease
- Hepatitis C
- HTLV-1 infection
- Infiltrates (amyloidosis; haemochromatosis)
- Cystic fibrosis
- Others

Dehydration
- Diabetes mellitus
- Diabetes insipidus
- Renal failure
- Haemorrhage
- Other causes of fluid loss or deprivation

HIV, human immunodeficiency virus; HTLV-1, human T-lymphotropic virus 1.

that also causes fluctuating hearing loss and tinnitus (ringing in the ears); or perilymph fistula – a leakage of inner ear fluid to the middle ear. It can follow head injury, physical exertion or, rarely, be without a known cause. Benign paroxysmal positional vertigo (a brief intense sensation of vertigo caused by a specific positional change of the head), labyrinthitis (an infection of the inner ear) and vestibular neuronitis (a viral infection of the vestibular nerve) are other causes. Systemic disorders (vascular disorders or blood flow disorders) may be implicated.

DROOLING (SEE SIALORRHOEA)

DRY MOUTH

Important causes of dry mouth are drugs, irradiation of the major salivary glands, Sjögren syndrome and infections (Box 4.1). If it is a complaint when salivary flow is normal, it may be psychogenic. Smoking and alcohol use aggravate xerostomia.

DYSPHAGIA

Cranial nerves IX to XII, and the pharyngeal muscles in particular, are essential to swallowing. Dysphagia is difficulty in swallowing; pain may be associated. Dysphagia has many causes (Box 4.2).

DYSPNOEA

Dyspnoea is difficulty in breathing. Causes include cardiac and respiratory disorders and anaemia. Functional causes include anxiety, panic disorders and hyperventilation. Dyspnoea is typically exacerbated by exercise, but may occur at rest and persist or worsen when lying down (orthopnoea). Paroxysmal nocturnal dyspnoea (cardiac asthma) is a sudden attack of severe dyspnoea due to pulmonary oedema that wakes the patient from sleep with a terrifying sensation of suffocation.

DYSRHYTHMIAS (SEE ARRHYTHMIAS)

DYSURIA

Dysuria is the sensation of pain or burning on urination. It is more common in women than in men, and then bacterial cystitis (usually after intercourse) is the commonest cause. In men dysuria is also usually a result of urinary tract infection – in younger patients usually due to a sexually transmitted organism such as *Chlamydia trachomatis*. In those over 35 years, coliform bacteria predominate and infection results from urinary stasis secondary to prostatic hyperplasia.

Dysuria in either sex may occasionally be caused by renal calculus, genitourinary malignancy, spondyloarthropathy and medications.

EARACHE

Earache (otalgia) is commonly due to middle ear infection (otitis media) and is especially common in children, often following a sore throat or cold. There is severe pain, often a temporary loss of hearing and, with severe infections, the ear drum may perforate causing a leakage of pus from the ear. Tumours in the middle ear are uncommon but include cholesteatoma.

As aircraft descend, pressure rises even in the normal middle ear, and this can cause excruciating pain.

Pain may be referred to the ear from elsewhere, such as tongue cancer, the antra, dental abscesses and temporomandibular disorders.

ENCOPRESIS

Encopresis is the soiling of underwear with stool by children who are past the age of toilet training but it is not considered a medical condition unless the child is at least 4 years old. A total of 1–2% of children younger than 10 years are affected by

---

Box 4.2 Causes of dysphagia

Psychogenic
- Globus hystericus

Organic
- **Mouth**
- Xerostomia
- Inflammatory or neoplastic lesions
- **Pharynx**
- Inflammatory or neoplastic lesions
- Foreign bodies
- Sideropenic dysphagia (Paterson–Brown-Kelly syndrome)
- Pouch
- **Oesophagus**
- Benign stricture
- Inflammatory or neoplastic lesions
- Scleroderma
- External pressure from mediastinal lymph nodes

Neurological and Neuromuscular Causes
- Achalasia
- Cerebellar disease
- Cerebral palsy
- Cerebrovascular accidents
- Cerebrovascular disease (pseudobulbar palsy)
- Dermatomyositis
- Diphtheria
- Guillain–Barré syndrome
- Motor neuron disease
- Muscular dystrophies
- Myasthenia gravis
- Myopathies
- Parkinson disease
- Poliomyelitis
- Syringobulbia

---

encopresis, many more boys than girls. A large amount of hard stool is in the intestine, and stool leaks around this mass and out through the anus. The best way to prevent encopresis is to prevent constipation with a varied diet with plenty of fruits and vegetables and wholegrain bread and cereals.

EPILEPSY (SEE CH. 13)

EPISTAXIS (NOSEBLEEDS)

Most nosebleeds are caused by minor nose injuries, the common cold, or by nose picking, vigorous nose blowing or sneezing. Rarely it may be caused by a foreign body lodged in the nose, barotrauma, chemical irritants, drugs (e.g. anticoagulants or NSAIDs), maxillofacial or nasal surgery, hereditary telangiectasia or thrombocytopenia.

EROSION OF TEETH

Tooth erosion can result from exposure to dietary acidic sources (carbonated drinks, citrus fruits and juices, pickles, vinegar, or some drugs, e.g. chewable vitamin C); regurgitated gastric contents (anorexia nervosa, bulimia, gastro-oesophageal reflux or alcoholism); industrial sources (various acids); or other sources (e.g. swimming pool water).

EXOPHTHALMOS (SEE PROPTOSIS)

FAINTING (VASOVAGAL SYNCOPE)

Vasovagal syncope is a reflex mediated by autonomic nerves in which there is splanchnic and skeletal muscle vasodilatation, bradycardia and subsequent diminished cerebral blood flow, leading to loss of consciousness. Fainting can be precipitated by psychological factors (e.g. pain, or fear at the sight of an injection needle or blood); postural changes; hypoxia or carotid sinus syndrome. The latter is usually seen in elderly patients in whom mild pressure on the neck causes a vagal reaction leading to syncope with bradycardia or cardiac arrest.
Vasovagal syncope is treated by lying down with the legs raised (Ch. 01).

FACIAL SENSORY LOSS (SEE CH. 13)

FACIAL PARALYSIS (SEE CH. 13)

FEVER (PYREXIA)

Normal body temperature (37°C) has a diurnal rhythm, being lower in the morning before dawn and higher in the afternoon. It is maintained by temperature control activities that balance heat loss and production. An abnormal rise in body temperature is caused by either hyperthermia or fever. In fever, the body temperature controls are functioning correctly, but the hypothalamic set point is elevated by exogenous or endogenous pyrogens and temperature rises as the body responds to cytokines such as inter-leukin-1 produced by micro-organisms or immunocytes.

The main causes of fever include: infections, tumours, reactions to drugs (e.g. chemotherapy drugs, biological response modifiers, and antibiotics such as vancomycin and amphotericin), neuroleptic malignant syndrome, reactions to blood transfusions, connective tissue disorders, cerebrovascular accidents, graft-versus-host disease.

Fever may be complicated in children under 6 years, by seizures (febrile convulsions) and – in older persons when the hypothalamus temperature-regulating centres may function poorly – by arrhythmias, heart failure, cerebral hypoxia and confusion.

GASTROINTESTINAL BLEEDING

Bleeding in the digestive tract can be the result of many different conditions, some of which are life threatening. Bleeding can sometimes be unnoticed (occult or hidden bleeding), but the faecal occult blood test (FOBT) checks stool samples for traces of blood, detecting bleeding from almost anywhere in the digestive tract, and it can also be positive after taking medications that irritate the tract. Causes of gastrointestinal bleeding apart from drugs such as NSAIDs include lesions in: the oesophagus (oesophagitis (hiatus hernia), varices, tears (Mallory–Weiss syndrome, after severe vomiting), cancer); the stomach (ulcers, gastritis, cancer); the small intestine (duodenal ulcer, inflammatory bowel disease); and the large intestine and rectum (haemorrhoids, infections, ulcerative colitis, diverticular disease, polyps or cancer).

The clinical appearance of blood in the digestive tract depends upon the site and severity of bleeding. Blood originating from the rectum or lower colon is bright red. The stool may be mixed with darker blood if the bleeding is higher in the colon. Bleeding from the oesophagus, stomach or duodenum can cause black or tarry stools (melaena). Vomited blood may be bright red or have a coffee-grounds appearance.

Endoscopy facilitates examination of the oesophagus, stomach, duodenum (oesophagoduodenoscopy), colon (colonoscopy) and rectum (sigmoidoscopy), and permits biopsies.

Magnetic resonance imaging (MRI), computed tomography (CT), barium radiography, angiography, radionuclide scans and ultrasound can also be used to locate sources of chronic occult GI bleeding.

GINGIVAL SWELLING

Gingival swelling may be localized or generalized and is occasionally due to a systemic syndrome (Box 4.3).

HAEMATEMESIS

Haematemesis (blood in the vomit) typically results from the regurgitation of blood from the upper gastrointestinal tract (mouth, pharynx, oesophagus, stomach and small intestine). It may be difficult to distinguish it from coughing up blood (from the lung) or a nosebleed (bloody post-nasal drainage). Conditions that cause haematemesis can also cause blood in the stool, and include bleeding ulcer(s), neoplasms, angiomas or varices in the stomach, duodenum, or oesophagus; prolonged and vigorous retching, which may tear small blood vessels of the throat or oesophagus; drugs; and ingested blood (e.g. swallowed after a nosebleed) or gastroenteritis.

HAEMATURIA

The presence of blood in the urine should never be ignored. It typically originates in the urinary tract (urethra, bladder or ureter) but, in women, blood coming from the vagina may appear in the urine, and in men a bloody ejaculate is usually due to a prostate disorder. Causes of haematuria include: haematological disorders (e.g. coagulopathies, sickle cell disease, renal vein thrombosis, or the thrombocytopenias); renal and urinary tract diseases (calculi, benign familial haematuria, infection, tumour, renal vein thrombosis, systemic lupus

Box 4.3 Causes of gingival enlargement

Generalized

Congenital

- Hereditary gingival fibromatosis and related disorders
- Mucopolysaccharidosis I–H
- Fucosidosis
- Aspartylglycosaminuria
- Leprechaunism (Donohue syndrome)
- Pfeiffer syndrome
- Infantile systemic hyalinosis
- Primary amyloidosis
- Hypoplasminogenaemia

Acquired

HAEMATOLOGICAL

- Acute myeloid leukaemia
- Pre-leukaemic leukaemia(s)
- Aplastic anaemia
- Vitamin C deficiency

DRUGS

- Phenytoin
- Ciclosporin
- Calcium-channel blockers

Localized

Congenital

- Fabry syndrome (angiokeratoma corporis diffusum universale)
- Cowden syndrome (multiple hamartoma and neoplasia syndrome)
- Tuberous sclerosis
- Sturge–Weber angiomatosis
- Congenital gingival granular cell tumour

Acquired

EPULIDES

- Pregnancy epulis
- Fibrous epulis
- Giant-cell epulis (e.g. secondary to primary hyperparathyroidism)

GRANULOMATOUS CONDITIONS

- Pyogenic granuloma
- Sarcoidosis
- Crohn disease
- Orofacial granulomatosis
- Wegener granulomatosis

INFECTIONS WITH HUMAN PAPILLOMAVIRUS (HPV)

- Papilloma
- Condyloma
- Warts
- Heck disease

TUMOURS

- Squamous cell carcinoma
- Lymphomas
- Langerhans cell tumours
- Multiple myeloma
- Kaposi sarcoma
- Plasmacytomas
- Other primary and secondary neoplasms

erythematosus, haemolytic–uraemic syndrome, anaphylactoid (Henoch–Schönlein) purpura, polycystic kidney disease, glomerulonephritis, congenital anomalies); prostatitis; hypercalciuria (increased amounts of calcium in the urine); urethral ulceration or meatal stenosis; trauma (fracture of the pelvis, renal trauma, urethral trauma, surgical procedures, including catheterization, circumcision, surgery, and biopsy); drugs (anticoagulants, cyclophosphamide, metyrosine, oxyphenbutazone, phenylbutazone, thiabendazole).

HAEMOPTYSIS

Haemoptysis is the expectoration or spitting up of blood or bloody mucus from the lungs. It may confused with bleeding from mouth, nose, throat or gastrointestinal tract. Haemoptysis is a potentially serious complaint; its causes, apart from a simple recent nosebleed and irritation of the throat from violent coughing, may include pulmonary infection, bronchitis, bronchiectasis, cancer, embolus, oedema, cystic fibrosis, diagnostic tests (bronchoscopy, laryngoscopy, biopsy, mediastinoscopy, or spirometry), and systemic lupus erythematosus.

HALITOSIS

Volatile sulphur compounds (VSC) are at least partly responsible for oral malodour.

Oral malodour is common on awakening (morning breath), and is transient and rarely of any special significance, probably resulting from increased microbial metabolic activity during sleep aggravated by a physiological reduction in salivary flow, lack of nocturnal physiological oral cleansing (e.g. movement of the facial and oral muscles) and variable oral hygiene procedures prior to sleep. Starvation can lead to a similar malodour.

Malodour at other times may be due to ingestion of certain food and drinks, such as spices, garlic, onion, durian, cabbage, cauliflower and radish, or of habits such as smoking tobacco or drinking alcohol, and is usually transient. It is considered to arise both from intraoral (food debris) and extraoral (respiratory) origins.

Halitosis is frequently due to oral infection (such as the tongue flora or periodontal disease). Anaerobes are numerous and frequently produce VSC. The main causes of halitosis are shown in Table 4.4.

HEADACHE (SEE CH. 13)

HEART FAILURE (SEE CH. 05)

Heart failure is usually the result of cardiac disease, but an otherwise normal heart can fail as a consequence of overload (eg. severe analmis). The common causes are ischaemic heart disease, hypertension, valve disease and chronic obstructive pulmonary disease. Failure can predominantly affect either the left or right side of the heart, but left-sided heart failure is more common. Failure of one side of the heart usually leads to failure of the other. Right-sided failure often follows left-sided failure, particularly when there is mitral stenosis, and causes congestive cardiac failure.

HEPATOMEGALY

Hepatomegaly is enlargement of the liver beyond its normal size. The lower edge of the liver normally comes just to the lower edge of the ribs (costal margin) on the right side and it cannot be palpated. The diagnosis must be confirmed by imaging.

Table 4.4 Main causes of halitosis

Causes	Examples
Plaque-related gingival and periodontal disease	Gingivitis, periodontitis, acute necrotizing ulcerative gingivitis, pericoronitis, abscesses
Oral ulceration	Systemic disease (inflammatory/infectious disorders, cutaneous, gastrointestinal and haematological disease), malignancy, local causes, aphthae, drugs
Hyposalivation	(e.g. from drugs, Sjögren syndrome, radiotherapy, chemotherapy)
Tongue coating	Poor hygiene
Wearing dental appliances	Poor hygiene
Dental conditions	Food packing
Bone diseases	Jaw dry sockets, osteomyelitis, osteonecrosis, malignancy
Respiratory system	Sinusitis Antral malignancy Cleft palate Foreign bodies in the nose Nasal malignancy Tonsilloliths Tonsillitis Pharyngeal malignancy Lung infections Bronchitis Bronchiectasis Lung malignancy
Gastrointestinal tract	Oesophageal diverticulum Gastro-oesophageal reflux disease Malignancy
Metabolic disorders (blood-borne)	Acetone-like smell in uncontrolled diabetes Uraemic breath in renal failure Foetor hepaticus in liver disease Trimethylaminuria (fish odour syndrome) Hypermethioninaemia Cystinosis
Drugs (blood-borne)	Amphetamines Chloral hydrate Cytotoxic agents Dimethyl sulphoxide (DMSO) Disulfiram Nitrates and nitrites Phenothiazines Solvent abuse
Psychogenic causes	

Causes of hepatomegaly include infection (viral, bacterial or parasitic), e.g. viral hepatitis, infectious mononucleosis; malignancy (leukaemias, tumour metastases, neuroblastoma, hepatocellular carcinoma); anaemias; storage diseases (Niemann–Pick disease, hereditary fructose intolerance, glycogen storage disease; heart failure, congenital heart disease; toxins (e.g. alcohol); primary biliary cirrhosis, sarcoidosis, sclerosing cholangitis, haemolytic–uraemic syndrome or Reye syndrome.

HIRSUTISM (HYPERTRICHOSIS)

Excessive growth of dark, coarse body hair in women (and children) is called hirsutism, and typically appears in a distribution pattern normally seen in adult males. Excessive facial hair is usually the most troublesome aspect. Signs of masculinization, such as deepening of the voice, increased muscle mass, decreased breast size, increased size of genitals, and menstrual irregularities, may be associated with hirsutism.

Common causes of hirsutism include: genetic, endocrine abnormalities (polycystic ovarian syndrome, Cushing syndrome, adrenocortical carcinoma, congenital adrenal hyperplasia, or precocious puberty, pregnancy, menopause, ovarian tumour or cancer, ovarian overproduction of androgens) or drugs (aminoglutethimide, ciclosporin, phenytoin, drugs containing androgens, glucocorticoids, metoclopramide, and minoxidil).

HOARSENESS

Hoarseness is usually due to acute laryngitis, a self-limiting condition secondary to a viral upper respiratory infection such as a cold. Chronic laryngitis is the commonest cause of persistent hoarseness where the predisposing factors are usually smoking and voice abuse. However, any patient with hoarseness persisting for over 1 month should be investigated for trauma to the vocal cords (from persistent shouting or singing – singer's nodules); thyroid cancer; laryngeal cancer; surgical damage to the vagus or recurrent laryngeal nerve during thyroid or cardiovascular surgery; and psychological problems.

HOSTILITY

Hostile (acutely disturbed) patients can totally disrupt their environment and harm those with whom they come into contact. Frequently the cause is drunkenness, drug intoxication or an acute psychosis. Otherwise, the disorder may be due to infections, or withdrawal of drugs such as alcohol or other drugs of abuse. If the patient appears unresponsive to reason, no treatment should be attempted, but the physician or psychiatrist should be contacted.

No attempt should be made to sedate the patient: benzodiazepines usually worsen violently psychotic behaviour and adequate doses of phenothiazines such as chlorpromazine can cause severe hypotension. If the patient becomes violent, the police have to be called to restrain the patient; ambulance personnel cannot usually manage such cases. The usual treatment, once the patient has been forcibly restrained, is to give haloperidol by injection.

HYPERPIGMENTATION

Most pigmentation is racial in origin. Local pigmentations such as a tattoo are common. Systemic causes of pigmentation are rare (Box 4.4).

Box 4.4 Causes of hyperpigmentation

Congenital
- Racial (even in some Caucasians)
- Naevi
- Syndromes
  - Peutz–Jeghers syndrome: oral and perioral hyperpigmentation with small intestine polyps
  - Carney complex: lentiginosis due to adrenal disease, and multiple neoplasia such as myxomas of skin, heart and breast, schwannomas, pituitary adenomas, testicular and thyroid tumours
  - Laugier–Hunziker syndrome: oral and perioral hyperpigmentation with nail pigmentation
  - NAME syndrome (naevi, atrial myxoma, myxoid neurofibromata and ephelides)
  - LAMB syndrome (lentigines, atrial myxoma, mucocutaneous myxoma, blue naevi)
  - LEOPARD syndrome: lentigenes with hypertrophic cardiomyopathy, or arterial dissections

Acquired
Endocrine or metabolic
- Addison disease
- ACTH therapy
- ACTH-producing tumours (lung cancer)
- Haemochromatosis
- Nelson syndrome

Neoplastic
- Melanoma
- Kaposi sarcoma

Foreign bodies
Drugs
- Smoking
- Antimalarials
- Cytotoxics (particularly busulfan)
- Oral contraceptives
- Phenothiazines
- Minocycline
- Zidovudine
- Clofazimine

Others
- HIV infection and AIDS

ACTH, adrenocorticotropic hormone; AIDS, acquired immune deficiency syndrome.

HYPERTHERMIA

Hyperthermia is an unusual rise in body temperature above normal, caused by a disorder in body temperature control mechanisms. A group of inherited muscle problems characterized by muscle breakdown following certain stimuli is termed malignant hyperthermia. Attacks can be precipitated by anaesthesia, extreme exercise, fever or certain drugs.

HYPERVENTILATION (SEE TACHYPNOEA)

HYPODONTIA

Hypodontia is the developmental absence of teeth and affects about 5% of the population. The teeth most commonly missing, apart from third molars, are the mandibular second premolars, maxillary lateral incisors and maxillary second premolars. Severe hypodontia is the absence of six or more teeth and can be a feature of ectodermal dysplasia, Down syndrome, hemifacial microsomia and van der Woude syndrome.

HYPOGLYCAEMIA

Hypoglycaemia (low blood sugar) is when blood glucose levels drop too low to fuel body activity. Hypoglycaemia causes the patient to feel weak, drowsy, confused, hungry, aggressive and dizzy. Pallor, headache, irritability, trembling, sweating, rapid heart beat, and a cold, clammy feeling are other signs and, in severe cases, unconsciousness or coma can result. Hypoglycaemia causes include diabetes (insulin or drug overdose, missing or delaying a meal, eating too little food for the amount of insulin taken); exercising too strenuously, particularly when associated with beta-blocker medication; prolonged fasting; certain foods and drinks (excess alcohol, aspirin (in some children), unripe Jamaican ackee fruit); liver disease; hormonal states (early pregnancy, insulinomas, growth hormone deficiency, breast cancer and adrenal cancer); or hereditary enzyme or hormone deficiencies (hereditary fructose intolerance (attacks of hypoglycaemia, marked by seizures, vomiting, and unconsciousness) or galactosaemia (also causes vomiting, weight loss, and cataracts).

HYPOTHERMIA

Cold exposure is the main cause of low body temperature (hypothermia). Conditions that may predispose include drugs, by blunting the response to cold (alcohol, anxiolytics, antidepressants, antiemetics, and some over-the-counter cold remedies cause vasodilatation and heat loss); illnesses that restrict activity (stroke or other causes of paralysis, severe arthritis, Parkinson disease, Alzheimer disease); or hypothyroidism.

IMPOTENCE

Impotence is the term used particularly for erectile dysfunction (ED), lack of sexual desire and ejaculation or orgasm problems. ED is the repeated inability to achieve or maintain an erection adequate for intercourse. Causes are injuries to the nerves or conditions that impair penile blood flow and include particularly trauma (to penis, spinal cord, prostate, bladder or pelvis), including from surgery (especially radical prostate surgery); psychological factors, including stress, anxiety, guilt, depression, low self-esteem, and fear of sexual failure; smoking; drugs (antihypertensives, antihistamines, antidepressants, tranquillizers, appetite suppressants and cimetidine); and various diseases (diabetes, renal, alcoholism, multiple sclerosis, atherosclerosis, neurological) or hormonal abnormalities, such as inadequate testosterone. Sildenafil citrate (Viagra) is effective treatment.

INSOMNIA (SEE CH. 13)

JAUNDICE

Jaundice (icterus) is the accumulation in the body and colouring of the skin and mucous membranes by bilirubin, if it appears in excessive amounts, or is not conjugated or excreted. Jaundice can be a manifestation of haemolytic anaemias, liver disease, biliary disease or pancreatic disorders (Chs 9).

LOW BLOOD PRESSURE

Orthostatic (postural) hypotension is a sudden fall in blood pressure when a person assumes a standing position. It can cause dizziness, light-headedness, blurred vision and syncope (temporary loss of consciousness). Orthostatic hypotension can follow prolonged bed rest or may be caused by hypovolaemia such as results from excessive use of diuretics, vasodilators or other drugs, or by dehydration, Addison disease or atherosclerosis, or dysautonomias such as in diabetes.

LYMPHADENOPATHY

Many diseases can cause lesions in the neck, but most commonly they are swellings and/or pain in the cervical lymph nodes. About one third of all lymph nodes are in the neck and the dental surgeon can often detect serious disease by examination of the neck.

A limited number of lymph nodes swell, usually because of infection in the area of drainage. The nodes are then often firm, discrete and tender, but mobile (lymphadenitis), and the focus of inflammation can usually be found in the drainage area, which is anywhere on the face, scalp and nasal cavity, sinuses, ears, pharynx and oral cavity.

Lymphadenopathy in the anterior triangle of the neck alone is often due to local disease, especially if the nodes are enlarged on only one side. Infection and malignancy in the drainage area are important causes. Metastatic infiltration causes the node to feel distinctly hard, and it may become bound down to adjacent tissues ('fixed') and, in advanced cases, may ulcerate through the skin.

Lymph nodes may also swell in systemic infections or disorders involving the immune system, and there is then usually involvement of more than one node, and often several in different sites. Most children or young people may have small palpable cervical, axillary and/or inguinal nodes. Most are caused by viral infections.

Lymph node enlargement may be due to several disparate causes including infections – lymphadenitis (inflammation of lymph nodes) is the most common cause of lymphadenopathy. The location of the affected nodes is usually related to the site of the underlying infection (Box 4.5).

Box 4.5   Causes of lymphadenopathy

Bacterial
- Dental, face or scalp infections
- Tuberculosis
- Syphilis
- Cat scratch disease
- Brucellosis

Viral
- Herpetic stomatitis
- Infectious mononucleosis
- Adenovirus infections
- HIV
- Cytomegalovirus

Parasitic
- Toxoplasmosis

Connective tissue disorders
- Rheumatoid arthritis
- Systemic lupus erythematosus

Lymphoid or reticuloendothelial disease
- Leukaemias
- Hodgkin disease
- Non-Hodgkin lymphomas

Neoplasms
- Metastases from any tumour in the drainage area
- Nasopharyngeal carcinoma
- Neuroblastoma
- Thyroid carcinoma, chronic lymphocytic thyroiditis
- Kaposi sarcoma
- Langerhans histiocytosis

Immunodeficiency syndromes and phagocytic dysfunction
- Chronic granulomatous disease
- Hyperimmunoglobulin E (Job) syndrome
- HIV/AIDS

Metabolic and storage diseases
- Gaucher disease
- Niemann–Pick disease
- Cystinosis

Haemopoietic diseases
- Sickle cell anaemia
- Thalassaemia
- Congenital haemolytic anaemia
- Autoimmune haemolytic anaemia

Drug-induced hypersensitivity syndrome
- Phenytoin
- Others (such as cephalosporins, penicillins or sulfonamides)

Immunological disorders
- Serum sickness
- Chronic graft-versus-host disease
- Benign sinus histiocytosis
- Angioimmunoblastic or immunoblastic lymphadenopathy
- Chronic pseudolymphomatous lymphadenopathy (chronic benign lymphadenopathy)
- Sarcoidosis, Crohn disease and orofacial granulomatosis
- Kawasaki disease (mucocutaneous lymph node syndrome)
- Angiolymphoid hyperplasia with eosinophilia, haemangioma, with eosinophilic infiltration and lymphoid hyperplasia
- Castleman disease (angiofollicular lymphoid hyperplasia or benign giant lymph node hyperplasia).
- Kikuchi syndrome (Ch. 37)

Table 4.5 Causes of coloured stools (apart from foods/drinks/drugs)

Black	Maroon	Red
Bleeding gastric ulcer Gastritis Oesophageal varices Mallory–Weiss tear Bleeding disorder	All the causes of black coloured stool Bleeding diverticulae Bleeding vascular malformation Intestinal infection (e.g. bacterial enterocolitis) Inflammatory bowel disease Colonic polyps Colonic cancer	All the causes of black or maroon coloured stool Haemorrhoids Anal fissures

MALABSORPTION

Malabsorption is difficulty in the digestion or absorption of nutrients from food, such as failure to absorb specific sugars, fats, proteins or other nutrients (such as vitamins). Diarrhoea, bloating or cramping, weakness, failure to thrive, frequent bulky stools, muscle wasting and a distended abdomen may result and, in children, malabsorption can affect growth and development. Causes of malabsorption include: intestinal, biliary or pancreatic disease (cystic fibrosis, biliary atresia, Whipple disease, Shwachman–Diamond syndrome); food allergies or intolerances (coeliac disease, lactose intolerance, bovine lactalbumin intolerance (cow's milk protein), soy milk protein intolerance); vitamin B_{12} malabsorption (pernicious anaemia, ileal disease, *Diphyllobothrium latum* (fish tapeworm) infestation); other parasites (*Giardia lamblia*, *Strongyloides stercoralis* (threadworm), *Necator americanus* (hookworm)); or rarely acrodermatitis enteropathica or abetalipoproteinaemia.

MALAISE

Malaise is a generalized feeling of discomfort, illness, uneasiness, fatigue or lack of well-being, often associated with a disease state. However, it is a non-specific symptom and can be due to almost any significant infection, cancer, or can occur with metabolic, endocrine or neurological disorders, and may develop slowly or rapidly depending on the nature of the disease.

MELAENA

Melaena is the passage of black, tarry and foul-smelling stools and usually indicates bleeding from the upper GI tract. Other substances such as black berries, iron or liquorice can cause black stools (false melaena), so that black stools should be tested for blood. Table 4.5 shows the causes of stools of various colour.

MENORRHAGIA

Menorrhagia is heavy regular bleeding over consecutive menstrual cycles ('periods'). The definition of heavy periods is the loss of 80 ml or more of blood, but passage of clots and overuse of sanitary towels or tampons may be suggestive.

Common causes of menorrhagia are dysfunctional uterine bleeding (DUB) and uterine fibroids. Other causes are endometriosis, clotting disorders and anticoagulants.

MOUTH ULCERS

Oral ulcers are common; most are traumatic or recurrent aphthae, but more serious causes must always be excluded. Particular care must be taken to exclude cancer, blood dyscrasias, infections, gastrointestinal or mucocutaneous disease (see Box 4.6 and Ch. 11).

MURMURS

Heart murmurs are caused by turbulence of blood flow through valves or ventricular outflow tracts. The prevalence of cardiac murmurs in the general population is very high, and some indicate cardiac disease. Functional (high-flow – also called physiological) murmurs are innocent murmurs that are heard in the absence of cardiac valvular disease. An example is an aortic systolic ejection murmur caused by a high cardiac output state as in athletes and anaemia. Another example is pregnancy, where the rise in cardiac output, especially when coupled with anaemia, can result in physiological ejection murmurs.

NAUSEA AND VOMITING

Nausea is the sensation leading to the urge to vomit; vomiting is the forced ejection of stomach contents through the oesophagus and out of the mouth. Causes of nausea and vomiting are varied, but may include unusual motion (e.g., sea-sickness), gastroenterological causes (infections, food poisoning, food allergies, gastroenteritis, pyloric stenosis); neuropsychiatric (emotional stress, labyrinthitis, motion sickness, migraine, bulimia, cyclic vomiting syndrome); morning sickness during pregnancy; drugs (alcohol, general anaesthesia, chemotherapy – most drugs can, in some people, cause nausea or vomiting). Complications of vomiting include dehydration, loss of electrolytes, peptic oesophagitis, haematemesis, Mallory–Weiss tear, and tooth erosion if vomiting is chronic. Apart from treating the underlying cause, antiemetic drugs may help.

NECK LUMPS

The lumps in the neck of most significance are enlarged cervical lymph nodes, but lumps may also be due to other pathology (Box 4.7).

NECK STIFFNESS

Neck pain and stiffness may originate from any neck structure or the shoulders and arms ranging from the cervical vertebrae to blood vessels, muscles and lymphatic tissue, but can have

Box 4.6 Causes of oral ulceration

Systemic causes
Blood diseases (Ch. 8)
- Leukopenias including HIV disease
- Leukaemias and myelodysplastic syndrome
- Deficiency states or anaemia
- Hypereosinophilic syndrome

Infections
VIRAL, MAINLY **(Ch. 21)**
- Herpes viruses
- Coxsackie viruses
- ECHO viruses

BACTERIAL
- Acute necrotizing gingivitis
- Syphilis
- Tuberculosis

FUNGAL
- Cryptococcosis
- Histoplasmosis
- Paracoccidioidomycosis
- Blastomycosis
- Zygomycosis
- Aspergillosis

PROTOZOAL
- Leishmaniasis

Gastrointestinal disease (Ch. 7)
- Coeliac disease
- Crohn disease
- Ulcerative colitis

Mucocutaneous diseases (Ch. 11)
- Lichen planus
- Chronic ulcerative stomatitis
- Pemphigus
- Pemphigoid
- Localized oral purpura
- Erythema multiforme
- Epidermolysis bullosa
- Dermatitis herpetiformis
- Linear IgA disease
- Behçet and Sweet syndromes

Connective tissue and other diseases (Ch. 16)
- Lupus erythematosus
- Reiter syndrome
- Vasculitides
- Giant cell arteritis
- Wegener granulomatosis
- Periarteritis nodosa

Malignant neoplasms
- Squamous cell carcinoma
- Others **(Ch. 22)**

Local causes
- Trauma
- Chemical irritation
- Burns
- Irradiation

Aphthae and aphthous-like ulcers
Drugs (see Ch. 29)

IgA, immunoglobulin A.

Box 4.7 Causes of neck lumps other than lymphadenopathy

Infections
- Abscess
- Actinomycosis

Cysts
- Thyroglossal
- Branchial
- Cystic hygroma
- Sebaceous cyst
- Dermoid cyst

Hamartomas
- Haemangioma/lymphangioma

Thyroid
- Goitre
- Nodules (and carcinoma)

Carotid
- Aneurysm
- Body tumour

Skin
- Lipoma
- Seroma
- Carcinoma
- Pharyngeal pouch

serious significance since they can also originate from meningeal irritation.

Causes include strain and spasm of the neck muscles; trauma (road traffic accidents); arthritis; meningitis, a potentially life-threatening condition, causing fever, neck stiffness, an aversion to light, and severe headache; and meningism – a non-infective syndrome, caused by meningeal irritation by, for example, an intracranial haemorrhage or tumour.

NOCTURIA

Nocturia is the passing of too much urine at night. Young people tend to excrete their daily urine output mostly in the day; older people commonly also pass urine once or twice at night. Causes of nocturia include in particular drinks too close to bedtime; insomnia or other sleep-related difficulties; urinary or prostatic disorders (e.g. benign prostate disease or cystitis); chronic kidney disease; diabetes; or cardiac failure.

NYSTAGMUS

A few irregular eye jerks are normal in some individuals when the eyes are deviated far to one side. Nystagmus is involuntary rapid back and forth repetitive eye movements, caused by abnormalities of function in the areas of the brain that control eye movements. Some cases are drug induced (see later).

Nystagmus may be congenital (the most common) when it is usually mild, does not change in severity, and is not associated with any other disorder. It may be caused by disease or injury later in life, most commonly by head injury or, in older people stroke, but any brain diseases such as multiple sclerosis or brain tumours, inner ear problems, or drugs can be responsible.

The most common form of nystagmus is rhythmic (jerk), which is usually horizontal, but can be vertical or rotary, and results from drug intoxication (barbiturates, phenytoin toxicity and alcohol intoxication); inner ear disease (Ménière disease); cerebellar disease; or brainstem disease.

OBESITY (SEE CH. 27)

OEDEMA

Oedema is the accumulation of fluid in the tissues. Injury or trauma, insect bite or sting, burns, allergic reactions or angioedema can cause oedema. Slight oedema of the legs is common in healthy persons especially in warm summer months, after prolonged standing and/or on long flights or car journeys.

Oedema may also be caused by more serious conditions. When venous pressure rises in cardiac failure, subcutaneous oedema gravitates to dependent parts; ankle oedema is seen in ambulant patients and sacral oedema in patients in bed. Oedema may be pitting (when pressing a finger against a swollen area for 10 s and then quickly removing it, an indentation is left that fills slowly) or non-pitting (no indentation is left). In pregnancy (pre-eclampsia – hypertension with albuminuria), oedema can appear between the 20th week of pregnancy and the end of the first week post-partum. Loss of plasma proteins from renal loss or malnutrition (causing the nephrotic syndrome) and medical treatments (body fluid overload, infiltration of an intravenous site, diagnostic tests, e.g. venogram) including drugs (corticosteroids, androgenic and anabolic steroids, oestrogens, antihypertensives, NSAIDs) are other causes.

PALMAR ERYTHEMA

Redness of the palms of the hands may be seen in cirrhosis, pregnancy, rheumatoid arthritis, systemic lupus erythematosus and hyperthyroidism.

PALPITATIONS

Palpitations are the consciousness of rapid heart action. Cardiac activity is controlled by the autonomic nervous system and is commonly sensed only by persons with abnormally heightened awareness of their body functions, as in anxiety states, or following exercise – when heart stroke volume or rate rise. Palpitations are most commonly caused by arrhythmias but also by disorders such as anaemia, aortic regurgitation or thyrotoxicosis. Palpitations accompanied by myocardial ischaemia-type chest pain probably indicate coronary artery disease. Inquiry into the rate and the rhythm of palpitations helps differentiate pathological from physiological, since palpitations due to an arrhythmia may be accompanied by weakness, dyspnoea or light-headedness.

Atrial or ventricular extrasystoles are often described as skipped beats, atrial fibrillation as total irregularity, while supraventricular or ventricular tachycardia is most often perceived as being rapid and regular and of sudden onset and termination.

PAPILLOEDEMA

Papilloedema is the swelling of the optic nerve as it enters the eye. The optic nerve anatomy makes it sensitive to even slight rises in cerebrospinal fluid (CSF) pressure; when the optic nerve is exposed to such pressure, or when it becomes inflamed, it can bulge (papilloedema). Papilloedema can also arise from local inflammation (optic neuritis); multiple sclerosis is the most common cause. Causes of raised CSF pressure and papilloedema are brain disease and raised intracranial pressure (e.g. haemorrhage, tumours, infections – brain abscess, meningitis or encephalitis); pseudotumour cerebri or benign intracranial hypertension (results from CSF overproduction). This is more common in women who are obese and of childbearing age, and seems to be triggered at times of hormone change, such as pregnancy, the start of contraceptive pill use, tetracycline use, the first menstrual period or menopause.

Symptoms related to papilloedema are caused by the raised pressure and include headache and nausea with vomiting. About 25% with advanced papilloedema also develop some visual symptoms such as recurring brief episodes in which the vision turns grey or 'blacks out', as if a veil has fallen over the eyes.

Ophthalmoscopy shows an elevated optic disc with a blurred margin, and there is a wider blind spot and narrowing of peripheral vision.

POLYDIPSIA

Polydipsia is an abnormal feeling of constant thirst. The most common cause of excessive thirst is the excessive intake of salty foods but the desire to drink excessively beyond a certain limit may reflect an underlying disease, either physical or emotional. Excessive loss of water and salt (as with water deprivation, profuse sweating, diarrhoea or vomiting, severe infections or widespread burns); fluid loss during exercise; bleeding sufficient to cause a significant fall in blood volume; drugs (including anticholinergics, demeclocycline, diuretics, lithium, phenothiazines); endocrine disorders (diabetes mellitus, Conn disease, Cushing disease, hyperthyroidism, diabetes insipidus); or cardiac, hepatic or renal failure are causes. Psychogenic causes are most commonly seen in women over age 30.

POLYURIA

Polyuria – the passing of abnormally large amounts (for an adult, at least 2.5 L per day) of urine – is fairly common and often first noticed at night.

Polyuria is to be expected if there is excessive fluid intake, particularly fluids containing caffeine or alcohol, too much salt or glucose (especially if diabetic), or with the use of diuretics. Other causes include diabetes mellitus or insipidus; psychogenic polydipsia; renal failure; sickle cell anaemia; and radiography using contrast media.

PROPTOSIS

Proptosis is the anterior displacement of one or both eye globes within the bony orbit. The term exophthalmos is sometimes used, particularly when the proptosis is related to thyroid dysfunction. The normal amount of ocular protrusion as measured (with an exophthalmometer) from the lateral orbital rim to the corneal apex is 14–21 mm in adults: protrusion greater than 21 mm or a 2-mm difference is abnormal. On scans, proptosis is defined as globe protrusion > 21 mm anterior to the interzygomatic line on axial scans at the level of the lens.

Proptosis without displacement (axial) is due to intraconal, most commonly dysthyroid, eye disease. In this case, the protrusion is caused by inflammatory swelling of the small eye-moving muscles behind the globe. Thyroid exophthalmos may appear months or years after the onset of a thyroid disorder but may occasionally precede it. Tumours (such as glioma and meningioma of the optic nerve and cavernous haemangioma) may also be responsible.

Proptosis with displacement (non-axial) is due to extraconal disease, most commonly lacrimal tumours or a mucocoele.

Pseudoproptosis is either the simulation of abnormal eye prominence, or a true asymmetry that is not the result of increased orbital contents. Causes include enlarged eye globe (high myopia, buphthalmos); extraocular muscle weakness or paralysis; contralateral enophthalmos; asymmetrical orbital size (congenital, post-irradiation, post-surgical); asymmetrical palpebral fissures (e.g. caused by ipsilateral eyelid retraction, scarring or facial nerve paralysis or contralateral ptosis).

PRURITUS (ITCHING)

Pruritus is a peculiar tingling or uneasy irritation of the skin which causes a desire to scratch the affected part. There are many causes such as localized skin irritation from insect bites and stings. Localized or generalized causes include chemical irritation such as from stinging nettle or poison ivy; environmental causes (drying, sunburn); or urticaria.

Parasites (e.g. lice) or skin conditions (e.g. lichen planus, dermatitis herpetiformis) are causes. Less commonly, pruritus is caused by infectious diseases (chickenpox), pregnancy, allergic reactions, kidney disease, jaundice, drug or medications (penicillin, sulfonamides, gold, griseofulvin, isoniazid, opiates, phenothiazines or vitamin A) or contact irritants (such as soaps, chemicals or wool).

Pruritus (itching) ani is a common and troublesome complaint which can result from such causes as haemorrhoids or irritable bowel syndrome; fistulas or fissures; mucocutaneous diseases such as lichen planus; or infections such as candidosis or worms.

PTOSIS

Ptosis is drooping eyelids, caused by weakness of the muscle responsible for raising the eyelid (levator palpebrae superioris), damage to the nerves which control those muscles, or laxity of the skin of the upper eyelids. Congenital ptosis is most commonly due to a defect in the levator palpebrae superioris or rare myopathies (e.g. myotonica congenita). Marcus Gunn 'jaw-winking' syndrome is ptosis usually in one eye only and due to the lid partially opening as the jaw opens because of an abnormal nerve connection.

Ptosis can be acquired through age-related defects of the eyelid muscles and nerves, damage to the sympathetic nerve supply or the oculomotor nerve. A mechanical defect caused by anything that increases the weight of the eyelid, such as a cyst, may also cause ptosis.

PUPIL ANOMALIES

The pupils normally are equal in size, and they constrict on exposure to bright light and on accommodation for near objects. Light shone in one eye causes pupillary constriction in that eye (direct light reflex) and also in the unexposed eye (indirect or consensual reflex).

Pupil size is determined by dilator fibres (the sympathetic nerve supply from the superior cervical ganglion runs along the internal carotid artery and joins the ophthalmic division of the trigeminal nerve and the long ciliary nerves) and the sympathetic nerve supply is also partially responsible for contraction of the levator palpebrae superioris muscle (raising the upper eyelid). Pupil size is also determined by constrictor fibres (the parasympathetic supply runs with the oculomotor nerve). Pupil constriction (miosis) can be caused by a lesion of the sympathetic supply, and dilatation (mydriasis) by a IIIrd nerve lesion (Fig. 4.2). The most important cause of an abnormally dilated pupil is a rise in intracranial pressure where the pupil also becomes non-reactive owing to pressure on the oculomotor nerve (Table 4.6).

PURPURA

Purpura is abnormal bruising with small bleeds into the skin (petechiae) or larger bleeds (ecchymoses), and bleeding from mucosae (epistaxes – nosebleeds – and gingival bleeding).

Causes of purpura include *purpura simplex* (easy bruising), the most common vascular bleeding disorder, due to excessive vascular fragility and usually seen in women in whom the platelet count and tests of platelet function, blood coagulation and fibrinolysis are normal. Bruises develop without known trauma on the thighs, buttocks, and upper arms, and are typically small.

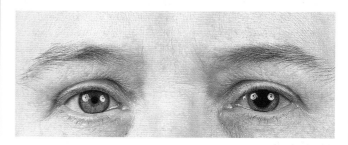

Fig. 4.2 Mydriasis

Table 4.6 Causes of pupillary abnormalities

Pupils	Other signs	Significance
Constricted bilaterally	+/- signs of drug abuse	Opiate use
Constricted bilaterally, unequal, react to accommodation but not light	–	Argyll Robertson pupils – neurosyphilis, multiple sclerosis, diabetes mellitus, sarcoid, brain tumour, amyloid, trauma, Lyme disease
Constricted unilaterally	Ptosis, absence of facial sweating, enophthalmos sometimes	Horner syndrome – damage to sympathetic fibres, usually in neck (e.g. by trauma, or bronchial carcinoma)
Dilated unilaterally	Ptosis	IIIrd nerve lesion
Dilated unilaterally and react slowly to light or convergence	Ankle or knee jerks may be absent	Usually benign Adie (Holmes–Adie) pupil
Dilated bilaterally and reactive	+/- signs of drug abuse	Cocaine or other drug use
Dilated bilaterally and unreactive	+/- Headaches	Raised intracranial pressure

Senile purpura is a common disorder affecting older patients mainly on the extensor surfaces of the hands and forearms, particularly in those who have had excessive sun exposure. Lesions appear without known trauma as dark purple ecchymoses and slowly resolve over several days, leaving a brownish discoloration caused by deposits of haemosiderin. The condition has no serious consequences. Angina bullosa haemorrhagica may be a localized form of purpura seen in the mouth or throat (see page 11).

Thrombocytopenia is the most important systemic cause of purpura (Ch. 8).

RAISED INTRACRANIAL PRESSURE

Normal intracranial pressure (ICP) for an adult at rest is 7–15 mmHg supine, becoming negative (-10 mmHg) in the vertical position. Changes in ICP are attributed to volume changes in one or more of the constituents contained in the cranium. Any expansion of cranial contents causes a rise of ICP which tends to impede the venous return from the brain and further to increase the pressure. Cerebral blood flow is thus diminished even though the raised CSF pressure causes a reflex rise in systemic blood pressure in an attempt to improve cerebral blood flow.

Raised ICP can be fatal as the pressure can cause herniation of the brain (displacement of part of the brain from one dural compartment to another) and pressure is exerted on the brainstem and medullary respiratory and cardiac control centres (called 'coning').

Causes of raised ICP include hydrocephalus, intracranial haemorrhage (after head injury), space-occupying lesions (abscess, tumour or haematoma), oedema (trauma, malignant hypertension, vascular lesions or tumours of the brain), or obstruction to the flow of CSF (blockage of the aqueduct of Sylvius, or subarachnoid adhesions due to meningitis).

Idiopathic intracranial hypertension, sometimes called benign intracranial hypertension or pseudotumour cerebri, occurs in the absence of a tumour or other disease affecting the brain or meninges.

Characteristic symptoms of raised ICP are headache, transient visual changes or loss in one or both eyes usually lasting seconds, pulse synchronous tinnitus (a 'whooshing noise'), diplopia and visual loss. Signs include papilloedema (bulging of the optic disc with engorgement of its vessels seen by ophthalmoscopy); restlessness (in the unconscious patient); vomiting; decreasing consciousness; rising blood pressure and slowing of the pulse; dilatation of the pupil on the side of the lesion with diminished reaction to light, and loss of visual acuity and fields. Diplopia (double vision), if present, may be due to abducens palsy.

Lumbar puncture is contraindicated if intracranial pressure is raised as it can precipitate brain herniation and death by coning. The possibility of herniation is suggested by signs of raised ICP, particularly pupil dilatation and reduced reactivity to light caused by stretching of the oculomotor nerves.

RAISED INTRAOCULAR PRESSURE

Normal intraocular pressure is between 12 and 21 mmHg. Glaucoma is a group of diseases of raised intraocular pressure that can lead to damage to the eye's optic nerve and result in blindness (Table 4.7). Atropine, scopolamine and glycopyrrolate are contraindicated, especially in open-angle glaucoma.

RED EYE

There are many causes of red eye (Fig. 4.3) ranging from simple superficial inflammation (conjunctivitis) to more serious corneal ulceration, uveitis (inflammation of iris, ciliary body and choroids) to acute glaucoma – a medical emergency.

RED LESIONS IN THE MOUTH

Many oral mucosal red lesions are due to: infections or are inflammatory with no identified infectious agent (sarcoid, Crohn disease); vascular anomalies (e.g. telangiectasias); or mucosal atrophy (desquamative gingivitis, erythroplasia or due to a deficiency state). Lichen planus, lupus erythematosus and candidosis may cause red or white lesions (Ch. 11). Red lesions are sometimes due to Kaposi sarcoma or Wegener granulomatosis.

Table 4.7 Types of glaucoma

Type	Features	Treatment
Open-angle	Most common. The angle that allows fluid to drain out of the anterior chamber is *open*. However, the fluid passes too slowly through the mesh-work drain. Optic nerve damage and narrowed side vision develop. Risk groups include people of African heritage over age 40, anyone over age 60 and family history of glaucoma	Drugs or laser trabeculo-plasty
Low-tension or normal-tension	Optic nerve damage and narrowed side vision develop unexpectedly in people with normal eye pressure	Drugs or laser trabeculo-plasty
Closed-angle	The fluid at the front of the eye cannot reach the angle and leave, because the angle gets blocked by part of the iris. Without treatment, the eye can become blind within 48 h	A medical emergency. Immediate laser treatment
Congenital	Defects in the angle of the eye that slow the normal drainage of fluid	Surgery
Secondary glaucomas	Develops as a complication of other medical conditions, cataracts, uveitis, eye surgery, injuries, or tumours	Various

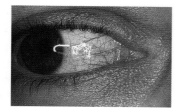

Fig. 4.3 Red eye

SALIVARY SWELLING

The most common cause of salivary swelling is mumps (Ch. 21), which usually affects children and typically causes bilateral painful swellings, but there are many other causes (Box 4.8). Salivary obstruction as by a calculus (stone) is the common cause of a unilateral swelling. Neoplasms (usually pleomorphic adenoma) must be considered, particularly when there is a persistent unilateral swelling in older patients. Painless bilateral salivary swelling is usually due to sialadenosis (sialosis) and to autonomic dysfunction; it is thus a rare feature of alcoholic cirrhosis, diabetes mellitus, acromegaly, starvation or bulimia, or may be idiopathic. Sjögren syndrome may also cause salivary gland swelling (Box 4.8).

SCIATICA

Sciatica is pain down the leg, caused by irritation of the sciatic nerve, the main nerve to the leg. The pain travels below the knee and may involve the foot, and there may be numbness and weakness of the lower leg muscles.

Box 4.8 Causes of salivary gland swelling

Inflammatory
- Mumps
- Bacterial ascending sialadenitis
- Obstructive sialadenitis
- Allergic sialadenitis (e.g. to iodides or chlorhexidine)
- Sjögren syndrome
- Sarcoidosis
- HIV infection
- Tuberculosis and non-tuberculous mycobacteriosis
- Actinomycosis
- Toxoplasmosis

Neoplastic
- Pleomorphic adenoma and many others

Endocrine and metabolic
- Alcoholic and other types of cirrhosis
- Diabetes mellitus
- Acromegaly
- Malnutrition or bulimia
- Cystic fibrosis
- Chronic renal failure
- Amyloidosis
- Haemochromatosis

Drugs (rarely)
- Isoprenaline
- Phenylbutazone
- Iodides
- Chlorhexidine

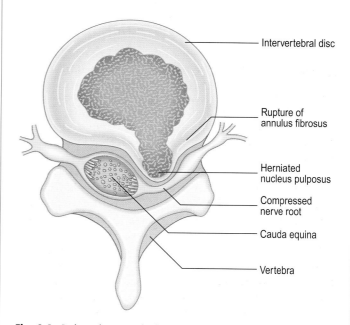

Fig. 4.4 Prolapsed intervertebral disc ('slipped disc')

The most common cause is a 'slipped disc' (a prolapsed intervertebral disc or herniated nucleus pulposus). Pressures within intervertebral discs can be high on bending or twisting, even without carrying a load. If part of the fibrous outer ring of the disc is weak, the softer nucleus pulposus centre may push its way through, and if it presses against a nerve it causes symptoms. Sciatica occurs when the herniated disc presses against the sciatic nerve (Fig. 4.4).

Computed tomography or MRI scans determine whether an operation will help cure the sciatica. Simple analgesics, such as pasacetamol or ibuprofen, help. Activities likely to put unnecessary strain on the back should be avoided. In the minority of cases in which sciatica does not settle, or complications arise, surgery is needed.

SIALORRHOEA (HYPERSALIVATION)

Normally, any excess of saliva is swallowed and causes no symptoms. In infants, and in patients who have learning impairment, poor neuromuscular coordination, or who have pharyngeal or oesophageal obstruction, drooling is common without any true overproduction of saliva.

Hypersalivation is rare, although it may be induced by lesions or foreign bodies in the mouth, by drugs such as anticholinesterases or clozapine, or rarely by rabies. However, there is often no objective evidence for the complaint and it has a psychogenic basis.

Hypersalivation or drooling may be controllable with antimuscarinic agents such as propantheline bromide. If very severe, surgical relocation of the parotid duct such that it discharges into the pharynx may be effective, and the submandibular duct can also be moved.

SNEEZING (STERNUTATION)

Sneezing is a sudden, forceful, involuntary burst of air through the nose and mouth, almost invariably caused by irritation to the mucous membranes of the nose or throat. Rarely a sign of serious disease, sneezing typically is caused by allergy or hay fever, upper respiratory tract infections, opioid withdrawal or corticosteroid inhalation.

SNORING

Snoring is caused by obstructed breathing; the sound is usually made by the palate vibrating when the muscles relax, narrowing the airway. Snoring is usually normal, of unknown cause and not an indication of any underlying disorder. Excess alcohol or sedation can contribute. However, snoring can also be a sign of the *sleep apnoea syndrome*, with chronic nasal congestion or obstruction by enlarged tonsils and adenoids – or more serious pathology. Snoring may often be reduced by avoiding too much alcohol or sedation at bedtime, avoiding sleeping flat on the back, and by weight loss.

SORE THROAT

A sore throat is discomfort, pain or scratchiness in the throat, often associated with pain on swallowing. Sore throats are common, especially in children between the ages of 5 and 10, most often caused by upper respiratory viruses (Ch. 14). Streptococcal throat is the most common bacterial cause and can occasionally lead to rheumatic fever, so antibiotics are indicated. Other causes of sore throat include trauma (fish, chicken bone

---

Box 4.9 Causes of splenomegaly

Infections
- Malaria (worldwide the most common cause)
- Infectious mononucleosis
- Cytomegalovirus infection
- Other viral infections
- Parasitic infections
- Cat scratch disease
- Bacterial infections

Liver diseases
- Cirrhosis (portal vein obstruction, portal hypertension)
- Sclerosing cholangitis
- Wilson disease
- Biliary atresia
- Cystic fibrosis

Haemolytic anaemias
- Thalassaemia
- Haemoglobinopathies
- G6PD deficiency
- Idiopathic autoimmune haemolytic anaemia
- Immune haemolytic anaemia

Malignant disease
- Leukaemia
- Lymphoma
- Hodgkin disease

Other causes
- Sarcoidosis
- Sickle cell splenic crisis
- Banti syndrome
- Felty syndrome

G6PD, glucose-6-phosphate dehydrogenase.

or other foreign substance stuck in the throat, endotracheal intubation, or local surgery, such as tonsillectomy and adenoidectomy). Occasionally more serious pathology underlies the complaint.

SPLENOMEGALY

Splenomegaly is enlargement of the spleen beyond its normal size. The spleen is involved in the production and maintenance of erythrocytes and the production of certain immunocytes, and may be affected and enlarged by many conditions involving the blood or lymph system, and by infection, liver disease, haemolytic anaemias, malignancies and parasites. Causes of splenomegaly can include those listed in Box 4.9.

Rupture of the enlarged spleen is possible and usually due to trauma.

STROKE (CEREBROVASCULAR ACCIDENT; CVA) (SEE CH. 12)

STUTTERING

Stuttering (stammering) is a speech disorder in which the normal flow of speech is disrupted by frequent repetitions or prolongations of speech sounds, syllables or words, or by an

---

Box 4.10 Causes of sweating

- Exercise
- Fevers
- Menopause
- Malignant disease
  - Breast cancer
  - Prostate cancer
  - Hodgkin disease
  - Phaeochromocytoma
  - CNS tumours
  - Endocrine tumours
- Drugs
  - Tamoxifen
  - Opioids
  - Antidepressants
  - Steroids
  - Recreational drugs
- Hypothalamic disease
- Sweating disorders (hyperhidrosis)

CNS, central nervous system.

Box 4.11 Causes of tachypnoea

Psychological states
- Anxiety
- Stress
- Where there is a psychological advantage in having a sudden dramatic illness

Drug use
- Stimulant use
- Drugs (e.g. aspirin overdose)

Respiratory disorders
- Asthma
- Chronic obstructive pulmonary disease
- Pneumonia
- Pulmonary fibrosis
- Pleurisy
- Pulmonary embolism

Cardiac disease
- Congestive heart failure
- Coronary artery disease
- Valvular disease

Severe pain

Ketoacidosis and similar medical conditions

---

individual's inability to start a word. Stuttering usually has a genetic basis but other causes can be neurogenic – following a stroke or other brain injury, or psychogenic, particularly anxiety. Stuttering may be accompanied by rapid eye blinks, lip and/or jaw tremors or other movements. Certain situations, such as lecturing, talking on the telephone or being interviewed, tend to aggravate the stuttering, whereas other situations, such as singing or speaking alone, often improve it.

SWEATING

Sweating is a heat-regulatory mechanism, mediated by the hypothalamus, when in a warm environment or exercising. The evaporation of sweat, produced by sweat glands in the skin, leads to heat loss. Other causes of sweating are shown in Box 4.10.

SYNCOPE

Syncope is a feeling of faintness, dizziness or light-headedness (pre-syncope), or loss of consciousness (syncope), due to a sudden decline in blood flow to the brain. Syncope can affect otherwise healthy people but may also be caused by an irregular cardiac rate or rhythm, or by changes of blood volume or distribution. The main causes include: vasovagal attack (fainting, see Ch. 1); respiratory (severe coughing causing vagal stimulation); cardiac (arrhythmias, heart block, aortic stenosis); paralytic – in the elderly, especially those taking drugs such as phenothiazines, levodopa, hypotensive agents, tricyclics or benzodiazepines; brainstem – owing to migraine or vertebrobasilar disease, usually in the elderly; and carotid sinus syndrome – an exaggerated baroreceptor response resulting in periods of inappropriately high vagal tone and sympathetic suppression. The diagnosis is frequently made in men over 50, and patients with atherosclerosis and hypertension. Syncope may also be caused by turning or pressing on the neck.

TACHYCARDIA (SEE CH. 5)

TACHYPNOEA

Tachypnoea or hyperventilation is excessive, rapid and deep breathing, resulting in a fall in the carbon dioxide level in the blood. Hyperventilation is not uncommon in young adults, especially in women, usually when nervous and tense. It can also be a symptom of other disorders. Causes of tachypnoea include those shown in Box 4.11.

TASTE DISORDERS (SEE CH. 12)

TEETHING

Restlessness, irritability, finger-sucking, gum-rubbing and drooling may be associated with the eruption of deciduous teeth.

Teething is traditionally blamed for a variety of other signs and symptoms in infancy, but is not responsible for diarrhoea, fever, convulsions or other systemic disorders. These have systemic causes, usually infections – often herpetic stomatitis.

TOOTH DISCOLORATION

Most causes of discoloration of several teeth are extrinsic stains. Discoloration of isolated teeth is commonly related to caries or trauma. Fluorosis, tetracyclines or congenital defects of enamel or dentine may cause brown or white intrinsic discoloration of most or all teeth; biliary atresia may cause green teeth, and erythropoietic porphyria may cause red teeth (Table 4.8).

Table 4.8	Causes of discoloration of teeth
Extrinsic	**Intrinsic**
Most teeth affected	
Smoking, beverages, e.g. tea Drugs, e.g. iron, chlorhexidine, minocycline Poor oral hygiene, betel chewing	Tetracycline, fluorosis, amelogenesis imperfecta, dentinogenesis imperfecta, kernicterus, biliary atresia, porphyria
One or a few teeth affected	
As above	Trauma, caries, resorption

TINNITUS

Tinnitus is a ringing, roaring or other sound inside the ears. Tinnitus may be caused by ear problems (wax, infection, Ménière disease); neurological causes; or aspirin or certain antibiotics (aminoglycosides mainly). However, the reason for the tinnitus often cannot be found. Tinnitus can fluctuate or can resolve spontaneously, but is frequently untreatable.

TIREDNESS

Tiredness is a feeling of lack of energy, fatigue or weariness. Fatigue represents a normal response to physical exertion, emotional stress or lack of sleep, but can also be a non-specific symptom of a psychological or physiological disorder. In many cases, fatigue is related to boredom, unhappiness, disappointment, lack of sleep or hard work. Because fatigue is such a common complaint and is often caused by psychological problems, its potential seriousness is often overlooked.

Pathological (illness-related) fatigue is not relieved by rest, adequate sleep or removal of stressful factors. An example is the so-called *chronic fatigue syndrome*.

The pattern of fatigue may help delineate its underlying cause: individuals who arise in the morning rested but, with activity, rapidly fatigue may have a disease, while individuals who awaken fatigued and the level of fatigue remains constant throughout the day may be suffering from depression. Other causes are shown in Box 4.12.

TREMOR

Tremor is an unintentional, somewhat rhythmic, involuntary muscle movement involving to-and-fro movements (oscillations) of one or more parts of the body, most commonly affecting the hands. Tremor may also affect the arms, head, face, vocal cords, trunk and legs (see Table 4.9). Caffeine (in substances such as coffee and carbonated beverages) and other stimulants should be avoided because they commonly worsen a tremor, as may emotion, stress, fever or physical exhaustion.

The most common form of tremor occurs in otherwise healthy people; this is essential tremor (no known cause). Tremor may also be caused by drugs (e.g. alcohol, amphetamines, caffeine, corticosteroids, ciclosporin, lithium, major tranquillizers and

Box 4.12	Causes of tiredness

- Excessive physical exertion
- Poor nutrition
- Infections (e.g. tuberculosis, bacterial endocarditis, HIV, hepatitis, influenza and mononucleosis) Chronic fatigue syndrome
- Psychological disorders
  - Anxiety and depression
  - Chronic boredom
  - Grief
  - Sleep disorders, such as insomnia
  - Stress
- Anaemia
- Endocrinopathies (e.g. diabetes, hypothyroidism, Addison disease, acromegaly)
- Drugs such as antihistamines, antihypertensives, sedatives, or diuretics
- Chronic disease (e.g. cancer, rheumatoid arthritis, systemic lupus erythematosus)
- Most types of surgery
- Cardiac failure

Table 4.9	Different types of tremor
Type	**Causes**
Contraction tremors (e.g. making a tight fist while the arm is resting and supported)	Essential tremor, cerebellar disease, hyperthyroidism, drugs such as caffeine and anticholinergic agents
Intention (action or kinetic) tremors (e.g. finger to nose test)	Cerebellar disorders and alcohol
Posture tremors (e.g. with the arms raised against gravity)	Essential tremor, physiological tremor, tremor with basal ganglia disease (as in Parkinsonism), cerebellar disease, peripheral neuropathy, post-traumatic, and alcoholic
Resting tremors (e.g. when the hands are lying on the lap)	Parkinsonism, antipsychotic drugs, essential tremor

valproic acid); poisoning (e.g. mercury); neurological disorders (e.g. Parkinson disease, multiple sclerosis, cerebellar disease); psychogenic reactions; or metabolic disorders (hypoglycaemia, hyperthyroidism, liver failure).

URINARY INCONTINENCE

Urinary incontinence is an inability to hold urine until a lavatory is reached. It results from an underlying medical condition and is often only temporary. Women, particularly older women, experience incontinence twice as often as men, because of problems associated with pregnancy and childbirth, and the menopause. Both women and men can become incontinent from neurological injury, birth defects, strokes, multiple sclerosis and physical problems associated with ageing.

Stress incontinence results from physical changes from pregnancy, childbirth and the menopause, and causes incontinence when coughing, laughing, sneezing or other movements put pressure on the bladder.

Urge incontinence is caused by inappropriate bladder contractions, which result from overactive nervous control of the bladder. Urine is lost for no apparent reason while suddenly feeling the need or urge to urinate. Urge incontinence can mean that the bladder empties during sleep, after drinking a small amount of water, or when touching water or hearing it running (as when washing dishes or hearing someone else taking a shower). Involuntary actions of bladder muscles can occur due to damage to the nerves of the bladder, to the nervous system (spinal cord and brain), or to the muscles themselves as in multiple sclerosis, Parkinson disease, Alzheimer disease, stroke and injury.

Functional incontinence appears in people who have problems thinking, moving or communicating that prevent them from reaching a lavatory fast enough, as in Alzheimer disease. A person in a wheelchair may be blocked from getting to a lavatory in time.

Overflow incontinence is seen when the bladder is always full because of weak bladder muscles or a blocked urethra (e.g. prostatic disease), so that it leaks urine frequently. Nerve damage from diabetes or other diseases can lead to weak bladder muscles; tumours and urinary stones can block the urethra.

VERTIGO (SEE DIZZINESS)

VISUAL IMPAIRMENT

Visual impairment may be suspected if a patient has overcautious driving habits; finds lighting either too bright or too dim; has frequent spectacle prescription changes; holds books or reading material close to face or at arm's length; squints or tilts the head to see; has difficulty in recognizing people; changes leisure time activities, personal appearance or table etiquette; moves about cautiously or bumps into objects; or acts confusedly or is disoriented.

Blindness or defects of visual fields can be caused by ocular, optic nerve or cortical damage, but the type of defect varies according to the site and extent of the lesion. A complete lesion of one optic nerve causes that eye to be totally blind. There is no direct reaction of the pupil to light (loss of constriction) and, if a light is shone into the affected eye, the pupil of the unaffected eye also fails to respond (loss of the consensual reflex). However, the nerves to the affected eye responsible for pupil constriction run in the IIIrd cranial nerve and should be intact. If, therefore, a light is shone into the *unaffected eye*, the pupil of the affected eye also constricts, even though that eye is sightless.

Lesions of the optic tract, chiasma, radiation or optic cortex cause various visual field defects involving both visual fields but without total field loss on either side.

Visual field examination (perimetry) tests the total area where objects can be seen in the peripheral vision while the eye is focused on a central point. Confrontation visual field examination is a quick and basic evaluation of the visual field done by an examiner sitting directly in front of the patient who is asked to look at the examiner's eye and tell when they can see the examiner's hand. Tangent screen examination involves the patient looking at a central target and telling the examiner when an object brought into the peripheral vision can be seen.

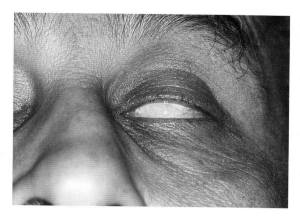

Fig. 4.5   Complete blindness; an opaque eye

Automated perimetry is when the patient sits in front of a computer-driven programme, which flashes small lights at different locations, and presses a button whenever the lights in the peripheral vision are seen. An ophthalmological opinion should always be obtained if there is any suggestion of a visual field defect.

Vision is tested by visual acuity testing using the Snellen eye chart or another standard eye chart. This has a series of letters or letters and numbers, with the largest at the top. As the person being tested reads down the chart, the letters gradually become smaller. When checking visual acuity, one eye is covered at a time and the vision of each eye is recorded separately, as well as both eyes together. Normal vision is 20/20, which means that the eye being tested can read a certain size letter when it is 20 feet away. If a person sees 20/40, then at 20 feet from the chart that person can read letters that a person with 20/20 vision could read from 40 feet away. The 20/40 letters are twice the size of 20/20 letters; however, if 20/20 is considered 100% visual efficiency, 20/40 visual acuity is 85% efficient. For people who have worse than 20/400 vision, a different eye chart can be used. It is common to record vision worse than 20/400 as count fingers (CF at a certain number of feet), hand motion (HM at a certain number of feet), light perception (LP) or no light perception (NLP). Legal blindness: in the UK, the statutory definition of 'blind' is 'so blind as to be unable to perform any work for which eyesight is essential' (the Blind Persons Act 1920). There is no statutory definition of 'partial sight', although the guideline is 'substantially and permanently handicapped by defective vision caused by congenital defect, illness, or injury' (the National Assistance Act 1948).

Ophthalmoscopy/fundoscopy: after the pupils have been dilated, direct ophthalmoscopy provides a wider magnified view of the retina. *Tonometry* measures pressure inside the eye and is one of several tests necessary to detect glaucoma. *Slit-lamp examination* allows examination of the front of the eye. *Phoroptery* detects refractive errors.

Visual impairment can vary from limitations in sight for distance, colour, size or shape to full blindness (Fig. 4.5). It is an important disability that invariably restricts activity to some degree. Most visual impairment is caused by disease or malnutrition. The main causes include:

- cataracts (48%)
- glaucoma (12%)

- uveitis (10%)
- age-related macular degeneration (9%)
- trachoma (4%)
- corneal opacity (5%)
- diabetic retinopathy (5%).

Cataracts, a common cause of visual impairment in the elderly, are lens opacities that are more common in diabetes or after excess exposure to sunlight, ionizing irradiation or corticosteroids.

Visual defects are also among the most common genetic disorders and congenital blindness may be associated with other handicaps such as epilepsy.

Clearly communication is best verbally, though, for the partially sighted, writing matter can sometimes be used but must be in large, bold, black type on a white background.

Adaptive technology that may help includes adaptations around the home as well as large print books, books on tape and Braille, and low vision and blindness-related products.

VITILIGO

Vitiligo is loss of skin pigmentation (Fig. 4.6), which can be dramatically unaesthetic. It is usually an autoimmune disorder.

WEIGHT LOSS

The main causes of involuntary weight loss apart from malnutrition are diabetes, hyperthyroidism, eating disorders, cancer (e.g. lung, gastrointestinal), infections (e.g. HIV disease, tuberculosis), depression and drugs.

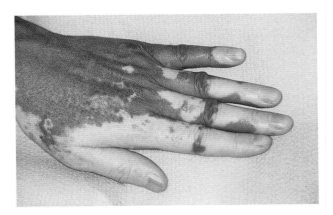

Fig. 4.6 Vitiligo

WHITE LESIONS IN THE MOUTH

Most white oral lesions are due to local causes, such as keratoses caused by irritation, or idiopathic leukoplakia. Rare congenital causes include white sponge naevus (can involve the vagina and anus), dyskeratosis congenita and pachyonychia congenita.

Candidosis may cause white or red lesions (Ch. 21). Lichen planus and lupus erythematosus are discussed in Ch. 11. Cancer may present as a white lesion.

SECTION B

ORGAN SYSTEMS MEDICINE

The cardiovascular system is a blood transportation network comprising the heart and blood vessels. The heart is vital to life, as its essential function is pumping oxygenated blood to the brain and vital organs. Blood becomes oxygenated in the lungs and travels in the pulmonary vein to the heart at the left atrium, from where it flows to the left ventricle through the mitral valve. Blood leaves the left ventricle through the aortic valve to the aorta (the body's main artery) and is distributed via arteries throughout the body, is collected into veins and returns via the venae cava to the right atrium. Thus the left ventricle is the most powerful chamber as it has to move blood all around the body. Arteries branch to arterioles and then to capillaries to transport oxygen to the tissues (Fig. 5.1). Oxygen is transported on the red blood-cell pigment haemoglobin, which colours the blood red. Capillaries release oxygen to the tissues and collect carbon dioxide as a waste product. A vast venous network collects blood and carbon dioxide from all the tissues and returns it to the heart. Veins transport blood eventually back through the superior vena cava and the inferior vena cava to the right atrium of the heart and generally carry deoxygenated blood (Fig. 5.2). This then flows through the tricuspid valve to the right ventricle. Blood leaves the right ventricle through the pulmonary valve to the pulmonary artery and thence to the lungs where it takes up oxygen. The heart thus consists of four chambers: two ventricles and two atria. It is centrally located in the chest (thorax) but, because the left ventricle is larger, the heart beat (apex beat) is found to the left side (Fig. 5.3).

The heart rate and force of contraction are controlled by nerves (mainly vagus and sympathetic) and hormones (especially adrenaline, which increases both rate and force). Anxiety and exercise can increase the pulse rate and force of the heartbeat.

HEART DISEASES

Heart disease is a major killer: in the USA possibly one person dies from heart disease every 30 s. It also causes significant morbidity and disability in many aspects of life, including effects on entitlement to drive a motor vehicle. There is a wide range of disorders that can affect the heart (Box 5.1).

CONGENITAL HEART DISEASE (CHD)

Congenital heart defects are the most common type of heart problem in children, present in about 1% of live births. CHD includes a wide variety of structural defects that can lead to

malfunction such as arrhythmias or flow problems. Lesions may involve the heart or adjacent great vessels, in isolation or in a variety of combinations. Vessel or valve stenosis or obstruction and septal defects strain the myocardium. CHD may be: cyanotic ('blue babies'), where there is right-to-left shunting, and in general these are more severe defects; or acyanotic, which is generally less severe. Cyanosis and hypoxia can lead to neurological deficits and polycythaemia (with hypercoagulability and thrombosis), and systemic infections (e.g. brain abscess). The types of CHD are summarized in Table 5.1. Approximately 20% of patients with CHD have other congenital anomalies.

Often the cause of CHD is unidentified but some have a genetic cause (e.g. Down syndrome; see Ch. 28). There are many other causes (Table 5.2; Appendix 5.1 and 5.2) and syndromes (e.g. oesophageal atresia and heart disease, and forearm/digit abnormalities and atrial septal defect; ASD).

The main acquired causes of CHD are maternal infections – congenital rubella, herpes or cytomegalovirus infection, which can cause patent ductus arteriosus (PDA), pulmonary stenosis, ventricular septal defect (VSD) and coarctation of the aorta; maternal drug use (e.g. alcohol, anticonvulsants, lithium,

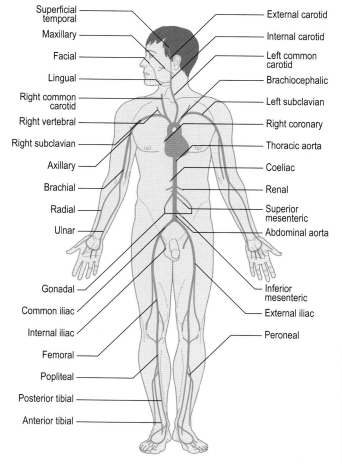

Fig. 5.1 Major arteries

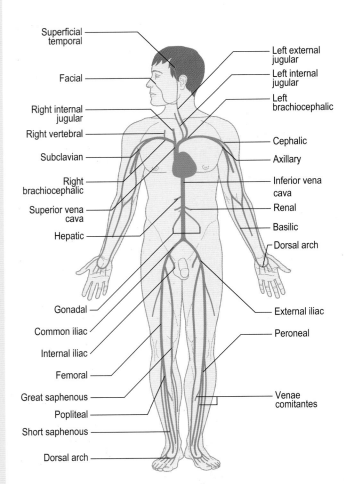

Fig. 5.2 Major veins

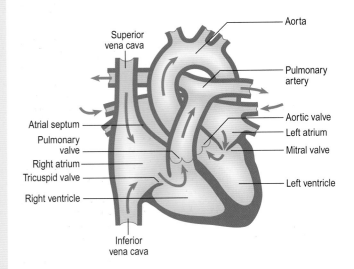

Fig. 5.3 Cardiac anatomy

Box 5.1 Causes of cardiovascular disease

Organic disease of the heart

- Myocardial
  - Overload secondary to hypertension or valve disease[a]
  - Coronary (ischaemic) heart disease[a]
  - Cardiomyopathies
- Endocardial
  - Rheumatic heart disease
  - Congenital anomalies[a]
  - Infective endocarditis
- Pericardial
  - Pericarditis
  - Pericardial effusion

Functional disorders

- Due to hypertension[a]
- Due to abnormalities in heart rate
  - Tachycardias
  - Bradycardias
  - Other arrhythmias
- Changes in circulatory volume
  - Hypervolaemia (shock syndrome)
  - Hypervolaemia (circulatory overload)
  - Others

[a]Common causes of heart failure

Table 5.1   Types of congenital heart disease (see Table 5.2)

CYANOTIC	ACYANOTIC	
	With no shunt	**With left to right shunt**
Eisenmenger syndrome	Aortic stenosis (AS)	Atrial septal defect (ASD)
Fallot tetralogy	Bicuspid aortic valve	Patent ductus arteriosus (PDA)
Pulmonary atresia (PA)	Coarctation of the aorta	Ventricular septal defect (VSD)
Pulmonary valve stenosis	Dextrocardia	
Total anomalous venous drainage	Mitral valve prolapse	
Transposition of the great vessels		
Tricuspid atresia (TA)		

CLINICAL FEATURES OF CONGENITAL HEART DISEASE

Cyanotic CHD is in general a much more severe defect (Fig. 5.4), which can lead to cardiac failure or be fatal or life-threatening without surgical intervention. Cyanosis (caused by > 5 g of reduced haemoglobin per decilitre of blood) results from shunting deoxygenated blood from the right ventricle into the left side of the heart and the systemic circulation (*right-to-left shunt*), and leads to chronic hypoxaemia (Fig. 5.5). Patients may crouch in an effort to improve venous return, but eventually polycythaemia develops – with haemorrhagic or thrombotic tendencies. Finger- and toe-clubbing are associated with cyanotic CHD, but does not appear until about 3 months

recreational drugs, thalidomide and warfarin); or systemic disease, for example systemic lupus erythematosus and Sjögren syndrome (which can cause heart block), and diabetes (which has an increased incidence of VSD, coarctation and transposition of the great arteries and/or a characteristic hypertrophic cardiomyopathy); and, rarely, maternal irradiation.

Table 5.2 Main features of congenital heart disease (CHD)

CHD	Main pathology/location	Main features
Aortic stenosis	Narrowing of the aortic valve	Angina, dyspnoea and syncope. Balloon valvuloplasty or surgery may be indicated
Atrial septal defect (ASD)	Usually near foramen ovale and termed a secundum defect. Associated in 10–20% with mitral valve prolapse	Initially acyanotic, with survival into middle age in most cases and therefore is the most common CHD presenting in adults. In the absence of surgical correction, right ventricular failure eventually develops. Usually repaired by primary closure, or pericardial or Dacron patch
Bicuspid aortic valve	Valve is bicuspid instead of tricuspid. Often associated with other left-sided lesions (e.g. coarctation of the aorta or interrupted aortic arch)	Usually asymptomatic, even in athletes, but there is a high risk of infective endocarditis
Coarctation of the aorta	In aorta beyond the origin of the subclavian arteries	Normal blood supply to the head, neck and upper body but restricted to lower body. Surgery is indicated
Ebstein anomaly	Congenital abnormality of the tricuspid valve, usually associated with ASD	Ebstein anomaly is mild in most and surgery is needed only if the tricuspid valve leaks severely enough to result in heart failure or cyanosis
Eisenmenger syndrome or reaction	This is the process in which a left-to-right shunt in the heart causes increased flow through the pulmonary vasculature (and pulmonary hypertension) which, in turn, causes increased pressures in the right heart and reversal into a right-to-left shunt	Ventricular or atrial septal defects, patent ductus arteriosus and more complex types of acyanotic heart disease can underlie this. Initially there is pulmonary hypertension, polycythaemia and a hyperviscosity syndrome with haemorrhagic and thrombotic tendencies. Later there is right ventricular hypertrophy and cyanosis. Anticoagulants and pulmonary vasodilators (e.g. bosentan) may be indicated
Fallot tetralogy	Ventricular septal defect, pulmonary stenosis, right ventricular hypertrophy and an aorta that overrides both ventricles	Cyanosis progressive from birth. Chronic hypoxia causes decreased neurological function. Episodes of acute hypoxia from infundibular spasm are life threatening. Polycythaemia causes hypercoagulability and thrombosis. Right-to-left shunting is associated with a higher incidence of systemic infection such as a brain abscess. Surgery is indicated
Mitral valve prolapse (floppy mitral valve; Barlow syndrome)	The most common CHD, affecting 5–10% of the population. Seen mainly in women. Strong hereditary tendency. Seen especially in Marfan, Ehlers–Danlos and Down syndromes. May be associated with polycystic kidney disease and panic disorder	May cause no symptoms but, if there is mitral regurgitation, some patients develop pain, irregular or racing pulse, or fatigue and heart failure
Patent ductus arteriosus (PDA)	A persistent opening (normally closed by the third month of life) between aorta and pulmonary artery, common in prematurity and maternal rubella	Shunt is left to right, initially acyanotic, and typical complication is right ventricular failure. Closure can be promoted in early infancy by giving intravenous indometacin, a prostaglandin inhibitor
Pulmonary atresia	No pulmonary valve exists, so blood cannot flow from the right ventricle into the pulmonary artery and to the lungs. The right ventricle is not well developed. The tricuspid valve is often poorly developed. An ASD allows blood to exit the right atrium, so the baby is cyanotic. The only source of lung blood flow is the PDA	Early treatment often includes using a drug to keep the PDA from closing, and surgery to create a shunt between the aorta and the pulmonary artery
Pulmonary stenosis	Narrowing of the pulmonary valve	Symptoms are breathlessness and right ventricular failure. Balloon valvuloplasty or surgery may be indicated
Transposition of the great vessels	Reversal of pulmonary artery and aorta origins	Cyanosis and breathlessness from birth, with early congestive cardiac failure and death in infancy unless there are associated defects providing sufficient collateral circulation (such as a patent interventricular septum or PDA)
Tricuspid atresia	Absence of the tricuspid valve means no blood can flow from the right atrium to the right ventricle. Thus the right ventricle is small. Survival depends on there being an ASD and usually a ventricular septal defect	A surgical shunting procedure is often needed to increase the lung blood flow and reduce cyanosis. Some children may need pulmonary artery banding to *reduce* blood flow to the lungs. Others may need a more functional repair (Fontan procedure)
Ventricular septal defect (VSD)	One of the most common CHD. Ranges from a pinhole compatible with survival at least into middle age, to a large defect causing death in infancy if untreated. 90% of children with VSD have an additional cardiac defect	Initially left-to-right shunt but, with right ventricular hypertrophy, shunt may eventually reverse with late-onset cyanosis. Right ventricular failure may develop. Usually repaired by primary closure, or a pericardial or Dacron patch

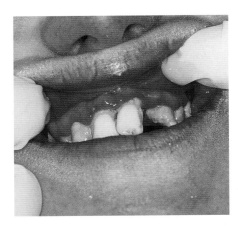

Fig. 5.4 Central cyanosis in a child with a congenital heart defect, showing purple lips and gingivae

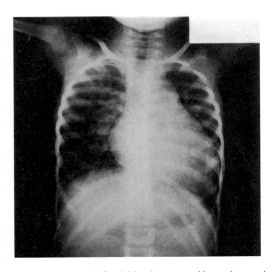

Fig. 5.5 Chest radiograph of a child with congenital heart disease showing gross cardiac enlargement (the heart normally occupies less than half the width of the chest)

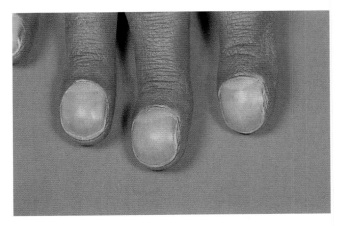

Fig. 5.6 Finger-clubbing in a patient with Fallot tetralogy. Finger-clubbing can be found in several different disorders, particularly cyanotic heart disease, chronic respiratory disease, lung cancer, Crohn disease, etc., but is sometimes benign and hereditary

---

Box 5.2 Possible complications in coronary heart disease

- Bleeding tendency
- Cardiac failure
- Cyanosis
- Fatigue
- Growth retardation
- Infections (e.g. brain abscess, endocarditis)
- Polycythaemia
- Pulmonary oedema

---

of age (Fig. 5.6). In the absence of treatment, 40% of children with cyanotic CHD die within the first 5 years.

Pulmonary hypertension and, eventually, right ventricular hypertrophy may be seen where the shunt is *left to right* and some of the output of the left ventricle is recirculated through the lungs. The shunt may eventually reverse and then cyanosis develops. Patients with CHD are liable to a range of complications (Box 5.2).

GENERAL MANAGEMENT

An obstetric ultrasound scan is often used to screen pregnant women at around 20 weeks for signs of CHD in their unborn babies. Most defects, however, are well tolerated *in utero* and it is only after birth that the impact of the anatomic and subsequently haemodynamic abnormality becomes evident. In young children, chest radiography may show cardiomegaly. Electrocardiography (ECG) may demonstrate an abnormal cardiac axis, ventricular hypertrophy and strain depending on the lesion present. CHD is most commonly diagnosed through echocardiography, which

has superseded intracardiac catheter studies, and confirmed by cardiac magnetic resonance imaging (MRI).

Early correction of the congenital defect, often by transvenous catheter techniques, is the treatment of choice. More complex defects may require an operation. Medical treatment may be needed for the management of pulmonary oedema, heart failure, polycythaemia, infection or emotional disturbances.

Modern surgical and medical care helps children survive into adult life and patients are then often called adult or 'grown-up' CHD. Nevertheless, complications observed in adults who were previously thought to have had successful repair of CHD include arrhythmias, valve disorders and cardiac failure, and residual defects can still predispose to complications such as infective endocarditis.

DENTAL ASPECTS

All dental surgery staff should be certified in basic cardiopulmonary resuscitation (CPR), and the entire team should rehearse emergency protocol procedures regularly (Ch. 1). Patients with heart disease should take their medications as usual on the day of the dental procedure, and should bring all their medications to the dental office for review at the time of the first appointment. The most important aspect for dentists to consider is how well the patient's heart condition is compensated. Patients with stable heart disease receiving atraumatic treatment under local anaesthesia (LA) can receive treatment in the dental surgery. Since cardiac events are most likely to occur in the early morning, patients with cardiac disease should be treated in the late morning or early afternoon appointments. The dentist and team should provide dental care with a stress-reduction protocol and with good analgesia, limiting the dosage of epinephrine.

An aspirating syringe should be used to give a LA, since adrenaline/epinephrine in the anaesthetic entering a vessel may theoretically raise the blood pressure or precipitate arrhythmias. Gingival retraction cords containing adrenaline/epinephrine should be avoided. Conscious sedation preferably with nitrous oxide can be given with the approval of the physician. General anaesthesia (GA) is a matter for expert anaesthetists in hospital.

Congestive cardiac failure may complicate management. In cyanotic CHD there may also be polycythaemia-related bleeding tendencies caused by thrombocytopenia, platelet dysfunction, coagulation defects (from liver hypoxia – causing reduced vitamin K-dependent factors), and excessive fibrinolytic activity. Thus platelets may be reduced, and the haematocrit, prothrombin time (PT) and activated partial thromboplastin time (APTT) increased. Occasionally there is a thrombotic tendency. A special hazard in some types of CHD is the development of cerebral abscess, occasionally due to oral bacteria. Leukopenia may be a factor in some right-to-left shunts. There may be susceptibility to infective endocarditis.

Oral abnormalities can be associated with cyanotic CHD and may include:

- delayed eruption of both dentitions
- greater frequency of positional anomalies
- enamel hypoplasia – the teeth often have a bluish-white 'skimmed milk' appearance and there is gross vasodilatation in the pulps
- greater caries and periodontal disease activity, probably because of poor oral hygiene and lack of dental attention
- after cardiotomy, transient small white non-ulcerated mucosal lesions of unknown aetiology may appear.

CONGENITAL HEART DISEASE IN OTHER SYNDROMES

Down syndrome (see Ch. 28)

Noonan syndrome

Noonan syndrome, usually an autosomal dominant trait, is characterized by short stature, unusual facies, chest deformity, learning disability, cryptorchidism in males and CHD. The commonest cardiac lesions are pulmonary stenosis, septal defects and hypertrophic cardiomyopathy.

Facial features may include an elongated mid-face height, hypertelorism, retrognathia, a lower nasal bridge and nasal root, a wider mouth, a more prominent upper lip and low-set ears. Abnormal vision and hearing are common. Other associations include hepatosplenomegaly and an abnormal bleeding tendency associated with low levels of clotting factors (particularly XI and XII), and associations with cherubism, jaw giant-cell lesions and neurofibromatosis.

Hypercalcaemia–supravalvular aortic stenosis syndrome (Williams syndrome)

Williams syndrome comprises, in its rare complete form, infantile hypercalcaemia, elfin facies, learning disability and CHD. Most cases appear to be sporadic. These children may be sociable and talkative ('cocktail party manner'). Hypercalcaemia typically remits in infancy but leaves growth deficiency, osteosclerosis and craniostenosis. Cardiovascular lesions include supravalvular subaortic stenosis or other abnormalities, and may contraindicate GA. Also, masseter spasm has been reported during GA with halothane and suxamethonium, but it is not malignant hyperthermia. Dental defects may include hypodontia, microdontia and hypoplastic, bud-shaped teeth. The upper arch may be disproportionately wide and overlap the lower.

ACQUIRED HEART DISEASE

GENERAL ASPECTS

Ischaemic heart disease (IHD; coronary artery disease; CAD) is the most common and important cardiac disease and the major killer in the developed world. Functional disorders, where there is no organic disease of the heart itself, can also cause circulatory failure, as in shock. A variety of common extracardiac diseases can aggravate heart disease, particularly if there is impaired oxygenation, as in severe anaemia.

CLINICAL FEATURES

Serious heart disease is not always symptomatic, and patients can die suddenly from myocardial infarction (MI) despite having experienced neither chest pain nor any other symptom. Also, many patients with manifest cardiac disease can have signs and symptoms effectively controlled so that they may superficially appear well. Often, only the drug history gives a clue to the nature of any cardiac illness. Common clinical features of cardiac disease include breathlessness, chest pain, palpitations and cyanosis, while signs may be seen on the hands (clubbing, cyanosis), or from measuring the blood pressure, from palpation of the pulse, or from listening to the heart (auscultation).

GENERAL MANAGEMENT

The heart rate, force of contraction and rhythm can be assessed from palpation of the pulse; disturbances of rhythm may signify cardiac disease.

The blood pressure (BP) is measured by sphygmomanometry. The finding of either normal levels (pressures of 120 mmHg systolic and 80 mmHg diastolic) or grossly raised levels (> 160/90 mmHg for a male of 45 years or over) is informative. However, these must be checked on further occasions as the BP frequently increases in anxiety. In an injured patient, a falling BP is also a danger sign that must not be ignored, since it implies a serious complication such as haemorrhage or shock.

Experienced cardiologists can identify by auscultation the vast majority of innocent functional murmurs from the serious murmurs of aortic stenosis, mitral regurgitation, tricuspid regurgitation, pulmonary stenosis, ventricular septal defects and hypertrophic cardiomyopathy.

Other investigations include blood assays of cardiac enzymes (troponin, troponin T, creatine kinase), which are raised after cardiac damage such as a myocardial infarct. Chest radiography (CXR) helps detect heart enlargement (e.g. in cardiac failure or hypertension). Electrocardiography, invaluable for the diagnosis of arrhythmias and of IHD, is a graphic tracing of the variations in electrical potential caused by the excitation of the atria (Fig. 5.7).

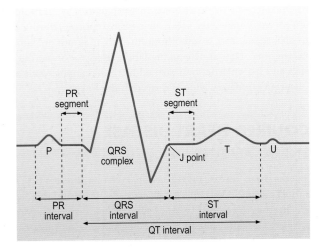

Fig. 5.7 Normal ECG tracing

The QRS deflections are due to excitation (depolarization) of the ventricles. The T wave is due to recovery of the ventricles (repolarization). Doppler echocardiography (cardiac ultrasonography) is a valuable non-invasive imaging tool for the heart, helpful in establishing a specific diagnosis and estimating the severity of various diseases by evaluating cardiac chamber size, wall thickness, wall motion, valve configuration and motion, and the proximal great vessels. This technique also provides a sensitive method for detecting pericardial and pleural fluid accumulation, and can allow identification of mass lesions within and adjacent to the heart. Cardiac MRI, scans using thallium-201 or technetium-99, or positron emission tomography (PET) using ^{18}F-deoxyglucose (FDG) are also extremely useful.

Medical treatments are available to control many cardiac disorders, but surgery may be required, especially for IHD.

DENTAL ASPECTS

Management implications in oral health care depend mainly on the type of intervention and the degree of cardiovascular risk (Table 5.3).

Table 5.3 Predictors of high cardiovascular risk

Very high risk	Medium risk	Low risk
MI in previous month	Mild angina	Old age
Unstable or severe angina	Myocardial infarction more than 1 month previously	ECG abnormalities only
Atrioventricular block	Compensated heart failure	Atrial fibrillation
Ventricular arrhythmias		Stroke
Severe cardiac valvular disease		Uncontrolled hypertension
Advanced heart failure		

ECG, electrocardiogram; MI, myocardial infarction.

Patients should receive short, minimally stressful appointments: anxiety, exertion and pain should be minimized. Endogenous adrenaline/epinephrine levels peak during morning hours and adverse cardiac events are most likely in the early morning, so late morning appointments are recommended. Cardiac monitoring is desirable in many instances (Figs 5.8 and 5.9).

General anaesthesia for dental care in cardiac patients should be avoided unless essential. Effective painless LA is essential. An aspirating syringe should be used since adrenaline/epinephrine in the anaesthetic may get into the blood and may (theoretically) raise the blood pressure and precipitate arrhythmias. BP tends to rise during oral surgery under LA, and adrenaline/epinephrine theoretically can contribute, but this is usually of little practical importance. However, adrenaline/epinephrine-containing LA should not be given in excessive doses to patients taking beta-blockers, as this may induce hypertension and cardiovascular complications. *Note:* A woman on beta-blockers, who was (inexcusably) given 16 dental cartridges of LA, died from lidocaine overdosage, *not* from accelerated hypertension. Gingival retraction cords containing adrenaline/epinephrine should be avoided wherever possible.

A range of cardiovascular drugs can influence oral health care (Table 5.4), while drugs used in dentistry can interact with cardiac drugs.

Aspirin may cause sodium and fluid retention, which may be contraindicated in severe hypertension or cardiac failure. Indometacin

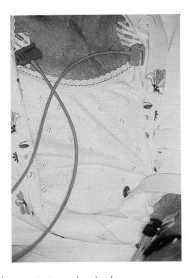

Fig. 5.8 Cardiac monitoring – chest leads

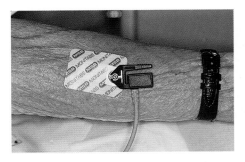

Fig. 5.9 Cardiac monitoring – arm lead

Table 5.4 Cardiovascular drugs: potential effects on oral health care

Group	Examples	Possible reaction
Alpha-blockers	Prazosin	Orthostatic hypotension
Alpha/beta-blockers	Carvedilol	Enhance pressor response to adrenaline/epinephrine
ACE inhibitors	Enalapril, Perindopril	Indometacin impairs
Antiplatelets	Disopyramide Clopidogrel Eptifibatide	Erythromycin enhances Bleeding tendency
Beta-blockers (non-cardioselective)	Nadolol, Propanolol	Enhance pressor response to adrenaline/epinephrine
Digitalis glycosides	Various	LA vasoconstrictor may induce arrhythmias Gag reflex increased
Statins	Simvastatin, Atorvastatin	Muscle damage increased by macrolides (erythromycin, clarithromycin and telithromycin) and azoles (fluconazole, itraconazole, ketoconazole, miconazole) but rosuvastatin, pravastatin and fluvastatin do not appear to have this problem

ACE, angiotensin-converting enzyme; LA, local analgesia.

may interfere with antihypertensive agents. Macrolides and azoles may cause statins to produce increased muscle damage.

An association between periodontal disease and cardiovascular disease has been suggested, but recent evidence-based reviews question this association.

ATHEROMA, AND ISCHAEMIC OR CORONARY HEART DISEASE

General aspects

Atheroma (atherosclerosis; arteriosclerosis) is characterized by the accumulation of cholesterol and lipids in the intima of arterial walls, and can lead to thromboses (clots), which sometimes break off and move within the vessels to lodge in and occlude small vessels (embolism). Atheroma can thus lead to IHD with angina, myocardial infarction, cerebrovascular disease and stroke (Table 5.5). It also affects other arteries and can cause, for example, ischaemic pain in the calves whilst walking – intermittent claudication – seen especially in young smokers when it is termed Buerger disease. In Western populations, atheroma may affect up to 45% of young adult males, and IHD affects at least 20% and increasingly thereafter, and accounts for about 35% of total mortality in Britain and the USA.

Atheroma results from a combination of genetic and lifestyle factors. Irreversible (fixed) risk factors include increasing age, male gender and family history of atheroma. Potentially reversible (modifiable) risk factors for atheroma include:

- cigarette smoking
- blood lipids

Table 5.5 Main sites and results of atheroma

Site	Consequence	Possible clinical syndromes
Coronary arteries	Coronary artery disease	Impairs oxygenation and can lead to chest pain (angina), arrhythmias or myocardial infarction
Carotid and other cerebral arteries	Cerebrovascular disease	Stroke or transient ischaemic attacks
Peripheral arteries	Peripheral vascular disease	Impaired oxygenation, pain (intermittent claudication) and sometimes gangrene

Table 5.6 Risk and protective factors for atheroma

Primary risk factors	Secondary risk factors	Unclear factors	Protective factors
High LDL	Low LDL	Low dietary fibre	Raising HDL to LDL ratio
Hypertension	Diabetes	Soft water	More exercise
Smoking	Obesity	High plasma fibrinogen	Moderate red wine or other alcohol
	Family history of CAD	Raised blood factor VII	
	Physical inactivity	Raised lipoprotein levels	
	Type A personality	Homocystein levels	
	Gout	Folate levels	
	Ethnic (Asians)	Creactive protein levels	
	Male gender		
	Increasing age		
	Low social class		
	Chronic renal failure		

CAD, coronary artery disease; HDL, high-density lipoproteins; LDL, low-density lipoproteins.

- hypertension
- diabetes mellitus
- obesity and lack of exercise
- the metabolic syndrome (Table 5.6; see Ch. 23).

High blood cholesterol is one of the major risk factors for IHD. Low-density lipoproteins (LDLs) are associated with a high risk of atheroma, whilst high-density lipoproteins (HDLs) appear to be anti-atherogenic (Table 5.7).

Atheroma is a disease predominantly of males, particularly of affluent societies, linked to smoking, lack of exercise, hypertension and hyperlipidaemia. Dietary fat is processed by the liver to form four main lipoproteins – chylomicrons,

Table 5.7 Blood lipids

	Total cholesterol	LDL ('bad') cholesterol	Lipid HDL ('good') cholesterol	Triglycerides
Significance of high level	May indicate atheroma	Main source of atheroma	Inhibits atheroma. Less than 40 mg/dl considered a major risk factor for CAD	May indicate atheroma
Target blood levels for health	Less than 200 mg/dl	Less than 100 mg/dl	Levels of 60 mg/dl or more	Less than 150–199 mg/dl

CAD, coronary artery disease; HDL, high-density lipoprotein; IHD, ischaemic heart disease; LDL, low-density lipoprotein.

very-low-density lipoproteins (VLDL), LDLs and HDLs. VLDL reforms to LDL, and it is these fats that are incorporated into atherosclerotic plaque and associated with a high risk of CAD. By contrast, HDLs clear cholesterol from the blood via the liver, appear to be anti-atherogenic, and are associated with a lower risk of CAD (Table 5.7). Cholesterol may be raised genetically, and with increasing age in both sexes. Before the menopause, women have lower total cholesterol levels than men of the same age but, after the menopause, women's LDL levels tend to rise with inactivity and being overweight, with a low fruit and vegetable diet, with smoking and with other diseases such as hypertension and diabetes.

There is a higher incidence of CAD in patients with diabetes, hyperlipidaemia, the metabolic syndrome and hypothyroidism. Hyperlipidaemia and hypertension seem to be linked, and immigrants from the Indian subcontinent have a higher than average morbidity and mortality from CAD. Apolipoprotein E genotyping may help confirm a diagnosis of type III hyperlipoproteinaemia (also known as dysbetalipoproteinaemia), to evaluate a possible genetic cause of atheroma. Periodontal disease could be an independent risk factor for CAD, because oral bacteria, inflammatory mediators and endotoxaemia might contribute. Other infectious agents implicated have included *Chlamydia pneumoniae*, *Helicobacter pylori* and cytomegalovirus, but the associations have not been proven.

Clinical features

Atheroma has a patchy distribution and, depending on the site and extent of disease, can give rise to a variety of clinical presentations (Table 5.5). Atheromatous plaques may rupture and 'heal' spontaneously. Alternatively a platelet–fibrin thrombus (clot) may form, break up and travel in the bloodstream (thromboembolism) with potentially life-threatening consequences.

Coronary artery disease is due to occlusion of the coronary arteries and leads to angina pectoris (pain arising from the myocardial oxygen demand exceeding the supply). Rare causes of CAD include embolism and coronary artery spasm. Patients with CAD are at greatest risk from myocardial infarction, which, if severe, causes cardiac arrest with acute failure of the whole circulation, loss of cerebral blood supply and often death within a few minutes. MI differs from angina in that it causes more severe and persistent chest pain, which is not

> **Box 5.3 Lifestyle recommended for lowering the risk of ischaemic heart disease**
>
> - Healthy weight
> - Stopping smoking
> - Moderate alcohol consumption
> - Regular exercise (e.g. brisk walking for at least 30 min daily)
> - Fresh fruit and vegetable intake of at least five servings a day
> - Grain intake of at least six servings a day with at least 1/3 whole grain

controlled by rest; it leads to irreversible cardiac damage or sudden death.

A chronically reduced blood supply to the myocardium progressively damages the heart and may lead to cardiac arrhythmias and cardiac failure.

Prevention

The primary aim is to prevent or reduce progression of coronary atheroma by lifestyle changes as shown in Box 5.3.

Coronary artery disease prophylaxis is by lowering cholesterol levels that are too high. If the total cholesterol is 200 mg/dl or more, or if HDL is less than 40 mg/dl, a lipoprotein profile should be done after a 9–12-h fast. Abnormal cholesterol levels can be altered by: improving diet (reducing saturated fat and cholesterol); losing weight, which can help lower LDL and total cholesterol levels, as well as raise HDL and lower triglyceride levels; greater physical activity, which can help lower LDL and raise HDL levels and also helps weight loss; stopping cigarette smoking; controlling hypertension; taking drugs to lower LDL cholesterol if it is 130 mg/dl or more – statins (simvastatin, pravastatin, etc.) which inhibit the production *de novo* of cholesterol via hydroxymethylglutaryl coenzyme A (HMG-CoA) reductase; taking bile acid sequestrants (colesevelam) or resins (cholestyramine, colestipol), nicotinic acid-related drugs (nicotinic acid and acipimox); and by taking a diet high in marine triglycerides (and omega-3 fatty acids) and fruit and vegetables. Fibrates (clofibrate, fenofibrate, gemfibrozil) may be alternatives to statins. Fish such as salmon, tuna and mackerel containing omega-3 fatty acids offer protection against CAD by reducing inflammation. Polyunsaturated fatty acids of the omega-3 type are present as alpha-linolenic acid, mainly in certain vegetable sources such as soybean, canola oil and English walnuts, and in fish oils as eicosapentaenoic acid (EPA) and docosahexaenoic acid (DHA). Fruits and vegetables, and other foods high in antioxidants, are associated with a lower risk of CAD. Moderate red wine consumption is also associated with lower CAD mortality (possibly because of the contained antioxidant resveratrol), and eating less salt may reduce the chances of developing high BP.

General management

The diagnosis of CAD may be suggested by the history. Resting ECG may help but, if normal, exercise ECG is indicated. Use of a radionuclide such as thallium-201 or MIBI (2-methoxy isobutyl isonitrile; sestamibi) can enhance the sensitivity. Myocardial perfusion scans (thallium-201) may reveal ischaemic areas which show as 'cold spots' during exercise. Coronary arteriography (angiography) demonstrates the anatomy and patency of the arteries and also allows for intervention if necessary (percutaneous coronary intervention; PCI). Placement of stents may correct any stenosis (angioplasty).

The most effective ways to treat patients with IHD include the lifestyle changes described above, particularly stopping smoking. Drugs that may help include antiplatelet drugs (aspirin or clopidogrel) to prevent thrombosis; beta-blockers (atenolol, metoprolol, etc.) to lower the blood pressure; angiotensin-converting enzyme (ACE) inhibitors (enalapril, fosinopril, etc.) to lower peripheral resistance and cardiac workload, and hence blood pressure, and statins to lower blood cholesterol. Statins may cause muscle damage, sleep disturbances, memory loss, depression, sexual dysfunction or interstitial lung disease. Other measures include good control of blood glucose levels in diabetics.

Pain relief and prophylaxis of angina is with nitroglycerine (glyceryl trinitrate) 0.3–0.6 mg sublingually during attacks, or before anticipated physical activity or stress. Long-acting nitrates (e.g. isosorbide dinitrate) may help prevent attacks.

When CAD is extensive and an individual's symptoms are worsening despite general measures and optimal medical management, cardiac revascularization techniques should be considered. These include: *coronary angioplasty* – stents may be placed percutaneously (PCI) to re-establish coronary blood flow and improve myocardial perfusion; or *coronary artery bypass graft (CABG)* – to bridge severe obstructions in the coronary blood vessels.

Dental aspects

Stress, anxiety, exertion or pain can provoke angina and, therefore, patients should receive dental care in short, minimally stressful appointments in the late morning. Effective painless LA is essential. An aspirating syringe should be used since adrenaline/epinephrine in the LA may enter the blood and may (theoretically) raise the BP and precipitate arrhythmias. Adrenaline/epinephrine-containing LA should not be given in excessive doses to patients taking beta-blockers, since the interaction may induce hypertension and cardiovascular complications if excessively large doses are given. Gingival retraction cords containing adrenaline/epinephrine should be avoided.

Conscious sedation should be deferred for at least 3 months for patients after MI, recent-onset angina, unstable angina or recent development of bundle branch block and, in any case, should be given in hospital. GA should be avoided wherever possible and at least deferred for 3 months after MI.

Drugs may affect dental care (Table 5.4). Angina can rarely cause pain in the mandible, teeth or other oral tissues. Patients with CAD appear to have more severe dental caries and periodontal disease than the general population. Whether these infections bear any causative relationship to heart disease remains controversial but periodontal disease could be an independent risk factor, because oral bacteria, inflammatory mediators and endotoxaemia might contribute.

ANGINA PECTORIS

Angina pectoris is the name given to episodes of chest pain caused by myocardial ischaemia secondary to CAD. It affects around 1% of adults and its prevalence rises with increasing age. The severity and prognosis of angina depends upon the degree of coronary artery narrowing and has a varied clinical presentation. The usual underlying causes are atherosclerotic plaques that rupture with resulting platelet activation, adhesion and aggregation, and thrombosis impeding coronary artery blood flow (or, if this is complete occlusion, myocardial infarction). Arterial spasm alone may, rarely, be responsible.

The mortality rate in angina is about 4% per year, the prognosis depending on the degree of coronary artery narrowing.

Clinical features

The most common precipitating causes of angina pain are physical exertion (particularly in cold weather); emotion (especially anger or anxiety); and stress caused by fear or pain, leading to adrenal release of catecholamines (adrenaline/epinephrine and norepinephrine) and consequent tachycardia, vasoconstriction and raised blood pressure. Consequently an increased cardiac workload is accompanied by a paradoxical drop in blood flow and myocardial ischaemia occurs resulting in angina. This is often an unmistakable pain described as a sense of strangling or choking, or tightness, heaviness, compression or constriction of the chest, sometimes radiating to the left arm or jaw *but relieved by rest* (Box 5.4).

Patients may have repeated attacks of angina over a long period, or have a MI soon after the first one or two attacks. Many patients also have painless myocardial ischaemia, as shown by arteriography (angiography) and exercise ECG changes. Some have hyposensitivity to pain. Variants of angina are shown in Box 5.5.

Box 5.4 Features of angina

- Chest pain described as a pressure sensation, fullness or squeezing in the mid-portion of the thorax, relieved by rest or glyceryl trinitrate
- Radiation of chest pain into the jaw/teeth, shoulder, arm, and/or back
- Occasionally associated dyspnoea or shortness of breath, epigastric discomfort or sweating

General management

The diagnosis is primarily clinical: occasionally gastro-oesophageal reflux disease (GORD) and chest wall disease mimic angina, and neither physical examination nor investigations are are necessarily abnormal. Investigations may include especially resting ECG, which typically shows ST segment depression with a flat or inverted T wave, but is usually normal between episodes of angina. Exercise ECG testing is positive in approximately 75% of people with severe CAD. Myocardial perfusion scans (thallium-201) highlight ischaemic myocardium. Coronary angiography can assess coronary blood flow in diagnostically challenging cases.

Risk factors for CAD (cigarette smoking, physical inactivity, obesity, hypertension, diabetes, hypercholesterolaemia) should be identified and corrected. Prognostic therapies for angina include aspirin (inhibits platelet aggregation by preventing the synthesis of thromboxane A_2); glycoprotein IIb/IIIa receptor inhibitors (e.g. clopidogrel), which prevent adherence of fibrinogen to platelets and reduce thrombus formation; and lipid-lowering drugs, which reduce mortality rates in patients with CAD.

During acute episodes of angina, pain is relieved by oxygen, sublingual glyceryl trinitrate (GTN) and reducing anxiety. The pain, though relieved by rest, is ameliorated more quickly by nitrates – usually GTN (nitroglycerin) – which act by lowering the peripheral vascular resistance and lowering the oxygen demands of the heart. Most patients use this in the buccal sulcus or sublingually, as a spray or tablet. Other nitrates, calcium-channel blockers and occasionally potassium-channel activators such as nicorandil may also be used. Nitrates are not used to relieve an angina attack if the patient has recently taken sildenafil as there may be a precipitous fall in blood pressure; analgesics should be used.

When angina is frequent, long-acting nitrates (isosorbide mononitrate), beta-adrenergic blocking drugs (atenolol), and calcium antagonists (amlodipine) are used. Drugs used to prevent thrombosis in unstable angina in particular include: aspirin, which acetylates platelet cyclo-oxygenase (COX), and thereby inhibits platelet function for about 7 days, and is more effective when used with clopidogrel; glycoprotein IIb and IIIa inhibitors, such as abciximab, to prevent adherence of fibrinogen to receptors on platelets and block their aggregation; and low-molecular-weight heparin. In angina that does not respond to drugs, PCI procedures or by-pass grafts may be indicated.

Percutaneous transluminal coronary angioplasty (PTCA) aims to open up the coronary blood flow by inserting a balloon-tipped catheter through the groin up into the area of arterial blockage. However, 40–50% of arteries block again within 6 months though this may be partially prevented with clopidogrel, aspirin or other antiplatelet drugs. PTCA has a lower morbidity than coronary by-pass. Stents (miniature wire coils) may be inserted at the time of angioplasty to keep arteries open. However, re-narrowing (restenosis) follows in about 25% of patients. Stents coated with sirolimus, a potent immunosuppressive, reduce this restenosis. Minute amounts of beta radiation in vascular brachytherapy (intravascular brachytherapy or endovascular brachytherapy) can inhibit or reduce restenosis.

Coronary artery bypass grafts (CABG) are vascular grafts made to bridge the obstructions in the coronary blood vessels. Saphenous veins (from the leg) are placed, accessing the heart by full sternotomy. Minimally invasive CABG uses arteries such as the internal mammary artery without the need for full sternotomy. CABG results in a 5-year survival of over 85%, and a 10-year survival of around 70%.

Car drivers should avoid driving for 1 week after PTCA, or pacemaker insertion, and for 1 month after MI, CABG or when they have unstable angina. Patients with implantable defibrillators usually lose their driving licence but may regain it if they are shock-free for at least 6 months.

Dental aspects

Pre-operative GTN and sometimes oral sedation (e.g. temazepam) are advised. Dental care should be carried out with minimal anxiety, and oxygen saturation, blood pressure and pulse monitoring. Effective LA is essential. Ready access to medical help, oxygen and nitroglycerin is crucial.

If a patient with a history of angina experiences chest pain in the dental surgery, dental treatment must be stopped, the patient should be given GTN sublingually and oxygen, and be kept sitting upright. Vital signs should be monitored. The pain should be relieved in 2–3 min; the patient should then rest and be accompanied home.

If chest pain is not relieved within about 3 min, MI is a possible cause (see later) and medical help should be summoned. Pain that persists after three doses of nitroglycerin given every 5 min, that lasts more than 15–20 min, or that is associated with nausea, vomiting, syncope or hypertension is highly suggestive of MI. If pain persists, the patient should continue oxygen, and *chew* 300 mg of aspirin (Ch. 1).

Tricyclic antidepressants are best avoided as they can disturb cardiac rhythm. Sumitriptan is contraindicated as it may cause coronary artery vasoconstriction.

Angina is a rare cause of pain in the mandible, teeth or other oral tissues, or pharynx. Drugs used in the care of patients with angina may cause oral adverse effects such as lichenoid lesions (calcium-channel blockers), gingival swelling (calcium-channel blockers) or ulcers (nicorandil).

Conscious sedation should be deferred for at least 3 months in patients with recent-onset angina, unstable angina or recent development of bundle branch block and, in any case, it should be given in hospital.

General anaesthesia should be deferred for at least 3 months in patients with recent-onset angina, unstable angina or recent development of bundle branch block and, in any case, must be given in hospital. Intravenous barbitures are particularly dangerous.

STABLE ANGINA

For anything but minor treatment under LA, the physician should be consulted and consideration should be given to any other complicating factors such as beta-blocker therapy, hypertension or cardiac failure. Other medication should not be interfered with. Before dental treatment, patients with stable angina should be reassured and possibly sedated with oral diazepam. Prophylactic administration of GTN may be indicated if the patient has angina more than once a week.

UNSTABLE ANGINA

Elective dental care should be deferred until a physician has agreed to it, because of the risk of infarction. Pre-operative GTN sublingually or by inhalation should be given, together with relative analgesia monitored by pulse oximetry, and LA; however, such patients are best cared for in a hospital, as intravenous nitrates may be indicated.

Emergency dental care should be the least invasive possible, using pre-operative GTN sublingually or by inhalation, together with relative analgesia monitored by pulse oximetry and LA; however, such patients are best cared for in a hospital environment, as coronary vasodilators may be indicated intravenously. Other medication should not be interfered with.

POST-ANGIOPLASTY

Elective dental care should be deferred for 6 months; emergency dental care should be in a hospital setting.

PATIENTS WITH CORONARY ARTERY BYPASS GRAFT

Patients should not receive an adrenaline/epinephrine-containing LA, since it may possibly precipitate arrhythmias. For the first couple of weeks after surgery, the patient may feel severe pain when reclining in the dental chair as a side-effect of the surgery.

PATIENTS WITH VASCULAR STENTS THAT ARE SUCCESSFULLY ENGRAFTED

The main points have been discussed earlier. It may be prudent to provide antibiotic coverage if emergency dental treatment is required during the first 6 weeks post-operatively. Elective dental care should be deferred. Patients may require long-term anticoagulant medication. Appropriate action is required to deal with any bleeding tendencies (Ch. 00), but most patients are on aspirin or clopidogrel rather than warfarin.

MYOCARDIAL INFARCTION

General aspects

Myocardial infarction (coronary thrombosis or heart attack) results from the complete occlusion (blockage) of one or more coronary arteries. It arises when atherosclerotic plaques rupture

causing platelet activation, adhesion and aggregation with subsequent thrombus formation within the coronary circulation. Angina may progress to MI but fewer than 50% of patients with MI have any preceding symptoms.

Clinical features

Myocardial infarction most commonly presents with central chest pain similar to that of angina *but is not relieved by rest or with sublingual nitrates*. MI may appear without warning or is sometimes precipitated by exercise or stress. The pain is often unmistakable and described as an unbearably severe sense of strangling or choking, or tightness, heaviness, compression or constriction of the chest. It sometimes radiates to the left arm or jaw. Sometimes MI is preceded by angina, often felt as indigestion-like pain (Box 5.6). It can persist for hours, if death does not supervene.

Box 5.6 Features of myocardial infarction

- Chest pain described as a pressure sensation, fullness or squeezing in the mid-portion of the thorax
- Radiation of chest pain into the jaw/teeth, shoulder, arm, and/or back
- Associated dyspnoea or shortness of breath
- Associated epigastric discomfort with or without nausea and vomiting
- Associated diaphoresis or sweating
- Syncope or near-syncope without other cause
- Impairment of cognitive function without other cause

The pain of MI may sometimes start at rest, and is not relieved by nitrates. Vomiting, facial pallor, sweating, restlessness, shortness of breath and apprehension are common. Other features may include breathlessness, cough and loss of consciousness, but the clinical picture is variable and fewer than 50% of patients with an MI have any warning premonitory symptoms.

Approximately 10–20% of individuals, however, have silent (painless) infarctions and the first sign may be the catastrophic onset of left ventricular failure, shock, loss of consciousness and death.

Death soon after the onset of the chest pain is common, often from ventricular fibrillation or cardiac arrest. Less often, there is sudden cardiac death characterized by immediate collapse without premonitory symptoms, and loss of pulses. In such cases, the precipitating event is a severe arrhythmia such as ventricular fibrillation. Up to 50% of patients die within the first hour of MI and a further 10–20% within the next few days.

The prognosis of MI may be judged based on the Killip classification (Table 5.8).

Cardiac failure and arrhythmias may develop in survivors and the chances of re-infarction are high in the immediate post-infarction weeks. Valvular dysfunction and myocardial rupture may complicate a MI. Dressler syndrome is a form of pericarditis complicating MI, also known as post-myocardial infarction syndrome and post-cardiotomy pericarditis.

General management

Myocardial infarction is diagnosed mainly from clinical features supported by ECG (Fig. 5.10) and changes in serum levels of enzymes termed 'cardiac enzymes' (Box 5.7).

Table 5.8 Killip classification of acute myocardial infarction

Killip class	Defining features	Mortality rate (%)
I	No clinical signs of heart failure	6
II	Rales or crackles in the lungs, an S_3 gallop and elevated jugular venous pressure	17
II	Frank acute pulmonary oedema	38
IV	Cardiogenic shock or hypotension (systolic blood pressure < 90 mmHg), and evidence of peripheral vasoconstriction (oliguria, cyanosis or sweating)	81

Table 5.9 Serum enzyme level changes after myocardial infarction

Enzyme	Abbreviation	Number of days after MI that maximum rise seen
Troponin T (troponin 1)	TT	0.5–1.0
Creatine kinase MB	CK-MB	1.5
Aspartate transaminase	AST	2.0
Lactic dehydrogenase	LDH	3.0

MI, myocardial infarction.

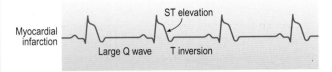

Fig. 5.10 Myocardial infarction electrocardiogram tracings: large Q, ST elevation, inverted T

Box 5.7 Myocardial infarction – diagnosis

- Severe unremitting chest pain
- Collapse
- Changes in heart rate
- Arrhythmias
- Hypotension
- Shock
- Electrocardiogram changes
- Rise in serum 'cardiac' enzymes (see Table 5.9)
- Fever and leukocytosis

Box 5.8 Immediate treatment of myocardial infarction (see Ch.1)

- Alert emergency services (if in community) or cardiac arrest team (if in hospital)
- Aspirin (300 mg); to be chewed. Clopidogrel
- Rest and reassure
- Pain relief: opioid analgesia (diamorphine) is usually necessary, preferably by slow intravenous injection (2 mg/min) or up to 15 mg i.m. according to the size of the patient, plus cyclizine 50 mg. Alternatively, nitrous oxide with at least 28% oxygen should be given to relieve pain and anxiety. Pentazocine is contraindicated as it can cause dysphoria and raises pulmonary arterial pressure. It is less effective than morphine, even when given by injection, but does not relieve and may even increase anxiety
- Oxygen or nitrous oxide with at least 28% oxygen by face mask or intranasally
- Primary percutaneous intervention, or thrombolysis – streptokinase/tissue plasminogen activator (t-PA), alteplase, reteplase or tenecteplase – to dissolve the coronary thrombus provided the patient is not at risk of a life-threatening haemorrhage
- Insulin infusion to prevent a stress hyperglycaemia (high blood sugar level)
- Glyceryl trinitrate infusion to relief pain and prevent pulmonary oedema (fluid accumulation within the lungs)
- Prompt treatment of complications, particularly cardiac arrhythmias, including the initiation of cardiopulmonary resuscitation

In the first few hours, T waves become abnormally tall (hyperacute with the loss of their normal concavity) and ST segments begin to rise. Pathological Q waves may appear within hours or may take longer than 24 h. Thus the characteristic pattern of MI is a normal or raised ST segment, with hyperacute T and acute Q waves (Fig. 5.10). By 24 h, the T wave becomes inverted as the ST elevation begins to resolve. Long-term ECG changes include persistent Q and T waves.

Damaged (infarcted) cardiac muscle releases several enzymes into the blood – troponin T (TT); cardiac-specific creatine kinase (CK-MB), aspartate transaminase (AST) and lactic dehydrogenase (LDH). The earliest changes are in cardiac TT, an enzyme expressed only in the myocardium, not other muscle, and which can be detected in the blood 3–6 h after onset of the chest pain of MI, reaching peak levels within 16–25 h. TT is also useful for the late diagnosis of MI because elevated concentrations can be detected from blood even 5–8 days after onset (Table 5.9).

Myocardial infarction requires immediate hospital admission and treatment (halves the mortality rate). Management aims to relieve pain, limit the myocardial damage (infarct size) and prevent/treat complications. Immediate treatment of MI is shown in Box 5.8 (see also Ch. 1).

Ventricular fibrillation is the most common cause of death and nearly 50% of deaths are in the first hour. Immediate defibrillation and cardiopulmonary resuscitation can be life saving (Ch. 1). In the convalescent stage, ACE inhibitors or beta-blockers, particularly atenolol or metoprolol, can lessen mortality and reduce the risk of recurrence. Early mobilization, a cardiac rehabilitation programme and correction of risk factors for CAD (as in the management of angina) are indicated. Mechanical circulatory support (MCS) may be used for treatment of patients with severe cardiogenic shock, over a period of several days up to months before heart transplantation. A multicentre automatic defibrillator implantation trial II (MADIT II) showed a 30% relative risk reduction in all-cause mortality with the prophylactic use of an automatic implantable cardiac defibrillator (AICD) in patients post-MI. The National Institute for Health and Clinical Excellence (NICE) also recommends the use of AICD in people having survived a cardiac arrest due to either ventricular tachycardia (VT) or ventricular fibrillation (VF).

NON-ST-SEGMENT ELEVATION MYOCARDIAL INFARCTION (NSTEMI)

At least 50% of survivors of attacks of sudden cardiac death have no evidence from the ECG or serum enzyme levels of myocardial damage and the pathogenesis appears not to be the same as in typical MI, so the term non-ST-segment elevation MI (NSTEMI) is used for such acute coronary syndromes. For NSTEMI, glycoprotein IIb/IIIa inhibitors are given.

Dental aspects

Dental intervention after MI can precipitate arrhythmias or aggravate cardiac ischaemia, and this is more likely the more severe the MI, the closer in time to the actual infarct and when there are cardiac complications. The severity of a MI is suggested by the resulting disability, by the length of the acute illness and whether or not the patient was hospitalized; nevertheless, it is important to consult the patient's physician before undertaking operative treatment. In general, patients within 6 months of an MI (recent MI) are at greatest risk of further MI, chest pain or arrhythmias or other complications and have generally been classed as ASA class IV. A level of re-infarction of 50% has been reported in major surgery done during this period; therefore, higher risk procedures such as elective surgery should be deferred. Simple emergency dental treatment under LA may be given during the first 6 months after MI but the opinion of a physician should be sought first. Symptomatic patients with previous older MI (more than 6 months and under 12 months) can normally have elective simple dental care carried out safely, but it is wise to minimize pain and anxiety. Higher risk procedures such as elective surgery may need to be deferred since a level of re-infarction of 20% has been reported in major surgery and about 5% in minor surgery done during this period. Asymptomatic previous but older MI (more than 12 months) patients can normally have elective dental care carried out safely, but it is wise to minimize pain and anxiety. A level of re-infarction of 5% has been reported in major surgery done during this period.

The level of risk will depend on the type of intervention; surgery is a higher risk than conservative dentistry. Anxiety and pain must be minimized, and the physician may advocate pre-operative use of GTN. Effective LA, possibly supplemented with relative analgesia, and monitoring of BP, ECG, pulse and oxygen saturation are indicated. There must be ready access to oxygen and medical help. Dental procedures should be stopped if there is chest pain, dyspnoea, a rise in heart rate of 40 beats/min or more, a rise in the ST-segment displacement of above 0.2 mV on ECG, arrhythmias, or a rise in systolic BP > 20 mmHg.

Heart block resulting from damage to the conduction tissues by an MI may necessitate insertion of a cardiac pacemaker and result in other complications, as discussed later.

The incidence of MI after GA in patients with documented pre-operative MI is up to eight times that of patients with no previous history. Nearly 30% of patients having a GA within 3 months of an infarct have another in the first post-operative week and at least 50% die. Elective surgery under GA should therefore be postponed for at least 3 months and preferably a year since the prognosis of recurrent MI is also influenced by the time after the first attack.

After mechanical circulatory support, management is complicated by a combination of anticoagulant and antiplatelet medication, and sometimes increased risk of thromboembolic events and infections. Elective interventions should be postponed.

Patients with automatic implantable cardioverter defibrillators do not need antibiotic cover to prevent endocarditis. Adrenaline/epinephrine or other vasoconstrictors should be used with caution (lower dose and careful monitoring) in patients with AICDs and there are certain procedures where interference with an AICD is likely (especially MRI), or a possibility (Table 5.10).

HYPERTENSION

General aspects

Hypertension is a persistently raised blood pressure. The BP is the product of cardiac output and peripheral resistance and is dependent on the heart and vasculature, autonomic nervous system, endocrine system and kidneys. In general, the BP rises with age. Regulatory mechanisms, though unclear, involve baroreceptors in various organs that detect changes in BP,

Table 5.10 Automatic implantable cardiac defibrillator (AICD) interference with medical/dental procedures

Procedures that are safe from interfering with AICD	Procedures where interference with AICD can be reduced when safety measures are taken	Procedures where interference with an AICD is *likely*
Diagnostic radiographs, CT (or CAT) scans. If the ICD is placed in the upper chest area, the radiography equipment may be adjusted to lessen pressure on the defibrillator Dental procedures and equipment such as dental drills, ultrasonic scalers or endosonic instruments, and dental radiographs Fluoroscopy	Transcutaneous electrical nerve stimulation (TENS) Ultrasound for diagnostic or therapeutic purposes: keep the transducer head 10 in (25 cm) from the defibrillator	**MRI is contraindicated** for a person with a defibrillator. Even when the MRI scanner is turned off, a strong magnetic field surrounds it and may affect a defibrillator External defibrillation – if needed, the health care professional should not place the paddles directly over the defibrillator Diathermy, electrocautery, lithotripsy, radiation therapy

CAT, computed axial tomography; CT, computed tomography; ICD, implantable cardiac defibrillator; MRI, magnetic resonance imaging.

and adjust it by altering both the heart rate and force of contractions, as well as the peripheral resistance. Other factors are the kidney renin–angiotensin system, which responds to BP fall by activating the vasoconstrictor angiotensin II, and the adrenocortical release of aldosterone in response to angiotensin II, causing fluid retention via the kidney – increasing sodium retention and potassium excretion. The most potent vasoconstrictor is endothelin-1, released by vascular endothelium in response to expansion of plasma volume, hypoxia or growth factors, and which regulates vascular tone. Nitric oxide (NO) modulates vasodilator tone in the control of BP.

The BP is lowest at night and highest first thing in the morning. Since the BP rises with anxiety, measurements should be made with the patient relaxed and fully at rest. The BP is measured with a sphygmomanometer (Box 5.9), in units of millimetres of mercury (mmHg).

Box 5.9 Manual technique for recording blood pressure

1 Alcohol and smoking should be avoided for 30 min before measurement
2 Allow the patient to sit at rest for as long as possible
3 Place sphygmomanometer cuff on right upper arm with about 3 cm of skin visible at the antecubital fossa: the bladder should encircle at least two-thirds of the arm
4 Palpate right brachial pulse
5 After 5 min, inflate the cuff slowly to about 200–250 mmHg, or until the pulse is no longer palpable
6 Deflate cuff slowly while listening with stethoscope over the brachial artery over skin on inside of arm below cuff
7 Record the systolic pressure as the pressure when the first tapping sounds appear (Korotkoff sounds)
8 Deflate cuff further until the tapping sounds become muffled (diastolic pressure) and then disappear
9 Repeat; record blood pressure as systolic/diastolic pressures

---

Hypertension may be defined as an elevated BP of at least 140/90 mmHg, based on at least two readings on separate occasions. Indeed, the Seventh Report of the Joint National Committee on Prevention, Detection, Evaluation, and Treatment of High Blood Pressure in 2003 defined a BP of 120/80 to 139/89 mmHg as pre-hypertension – a designation chosen to identify individuals at high risk of developing hypertension. The National Heart, Lung and Blood Institute (NHLBI) has even recommended 'pre-hypertension' to begin when BP is 115/75 mmHg. The BP will vary depending on age, gender, ethnicity, environment, emotional state and activity. The BP tends to increase with age.

Some 40% of adults in the developed world have hypertension but in more than 90% the cause is unknown and this is then termed 'primary', 'idiopathic' or 'essential' hypertension. In 1–2% of hypertensive patients, an identifiable cause is present and this is termed 'secondary' hypertension. Aetiological factors are shown in Table 5.11.

Lifestyle factors that can raise the BP include stress, obesity, salt intake, smoking, alcohol, illicit drugs (cocaine, amphetamines) or prescribed drugs (immunosuppressives, glucocorticoids, mineralocorticoids, anabolic steroids) but other factors can lower the BP (Table 5.12).

Table 5.11 Causes of hypertension

Secondary hypertension	Idiopathic (essential) hypertension
Renal disease (80% of cases) – renal artery disease, pyelonephritis, glomerulonephritis, polycystic disease, post-transplant	Genetic predisposition High alcohol intake High salt intake; not widely accepted High basal metabolic index (BMI) Insulin resistance Sympathetic overactivity: 40% of hypertensive patients have raised catecholamines (adrenaline/epinephrine and norepinephrine)
Endocrine conditions — pregnancy, Cushing syndrome and corticosteroid therapy, hyperaldosteronism, phaeochromocytoma, acromegaly	
Cerebral disease — cerebral oedema (mainly strokes, head injuries or tumours)	
Coarctation of aorta Hypertension in upper half of body only	
Drugs — oral contraceptive pill; corticosteroids, non-steroidal anti-inflammatory drugs Liquorice	
Sleep apnoea	

Table 5.12 Lifestyle risk factors modifying hypertension

Factors raising blood pressure	Factors lowering blood pressure
Obesity	No obesity
High dietary salt intake	Low salt intake
Excess alcohol	Low alcohol intake
Smoking	Stopping smoking
Excessive physical inactivity	Physical activity
Stress/anxiety	Relaxation
	High-fibre diet
	Omega-3 fatty acids
	Fruit and vegetables
	Supplemental potassium

Long-standing hypertension accelerates atheroma and predisposes to: coronary artery disease; cerebrovascular disease; chronic kidney disease (hypertensive nephrosclerosis is the term given to long-term essential hypertension, hypertensive retinopathy, left ventricular hypertrophy, minimal proteinuria and progressive renal insufficiency); peripheral vascular disease and hypertensive retinopathy leading to retinal haemorrhages, retinopathy or optic neuropathy and blindness. Hypertension shortens life by 10–20 years. The risk of these sequelae is greater in people who also have diabetes and cardiac or renal disease.

Clinical features

At least one-third of people who are hypertensive are asymptomatic or have only trivial complications such as epistaxes. Hypertension however, affects the brain, heart, eyes and kidneys, with complications that include particularly coronary artery disease, MI and heart failure (Table 5.13).

General management

Hypertension is diagnosed by standardized serial BP measurements. Investigations to identify a 'secondary' cause and assess end-organ damage include: chest radiography (cardiomegaly is suggestive of hypertensive heart disease); ECG (may indicate IHD); serum urea and electrolytes (deranged in hypertensive renal disease and endocrine causes of secondary hypertension); urine Stix testing (blood and protein suggests renal disease).

Acute emotion, particularly anger, fear and anxiety, can cause great rises in catecholamine output and transient rises in BP and should, therefore, be avoided or controlled. Treatment of hypertension reduces the risk of stroke, heart failure and renal failure. It has less of an effect on ischaemic cardiac events. Hypertension and its complications can be modulated by various lifestyle factors (Table 5.13): relaxation, weight loss, high-fibre diet, reduction in salt intake, restricting alcohol consumption, restricting caffeine intake, stopping smoking and taking more exercise. Antihypertensive therapy is used with the goal of using the minimum dose of drugs commensurate with achieving the desired BP, currently optimal at < 140/80 mmHg, and with minimal adverse effects. Therapy is urgently indicated where the systolic pressure exceeds 200 mmHg, or the diastolic 110 mmHg, and is indicated at lower levels particularly if there are vascular complications, diabetes or end-organ damage such as renal impairment. A large number of antihypertensive drugs are available (Table 5.14).

Diuretics such as bendrofluazide, angiotensin-converting enzyme inhibitors such as enalapril or perindopril, and calcium-channel blockers, are now commonly used as first-line antihypertensives. A single agent (monotherapy) is used initially but combination therapy may be needed in more resistant cases for adequate BP control. The most effective drug combinations include a beta-blocker or ACE inhibitor with a diuretic, or a beta-blocker with a calcium antagonist (channel blocker).

Adrenergic inhibitors, particularly beta-blockers such as atenolol, are the usual alternative antihypertensive drugs but may cause bradycardia and should not be used in patients with asthma or chronic obstructive pulmonary disease. Alpha-blockers may also be used. The main drawback of ACE inhibitors is that patients may develop a cough. Calcium-channel blockers can cause peripheral oedema. Adverse effects of antihypertensive treatment can sometimes be troublesome and treatment has to be tailored to each patient's response (Table 5.15).

Table 5.13 Features of advanced hypertension

Symptoms	Signs
Headaches	Hypertension on testing
Visual disorders	Retinal changes
Tinnitus	Left ventricular hypertrophy
Dizziness	Proteinuria
Angina	Haematuria

Table 5.14 Antihypertensive drugs

Antihypertensive agents	Examples
Alpha-adrenergic blockers	Doxazosin, prazosin
Angiotensin-converting enzyme (ACE) inhibitors	Captopril, enalapril, ramipril
Angiotensinogen II receptor blockers (ARBs)	Candesartan, losartan
Beta-adrenergic blockers	Atenolol, propranolol
Calcium-channel blockers	Amlodipine, nifedipine, verapamil, diltiazem
Diuretics	Bendroflumethiazide, indapamide, furosemide, amiloride, spironolactone
Sympatholytics	Clonidine, methyldopa
Vasodilators	Hydralazine, minoxidil

Table 5.15 Adverse effects from antihypertensive and other cardioactive drugs

Group	Comments and adverse effects	Possible oral effects
Alpha-adrenergic blockers	Thrombocytopenia	Dry mouth
Angiotensin-converting (ACE) enzyme inhibitors	First dose may cause sudden fall in blood pressure May impede renal function, especially if NSAIDs also given Cough, angioedema	Burning sensation or ulceration or loss of taste Angioedema Dry mouth Sinusitis with quinapril, lichenoid reactions
Angiotensin II receptor blockers (ARBs)	Generally well tolerated	Facial flushing Taste disturbance Gag reflex Dry mouth Lupoid reactions
Beta-blockers	Bronchospasm Contraindicated in asthma Avoid in heart failure or heart block Muscle weakness Lassitude Disturbed sleep	Dry mouth Lichenoid lesions Paraesthesiae
Calcium-channel blockers	Headache and flushing Swollen legs	Gingival swelling, most with nifedipine (30% are affected) Salivation with nicardipine Angioedema
Centrally acting antihypertensives (largely obsolete)	Cass effects Halmolysis Hepatitis	Dry mouth
Diuretics	Hypovolaemia Electrolyte changes	Dry mouth Erythema multiforme Lichenoid lesions
Potassium-channel blockers	Headache, may cause flushing	Ulceration
Vasodilators	Lupoid reactions	

NSAIDs, non-steroidal anti-inflammatory drugs.

...ELERATED (MALIGNANT) HYPERTENSION

...rated hypertension typically affects young adults, espe-...lly those of African or Afro-Caribbean heritage and, like essential hypertension, often causes no symptoms until complications develop. It may present with headaches, visual impairment, nausea, vomiting, fits (seizures) or acute cardiac failure. The chief complication is severe ischaemic damage to the kidneys and renal failure, which can be fatal within 1 year of diagnosis. Other causes of death are cardiac failure or cerebrovascular accidents. Life-threatening accelerated hypertension requires urgent hospital admission with the aim to reduce the BP slowly with oral antihypertensives. Rarely, intravenous antihypertensives (sodium nitroprusside) are used but a sudden drop in BP may result in a stroke (cerebral infarction). Vigorous treatment, if started before renal damage is too far advanced, can greatly improve the life expectancy. About 50% of such patients can now expect to live for at least 5 years.

Dental aspects of hypertension

Blood pressure should be controlled before elective dental treatment or the opinion of a physician should be sought first (Table 5.16).

Dental management can be complicated, since the BP rises even before a visit for dental care; pre-operative reassurance is important and sedation using temazepam may be helpful. Endogenous adrenaline/epinephrine levels peak during the morning hours and adverse cardiac events are most likely in the early morning. Patients therefore are best treated in the late morning. Patients with stable hypertension may receive dental care in short, minimally stressful appointments. It is essential to avoid

anxiety and pain, since endogenous adrenaline/epinephrine released in response to pain or fear may induce arrhythmias. Adequate analgesia must be provided. Both the pain threshold and tolerance are higher in hypertensive than normotensive subjects; the mechanism is unclear but drug treatment of the hypertension normalizes the pain perception. An aspirating syringe should be used to give a LA, since epinephrine (adrenaline) in the anaesthetic given intravenously may (theoretically) increase hypertension and precipitate arrhythmias. Blood pressure tends to rise during oral surgery under LA, and epinephrine (adrenaline) theoretically can contribute to this, but this is usually of little practical importance. Under most circumstances, the use of adrenaline/epinephrine in combination with LA is not contraindicated in the hypertensive patient unless the systolic pressure is over 200 mmHg and/or the diastolic is over 115 mmHg. Epinephrine (adrenaline)-containing LA should not be given in large doses to patients taking beta-blockers, since interactions between adrenaline/epinephrine and the beta-blocking agent may induce hypertension and cardiovascular complications. Lidocaine should be used with caution in patients taking beta-blockers. Adrenaline/epinephrine effects may be reversed in patients taking alpha-blockers causing vasodilation. Gingival retraction cords containing adrenaline/epinephrine should be avoided.

Conscious sedation may be advisable to control anxiety. Continuous BP monitoring is indicated. Raising the patient suddenly from the supine position may cause postural hypotension and loss of consciousness if the patient is using antihypertensive drugs such as thiazides, furosemide or a calcium-channel blocker.

All antihypertensive drugs are potentiated by GA agents, which can induce dangerous hypotension. Intravenous barbiturates in particular can be dangerous in patients on antihypertensive therapy, but halothane, enflurane and isoflurane may also cause hypotension in patients on beta-blockers. However, antihypertensive drugs should not be stopped, since rebound hypertension can result, and the risks of cerebrovascular accidents and cardiovascular instability that result from withdrawal of antihypertensive medication and rebound hypertension outweigh the dangers of drug interactions, which to some extent are predictable and manageable by an expert anaesthetist. Therefore, antihypertensive treatment is usually maintained, but the management of such patients is a matter for the specialist anaesthetist in hospital. A severely reduced blood supply to vital organs can be dangerous even in a normal person, but in the chronically hypertensive patient the tissues have become adapted to the raised blood pressure, which becomes essential (hence the term 'essential hypertension') to overcome the resistance of the vessels and maintain adequate perfusion. A fall in blood pressure below the critical level needed for adequate perfusion of vital organs, particularly kidneys, can therefore be fatal. Hypertension may be a contraindication to GA if complicated by cardiac failure, coronary or cerebral artery insufficiency or renal insufficiency. Chronic administration of some diuretics such as furosemide may lead to potassium deficiency, which should, therefore, be checked pre-operatively in order to avoid arrhythmias and increased sensitivity to muscle relaxants such as curare, gallamine and pancuronium.

The management of hypertensive patients may also be complicated by disease such as cardiac or renal failure. Systemic

---

Table 5.16 Hypertension; ASA (American Society of Anesthesiologists) grading and dental management considerations

Blood pressure (mmHg; systolic, diastolic)	ASA grade	Hypertension stage	Dental aspects
< 140, < 90	I	–	Routine dental care
140–159, 90–99	II	1	Recheck BP before starting routine dental care
160–179, 95–109	III	2	Recheck BP and seek medical advice before routine dental care Restrict use of adrenaline/epinephrine Conscious sedation may help
> 180, > 110	IV	3	Recheck BP after 5 min quiet rest Medical advice before dental care Only emergency care until BP controlled Avoid vasoconstrictors

BP, blood pressure.

corticosteroids may raise the blood pressure and antihypertensive treatment may have to be adjusted accordingly. Some NSAIDs (indometacin, ibuprofen and naproxen) can reduce the efficacy of antihypertensive agents.

There are no recognized oral manifestations of hypertension but facial palsy is an occasional complication of malignant hypertension. Antihypertensive drugs can sometimes cause orofacial side-effects, such as xerostomia, salivary gland swelling or pain, lichenoid reactions, erythema multiforme, angioedema, gingival swelling, sore mouth or paraesthesiae (Table 5.15). Clonidine in particular can cause xerostomia.

HYPOTENSION

Hypotension is uncommon but can have many causes (Table 5.17). Raising the patient suddenly from the supine position may cause postural (orthostatic) hypotension and loss of consciousness.

Table 5.17 Causes of orthostatic hypotension

Primary autonomic causes	Secondary autonomic causes	Non-autonomic causes
Familial dysautonomia (Riley–Day syndrome)	B vitamin deficiency	Hypovolaemia
Pure autonomic failure (idiopathic orthostatic hypotension)	Alcoholism	Ageing
Shy–Drager syndrome	Diabetes	Prolonged bed rest
Dopamine	Parkinsonism	Pregnancy
Beta-hydroxylase deficiency	Porphyria	Drugs (e.g. antihypertensives)

CARDIOMYOPATHIES

General aspects

Cardiomyopathy means (from the Latin), a heart muscle disease; alcoholism is the most common of the many causes. Extrinsic or specific cardiomyopathies include those associated with coronary artery disease; congenital heart disease; nutritional diseases; hypertension; valvular cardiac disease; inflammatory diseases; or systemic metabolic disease. Intrinsic cardiomyopathy has a number of causes including *drug* and *alcohol* toxicity, certain *infections* (including *hepatitis* C), and various *genetic* and *idiopathic* causes. Four separate and distinct types of intrinsic cardiomyopathy are recognized (Box 5.10).

Box 5.10 Intrinsic cardiomyopathies

- Arrhythmogenic right ventricular cardiomyopathy (ARVC)
- Dilated cardiomyopathy (DCM)
- Hypertrophic cardiomyopathy (HCM)
- Restrictive cardiomyopathy (RCM), the least common form, can be idiopathic or secondary to radiation therapy or to rare disorders such as endomyocardial fibrosis (tropical hypereosinophic syndrome), infiltrative disorders (amyloidosis, sarcoidosis), and metabolic disorders (Gaucher disease, mucopolysaccharidoses, Fabry disease, carcinoid syndrome)

Most affected individuals have a normal quality and duration of life. A minority, however, have significant symptoms and there is sometimes a risk of sudden death. People with cardiomyopathy are at risk from arrhythmias and sudden cardiac death.

Clinical features

Frequently, there are no symptoms until complications develop. Congestive cardiac failure with atrial fibrillation or other serious complications (mitral regurgitation, angina, sudden death or infective endocarditis) can result. Exercise-induced sudden death is a constant risk.

General management

Medical care prolongs life to a variable degree and aims to ameliorate symptoms.

Medication, implanted pacemakers, defibrillators or ventricular assist devices (VADs), ablation or transplantation often become necessary.

Dental aspects

Adrenaline/epinephrine should be used in limited amounts, and nitroglycerin or similar drugs are contraindicated. If angina pectoris, myocardial infarction or fibrillation occurs, oxygen should be given and preparations made to perform cardiopulmonary resuscitation and to activate the emergency response system.

Conscious sedation with nitrous oxide and oxygen may be used if necessary, with the approval of the physician. Patients with cardiomyopathy are a poor risk for GA because of alcoholism, arrhythmias, cardiac failure or myocardial ischaemia.

ARRHYTHMIAS (DYSRHYTHMIAS)

Normally, the heart chambers (atria and ventricles) contract in a coordinated manner initiated by an electrical signal in the sinoatrial node (sinus node or SA node), a small mass of heart tissue with characteristics of both muscle and nerve located in the right atrial wall. The electrical signal is conducted through the atria, stimulating them to contract, and then passes through the atrioventricular node (AV node), where the impulse transmission to the ventricles is delayed transiently while the atria complete their contraction (consistent with the P wave on the ECG) and empty their blood into the ventricles (these are already partially filled with blood which had passively drained from the large veins – vena cava on the right side and the pulmonary veins on the left side – into the atria during diastole). Once the impulse leaves the AV node, it descends in the interventricular septum via the bundle of His and reaches the Purkinje fibres of the ventricle walls, causing them to contract (i.e. the ventricular component of systole) as noted on the ECG by the presence of the QRS complex.

Following excitation and depolarization, the conductive tissue repolarizes to be ready for the next pulse. In adults, the heart beats regularly and the resting rate ranges from 60 to 100 beats per minute. In children the rate is much faster.

General and clinical aspects

Arrhythmia is a term for any of a large and heterogeneous group of conditions in which there is abnormal electrical activity in the heart. However, sinus arrhythmia is not a true arrhythmia but a normal phenomenon of mild acceleration and slowing of the heart rate that occurs with breathing in and out; it is usually quite pronounced in children, and lessens with age.

Up to 15% of the population have arrhythmias: the heart beat may be too fast or too slow, and may be regular or irregular. Extrasystoles are the most common arrhythmia. Arrhythmias may be provoked by stress or catecholamines, or some illegal, prescription and over-the-counter drugs, as well as alcohol, tobacco, foods and other substances (Table 5.18).

Table 5.18 Arrhythmia-inducing drugs and foods

Tachycardias	Bradycardias	Other arrhythmias
Alcohol	Beta-blockers	Alcohol
Atropine	Calcium channel blockers	Amphetamines
Caffeine	Digitalis	Atropine
Epinephrine (adrenaline)	Morphine	Cocaine
Nicotine		Digitalis
		Adrenaline/epinephrine Procainamide Quinidine Tricyclics

Arrhythmias may also arise from cardiac, respiratory, autonomic or endocrine disease, fever, hypoxia or electrolyte disturbances. Surgery is sometimes implicated; the trigeminocardiac reflex (TCR), which may be associated with maxillofacial surgery, consists of bradycardia, hypotension, apnoea and gastric hypermotility. Central stimulation of the trigeminal can cause reflex bradycardic responses during maxillofacial or ocular surgical procedures or neurosurgery, but some have followed oral or perioral procedures. The parasympathetic supply to the face is carried in the trigeminal nerve; alternative afferent pathways must exist via the maxillary and/or mandibular divisions, in addition to the commonly reported pathway via the ophthalmic division of the trigeminal in the classic oculocardiac reflex. The efferent arc involves the vagus.

Cardiac surgery may also be followed by arrhythmias: junctional ectopic tachycardia is then the most common arrhythmia, presumed to be initiated from a small focus of abnormal automaticity somewhere in the AV node or bundle of His.

Thus the significance of arrhythmias varies from the fatal to inconsequential (Table 5.19), some being regarded as variants of normal, others may be merely annoying – such as an abnormal awareness of heartbeat (palpitations). Some reduce cardiac efficiency and output and cause palpitations with dyspnoea, angina or syncope; some are life-threatening and can lead to cardiac arrest; and others cause no symptoms but still predispose to potentially life-threatening complications such as stroke and transient ischaemic attacks.

Table 5.19 Arrhythmias of different level of risk to the patient

USUAL LEVEL OF RISK			
High	**Medium**	**Low**	**None**
Atrial fibrillation	Atrial arrhythmias which are symptomatic or under treatment	Atrial arrhythmias which are asymptomatic and not under treatment	Bradycardia in athletes
Bradycardia plus other arrhythmia	Drug-induced arrhythmias	Premature ventricular beats	Extrasystoles (atrial)
Bradycardia plus pacemaker	Pacemaker		
Irregular pulse ventricular extrasystoles	Paroxysmal supraventricular tachycardia		
Irregular pulse plus bradycardia	Ventricular arrhythmias which are symptomatic or under treatment		
Tachycardia plus other arrhythmia			
Ventricular fibrillation			
Ventricular tachycardia			
Wolf–Parkinson–White syndrome			

Types of arrhythmia

Extrasystoles (ectopics) are essentially extra beats, or contractions, which occur when there is electrical discharge from somewhere in the heart other than the SA node. Extrasystoles in themselves usually do not cause any problems but they can sometimes be a feature of cardiac disease. Also, extrasystoles occurring during exercise and in the recovery period after exercise, *in people with otherwise apparently normal hearts*, can have some increased mortality risk.

Atrial extrasystoles (premature atrial contractions; PACs) are common in healthy people with normal hearts, especially with advancing age, but can also occur when there is increased pressure on the atria such as in cardiac failure or mitral valve disease and, in such cases, may occur prior to the development of atrial fibrillation. They are exacerbated by alcohol and caffeine (as a former UK Prime Minister found!) (see Table 5.18). Atrial extrasystoles may be of little consequence.

Ventricular extrasystoles occur when the discharge arises from the ventricles and, though they can occur in people with normal hearts, they are more commonly found in those with heart disease. Ventricular extrasystoles are the commonest type of arrhythmia arising after myocardial infarction and may also occur in severe left ventricular hypertrophy, hypertrophic cardiomyopathy and congestive cardiac failure. Ventricular extrasystoles usually have no significance but, rarely, they may induce ventricular fibrillation and can cause sudden cardiac death. The British Heart Foundation in 2005 stated that ventricular ectopics, in the absence of structural heart disease or a family history of sudden death, are benign and do not require specialist intervention or specific drug therapy.

Arrhythmias may be classified by rate (tachycardia, bradycardia), mechanism (automaticity, re-entry, fibrillation) or site of origin.

Tachycardias

Tachycardia is a heart rate faster than 100 beats per minute. It may result in palpitation, but is not *necessarily* an arrhythmia. *Sinus tachycardia* is an increased heart rate as a normal response to exercise or emotional stress, mediated by the sympathetic nervous system and catecholamines on the SA node. Hyperthyroidism and ingested or injected substances such as caffeine, cocaine, ectasy, amphetamines, or caffeine can produce or exaggerate this effect.

Supraventricular tachycardias

Tachycardia can also result from the addition of abnormal impulses to the normal cardiac cycle by automaticity, re-entry or by triggered activity. Automaticity refers to a cardiac muscle cell firing off an impulse on its own and it can be provoked by hypoxia or the sympathetic nervous system and catecholamines. Only the specialized cells of the 'conduction system' (the SA node, AV node, bundle of His and Purkinje fibres) can usually cause such an impulse. The SA node has a higher automaticity (a faster pacemaker) than the rest of the heart, and therefore is usually the one to start this type of tachycardia. An ectopic focus can also produce a sustained abnormal rhythm.

Re-entry arrhythmias occur when an electrical impulse travels in a circle within the heart, rather than moving outward and then stopping, and can produce a sustained abnormal rhythm, such as atrial flutter, supraventricular tachycardia, ventricular tachycardia or, when an entire chamber of the heart is involved in multiple micro-re-entry circuits, it is said to fibrillate.

Triggered activity is caused by after-depolarizations that reach activation threshold. This can be a mechanism for atrial and ventricular arrhythmias. It is related to the flow of calcium in and out of cells and sometimes responds to calcium-channel blockers.

Atrioventricular nodal re-entrant tachycardia is the most common cause of paroxysmal supraventricular tachycardia (PSVT) and occurs most often in young people and infants. Risks include excessive smoking, caffeine and alcohol use, and digitalis toxicity. PSVT may remit spontaneously but can recur. Electrical cardioversion (shock) is successful in conversion of PSVT to a normal sinus rhythm in many other cases. Another way to convert a PSVT rapidly is to administer adenosine or verapamil.

Other supraventricular tachycardias are due to accessory pathways. If this pathway conducts anterogradely and can be seen on the 12-lead ECG, it is called Wolff–Parkinson–White (WPW) syndrome – a syndrome of ventricular pre-excitation due to an accessory conduction pathway (the bundle of Kent). It can cause both narrow and broad complex tachycardias via

a re-entrant mechanism. It is associated with atrial fibrillation, which can result in a very rapid tachycardia and, in rare instances, result in ventricular fibrillation. Radiofrequency ablation is the treatment of choice.

Atrial fibrillation (AF) is common, with a prevalence of 0.5–1.0% in the general population. This is tenfold greater in those over 65, however. AF is a common end point for many cardiac diseases that cause atrial myocyte damage and fibrosis, but can be part of the ageing process. AF is associated with thrombus formation, particularly in the left atrial appendage. Both aspirin and warfarin have been shown to reduce the consequent stroke risk but a patient's absolute risk depends on other risk factors like age, left ventricular function, hypertension and previous thromboembolic event. After managing stroke risk, the basis of treatment of AF is either to control the ventricular rate with drugs that block the AV node or to try to maintain sinus rhythm.

Ventricular tachycardias

Ventricular tachycardia is usually the result of structural heart disease, most commonly related to previous myocardial infarction and is dangerous as it can result in chest pain, cardiac failure, syncope or ventricular fibrillation. Ventricular fibrillation is the most serious arrhythmia and the most common cause of sudden death, typically a consequence of myocardial infarction or structural heart disease, occasionally of idiopathic fibrosis affecting the conduction mechanism, thyrotoxicosis, halothane anaesthesia, or adrenaline/epinephrine, cocaine or digitalis overdosage. Ventricular fibrillation is effectively a type of cardiac arrest and is imminently life threatening.

Bradycardias

Bradycardia is a slow cardiac rhythm (< 60 beats per minute). This may be caused by a slowed electrical signal from the SA node (sinus bradycardia), a pause in the normal activity of the SA node (sinus arrest), or blocking of the impulse between the atria and ventricles (AV block or heart block). Mild heart block may only be detectable as PR prolongation on an EGG (first-degree heart block). Second-degree heart block (Type 1 second-degree heart block (Mobitz I or Wenckebach) or Type 2 second-degree heart block (Mobitz II) may be symptomatic. Third-degree heart block (complete heart block), when the ventricle contracts at its intrinsic rate of about 30–40 per minute, causes severely reduced cardiac output with pallor or cyanosis, dyspnoea and syncopal (Stokes–Adams) attacks. Among the more common causes of heart block are IHD, drugs (especially digitalis), surgery, connective tissue disorders, including Sjögren syndrome and, in the past, rheumatic fever.

Bradycardia may be unimportant in a young person and is often found in athletes. Bradycardia in an older person, however, especially when associated with heart disease, can cause sudden loss of consciousness (syncope).

General management of arrhythmias

Although palpation of pulse and cardiac auscultation may help, an ECG is the best way to diagnose and assess the risk of any given arrhythmia.

Supraventricular tachycardias can often be slowed or stopped by physical manoeuvres (vagal manoeuvres, such as pressure on the neck), which increase parasympathetic stimulation to the heart, thereby inhibiting electrical conduction through the AV node. Most tachycardias respond well to antiarrhythmic drugs (Table 5.20 and Appendix 5.3). Cardiac ablation, defibrillation or cardioversion may otherwise be needed (see later; Table 5.21). Anticoagulants (warfarin and heparins) and antiplatelet drugs (e.g. aspirin) are often also used to reduce the risk of clotting.

Table 5.20   Antiarrhythmic agents

| Type of arrhythmia | EXAMPLES OF DRUGS USED | |
	Main	Others
Supraventricular	Verapamil	Adenosine, digoxin, beta-blockers
Supraventricular and ventricular	Disopyramide	Amiodarone, beta-blockers, flecainide, procainamide, propafenone
Ventricular	Lidocaine	Mexiletine, moracizine

Catheter ablation is the treatment of choice for most simple arrhythmias and also has an important role with more complex rhythm disorders (e.g. atrial fibrillation and ventricular tachycardia). Catheter ablation uses flexible catheters introduced under radiographic guidance via the blood vessels and directed to the heart to destroy cardiac tissue that gives rise to abnormal electrical signals causing arrhythmias. A burst of radiofrequency energy or cautery with heat, cold, electrical or laser probes allows abnormal areas of conduction to be located and destroyed.

Electric shock across the heart (defibrillation or cardioversion), either externally to the chest or internally to the heart via implanted electrodes, may be needed.

Defibrillation is the application of a shock that is *not synchronized*; it is needed for the chaotic rhythm of ventricular fibrillation and for pulseless ventricular tachycardia. *Cardioversion* is the application of a shock *synchronized* to the underlying heartbeat and is used for treatment of supraventricular tachycardias, such as atrial tachycardia, including atrial fibrillation.

Defibrillation or cardioversion may also be accomplished by an automatic *implantable cardioverter–defibrillator*, an electronic device that is the most successful treatment to prevent ventricular fibrillation and 99% effective in stopping life-threatening arrhythmias. An AICD continuously monitors the heart rhythm, automatically functions as a pacemaker for heart rates that are too slow, and delivers life-saving shocks if a dangerous rhythm is detected. Because AICDs must be built to both pace and deliver shocks, they are larger than pacemakers and their batteries do not last as long.

Bradycardias may be treated by cardiac pacing with a pacemaker – a small implanted electronic device which has a pulse generator and one (monopolar) or, more usually now, two (bipolar) electrode leads and is powered by lithium batteries. Modern pacemakers are bipolar, implanted transvenously

Table 5.21   Treatment of arrhythmias

Heart rhythm changes	Usual treatments
Atrial fibrillation (AF)	Cardioversion Digoxin Anticoagulants advocated
Atrial tachycardia	–
Bradycardia (pathological)	Atropine may be indicated May need a pacemaker
Extrasystoles	–
Paroxysmal supraventricular tachycardia (SVT)	Vagal pressure or intravenous adenosine Cardiac glycosides or verapamil may be needed
Sinus tachycardia	–
Ventricular fibrillation (VF)	Defibrillation For acute VF, flecainide and disopyramide are indicated. Lidocaine is the usual treatment but bretyllium, or mexilitine, may be required Implantable cardioverter defibrillators may be used
Ventricular tachycardia	Cardioversion Lidocaine
Wolff–Parkinson–White syndrome	Medications, or catheter ablation to destroy the abnormal pathway

via the subclavian or cephalic vein and typically sited in the right ventricle, or on the chest wall either within the pectoral muscle or underneath the skin, or in the abdominal wall. Most work mainly on demand and are rate-adaptive and can be programmed to adjust the rate of heartbeat by tracking sinus node activity or by responding to sensors that monitor body motion and depth or rate of respiration. Adjustments to the pacemaker can be made non-invasively, using a specially designed radiofrequency programmer, with a wand placed on the skin over the implanted device. Pacemakers and batteries last for 6–10 years. Patients should carry a pacemaker registration card bearing details of the make and model.

Interference with pacemakers/defibrillators

High-frequency external electromagnetic radiation, ionizing radiation, ultrasonic and electromagnetic interference from a wide range of sources can interfere with the sensing function of pacemakers and of implantable cardioverter–defibrillators, and may induce fibrillation (Table 5.22).

The responses of the pacemaker to interference are varied, and usually temporary. They are only seen while the patient remains in the range of the source of interference; moving away from the source of interference will usually return the pacemaker to normal behaviour. The response largely depends on the interference signal characteristics and includes a single-beat inhibition (where the pacemaker may not pace the heart for a single cardiac cycle), total inhibition (where the pacemaker ceases to pace the heart), asynchronous pacing (where the pacemaker paces the heart at a fixed rate), rate rise or erratic pacing rate. In extreme cases, where the interference

Table 5.22 Sources of possible interference with cardiac pacemaker function

Sources	Electrically coupled	Magnetic	Galvanic	Ultrasonic	Ionizing radiation
Medical	Electrical appliances – particularly those with large motors and/or large power supplies. Problems more likely if appliance is in poor working condition, with motors or relays that are arcing or sparking	Magnetic resonance imaging (MRI)	Defibrillation/cardioversion Electrocautery Diathermy TENS (transcutaneous electrical nerve stimulation)	Ultrasound equipment (see text) Lithotripsy	Radiotherapy
Non-medical	Gasoline (petrol)-powered lawn mowers Gasoline (petrol)-powered saws High-voltage power lines Ham radios Arc welders Cellular (mobile) phones High-power automobile ignition systems Metal detectors	Close proximity to powerful and large loudspeakers Induction furnaces, such as those used in the steel industry Large generators, such as those used in the power industry Electromagnets of the type used in car-wrecking yards	Workplace situations (e.g. in the electrical/computer manufacturing industry) Domestic situations (e.g. current leakage due to defective or poorly maintained house or appliance wiring)	Ultrasound equipment	Ionizing radiation sources
Comments	Interference requires no direct contact with the patient[a]	Interference requires no direct contact with the patient[a]	Interference requires that the pacemaker patient be in direct contact with an electrical current[a] Disengaging contact from the source of interference will usually return the pacemaker to normal behaviour		

[a]The likelihood of interference from these sources of interference increases with the strength of the source and with the proximity of the pacemaker to the source.

is of a sufficiently high magnitude, it is possible for the pacemaker circuitry to be damaged, leading to persistently abnormal pacing.

Modern bipolar pacemakers have improved titanium-insulated interference-resistant circuitry and the risk of electromagnetic interference is very small. The chief and real hazard is with MRI because of the static magnetic, alternating magnetic and radiofrequency fields (Table 5.22).

Some dental electrical devices capable of generating electromagnetic radiation may pose a low-grade threat to dental patients *but usually only if the devices are placed very close to the pacemaker* (Table 5.23).

The pacemaker's stainless steel metal casing, and some of its components, can trigger security devices, but the pacemaker function is *not* significantly affected. Brief exposure of a pacemaker to electromagnetic antitheft or surveillance devices, typically found in airports, shops and libraries, causes no significant disruption of function. Digital mobile phones, and even television transmitters and faulty or badly earthed equipment, may cause interference, but the risk is very small and only when used close to the pacemaker. For most digital phones and for most pacemakers now in use, electromagnetic interference does not have an effect if the phone is more than about 6 inches from the implanted pacemaker.

Domestic electrical appliances – even remote controls, CB radios, electric blankets, heating pads, shavers, sewing machines, kitchen appliances and microwave ovens – are safe. However, some old microwave ovens (20 years or older) may leak and cause temporary confusion to a pacemaker.

Table 5.23 Oral health care equipment effects on cardiac pacemakers

Procedures where interference is unlikely	Procedures where interference is likely
Amalgamator	Diathermy units
Composite curing lights	Electronic dental analgesia units
Dental chair or light	Electrosurgical units
Dental handpieces	Ferromagnetic (magnetostrictive) ultrasonic scalers
Dental radiography unit	Lithotripsy units
Electric toothbrushes	Magnetic resonance imaging (MRI)
Electronic apex locators	TENS (transcutaneous electrical nerve stimulation) units
Electronic pulp testers	Ultrasonic instrument baths
Microwave ovens	
Piezoelectric ultrasonic scalers	
Sonic scalers	

If a pacemaker does shut off, all possible sources of interference should be switched off and the patient given cardiopulmonary resuscitation in the supine position. Artificial respiration should force the heart to resume its rhythm and the pacemaker to start up again.

An implanted cardioverter defibrillator by contrast will not only trigger airport security alarms but also the use of strong magnets over the device may adversely affect its function and even render it non-operational. Patients with implantable cardioverter–defibrillators do not need antibiotic cover to prevent endocarditis. Adrenaline/epinephrine or other vasoconstrictors should be used with caution (lower dose and careful monitoring) in patients with AICDs.

Dental aspects

Most sudden cardiac arrests come during peak endogenous adrenaline/epinephrine levels (8–11 am) and thus appointments are best made for late morning or early afternoon.

Syncope can result from bradycardia, heart block or atrial tachycardia, and may need to be distinguished from a simple fainting attack by the slowness or irregularity of the pulse. Otherwise the initial treatment is the same.

Ventricular fibrillation is clinically indistinguishable from asystole and is one of the most serious emergencies that may have to be managed in the dental surgery (see Ch. 1). Patients with atrial fibrillation may be treated with anticoagulants, which influence operative care (Ch. 8).

Arrhythmias can be induced, particularly in the elderly and patients with coronary artery disease or aortic stenosis, by:

- manipulation of the neck, carotid sinus or eyes (vagal reflex)
- local analgesia (rarely)
- supraventricular or ventricular ectopics, which may develop during dental extractions or minor pre-prosthetic surgery, but these are rarely significant
- drugs – GA agents, especially halothane (isoflurane is safer), digitalis, and erythromycin or azole antifungal drugs, in patients taking terfenadine, cisapride or astemizole.

An aspirating syringe is advised. Adrenaline/epinephrine accidentally entering a blood vessel may (theoretically) increase hypertension and precipitate arrhythmias. Blood pressure tends to rise during oral surgery under LA, and epinephrine (adrenaline) theoretically can contribute to this but this is usually of little practical importance.

Adequate analgesia is essential. Pain can cause far greater outpouring of endogenous adrenaline/epinephrine than that from the LA.

Vasoconstrictors such as adrenaline/epinephrine or levonordefrin may raise blood pressure or lead to unanticipated atrial or ventricular arrhythmias including fibrillation or even asystole. In large doses they may adversely interact with digoxin, non-selective beta-adrenergic-blocking drugs, antidepressants or cocaine. There appears to be no advantage in using levonordefrin rather than adrenaline/epinephrine.

Adrenaline/epinephrine-containing LA should not be given in large doses to patients taking beta-blockers. Interaction between adrenaline/epinephrine and the beta-blocking agent may induce hypertension and cardiovascular complications. Mepivacaine 3% is thought to be preferable to lidocaine.

Intraosseous or intraligamental injections with LA agents containing vasoconstrictor should usually be avoided to prevent excessive systemic absorption. Gingival retraction cords containing adrenaline/epinephrine should be avoided.

Cardiac pacemakers usually now have two (bipolar) electrode leads and present few problems for dental treatment. In patients with pacemakers, MRI, electrosurgery diathermy and transcutaneous nerve stimulation are contraindicated.

Pacemaker single-beat inhibition of little consequence may occasionally be caused by dental equipment such as piezoelectric ultrasonic scalers and ultrasonic baths, older ferromagnetic ultrasonic scalers, pulp testers, electronic apex locators, dental induction casting machines, belt-driven motors in dental chairs, and older radiography machines. Modern piezoelectric scalers have no significant effect, but activity rate-responsive devices may exhibit faster pacing rates.

The only safe procedure under such circumstances is to avoid the use of all such equipment whenever a patient with a pacemaker is being treated, as it is difficult to assess the level of risk in any individual patient. Patients should be treated in the supine position; electrical equipment kept over 30 cm away; and rapid, repetitive switching of electrical instruments avoided. Diagnostic radiation and ultrasonography have no effect on pacemakers, even with cumulative doses, but faulty equipment may cause problems.

Patients with permanent pacemakers do not need antibiotic cover to prevent endocarditis. If a temporary transvenous pacemaker is present, however, the physician should be consulted first.

Automatic implantable cardiac defibrillators may activate without significant warning, possibly causing the patient to flinch, bite down or perform other sudden movements that may result in injury to the patient or clinician. Some patients with AICDs may lose consciousness when the device is activated. This is less likely with newer devices, which initially emit low-level electrical bursts followed by stronger shocks if cardioversion does not follow immediately. Patients with AICDs do not need antibiotic cover.

Adrenaline/epinephrine or other vasoconstrictors should be used with caution (lower dose and careful monitoring) in patients with pacemakers and AICDs.

Concerning conscious sedation, the physician should decide whether this is acceptable for any given patient. GA is generally to be avoided. If unavoidable, it is a matter for an expert anaesthetist in hospital.

Several anti-arrhythmic drugs can cause oral lesions. Verapamil, enalapril and diltiazem can cause gingival hyperplasia, some beta-blockers may rarely cause lichenoid ulceration and procainamide can cause a lupus-like reaction.

Patients with pacemakers are usually advised to avoid elective dental care within the first few weeks after receiving the pacemaker.

THYROID-RELATED HEART DISEASE (SEE ALSO CH. 6)

General aspects

Hyperthyroidism raises the metabolic rate and activity of the heart, and sensitizes the myocardium to sympathetic activity. The heart may be unable to meet the greater demands resulting from the raised metabolic activity of the rest of the body, particularly in the elderly.

Hypothyroidism slows the metabolic rate and activity of the heart and other tissues.

Clinical features

Untreated thyrotoxicosis causes tachycardia and a tendency to arrhythmias, which can lead to cardiac failure or myocardial infarction, especially in the elderly.

Hypothyroidism slows the heart rate and myxoedema patients may have hypercholesterolaemia associated with atheroma. Ischaemic heart disease often develops but is unusual in that it predominantly affects women.

General management

Beta-blockers are useful to control hyperthyroid heart disease.

Dental aspects

Patients with uncontrolled hyperthyroidism can sometimes be difficult to manage, as a result of heightened anxiety, hyperexcitability and excessive sympathetic activity.

Effective analgesia must be provided. An aspirating syringe should be used to give a LA, and LA-containing adrenaline/epinephrine should in theory be avoided, because of the possible risk of dangerous arrhythmias. However, there seems little clinical evidence for this and the risk is probably real only if an overdose is given. There is no evidence that prilocaine with felypressin is any safer.

Gingival retraction cords containing adrenaline/epinephrine should be avoided.

Conscious sedation preferably with nitrous oxide and oxygen may be beneficial by calming the patient. The same reservations about GA apply to patients with uncontrolled thyroid heart disease as to those with other dangerous heart diseases.

Hypothyroid patients may be at risk in the dental surgery if they have CAD. Sjögren syndrome is occasionally associated. In severe myxoedema, diazepam and other CNS depressants can precipitate coma.

PULMONARY HEART DISEASE (COR PULMONALE)

General aspects

Cor pulmonale is heart disease resulting from the excessive load imposed on the right ventricle by diseases of the lungs or pulmonary circulation, especially chronic obstructive pulmonary (airways) disease (COAD, COPD; Ch. 15).

Clinical features

Right ventricular hypertrophy may lead to right-sided failure with systemic venous congestion and persistent hypoxia. In the early stages, there is dyspnoea, a chronic cough, wheezing and often cyanosis. Later there is also ankle oedema and ascites.

General management

Oxygen, diuretics, vasodilators, salbutamol and ipratropium are among the measures that may be needed.

Dental aspects

Ipratropium can cause a dry mouth.

Local analgesia is the main means of pain control. Conscious sedation with diazepam or midazolam is contraindicated because of their respiratory depressant action in a hypoxic patient. Nitrous oxide and oxygen may be acceptable. Intravenous barbiturates are also contraindicated because of their respiratory depressant effect.

VALVULAR HEART DISEASE
RHEUMATIC FEVER

General aspects

Rheumatic fever sometimes follows a sore throat caused by certain strains of beta-haemolytic streptococci (*Streptococcus pyogenes*). Rheumatic fever is now a very rare disease in the Western world but is common in countries such as the Indian subcontinent, the Middle East and some of the Caribbean islands. Children between 5 and 15 years are predominantly affected.

Rheumatic fever may occasionally be followed by chronic rheumatic carditis with permanent cardiac valvular damage. The inflammatory reaction of rheumatic carditis appears to result from immunological cross-reactivity with streptococcal antigens and immunologically mediated tissue damage, which may lead, after the lapse of years, to fibrosis and distortion of the cardiac valves (chronic rheumatic heart disease).

Clinical features

A sore throat may be followed after about 3 weeks (2–26 weeks) by an acute febrile illness with pain flitting from one joint to another (migratory arthralgia). Usually there is resolution within 6–12 weeks without apparent after-effects. Pain in the large joints (which gives rheumatic fever its name) is conspicuous, but heals without permanent damage in about 3 weeks.

Other effects may include: cerebral involvement – causing spasmodic involuntary movements (Sydenham chorea, St Vitus dance); a characteristic rash (erythema marginatum); lung involvement and subcutaneous nodules (usually around the elbows).

The most serious cardiac complication is subendocardial inflammation, particularly along the lines of closure of the mitral and aortic valve cusps, resulting in the formation of minute fibrinous vegetations and later scarring. There is usually little detectable effect on cardiac function in the acute phase but, in unusually severe cases, myocarditis can cause death from cardiac failure. The essential features of chronic rheumatic heart disease are fibrotic stiffening and distortion of the heart valves, often causing mitral stenosis. This is essentially a mechanical, haemodynamic disorder, in which the defective valves may become infected at any time, leading to infective endocarditis. Cardiac failure can develop, often after many years.

General management

The clinical manifestations of acute rheumatic fever are so variable that the diagnosis is made only if at least two of the major criteria are fulfilled (Table 5.24).

Table 5.24 Rheumatic fever: diagnostic criteria

Major	Minor
Carditis	Pyrexia
Polyarthritis	Arthralgia
Chorea	Previous rheumatic fever
Erythema marginatum	ESR and CRP raised
Subcutaneous nodules	Characteristic ECG changes

CRP, C-reactive protein; ECG, electrocardiogram; ESR, erythrocyte sedimentation rate.

Preceding streptococcal infection is confirmed by a high or rising titre of antistreptolysin O antibodies (ASOT), which is suggestive, but not diagnostic, of rheumatic fever, but a low ASOT virtually excludes the diagnosis.

Streptococcal sore throat is an indication for treatment with antibiotics, usually penicillin. Prompt antimicrobial treatment (within 24 h of onset) prevents the development of rheumatic fever in most cases. Complications such as cardiac failure are treated along conventional lines. Chorea may recur during pregnancy or in patients taking the contraceptive pill, but does not indicate recurrent carditis.

After an attack of rheumatic carditis, there is a risk of recurrence and continuous antibiotic prophylaxis becomes necessary to lessen the risk of permanent cardiac damage. The drug of choice is usually oral phenoxymethyl penicillin until the age of 20. For those allergic to penicillin, sulfadimidine should be given.

In the past, approximately 60% of children who survived acute rheumatic fever developed a cardiac lesion detectable after 10 years, but heart failure frequently took 10 or more years to develop. However, such complications have become increasingly rare in the developed world and chronic rheumatic heart disease is only likely to be seen now in the middle-aged and some immigrants. The mitral valve is usually affected, either alone (60–70%), or with the aortic valve in a further 20%. The aortic valve alone is affected in only 10%. Valve narrowing (stenosis) and regurgitation (incompetence) are associated in varying degrees. The earliest sign of valve damage is a murmur. Later effects, particularly enlargement of the heart, may be detected clinically, radiographically and by ECG and echocardiography changes. Treatment is by mitral balloon valvuloplasty, using an Inoue balloon.

Dental aspects

Acute rheumatic fever patients are exceedingly unlikely to be seen during an attack but emergency dental treatment may be necessary. Most patients with chronic rheumatic fever are anticoagulated; treatment can be done under LA in consultation with the physician. Conscious sedation with nitrous oxide may be given if cardiac function is good and with the approval of the physician.

KAWASAKI DISEASE (MUCOCUTANEOUS LYMPH NODE SYNDROME)

General aspects

Kawasaki disease is an acute febrile illness with lymphadenopathy and desquamation of lips, fingers and toes, simulating scarlet fever and erythema multiforme. It is now a considerably more common cause of severe childhood heart disease in many countries than rheumatic fever. It is considerably more prevalent in Japanese and Korean people.

Although an infection is probably causal, presumably in persons of certain genetic backgrounds, no agent has yet been consistently isolated. Superantigens (bacterial toxins that stimulate T lymphocytes) are another possible cause. The main pathological process is a widespread vasculitis, which can, in approximately 25%, affect the coronary arteries – with aneurysm formation.

Clinical features

Eighty per cent of affected children are aged less than 5 years, with a male preponderance in a ratio of more than 2 to 1.

Fever lasting at least 5 days, erythema and oedema of the extremities followed by desquamation, a polymorphous rash, labial and oral mucosal erythema, cervical lymphadenopathy, conjunctival injection and mood changes (extreme misery) are seen. The mortality is 5–10%, death mainly being from myocardial infarction secondary to aneurysmal thrombus formation.

General management

Erythrocyte sedimentation rate (ESR) and C-reactive protein (CRP) are elevated; liver function is abnormal; there may be pyuria, and normocytic anaemia. Ultrasonography may show enlarged gallbladder; ECG and echocardiography may show abnormalities; and lumbar puncture may show aseptic meningitis.

Patients should be admitted to hospital for intravenous gammaglobulin treatment. Aspirin or systemic steroids are usually also given.

Dental aspects

Characteristic oral changes include a strawberry tongue, labial oedema, crusting or cracking of the lips, pharyngitis, oropharyngeal erythema and cervical lymphadenopathy – usually unilateral but occasionally massive. Facial palsy is sometimes seen, but is self-limiting and usually associated with cardiovascular disease. Treatment is unlikely to be given to a young child in the acute phase but, for a dental emergency, LA may be given. Conscious sedation is inappropriate and GA is contraindicated.

DRUG-INDUCED CARDIAC VALVULAR LESIONS

Use of a combination of the appetite suppressants fenfluramine and phentermine has been associated with a risk of cardiac valve regurgitation, particularly aortic regurgitation. All patients who have taken these drugs for longer than 3 months should have a clinical examination and, if any abnormality is detected, should be referred to a cardiologist for echocardiography.

CARDIAC VALVE SURGERY

Heart valve defects may be corrected by valvotomy, grafts or prosthetic valves.

Patients scheduled for cardiac surgery should ideally have excellent oral health established before operation. Generally speaking, teeth with a poor pulpal or periodontal prognosis are best removed, particularly before a valve replacement, major surgery for congenital anomalies or a heart transplant. Teeth with no more than shallow caries and periodontal pocketing should be conserved.

Elective dental care should be avoided for the first 6 months after cardiac surgery. Some patients are on anticoagulant treatment, immunosuppression or other drugs, or may also have a residual lesion. Prosthetic valves are particularly susceptible to infective endocarditis and there is then a high mortality rate. Endocarditis within the first 6 months is usually by *Staphylococcus aureus*, rarely of dental origin and has a mortality rate of around 60%.

INFECTIVE (BACTERIAL) ENDOCARDITIS

General aspects

Infective endocarditis (IE) is a rare but potentially life-threatening infection, predominantly affecting damaged heart valves. Individuals who have had uncomplicated myocardial infarcts, coronary angioplasty, coronary artery bypass grafts and cardiac pacemakers inserted do not have an increased risk of developing IE. Natural heart valves (native valve endocarditis) sometimes damaged by disease (e.g. rheumatic carditis) are usually affected by IE, but it can also affect people with congenital heart disease or after valve surgery (Table 5.25).

Table 5.25 Main groups affected by infective endocarditis	
Aetiology	Approximate % of all cases of infective endocarditis
No obvious cardiac valve disease	40
Chronic rheumatic heart disease	30
Congenital heart disease	10
Prosthetic cardiac valves	10
Intravenous drug abuse	10

Cardiac valves already damaged by infective endocarditis, or prosthetic cardiac valves (prosthetic valve endocarditis), are particularly at risk of infection (Box 5.11).

Platelet–fibrin deposits may form along the free margins of valves, where there is turbulent blood flow, forming sterile vegetations (aseptic thrombotic endocarditis), which may become infected with micro-organisms resulting in large friable vegetations (IE). Most bacteraemias are transient, self-limiting and not associated with any systemic complications.

> **Box 5.11 Patients at highest risk from infective endocarditis**
> - Prosthetic valves
> - Previous infective endocarditis
> - Complex cyanotic congenital heart disease – e.g. tetralogy of Fallot, TGA (transposition of great arteries) or Gerbode defect
> - Surgically constructed systemic–pulmonary shunts or conduits
> - Mitral valve prolapse with regurgitation or thickened leaflets

The factors which determine the development of IE are complex, but a susceptible surface (damaged endocardium) and high bacterial loads in the circulation appear to be important. Oral viridans streptococci (*Streptococcus mutans* and *sanguis*) from plaque enter the bloodstream (bacteraemia) during chewing, oral hygiene, tooth extractions and other oral procedures. They have complex attachment mechanisms, which enable them to adhere to damaged endocardium. Other micro-organisms are also implicated, particularly *Staphylococcus aureus* and enterococci. Very few healthy ambulant patients, probably less than 5%, acquire IE as a result of dental treatment, and it is also clear that bacteria enter the blood from the mouth (and other sites) on inumerable occasions unrelated to operative intervention, but usually cause no harm. In statistical terms, the chance of dental extractions causing IE, even in a patient with valvular disease, may possibly be as low as 1 in 3000.

Intravascular access devices, such as central intravenous lines, Hickman lines or Uldall catheters, often become infected but there is also no evidence for a dental focus for such infections.

An uncommon but dangerous type of right-sided infective endocarditis in a previously healthy heart results from intravenous drug abuse when highly virulent bacteria such as staphylococci can be introduced from the skin into the bloodstream with the addict's needle.

Clinical features

The clinical features of infective endocarditis are highly variable, often with an insidious onset, but should be considered in any individual presenting with fever and a new or changing heart murmur. IE cases range from fulminatingly acute to chronic.

Pallor (anaemia) or light (café-au-lait) pigmentation of the skin, joint pains and hepatosplenomegaly are typical, but the main effects of endocarditis are progressive heart damage (valve destruction and heart failure). Increasing disability is associated with changing cardiac murmurs indicative of progressive heart damage, infection or embolic damage of many organs, especially the kidneys (fever, malaise, night sweats and weight loss). Release of emboli can have widespread effects (on brain, lungs, spleen and kidneys), ranging from loss of a peripheral pulse to (rarely) sudden death from a stroke. Embolic phenomena include haematuria, cerebrovascular occlusion, petechiae or purpura of skin and mucous membranes, and splinter haemorrhages under the fingernails. Roth spots are small retinal haemorrhages. Immune complex formation from the antigens and resultant antibodies can lead to vasculitis, arthritis, retinal and renal damage. Osler's nodes are small, tender vasculitic lesions in the skin.

General management

Diagnosis is based on changing murmurs, ECG (may show conduction abnormalities), echocardiography (may identify vegetations and enables assessment of valvular and cardiac function) and blood culture. This is essential on suspicion and must be carried out before antimicrobial treatment is started; at least three samples of blood should be taken aseptically, at half-hourly intervals to increase the chances of obtaining a positive culture. Urine Stix may detect microscopic haematuria. Serological testing helps identify atypical organisms (e.g. *Legionella*).

Without treatment, IE is fatal in approximately 30% of cases, so the patient should be admitted to hospital for intravenous antibiotic therapy, usually benzylpenicillin and gentamicin. If staphylococcal endocarditis is suspected, vancomycin should be substituted in place of penicillin. In severe cases, such as prosthetic valve endocarditis, early removal of the infected valve and insertion of a sterile replacement may be needed.

Dental aspects

Patients at risk of endocarditis should receive intensive preventive dental care to minimize the need for dental intervention. However, this aspect of care is frequently neglected; a very high proportion of patients attending cardiology clinics have periodontal disease. There is no reliable evidence to suggest that oral hygiene aids such as electric toothbrushes or water-piks or similar devices pose a risk.

In many countries there are national guidelines on the use of antimicrobial prophylaxis against IE, if dental interventions are needed. However, the efficacy of such antimicrobial prophylaxis has been questionable, and antibiotic prophylaxis is no longer mandatory for IE-susceptible patients who are to undergo dental care (Box 5.12).

There is always a risk of adverse reactions to the antimicrobial (such as anaphylaxis), which can approach 5% and can be as high from oral amoxicillin as from intramuscular administration. Estimates suggest that deaths from anaphylaxis to antibiotics are possibly five to six times more likely than deaths from IE.

Medicolegal and other considerations suggest that one should act on the side of caution in relation to antibiotic prophylaxis of infective endocarditis, as in the following.

Box 5.12 Reasons for abandoning the use of antibiotic prophylaxis for endocarditis

- Dental treatment is a proven cause of only very few cases of infective endocarditis. A US study demonstrated that in the 3 months preceding diagnosis of endocarditis, dental treatment was no more frequent than in non-infected age- and sex-matched controls. The study concluded that very few cases of endocarditis would be prevented even if antibiotic prophylaxis was provided for dental procedures and was 100% effective. Another study concluded that, if antibiotic prophylaxis was 100% effective and provided for all at-risk patients receiving dental treatment, only a small fraction of cases (5.3%) would be potentially prevented
- Prophylactic antibiotic regimens fail in some instances
- Adverse reactions to antimicrobials are possible
- The cost-effectiveness of prophylaxis is questionable
- There is an increased risk of resistant bacteria in society

---

- Fully inform and discuss with the patient.
- Take medical advice in any case of doubt.
- In countries where there are national guidelines on antimicrobial prophylaxis against IE, it is mandatory for medicolegal reasons to give such prophylaxis to patients at risk. For example, in 2007 the ADA (American Dental Association), endorsed by the Infectious Diseases Society of America and Pediatric Infectious Diseases Society, recommended prophylaxis, but in only high-risk circumstances:

- history of IE
- artificial heart valves
- certain specific, serious congenital heart conditions, namely
  a unrepaired cyanotic congenital heart defects, including palliative shunts and conduits
  b completely repaired congenital heart defects with prosthetic material or device, whether placed by surgery or by catheter intervention, during the first 6 months after the procedure (prophylaxis is recommended for first 6 months because endothelialization of prosthetic material occurs within 6 months after the procedure)
  c repaired congenital heart defect with residual defects at the site or adjacent to the site of a prosthetic patch or prosthetic device (which inhibit endothelialization)
  d cardiac transplantation recipients who develop heart valve dysfunction.

In the UK over the years, a number of regimens have been suggested for endocarditis cover. The British Society for Antimicrobial Chemotherapy (BSAC) in 1992 recommended cover for all procedures associated with bleeding. The British Cardiac Society/ Royal College of Physicians (BCS/RCP) in 2004 suggested antibiotic prophylaxis for all bacteraemic dental procedures and for a large range of cardiac defects and/or surgery. In 2006, BSAC recommended antibiotic prophylaxis in only three (high-risk) circumstances:

- previous IE
- prosthetic valves
- surgically constructed pulmonary shunts or conduits.

Subsequently, the UK National Institute for Health and Clinical Excellence (NICE) issued the following recommendations in 2008, *completely removing the need for antibiotic prophylaxis in relation to dentistry.*
Antibiotic prophylaxis is not recommended for patients at risk of endocarditis undergoing dental procedures. Patients at risk of endocarditis should achieve and maintain high standards of oral health. NICE recommended that patients at risk for endocarditis should receive intensive preventive oral health care, to try and minimise the need for dental intervention.

See also Appendix 5.4.

CARDIAC FAILURE
GENERAL ASPECTS

Not to be confused with cardiac *arrest*, cardiac or heart failure is when any structural or functional impairment of the pumping action of the heart leads to blood output insufficient to meet body demands. Lack of tissue and organ perfusion with congestion results, and thus the term 'congestive cardiac failure' is often used. Cardiac failure is the leading cause of hospitalization in people older than 65 and it is associated with an annual mortality rate of 10%. The most common cause of cardiac failure is IHD but there are many others (Table 5.26).

Table 5.26	Main causes of heart failure	
Left-sided mainly	**Right-sided mainly**	**Biventricular**
Ischaemic heart disease Aortic valve disease Mitral valve disease Hypertension	Chronic obstructive pulmonary disease Pulmonary embolism	Ischaemic heart disease Aortic valve disease Mitral valve disease Hypertension Cardiomyopathies Hyperthyroidism Chronic anaemias Arrhythmias

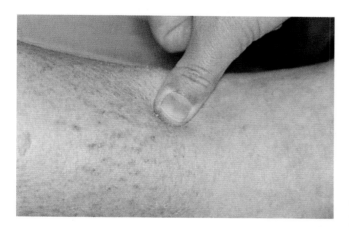

Fig. 5.11 Pressure on ankle in a person with suspected ankle oedema

CLINICAL FEATURES

Features depend on which side of the heart, left or right, is predominantly involved and on the type of failure, either diastolic or systolic. Congestive heart failure is often undiagnosed owing to a lack of a universally agreed definition and difficulties in diagnosis, particularly when the condition is considered 'mild'. Symptoms can be few until activity becomes limited with breathlessness (dyspnoea), cyanosis and dependent oedema (usually swollen ankles or sacral oedema; Figs 5.11 and 5.12).

Left-sided heart failure results in damming of blood back from the left ventricle to the pulmonary circulation with pulmonary hypertension, pulmonary oedema and dyspnoea. Lying down worsens pulmonary congestion, oedema and dyspnoea (orthopnoea). It also makes respiration less efficient, and cyanosis likely, because the abdominal viscera move the diaphragm higher and reduce the vital capacity of the lungs. Coughing is another typical consequence: the sputum is frothy and, in severe cases, pink with blood. In the more advanced stages of left-sided heart failure, there is inadequate cerebral oxygenation leading to symptoms such as loss of concentration, restlessness and irritability or, in older people, disorientation.

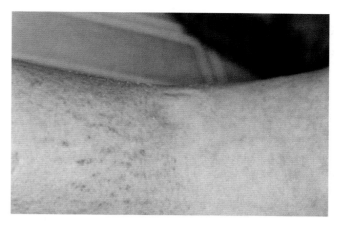

Fig. 5.12 Pitting oedema, indicating oedema and probable cardiac failure

Right-sided heart failure causes congestion of the main venous systems and thus affects primarily the liver, gastrointestinal tract, kidneys and subcutaneous tissues. It presents with peripheral (dependent) oedema, fatigue and hepatomegaly due to passive congestion, causing abdominal discomfort and, in severe cardiac failure, raised portal venous pressure, which also leads to escape of large amounts of fluid into the peritoneal cavity (ascites).

Failure of one side of the heart usually leads to failure of the other – biventricular failure. The pulse may then become rapid and irregular, particularly if there is atrial fibrillation and, in extreme cases, patients are cyanotic, polycythaemic, dyspnoeic at rest and oedematous with pulmonary oedema and distension of the neck veins (raised jugular venous pressure). Arrhythmias and sudden death may result.

The American College of Cardiology/American Heart Association has defined four stages in the progression of cardiac failure (Table 5.27).

Table 5.27	American College of Cardiology/American Heart Association stages of heart failure
Stage	**Features**
A	High risk of failure in the future but no structural heart disorder
B	Structural heart disorder but no symptoms
C	Previous or current symptoms of heart failure in the context of an underlying structural heart problem, but managed with medical treatment
D	Advanced disease requiring hospital-based support, heart transplant or palliative care

GENERAL MANAGEMENT

Heart failure is diagnosed clinically and by chest radiography (cardiomegaly), echocardiography, ECG and biochemistry. Echocardiography determines the *stroke volume* (SV; the amount of blood that exits the ventricles with each heartbeat), the *end-diastolic volume* (EDV; the amount of blood at the end of diastole), and the SV in proportion to the EDV (the *ejection fraction*; EF). Normally, the EF should lie between 50 and 70% but, in cardiac failure, it is < 40%.

A raised *B-type natriuretic peptide* (BNP) is a specific test indicative of cardiac failure. There may be abnormal liver and renal function tests, hyponatraemia and alkalosis.

Heart failure is managed by treating the symptoms and signs by reducing the heart workload, and correcting precipitating factors such as hypertension, anaemia, valvular disease and thyrotoxicosis. General measures may include rest, stress reduction, control of hypertension, weight loss, stopping smoking, and salt restriction. Angiotensin-converting enzyme inhibitors (ACEi; such as enalapril, ramipril, quinapril, perindopril, lisinopril and benazepril) or angiotensin II receptor blockers or sartans (e.g. valsartan, telmisartan, losartan, irbesartan and olmesartan) are first-line therapies, delaying progression of failure and reducing mortality. They also improve myocardial contractility, tissue and organ perfusion and oxygenation. Vasodilators, particularly isosorbide dinitrate plus hydralazine, may be valuable for people who fail to respond to ACEi.

Diuretics (mainly loop diuretics such as furosemide or bumetanide) increase sodium and water excretion. Betablockers may be indicated for patients with systolic heart failure due to left ventricular systolic dysfunction after stabilization with ACEi and diuretics. Recombinant BNP (nesiritide) is indicated for patients with acute heart failure who have dyspnoea at rest. Antagonists of vasopressin receptor (tolvaptan and conivaptan) and aldosterone receptor (spironolactone and eplerenone) are newer therapies. Phosphodiesterase inhibitors (enoximone or milrinone) may help to support cardiac function. Digoxin may help when failure is associated with atrial fibrillation.

Supplemental oxygen may be required and surgery (heart transplantation) is occasionally used to treat severe cardiac failure. New technologies include:

- heart pump – a left ventricular assist device, implanted into the abdomen and attached to the heart, which helps it pump
- biventricular cardiac pacemaker, which sends specifically timed electrical impulses to the ventricles for cardiac resynchronization therapy
- xenotransplantation – genetically manipulated pig hearts transplanted into humans
- artificial hearts – the first all-mechanical artificial hearts have already been implanted in humans.

DENTAL ASPECTS

For patients with poorly controlled or uncontrolled cardiac failure (worsening dyspnoea with minimal exertion, dyspnoea at rest, or nocturnal angina), medical attention should be obtained before any dental treatment. Elective dental treatment should be delayed until the condition has been stabilized medically. Emergency dental care should be conservative, principally with analgesics and antibiotics.

Routine dental care can usually be provided for patients with mild controlled cardiac failure with little modification. Appointments for patients with cardiac failure should be short and in the late morning. Endogenous adrenaline/epinephrine levels peak during the morning hours and cardiac complications are most likely in the early morning.

The dental chair should be kept in a partially reclining or erect position. It is dangerous to lay any patient with left-sided heart failure supine, as this may severely worsen dyspnoea.

Pain and anxiety may precipitate arrhythmias, angina or heart failure and thus effective analgesia must be provided. Lidocaine or prilocaine can be used but bupivacaine should be avoided as it is cardiotoxic. An aspirating syringe should be used to give the LA. Adrenaline/epinephrine may theoretically increase hypertension and precipitate arrhythmias. Blood pressure tends to rise during oral surgery under LA, and adrenaline/epinephrine can theoretically contribute, but this is usually of little practical importance. Adrenaline/epinephrine-containing LA should not be given in large doses to patients taking beta-blockers. Interactions between adrenaline/epinephrine and the beta-blocker may induce hypertension if excessive doses of the LA are given. Gingival retraction cords containing adrenaline/epinephrine should be avoided. Cardiac monitoring is desirable and supplemental oxygen should be readily available.

Conscious sedation can usually safely be used. However consideration must be given to the underlying cause of the cardiac failure (Table 5.26). GA is contraindicated in cardiac failure until it is under control. Care should be taken after GA since there is a predisposition to venous thrombosis and pulmonary embolism.

Some drugs may complicate dental treatment (Table 5.28).

Table 5.28 Cardiac failure treatment drugs in oral health care

Medical drug	Oral complication, or complication that may disturb dental care	Drug used in dentistry to be used with caution	Possible complication
ACE inhibitors (ACEi)	Coughing Erythema multiforme, angioedema, burning mouth	Itraconazole NSAIDs other than aspirin	Can aggravate cardiac failure Increases the risk of renal damage from ACEi
Digitalis	ECG changes (e.g. ST-segment depression during dental extractions) Vomiting	Erythromycin Tetracycline	May induce digitalis toxicity by impairing its gut flora metabolism May induce digitalis toxicity by impairing its gut flora metabolism
Diuretics	Orthostatic hypotension	Carbamazepine	Hyponatraemia

NSAIDs, non-steroidal anti-inflammatory drugs.

CARDIAC TRANSPLANTATION (HEART TRANSPLANTATION)

GENERAL ASPECTS

Heart transplantation uses a heart that has usually come from a brain-dead organ donor (*allograft*). The recipient patient's own heart may either be removed (*orthotopic procedure*) or, less commonly, left *in situ* to support the donor heart (*heterotopic procedure*; Fig. 5.13). Survival after cardiac transplantation is improving (Table 5.29) and some patients have survived for around 30 years. Heart–lung transplants are also increasingly used. The outcomes using a heart from another species (*xenograft*), or an *artificial heart*, have been less successful.

Heart transplantation is increasingly used to treat patients with otherwise uncontrollable cardiac failure, especially cardiomyopathy, congenital heart disease, coronary artery disease, heart valve disease and life-threatening arrhythmias.

All transplant recipients require lifelong immunosuppression to prevent a T-cell, alloimmune rejection response, usually with ciclosporin, mycophenolate or azathioprine, corticosteroids and antithymocyte globulin, or tacrolimus.

Patients may be anticoagulated or taking aspirin and dipyridamole to reduce platelet adhesion and prolong the bleeding time. They are often given a statin to minimize the risk of atheroma in the transplanted heart.

Since the vagus nerve is severed during the transplant operation, the donated heart will beat at around 100 beats per minute until nerve regrowth occurs. There is evidence of increased cardiac sensitivity to catecholamines such as adrenaline/epinephrine. Owing to the absence of innervation, angina is rare and patients may experience 'silent' myocardial infarction or sudden death.

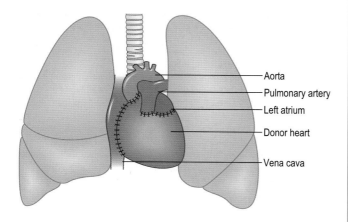

Fig 5.13 Heart transplantation

Aorta

Pulmonary artery

Left atrium

Donor heart

Vena cava

Table 5.29 Average survival of patients after cardiac transplant			
At year	1	3	5
% survival	> 80	> 75	> 70

DENTAL ASPECTS, IN ADDITION TO THOSE DISCUSSED IN CH. 35

A meticulous pre-surgery oral assessment is required and dental treatment undertaken with particular attention to establishing optimal oral hygiene and eradicating sources of potential infection. Dental treatment should be completed before surgery.

For 6 months after surgery, elective dental care is best deferred. If surgical treatment is needed during 6 months after surgery, or until the ECG is normal, antibiotic prophylaxis against endocarditis (see Infective endocarditis) may be requested by the surgeons.

It has been suggested that heart transplant patients cannot show any vasovagal reaction because the donor heart is completely deprived of any vagal or sympathetic innervation. However, episodes of vasovagal syncope in heart transplant patients undergoing periodontal surgery have been reported.

Local analgesia without adrenaline/epinephrine is indicated.

VASCULAR SURGERY

Bypass grafts to the aorta and lower limb vasculature (femoro-popliteal bypass) are often made of synthetic materials. They remain non-endothelialized and liable to infection, typically with *Staphylococcus epidermidis*. There is no evidence for odontogenic infection of such grafts, and no good evidence that antimicrobial prophylaxis should be given for dental procedures.

Magnetic resonance imaging is contraindicated where ferromagnetic vascular clips have been placed.

Patients undergoing vascular surgery have a high incidence of periodontal disease.

FURTHER READING

Academy report, 2002. Periodontal management of patients with cardiovascular diseases. J Periodontol 73, 954–968.

Auluck, A., Manohar, C., 2006. Haematological considerations in patients with cyanotic congenital heart disease. Dental Update 33, 617–622.

Bader JD. Bonito AJ, Shugars DA. Cardiovascular effects of epinephrine on hypertensive dental patients. Agency for Healthcare Research and Quality Evidence Report 48, 2002.

Bajorek, B.V., Krass, I., Ogle, S.J., Duguid, M.J., Shenfield, G.M., 2005. Optimizing the use of antithrombic therapy for atrial fibrillation in older people: a pharmacist-led multidisciplinary intervention. J Am Geriatr Soc 53, 1912–1920.

Becker, R.C., Meade, T.W., Berger, P.B., et al., 2008. The primary and secondary prevention of coronary artery disease: American College of Chest Physicians evidence-based clinical practice guidelines, 8th edn. Chest 133 (6 Suppl), 776S–814S.

Beirne, O.R., 2005. Evidence to continue oral anticoagulant therapy for ambulatory oral surgery. J Oral Maxillofac Surg 63, 540–545.

Blanchaert Jr., R.H., 1999. Ischemic heart disease. Oral Surg Oral Med Oral Pathol Oral Radiol Endod 87, 281–283.

Bodenheimer, M.M., 1996. Noncardiac surgery in the cardiac patient; what is the question?. Ann Intern Med 124, 763–766.

Brand, H.S., Gortzak, R.A., Palmer-Bouva, C.C., Abraham, R.E., Abraham-Inpijn, L., 1995. Cardiovascular and neuroendocrine responses during acute stress induced by different types of dental treatment. Int Dent J 45, 45–48.

Campbell, J.H., Alvarado, F., Murray, R.A., 2000. Anticoagulation and minor oral surgery: should the anticoagulation regimen be altered?. J Oral Maxillofac Surg 58, 131–136.

Campbell, R.L., Langston, W.G., Ross, G.A., 1997. A comparison of cardiac rate-pressure product and pressure-rate quotient with Holter monitoring in patients with hypertension and cardiovascular disease: a follow-up report. Oral Surg Oral Med Oral Pathol Oral Radiol Endod 84, 125–128.

Carmona, I.T., Dios, P.D., Scully, C., 2002. An update on the controversies in bacterial endocarditis of oral origin. Oral Surg Oral Med Oral Pathol Oral Radiol Endod 93, 660–670.

Carmona, I.T., Dios, P.D., Scully, C., 2007. Efficacy of antibiotic prophylactic regimens for the prevention of bacterial endocarditis of oral origin. J Dent Res 86, 1142–1159.

D'Aiuto, F., Parkar, M., Tonetti, M.S., 2007. Acute effects of periodontal therapy on bio-markers of vascular health. J Clin Periodontol 34, 124–129.

Falk, R.H., 2001. Atrial fibrillation. N Engl J Med 344, 1067–1078

Friedlander, A.H., Yoshikawa, T., Chang, D.S., Feliciano, Z., Scully, C., 2009. Atrial fibrillation: pathogenesis, medical-surgical management and dental implications. Jounrnal of the American Dental Association 140: 167–177.

Fuster, V., Ryden, L.E., Cannom, D.S., et al., and the American College of Cardiology/American Heart Association Task Force on Practice Guidelines; European Society of Cardiology Committee for Practice Guidelines; European Heart Rhythm Association; Heart Rhythm Society, 2006. Guidelines for the Management of Patients with Atrial Fibrillation: a report of the American College of Cardiology/American Heart Association Task Force on Practice Guidelines and the European Society of Cardiology Committee for Practice Guidelines (Writing Committee to Revise the 2001 Guidelines for the Management of Patients With Atrial Fibrillation): developed in collaboration with the European Heart Rhythm Association and the Heart Rhythm Society. Circulation 114, e257–e354.

Gibson, R.M., Meechan, J.G., 2007. The effects of antihypertensive medication on dental treatment. Dent Update 34, 70–78.

Goldstein, L.B., Adams, R., Alberts, M.J., et al., 2006. American Heart Association; American Stroke Association Stroke Council. Primary prevention of ischemic stroke: a guideline from the American Heart Association/American Stroke Association Stroke Council: cosponsored by the Atherosclerotic Peripheral Vascular Disease Interdisciplinary Working Group; Cardiovascular Nursing Council; Clinical Cardiology Council; Nutrition, Physical Activity, and Metabolism Council; and the Quality of Care and Outcomes Research Interdisciplinary Working Group. Circulation 113, e873–e923 [Erratum in Circulation 2006; 114, e617].

Gottdiener, J.S., Arnold, A.M., Aurigemma, G.P., et al., 2000. Predictors of congestive heart failure in the elderly: the Cardiovascular Health Study. J Am Coll Cardiol 35, 1628–1637.

Gould, F.K., Elliott, T.S., Foweraker, J., et al., 2006. Guidelines for the prevention of endocarditis: report of the Working Party of the British Society for Antimicrobial Chemotherapy. J Antimicrob Chemother 58, 896–898.

Holmstrup, P., Poulsen, A.H., Andersen, L., Skuldbol, T., Fiehn, N.E., 2003. Oral infections and systemic diseases. Dent Clin North Am 47, 575–598.

Hylek, E.M., Regan, S., Go, A.S., Hughes, R.A., Singer, D.E., Skates, S.J., 2001. Clinical predictors of prolonged delay in return of the international normalized ratio to within the therapeutic range after excessive anticoagulation with warfarin. Ann Intern Med 135, 393–400.

Jowett, N.I., Cabot, L.B., 2000. Patients with cardiac disease; considerations for the dental practitioner. Br Dent J 189, 297–302.

Kistler, P.M., 2007. Management of atrial fibrillation. Aust Fam Physician 36, 506–511.

Lessard, E., Glick, M., Ahmed, S., Saric, M., 2005. The patient with a heart murmur. Evaluation, assessment and dental considerations. J Am Dent Assoc 136, 347–356.

Lip, G.Y., Tse, H.F., 2007. Management of atrial fibrillation. Lancet 370, 604–618.

Little, J.W., 2000. The impact on dentistry of recent advances in the management of hypertension. Oral Surg 90, 591–599.

Lund, J.P., Drews, T., Helzer, R., Reichart, P.A., 2002. Oral surgical management of patients with mechanical circulatory support. Int J Oral Maxillofac Surg 31, 629–633.

Mahmood, M., Malone, D.C., Skrepnek, G.H., et al., 2007. Potential drug-drug interactions within Veterans Affairs medical centers. Am J Health Syst Pharm 64, 1500–1505.

Mead, G.E., Elder, A.T., Flapan, A.D., Kelman, A., 2005. Electrical cardioversion for atrial fibrillation and flutter. Cochrane Database Syst Rev 3 CD002903.

Miloro, M., 2000. Congestive heart failure. Oral Surg 90, 9–11.

National Collaborating Centre for Chronic Conditions, 2006. Atrial fibrillation: national clinical guideline for management in primary and secondary care. Royal College of Physicians, London.

Niederman, R., Joshipura, K., 2000. Cause célèbre; oral health and heart disease. Evid Based Dent 2, 59–60.

Oliver, R., Roberts, G.J., Hooper, L., 2004. Penicillins for the prophylaxis of bacterial endocarditis in dentistry. Cochrane Database Syst Rev 2 CD003813.

Perez-Gomez, F., Iriarte, J.A., Zumalde, J., et al., 2007. Antithrombotic therapy in elderly patients with atrial fibrillation: effects and bleeding complications: a stratified analysis of the NASPEAF randomized trial. Eur Heart J 28, 996–1003.

Research Science and Therapy Committee, 2000. Sonic and ultrasonic scalers in periodontics. J Periodontol 71, 1792–1801.

Roberts, H.W., Mitnisky, E.F., 2001. Cardiac risk stratification for postmyocardial infarction in dental patients. Oral Surg 91, 676–681.

Rustemeyer, J., Bremerich, A., 2007. Necessity of surgical dental foci treatment prior to organ transplantation and heart valve replacement. Clin Oral Invest 11, 171–174.

Saffitz, J.E., 2006. Connexins, conduction, and atrial fibrillation. N Engl J Med 354, 2712–2714.

Saxena, R., Koudstaal, P.J., 2004. Anticoagulants versus antiplatelet therapy for preventing stroke in patients with nonrheumatic atrial fibrillation and a history of stroke or transient ischemic attack. Cochrane Database Syst Rev 4 CD000187.

Schauer, D.P., Moomaw, C.J., Wess, M., Web, T., Eckman, M.H., 2005. Psychosocial risk factors for adverse outcomes in patients with nonvalvular atrial fibrillation receiving warfarin. J Gen Intern Med 20, 1114–1119.

Scully, C., Chaudhry, S., 2006. Aspects of Human Disease 1. Atheroma and coronary artery (ischaemic heart) disease Dental Update 33; 251.

Scully, C., Chaudhry, S., 2006. Aspects of Human Disease 2. Angina pectoris Dental Update 33; 317.

Scully, C., Chaudhry S., 2006. Aspects of Human Disease 3. Myocardial infarction Dental Update 33; 381.

Scully, C., Chaudhry S., 2006. Aspects of Human Disease 4. Hypertension Dental Update 33; 443.

Scully, C., Chaudhry S., 2006. Aspects of Human Disease 5. Infective endocardius Dental Update 33; 509.

Scully, C., Chaudhry S., 2006. Aspects of Human Disease 6. Congenital Heart Disease Dental Update 33; 573.

Scully, C., Ettinger, R., 2007. The influence of systemic diseases on oral health care in older adults. JADA 138 (Suppl), 7S–14S.

Scully, C., Wolff, A., 2002. Oral surgery in patients on anticoagulant therapy. Oral Surg Oral Med Oral Pathol Oral Radiol Endod 94, 57–64.

Scully, C., Roberts, G., Shotts, R., 2001. The mouth in heart disease. Practitioner 245, 432–437.

Scully, C., Diz Dios, P., Kumar, N., 2007. Special care in dentistry: handbook of oral healthcare. Churchill Livingstone Elsevier, Edinburgh.

Seymour, R.A., Whitworth, J.M., 2002. Antibiotic prophylaxis for endocarditis, prosthetic joints, and surgery. Dent Clin North Am 46, 635–651.

Sirois, D.A., Fatahzadeh, M., 2001. Valvular heart disease. Oral Surg Oral Med Oral Pathol Oral Radiol Endod 91 (1), 15–19.

Snow, V., Weiss, K.B., LeFevre, M., et al., and AAFP Panel on Atrial Fibrillation and ACP Panel on Atrial Fibrillation, 2003. Management of newly detected atrial fibrillation: a clinical practice guideline from the American Academy of Family Physicians and the American College of Physicians. Ann Intern Med 139, 1009–1017.

Stecksén-Blicks, C., Rydberg, A., Nyman, L., Asplund, S., Svanberg, C., 2004. Dental caries experience in children with congenital heart disease: a case-control study. Int J Paediatr Dent 14, 94–100.

Stevenson, H., Longman, L.P., Randall, C., Field, E.A., 2006. The statins; drug interactions of significance to the dental practitioner. Dent Update 33, 14–20.

Stroke Risk in Atrial Fibrillation Working Group, 2007. Independent predictors of stroke in patients with atrial fibrillation. A systematic review. Neurology 69, 546–554.

Tempe, D.K., Virmani, S., 2002. Coagulation abnormality in patients with cyanotic congenital heart disease. J Cardiothoracic Vasc Anaesth 16, 752–756.

Tomás Carmona, I., Álvarez, M., Limeres, J., et al., 2007. A clorhexidine mouthwash reduces the risk of post-extraction bacteraemia. Infect Control Hosp Epidemiol 28, 577–582.

Tonetti, M.S., D'Aiuto, F., Nibali, L., et al., 2007. Treatment of periodontitis and endothelial function. N Engl J Med 356, 911–920.

Webster, K., Wilde, J., 2000. Management of anticoagulation in patients with prosthetic heart valves undergoing oral and maxillofacial operations. Br J Oral Maxillofac Surg 38, 124–126.

Wilson, W., Taubert, K.A., Gewitz, M., et al., 2007. Prevention of infective endocarditis. Guidelines from the American Heart Association. J Am Dent Assoc 138, 739–745, 747–60.

Woods, K., Douketis, J.D., Kathirgamanathan, K., Yi, Q., Crowther, M.A., 2007. Low-dose oral vitamin K to normalize the international normalized ratio prior to surgery in patients who require temporary interruption of warfarin. J Thromb Thrombolysis 24, 93–97.

Ziv, O., Choudhary, G., 2005. Atrial fibrillation. Prim Care Clin Office Pract 32, 1083–1107.

Appendix 5.1 Genetic syndromes with associated cardiac defects

Names of disorder	Further information
Chromosomal disorders	
Down	Ch. 28
Edward	Ch. 28
Patau	Ch. 28
Turner (XXY)	Ch. 28
XXXY	Learning disability: hypogonadism
XXXXX	Learning disability: small hands
Hereditary disorders	
Ehlers–Danlos	Ch. 16
Marfan	Ch. 16
Osteogenesis imperfecta	Ch. 16
The mucopolysaccharidoses (Hurler and related syndromes)	Ch. 23
Ellis–van Creveld	Ch. 37
TAR	Thrombocytopenia: absent radius
Holt–Oram	Hypoplastic clavicles: upper limb defect
Multiple lentigenes	Basal cell naevi: rib defects
Rubenstein–Taybi	Broad thumbs and toes: hypoplastic maxilla

Appendix 5.2 Main CHD that may be associated with various eponymous syndromes

Syndrome	Defects
Down	Atrioventricular defect and also PDA and Fallot tetralogy
Ehlers–Danlos	Mitral valve prolapse
Friedreich	Hypertrophic cardiomyopathy
Holt–Oram	ASD, VSD
Klinefelter	ASD
Marfan	Mitral valve prolapse, aortic regurgitation
Noonan	Pulmonary stenosis, sometimes Fallot tetralogy
Turner	Coarctation, aortic stenosis
Williams	Supravalvular aortic stenosis

ASD, atrial septal defect; CHD, congenital heart disease; PDA, patent ductus arteriosus; VSD, ventricular septal defect.

Appendix 5.3 Vaughan–Williams classification of anti-arrhythmic agents

Mechanism	Class	Examples	Main uses
Membrane stabilizing (sodium-channel blockers)	Ia	Disopyramide Procainamide Quinidine	Ventricular arrhythmias Wolff–Parkinson–White syndrome
	Ib	Lidocaine Phenytoin	Ventricular tachycardia Atrial fibrillation
	Ic	Flecainide Propafenone	Paroxysmal atrial fibrillation
Beta-blockers	II	Atenolol Metoprolol Propranolol Sotalol Timolol	Tachyarrhythmias
Unknown	III	Amiodarone Dofetilide Nibentan Sotalol	Atrial fibrillation Ventricular tachycardias Wolff–Parkinson–White syndrome
Calcium-channel blockers	IV	Diltiazem Verapamil	Paroxysmal supraventricular tachycardia Atrial fibrillation

Appendix 5.4 Endocarditis

Do patients undergoing dental procedures require endocarditis prophylaxis?

[Reproduced with permission from UK Medicines Information (UKMi) pharmacists for NHS healthcare professionals]

BACKGROUND

Infective endocarditis is an inflammation of the inner lining of the heart (endocardium), particularly affecting the heart valves and caused mainly by bacterial infection. Patients with structural abnormalities of the heart, hypertrophic cardiomyopathy, replacement heart valves or with a history of infective endocarditis are considered to be at risk of developing infective endocarditis.

Traditionally, prophylactic antibiotics have been given to patients at risk of infective endocarditis before undergoing dental procedures. Typically, three grams of oral amoxicillin would be taken one hour beforehand. The rationale for using antibiotics was that dental procedures lead to increased numbers of bacteria in the blood (bacteraemia) and it was assumed that bacteraemia was a key factor in the development of infective endocarditis.

In recent years, there have been conflicting guidelines as to which patients and dental procedures warranted the use of prophylactic antibiotics (1, 2, 3). This led to confusion for health professionals and patients. The National Institute for Health and Clinical Excellence (NICE) has now issued definitive, evidence-based guidance on the prophylaxis of infective endocarditis (4). This guidance has been adopted nationally and is reflected in the current British National Formulary, published March 2008 (5).

ANSWER

Antibiotic prophylaxis is *not* recommended for the prevention of infective endocarditis in adults or children undergoing any dental procedure (4).

The basis for this recommendation is:

- There is no consistent association between dental procedures and an increased risk of infective endocarditis;
- Bacteraemia associated with dental procedures is no greater than that from toothbrushing; Regular toothbrushing almost certainly presents a greater risk of infective endocarditis than a single dental procedure because of repetitive exposure to bacteraemia;
- Antibiotics are not proven to reduce the risk of infective endocarditis;
- Antibiotics are themselves not without risk and can cause fatal anaphylaxis.

Patients who previously received endocarditis prophylaxis for dental procedures will require a clear explanation as to why prophylaxis is no longer recommended. A summary of the NICE guideline for patients (6) and a 'quick reference leaflet' (7) are available online. Printed copies can be ordered from NICE Publications via 0845 003 7783 or publications@nice.org.uk (quote reference numbers N1488 and N1487 when ordering the patient summary and quick reference leaflet, respectively).

NICE states that healthcare professionals should offer clear and consistent advice to patients on four points, details of which are on page 2 of this document.

The NICE summary for patients (6) includes a list of questions that patients might ask their healthcare team; answers are suggested on page 3 of this document.

ADVICE FOR HEALTHCARE PROFESSIONALS TO OFFER TO PATIENTS

Patients at risk of infective endocarditis should be reassured that antibiotic prophylaxis is no longer recommended and offered information regarding:

THE BENEFITS AND RISKS OF ANTIBIOTIC PROPHYLAXIS, AND AN EXPLANATION OF WHY ANTIBIOTIC PROPHYLAXIS IS NO LONGER RECOMMENDED

Patients at risk of infective endocarditis have traditionally received prophylactic antibiotics prior to dental procedures. Procedures that disturb bacteria in the mouth increase the number of bacteria in the blood (bacteraemia). High levels of bacteraemia have been shown (in animal models) to increase the risk of infective endocarditis. On this basis, it was considered prudent to provide antibiotic prophylaxis to reduce bacteraemia in patients considered to be at risk of infective endocarditis. Over recent years, there have been conflicting guidelines as to which patients required antibiotic prophylaxis and for which dental procedures.

NICE has reviewed the evidence regarding infective endocarditis and concluded that there is no clear association between dental procedures and infective endocarditis. Evidence shows that levels of bacteraemia associated with dental procedures are no greater than those associated with regular toothbrushing. The risk of infective endocarditis is almost certainly greater from toothbrushing than from a single dental procedure due to repeated exposure to bacteraemia.

Antibiotic prophylaxis given before dental procedures has not been shown to eliminate bacteraemia or to reduce the risk of infective endocarditis and is associated with risks of its own. Antibiotics can cause adverse reactions including fatal anaphylaxis. Using antibiotics when not indicated puts patients at risk from adverse effects and can increase bacterial resistance to antibiotics. For all these reasons, antibiotic prophylaxis is no longer recommended for the prevention of infective endocarditis in patients undergoing dental procedures.

THE IMPORTANCE OF MAINTAINING GOOD ORAL HEALTH

Maintaining good oral health reduces the numbers of bacteria in the mouth and helps prevent tooth decay and gum disease. Patients should be advised to keep their mouth and teeth clean with twice-daily toothbrushing, to have regular dental check-ups and not to let any dental problems such as abscess or gum disease go untreated.

SYMPTOMS THAT MAY INDICATE INFECTIVE ENDOCARDITIS AND WHEN TO SEEK EXPERT ADVICE

Infective endocarditis is rare and patients are unlikely to develop it. Early symptoms of infective endocarditis are similar to flu-symptoms: fever, night sweats and chills, weakness and tiredness, and also breathlessness, weight loss and joint pain. Patients at risk of infective endocarditis should be advised to see a GP if they have such symptoms for longer than a week (8).

THE RISKS OF UNDERGOING INVASIVE PROCEDURES, INCLUDING NON-MEDICAL PROCEDURES SUCH AS BODY PIERCING OR TATTOOING

Bacteraemia can develop following piercing or tattooing, particularly if non-sterile equipment or techniques are involved. Patients at risk of infective endocarditis should be discouraged from having procedures such as piercing or tattooing (8).

People with the following cardiac conditions are considered to be at risk of developing infective endocarditis and would have received antibiotics for endocarditis prophylaxis in the past:

- Previous infective endocarditis,
- Replacement heart valve,
- Structural congenital heart disease (but not isolated atrial septal defect, fully repaired septal defect, fully repaired patent ductus arteriosus or congenital heart disease repaired with closure devices that are judged to be endothelialised),
- Valvular heart disease with stenosis or regurgitation,
- Hypertrophic cardiomyopathy.

QUESTIONS PATIENTS MAY ASK

IN THE PAST I HAVE BEEN GIVEN ANTIBIOTICS TO PREVENT INFECTIVE ENDOCARDITIS FOR THE SAME DENTAL PROCEDURE BUT HAVE NOT BEEN OFFERED THEM NOW. WHY HAS THIS CHANGED?

In the past, guidelines recommended that people at risk of infective endocarditis were given prophylactic (preventative) antibiotics before certain procedures. The National Institute for Health and Clinical Excellence (NICE) has reviewed the evidence regarding infective endocarditis and concluded that prophylactic antibiotics are *not* required for dental procedures.

To understand why the guidelines have changed, it is helpful to know why antibiotics were recommended in the first place: Dental procedures (such as scaling or tooth extraction) disturb bacteria in the mouth and these bacteria can then enter the bloodstream. It was thought that the rise in the number of bacteria in the bloodstream (bacteraemia) that occurred following dental procedures increased the risk of getting endocarditis, and antibiotics were given to combat this rise.

NICE has found that the levels of bacteria in the bloodstream associated with dental procedures are no higher than those associated with toothbrushing. So, patients undergoing dental procedures are not at any greater risk of getting endocarditis than they are from brushing their teeth. The bacteria that enter the bloodstream are killed by the body's immune system.

Antibiotics can cause side effects, some of which can be very serious, or even fatal. Taking antibiotics when they are not needed puts patients at unnecessary risk. Because antibiotics have not been shown to reduce the chance of getting endocarditis, and because dental procedures are no longer thought to be a cause of endocarditis, taking antibiotics before dental procedures is no longer recommended.

I'VE USED A CHLORHEXIDINE MOUTHWASH WHEN I HAVE HAD DENTAL TREATMENT IN THE PAST. IS THIS HELPFUL?

Chlorhexidine mouthwash is not recommended to prevent infective endocarditis. It has not been shown to reduce the chance of getting endocarditis and, as explained above, dental procedures are no longer thought to be a cause of endocarditis.

IS THERE SOME WRITTEN MATERIAL (LIKE A LEAFLET) ABOUT INFECTIVE ENDOCARDITIS THAT I CAN HAVE?

The British Heart Foundation has information about infective endocarditis on its website. Go to the home page (www.bhf.org.uk) and type 'endocarditis' in the search box at the top of the screen.

WHAT CAN I DO TO IMPROVE MY ORAL HEALTH?

Keep your teeth and mouth clean with twice-daily toothbrushing. Visit your dentist for regular check-ups and don't let any dental problems such as a dental abscess or gum disease go untreated.

WHAT ARE THE SYMPTOMS OF INFECTIVE ENDOCARDITIS? WHAT SHOULD I DO IF I THINK I HAVE IT?

Infective endocarditis is very rare. Symptoms are flu-like, and include fever, night sweats and chills, weakness and tiredness as well as breathlessness, weight loss and joint pain. It is very unlikely that you will ever suffer from endocarditis but if you are at risk (e.g. if you have a replacement heart valve, valvular heart disease or hypertrophic cardiomyopathy) and have flu-like symptoms for longer than a week you should see a GP.

WHAT DO I DO IF I THINK I HAVE AN INFECTION?

Guidelines for the *treatment* of infections have not changed. If you think you have an infection, contact a healthcare professional (e.g. pharmacist, GP, dentist or optician) as you would normally.

NICE provides guidance for the NHS in England and Wales. Further information about NICE, its work and how it reaches decisions is available online at www.nice.org.uk/aboutguidance.

SUMMARY

Antibiotic prophylaxis is not recommended for the prevention of infective endocarditis in patients undergoing dental procedures.

LIMITATIONS

This document does not relate to the use of pre-procedural antibiotics to prevent infections other than infective endocarditis.

DISCLAIMER

- Medicines Q&As are intended for healthcare professionals and reflect UK practice.
- Each Medicines Q&A relates only to the clinical scenario described.
- Medicines Q&As are believed to accurately reflect the medical literature at the time of writing.
- See www.nelm.nhs.uk for full disclaimer.

REFERENCES

1. Joint Formulary Committee. British National Formulary, 54th edition. London: British Medical Association and Royal Pharmaceutical Society of Great Britain; 2007. Chapter 5.1, Table 2: Summary of antibacterial prophylaxis (page 279).
2. Ramsdale DR, Turner-Stokes L, Advisory Group of the British Cardiac Society Clinical Practice Committee, et al. Prophylaxis and treatment of infective endocarditis in adults: a concise guide. Clin Med 2004;4:545–550.
3. Gould FK, Elliott TSJ, Foweraker J et al. Guidelines for prevention of endocarditis: report of the Working Party of the British Society for Antimicrobial Chemotherapy. J Antimicrob Chemother 2006;57:1035–1042. Accessed on 8/4/2008 at: http://jac.oxfordjournals.org/cgi/reprint/dkl121v1
4. National Institute for Health and Clinical Excellence. Prophylaxis against infective endocarditis. March 2008 (NICE Clinical Guideline No.64). Accessed on 8/4/2008 at: NICE full guideline www.nice.org.uk/nicemedia/pdf/CG64NICEguidance.pdf (107 pages) and NICE appendices to the full guideline www.nice.org.uk/nicemedia/pdf/CG64Appendices.pdf (270 pages)
5. Joint Formulary Committee. British National Formulary, 55th edition. London: British Medical Association and Royal Pharmaceutical Society of Great Britain; 2007. Chapter 5.1, Table 2: Summary of antibacterial prophylaxis (page 283).
6. National Institute for Health and Clinical Excellence. Understanding NICE guidance: information for people who use NHS services. Preventing infective endocarditis. Reference N1488. Accessed on 8/4/2008 at: www.nice.org.uk/nicemedia/pdf/CG64UNG.pdf
7. National Institute for Health and Clinical Excellence. Prophylaxis against infective endocarditis. Quick reference guide. Reference N1487. Accessed on 8/4/2008 at: www.nice.org.uk/nicemedia/pdf/CG64PIEQRG.pdf
8. British Heart Foundation. Infective endocarditis: the facts. Accessed on 8/4/2008 at: www.bhf.org.uk/yheart/default.aspx?page=175

QUALITY ASSURANCE

PREPARED BY
Karoline Brennan, North West Medicines Information Centre

DATE PREPARED
April 2008

CHECKED BY
Christine Randall, North West Medicines Information Centre

DATE OF CHECK
April 2008

ENDOCRINOLOGY

> - Diabetes is common, the main endocrine disorder and is increasing
> - Hypoglycaemia must be avoided

The endocrine system is widespread and consists of glands that exert their effects by means of chemicals (hormones) secreted into the blood circulation (Fig. 6.1). Hormones are chemical messengers of various types, which act usually at some distance from their source, and can be classified according to their main function.

Nervous and endocrine control mechanisms normally maintain body homeostasis, coordinated via the neuroendocrine system, most apparent in the hypothalamus. The hypothalamus, along with the pituitary gland controls many other endocrine functions.

ENDOCRINE RESPONSES

Pregnancy and the menopause are important states with endocrine changes discussed elsewhere (see Ch. 00). It is common to see endocrine disorders in people who overexercise or who are anorectic, starving, stressed or ill (Table 6.1).

ENDOCRINE DISORDERS

Endocrine glands can overproduce (hyperfunction) or underproduce (hypofunction) their hormones. Endocrine disorders (endocrinopathies) may be caused by hormone excess (e.g. primary hyperparathyroidism), by diminished hormone release (e.g. hypothyroidism) or by hormone resistance (e.g. type 2 diabetes).

The function of an endocrine gland can be assessed by measuring: the hormone in the blood plasma (many have a circadian rhythm – the level varies throughout the 24 h); the hormone or its metabolite in the urine; or dynamic tests of hormone secretion or regulation – by suppressing (tests hormone excess) or stimulating (tests hormone deficiency) hormone release; levels of hormone receptors, or effects on the target tissues.

The most common and important specific endocrine disorder is diabetes mellitus, but the hypothalamus is the conductor of the endocrine 'orchestra' (Table 6.2).

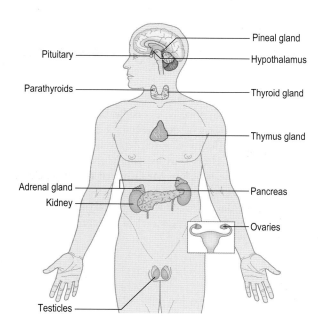

Fig. 6.1 Main endocrine glands (hormones are also produced by other tissues).

Table 6.1 Endocrine responses to severe stress or illness

HORMONE		
Plasma levels rise	**Plasma levels fall**	**Resistance increases**
Epinephrine Glucagon Glucocorticoids and adrenocorticotropic hormone Growth hormone Prolactin	Luteinizing hormone and follicle-stimulating hormone Sex steroids Thyroid hormones and thyroid-stimulating hormone	Insulin

Table 6.2 Hormones-classified by function

Electrolyte/fluid/vascular	Metabolic	Liver and digestive	Reproductive	Stress
Aldosterone Androstenedione Bradykinin Calcitonin Erythropoietin Neurotensin Vasopressin (antidiuretic hormone)	Adrenaline (epinephrine) and noradrenaline (norepinephrine) Cortisol Growth hormone Glucagon Insulin Parathyroid hormone Thyroid hormone	Cholecystokinin Gastrin Vasoactive intestinal peptide	Aetiocholanolone Chorionic gonadotropin Oestradiol Oestriol Oestrone Progesterone Prolactin Testosterone	Adrenaline (epinephrine) and noradrenaline (norepinephrine) Adrenocorticotropic hormone Corticosterone Growth hormone Hydrocortisone (cortisol)

HYPOTHALAMUS AND PITUITARY GLAND

The hypothalamus is the part of the brain that controls many other endocrine glands, via pituitary function and hypophysiotropic hormones sometimes termed 'releasing factors'.

The anterior pituitary (adenohypophysis) originates as an outgrowth from the stomatodeum (Rathke pouch) and, although anatomically distinct from the hypothalamus, falls under its influence by factors passing through a portal venous system (Fig. 6.2). Hypothalamic hormones which act on the anterior pituitary gland include *thyrotropin-releasing hormone* (TRH), *gonadotropin-releasing hormone* (GnRH), *growth hormone-releasing hormone* (GHRH), *corticotropin-releasing hormone* (CRH) and *somatostatin* (Table 6.3).

The posterior pituitary (neurohypophysis) is a downgrowth from the base of the brain connected with the hypothalamus by neurons. Two hypothalamic hormones act on the posterior pituitary gland – *antidiuretic hormone* (ADH) and *oxytocin*.

The hypothalamus is under the control of higher centres in the brain, and inhibited by the hormone somatostatin (octreotide). Feedback control influences the amount of hypothalamic hypophysiotropic hormone secreted. *Dopamine* inhibits pituitary release of *prolactin* (PRL).

Pituitary hyperfunction is sometimes caused by pituitary tumours, usually microadenomas (smaller than 1 cm), which can have pressure effects on adjacent structures such as the rest of the anterior pituitary gland, and the optic chiasma (Fig. 6.3), causing headaches and visual defects as well as effects on hormone release. Around 50% of pituitary adenomas are hormone-secreting – half producing prolactin, the rest producing growth hormone, or adrenocorticotropic hormone (ACTH) or thyroid-stimulating hormone (TSH).

Pituitary hormones, used to stimulate growth, have been implicated in the transmission of some cases of iatrogenic Creutzfeldt–Jakob disease (Ch. 13).

POSTERIOR PITUITARY HYPOFUNCTION

Diabetes insipidus

General aspects

Diabetes insipidus is a rare disease caused by lack of antidiuretic hormone effect. Rarely, this is because of renal insensitivity to ADH (nephrogenic diabetes insipidus – a rare X-linked disorder affecting renal tubular ADH receptors, or due to hypercalcaemia, hypokalaemia, renal disease or drugs such as lithium), more commonly because of reduced ADH secretion – cranial diabetes insipidus, which is caused by head injuries (when it may be temporary), a tumour (usually craniopharyngioma), infiltration or vascular disease in the region of the hypothalamus or pituitary, or it may be idiopathic.

Clinical features

Diabetes insipidus is characterized by an excessive volume of dilute urine (polyuria), and persistent thirst and drinking (polydipsia). *Cranial* diabetes insipidus may also cause pressure on the optic chiasma leading to visual or cranial nerve defects, or raised intracranial pressure and headaches.

General management

The diagnosis is established by assessing the relation of plasma to urine osmolality and by demonstrating an inability to concentrate the urine during a water-deprivation test. The local extent of disease is assessed by imaging (skull radiography and magnetic resonance imaging; MRI), visual field charting and tests of anterior pituitary function.

Diabetes insipidus is treated with the ADH-like peptide desmopressin or antidiuretic drugs such as chlorpropamide or carbamazepine.

Dental aspects

Local anaesthesia (LA) is the most satisfactory means of pain control. Conscious sedation may be needed to control anxiety. Dentistry is usually uncomplicated by this disorder except for dryness of the mouth.

Carbamazepine used in the treatment of trigeminal neuralgia may have an additive effect with other drugs used to treat diabetes insipidus. Transient diabetes insipidus can be a complication of head injury. But head injury can also cause the opposite effect – excessive ADH levels.

Syndrome of inappropriate antidiuretic hormone secretion (SIADH)

Excessive ADH levels may be caused by: maxillofacial injury or even elective maxillofacial surgery, head injury or intracranial lesions; general anaesthesia (GA); pain; fits; smoking; tumours (especially some lung cancers); or drugs (carbamazepine, chlorpropamide, vinca alkaloids).

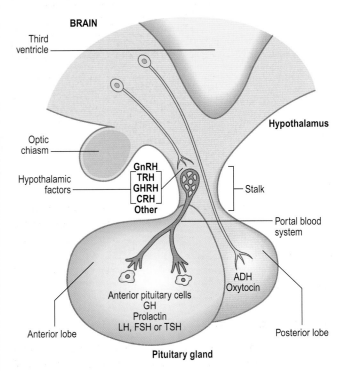

Fig. 6.2 Hypothalamo-pituitary control

Table 6.3 Hypothalamic hormones

Hypothalamic hormone	Primary activities	Effects
Thyrotropin-releasing hormone (TRH)	Stimulates pituitary release of thyroid-stimulating hormone (TSH) and prolactin (PRL)	Stimulates thyroid hormone synthesis and release
Gonadotropin-releasing hormone (GnRH)	Stimulates pituitary release of luteinizing hormone (LH) and follicle-stimulating hormone (FSH)	LH stimulates follicle to secrete oestrogen in the first half of menstrual cycle, triggers the completion of meiosis and egg release (ovulation) in mid-cycle and stimulates the empty follicle to develop into corpus luteum, which secretes progesterone during the latter half of the cycle. LH acts on testes interstitial cells stimulating them to synthesize and secrete testosterone. FSH acts on follicle to stimulate it to release oestrogens and on spermatogonia, stimulating (with the aid of testosterone) sperm production
Growth hormone-releasing hormone (GHRH)	Stimulates pituitary release of growth hormone (GH)	Growth (also diabetogenic)
Corticotropin-releasing hormone (CRH)	Stimulates pituitary release of adrenocorticotropic hormone (ACTH)	Stimulates glucocorticoid synthesis and release
Somatostatin	Inhibits pituitary release of TSH and GH	Pituitary control
Antidiuretic hormone (ADH)	Promotes water absorption in renal tubules	Water control
Oxytocin	Stimulates uterine contraction and breast milk ejection	Lactation

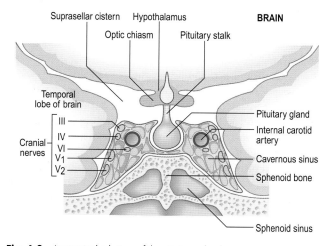

Fig. 6.3 Anatomical relations of the pituitary gland

Table 6.4 Hypopituitarism: clinical effects

Sequence of hormone deficiencies		Effects
1	LH FSH	Impotence
		Amenorrhoea
		Infertility
		Loss of pubic hair
2	GH	Impaired growth in children
3	Prolactin	Failure of lactation if postpartum (Sheehan syndrome)
4	ACTH	Hypoadrenocorticism
5	TSH	Hypothyroidism

ACTH, adrenocorticotropic hormone; FSH, follicle-stimulating hormone; GH, growth hormone; LH, luteinizing hormone; TSH, thyroid-stimulating hormone.

Inappropriate ADH secretion causes water retention, overhydration, confusion, behavioural disturbances, ataxia and dysphagia. Diagnosis is by finding hyponatraemia with concentrated urine and high plasma and urinary ADH, and an abnormal water excretion test.

Patients with SIADH are treated with fluid restriction, corticosteroids or demeclocycline.

ANTERIOR PITUITARY HYPOFUNCTION

General aspects

The usual causes of hypopituitarism are local hypothalamic or pituitary lesions, such as tumours, or irradiation (similar factors to those causing cranial diabetes insipidus) or infarction of the pituitary following postpartum haemorrhage (Sheehan syndrome).

Clinical features

The results of hypopituitarism (Table 6.4) are essentially hypofunction of the target glands, (the gonads, thyroid and/or adrenal cortex) with soft skin, hypotension, hypoadrenalism and hypothyroidism.

Multiple (pan-hypopituitarism) hormone deficiencies can result (Fig. 6.4).

General management

Hormone substitution therapy (corticosteroids and thyroxine) is needed. Surgery may be needed if there are tumours, cranial nerve defects or hydrocephalus.

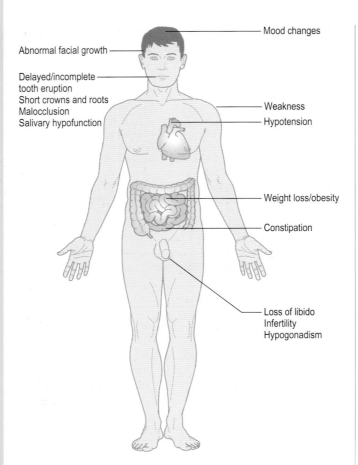

Mood changes

Abnormal facial growth

Delayed/incomplete
tooth eruption
Short crowns and roots
Malocclusion
Salivary hypofunction

Weakness

Hypotension

Weight loss/obesity

Constipation

Loss of libido
Infertility
Hypogonadism

Fig. 6.4 Hypopituitarism

Dental aspects

Patients are at risk from adrenal crisis (Ch. 1), and hypopituitary coma, which is precipitated by stress (trauma, surgery, GA, sedatives or hypnotics, or infection), much in the way that an adrenal crisis may be.

Hypopituitary coma should be treated by laying the patient flat and giving an immediate intravenous injection of 200 mg hydrocortisone sodium succinate. Blood should be taken for assay of glucose, thyroid hormones and cortisol, and 25–50 g dextrose should be given intravenously if there is hypoglycaemia (defined as a blood glucose < 3.0 mmol/L). Oxygen should be given by face mask, medical assistance summoned and emergency admission to hospital arranged.

Gonadotropin (GnRH) deficiency

Hyposecretion of GnRH may be seen most commonly in intense physical training or anorexia nervosa, rarely in syndromes (Box 6.1).

Kallman syndrome (hypogonadotropin eunuchoidism) is the most frequent form of isolated gonadotropin deficiency – a rare X-linked recessive disease caused by a defect in a cell adhesion protein that participates in the migration of the GnRH neurons. These normally originate in olfactory tissues and migrate to the hypothalamus. Impaired sense of smell is caused by the absence of the olfactory bulbs. Kallman syndrome mainly affects males and becomes apparent when they

Box 6.1 Gonadotropin deficiency syndromes

- Kallman
- Laurence–Moon–Biedl
- Moebius
- Praeder–Labhart–Willi
- Rud
- Syndromes of cerebellar ataxia

fail to develop secondary sexual characteristics. Thus, hypogonadism and anosmia, with underdeveloped genitalia and sterile gonads, are classic presentations. Treatment involves oestrogen or testosterone replacement, and pulsatile GnRH injections.

ANTERIOR PITUITARY HYPERFUNCTION

Growth hormone excess: gigantism and acromegaly

General aspects

Overproduction of growth hormone by an anterior pituitary adenoma causes gigantism before the epiphyses have fused, and acromegaly thereafter.

Clinical features

In gigantism, all the organs, soft tissues and skeleton enlarge, leading to excessively tall stature, thickening of the soft tissues with prominence of the supraorbital ridge, coarse oily skin, thick spade-like fingers and deepening of the voice.

In acromegaly, only those bones with growth potential, particularly the mandible, can enlarge. There is thickening of the soft tissues and the hands become large and spade-like. Acromegaly is one of the few endocrine diseases that should be instantly recognized – even in a passer-by – by the gross prognathism and the thickened facial features and hands (Fig. 6.5).

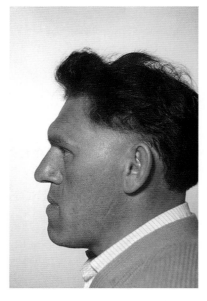

Fig. 6.5 Acromegaly showing prominent supraorbital ridges and prognathism

In both gigantism and acromegaly, local pressure effects from the pituitary tumour may cause hypopituitarism plus compression of the optic chiasma and visual field defects and raised intracranial pressure with severe headaches.

Growth hormone disorders may be complicated by diabetes mellitus, hypertension, cardiomyopathy, sleep apnoea, hypercalcaemia and osteoarthritis (Fig. 6.6). Life expectancy is also shortened by diseases such as colonic carcinoma.

General management

Family photographs may clearly demonstrate the increasingly coarse features. Skull radiography, computed tomography (CT) and MRI scans (for pituitary – sella turcica – enlargement) are indicated. Sella enlargement is also sometimes due to other causes, such as hypothalamic masses or cysts or the empty sella syndrome (this is caused by herniation of a sac of leptomeninges into the sella). Rhinorrhoea may warrant surgical correction, but no other treatment is needed.

Other investigations in growth hormone excess are visual field assessment (to detect optic chiasma involvement), glucose tolerance tests (to exclude diabetes and to assess the plasma growth hormone response), levels of growth hormone and insulin-like growth factor 1 (IGF-1), and assessment of function of the remaining pituitary.

The pituitary adenoma may be resected trans-sphenoidally or the whole gland may have to be irradiated (e.g. by transnasal yttrium). Hypopituitarism or diabetes insipidus follows such treatment.

Bromocriptine or octreotide (an analogue of the hypothalamic release-inhibiting hormone somatostatin) may also help treatment.

Dental aspects

Local analgesia is suitable. Conscious sedation may be given, if necessary, provided the airway is clear. GA may be hazardous because of complications (see later).

Dental management may be complicated by:

- Blindness, diabetes mellitus, hypertension, cardiomyopathy, arrhythmias and hypopituitarism.
- Kyphosis and other deformities affecting respiration may make GA hazardous. The glottic opening may be narrowed and the cords' mobility reduced. A goitre may further embarrass the airway.
- Rarely, acromegalics develop Cushing syndrome or hyperparathyroidism due to associated multiple endocrine adenoma syndrome.

Mandibular enlargement leads to prognathism (class III malocclusion) with spacing of the teeth and thickening of all soft tissues, but most conspicuously of the face. Orthognathic

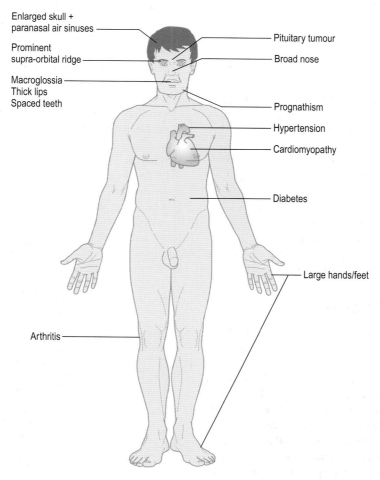

Enlarged skull + paranasal air sinuses

Prominent supra-orbital ridge

Macroglossia
Thick lips
Spaced teeth

Pituitary tumour

Broad nose

Prognathism

Hypertension

Cardiomyopathy

Diabetes

Large hands/feet

Arthritis

Fig. 6.6 Acromegaly

surgery may be needed and fatalities have followed such surgery in the past, because of airways obstruction. The paranasal air sinuses are enlarged and the skull thickened. Sialosis may develop.

PANCREAS

All carbohydrate eaten is digested into glucose, which passes from the stomach and intestine into the blood and is the main source of energy. Glucose homeostasis depends mainly on the pancreatic hormones insulin (from the beta-cells of the islets of Langerhans) and glucagon from the alpha-cells in the islets.

Insulin facilitates glucose transport into cells and thus lowers blood sugar (glucose) levels. Glucagon stimulates the liver to convert glycogen into glucose, thus raising glucose levels and having the opposite effect to insulin (Fig. 6.7). The beta-cells also produce amylin, which modulates gastric emptying and satiety and decreases the postprandial rise in glucagon. Also involved in glucose homeostasis are gastric inhibitory polypeptide (GIP) and glucagon-like peptide 1 (GLP-1) – small intestine hormones (incretins) secreted when eating. GLP-1 has a glucose-lowering effect via stimulation of insulin production and inhibition of glucagon (as well as preserving pancreatic beta-cell function, slowing gastric emptying and suppressing food intake). Several other hormones that can influence glucose include catecholamines (adrenaline and noradrenaline), corticosteroids, thyroid hormone and growth hormone.

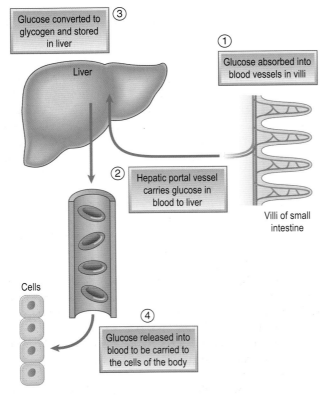

Fig. 6.7 Glucose absorption and homeostasis

DIABETES MELLITUS

General aspects

Diabetes mellitus (DM) is a disorder caused by an absolute or relative lack of insulin: there can be a low output of insulin from the pancreas, or the peripheral tissues may resist insulin. In diabetes, with insulin lacking or its action blocked, glucose cannot enter cells and, without energy, weakness results. Glucose also then accumulates in the blood (hyperglycaemia) and spills over into the urine (glucosuria), taking with it, osmotically, a large amount of water (polyuria). This leads to dehydration and thus thirst and the need to drink excessively (polydipsia). As glucose is then no longer a viable energy source, fat and protein stores are metabolized with weight loss, peripheral muscle wasting and, in type 1 diabetes, the production of ketone bodies (acetoacetate, β-hydroxybutyrate and acetone). In severe cases, ketone bodies may be detected on the breath (in particular acetone) and accumulate in the blood (ketonaemia) as well as be excreted in the urine (ketonuria). The resultant metabolic ketoacidosis leads to a compensatory increase in respiratory rate (hyperventilation) and a secondary respiratory alkalosis.

Chronic hyperglycaemia causes microvascular complications, and atherosclerosis, and is a leading cause of death and disability.

Diabetes affects about 3–4% of the general population but may be recognized in only 75% of those individuals, yet it is a leading cause of death and disability. Worldwide, about 246 million people are affected. Risk factors for diabetes include family history (the risk of developing diabetes rises if a close relative, such as a parent or sibling, has the disease); being overweight; inactivity; age (the risk of developing type 2 diabetes rises with age, especially after age 45) and race. Genetics has a role. Type 1 diabetes is more common in Caucasians and in European countries, such as Finland and Sweden. Type 2 diabetes is especially common in people of African heritage, Asians and Hispanics, and has a stronger genetic background. Diabetes affects up to one-third of the elderly from the Asian subcontinent. Among the Pima Indians in USA and in Nauru in the Pacific, around half of all adults have type 2 diabetes – the highest rates in the world. The prevalence of diabetes appears to be rising, mainly as more children and adolescents become overweight. In contrast, fewer diabetics remain undiagnosed, and associated ischaemic heart disease and retinal disease are falling.

Diabetes may be primary, or secondary to some other factor(s) as shown in Table 6.5. Type 2 is by far the most common type of diabetes (Table 6.6).

Table 6.5	Classification of diabetes mellitus
Primary	Type 1 – insulin-dependent (IDDM); juvenile onset Type 2 – non-insulin-dependent (NIDDM); maturity onset
Secondary	Drugs (corticosteroids, thiazide diuretics, beta-blockers) Endocrine disorders (phaeochromocytoma, acromegaly, Cushing syndrome) Pancreatic disease (pancreatitis), haemochromatosis Pregnancy (gestational diabetes) usually represents type 2 diabetes exposed by the increased insulin resistance of pregnancy

Table 6.6 Types of diabetes mellitus

Type	Formerly called	Typical time of onset	% of all diabetes	Aetiopathogenesis	Autoantibodies	Other factors
1	Insulin-dependent (IDDM)	Juvenile onset	5–10	Insulin deficiency	Islet cell antibodies in up to 90%	Genetic; HLA DR3/4 in 95%. Viruses (mumps or Coxsackie) affect beta-cells: implicated in autoimmune disease
2	Non-insulin-dependent (NIDDM)	Maturity onset	90–95	Insulin resistance	None	Overweight, often family history of diabetes; no HLA association. Subtypes result from mutations in gluco-kinase gene, changes in insulin signalling, defective phosphatidylinositol kinases or other mechanisms
3	Gestational diabetes	Appears usually in second or third trimester of pregnancy	Rare	Affects up to 5% of pregnant women. Placental hormones interfere with insulin	None	Most common in people of African heritage or with a family history of diabetes. Increased risk of type 2 diabetes later

Type 1 diabetes – formerly termed insulin-dependent (IDDM) or juvenile-onset diabetes – is most commonly diagnosed at about 12 years of age and commonly presents before the third decade, but can appear at any age. Associated with other organ-specific autoimmune diseases, it is characterized by antibodies directed against insulin and the pancreatic islets of Langerhans. It may have a viral (possibly Coxsackie or rubella) aetiology. Latent autoimmune diabetes in adults (LADA) is essentially a slow presentation of type 1 diabetes, which is seen in slimmer patients who progress quickly to insulin requirement. Anti-GAD (glutamic acid decarboxylase) antibodies may be helpful in the diagnosis.

Type 2 diabetes – formerly termed non-insulin-dependent (NIDDM) or maturity-onset diabetes – accounts for 80–90% of diabetics. Generally it occurs in genetically predisposed individuals over the age of 40 who are typically overweight. Patients are insulin resistant and have diminished beta-cell function. Maturity-onset diabetes of the young (MODY) is caused by autosomal dominant mutations and so there is vertical transmission of diabetes within families. The phenotype varies from mild glucose intolerance to insulin-requiring diabetes, typically diagnosed before the age of 25 years.

Gestational diabetes is basically an insulin-resistant state exposing future risk of type 2 diabetes (Table 6.6).

Clinical features

Patients with diabetes may be asymptomatic and detected on routine or opportunistic screening, or present in a variety of ways related to severity and degree of onset (Table 6.7).

Lethargy is the most common symptom but hyperglycaemia, polyuria and thirst (polydipsia) are prominent. Since glucose is lost as an energy source in type 1 diabetes, fats must be metabolized, leading to weight loss from fat breakdown to fatty acids and ketone bodies, which appear in the blood causing acidosis and hyperventilation, and in the urine (ketonuria) and to some extent in the breath (acetone). Overproduction of acetoacetate is converted to the other ketone bodies, hydroxybutyrate and acetone. Diabetes is also associated with immune deficiencies, particularly polymorph dysfunction, leading to susceptibility to infections (mainly skin infections and mucosal candidosis; Fig. 6.8).

Table 6.7 Acute and chronic presenting features of diabetes mellitus

Acute	Chronic
Thirst	Thirst
Polyuria and polydipsia	Polyuria and polydipsia
Weight loss and weakness	Weight loss and weakness
Lethargy	Lethargy
Confusion/aggression/ behavioural changes	Irritability
Abdominal pain	Recurrent skin, oral and genital infections
Nausea and vomiting	Visual deterioration
Ketoacidosis	Paraesthesia (hands and feet)
Dehydration	
Renal failure	
Coma	

Type 1 diabetes develops most often in children and young adults, generally before the age of 25. Symptoms usually develop over a short period. Excessive thirst and urination, constant hunger, weight loss, blurred vision and extreme fatigue are typical. Life-threatening diabetic coma (diabetic ketoacidosis) is a significant risk. Insulin is required daily for treatment, for life, and diet must be controlled. Hypoglycaemia is a risk.

Type 2 diabetes develops most often in overweight patients. Symptoms usually develop gradually. Fatigue, frequent urination, unusual thirst, weight loss, blurred vision, frequent infections, and slow healing of wounds or sores are seen. Most patients with type 2 diabetes can be managed on diet and oral hypoglycaemic drugs. Many will eventually need insulin, but are often resistant. About 80% of people with type 2 diabetes have the *metabolic syndrome* that includes obesity, elevated blood pressure and high levels of blood lipids (Ch. 23).

Maturity-onset diabetes of youth is a rare, dominantly inherited form of type 2 diabetes that usually affects people below the age of 25 years.

Factors that affect the blood glucose level are shown in Box 6.2.

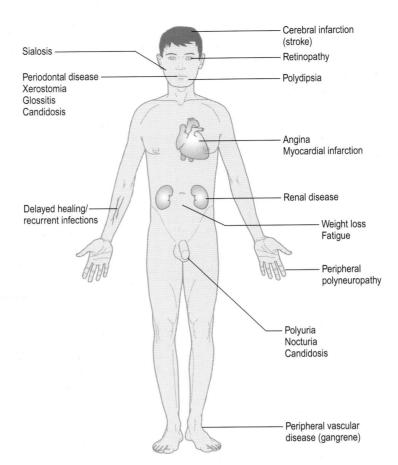

Sialosis

Periodontal disease
Xerostomia
Glossitis
Candidosis

Delayed healing/
recurrent infections

Cerebral infarction
(stroke)

Retinopathy

Polydipsia

Angina
Myocardial infarction

Renal disease

Weight loss
Fatigue

Peripheral
polyneuropathy

Polyuria
Nocturia
Candidosis

Peripheral vascular
disease (gangrene)

Fig. 6.8   Diabetes mellitus

Box 6.2 Factors that affect the blood glucose level

- Food – carbohydrates raise blood glucose, which is highest 1–2 h after a meal
- Exercise and physical activity lower blood glucose.
- Medications: insulin and oral diabetes medications lower blood glucose. (Steroids, thiazides, beta-blockers and niacin may raise blood glucose)
- Illnesses such as infections can raise blood glucose
- Alcohol – even about 2 units can cause blood glucose to fall
- Hormones – oestrogen typically increases cells' response to insulin, and progesterone makes them more resistant

Table 6.8   Causes of hypoglycaemia

Common (diabetics)	Rare (non-diabetics)
Excess insulin or hypoglycaemic drug	Insulinoma
Missed meal	Hepatic disease
Unaccustomed exercise	Hypoadrenocorticism
Alcohol (the effect of which is delayed)	Hypopituitarism
	Functional hypoglycaemia
	Beta-blockers

Acute complications of diabetes

Diabetes can lead to coma. Hypoglycaemic coma is the main acute complication of diabetes, is growing in frequency with the trend towards tighter metabolic control of diabetes, and is usually the result of one or more of the above factors. Less common causes are shown in Table 6.8. Many insulin-treated patients are liable to hypoglycaemia, due to an imbalance between food intake and usage, and insulin therapy. Hypoglycaemia can be of rapid onset, and may resemble fainting. There is adrenaline release, leading to a strong and bounding pulse, sweaty skin, and often anxiety, irritability and disorientation, before consciousness is lost. Occasionally the patient may convulse.

Treat first (Table 6.9): hypoglycaemia must be quickly corrected with glucose or brain damage can result. Glucose will cause little harm in hyperglycaemic coma but will improve hypoglycaemia. Never give insulin since this can cause severe brain damage or kill a hypoglycaemic patient. Assess the glucose level with a testing strip.

If the patient is conscious, give glucose solution or gel (GlucoGel) immediately by mouth or 10 g sugar but, if the patient is comatose, give 10–20 ml of 20–50% sterile dextrose intravenously or, if a vein cannot readily be found, glucagon 1 mg intramuscularly. On arousal, the patient should also be given glucose orally, usually in the form of longer-acting carbohydrate (e.g. bread, biscuits).

Other diabetics are difficult to control (brittle diabetes – a term usually given to adolescent girls who may be self-harming) and more prone to ketosis, severe acidosis and hyperglycaemia (diabetic coma), the result of a relative or absolute deficiency of insulin. In patients under treatment, it may be precipitated by factors such as infections.

Hyperglycaemic coma usually has a slow onset over many hours, with deepening drowsiness (but unconsciousness is rare, so an unconscious diabetic should always be assumed to be hypoglycaemic), signs of dehydration (dry skin, weak pulse, hypotension), acidosis (deep breathing) and ketosis (acetone smell on breath and vomiting) only in type 1 diabetes. If it is certain that collapse is due to hyperglycaemic ketoacidotic coma, the first priority is to establish an intravenous infusion line. This enables rapid rehydration to correct dehydration and electrolyte (especially potassium) losses, and the administration of insulin. Blood should be taken for baseline measurements of glucose, electrolytes, pH and blood gases. Raised plasma ketone body levels can be demonstrated with a testing strip such as Ketostix (Ames). Insulin is then started, such as 20 units i.m. stat. Medical help should be obtained as soon as possible.

Coma in a diabetic patient, though usually due to hypo- or hyperglycaemia, may have other causes such as myocardial infarction (Ch. 5).

Chronic complications of diabetes

Diabetes is associated with long-term microvascular and macrovascular complications that can affect almost every part of the body (Table 6.10). Diabetes is a leading cause of death and disability due to premature cardiovascular disease: the risk of myocardial infarction is at least tripled. Renal and retinal complications are also incapacitating, as is gangrene of toes.

Smoking increases the risk of many chronic complications. Phagocytic defects contribute to an immune defect and liability to infections. Babies born to women with diabetes are often large and sometimes have birth defects. Occasionally there are associations of type 1 diabetes with autoimmune disorders, especially Addison disease. There may be a predilection to oral cancer.

General management

Glycosuria is *usually* indicative of diabetes, but absence of glycosuria does not completely exclude it, and confirmation by blood glucose levels is essential. Diagnosis is from the presence of raised blood (venous plasma) glucose level (Table 6.11).

Table 6.9 Hypoglycaemic and hyperglycaemic comas and their treatment

Hypoglycaemic coma	Hyperglycaemic coma
Diabetes usually known	Diabetes may be unrecognized
Too much insulin or too little food, or too much exercise or alcohol	Too little insulin, infection, or myocardial infarct
Adrenaline release causes: Sweaty warm skin Rapid bounding pulse Dilated (reacting) pupils Anxiety, tremor, aggression Tingling around mouth	Acidosis in some variants causes: Vomiting Hyperventilation Ketonuria Acetone breath
Cerebral hypoglycaemia causes: Confusion, disorientation, aggression Headache Dysarthria Unconsciousness Focal neurological signs (e.g. fits)	Osmotic diuresis and polyuria cause: Dehydration Hypotension Tachycardia Dry mouth and skin Abdominal pain
Management	
Take blood for baseline glucose, electrolytes, urea, Hb and PCV	
If conscious, give Hypostop (GlucoGel) or 25 g glucose orally (2 teaspoons sugar, 3 lumps sugar, 3 Dextrosol tablets, 60 ml Lucozade, 15 ml Ribena, 90 ml cola drink (*not* 'diet' variety) or 1/3 pt milk)	Put up infusion to rehydrate and give insulin
If comatose, give 20 mg 20% or 50% dextrose i.v. and on arousal 25 mg orally	
If i.v. injection impossible, give glucagon 1 mg i.m.	
Call ambulance (Ch.1)	

Table 6.10 Chronic complications of diabetes

Cardiovascular	Atherosclerosis leading to ischaemic heart disease, cerebrovascular disease and peripheral gangrene
	Cardiorespiratory arrest
Renal	Renal damage and failure
Ocular	Retinopathy
	Cataracts
Neuropathies	Peripheral polyneuropathy
	Mononeuropathies
	Autonomic neuropathy (postural hypotension)
Infections	Candidosis
	Staphylococcal infections
	Systemic mycoses (rarely)

Table 6.11 Glucose assays in the diagnosis of diabetes

Test	Confirms diabetes[a]	Excludes diabetes
Fasting plasma glucose (after a person has fasted for 8 h)	> 7.0 mmol/L	< 6 mmol/L
Random blood glucose (taken any time of day)	≥ 11.1 mmol/L	< 8 mmol/L[b]
Plasma glucose taken 2 h after a person has consumed a drink containing 75 g of glucose in oral glucose tolerance test (OGTT)	> 11.1 mmol/L[a]	< 11.1 mmol/L

[a]If associated with symptoms, or abnormal on repeat testing.
[b]Must be checked with fasting glucose.

A diagnosis of diabetes is made when any one of the above three tests (glycosutia random and fasting blood glucose) is positive, with a second test positive on a different day (not needed if symptomatic). *Pre-diabetes* is the term given when there is either of the following.

- An impaired glucose tolerance (IGT) test – blood glucose during the oral glucose tolerance test is higher than normal but not high enough for a diagnosis of diabetes (7.8–11.0 mmol/L).
- An impaired fasting glucose (IFG; impaired fasting glycaemia) – fasting plasma glucose is higher than normal (6.1–6.9 mmol/L) but less than the level confirming the presence of diabetes.

Patients with IGT and IFG are more likely to develop type 2 diabetes, and have an increased risk of cardiovascular disease.

Diabetes prevention

- Weight reduction and greater physical activity.
- Diet may help diabetic control; recommendations are to:
-eat more starches such as bread, cereal and starchy vegetables. eat five portions of fruits and vegetables every day. Soluble fibres found mainly in fruits, vegetables and some seeds, are especially useful by helping to slow down or reduce intestinal absorption of glucose. Legumes, such as cooked kidney beans, are among the highest soluble-fibre foods. Other fibre-containing foods, such as carrots, also have a positive levelling effect on blood glucose.
-eat fewer sugars and sweets.

Treatment

Diabetic control should attempt to maintain blood glucose levels as normal as possible, to minimize microvascular complications.

Treatment objectives are:

- reduction of hyperglycaemia – to alleviate presenting symptoms
- prevention of hypoglycaemia and other acute complications
- maintenance of near-normal blood glucose levels to prevent chronic complications
- reducing other cardiovascular risk factors (smoking, exercise, hypertension and lipids).

Individuals should be educated with regard to the importance of good long-term diabetic control and have a thorough knowledge of the disease. The progressive nature of diabetes, its complications and management aims should be well understood. Patients should also be aware of the range of diabetic services available and how to make appropriate use of them. A multidisciplinary team approach is required for their effective management. Meals should be at regular intervals, with a high fibre and relatively high carbohydrate content but avoiding sugars, and with a caloric intake strictly related to physical activity. Lifestyle changes such as exercise, diet, fasting, travel (including changing time zones) and changes in working practices can impact on diabetic control. All diabetics should carry a card indicating the diagnosis, treatment schedule and physician in charge and should be encouraged to wear a Medic-Alert type device.

Urine testing has little or no place in assessment or control of diabetes. Control is assessed by blood glucose levels and used to guide medication. A glucometer allows glucose readings to be taken easily by the patient at home. Fasting glucose < 6 mmol/L is normal. Long-term assessment of glucose control is made by estimation of the blood level of glycosylated haemoglobin (HbA1c). HbA1c is normal adult haemoglobin that binds glucose, remains in the circulation for the life of the erythrocyte and therefore acts as a cumulative index of diabetic control over the preceding 3 months; the higher the glycosylated haemoglobin level, the greater the risk of chronic complications. Patients should have an HbA1c test every 3–6 months; glycosylated haemoglobin below 4.8% of total haemoglobin is normal. Fructosamine is an alternative assay of long-term diabetic control.

Optimum control would be to aim to keep blood glucose levels at 4–7 mmol/L before meals (preprandial) and at no higher than 10 mmol/L 2 h after meals (postprandial) and HbA1c (long-term glucose level) optimally at 7% or less.

Type 1 diabetes

Basic treatment of type 1 diabetes is subcutaneous insulin administration, the amount being balanced against food intake and daily activities, and home blood glucose testing. The types of insulin used include those shown in Table 6.12. Insulin may be of human or animal (pork or beef) origin, and comes in various forms: short-acting, intermediate-acting or long-acting insulins; insulin analogues have been modified so as to produce very rapid-onset and very long duration of activity.

Modern highly purified animal insulins are safe, effective and reasonably reproducible in their actions. Human insulins,

Table 6.12 Different insulins

Type	Origin	Examples	Effect starts in (min)	Effect lasts (h)
Rapid-acting	Analogue	Lispro Aspart Glulisine	15	4–6
Short-acting	Human	Soluble insulin Actrapid	30–60	6–8
Intermediate	Human isophane	Humulin I Insulatard	60–120	10–14
Long-acting	Analogue Bovine insulin zinc suspension Bovine protamine zinc insulin	Glargine Detemir Hypurin bovine lente Hypurin bovine protamine zinc	120	24

Biphasic insulins are mixtures of short-acting and intermediate-acting insulins in different proportions, such as 30/70, 50/50. Examples are NovoMix 30, Humulin M3, Insuman Comb and Humalog Mix25.

prepared usually by genetic engineering, are similar to highly purified pork insulins. There may also be cultural and religious issues to consider. All insulin therapy is associated with the risk of hypoglycaemia, but there is no evidence that this is worse with human rather than animal insulins. Genetically modified insulin *analogues* may provide advantages in patients with problematic hypoglycaemia but are expensive and there are no long-term safety data.

Insulin is given by injection. There is no single standard for patterns of insulin administration. The dose varies widely between patients and also depends on the type of preparation, diet and exercise. Infections or traumas also raise insulin requirements. The first line would be basal bolus (see later) with others going on to twice-daily fixed mixtures (biphasic insulins), which would include a rapid-acting insulin analogue (e.g. NovoMix 30). Neutral insulins purified to be virtually non-antigenic (monocomponent insulins) and human (recombinant) insulins have been introduced.

The following three insulin regimes are in common use.

1. Twice-daily doses of short- and intermediate-acting insulin, often pre-mixed, given before breakfast and before the evening meal. The short-acting doses cover the insulin needs of the morning and evening. The intermediate-acting doses cover the afternoon and overnight.

2. Three times a day dosing; short-acting and intermediate-acting insulin before breakfast, short-acting insulin before the evening meal and intermediate-acting insulin before bed.

3. Multiple daily doses: short-acting insulin used before each main meal and an intermediate- or long-acting insulin used before bedtime to give coverage overnight.

Type 2 diabetes

Basic treatment of type 2 diabetes is by controlled eating and physical activity, and home blood glucose testing. In some patients, hypoglycaemic drugs may also be needed (Table 6.13), which may be used as monotherapy or in certain combinations such as dual therapy (e.g. metformin plus a sulfonylurea or sitagliptin; or a glitazone plus sitagliptin).

Intensive control of blood glucose and blood pressure lowers the risk of blindness, renal disease, stroke and myocardial infarction. Gastric bypass surgery provides long-term control for obesity and diabetes in adult-onset diabetes, and also alleviates some of the complications.

Emerging treatments

Combined kidney and pancreas transplantation is used for renal failure from type 1 diabetes in persons who are otherwise in acceptable health. Most people who receive a donor pancreas fall into this group. Approximately 85% of people who receive a combined kidney and pancreas transplant no longer require insulin a year after surgery. Pancreatic transplantation can be associated with all the problems that accompany immunosuppression (Ch. 35).

Islet cell transplantation is now considered treatment rather than research, and offers a less invasive, expensive and risky option than a pancreas transplant.

Dental aspects

There are no specific oral manifestations of diabetes mellitus but, even if well controlled, patients are predisposed to infections, and diabetics have more severe periodontal disease than

Table 6.13 Hypoglycaemic drugs other than insulin

Drug group	Route of administration	Examples	Mode of action and comments
Biguanides	Oral	Metformin	Decrease target tissue insulin resistance, affect the absorption and metabolism of glucose and reduce appetite but can induce lactic acidosis
Glitazones (thiazolidinediones)	Oral	Pioglitazone Rosiglitazone	Help overcome insulin resistance by binding to the adipocyte receptor. Mainly used in addition to metformin/sulfonylurea. Contraindicated in heart failure, ischaemic heart disease or peripheral vascular disease. May increase bone fracture risk
Incretins (dipeptidyl peptidase-4 inhibitors)	Oral	Saxagliptin Sitagliptin Vildagliptin	Impede breakdown of endogenous incretin glucagon-like peptide 1 (GLP-1) thus stimulating insulin secretion, but rarely causing hypoglycaemia
Incretin mimetics	Injected	Exenatide (twice daily) Liiaglutide (once daily)	GLP-1 mimetics may produce nausea but have the advantage over other drugs of not producing weight gain
Intestinal alpha-glucosidase inhibitors	Oral	Acarbose Miglitol	Slightly delay intestinal breakdown of oligosaccharides to glucose and monosaccharides
Meglitinides	Oral	Nateglinide Repaglinide	Stimulate insulin release. Preprandial glucose regulators
Sulfonylureas	Oral	Gliclazide Glipizide Gliquidone Glimepiride Glibenclamide (infrequently used and not in elderly)	Stimulate the release of insulin from the pancreas. More likely than metformin to cause hypoglycaemia. May enhance, or be enhanced by, aspirin, anticoagulants, monoamine oxidase inhibitors, beta-blockers or clofibrate
Synthetic amylin	Injected	Pramlintide	Adjunct for use in type 2 or type 1 diabetes. Danger of hypoglycaemia

controls. Severe periodontitis may also upset glycaemic control. If diabetic control is poor, oral candidosis can develop and cause, for example, angular stomatitis. Severe diabetes with ketoacidosis predisposes to and is the main cause of mucormycosis originating in the paranasal sinuses and nose (Ch.).Severe dentoalveolar abscesses with fascial space involvement in seemingly healthy individuals may indicate diabetes. Any such patients should be investigated to exclude it and other immune defects.

In patients with insulin-treated diabetes, circumoral paraesthesia is a common and important sign of impending hypoglycaemia. Neuropathy may occasionally cause cranial nerve deficits and occasionally there is swelling of the salivary glands (sialosis) due to autonomic neuropathy. Temporary lingual and labial paraesthesia may follow the removal of mandibular third molar teeth. A burning mouth sensation in the absence of physical changes may be possible. A dry mouth may result from dehydration. The 'Grinspan syndrome' (diabetes, lichen planus and hypertension) may be the result of purely coincidental associations of common disorders probably related to drug use.

Diabetes may have significant complications, such as hypoglycaemia, visual impairment, renal failure, gangrene, stroke or myocardial infarction, which can significantly influence oral health care. The main hazard is hypoglycaemia, as dental disease and treatment may disrupt the normal pattern of food intake. Prevent this by planning, such as by administering oral glucose just before the appointment if a patient has taken his or her medication but has not had the appropriate meal. Furthermore, particularly before surgical procedures, the patient's blood glucose level may be tested using a point of care device prior to treatment, and oral glucose given if the level is too low – less than about 5 mmol/L (180 mg/dl). If normal eating will not be resumed at lunchtime, a post-operative blood glucose level may be taken and further glucose given.

In a well-controlled diabetic patient, providing that normal diet has, and can, be taken, it is feasible to carry out even minor surgical procedures, such as simple single extractions under LA, as long as the procedure is carried out within 2 h of breakfast and the morning insulin injection, with no change in the insulin regimen. More protracted procedures, such as multiple extractions, must only be carried out in hospital. Poorly controlled diabetics (whether type 1 or 2) should also be referred for improved control of their blood glucose before non-emergency treatment is performed.

Drugs should be sugar-free, avoiding those that can disturb diabetic control: steroids, which increase blood glucose; and doxycycline, tetracyclines and ciprofloxacin, which enhance insulin hypoglycaemia. Acetaminophen/paracetamol or codeine are the analgesics of choice. Non- steroidal anti-inflammatory drugs (NSAIDs) should be used with caution in view of renal damage and risk of gastrointestinal bleeding, especially as many diabetics are already on low-dose aspirin for prophylaxis of ischaemic heart disease. The dentist should manage infections aggressively, as people with diabetes may be immunocompromised (Ch. 20). Amoxicillin is the antibiotic of choice.

Local analgesia can usually be safely used in diabetics; the dose of adrenaline is unlikely to increase blood glucose levels significantly. Conscious sedation with benzodiazepines can usually be safely used. Autonomic neuropathy in diabetes can cause orthostatic hypotension; therefore the supine patient should be slowly raised upright in the dental chair. Routine non-surgical procedures or short minor surgical procedures under LA can be carried out with no special precautions apart from ensuring that treatment does not interfere with eating.

For surgical procedures, the essential requirement is to avoid hypoglycaemia but to keep hyperglycaemia below levels which may be harmful because of delayed wound healing or phagocyte dysfunction. The desired whole blood glucose level is therefore 3–5 mmol/L. For major surgery, intermediate insulins are usually omitted and an intravenous infusion is given containing glucose to which, according to the level of plasma glucose, regularly measured, soluble (regular) insulin can be added as required. The effects of stress and trauma may raise insulin requirements and precipitate ketosis.

Diabetics on insulin

In a well-controlled insulin-dependent diabetic, providing that a normal diet can be taken and that the procedure is carried out within 2 h of breakfast and the morning insulin injection, with no change in the insulin regimen, it is feasible to carry out minor surgical procedures (e.g. simple single extractions under LA, or minor operations under GA in hospital) by operating early in the morning and withholding both food and insulin from the previous midnight, until after the procedure.

More protracted procedures, such as multiple extractions, must only be carried out in hospital, with the following precautions.

- Pre-operative assessment (Table 6.14): before the operation, the patient should be put on soluble insulin and stabilized. Insulin may need to be given twice or three times daily, and control is confirmed by estimation of blood glucose (fasting, midday and before the evening meal).
- The operation should be carried out early in the morning and booked first in the list, so that any delays in the operation schedule will not impair diabetic control.
- At 8.00–9.00 am blood should be taken for glucose estimation and an intravenous infusion set up giving glucose 10 g, soluble insulin 2 units and potassium 2 mmol/h (GIK infusion), until normal oral feeding is resumed – at which time the patient can be returned to the pre-operative insulin regimen.
- Blood glucose should be monitored at 2–4-hour intervals until the patient is feeding normally.
- The patient is put on an insulin sliding scale from the morning of the day of operation until the normal feeding regimen is possible.

General anaesthesia for the diabetic patient may be complicated especially by hypoglycaemia, chronic renal failure, ischaemic heart disease or autonomic neuropathy. Severe autonomic neuropathy can lead to postural hypotension and impaired ability to respond to hypoglycaemia, and carries a risk of cardiorespiratory arrest under GA.

Diabetics controlled by diet alone

These diabetics have no liability to ketosis and, if well controlled, can frequently tolerate minor surgical procedures, such as single extractions under LA. A brief GA can be given without

Table 6.14 Management of diabetes requiring general anaesthesia

	Non-insulin-dependent diabetes*a*	Insulin-dependent diabetes	
	Minor operations (e.g. few extractions)	Major operations (e.g. maxillofacial surgery)	Any operation
Pre-operative	Stop biguanides	Stabilize on at least twice-daily insulin for 2–3 days pre-operatively. One day pre-operatively use only short-acting insulin (Actrapid soluble or neutral)	
Perioperative	Omit oral hypoglycaemic. Estimate blood glucose level	Do not give sulfonylurea or subcutaneous insulin on day of operation. Estimate blood glucose level. Set up intravenous infusion of 10% glucose 500 ml containing Actrapid or Leo neutral insulin 10 units plus KCl 1 g at 8.00 am. Infuse over 4 h. Estimate blood glucose and potassium levels 2-hourly. Adjust insulin and potassium to keep glucose at 5–10 mmol/L and normokalaemic	
Post-operative	Estimate blood glucose 4 h post-operatively	Continue infusion 4-hourly. Estimate blood glucose 4-hourly. Estimate potassium 8-hourly	
On resuming normal diet	Start sulfonylurea or other usual regimen	Stop infusion. Start Actrapid or Leo neutral insulin and continue over the next 2 days. Start sulfonylurea. Start normal insulin regimen	

*a*If well controlled, otherwise treat as insulin dependent.

special precautions apart from monitoring the blood glucose before the operation and on recovery, at 2-hourly intervals. The anaesthetic must be given in hospital and, if ketonuria develops, blood glucose levels can be rapidly estimated. Diabetics requiring more major surgery should be admitted to hospital pre-operatively for assessment and possible stabilization with insulin. The blood glucose should be monitored during and after operation.

There is no good evidence to support the belief that well-controlled or even moderately well-controlled, non-ketotic diabetic patients are prone to infection when undergoing uncomplicated dentoalveolar surgery. Routine administration of prophylactic antibiotics should be considered only in situations where prophylactic antimicrobials would be used for a non-diabetic patient.

Poorly controlled diabetics (whether type 1 or 2), with raised fasting glucose levels, should be referred for improved control of their blood glucose before elective surgery is performed. If emergency surgery is needed, then prophylactic antibiotics are recommended.

Diabetics controlled by diet and oral hypoglycaemics

Patients controlled by oral hypoglycaemic drugs may tolerate minor oral surgical procedures under LA, provided that normal meals are not interrupted. Well-controlled patients can safely have short simple procedures carried out under GA in hospital without insulin, but the blood glucose should be monitored 2-hourly.

If diabetic control is poor, if the patient is on large doses of drugs or if more major surgery is planned, a suggested regimen is as follows:

- Pre-operative assessment and stabilization.
- Metformin must be stopped at least 2 days pre-operatively because of the risk of lactic acidosis if contrast media are being used.
- At 8.00–9.00 am on the day of operation, blood is taken for glucose estimation and an intravenous infusion line is put up.

- Infusion of 10% glucose (500 ml) containing 10 mmol potassium chloride and insulin 5 units (if the blood glucose is < 6 mmol/L) or insulin 10 units (if the blood glucose is > 6 mmol/L) appears to be satisfactory. The blood glucose is monitored regularly and this regimen is continued at 100 ml/h until normal food can be taken orally.
- The infusion is then stopped and the oral hypoglycaemic restarted.

ADRENAL CORTEX

The hypothalamus is in overall control of adrenocortical function by producing factors that stimulate the pituitary to release adrenocorticotropic hormone (Fig. 6.9). ACTH arises from a

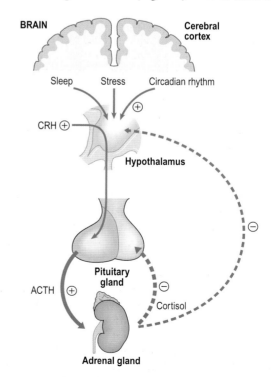

Fig. 6.9 Adrenal control homeostasis.
CRH Corticotrophin releasing hormone ACTH Adrenocorticotrophic hormone

precursor, pro-opiomelanocortin, and is released in response to hypothalamic corticotropin-releasing hormone (CRH), with a diurnal rhythm (peak early morning, nadir on retiring). Circulating corticosteroids have a negative feedback control on hypothalamic activity and ACTH production. There is thus a hypothalamic–pituitary–adrenocortical axis. Glucocorticoid production is stimulated by ACTH (corticotropin) from the anterior pituitary gland, and cortisol exerts a negative feedback on the pituitary and hypothalamus. The adrenal cortex produces a series of corticosteroids, mainly cortisol (hydrocortisone) and corticosterone (the glucocorticoids), and aldosterone (the mineralocorticoid).

Corticosteroids are an essential part of the body's response to stresses such as trauma, infection, GA or operation, pain, stress, fever, burns and hypoglycaemia. At such times, there is normally raised adrenal corticosteroid production and the size of the response is proportional to the degree of stress.

Mineralocorticoid (aldosterone) production is regulated mainly by the renin–angiotensin system, renal blood pressure and sodium and potassium levels. Renin, an enzyme that converts angiotensinogen to angiotensin 1, is produced by the renal juxtaglomerular apparatus in response to low sodium or renal perfusion (Fig. 6.10). Angiotensin 1 is converted by angiotensin-converting enzyme in the lung parenchyma, to the active angiotensin 2, which stimulates aldosterone release. Aldosterone acts on the kidney to promote sodium retention, potassium excretion and fluid retention, and causes vasoconstriction and thirst.

Atrial natriuretic peptide, synthesized by myocytes in the right atrium and ventricles, causes sodium loss and thus counters the effect of aldosterone.

ADRENOCORTICAL DISORDERS

Adrenocortical hyperfunction may lead to release of excessive:

- glucocorticoids (Cushing disease)
- mineralocorticoids (Conn syndrome or hyperaldosteronism) or
- androgens (congenital adrenal hyperplasia).

CUSHING DISEASE

General aspects

Cushing disease is caused by excess glucocorticoid production by adrenal hyperplasia secondary to excess ACTH production by pituitary basophil adenomas. It is occasionally caused by ectopic ACTH from adrenal or other tumours such as small-cell lung carcinomas or carcinoid tumours. A similar clinical picture results where there is ectopic production by a tumour (usually a bronchial carcinoid tumour) of CRH.

Cushing syndrome is clinically similar but is caused by primary adrenal disease (adenoma or rarely carcinoma or micronodular bilateral hyperplasia). However, most cases of Cushing syndrome have been found to be due to microadenomas of the pituitary, so that the terms Cushing disease and Cushing syndrome are in effect synonymous.

A similar clinical picture is produced by corticosteroid therapy or rarely by the multiple endocrine adenoma syndromes (see later).

Clinical features

These are listed in Box 6.3. The most obvious feature is central obesity, affecting the abdomen and also the face (moon face; Fig. 6.11). Facial photographs from the past and more recently may show the development of moon face, interscapular

> **Box 6.3 Hyperadrenocorticism: clinical features**
>
> - Weakness
> - Weight gain
> - Truncal obesity
> - Hypertension
> - Hirsutism
> - Amenorrhoea
> - Cutaneous striae
> - Personality changes

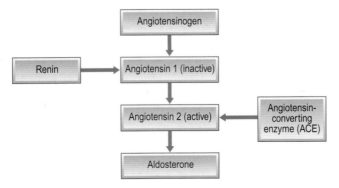

Fig. 6.10 Blood pressure regulation via aldosterone production

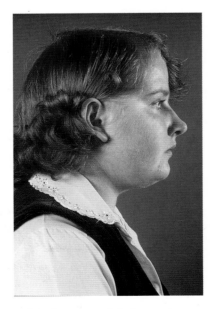

Fig. 6.11 Moon face in a patient with Cushing syndrome

region (buffalo hump) and trunk, but with relative sparing of the limbs. Hypertension is common. Breakdown of proteins with conversion to glucose (gluconeogenesis) leads to hyperglycaemia and possibly diabetes mellitus, osteoporosis, muscle weakness, thinning of the skin, purpura and purplish skin striae (Fig. 6.12). Other features may include hirsutism and acne, oligomenorrhoea, infections and psychoses (Fig. 6.13).

General management

The main differential diagnoses are from severe depression and alcoholism.

The diagnosis is confirmed by a raised plasma cortisol level and absence of the normal diurnal variation in cortisol levels, normally highest in the morning around 8.00 am and lowest at midnight. Another useful screening test is to measure plasma cortisol at 8.00–9.00 am after giving 1 mg dexamethasone orally at midnight to suppress the adrenal glands temporarily; in health, cortisol levels fall but in Cushing syndrome there is no such fall (low-dose overnight dexamethasone suppression test).

Localization of the cause as adrenal, pituitary or ectopic tumour relies on the corticotropin-releasing hormone stimulation test, which depends on the fact that the pituitary responds to CRH, whereas adrenal and other tumours producing ectopic ACTH do not. Baseline plasma ACTH and cortisol levels are first obtained, CRH is then given and an exaggerated rise in ACTH and cortisol levels is given by patients with pituitary Cushing but not by patients with other types of Cushing syndrome. Other special dexamethasone tests or sampling from the inferior petrosal sinus are needed to distinguish pituitary from adrenal causes of Cushing syndrome. Other diagnostic aids include pituitary MRI, tomography of the sella turcica, abdominal CT and adrenal ultrasound scans.

In Cushing disease, the pituitary tumour is treated by transsphenoidal microadenectomy and then, for those not cured, by pituitary irradiation or an yttrium implant. Cyproheptadine or sodium valproate is sometimes used where surgery is inappropriate.

In Cushing syndrome, the adrenal gland is usually irradiated or excised (adrenalectomy), though ketoconazole, mitotane, aminoglutethimide or metyrapone can also be effective. Some patients subjected to bilateral adrenalectomy develop pituitary ACTH-producing adenomas with hyperpigmentation and symptoms related to the pituitary tumour (Nelson syndrome). Cushing syndrome secondary to carcinoma of the bronchus is not controllable by surgery but metapyrone, an inhibitor of hydroxylation in the adrenal cortex, can relieve symptoms.

Steroid replacement is subsequently necessary in treated Cushing disease/syndrome. Subacute adrenal insufficiency develops if corticosteroid dosage is reduced too quickly after replacement therapy in post-surgical patients with Cushing syndrome. Features include lethargy, abdominal pain, hypotension, and psychological disturbances, and a characteristic sign is scaly desquamation of the facial skin, particularly of the forehead.

Dental aspects

Local analgesia is preferred for pain control. Conscious sedation can be given, preferably with nitrous oxide and oxygen. GA must be carried out in hospital.

Management complications may include:

- the need for corticosteroid cover; patients, once treated, are maintained on corticosteroid replacement therapy and

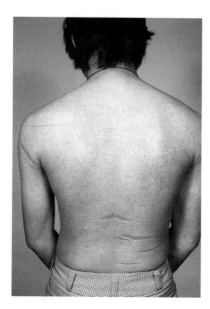

Fig. 6.12 Systemic corticosteroid therapy causes several complications, including cutaneous striae as shown here

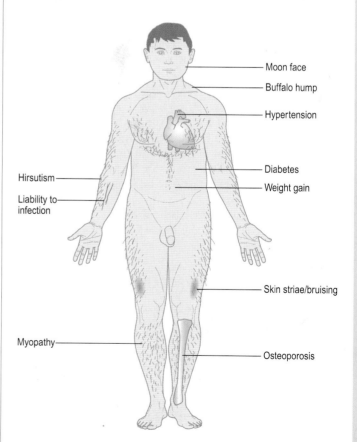

Moon face

Buffalo hump

Hypertension

Diabetes

Weight gain

Hirsutism

Liability to infection

Skin striae/bruising

Myopathy

Osteoporosis

Fig. 6.13 Cushing syndrome

then are at risk from an adrenal crisis if subjected to operation, anaesthesia or trauma

- hypertension
- cardiovascular disease
- diabetes mellitus
- psychosis
- vertebral collapse or myopathy causing limited mobility
- multiple endocrine adenomatosis (MEA I; see later).

There are no specific oral manifestations of Cushing disease, but patients have been referred for a suspected dental cause of the swollen face.

HYPERALDOSTERONISM

General aspects

Primary hyperaldosteronism (Conn syndrome) arises from an adrenal cortex benign tumour or hyperplasia. Secondary hyperaldosteronism arises from activation of the renin–angiotensin system in cirrhosis, nephrotic syndrome, severe cardiac failure or renal artery stenosis.

Clinical features

High aldosterone secretion leads to potassium loss (hypokalaemia) – causing muscle weakness and cramps, paraesthesia, polyuria and polydipsia, and, since it is associated with a metabolic alkalosis, may lead to tetany – and sodium retention (causing hypertension but rarely oedema).

General management

Amiloride, or the aldosterone antagonist spironolactone, is given until the affected adrenal gland can be excised.

Dental aspects

Local analgesia is used for pain control. Conscious sedation may be helpful, especially if there is hypertension. GA must as always be carried out in hospital. In the untreated patient, hypertension and muscle weakness are the main complications. Competitive muscle relaxants may be dangerous, as they can cause profound paralysis.

If bilateral adrenalectomy has been carried out, the patient is at risk from collapse during dental treatment and therefore requires corticosteroid cover.

ADRENOCORTICAL HYPOFUNCTION

Adrenocortical hypofunction can lead to hypotension, shock and death if the individual is stressed, for example by operation, infection or trauma.

Adrenocortical hypofunction is due most commonly to adrenocorticotropic hormone (corticotropin) deficiency caused by the suppression of adrenocortical function following the use of systemic corticosteroids (secondary hypoadrenocorticism); occasionally by acquired adrenal disease (primary hypoadrenocorticism); and rarely, due to a congenital defect in corticosteroid biosynthesis (congenital adrenal hyperplasia; Table 6.15).

Table 6.15 Causes of adrenal insufficiency

Patient on systemic corticosteroids	Adrenal disorders	Hypopituitarism
Trauma	Addison disease	
Operation	Post-adrenalectomy	
General anaesthesia	Waterhouse–Friderichsen syndrome (adrenal haemorrhage caused by septicaemia, anticoagulants or epilepsy)	
Infection	Congenital adrenal hyperplasia	

Primary hypoadrenocorticism (Addison disease)

Primary hypoadrenocorticism is rare and caused by autoantibodies to the adrenal cortex, causing adrenocortical atrophy and failed hormone secretion – cortisol (hydrocortisone) and aldosterone. Patients also have a higher incidence of other endocrine deficiencies (see later), vitiligo and, occasionally, chronic mucocutaneous candidosis.

Primary hypoadrenocorticism occasionally has other adrenal causes (though the term *primary* is then really a misnomer) such as tuberculosis, histoplasmosis (particularly secondary to human immunodeficiency virus infection), malignancy, haemorrhage, sarcoidosis, or amyloidosis or adrenalectomy for metastatic breast cancer.

Clinical features

Lack of cortisol predisposes to hypotension and hypoglycaemia, but stimulates the hypothalamopituitary axis causing release of pro-opiomelanocortin which has ACTH and melanocyte-stimulating hormone (MSH) activity and can cause hyperpigmentation. Lack of aldosterone leads to sodium depletion, reduced extracellular fluid volume and hypotension (Fig. 6.14).

The lack of adrenocortical reserve makes patients vulnerable to any stress such as infection, trauma, surgery or anaesthesia, though they may be asymptomatic otherwise. An acute adrenal crisis (Addisonian crisis or shock) is thus characterized by collapse, bradycardia, hypotension, profound weakness, hypoglycaemia, vomiting and dehydration.

Patients with hypoadrenocorticism also suffer from fatigue and weakness, lethargy, weight loss, anorexia, nausea, vomiting, diarrhoea, hyperpigmentation, dizziness and postural hypotension (Box 6.4).

Box 6.4 Hypoadrenocorticism: clinical features

- Anorexia, nausea and vomiting
- Hypotension
- Skin and mucosal pigmentation
- Weakness
- Weight loss

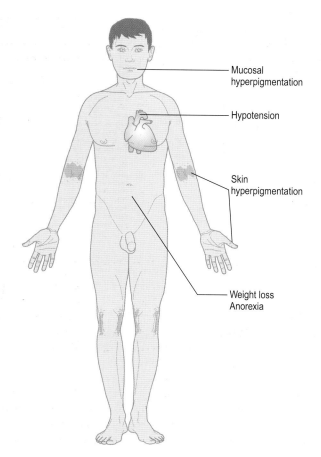

Fig. 6.14 Hypoadrenocorticism

Labels on figure:
- Mucosal hyperpigmentation
- Hypotension
- Skin hyperpigmentation
- Weight loss Anorexia

General management

Diagnosis of hypoadrenocorticism is confirmed by: hypotension; sometimes low plasma sodium and raised potassium; plasma glucose assay (hypoglycaemia is common); and low plasma cortisol levels and depressed cortisol responses to ACTH stimulation. Blood for plasma cortisol estimation (10 ml in a lithium heparin tube, or plain tube) should be taken at 8.00 or 9.00 am. In hypoadrenocorticism the basal plasma cortisol level is usually lower than 6 mg/100 ml (170 nmol/L), often lower than 100 nmol/L. In early hypoadrenocorticism, the cortisol levels may still be in the low normal range and therefore a short ACTH stimulation test is indicated. Plasma is collected before and 30 min after 250 mg of tetracosactrin (synthetic ACTH; Synacthen) is injected intramuscularly or intravenously. In health, the plasma cortisol level normally doubles from at least 200 nmol/L to more than 500 nmol/L after tetracosactrin. In hypoadrenocorticism, the basal cortisol level is low and does not rise by more than 200 nmol/L after tetracosactrin is given.

Estimation of serum ACTH levels differentiates primary (ACTH raised, usually above 200 ng/L) from secondary (ACTH low or normal) hypoadrenocorticism.

Serum should be tested for autoantibodies to various tissues, especially endocrine glands, and other investigations may be needed, including radiography or CT or MRI scans of the skull (for pituitary abnormalities), chest (for tuberculosis) or abdomen (for adrenal calcification suggestive of tuberculosis or a mycosis).

Most patients are treated with oral hydrocortisone and fludrocortisone.

Dental aspects

The risk of precipitating hypotensive collapse is such that corticosteroids must be given pre-operatively. This is discussed more fully below (see Systemic corticosteroid therapy). Conscious sedation should generally be avoided unless the patient has had corticosteroid cover. GA is obviously a matter for the expert anaesthetist in hospital.

Brown or black pigmentation of the mucosa is seen in over 75% of patients with Addison disease, but is not a feature of corticosteroid-induced hypoadrenocorticism or of hypo-adrenocorticism secondary to hypothalamopituitary disease. Hyperpigmentation is related to high levels of MSH and affects particularly areas normally pigmented or exposed to trauma (e.g. in the buccal mucosa at the occlusal line, or the tongue, but also the gingivae). Other causes of oral pigmentation (Ch. 11; especially racial pigmentation) are far more common and need to be differentiated. Addison disease is a rare cause but must be considered, particularly if there is hypotension, weakness, weight loss, anorexia, nausea, vomiting or abdominal pain.

Acute adrenal insufficiency has several causes (Table 6.15) and is managed as in Ch. 1.

AUTOIMMUNE POLYENDOCRINOPATHY SYNDROME (SEE LATER)

SYSTEMIC CORTICOSTEROID THERAPY

General aspects

Corticosteroids are used frequently to suppress inflammation, to suppress graft rejection and occasionally to replace missing hormones (in Addison disease or after adrenalectomy; Table 6.16). Steroids have different potencies (Table 6.17).

Corticosteroids are an essential part of the body's response to stresses such as trauma, infection, GA or operation. At such times there is normally an enhanced adrenal corticosteroid

Table 6.16 Some uses of systemic corticosteroids	
Adrenal insufficiency	Addison disease Adrenalectomy Hypopituitarism
Allergic disorders	Asthma
Blood dyscrasias	Idiopathic thrombocytopenia Lymphocytic leukaemia Lymphoma
Connective tissue disorders	Rheumatoid arthritis (rarely) Systemic lupus erythematosus
Gastrointestinal disorders	Ulcerative colitis Crohn disease
Mucocutaneous diseases	Pemphigus
Post-transplantation	Any organ transplant
Renal disorders	Nephrotic syndrome Renal transplants

">

6

ENDOCRINOLOGY

Table 6.17 Approximate potencies of systemic corticosteroids relative to cortisol[a]

Short-acting		Medium-acting		Long-acting	
Cortisone	1	Triamcinolone	5	Betamethasone	25
Methylpred-nisolone	5			Dexamethasone	30
Prednisolone	4				
Prednisone	4				

[a]Cortisol (hydrocortisone) = 1.

response related to the degree of stress. In patients given exogenous steroids, the enhanced adrenal corticosteroid response may not follow.

Corticosteroids have a negative feedback control on hypothalamic activity and ACTH production and there is thus suppression of the HPA axis and the adrenals may become unable to produce a steroid response to stress. When the adrenal cortex is unable to produce the necessary steroid response to stress, acute adrenal insufficiency (adrenal crisis) can result, with rapidly developing hypotension, collapse and possibly death.

Suppression of the HPA axis becomes profound if corticosteroid treatment has been prolonged and/or the dose of steroids exceeds physiological levels (more than about 7.5 mg/day of prednisolone). Adrenal suppression is less when the exogenous steroid is given on alternate days or as a single morning dose (rather than as divided doses through the day). Corticotropin (ACTH) has been used in the hope of reducing adrenal suppression, but the response is variable and unpredictable, and wanes with time.

However, adrenal function may even be suppressed for up to a week after cessation of steroid treatment lasting only 5 days. If steroid treatment is for longer periods, adrenal function may be suppressed for at least 30 days and perhaps for 2–24 months after the cessation of treatment. Patients on, or who have been on, corticosteroid therapy within the past 30 days may be at risk from adrenal crisis, and those who have been on them during the previous 24 months may also be at risk, if they are not given supplementary corticosteroids before and during periods of stress such as operation, GA, infection or trauma. Patients who have used systemic corticosteroids should be warned of the danger and should carry a steroid card indicating the dosage and the responsible physician (Fig. 6.15). Metal bracelets or necklaces with the diagnosis engraved on them are available, for example from Medic-Alert Foundation, 9 Hanover Street, London W1R 9HF, UK (see Ch. 2).

However, the frequency and extent of the adrenocortical suppression (and the need for supplementary corticosteroids before and during periods of stress) is unclear and has been questioned. Although the evidence for the need for steroid cover may be questionable, medicolegal and other considerations suggest that one should act on the side of caution and fully inform and discuss with the patient, take medical advice in any case of doubt and give steroid cover unless confident that collapse is unlikely.

I am a patient on—

STEROID TREATMENT

which must not be stopped abruptly

and in the case of intercurrent illness may have to be increased

full details are available from the hospital or general → practitioners shown overleaf

STC1

INSTRUCTIONS

1 DO NOT STOP taking the steroid drug except on medical advice. Always have a supply in reserve.

2 In case of feverish illness, accident, operation (emergency or otherwise), diarrhoea or vomiting the steroid treatment MUST be continued. Your doctor may wish you to have a LARGER DOSE or an INJECTION at such times.

3 If the tablets cause indigestion consult your doctor AT ONCE.

4 Always carry this card while receiving steroid treatment and show it to any doctor, dentist, nurse or midwife whom you may consult.

5 After your treatment has finished you must still tell any new doctor, dentist, nurse or midwife that you have had steroid treatment.

Fig. 6.15 Steroid warning card. This is a blue card that should be carried at all times by patients on systemic corticosteroids in view of the danger of an adrenocortical crisis and collapse if the patient is subject to trauma, stress or anaesthesia. (By permission of the Controller of Her Majesty's Stationery Office)

Table 6.18 Complications of systemic corticosteroid therapy

Cardiovascular	Cerebrovascular accidents Hypertension Myocardial infarction
Dermatological	Acne Bruising Hirsutism Striae
Gastrointestinal	Peptic ulcer
Immunosuppressive	Increased susceptibility to infections Neoplasms long-term
Neurological	Cataracts Mood changes Psychosis
Metabolic	Fat redistribution (moon face and buffalo hump) Growth retardation Hypothalamic–pituitary–adrenal suppression Impaired glucose tolerance or diabetes mellitus Loss of sodium and potassium Muscle weakness Osteoporosis Weight gain

Clinical features

Long-term systemic use of corticosteroids can cause many other adverse effects, often beginning soon after the start of treatment, and can cause significant morbidity or mortality (Table 6.18), including immediately obvious effects such as Cushingoid weight gain around the face (moon face) and upper back (buffalo hump) and hirsutism. Other possible complications are shown in Table 6.18.

General management

Complications may be reduced but not abolished if steroids are given on alternate days. In order to minimize the effects above, patients on systemic steroids are usually monitored and given drugs prophylactically as below.

- There should be no contraindications such as hypertension (see Ch. 5), diabetes or latent tuberculosis.
- The smallest effective steroid dose should be given, best in the morning on alternate days.
- Systemic corticosteroids cause the greatest risk of adrenocortical suppression, so topical steroids should always be used in preference, provided that the desired therapeutic effect is achievable. However, there can even be adrenocortical suppression from extensive application of steroid skin preparations, particularly if occlusive dressings are used, or from some use in the mouth if ulceration is extensive and potent steroids are used.
- The patient must be given a warning card and told of the dangers of withdrawal, and side-effects. There should never be abrupt withdrawal of the steroid. The dose should be raised if there is illness, infection, trauma or operation.
- Weight, chest radiography, bone mineral density, blood pressure and blood glucose baseline measures should be taken and these parameters monitored.
- Ranitidine and calcitriol or didronel are often given.

Dental aspects

Cortisol is the major glucocorticoid in humans and is involved in metabolic processes, vascular tonicity, inflammatory responses and the control of response to stresses such as trauma, infection, GA or surgery. Secretion from the adrenals is regulated via the HPA axis by involving ACTH. In patients given exogenous corticosteroids (steroids), this feedback response may not occur and acute adrenal insufficiency (adrenal crisis) may result as the adrenal cortex is unable to produce the necessary steroid response to stress.

Suppression of the HPA axis becomes deeper if treatment with exogenous steroids is prolonged and the dose exceeds physiological levels (over 7.5 mg/day of prednisolone).

Adrenal suppression is likely if the patient is currently on daily systemic corticosteroids at doses of 10 mg prednisolone or above, or has been in the last 3 months.

Adrenocortical function may be suppressed if:

- the patient is currently on daily systemic corticosteroids at doses above 5 mg prednisolone
- corticosteroids have been taken regularly during the previous 30 days
- corticosteroids have been taken for more than 1 month during the past year.

During intercurrent illness or infection, after trauma, or before operation or anaesthesia, these patients may require a higher steroid dosage. Steroid supplementation should be considered before stressful procedures. It is recognized that dentoalveolar or maxillofacial surgery may result in stress, but most other forms of dental treatment cause little response. The blood pressure must be carefully monitored during the operative care and recovery. Although the evidence for this may be questionable, medicolegal and other considerations suggest that one should act on the side of caution and give steroid cover unless confident that collapse is unlikely.

The blood pressure must be carefully watched during surgery and especially during recovery, and steroid supplementation given immediately if the blood pressure starts to fall. Dentoalveolar or maxillofacial surgery may result in stress and a cortisol response, but most other forms of dental treatment cause little response.

Minor operations under LA may be covered by giving the usual oral steroid dose in the morning and giving oral steroids 2–4 h pre- and post-operatively (25–50 mg hydrocortisone or 20 mg prednisolone or 4 mg dexamethasone) or by giving intravenous 25–50 mg hydrocortisone immediately before operation (Table 6.19). Intravenous hydrocortisone must be immediately available for use if the blood pressure falls or the patient collapses.

Cover for major operations can be provided by giving at least 25–50 mg hydrocortisone sodium succinate intramuscularly or intravenously (with the pre-medication) and then 6-hourly for a further 24–72 h (Table 6.19). Corticosteroids given by intramuscular injection are more slowly absorbed and reach lower plasma levels than when given intravenously or orally.

In 1998, Nicholson et al. reviewed all the available evidence and published new recommendations for steroid cover, where hydrocortisone supplementation is given intravenously. Patients who have taken steroids in excess of 10 mg prednisolone, or equivalent, within the last 3 months should be considered for supplementation. Patients who have not received steroids for more than 3 months are considered to have full recovery of the HPA axis and require no supplementation. Nicholson's guidelines are not universally accepted amongst the dental profession as they require intravenous administration of steroids. For this reason, regimens such as doubling the normal daily oral steroid dose on the day of procedure (Gibson and Ferguson, 2004) are more commonly used.

Drugs, especially sedatives and general anaesthetics, are a hazard and it is extremely important to avoid hypoxia, hypotension or haemorrhage. Patients may also require special management as a result of diabetes, hypertension, poor wound healing or infections. Aspirin and other NSAIDs should be avoided as they may increase the risk of peptic ulceration. Osteoporosis introduces the danger of fractures when handling the patient.

Topical corticosteroids for use in the mouth are unlikely to have any systemic effect but predispose to oral candidosis. Susceptibility to infection is increased by systemic steroid use (see later) and there is a predisposition to herpes virus infections (particularly herpes simplex). Chickenpox is an especial hazard to those who are not immune and fulminant disease can result. Passive immunization with varicella zoster immunoglobulin is indicated for non-immune patients on systemic corticosteroids (or who have been on them within the previous 3 months), if exposed to chickenpox or zoster. Immunization should be given within 3 days of exposure.

Wound healing is impaired and wound infections are more frequent. In addition to careful aseptic surgery, prophylactic antimicrobials may be indicated.

Long-term and profound immunosuppression may lead to the appearance of hairy leukoplakia, Kaposi sarcoma, lymphomas, lip cancer or oral keratosis or other oral complications (Ch. 35).

Corticosteroids can also mask the presence of many serious diseases that may influence dental care as well as causing suppression of the adrenocortical response to stress (see Table 6.19 for management).

Table 6.19 Suggested management of patients with a history of systemic corticosteroid therapy

	No steroids for previous 12 months	Steroids taken during previous 12 months	Steroids currently taken
Conservative dentistry or dentoalveolar surgery (e.g. single extraction under LA)	No cover required	Give usual oral steroid dose in morning or hydrocortisone[a] 25–50 mg i.v. pre-operatively	Double oral steroid dose in morning or hydrocortisone[a] 25–50 mg i.v. pre-operatively. Continue normal steroid medication post-operatively
Intermediate surgery (e.g. multiple extractions, or surgery under GA)	Consider cover if large doses of steroid were given. Test adrenocortical function (ACTH stimulation test)	Give usual oral steroid dose in morning plus hydrocortisone[a] 25–50 mg i.v. pre-operatively and i.m. 6-hourly for 24 h	Double oral steroid dose in morning plus hydrocortisone[a] 25–50 mg i.v. pre-operatively and i.m. 6-hourly for 24 h. Then continue normal medication
Maxillofacial surgery or trauma	Consider cover if large doses of steroid were given. Test adrenocortical function (ACTH stimulation test)	Give usual oral steroid dose in morning plus hydrocortisone[a] 25–50 mg i.v. pre-operatively and i.m. 6-hourly for 72 h	Double oral steroid dose in morning plus hydrocortisone[a] 25–50 mg i.v. pre-operatively and i.m. 6-hourly for 72 h. Then continue normal medication

[a]Hydrocortisone sodium succinate (e.g. Efcortelan soluble) or phosphate given immediately pre-operatively and blood pressure monitored.
ACTH, adrenocorticotropic hormone; GA, general anaesthesia; LA, local anaesthesia.

SECONDARY ADRENOCORTICAL INSUFFICIENCY

Secondary adrenocortical insufficiency can also be caused by ACTH deficiency as a result of hypothalamic or pituitary disease. It is then associated with other endocrine defects, but *no* hyperpigmentation (ACTH levels are low) and blood pressure is virtually normal (aldosterone secretion is normal).

CONGENITAL ADRENAL HYPERPLASIA

Congenital adrenal hyperplasia is the term given to a group of rare autosomal recessive inborn errors of corticosteroid metabolism characterized by defects in 21-hydroxylase or 11-hydroxylase, resulting in lack of cortisol (adrenal insufficiency) and androgen excess. Male precocious puberty or female ambiguous genitalia can result.

POLYCYSTIC OVARY SYNDROME (PCOS)

Polycystic ovary syndrome (PCOS) presents with hirsutism, acne, oligomenorrhoea and subfertility. Other features include obesity, acanthosis nigricans and hypertension (and premature balding in male relatives).

ADRENAL MEDULLA

The adrenal medulla secretes the catecholamines norepinephrine (noradrenaline) and epinephrine (adrenaline) in response to hypotension, hypoglycaemia and other stress, their release being regulated by the central nervous system.

PHAEOCHROMOCYTOMA

General aspects

Phaeochromocytomas are rare, usually benign tumours, most commonly in the adrenal medulla (producing epinephrine) but others arise in other neuroectodermal tissues such as paraganglia or the sympathetic chain and produce norepinephrine or dopamine. Ten per cent of phaeochromocytomas are familial, 10% are bilateral, 10% are outside the adrenals and 10% are malignant. Phaeochromocytomas may occasionally be associated with other tumours – neurofibromatosis; endocrine tumours, particularly medullary carcinoma of the thyroid and hyperparathyroidism [multiple endocrine adenomatosis: MEA II or III (see later)]; von Hippel–Lindau disease (cerebelloretinal haemangioblastomatosis); and gastric leiomyosarcoma, pulmonary chondroma and testicular tumours (Carney triad).

Clinical features

Typical features are episodes of anxiety, headache, epigastric discomfort, palpitations, tachycardia, arrhythmias, hypertension, sweating, pyrexia, flushing and glycosuria.

General management

Plasma catecholamines (collected at rest in the supine position) may be raised but are less reliable than urinary assays. Diagnosis is supported by finding excessive urinary catecholamines and their metabolites such as vanillylmandelic acid (VMA) or metanephrines. The tumour is located by CT, MRI, venous catheterization, arteriography, ultrasonography and radionuclide scanning such as MIBG (^{131}I-meta-iodobenzylguanidine). The tumour is excised after the blood pressure has been controlled with an alpha-blocking agent (e.g. phenoxybenzamine) and a beta-blocker.

Dental aspects

Acute hypertension and arrhythmias may complicate dental treatment. Elective treatment should therefore be deferred until after surgical treatment of the phaeochromocytoma. If emergency care is required, the blood pressure should first be controlled with alpha- (such as phenoxybenzamine or prazosin) and then beta-adrenergic (such as propanolol) blockers.

Patients who have had adrenal surgery may suffer from hypo-adrenocorticism, since the adrenal cortex is inevitably damaged at operation. These patients therefore require steroid cover at operation. Local analgesia is then generally safe and epinephrine in modest amounts is unlikely to have any significant adverse effect. Conscious sedation may be desirable to control anxiety and endogenous epinephrine production.

General anaesthesia must only be given in hospital; neuro-leptanalgesia using a combination such as droperidol, fentanyl and midazolam may be the most satisfactory choice.

Phaeochromocytoma is occasionally associated with oral mucosal neuromas (MEA III syndrome; see later).

THYROID GLAND

The thyroid gland is under the influence of thyroid-stimulating hormone (TSH or thyrotropin) from the pituitary gland, which is itself regulated by thyrotropin-releasing hormone (TRH) from the hypothalamus. Thyroid hormones stored as iodide-rich 'thyroid colloid', are thyroxine (T4; tetraiodothyronine), which has a half-life of 1 week, and is converted to tri-iodothyronine (T3) – the active form, which has a half-life of 1 day. Thyroid hormones feed back to the hypothalamus and pituitary to regulate TSH release.

Thyroid hormones act on metabolism by regulating protein synthesis via effects on gene transcription and mRNA stabilization and have profound effects on the sensitivity of tissues to catecholamines, as well as on mitochondrial oxidative activity, synthesis and degradation of proteins, differentiation of muscle fibres, capillary growth and levels of antioxidant compounds.

Thyroid function tests (Table 6.20) include serum levels of T4 and T3. Free T4 and free T3 provide a better assessment of the thyroid status than do total T4 and T3 since about 95% of thyroid hormones is bound to plasma proteins, especially thyroid-binding globulin (TBG) and thyroid–binding pre-albumin (TBPA).

Thyroid–stimulating hormone (TSH) levels can be assayed. Thyroid antibody tests, ultrasound and radio-iodine uptake using ^{131}I or ^{123}I are the other common thyroid function tests.

LINGUAL THYROID

The thyroid normally develops as a downgrowth from the foramen caecum at the junction of the posterior third with the anterior two-thirds of the tongue. Rarely, ectopic thyroid tissue remains in this tract and may be seen as a lump in the midline between the foramen caecum and epiglottis, but has also been recorded in the oropharynx, infra-hyoid region, larynx, oesophagus, heart and mediastinum. A lingual thyroid is seen mainly in females, and is often asymptomatic but may cause dysphagia, airway obstruction or even haemorrhage. Hypothyroidism may be associated in about one-third of cases and, occasionally, the lingual thyroid becomes malignant. There is a raised incidence of thyroid disease in relatives.

A lingual thyroid may not be suspected until the lump in the tongue has been biopsied or excised and examined histologically. The diagnosis can be confirmed by iodine-123 or -131, or technetium-99 uptake in the tongue, by biopsy, by CT scanning without contrast or by MRI.

Treatment depends on the size of the lingual thyroid but thyroxine may be needed and, if the lump does not regress sufficiently, the lingual thyroid can be ablated, best by surgery, or, if the patient is unfit, by iodine-131, if normal functioning thyroid tissue is identified in the neck.

GOITRE

A goitre is an enlarged thyroid gland (Fig. 6.16). Most goitres are acquired and seen in Graves disease or thyroiditis (Box 6.5).

The cause of the goitre should be sought. A rare cause of goitre is a medullary carcinoma of the thyroid, which can be part of a multiple endocrine adenomatosis syndrome (MEA II and MEA III).

Table 6.20 Tests of thyroid function		
Test	**Hyperthyroidism**	**Hypothyroidism**
T4 serum level	↑	↓
T3 serum level	↑	↓
Free thyroxine index	↑	↓
T3 resin uptake	↑	↓
Serum TSH	↓	↑[a]
TRH test (release of TSH by TRH)	ND	↓
Radio-iodine uptake	↑[b]	ND
Thyroid autoantibodies	LATS	Thyroglobulin autoantibodies

[a]Depressed in pituitary hypofunction.
[b]Not suppressed by administration of T3.
Note: Basal metabolic rate not now used as a test.
LATS, long-acting thyroid stimulator; ND, not done; T3, tri-iodothyronine; T4, thyroxine (tetraiodothyronine); TRH, thyrotropin-releasing hormone; TSH, thyroid-stimulating hormone; arrows indicate raised (↑) or lowered (↓) values.

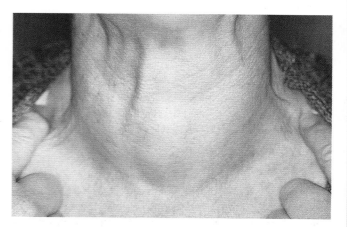

Fig. 6.16 Goitre

Box 6.5 Causes of goitre

Physiological
- Puberty
- Pregnancy

Low iodine intake or natural goitrogens (endemic goitre)

Drugs
- Thiouracil
- Carbimazole
- Potassium perchlorate
- Lithium
- Phenylbutazone

Thyroid disease
- Graves disease (toxic goitre)
- Dyshormonogenesis
- Carcinoma
- Hashimoto thyroiditis

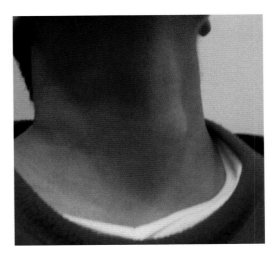

Fig. 6.17 Thyroid nodule

Thyroid function is assessed to determine whether it is normal (euthyroid), hyperactive (hyperthyroid) or hypoactive (hypothyroid).

Most goitres do not require surgery but this is indicated if there is a danger of airways obstruction (cough, voice changes, dyspnoea, tracheal deviation or dysphagia) or for cosmetic reasons.

Dental management in goitre may be influenced by abnormal thyroid function, by the underlying cause of the goitre or by complications such as respiratory obstruction.

THYROID NODULES

A nodule in the thyroid gland may represent a benign or malignant neoplasm (Fig. 6.17). Patients are examined with radio-iodine thyroid scans, ultrasound-guided needle biopsy and thyroid function tests. A nodule that takes up radio-iodine is termed a hot nodule and unlikely to be malignant, and more usually is an adenoma.

A nodule that fails to take up the radio-iodine is termed a cold nodule, and may be malignant, usually a papillary, follicular or medullary cell carcinoma. Needle biopsy is indicated.

HYPERTHYROIDISM

General aspects

Hyperthyroidism is usually associated with a diffuse goitre due to autoimmune disease (Graves disease, primary hyperthyroidism) when there are thyroid-stimulating autoantibodies against thyroid TSH receptor (TRAbs) and thyroid microsomal antibodies (TMAbs). Sometimes, a hyperfunctioning (toxic) multinodular goitre or nodule due to one or more thyroid adenomas produces excess thyroxine. Ninety per cent of the swellings are benign. Rarely, thyroiditis, thyroid hormone overdosage or ectopic thyroid tissue causes a goitre.

Clinical features

Hyperthyroidism may cause exophthalmos, eyelid lag and eyelid retraction (Box 6.6, Figs 6.18 and 6.19); it mimics the effects of epinephrine, and can cause anorexia, vomiting or diarrhoea, weight loss, anxiety and tremor, sweating and heat intolerance.

Box 6.6 Hyperthyroidism: typical clinical features

- Amenorrhoea
- Atrial fibrillation
- Diarrhoea
- Excess sweating
- Exophthalmos in some
- Gynaecomastia
- Heart failure
- Heat intolerance
- Increased appetite
- Irritability
- No hair loss
- No voice change
- Psychosis
- Tachycardia
- Tremor
- Warm moist skin
- Weight loss

Cardiac disturbances, particularly in older patients, include tachycardia, arrhythmias (especially atrial fibrillation) or cardiac failure.

Thyrotoxic periodic paralysis comprises attacks of mild to severe weakness, during which serum potassium levels are generally low.

Myasthenia gravis may occasionally be associated.

General management

The diagnosis is confirmed by raised serum levels of T3 and T4. Circulating thyroid microsomal antibodies (TMAbs), and thyroid stimulating hormone receptor antibodies (TRAbs) are found in 55% of patients with Graves disease. A scan or radioactive iodine uptake can differentiate causes of hyperthyroidism: subacute thyroiditis (low uptake) versus Graves disease (high uptake).

Hyperthyroidism can be treated with beta-blockers (achieve rapid control of many of the signs and symptoms by moderating sympathetic overactivity, but suddenly stopping beta-blocker treatment can precipitate a thyroid crisis within 4 h). Carbimazole, the usual antithyroid drug, can suppress the bone marrow and cause rashes. Iodine-131 is effective, but can result in hypothyroidism. There appears to be no risk of neoplastic

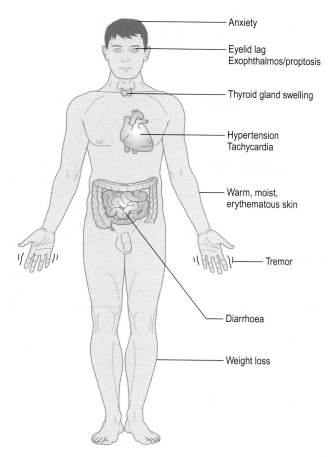

- Anxiety
- Eyelid lag Exophthalmos/proptosis
- Thyroid gland swelling
- Hypertension Tachycardia
- Warm, moist, erythematous skin
- Tremor
- Diarrhoea
- Weight loss

Fig. 6.18 Hyperthyroidism

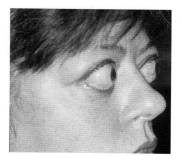

Fig. 6.19 Exophthalmos

change. Surgery is effective, but leads to hypothyroidism in about 30%. Hypoparathyroidism and recurrent laryngeal nerve palsy are rare complications.

In untreated patients with hyperthyroidism, pain, anxiety, trauma, GA, or premature cessation of antithyroid treatment may precipitate a thyroid (thyrotoxic) crisis, characterized by anxiety, tremor and dyspnoea, which can go on to ventricular fibrillation. Medical assistance is essential as treatment requires the use of potassium iodide and propylthiouracil, and propranolol or chlorpromazine.

Dental aspects

Patients with sympathetic overactivity in untreated hyperthyroidism can be anxious, irritable and may faint. LA is the main means of pain control: any risk from epinephrine exacerbating sympathetic overactivity is only theoretical and prilocaine with felypressin is not known to be safer than lidocaine. Conscious sedation is frequently desirable to control excessive anxiety. Benzodiazepines may potentiate antithyroid drugs, and therefore nitrous oxide, which is more rapidly controllable, is probably safer.

Povidone–iodine and similar compounds are best avoided. Carbimazole occasionally causes agranulocytosis, which may cause oral or oropharyngeal ulceration. Otherwise the treated thyrotoxic patient presents no special problems in dental treatment. However, after treatment of hyperthyroidism, the patient is at risk from hypothyroidism, which may pass unrecognized. This point must especially be borne in mind if a GA is required.

HYPOTHYROIDISM

General aspects

Hypothyroidism may be primary (due to thyroid disease) or secondary (due to hypothalamic or pituitary dysfunction). The common causes are thyroid loss from surgery or destruction by irradiation of the neck or thyroid gland. Autoimmune disease (Hashimoto thyroiditis), associated with autoantibodies to thyroglobulin and thyroid microsomes, and drugs such as amiodarone, carbimazole, lithium or radio-iodine may be implicated. Rare cases in the developed world are caused by iodine deficiency.

Clinical features

Hypothyroidism is often unrecognized. Subclinical hypothyroidism, with raised TSH but normal T4 levels, may be found in up to 10% of postmenopausal females. However, hypothyroidism can cause weight gain, lassitude, dry skin, myxoedema, loss of hair, cardiac failure or ischaemic heart disease, bradycardia, anaemia, neurological or psychiatric changes, hypotonia, cerebellar signs of ataxia, tremor, and dysmetria, polyneuropathy, cranial nerve deficits, entrapment neuropathy (e.g. carpal tunnel syndrome), myopathic weakness, dementia, apathy, mental dullness, irritability and sleepiness (Fig. 6.20).

Hoarseness and hypothermia and may be complicated by coma (Box 6.7). Sjögren syndrome (Ch. 16) may be associated. Congenital hypothyroidism (cretinism) has similar features, together with an enlarged tongue and learning impairment.

General management

The diagnosis is confirmed by demonstrating low serum T4 and T3 levels. TSH levels are raised in primary hypothyroidism and depressed in secondary hypothyroidism. Serum antibodies are detectable in Hashimoto thyroiditis – TMAbs in 95%, thyroglobulin antibodies (TGAbs) in 60%.

Symptomatic patients are managed with daily oral thyroxine sodium. Treatment is started slowly but, especially if there is evidence of ischaemic heart disease, angina, myocardial infarction or sudden death may be precipitated.

Dental aspects

The main danger is of precipitating myxoedema coma by the use of sedatives (including diazepam or midazolam), opioid analgesics (including codeine) or tranquillizers. These should

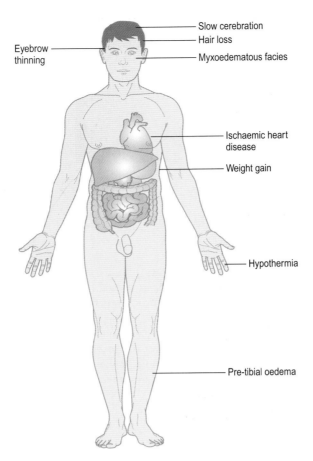

Eyebrow thinning

Slow cerebration
Hair loss
Myxoedematous facies

Ischaemic heart disease

Weight gain

Hypothermia

Pre-tibial oedema

Fig. 6.20 Hypothyroidism

Box 6.7 Hypothyroidism: typical clinical features

- Angina
- Bradycardia
- Cold intolerance
- Constipation
- Decreased appetite
- Decreased sweating
- Dry cold skin
- Hair loss
- Hoarseness
- Ischaemic heart disease
- Menorrhagia
- Periorbital oedema
- Psychosis
- Serous effusions
- Slow cerebration, poor memory
- Slow reactions
- Weight gain

---

therefore be either avoided or given in a low dose. LA is satisfactory for pain control. Conscious sedation can be carried out with nitrous oxide and oxygen. Diazepam or midazolam may precipitate coma.

General anaesthesia may be complicated because of possible ischaemic heart disease, the danger of coma, and the respiratory centre is also hypersensitive to drugs such as opioids or sedatives. GA, if unavoidable, should be delayed if possible until thyroxine has been started.

Associated problems may include hypoadrenocorticism, anaemia, hypotension, diminished cardiac output and bradycardia. Occasional associations include hypopituitarism and other autoimmune disorders such as Sjögren syndrome.

Povidone–iodine and similar compounds are best avoided.

PARATHYROIDS

The parathyroid glands are four pea-sized glands located on the back of the thyroid gland in the neck, which produce (PTH). Occasionally, congenitally ectopic parathyroid glands are embedded in the thyroid, the thymus or the chest. In most such cases, ectopic glands function normally.

Parathyroid hormone and vitamin D both act to control plasma calcium levels. PTH secretion is stimulated by a fall in the level of the plasma ionized calcium. PTH acts on the kidneys to increase renal reabsorption of calcium and impair phosphate reabsorption (Fig. 6.21). PTH enhances gastrointestinal absorption of calcium and promotes osteoclastic bone resorption causing a rise in the plasma level of calcium and of the osteoblastic enzyme alkaline phosphatase (Table 6.21). Both bone mineral and matrix are degraded, and the amino acids such as hydroxyproline thus released are not reused but are excreted in the urine.

HYPERPARATHYROIDISM

General aspects

Primary hyperparathyroidism is usually caused by a parathyroid adenoma and seen in post-menopausal women. Rare causes include carcinoma of the parathyroids.

Secondary hyperparathyroidism is a response to low plasma calcium caused by chronic renal failure or prolonged dialysis, or severe malabsorption, and is rising in frequency.

Tertiary hyperparathyroidism follows prolonged secondary hyperparathyroidism, which has become autonomous.

Clinical features

The main features (Box 6.8) include hypercalcaemia and renal disease (most patients have renal calcifications), skeletal disease (bone pain, pathological fractures, giant cell tumours, bone rarefaction), peptic ulceration, pancreatitis, hypertension and arrhythmias (Fig. 6.22). Therefore, the expression 'stones, bones and abdominal groans' sometimes applies.

Hyperparathyroidism may occasionally be familial and associated with tumours of other endocrine glands (MEA I, II and III).

General management

The diagnosis in primary hyperparathyroidism is confirmed by raised parathyroid hormone levels, raised serum calcium, low or normal phosphate level and normal or raised alkaline phosphatase. *Primary hyperparathyroidism* is treated by parathyroidectomy, but medical treatment such as active vitamin D hormone (1,25-dihydroxycholecalciferol; 1,25-DHCC) is useful in those with severe bone disease. *Secondary hyperparathyroidism* often responds to 1,25-DHCC but not to dietary vitamin D

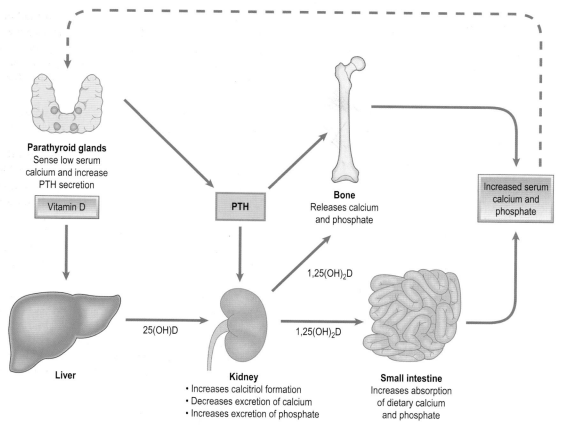

Fig. 6.21 Parathyroid vitamin D and calcium metabolism

Table 6.21	Parathyroid function tests				
	Calcium*a*	Phosphate*a*	Alkaline phosphatase	Urea*a*
Primary hyperparathyroidism					
Without bone lesions	↑	↓	N	N
With bone lesions	↑	N or ↓	↑	N or ↑
Secondary hyperparathyroidism					
Due to renal failure	N or ↓	N or ↑	N or ↑	↑
Due to malabsorption	N or ↓	↓	↑	N
Tertiary hyperparathyroidism					
With bone lesions	↑	N or ↓	↑	N or ↑
Without bone lesions	↑	↓	N	N or ↑
Hypoparathyroidism	↓	↑	N	N
Pseudohypoparathyroidism	↓	↑	N	N
Pseudo-pseudohypoparathyroidism	N	N	N	N
Vitamin D deficiency	↓	N or ↓	↑	N

*a*Serum concentrations.
Arrows indicate values above (↑) or below (↓) normal (N).

Box 6.8 Hyperparathyroidism: clinical features

- Bone resorption
- Nephrocalcinosis
- Peptic ulcer: pain
- Polyuria
- Psychiatric disorders
- Renal stones

(cholecalciferol). Parathyroidectomy may be needed. *Tertiary hyperparathyroidism* requires parathyroidectomy.

Calcimimetics, drugs which bind to the calcium-sensing receptors of the parathyroid glands and lower the sensitivity for receptor activation by extracellular calcium, diminish PTH release, and may become useful for the treatment of primary and secondary hyperparathyroidism.

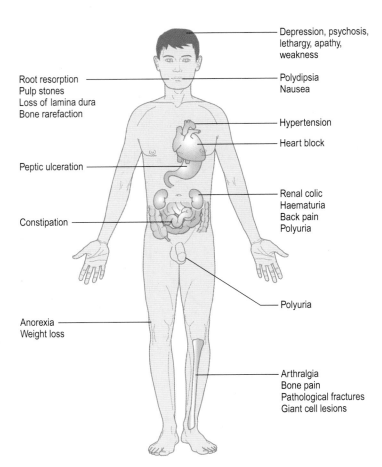

Depression, psychosis, lethargy, apathy, weakness

Polydipsia
Nausea

Hypertension

Heart block

Renal colic
Haematuria
Back pain
Polyuria

Polyuria

Arthralgia
Bone pain
Pathological fractures
Giant cell lesions

Root resorption
Pulp stones
Loss of lamina dura
Bone rarefaction

Peptic ulceration

Constipation

Anorexia
Weight loss

Fig. 6.22 Hyperparathyroidism ("stones, bones and abdominol groans")

Dental aspects

Dental changes in hyperparathyroidism include loss of the lamina dura and generalized bone rarefaction, but giant cell lesions are late and uncommon. Giant cell lesions of hyperparathyroidism (brown tumours) are rare but histologically indistinguishable from central giant cell granulomas of the jaws. If, therefore, a giant cell lesion is found, particularly in a middle-aged patient or in a patient with renal failure, parathyroid function should be investigated.

Local analgesia is the main means of pain control, especially if hypertension and arrhythmias are present. Conscious sedation is preferably with nitrous oxide and oxygen. GA may be complicated because of cardiovascular complications and sensitivity to muscle relaxants. Dental treatment in hyperparathyroidism may be complicated by renal disease, peptic ulceration, bone fragility or pluriglandular disease.

HYPOPARATHYROIDISM

General aspects

The most frequent cause of hypoparathyroidism is thyroidectomy, but it is relatively transient and typically resolves when the remaining parathyroid tissue undergoes compensatory hyperplasia. Rare cases of idiopathic hypoparathyroidism are congenital.

Clinical features

Low plasma calcium leads to muscle irritability and tetany, with facial twitching (Chvostek's sign; contracture of the facial muscles upon tapping over the facial nerve); carpopedal spasms (Trousseau's sign; contracture of the hand and fingers (*main d'accoucheur* – obstetrician's hand) on occluding the arm with a cuff); numbness and tingling of arms and legs, and even laryngeal stridor (Box 6.9 and Fig. 6.23).

Rare cases of idiopathic hypoparathyroidism may be associated with CATCH 22, or other endocrine defects – especially hypoadrenocorticism – associated with multiple autoantibodies (Table 6.23) and cataracts, calcification of the basal ganglia, defects of the teeth and, sometimes, chronic mucocutaneous candidosis.

Pseudohypoparathyroidism is characterized by normal or raised PTH secretion but unresponsive tissue receptors, and has clinical features similar to idiopathic hypoparathyroidism, but there is short stature and small fingers and toes, with a liability to develop cataracts, and no dental defects. Similar appearance in patients with normal biochemistry is termed pseudo-pseudohypoparathyroidism.

General management

Diagnosis is from low plasma calcium; phosphate is often raised (see Table 6.21). Replacement therapy includes vitamin D and calcium supplements.

Dental aspects

There may be facial paraesthesia and facial twitching caused by tetany (Chvostek's sign). Idiopathic (congenital) hypoparathyroidism may feature enamel hypoplasia, shortened roots

---

with osteodentine formation, delayed eruption and sometimes chronic mucocutaneous candidosis (Box 6.9).

Local analgesia is satisfactory. Conscious sedation can be given, preferably after replacement therapy. Dental management may be complicated by tetany, seizures, psychiatric problems or learning disability, hypoadrenocorticism, diabetes mellitus or other endocrinopathies or arrhythmias.

MULTIPLE ENDOCRINE ADENOMA SYNDROMES

Multiple endocrine adenoma (MEA) syndromes, also known as the multiple endocrine neoplasia (MEN) syndromes, are rare autosomal dominant diseases affecting several endocrine glands (Table 6.22) but are distinct from polyglandular autoimmune syndromes. All MEA syndromes feature parathyroid hyperplasia and hypercalcaemia. Their main relevance to dentistry is type III. In the latter, numerous small plexiform neuromas form in the oral mucosa, lips, eyelids and skin. The patient may also have a Marfanoid habitus and diarrhoea.

> **Box 6.9 Hypoparathyroidism: clinical features**
>
> - Acute pancreatitis
> - Candidosis[a]
> - Cataracts[a]
> - Constipation
> - Dental defects[a]
> - Epilepsy
> - Hypertension
> - Psychiatric disorders
> - Tetany
> - Weakness

[a]Only in some types of congenital hypoparathyroidism.

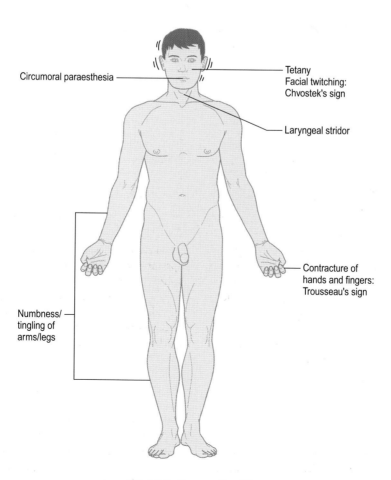

Fig. 6.23 Hypoparathyroidism

Circumoral paraesthesia

Tetany
Facial twitching:
Chvostek's sign

Laryngeal stridor

Contracture of
hands and fingers:
Trousseau's sign

Numbness/
tingling of
arms/legs

Table 6.22   Multiple endocrine adenoma syndromes

	MEA TYPE		
	I Werner syndrome	II (IIa) Sipple syndrome	III (IIb) Schmidt syndrome
Genetics	Menin gene	RET gene	RET gene
Adrenals	Adenoma	Phaeochromocytoma in 33%	Phaeochromocytoma in 70%
Pancreas	Nesidioblastoma, Zollinger–Ellison syndrome, insulinoma	–	–
Parathyroid	Hyperplasia	Hyperplasia	Hyperplasia
Pituitary	Adenoma (usually prolactinoma)	–	–
Thyroid	±	Medullary cell carcinoma in 75–100%[a] (calcitonin-secreting)	Medullary cell carcinoma in up to 80–100% (calcitonin-secreting)
Others	Carcinoid, lipomas, gastrinoma	Dermal neuroma	Oral mucosal neuromas, Marfanoid skeletal anomalies, visual disturbances

[a]Causes raised serum calcitonin levels and low serum calcium levels.

Table 6.23   Polyglandular autoimmune disease, type I and type II

	Type I	Type II
Female:male ratio	1.5:1	1.8:1
HLA associations findings	Not constant	B8 (A1)
Addison disease	100%	100%
Hypoparathyroidism	76%	–
Chronic mucocutaneous candidosis	73%	–
Alopecia	32%	0.5%
Malabsorption syndromes	22%	–
Gonadal failure	17%	3.6%
Pernicious anaemia	13%	0.5%
Chronic active hepatitis	13%	–
Autoimmune thyroiditis	11%	69%
Insulin-dependent diabetes	4%	52%

POLYGLANDULAR AUTOIMMUNE SYNDROMES

Polyglandular autoimmune syndromes feature multiple endocrine *deficiencies*, due to autoantibodies to the glands, most commonly Addison disease and hypoparathyroidism.

As shown in Table 6.23, chronic mucocutaneous candidosis is a very frequent feature in type 1. Its onset is frequently in infancy and it can precede any glandular deficiencies by 10 or more years. Occasionally this sequence is reversed, but in either case treatment of the glandular deficiency has no effect on the candidosis and vice versa.

Treatment of the hormone deficiencies is as described earlier.

HORMONE PRODUCTION BY TUMOURS

Tumours, especially bronchogenic carcinoma, can occasionally ectopically produce polypeptide hormones or other biologically active substances (see Appendix 6.1).

GONADS (SEE CH. 30)

USEFUL WEBSITES

http://www.medhelp.org/nadf/
http://www.endocrineweb.com/
http://www.diabetesnet.com/diabetes_treatments/diabetes_insulins.php
http://www.nlm.nih.gov/medlineplus/ency/article/001214.htm
http://diabetes.niddk.nih.gov/
http://www.glycosmedia.com/
http://www.diabetes.org.uk/

FURTHER READING

Alexander, R.E., Throndson, R.R., 2000. A review of perioperative corticosteroid use in dentoalveolar surgery. Oral Surg Oral Med Oral Pathol Oral Radiol Endod 90, 406–415.

Auluck, A., 2007. Diabetes mellitus: an emerging risk factor for oral cancer? J Can Dent Assoc 73, 501–503.

Barnett, A., 2007. Exenatide. Expert Opin Pharmacother 8, 2593–2608.

Blase, E., Taylor, K., Gao, H.Y., Wintle, M., Fineman, M., 2005. Pharmacokinetics of an oral drug (acetaminophen) administered at various times in relation to subcutaneous injection of exenatide (exendin-4) in healthy subjects. J Clin Pharmacol 45, 570–577.

Combettes, M., Kargar, C., 2007. Newly approved and promising antidiabetic agents. Therapie 62, 293–310.

Consensus Statement on the Worldwide Standardization of the Hemoglobin A1C Measurement, 2007. The American Diabetes Association, European Association for the Study of Diabetes, International Federation of Clinical Chemistry and Laboratory Medicine, and the International Diabetes Federation. Diabetes Care 30, 2399–2400.

Fiske, J., 2004. Diabetes mellitus and oral care. Dent Update 31, 190–198.

Gibson, N., Ferguson, J.W., 2004. Steroid cover for dental patients on long-term steroid medication: proposed clinical guidelines based upon a critical review of the literature. Br Dent J 197, 681–685.

Greenwood, M., Meechan, J.G., 2003. General medicine and surgery for dental practitioners. Part 6: The endocrine system. Br Dent J 195, 129–133.

Keene, J.R., Kaltman, S.I., Kaplan, H.M., 2002. Treatment of patients who have type 1 diabetes mellitus: physiological misconceptions and infusion pump therapy. J Am Dent Assoc 133, 1088–1092.

Lorenzo-Calabria, J., Grau, D., Silvestre, F.J., Hernandez-Mijares, A., 2003. Management of patients with adrenocortical insufficiency in the dental clinic. Med Oral 8, 207–214.

Manfredi, M., McCullough, M.J., Vescovi, P., Al-Kaarawi, Z.M., Porter, S.R., 2004. Update on diabetes mellitus and related oral diseases. Oral Dis 10, 187–200.

Mealey, B.L., Ocampo, G.L., 2000. Diabetes mellitus and periodontal disease. Periodontology 2007 (44), 127–153.

Mealey, B.L., Rose, L.F., 2008. Diabetes mellitus and inflammatory periodontal diseases. Curr Opin Endocrinol Diabetes Obes 15, 135–141.

Nicholson, G., Bunin, J.M., Hall, G.M., 1998. Peri-operative steriod supplementation. Anaesthesia 53,1091–1094.

Perry, R.J., McLaughlin, E.A., Rice, P.J., 2003. Steroid cover in dentistry: recommendations following a review of current policy in UK dental teaching hospitals. Dent Update 30, 45–47.

Pinto, A., Glick, M., 2002. Management of patients with thyroid disease: oral health considerations. J Am Dent Assoc 133, 849–858.

Scully, C., Chaudhry, S., 2007. Aspects of Human Disease 10. Diabetes Dental Update 34, 189.

Scully, C., 2009. Aspects of Human Disease 33. Pregnancy Dental Update 36, 253.

Scully, C., 2009. Aspects of Human Disease 35. Hyperthyroidism Dental Update 36, 381.

Scully, C., Diz Dios, P., Kumar, N., 2007. Special care in dentistry: handbook of oral healthcare. Elsevier, Edinburgh.

Seymour, R.A., 2003. Dentistry and the medically compromised patient. Surgeon 1, 207–214.

Skamagas, M., Breen, T.L., LeRoith, D., 2008. Update on diabetes mellitus: prevention, treatment, and association with oral diseases. Oral Dis 14, 105–114.

Soon, D., Kothare, P.A., Linnebjerg, H., et al., 2006. Effect of exenatide on the pharmacokinetics and pharmacodynamics of warfarin in healthy Asian men. J Clin Pharmacol 46, 1179–1187.

Vairaktaris, E., Spyridonidou, S., Goutzanis, L., et al., 2007. Diabetes and oral oncogenesis. Anticancer Res 27, 4185–4193.

Vernillo, A.T., 2001. Diabetes mellitus: relevance to dental treatment. Oral Surg Oral Med Oral Pathol Oral Radiol Endod 91, 263–270.

Appendix 6.1 Endocrine and metabolic effects of some cancers

Substance released	Tumours most commonly responsible[a]	Disease resulting	Features
Adrenocorticotropic hormone (ACTH)	Bronchial, carcinoid, pancreatic, parotid, phaeochromocytoma	Cushing syndrome	See text
Antidiuretic hormone (ADH)	Bronchial, Hodgkin disease, pancreatic	SIADH	See text
Catecholamines	Adrenal medulla	Phaeochromocytoma	Facial flushing
Erythropoietin	Adrenal, breast, bronchial, fibroids, hepatoma, phaeochromocytoma	Polycythaemia	See text
Gastrin	Pancreatic	Zollinger–Ellison syndrome	Diarrhoea, multiple small intestinal ulcers
Human chorionic gonadotropin (HCG)	Breast, hepatoblastoma, pancreatic	Precocious puberty	See text
Oestrogens	Adrenal, lung, testicular	Gynaecomastia	Gynaecomastia
Parathyroid hormone (PTH) and prostaglandins	Renal, almost any squamous cell carcinoma	Hypercalcaemia	Polyuria, polydipsia, psychosis, constipation, abdominal pain
Serotonin (5-hydroxytryptamine) and other vasoactive substances	Bronchial, ileocaecal	Carcinoid syndrome	Symptoms mainly if there are hepatic metastases, facial flushing, bronchospasm, diarrhoea. Right-sided valvular heart lesions (especially pulmonary stenosis)
Testosterone	Adrenal, ovarian		Hirsutism
Thyroid-stimulating hormone (TSH)	Trophoblastic	Hyperthyroidism	See text
Transforming growth factor (TGF)	Abdominal, breast	Acanthosis nigricans	See text

[a]Carcinomas unless otherwise stated.
SIADH, syndrome of inappropriate antidiuretic hormone secretion.

GASTROINTESTINAL AND PANCREATIC DISORDERS

OESOPHAGUS

The oesophagus has the single important function of carrying food, liquids and saliva from the mouth to the stomach, achieving this by an automatic process of coordinated contractions of its muscular lining (peristalsis), termed deglutition (swallowing).

Deglutition involves a complex and coordinated process initiated by sensory impulses from the oropharynx to the brainstem primarily through cranial nerves VII, IX and X. These come from stimulation of receptors on the fauces, tonsils, soft palate, base of the tongue and posterior pharyngeal wall.

The efferent (motor) function of swallowing is mediated by cranial nerves IX, X and XII. Cricopharyngeal sphincter opening is reflexive and starts when the bolus reaches the posterior pharyngeal wall before reaching this sphincter. Swallowing is divided into three phases: the first is voluntary, phases two and three are involuntary.

- *Phase one* is the voluntary collection and swallowing of the masticated food bolus. The next phases are involuntary.
- *Phase two* is passage of food through the pharynx into the beginning of the oesophagus.
- *Phase three* is the passage of food down into the stomach.

Swallowing and respiration are inextricably linked through structural and physiological coordination. Neurological damage, such as from a stroke, can lead to disturbed swallowing (dysphagia) and the risk of aspiration into the lungs.

The oesophagus is generally examined by endoscopy. The current 'gold standard' examination of swallowing is videofluoroscopy but it is often time-consuming and carries a small radiation risk.

REFLUX OESOPHAGITIS (GASTRO-OESOPHAGEAL REFLUX DISEASE)

General aspects

Gastro-oesophageal reflux disease (GORD) is the term used to describe a backflow of acid from the stomach into the oesophagus, one of the most common kinds of dyspepsia. GORD is predisposed to by gastrointestinal disorders (e.g. high acidity of gastric contents; impaired gastro-oesophageal motility) or extragastrointestinal conditions (obesity, stooping, large meals, smoking, alcohol).

Although at one time considered to be a result of hiatus hernia, the relationship between the symptoms and appearances on barium swallow is inconsistent. Hiatal hernias – also known as diaphragmatic hernias – form at the opening (hiatus) in the diaphragm where the oesophagus joins the stomach. The muscle tissue around the hiatus weakens, allowing the upper stomach to herniate through the diaphragm into the chest cavity. Hiatal hernias are found in about 25% of all people over age 50 – particularly in women and those who are overweight. Most hernias cause no symptoms but larger ones may allow food and acid to regurgitate into the oesophagus, which can cause chest pain ('heartburn').

Clinical features

The usual symptom heartburn, is an uncomfortable burning sensation behind the sternum, most commonly felt after a meal. Acid taste is common. In some individuals, reflux is frequent or severe enough to cause more significant problems and to be considered a disease. Complications may include stricture and iron-deficiency anaemia.

General management

Diagnosis can be confirmed by oesophageal pH monitoring. Conditions to differentiate include candidal oesophagitis, or chemical burns from acids or alkalis, non-steroidal anti-inflammatory drugs (NSAIDs), potassium chloride or tetracyclines.

Symptoms can often be effectively relieved by losing weight, raising the head of the bed by at least 4 inches at night and taking frequent small meals with antacids. Drugs typically effective include H_2-blockers (cimetidine, ranitidine or others), but proton-pump inhibitors such as omeprazole or lansoprazole are more effective.

Dental aspects

The gastric contents can have a pH as low as 1 and regurgitation, if chronic, can thus cause dental erosion. This is typically of the palatal aspects of the upper anterior teeth and premolars, and worse if there is impaired salivation. Some patients are convinced that other oral symptoms or diseases are caused by 'acid' but, apart from the few genuine cases with persistent regurgitation of gastric contents, this is no more than a folk myth, probably fostered by advertisements for antacids – for erosion, see also anorexia nervosa and bulimia (Ch. 27) and alcoholism (Ch. 34).

POST-CRICOID WEB

The association of post-cricoid dysphagia, upper oesophageal webs and iron-deficiency anaemia is known as the Plummer–Vinson syndrome (PVS) in the USA and the Paterson–Brown-Kelly syndrome in the UK. The term sideropenic dysphagia has also been used, since the syndrome can feature iron deficiency (sideropenia), but no anaemia. Postulated aetiopathogenic mechanisms include iron and nutritional deficiencies, genetic predisposition and autoimmune factors. The improvement in dysphagia after iron therapy provides evidence for an association between iron deficiency and post-cricoid dysphagia. Moreover, the decline in PVS seems to parallel an improvement in nutritional status, including iron supplementation. However, population-based studies have shown no relationship between post-cricoid dysphagia and anaemia or sideropenia.

If a web is suspected, endoscopy should be carried out carefully under direct vision through the upper oesophageal sphincter. The web typically appears as a thin mucosal membrane covered by normal squamous epithelium. Most webs are located along the anterior oesophageal wall in the shape of a crescent.

Although reports are inconsistent, patients with PVS seem to be at greater risk for hypopharyngeal, oesophageal and oral cancers.

Patients with PVS usually respond well to iron therapy, diet modification and, if necessary, oesophageal dilatation.

CANCER OF THE OESOPHAGUS

General aspects

Cancer of the oesophagus is usually squamous cell carcinoma in the upper and middle part of the oesophagus, or adenocarcinoma in the lower third. Oesophageal cancer is more frequent in older people and in men. Risk factors are shown in Box 7.1.

Box 7.1 Risk factors for oesophageal cancer

- Tobacco use
- Alcohol use
- Achalasia – failure of normal peristalsis and relaxation of oesophagogastric sphincter
- Barrett oesophagus – this premalignant condition may develop into adenocarcinoma
- Tylosis (autosomal dominant palmar–plantar hyperkeratosis)
- Systemic sclerosis
- Other types of irritation (e.g. swallowing lye or other caustic substances)
- Ethnicity – Chinese and Russian people appear predisposed

Clinical features

Early oesophageal cancer usually causes few or no symptoms but later features may include dysphagia, weight loss, pain (in the throat or back, behind the sternum or between the shoulder blades), hoarseness, chronic cough, vomiting or haemoptysis (coughing up blood).

Metastases are typically in the lymph nodes, liver, lungs, brain and bones.

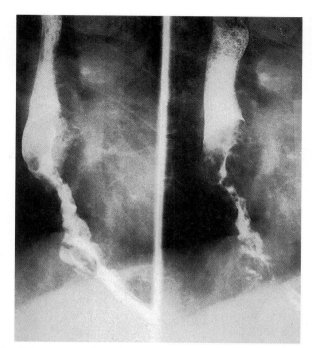

Fig. 7.1 Barium swallow radiography showing oesophageal carcinoma

General management

Diagnosis is confirmed by chest radiography, barium swallow (Fig. 7.1), oesophagoscopy (endoscopy), computed tomography (CT), magnetic resonance imaging (MRI) and biopsy. Bone scan and bronchoscopy may be needed.

Surgery is the most common treatment (oesophagectomy). Laser therapy or photodynamic therapy is sometimes used. Sometimes, a stent is used for palliation or a plastic tube or part of the intestine is used to remake the connection with the stomach.

Radiation therapy may be used alone or with chemotherapy as primary treatment or to shrink the tumour before surgery.

Dental aspects

Patients who have had oesophageal cancer have a greater chance of developing a second cancer in the head and neck area. Patterson–Brown-Kelly syndrome may be associated with a high risk of oral cancer. Rare patients have tylosis and oral leukoplakia.

THE STOMACH AND INTESTINES

Common symptoms of gastrointestinal disorders include nausea and vomiting, diarrhoea and constipation, though none is specific, and all have a wide range of causes (Ch. 4).

THE STOMACH

Gastric products include hydrochloric acid (secreted by parietal cells), pepsin (secreted by chief or peptic cells) and intrinsic factor (secreted by parietal cells). Gastric mucus contains

Table 7.1 Gastrointestinal hormones

Part of the gastrointestinal tract	Source	Hormones	Stimulus	Effects
Stomach	G cells	Gastrin	Gastric distension Amino acids	Secretion of gastric acid, pepsin, intrinsic factor
Small intestine	Duodenum and jejunum	Cholecystokinin/pancreozymin	Fats, amino acids, peptides	Pancreatic secretion, gallbladder contraction, gastric emptying delayed
	Duodenum and jejunum	Gastric inhibitory peptide	Glucose, fats, amino acids	Gastric acid secretion inhibited, insulin released, gut motility reduced
	Duodenum and jejunum	Motilin	Acid	Increased gut motility
	Duodenum and jejunum	Secretin	Acid	Pancreatic bicarbonate secretion, gastric emptying delayed
	Jejunum	Vasoactive intestinal peptide	Neural stimulation	Gastric acid and pepsin secretion inhibited, pancreatic and intestinal secretion stimulated
Pancreas	D cells	Somatostatin	Neural stimulation	Gastric and pancreatic secretion inhibited
	Pancreatic polypeptide cells	Pancreatic polypeptide	Proteins	Biliary and pancreatic secretion inhibited

several glycoproteins which, with bicarbonate, are produced by surface cells and protect the mucosa against erosion.

Hydrochloric acid secretion is stimulated by: hypoglycaemia and mediators including acetylcholine (muscarinic type receptor); gastrin (from G cells) and synthetic analogues of gastrin (pentagastrin); and histamine (from histaminocytes). Hydrochloric acid secretion is inhibited from higher centres and by low gastric pH and hormones – cholecystokinin, gastric inhibitory peptide (GIP) and secretin (Table 7.1).

Gastric acid secretion in response to various stimuli can be assessed by passing a nasogastric tube and measuring the volume, pH and acid concentration of the aspirate. The response to a meal is regulated by complex hormonal and neural (vagal) mechanisms (Table 7.1).

Peptic ulcer

General aspects

An ulcer is a break in the continuity of an epithelial surface. Peptic ulcer disease (PUD) develops in or close to acid-secreting areas in the stomach (gastric ulcer) or proximal duodenum (duodenal ulcer). PUD affects up to 15% of the general population, mostly men over the age of 45 years.

Helicobacter pylori, a spiral bacterium that lives in the stomach and duodenum, is the most common contributory cause to peptic ulcers. In the developed world, some 20–50% of normal adults are infected, but this is higher in poor socioeconomic circumstances, where it is found in 70–90%, though most carriers have no disease. Possible damaging actions of *H. pylori* include increased gastric acid secretion, loss of the mucous protective layer, increased secretion of pepsinogen and increased gastrin release.

Helicobacter pylori survives in the mucous lining, and resists gastric acid via the enzyme urease, which converts urea (abundant in the stomach from saliva and gastric juices) into bicarbonate and ammonia – both strong bases. The reaction of

urea hydrolysis is important for the diagnosis of *H. pylori* by the 'breath test'. *H. pylori* has another defence in that the immune response cannot reach it, and the polymorphs may release their destructive superoxide radicals on to the stomach lining cells, causing gastritis and perhaps eventually a peptic ulcer. *H. pylori* is found in the mouth, especially the gingival sulcus, and believed to be transmitted orofaecally. It is possible that *H. pylori* could be transmitted from the stomach to the mouth through gastro-oesophageal reflux and then be transmitted through oral contact.

Peptic ulcer disease is also associated with raised gastrin levels as in Zollinger–Ellison syndrome (a gastrin-producing tumour; high serum calcium provokes gastrin release) and chronic renal failure (poor gastrin metabolism). Other factors that predispose to peptic ulceration include NSAIDs, corticosteroids, smoking, alcohol, diet and stress. There are genetic influences: first-degree relatives have a threefold risk and there is an association with blood group O.

Clinical features

The main feature of PUD is epigastric pain, often relieved by antacids but many patients are symptomless or suffer only occasional dyspepsia. Some have no symptoms and the first sign of an ulcer may be one of the complications – haemorrhage, perforation or pyloric obstruction (stenosis) with vomiting.

General management

Patients less than 45 years old who present with typical ulcer symptoms should be screened for *H. pylori*. Older individuals require upper gastrointestinal endoscopy and multiple gastric biopsies are taken to exclude the presence of malignancy. Biopsy specimens are also tested for the presence of *H. pylori*. Studies of gastric acid or serum gastrin levels may be helpful and, if gastric outlet obstruction is suspected, a barium meal may be

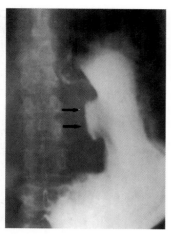

Fig. 7.2 Barium meal radiography showing gastric ulcer

diagnostically helpful (Fig. 7.2). The presence of *H. pylori* can be determined by breath test or biopsy, serologically, by lesional culture or stool test. The breath test is non-invasive, sensitive and specific, and involves ingesting ^{14}C-radiolabelled urea, and examining the breath for the released ^{14}C-radionuclide. The rapid urease test involves inoculating a piece of gastric biopsy into a gel containing urea and phenol red. If *H. pylori* is present and producing ammonia, the colour changes from yellow to pink.

Management of PUD involves conservative measures: dietary modification (frequent small meals with no fried foods); smoking cessation; and alcohol moderation.

Individuals who are *H. pylori* positive should be given 'triple therapy', usually for 7 days to eradicate infection. This normally is effective in over 90% with little risk of relapse and consists of a proton-pump inhibitor (esomeprazole, lansoprazole, omeprazole, pantoprazole or rabeprazole) and antibiotics (amoxicillin, clarithromycin and metronidazole). An additional reason to treat *H. pylori* infection is that it may lead to gastric cancer or mucosa-associated lymphoid tissue (MALT) lymphomas.

Peptic ulcer disease which is *H. pylori*-negative is usually associated with NSAID use. Drugs which block histamine (H_2) receptors, such as cimetidine and ranitidine, are therefore used to reduce gastric acid secretion. Prostaglandin analogues such as misoprostol promote healing in PUD and are indicated in patients from whom NSAIDs cannot be withdrawn.

Surgery is usually reserved for those with complications. Gastric ulcers may be managed by antrectomy with gastroduodenal anastomosis or partial gastrectomy; duodenal ulcers are rarely managed with vagotomy and pyloroplasty.

Dental aspects

Persistent regurgitation of gastric acid as a result of pyloric stenosis can cause severe dental erosion (perimylolysis), typically of the palatal aspects of the upper anterior teeth and premolars.

Gastric surgery may result in attacks of hypoglycaemia. After resection, deficiencies of vitamin B_{12}, folate or iron may cause ulcers, sore tongue or angular stomatitis. These should not be seen now except in the older generation.

Drugs that cause gastric irritation, or promote bleeding, and should not be given to patients with peptic ulcers include aspirin and other NSAIDs and corticosteroids.

Labial vascular anomalies may be associated with peptic ulcer disease.

Oral adverse effects from medications may include:

- dry mouth from proton-pump inhibitors, pirenzepine and sucralfate
- erythema multiforme from ranitidine
- loss of taste or erythema multiforme from omeprazole.

Helicobacter pylori may be transmitted in saliva. Dental staff do not appear to be at particular risk from infection. There are conflicting findings as to whether dental plaque or dentures are an important reservoir for *H. pylori* and significant in transmission of the organism. There may be an association with halitosis.

Antacids impede absorption of ciprofloxacin, erythromycin, metronidazole and tetracyclines. Cimetidine and omeprazole may delay clearance of lidocaine and benzodiazepines, but the effect is rarely clinically significant.

Cancer of the stomach

General aspects

The stomach is one of the most frequent sites of cancer, usually adenocarcinoma. Men are affected nearly twice as often as women. The aetiology of gastric cancer is unclear (Box 7.2).

Box 7.2 Risk factors for stomach cancer

- Genetic influences (carcinoma is common in Japanese people and where there is a positive history in first-degree relatives). The gene E-cadherin/CDH1 is responsible. Hereditary non-polyposis colorectal cancer (HNPCC; also known as Lynch syndrome) and familial adenomatous polyposis (FAP) are genetic disorders with a greatly increased risk of having colorectal cancer and a slightly increased risk of having stomach cancer. People who carry mutations of the inherited breast cancer genes *BRCA1* and *BRCA2* may also have a higher rate of stomach cancer.
- Male gender
- Older age
- Smoking
- Occupations – workers in coal, metal and rubber industries
- Atrophic gastritis
- Achlorhydria
- *Helicobacter pylori*
- Diet (smoked foods, salted fish and meat, and pickled vegetables; nitrates and nitrites are substances commonly found in cured meats)
- Pernicious anaemia
- Blood group A
- Obesity
- Previous stomach surgery
- Ménétrier disease (hypertrophic gastropathy)

Clinical features

Early symptoms of gastric cancer may closely mimic peptic ulcer. A common complaint is indigestion or vague upper abdominal pain. Later, there may be anorexia, loss of weight, nausea, vomiting, haematemesis or melaena (stools black and tarry with blood). Anaemia may develop.

The tumour spreads locally later to cause pain, and may obstruct the intestine to cause vomiting, or the bile duct to cause jaundice. Metastases are mainly to liver, peritoneum (causing ascites), lungs, bones or brain.

General management

The lesion may show on barium imaging and the diagnosis is usually confirmed by gastroscopy and biopsy, but is often delayed by the lack of early symptoms.

Most patients are treated by surgery, but it is frequently only palliative. The prognosis is poor, with about a 7% 5-year survival rate (Ch. 22).

Dental aspects

Anaemia or obstructive jaundice may complicate dental treatment. Oral effects of anaemia (glossitis, ulcers, angular stomatitis) can be an initial sign. It is important to remember that iron deficiency in a male usually results from chronic haemorrhage, often from the gastrointestinal tract, and then sometimes due to an ulcer or neoplasm in the stomach or large bowel.

Orofacial metastases from gastric carcinoma are uncommon, usually in the body of the mandible, and may cause swelling, pain, paraesthesia, loosening of teeth or sockets that fail to heal, or be found as ragged radiolucent areas, sometimes with resorption of tooth roots. Occasionally metastases from a gastric carcinoma may be first detected in a lower cervical (supraclavicular virchow) lymph node, usually on the left side (Troisier sign).

THE SMALL INTESTINE

The small intestine is the main site of digestion and absorption of food. Digestion depends on intestinal and pancreatic enzymes acting on food previously exposed to salivary amylase and gastric acid and pepsin.

Gastric intrinsic factor from the stomach parietal cells is needed for the absorption of vitamin B_{12}. This takes place in the terminal ileum. Iron and folate are absorbed in the duodenum, most other substances in the jejunum. Bile salts facilitate the absorption of fats and the fat-soluble vitamins (A, D, E and K).

Malabsorption is the main feature of small intestine disease and causes diarrhoea or steatorrhoea (fatty stools), and sometimes abdominal discomfort, and deficiency states leading to lassitude, weakness, loss of weight or failure to thrive, and anaemia.

Diseases of the small intestine of most significance include coeliac disease and Crohn disease. Other causes of problems include surgery, infestations and drugs.

Coeliac disease

Coeliac disease (CD; gluten-sensitive enteropathy; coeliac sprue, non-tropical sprue) is the most common genetic disease in Europe, where up to 1 in 250 people have coeliac disease. It is rarely found in African, Chinese or Japanese people. CD is strongly associated with genes on chromosome 6, on a genetic background of HLA-DQw2 or DRw3 and may have a familial tendency.

Coeliac disease is a hypersensitivity or toxic reaction of the small intestine mucosa to the gliadin component of gluten (prolamine), a group of proteins found in all forms of wheat (including durum, semolina, spelt, kamut, einkorn and faro), and related grains (rye, barley, triticale) and possibly oats. Ingestion of gluten causes destruction of jejunal villi (villous atrophy) and inflammation, leading to malabsorption. Coeliac disease may be associated with other autoimmune disorders (Box 7.3).

Box 7.3 Autoimmune disorders that may be associated with coeliac disease

- Dermatitis herpetiformis
- Immunoglobulin A (IgA) deficiency
- IgA nephropathy
- Insulin-dependent diabetes mellitus
- Primary biliary cirrhosis
- Systemic lupus erythematosus
- Thyroid disease

Clinical features

Coeliac disease is one of the great mimics in medicine. It may present at any age and many affected individuals are asymptomatic but coeliac disease can result in malabsorption (leading to growth retardation, vitamin and mineral deficiencies, which may result in anaemia, osteomalacia, bleeding tendencies and neurological disorders), abdominal pain, steatorrhoea and behavioural changes (Fig. 7.3). Intestinal lymphomas arise

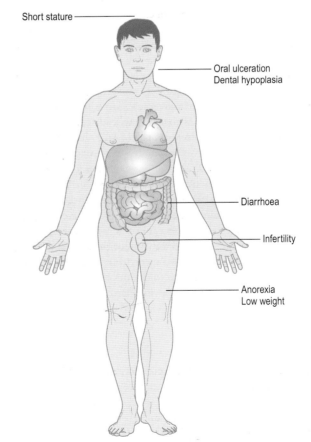

Fig. 7.3 Coeliac disease

Table 7.2 Serum antibodies, and antigens, in coeliac disease

	Antigens		Antibodies
Endomysium	Connective tissue stroma covering muscle fibres		IgA class antibodies appear in those with severe mucosal damage
Transglutaminase	Tissue transglutaminase – the protein cross-linking enzyme – is the endomysial antigen		IgA anti-tissue transglutaminase is 85% sensitive and 97% specific
Gliadin (gliaden)	Prolamins (glycoproteins) in wheat and several other cereals in the grass genus *Triticum*		ELISA test for gliadin antibodies is a reliable screening tool for evaluation of asymptomatic coeliac disease in pre-pubertal children. IgG antibody detection is more sensitive but less specific than IgA antibodies. Anti-gliadin antibodies lose specificity with age
Reticulin	Fibres composed of type III collagen		IgA class reticulin antibodies found in 60% of patients. IgG class reticulin antibodies occasionally also found in bullous dermatoses and in some normal subjects

ELISA, enzyme-linked immunosorbent assay; Ig, immunoglobulin.

in about 6% of individuals. Other food sensitivities or lactose intolerance may also be associated.

General management

It is important to diagnose coeliac disease and to institute a gluten-free diet, even in those with minimal symptoms, as early as possible in order to prevent long-term complications (especially intestinal lymphoma).

The clinical features are usually non-specific; investigations needed to establish the diagnosis include full blood count (anaemia is present in 50% of patients); haematinics (ferritin, vitamin B_{12} and folate levels may be low secondary to malabsorption); stool examination (24-h weight of stool – abnormal if greater than $300\,g$ – and the presence of excess fat (more than 6% of the amount of fat consumed)). Tolerance or measure of digestion/absorption tests include lactose tolerance and D-xylose tests.

Serum antibody screening is shown in Table 7.2.

Endoscopic biopsy of jejunal mucosa shows villous atrophy if positive, and is repeated after a gluten-free diet has been maintained for 3 months. In children the same procedure is used, except that an additional biopsy is carried out after a test challenge of gluten, as it is essential to establish the diagnosis with certainty from the outset, to encourage normal growth and to eliminate such conditions as post-infectious gastroenteritis, which can cause a histologically similar lesion. Similar jejunal changes are also seen in dermatitis herpetiformis.

Treatment of coeliac disease includes rectifying nutritional deficiencies, and a gluten-free diet for life. Instead of wheat flour, patients can use potato, rice, soy or bean flour and gluten-free bread, pasta and other products. Plain meat, fish, fruits and vegetables do not contain gluten. Patients require continued supervision, as it is often difficult to comply with such a diet, especially if eating away from home.

Dental aspects

Short stature associated with diarrhoea and enamel defects is particularly suggestive of early-onset coeliac disease. Anaemia may predispose to oral lesions, notably glossitis, burning mouth, angular stomatitis and ulcers. Coeliac disease may be found in up to 5% of patients with aphthous-like ulcers and should be suspected if there are any other symptoms suggesting small intestine disease.

Some untreated patients may have a bleeding tendency. Anaemia may complicate general anaesthesia (GA).

Inflammatory bowel disease

Inflammatory bowel disease (IBD) is a collective term for diseases that cause inflammation in the intestines and encompasses the spectrum of disease seen in Crohn disease and ulcerative colitis (UC; Table 7.3).

Table 7.3 Crohn disease and ulcerative colitis compared

	Crohn disease	Ulcerative colitis
Main site affected	Ileum	Colorectum
Other sites affected	Any part of the gastrointestinal tract, including the mouth	Terminal ileum
Pathology	Transmural granulomatous inflammation	Superficial inflammation
Abdominal pain	Prominent	Less prominent
Bloody diarrhoea	Less common	Prominent
Fistulae and abscesses	Possible	Rare
Colonic carcinoma risk	Increased	High
Iron deficiency	Common	Common
Folate deficiency	Common	Common
Other deficiencies	Vitamin B_{12} deficiency	Rare

These diseases are seen mainly in northern Europe and USA and in Caucasians. Genetic factors appear to influence disease susceptibility and patterns but environmental factors, possibly dietary factors, and infective agents may be at play. Antigens from commensal micro-organisms appear to trigger and maintain inflammation in a number of ways, with effector T cells (Th1, Th2, Th17) predominating and releasing interferon-gamma and interleukin-12 (IL-12), with other cytokines such as tumour necrosis factor alpha (TNFα), IL-1 and IL-6 being produced in response, by macrophages. Natural killer (NK) cells also contribute directly and via IL-13. Chemoattractants such as IL-8, macrophage inhibitory protein 1 (MIP1) and RANTES (regulated on activation normal T cells as secreted) recruit immunocytes to the area. Interactions between the nervous and immune systems may also play a role: activation of the enteric nervous system may reduce intestinal epithelial permeability, via several mediators including substance P, histamine, neurokinin, serotonin, vanilloids, *S*-nitrosoglutathione and vasoactive intestinal peptide (VIP). Emerging biological therapies are thus aimed at cytokines (e.g. adalimumab, certolizumab, infliximab), T-cell activation receptors (abatacept, visilizumab) or adhesion molecules (alicaforsen, MLN-02, natalizumab).

Crohn disease (regional enteritis or ileitis)

General aspects

Crohn disease appears to be a heterogeneous group of chronic inflammatory disorders seen mainly in Caucasians. About 20% of people with Crohn disease have a blood relative with some form of IBD, most often a brother or sister and sometimes a parent or child.

Microscopically, there is submucosal chronic inflammation with many mononuclear, IL-1-producing cells and non-caseating granulomas in the submucosa and lymph nodes. The inflammatory response is probably mediated by factors such as TNFα.

It has been hypothesized that Crohn disease involves augmentation of the Th1 response in inflammation. Susceptibility appears to be related in 15% to the *CARD15* gene, a locus on chromosome 16. The most recent gene implicated is the autophagy gene *ATG16L1*, which may hinder the body's ability to attack invasive bacteria. Possibly caused by commensal bacteria in persons with a genetically determined dysregulation of mucosal T lymphocytes, the micro-organisms involved are unknown but many have been implicated. *Mycobacterium avium* subspecies *paratuberculosis* is one incriminated, but is probably one of a variety of micro-organisms simply taking advantage of the damaged mucosa and inability to clear bacteria from the intestinal walls. Other workers have implicated a lack of *Faecalibacterium prausnitzii*. Diet, oral contraceptives, NSAIDs, isotretinoin and smoking have also been incriminated.

Clinical features

Crohn disease can affect any part of the gastrointestinal tract from top to tail (mouth to anus) but affects especially the ileocaecal region, typically with ulceration, fissuring and fibrosis of the wall. The manifestations depend on its severity and the site affected. Small intestinal involvement in Crohn disease may cause abdominal pain that often mimics appendicitis, with malabsorption or abnormal bowel habits. Alternating diarrhoea and constipation are typical (Fig. 7.4).

Colonic Crohn disease may mimic ulcerative colitis and frequently causes chronic perianal disease (Fig. 7.5). Complications of Crohn disease include weight loss, gastrointestinal obstruction, internal or external fistulas, perianal fissures, abscesses, arthralgia and sometimes sclerosing cholangitis or renal damage (renal stones or infections).

There is predisposition to large bowel carcinoma comparable with that in ulcerative colitis, and also a slight predisposition to small bowel carcinoma.

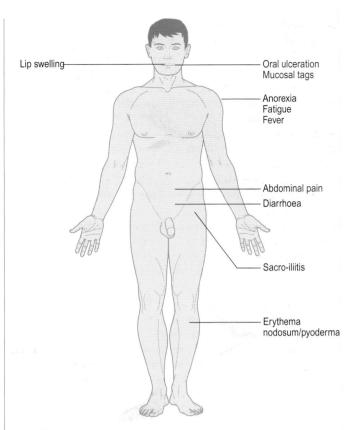

Fig. 7.4 Crohn disease

Lip swelling

Oral ulceration
Mucosal tags

Anorexia
Fatigue
Fever

Abdominal pain

Diarrhoea

Sacro-iliitis

Erythema
nodosum/pyoderma

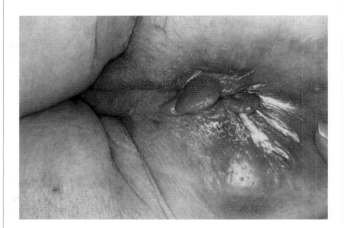

Fig. 7.5 Perianal tags in Crohn disease

General management

The major differential diagnoses include ulcerative colitis, tuberculosis, ischaemic colitis, infections, infestations such as giardiasis, and lymphoma. There are no specific diagnostic tests for Crohn disease but 60% have serum antibodies directed against *Saccharomyces cerevisiae*. Investigations include: blood count (anaemia is common); serum potassium, zinc and albumin (usually depressed); erythrocyte sedimentation rate (ESR), C-reactive protein (CRP) and seromucoid (often raised); plainfilm and contrast radiography (barium enemas of large and small bowel, or barium meal and follow-through); isotope leukocyte intestinal scans (may help to diagnose active disease);

ultrasound and CT; and endoscopy (sigmoidoscopy, colonoscopy) with mucosal biopsy (often shows typical granulomas).

A high-fibre diet is indicated and anaemia needs treatment. Treatment of Crohn disease includes sulfasalazine or newer 5-aminosalicylates (mesalazine or olsalazine) and corticosteroids locally (prednisolone, budesonide). Any of these may be supplemented with methotrexate/azathioprine. Aminosalicylates may cause headaches and blood dyscrasias, and regular blood counts are indicated. Everolimus may be used in unresponsive patients. Monoclonal antibodies directed against TNFα (adalimumab, certolizumab pegol or infliximab) may be beneficial but may have adverse effects.

Surgery (usually resection) becomes necessary at some stage in many patients with intestinal Crohn disease. However, nearly 50% relapse within 10 years of operation and, overall, such treatment is unsatisfactory.

Dental aspects

Dental management may be complicated by any of the problems associated with malabsorption or by corticosteroid or other immunosuppressive treatment. NSAIDs should be avoided. Antibiotics that could aggravate diarrhoea should be avoided; these include amoxicillin–clavulanate, erythromycin and clindamycin.

Oral lesions may be caused by Crohn disease itself or by associated nutritional defects and may include ulcers, facial or labial swelling (Fig. 7.6), mucosal tags or 'cobblestone' proliferation of the mucosa and angular stomatitis. Patients with atypical ulcers, especially when they are large, linear and ragged, or those with recurrent facial swellings, should have biopsy of the mucosa. Melkersson–Rosenthal syndrome (facial swelling, facial palsy and fissured tongue), cheilitis granulomatosa and orofacial granulomatosis may also be incomplete manifestations of Crohn disease, and some of these patients may have asymptomatic intestinal disease, or develop intestinal disease later.

A high prevalence of caries and periodontitis in Crohn disease has also been reported.

Orofacial granulomatosis

Orofacial granulomatosis (OFG) is the term given to granulomatous lesions similar to those of Crohn disease, found on oral biopsy, but where there is no detectable systemic Crohn disease, though this may be detected later. Th1 immunocytes produce IL-12 and RANTES/MIP-1α, and the granulomas. HLA typing may show HLA-A2 or HLA-A11.

Orofacial granulomatosis may sometimes result from reactions to some foods or medicaments such as cinnamonaldehyde and benzoates: up to 40% of patients may be positive to patch tests and half of these may respond to exclusion of dietary antigens (Table 7.4).

Table 7.4 Factors that have been implicated in orofacial granulomatosis

Foods/additives	Chemicals/metals	Micro-organisms
Benzoic acid	Cobalt	*Borrelia burgdorferi*
Butylated	Colophony	*M. paratuberculosis*
hydroxyanisole	Eugenol	*Saccharomyces*
Carbone piperitone	Formaldehyde	*cerevisiae*
Carvone	Isoeugenol	Spirochaetes
Chocolate	Nickel	
Cinnamaldehyde or	Oak moss absolute	
cinnamyl alcohol	Sodium metabisulfite	
Cocoa		
Dairy products		
Eggs		
Monosodium glutamate		
or glutamic acid		
Peanuts		
Piperitone		
Sorbic acid		
Sun Yellow		
Tartrazine		
Wheat		

Oral lesions of OFG include ulcers, facial or labial swelling, mucosal tags or 'cobblestone' proliferation of the mucosa. Gut Crohn disease and reactions to foods should be excluded by gastrointestinal investigations, and allergy tests are often indicated. If systemic Crohn disease can be excluded, patients still need to be kept under observation for its possible development later.

Exclusion of offending substances can be difficult but may help facial swelling resolve. Clofazimine, dapsone, thalidomide or intralesional injection of corticosteroids may also be needed.

Short bowel syndrome

Short bowel syndrome, where the small intestine is short, may be congenital or caused by surgery. Numerous metabolic defects, particularly vitamin and mineral deficiencies leading to osteomalacia and fractures, may result. Patients on home parenteral nutrition due to short bowel syndrome seem to have a high risk of developing systemic osteoporosis, including the jaws, but do not have a higher risk for deterioration of the dental or periodontal state.

THE PANCREAS

The pancreas is intimately associated with the common bile duct and performs exocrine and endocrine functions (Fig. 7.7). The exocrine pancreas produces digestive juices and the

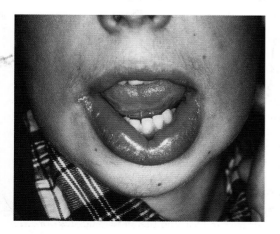

Fig. 7.6 Facial and labial swelling in Crohn disease

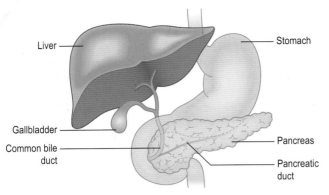

Fig. 7.7 Pancreatic anatomy

enzymes trypsinogen, chymotrypsinogen, amylase and lipase, which via the pancreatic duct enter the common bile duct and thence the small intestine. The pancreatic islets of Langerhans secrete hormones that regulate glucose metabolism (insulin and glucagon), along with pancreatic polypeptide, and soma-tostatin, which help control the function of other endocrine hormones (Ch. 6).

Acute pancreatitis

General aspects

Acute pancreatitis is mainly caused by gallstone disease, but may be precipitated by alcoholism, trauma, hypercalcaemia, hyperlipidaemia, viral infections such as mumps, endoscopic retrograde cholangiopancreatography or various other factors, or drugs. The last may include azathioprine, contraceptive pills, corticosteroids, furosemide or phenothiazines.

Clinical features

Acute pancreatitis causes acinar damage and activation of enzymes leading to local fat necrosis. Mild pancreatitis usually resolves in a few days. In fulminating pancreatitis, the patient is severely ill with retroperitoneal haemorrhage, pleural effusion and paralytic ileus. Systemic effects include severe abdomi-nal pain, nausea, vomiting, hypotension and shock. Possible complications are wide ranging (Box 7.4). The mortality rate is 15–25%.

Box 7.4 Complications of acute pancreatitis

- Abscess
- Acute renal failure
- Adult respiratory distress syndrome
- Disseminated intravascular coagulopathy
- Metabolic (hypocalcaemia, hyperbilirubinaemia and hyperglycaemia)
- Splenic vein thrombosis

General management

Raised serum levels of alkaline phosphatase, the transaminases, amylase and lipase, and radiology, MRI and ultrasonography aid the diagnosis.

Shock, metabolic complications and pain must be treated.

Dental aspects

Local anaesthesia is suitable if emergency treatment is required. Conscious sedation and GA are not feasible until after resolution.

Chronic pancreatitis

General aspects

Causes include gallstone disease and alcoholism particularly. Malnutrition, hyperparathyroidism, haemochromatosis, hyper-lipidaemia, carcinoma, cystic fibrosis and other factors may sometimes be implicated.

Clinical features

Chronic pancreatitis results in acinar atrophy and deterioration in both exocrine and endocrine function. Exocrine dysfunction causes a decline in the volume, bicarbonate content and enzyme content of pancreatic secretions. Endocrine dysfunction means that many patients develop abnormal glucose tolerance or frank diabetes. Chronic dull abdominal pain is punctuated by epi-sodes of acute pancreatitis. Weight loss is common, as are nau-sea, vomiting and pruritus.

General management

Diagnosis is assisted by finding raised serum levels of amylase and lipase. Pancrealauryl and para-aminobenzoic acid testing are used to assess exocrine function. Pancreatic steatorrhoea is suggested by high faecal fat and undigested meat fibres. Faecal levels of chymotrypsin are depressed. Radiography (CT) demonstrates pancreatic calcification, especially in alcoholic pancreatitis. Barium meal, duodenography, cholangiography and endoscopy (endoscopic retrograde cholangiopancreatogra-phy; ERCP) are diagnostically helpful.

Management includes analgesics, treatment of diabetes and the oral administration of pancreatic enzymes to aid digestion.

Dental aspects

Factors predisposing to or resulting from pancreatitis that might influence dental management include bleeding due to vitamin K malabsorption (Ch. 8), alcoholism (Ch. 34), diabetes mellitus (Ch. 6), hyperparathyroidism (Ch. 6), cystic fibrosis (Ch. 15) or narcotic abuse because of severe pain.

Local anaesthesia is satisfactory for pain relief. Conscious sedation may be given for control of anxiety. Oral ulceration can result from holding pancreatic enzyme in the mouth.

Pancreatitis has *rarely* arisen from an oral source of infection.

Pancreatic tumours

General aspects

Most pancreatic tumours originate in the exocrine duct (acinar cells) and nearly 95% are adenocarcinomas, usually involving the head of the pancreas. Pancreatic carcinoma appears to be rising in incidence and is now about one-tenth as common as bronchogenic carcinoma. A minority (less than 10%) of pan-creatic cancers result from an inherited tendency; the familial tendencies are a higher incidence in people with familial adenomatous polyposis, non-polyposis colonic cancer and familial breast cancer associated with the *BRCA2* gene. Periodontal inflammatory disease may also be implicated. Known risk factors are shown in Box 7.5.

> **Box 7.5 Risk factors for pancreatic cancer**
>
> - Betel chewing
> - Chronic exposure to petroleum compounds
> - Diets high in animal fat and low in fruits and vegetables
> - Heredity
> - Obesity and physical inactivity
> - Smoking (responsible for at least 30%)

Tumours that begin in the islet cells (endocrine tumours) are rare but these and others may release hormones (Table 7.5).

Clinical features

Pancreatic carcinoma frequently invades locally to cause biliary obstruction (causing jaundice), pancreatitis and diabetes mellitus. Extrapancreatic complications, such as peripheral vein thrombosis (thrombophlebitis migrans), pruritus, nausea and vomiting, are common.

General management

Plain radiography, CT, MRI, ultrasound, endoscopy (ERCP) or percutaneous transhepatic cholangiography may be of diagnostic help.

Pancreatic carcinoma is usually treated surgically, often with a bypass to relieve obstructive jaundice. Stenting may be used to relieve jaundice for as long as possible. The antimetabolite gemcitabine may help delay progress of advanced carcinoma.

Pancreatic carcinoma has the worst prognosis of any cancer, with a 1-year survival of 10% and a 5-year survival of 3% (see Ch. 22).

Dental aspects

In many cases the poor prognosis of pancreatic cancer may significantly influence the dental treatment plan. Biliary obstruction may lead to bleeding tendencies, especially if there are hepatic metastases. Diabetes mellitus may be an added complication. Periodontitis has been implicated as an association of pancreatic carcinoma.

Local anaesthesia is satisfactory. Conscious sedation may be given to relieve excessive anxiety. GA should not usually be considered because of the poor overall prognosis.

Pancreatic transplantation and simultaneous pancreas–kidney transplantation

General aspects

Pancreas transplantation is used to ameliorate type 1 diabetes and provide complete insulin independence. The pancreas usually comes from a cadaveric organ donor but living donor pancreas transplants have been performed. About 85% of pancreatic transplants are performed along with a kidney transplant (both organs from the same donor) in diabetic patients with renal failure, called a simultaneous pancreas–kidney transplant. About 10% of cases are performed after a previously successful kidney transplant (called a pancreas-after-kidney transplant); 5% are performed as pancreas transplant alone in non-uraemic patients with very labile and problematic diabetes.

Islet transplantation is an alternative newer method that also may ameliorate diabetes.

General management

All transplant recipients require lifelong immunosuppression to prevent a T-cell alloimmune rejection response.

Dental aspects in addition to those discussed in Ch. 35

A meticulous oral assessment is required before surgery, and dental treatment should be undertaken with particular attention to establishing optimal oral hygiene and eradicating sources of potential infection. Dental treatment should be completed

Table 7.5 Hormone-secreting pancreatic tumours

Tumour	Hormone released	Comments
Glucagonomas	Glucagon	Hyperglycaemia and abnormal glucose tolerance. Tumours are frequently malignant. Estimation of plasma glucagon levels differentiates glucagonomas from diabetes mellitus. Glucagon levels may also be raised in patients taking danazol. A major clinical feature is distinctive bullous or pustular skin and mouth lesions. Often also weight loss, anaemia and hypercholesterolaemia
Insulinomas	Insulin	Hypoglycaemia – the most common cause in those not taking insulin
Watery diarrhoea, hypokalaemia and achlorhydria (WDHA) syndrome	Vasoactive peptides	Hyperglycaemia, and watery diarrhoea, hypokalaemia and achlorhydria
Zollinger–Ellison syndrome	Gastrin	Diarrhoea and duodenal ulceration. May be part of the multiple endocrine adenoma syndrome (MEA or MEN I; Ch.6).

before surgery. For 6 months after surgery, elective dental care is best deferred.

If surgical treatment is needed during that period, antibiotic prophylaxis is probably warranted.

THE LARGE INTESTINE

The large intestine, between the terminal ileum and anus, consists of the caecum – a blind-ended pouch that carries a worm-like extension (the vermiform appendix) in humans; the colon, which forms most of the length of the large intestine and comprises ascending, transverse and descending segments; and the rectum – the short, terminal segment continuous with the anal canal.

The large intestine has two main functions: recovery of water and electrolytes (sodium and chloride), and the formation, storage and expulsion of faeces (stools).

Appendicitis

General aspects

Appendicitis is inflammation of the appendix, the cause of which is usually unknown but may follow a viral infection or obstruction. Appendicitis is most common in people aged 10–30.

Clinical features

Not all appendicitis causes symptoms but features may include pain in the right abdomen, nausea, vomiting, constipation, diarrhoea, abdominal swelling, anorexia and low fever that begins later. The pain usually begins near the umbilicus and moves down and into the right iliac fossa. The pain becomes worse when moving, taking deep breaths, coughing, sneezing and being touched (McBurney point).

General management

If untreated, an inflamed appendix can burst, causing peritonitis and even death, and is thus considered an emergency.

Diagnosis is based upon symptoms, examination, blood tests, such as a leukocyte count to check for infection, and urine tests to rule out a urinary tract infection. If a diagnosis of appendicitis is definite, surgery (appendicectomy) is indicated, sometimes via laparoscopic surgery. If the diagnosis of appendicitis is not certain, the patient may be watched and sometimes treated with antibiotics.

Irritable bowel syndrome

Irritable bowel syndrome (IBS; spastic colon; mucous colitis) may affect up to 30% of the population and is the most common cause of referrals to gastroenterologists. IBS causes recurrent abdominal pain together with increased tone and activity of the colon, and abnormal bowel habits and other symptoms. It may occur at any age and has a slight female predominance.

The cause of IBS is unclear but it may begin after an infection or stressful life event; there is often a positive family history, anxious personality type and history of migraine or psychogenic symptoms (Ch. 10). The protozoan *Dientamoeba fragilis* has

been implicated by some researchers. Cytokines (IL-1, IL-6 and TNF) and serotonin have been implicated.

Clinical features

Irritable bowel syndrome leads to crampy abdominal pain, flatulence, bloating and changes in bowel habit – constipation or diarrhoea, often with urgency (tenesmus). Additional gynaecological and urinary symptoms may be reported. Episodes may be precipitated by stressful life events or foods such as chocolate, caffeine, milk products, or large amounts of alcohol.

Examination may reveal some abdominal distension and tenderness. However, guarding or rebound tenderness of the abdomen along with blood or mucus per rectum suggest other organic disease.

General management

Irritable bowel syndrome is a diagnosis of exclusion. Investigations are tailored according to the patient's age, family history, severity and nature of symptoms in order to exclude coeliac disease inflammatory bowel disease or colonic cancer [(full blood count and haematinics); inflammatory markers (ESR); contrast radiography (barium studies); endoscopy and mucosal biopsy].

Stress reduction and a high-fibre diet may control symptoms. Anti-spasmodics (mebeverine, loperamide or an anti-muscarinic such as dicyclomine and peppermint oil) may help. Probiotics may have a role.

Cognitive behavioural therapy or antidepressants may be of benefit for patients with IBS who are clinically depressed. For severe cases that fail to respond to the above measures, it is important to reconsider the diagnosis and re-evaluate the patient's history and presentation: coeliac disease or IBD can be missed.

Dental aspects

Local anaesthesia is satisfactory for pain control. Conscious sedation may be needed because of these patients' anxious personalities. Orofacial manifestations may include psychogenic oral symptoms such as pain dysfunction syndrome, sore tongue or atypical facial pain.

Loperamide or dicyclomine may cause dry mouth.

Diverticular disease

General aspects

Diverticular disease includes both diverticulosis (small colonic pouches – diverticula – that bulge outward through weak spots of the large intestine) and diverticulitis (inflammation of these diverticula). Diverticular disease is most common in developed or industrialized countries, where it affects up to 25% of adults over middle age, and over 50% of those over 60 years. It may result from a low-fibre diet.

Clinical features

Left-sided diverticular disease (involving the sigmoid colon) is most common in the West, while right-sided diverticular disease is more prevalent in Africa and Asia. It may be asymptomatic, but is often accompanied by dyspepsia, abdominal pain, constipation and flatulence. Complications include infection (pericolic abscess), perforation and peritonitis, or fistula.

General management

Conditions to be excluded include IBD, IBS, cancer, and urological and gynaecological disorders. Management includes a high-fibre diet and reassurance. Antibiotics and surgery may be indicated if diverticulitis develops.

Dental aspects

There are no specific management problems in dentistry, although codeine should be avoided as it worsens constipation.

Ulcerative colitis

General aspects

Ulcerative colitis is an inflammatory bowel disease affecting part or the whole of the large intestine, most frequently the lower colon and rectum. Ulcerative colitis causes inflammation and ulcers in the superficial layers of the large intestine mucosa, followed by pseudopolyp formation. It most often affects people between the ages of 15 and 40 years.

The aetiology is unknown but autoimmunity, diet, sulphate-reducing bacteria, drugs such as isotretinoin and a genetic basis have been suggested. A role for *RUNX3* gene on chromosome 1 has been suggested but chromosomes 6, 16, 12, 14, 5, 19 and 3 have also been implicated. Psychosomatic symptoms are often associated.

Clinical features

Typical features are pain and diarrhoea with stools containing intermixed mucus, blood and pus, sometimes with systemic toxicity (fever, anorexia, weight loss, anaemia and raised ESR and CRP; Fig. 7.8). Disease with less than six bloody stools daily but no systemic toxicity is termed 'mild'; if there is toxicity, it is termed 'moderate'; and 'severe ulcerative colitis' is applied when there are more than six bloody stools daily plus toxicity.

Disease extension through the muscular layers may result in life-threatening toxic megacolon (the colon dilates and can perforate). The most serious complication is carcinoma of the colon which is up to 30 times more frequent than in the general population and most likely to develop in patients with early-onset colitis or with disease persisting for > 10 years.

Non-gastrointestinal features include arthralgia, conjunctivitis, uveitis, iritis, finger-clubbing, sacro-iliitis, skin disease (erythema nodosum and pyoderma gangrenosum), liver disease (primary sclerosing cholangitis), gallstones and renal calculi.

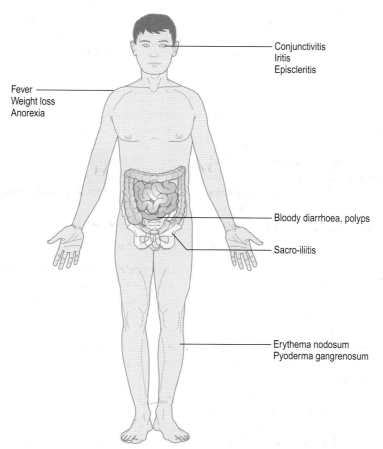

Conjunctivitis
Iritis
Episcleritis

Fever
Weight loss
Anorexia

Bloody diarrhoea, polyps

Sacro-iliitis

Erythema nodosum
Pyoderma gangrenosum

Fig. 7.8 Ulcerative colitis

THE STOMACH AND INTESTINES

Overproduction of platelets and some clotting factors may lead to thromboembolism. Various types of liver disease may complicate the condition.

General management

There are no specific diagnostic tests. Investigations include full blood count and haematinics; inflammatory markers (ESR); contrast radiography (barium studies); endoscopy and mucosal biopsy.

A high-fibre diet is indicated and any anaemia needs treatment. Medical therapy includes conservative measures (nutritional support) and drug therapy (Box 7.6).

Box 7.6 Management of ulcerative colitis

- Local corticosteroids (prednisolone) – often by enema
- Sulfasalazine or 5-aminosalicylates (balsalazide, mesalazine, olsalazine) to induce and maintain remission (aminosalicylates may cause headaches and blood dyscrasias and so regular blood counts are indicated)
- Tacrolimus, ciclosporin or infliximab
- Systemic steroids or azathioprine in acute exacerbations
- Surgery for failure of medical therapy or to treat complications from long-standing disease

---

The surgical options in UC depend on the extent of disease but generally consist of colectomy (excision of diseased bowel with either re-anastomosis or ileostomy construction) if symptoms are severe, the response to medical treatment is poor, or complications such as pyoderma gangrenosum or haemorrhage develop, or to eliminate the risk of malignant change. Unlike Crohn disease, surgery can be curative.

Dental aspects

Drugs that should be avoided include NSAIDs and antibiotics including amoxicillin–clavulanate, erythromycin and clindamycin which could aggravate diarrhoea.

Local anaesthesia is satisfactory and there are no objections to conscious sedation if needed. Management complications may include anaemia and those associated with corticosteroid therapy.

Oral manifestations in ulcerative colitis are rare but include pyostomatitis gangrenosum (chronic ulceration), pyostomatitis vegetans (multiple intraepithelial microabscesses), discrete haemorrhagic ulcers or lesions related to anaemia. Since uveitis, skin lesions and mouth ulcers can be found in ulcerative colitis, it is important to differentiate it from Behçet disease (Ch. 11).

Familial polyposis coli

Familial polyposis coli (FPC) is an autosomal dominant disease in which multiple adenomatous polyps affect the rectum and colon: carcinomatous change usually supervenes. FPC is a feature of Gardner syndrome, along with multiple exostoses and osteomas of the jaws. These also appear to be more common in patients with non-familial colorectal cancer than in the general population. Colectomy is indicated.

Carcinoma of the colon

General aspects

Carcinoma of the colon (colorectal cancer) is common. The peak incidence is in the sixth or seventh decades and the tumour usually forms in the rectum or pelvic (sigmoid) colon. A series of gene alterations can lead to adenomas and eventually, in some patients, to carcinoma. Risk factors are shown in Box 7.7.

Box 7.7 Risk factors for colonic carcinoma

- Cholecystectomy
- Diet low in fibre, fruit and vegetables, and high in red meat and fat
- Heredity; familial polyposis coli
- Inflammatory bowel disease
- Smoking

Long-term aspirin use lowers the risk of colonic cancer.

Clinical features

Carcinoma of the colon may cause abdominal pain, change in bowel habit, melaena, weight loss or complications such as anaemia, intestinal obstruction or perforation.

General management

Abdominal examination may reveal a mass. Sigmoidoscopy and sometimes faecal occult blood testing, MRI, ultrasound, barium enema (Fig. 7.9) and colonoscopy may be required.

Surgical resection is the usual treatment. Spread is frequently to the liver. The 5-year survival rate is overall about 30% (see Ch. 22). Radiotherapy may be useful for dealing with pain from recurrences. Chemotherapy may be used in advanced cancer: capecitabine, irinotecan, oxaliplatin, raltitrexed and possibly cetuximab, a chimerized (part mouse, part human) monoclonal antibody that targets epidermal growth factor receptor

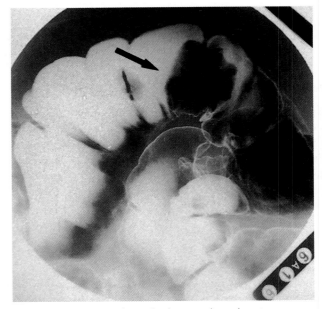

Fig. 7.9 Barium enema radiography showing colorectal carcinoma

(EGFr), which is associated with tumour cell growth in a number of EGFr-positive malignant tumours, including colorectal carcinoma.

Serial monitoring for serum carcinoembryonic antigen or serum or faecal M2-PK (M2-pyruvate kinase) antigen may help detect recurrences (Ch. 22). Metastatic carcinoma may be treated with bevacizumab and cetuximab.

Dental aspects

Local anaesthesia is satisfactory and acceptable. Conscious sedation can be given if needed. GA must be given by a specialist, particularly if complications have developed.

Anaemia resulting from chronic intestinal haemorrhage can complicate dental management or cause oral signs or symptoms.

Mandibular osteomas may be markers of an enhanced risk of colorectal cancer.

Antibiotic-associated (pseudomembranous) colitis

Most of the orally administered antimicrobials can cause diarrhoea, but clinically significant colitis is rare. Colitis following use of antibiotics is more likely to affect older or debilitated patients.

The most severe type of colitis is staphylococcal enterocolitis, usually caused by prolonged heavy doses of tetracyclines, particularly after bowel surgery. Now that the cause is recognized, this type of colitis has become rare.

Pseudomembranous colitis is caused more frequently by lincomycin and clindamycin than by other antibiotics, as a result of proliferation of toxigenic strains of clostridia, particularly *Clostridium difficile*. These are resistant to low concentrations of these antibiotics.

Clinically, antibiotic-associated colitis is characterized by painful diarrhoea and passage of mucus. In elderly debilitated patients especially, there is passage of blood and pseudomembranous material (necrotic mucosa), occasionally resulting in death. The diagnosis cannot be made from the presence of *C. difficile* in the stool, as 1–9% of hospital patients carry the bacterium, but only from sigmoidoscopy and biopsy.

Pseudomembranous colitis usually responds to metronidazole or oral vancomycin, plus cessation of the causal antibiotic.

Anal diseases

Because of the widespread habit of anal intercourse, the anus can show the signs of many sexually transmitted diseases. It is also a particularly important portal of entry for human immunodeficiency virus (HIV) infection because of the delicate lining of the anal canal. Carcinoma of the anus is rare, but more common in patients with HIV/acquired immune deficiency syndrome (AIDS) and often associated with human papillomavirus infection.

Haemorrhoids

General aspects

Haemorrhoids is a term that refers to a condition in which the veins around the anus or lower rectum are swollen and inflamed. Haemorrhoids may result from straining to pass stool. Contributory factors include pregnancy, ageing, chronic constipation or diarrhoea, and anal intercourse.

Clinical features

The most common symptom of internal haemorrhoids is bright red blood covering the stool, on toilet paper, or in the WC pan. Symptoms of external haemorrhoids may include irritation around the anus. Bleeding and/or itching, a painful swelling or hard lumps from thrombosed external haemorrhoids are other effects.

General management

Sigmoidoscopy or colonoscopy may be needed to rule out other causes of gastrointestinal bleeding such as colorectal cancer.

Application of a haemorrhoidal cream or suppository to the affected area relieves symptoms. A softer stool makes emptying the bowels easier and lessens the pressure on haemorrhoids.

Surgery may be needed, such as sclerotherapy, rubber band ligation, infrared coagulation or haemorrhoidectomy.

Peritonitis

The peritoneal cavity normally holds only 50 ml of fluid, which contains complement factors but few leukocytes, circulates in the peritoneal space and drains via the lymphatics.

Acute peritonitis is fairly uncommon, but is usually a serious infection with inflammation of the peritoneum that follows rupture of a viscus (e.g. appendix) or trauma. Chronic peritonitis develops in patients on continuous ambulatory peritoneal dialysis and in some intensive care patients.

Spontaneous bacterial peritonitis is an infection of ascites fluid in patients with cirrhosis, in which the source of the infection is not known. It is rare and *Streptococcus pneumoniae* is the most common pathogen, but there is rarely any obvious source of the infection.

Clinical features

Severe and generalized abdominal pain, vomiting, pyrexia, a rigid/board-like and tender abdomen and no bowel sounds are the main features.

Peritonitis can lead rapidly to hypovolaemic shock and death.

General management

Diagnosis is clinical supported by imaging and culture. Treatment includes urgent fluid administration, antibiotics and laparotomy/surgical debridement/drainage as required.

USEFUL WEBSITES

http://www.mayoclinic.com
http://www.niddk.nih.gov/health/digest/digest.htm
http://www.emedicine.com/derm/topic72.htm
http://digestive.niddk.nih.gov/ddiseases/pubs/celiac/index.htm
http://digestive.niddk.nih.gov/ddiseases/pubs/crohns/index.htm
http://digestive.niddk.nih.gov/ddiseases/pubs/colitis/index.htm

FURTHER READING

Baumgart, D.C., Sandborn, W.J., 2007. Inflammatory bowel diseases: cause and immunobiology. Lancet 369, 1627–1640.

Baumgart, D.C., Sandborn, W.J., 2007. Inflammatory bowel diseases: clinical aspects and established and evolving therapies. Lancet 369, 1641–1657.

Cornish, J.A., Tan, E., Simillis, C., Clark, S.K., Teare, J., Tekkis, P.P., 2008. The risk of oral contraceptives in the etiology of inflammatory bowel disease: a meta-analysis. Am J Gastroenterol 103, 2394–2400.

Hegarty, A., Hodgson, T., Porter, S., 2003. Thalidomide for the treatment of recalcitrant oral Crohn's disease and orofacial granulomatosis. Oral Surg Oral Med Oral Pathol Oral Radiol Endod 95, 576–585.

Kang, X., Zhang, L., Sun, J., et al., 2008. Prohibitin: a potential biomarker for tissue-based detection of gastric cancer. J Gastroenterol 43, 618–625.

Katz, J., Shenkman, A., Stavropoulos, F., Melzer, E., 2003. Oral signs and symptoms in relation to disease activity and site of involvement in patients with inflammatory bowel disease. Oral Dis 9, 34–40.

MacDonald, J.K., McDonald, J.W.D., 2006. Natalizumab for induction of remission in Crohn's disease. Cochrane Database Syst Rev 3, 1465–1458.

Miyagaki, H., Fujitani, K., Tsujinaka, T., et al., 2008. The significance of gastrectomy in advanced gastric cancer patients with non-curative factors. Anticancer Res 28 (4C), 2379–2384.

Moshkowitz, M., Horowitz, N., Leshno, M., Halpern, Z., 2007. Halitosis and gastroesophageal reflux disease: a possible association. Oral Dis 13, 581–585.

Rigoli, L., Romano, C., Caruso, R.A., et al., 2008. Clinical significance of NOD2/CARD15 and Toll-like receptor 4 gene single nucleotide polymorphisms in inflammatory bowel disease. World J Gastroenterol 14, 4454–4461.

Scheper, H.J., Brand, H.S., 2002. Oral aspects of Crohn's disease. Int Dent J 52, 163–172.

Schønnemann, K.R., Jensen, H.A., Yilmaz, M., Jensen, B.V., Larsen, O., Pfeiffer, P., 2008. Phase II study of short-time oxaliplatin, capecitabine and epirubicin (EXE) as first-line therapy in patients with non-resectable gastric cancer. Br J Cancer Aug 26 (Epub ahead of print).

Scully, C., 2001. Gastroenterological diseases and the mouth. Practitioner 245, 215–222.

Scully C, Chaudhry S, Aspects of Human Disease 11. Peptic ulcer disease (PUD) Dental Update 34; 253 (2007)

Scully C, Chaudhry S, Aspects of Human Disease 12. Inflammatory bowel disease (IBD) Dental Update 43; 317 (2007)

Scully C, Chaudhry S, Aspects of Human Disease 13. Coeliac disease (gluten-sensitive enteropathy) Dental Update 43; 381 (2007)

Scully C, Chaudhry S, Aspects of Human Disease 14. Irritable bowel syndrome (IBS) Dental Update 43; 453 (2007)

Silva, M.A.G.S., Damante, J.H., Stipp, A.C.M., Tolentino, M.M., Carlotto, P.R., Fleury, R.N., 2001. Gastroesophageal reflux disease; new oral findings. Oral Surg 91, 301–310.

Tilikaratne, W.M., Freysdottir, J., Fortune, F., 2008. Orofacial granulomatosis: review on aetiology and pathogenesis. J Oral Pathol Med 37, 191–195.

HAEMOSTASIS

Normal haemostasis depends on a complex interaction of blood vessels, platelets, fibrin coagulation and deposition, and fibrinolytic proteins (Fig. 8.1). The three reactions – primary, secondary and tertiary haemostasis – act simultaneously, not sequentially. Abnormal clotting is prevented by the endothelium providing a physical barrier and secreting products that inhibit platelets, including nitric oxide and prostaglandin I_2 (prostacyclin). Inhibitors limit haemostasis to the site of vessel injury and prevent overproduction of the clot, which could lead to pathological thrombosis.

PRIMARY HAEMOSTASIS (VASCULAR AND PLATELET ACTIVITY)

Primary haemostasis is by vasoconstriction after injury. This retards extravascular blood loss, and slows local blood flow, enhancing the adherence of platelets to exposed subendothelial surfaces and the activation of the coagulation process.

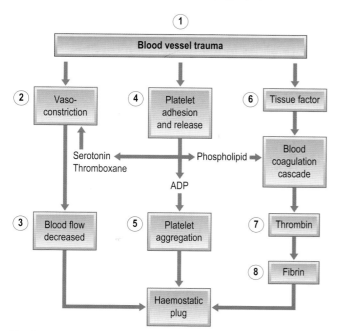

Fig. 8.1 Haemostasis

A primary platelet plug forms by platelet adhesion mediated by von Willebrand factor (vWF), which binds to a glycoprotein GP Ib in the platelet membrane (Fig. 8.2). Fibrinogen also binds platelets to the subendothelium by attaching to a platelet receptor.

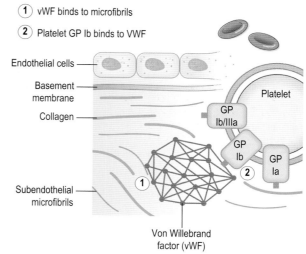

Fig. 8.2 Platelet plug formation

Adhesion of platelets to vessel walls causes them to change shape and activate surface collagen receptors and to release ADP and serotonin, thromboxane A_2 (TXA_2) and platelet activating factor (PAF). These are potent platelet-aggregating agonists and vasoconstrictors. Platelet activation and recruitment are also mediated by ADP and serotonin, enhanced by generation of thrombin through the coagulation cascade.

Abnormalities in primary haemostasis

Abnormalities in primary haemostasis (abnormal platelet number or function, abnormal vWF or defects in the blood vessel wall) result in haemorrhage from mucosal surfaces (epistaxis, melaena, haematuria), petechial or ecchymotic haemorrhages. Prolonged bleeding from wounds is usually limited by coagulation. However, if the defect is severe, bleeding more typical of disorders of secondary haemostasis can result (e.g. intracavity haemorrhage).

Primary haemostasis inhibitors

Primary haemostasis inhibitors are the natural inhibitors of platelet function, such as bradykinin, prostacyclin and nitric oxide, released by endothelial cells. Acquired inhibitors of platelet function are rare, whereas acquired inhibitors of vWF (platelet glycoprotein 1b, or GP1b) form in a variety of diseases and result in acquired von Willebrand disease (avWD).

More commonly, platelet function is inhibited intentionally by the administration of agents such as aspirin for the prevention of thrombosis.

Table 8.1 Blood coagulation factors

Factor	Name
I	Fibrinogen
II	Prothrombin
III	Thromboplastin
IV	Calcium
V	Proaccelerin
VI	–
VII	Proconvertin
VIII	Antihaemophilic factor
IX	Christmas factor (plasma thromboplastin component)
X	Stuart–Prower factor
XI	Plasma thromboplastin antecedent
XII	Hageman factor
XIII	Fibrin-stabilizing factor
Fitzgerald factor	High-molecular-weight kininogen
Fletcher factor	Prekallikrein

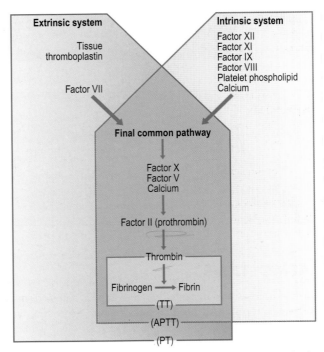

Fig. 8.3 Blood coagulation and assays. APTT activated partial thromboplastin time, PT prothrombin time, TT thrombin time

SECONDARY HAEMOSTASIS (BLOOD CLOTTING)

Secondary haemostasis is the formation of fibrin through the coagulation cascade (Table 8.1, Fig. 8.3). Platelets contribute by providing a phospholipid surface and receptors for binding coagulation factors. The coagulation cascade is traditionally separated into three pathways (intrinsic, extrinsic and common) involving blood coagulation factors acting as enzymes, which require activation and cofactors.

The extrinsic pathway, the main pathway for initiation of coagulation, is initiated by the generation/exposure of tissue factor (factor III), expressed by endothelial cells, subendothelial tissue and monocytes, with expression being upregulated by cytokines (TNF-alpha, interleukin-6). It also involves the tissue factor and factor VII complex, which activates factor X.

The intrinsic pathway, which amplifies coagulation, is stimulated by thrombin, through activation of factor XI, and involves high-molecular-weight kininogen, prekallikrein, factors XII, XI and IX, and factor VIII, which acts as a cofactor (with calcium and platelet phospholipid) for the factor IX-mediated activation of factor X. A minor route of stimulation of the intrinsic pathway (the alternative pathway) is the direct activation of factor IX by the tissue factor–factor VII complex.

The common pathway involves the factor X-mediated generation of thrombin from prothrombin (facilitated by factor V, calcium and platelet phospholipid ('prothrombinase complex'). Thrombin activates factors XI and VIII of the intrinsic pathway, which amplifies the coagulation cascade. Activated factor IX, together with activated factor VIII, calcium and phospholipid ('tenase complex'), amplify the activation of factor X, generating large amounts of thrombin.

Thrombin cleaves fibrinogen to form soluble fibrin monomers, which then spontaneously polymerize to form soluble fibrin polymer, and thrombin also activates factor XIII, which, together with calcium, serves to cross-link and stabilize the soluble fibrin polymer, forming cross-linked (insoluble) fibrin.

Thrombin promotes coagulation as a platelet agonist, promoting platelet aggregation, and also activating factors V and VIII – necessary cofactors for the 'prothrombinase' and 'tenase' complexes, respectively. Thrombin also activates factor XIII, essential for the cross-linking of the fibrin polymer, and inhibits fibrinolysis by generation of a thrombin-activatable fibrinolytic inhibitor (TAFI).

Drugs that act as anticoagulants (affecting coagulation) include warfarin, heparin and hirudin.

Abnormalities in the coagulation cascade

Defects in the coagulation cascade cause more serious bleeding than do defects of primary haemostasis. They include bleeding into cavities (chest, joints and cranium) and subcutaneous haematomas. Petechial haemorrhages are not seen.

Inhibitors of blood coagulation

The common pathway is rapidly inhibited by a lipoprotein-associated molecule, called tissue factor pathway inhibitor, thus allowing this pathway to generate only small amounts of thrombin. This is sufficient to amplify the coagulation cascade, but not enough to produce fibrin.

The main inhibitor of secondary haemostasis is antithrombin (AT; also called antithrombin III, or ATIII), an alpha2-globulin produced in the liver, that inhibits thrombin (factor IIa) and many activated coagulation proteins (including factors II, IX, X, XI and XII). Antithrombin complexes with thrombin; the complex is then removed by the monocyte–macrophage system. Heparin enhances antithrombin binding to thrombin and this is the basis for its use as an anticoagulant. *In vivo*, heparin is produced by degranulated mast cells or basophils and heparin-like glycosaminoglycans on endothelial cells. Heparin cofactor II is a specific thrombin antagonist, which, like AT, also requires heparin for activation, but in far greater concentrations.

Thrombin can be anticoagulant by binding to endothelial cell thrombomodulin to activate anticoagulant proteins C and S.

Protein C, a vitamin K-dependent protein produced in the liver, inactivates factors V and VIII. Protein S (named after Seattle where it was discovered), another vitamin K-dependent protein synthesized in endothelial cells, megakaryocytes and hepatocytes, facilitates the action of protein C.

The contact pathway is more important for activation of fibrinolysis and inflammation and modulation of vascular biology than it is for haemostasis. It consists of prekallikrein (Fletcher factor), high-molecular-weight kininogen (Williams–Fitzgerald factor) and factor XII (Hageman factor) and has important anticoagulant, profibrinolytic and pro-inflammatory roles.

TERTIARY HAEMOSTASIS (FIBRINOLYSIS)

Tertiary haemostasis is the formation of plasminogen and then plasmin, the main enzyme responsible for fibrinolysis, via t-PA. Other plasminogen activators include urokinase, factor XII and kallikrein. Activated factor XII and kallikrein can activate plasminogen into plasmin directly.

Factor XII and kallikrein produce bradykinin from high-molecular-weight kininogen in the contact portion of the intrinsic pathway of coagulation. Bradykinin and hypoxia stimulate release from endothelium of t-PA, which binds to plasminogen within the clot, converting it into plasmin, which lyses both fibrinogen and fibrin (soluble and cross-linked), releasing fibrin(ogen) degradation products.

Activation of fibrinolysis is triggered by the presence of fibrin, and tissue-type plasminogen activators (t-PA) at the site of fibrin formation, a process regulated by physiological inhibitors such as alpha2-antiplasmin, histidine-rich glycoprotein and plasminogen activator inhibitor.

HAEMOSTASIS INHIBITORS (INHIBITORS OF FIBRINOLYSIS)

Tertiary haemostasis inhibitors include thrombin-activated fibrinolytic inhibitor (TAFI), alpha2-antiplasmin and plasminogen activator inhibitor.

Amplification of the coagulation cascade from thrombin-mediated activation of factor XI leads to large amounts of thrombin and subsequent activation of TAFI, which prevents the binding of plasminogen to fibrin, thus inhibiting its conversion to plasmin. Alpha2-antiplasmin binds free plasmin (that not bound to fibrin) and causes its removal by the monocyte–macrophage system, preventing widespread fibrinolysis. Plasminogen activator inhibitors (PAI-1 and PAI-2) are released by endothelial cells and limit plasmin generation by binding to t-PA.

Drugs that inhibit fibrinolysis (anti-fibrinolytics) include epsilon aminocaproic acid and tranexamic acid.

POST-OPERATIVE BLEEDING

Plasminogen and plasminogen activator are present in the oral environment, since plasminogen is secreted into the saliva and t-PA arises from oral epithelial cells and gingival crevicular fluid. Oral surgery induces changes of fibrinolysis initially the fibrinolytic activity of saliva is weakened, due to inhibitors of fibrinolysis originating from the blood and the wound exudates but, when the bleeding and exudation abate, the fibrinolytic activity of saliva increases. This may contribute to bleeding.

Prolonged bleeding after dental extraction however, is one of the most common signs of haemorrhagic disease and may amount to a haemorrhagic emergency. It is sometimes the way by which the bleeding tendency is first recognized.

Faced with a bleeding patient, it is important to establish whether the situation is urgent and whether there could be a bleeding tendency, or if the patient is losing large quantities of blood, hypotensive (hypovolaemic) or bleeding internally.

MANAGEMENT OF POST-OPERATIVE BLEEDING

The precise site or origin of the bleeding must be discovered by cleaning out the mouth with swabs. Pressing firmly with a gauze pad over the socket for 10–15 min will usually stop the bleeding even in some bleeding tendencies but often only temporarily. Quicker and more effective is to suture the socket under local anaesthesia (LA). If the bleeding persists, consider a systemic cause such as:

- acquired deficiencies of haemostasis, such as anticoagulants or thrombocytopenia, or
- hereditary deficiencies of clotting factors (e.g. von Willebrand syndrome and haemophilia).

There could be a bleeding tendency if the bleeding is unexplained by the degree of trauma or there is a previous, or family, history of excessive bleeding such as:

- a previous diagnosis of a bleeding tendency
- bleeding for more than 36 h or restarting more than 36 h after operation (however, this could indicate an infection)
- admission to hospital to arrest bleeding
- blood transfusion for bleeding
- spontaneous bleeding (e.g. haemarthrosis, deep bruising or menorrhagia from little obvious cause)
- convincing family history of one of the above, combined with a degree of personal history
- treatment with significant drugs such as anticoagulants.

In emergencies an intravenous line must be established and plasma expanders or blood given. Blood transfusions were refused by Jehovah's Witnesses but their principles are being reconsidered, and alternatives to allogeneic blood are becoming available. In this group, blood loss may minimized, using aprotinin and tranexamic acid. Recombinant blood coagulation factors are acceptable to Jehovah's Witnesses (Ch. 30). Erythropoietin is acceptable, as often is intra-operative salvage of blood, or acute normovolaemic haemodilution (ANH; the preoperative removal of blood and replacement by crystalloid or colloid, followed by reuse of the patient's blood at operation).

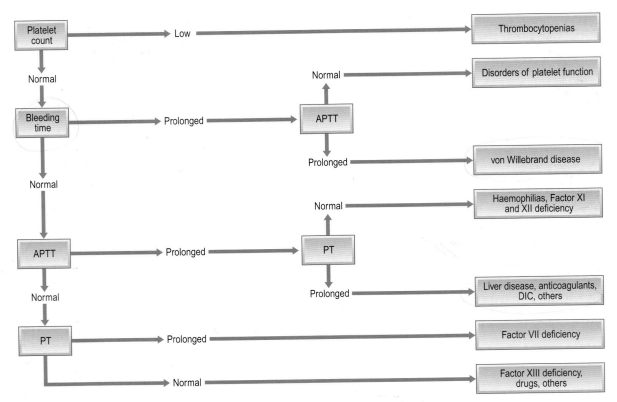

Fig. 8.4 Protocol for investigation of a bleeding disorder

Some will accept the use of Hemopure, a polymerized bovine haemoglobin.

Transfusions carry the risk of blood-borne viral infections (Chs. 9 and 21) and circulatory overload.

The platelet count provides a quantitative evaluation of platelet function. A normal platelet count should be 100 000–400 000 cells/mm³ (Fig. 8.4). A platelet count of < 100 000 cells/mm³ (thrombocytopenia) can be associated with major post-operative bleeding. The average lifespan of a platelet ranges from 7 to 12 days. The bleeding time is occasionally used to assess adequacy of platelet function. The test measures how long it takes a standardized skin incision to stop bleeding by the formation of a temporary haemostatic plug. The normal range of bleeding time depends on the way the test is performed, but is usually between 1 and 6 min. The bleeding time is prolonged in patients with platelet abnormalities or taking medications that affect platelet function.

The activated partial thromboplastin time (APTT) measures the effectiveness of the intrinsic pathway to mediate fibrin clot formation. It tests for all factors except for factor VII. The test is performed by measuring the time it takes to form a clot after the addition of kaolin, a surface activating factor, and cephalin, a substitute for platelet factor, to the patient's plasma. A normal APTT is usually 25–35 s. APTT is most often used by physicians to monitor heparin therapy.

The prothrombin time (PT) measures the effectiveness of the extrinsic pathway to mediate fibrin clot formation (Fig. 8.5). It is performed by measuring the time it takes to form a clot when calcium and tissue factor are added to plasma. A normal prothrombin time indicates normal levels of factor VII and those factors common to both the intrinsic and extrinsic

pathways (V, X, prothrombin, and fibrinogen). A normal prothrombin time is usually between 10 and 15 s. Prothrombin time is most often used by physicians to monitor oral anticoagulant therapy such as warfarin. The international normalized ratio (INR) is based on PT and was designed for patients on chronic anticoagulant therapy. It allows comparisons from one hospital to another. A patient with normal coagulation parameters has an INR of 1.0. The international normalized ratio is the prothrombin time (PT) ratio (patient's PT/control PT) that would have been obtained if an international reference thromboplastin reagent had been used and is recommended by the World Health Organization (WHO) for reporting PT values. In a person with a PT within the normal range, the INR is approximately 1. An INR above 1 indicates that clotting will take longer than normal. An INR of 2–3 is the usual therapeutic range for deep vein thrombosis, and an INR of up to 3.5 is required for patients with prosthetic heart valves.

BLEEDING DISORDERS

GENERAL ASPECTS

Bleeding disorders share common bleeding symptoms, including epistaxis and bleeding after surgery or wounds. The latter are often the first indication of a haemostatic defect. Defects in haemostasis, leading to bleeding disorders, can comprise defects in platelet activation and function, contact activation, the clotting proteins or excess antithrombin function. The more common causes include: aspirin, one tablet of which impairs platelet function for almost 1 week (however, this

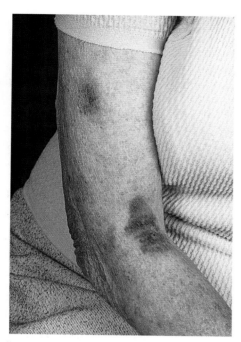

Fig. 8.5 Purpura in a patient with myeloid leukaemia

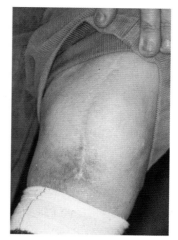

Fig. 8.6 Haemarthrosis in an older haemophiliac has caused crippling arthritis. His five brothers all succumbed to haemophilia at a time when factor VIII was unknown

rarely causes significant post-operative haemorrhage); warfarin, the most common anticoagulant, which interferes with clotting factor production, via vitamin K blockage; and von Willebrand disease, the most common inherited bleeding disorder.

CLINICAL FEATURES

Examination may reveal signs of purpura in the skin as in platelet disorders (Fig. 8.5). These include leukaemia and human immunodeficiency virus (HIV) disease. Signs of underlying disease such as anaemia and lymphadenopathy in leukaemia, for example, must also be looked for. Alternatively, purpura may be localized to the mouth (sometimes grandiloquently termed 'angina bullosa haemorrhagica') and not associated with any abnormal bleeding tendencies. Joint deformities from haemarthroses, characteristic of haemophilia, should also be looked for but are infrequently seen now (Fig. 8.6).

GENERAL MANAGEMENT

Table 8.2 shows comparative features of coagulation defects and platelet defects. An adequate history is the single most important part of the evaluation; physical examination is also necessary and laboratory tests are needed to confirm the diagnosis. An accurate diagnosis is essential in order to provide replacement therapy where appropriate, and to enable other management procedures to be organized. Patients may already be aware of having haemorrhagic disease and carry an appropriate medical card.

A history with any suggestion of a haemorrhagic tendency must be taken seriously. Nevertheless, patients can be remarkably capricious as to the information they provide and, in any case, can hardly be expected to know when bleeding can legitimately be regarded as 'abnormal'. Previous dental extractions provide a useful guide, but prolonged bleeding (up to 24–48 h) as an isolated episode is usually the result of local

Table 8.2	**Features of bleeding disorders**		
Platelet defects		**The purpuras**[a]	**Coagulation defects**
Gender affected		Females mainly	Males
Family history		Rarely	Usually positive
Nature of bleeding after trauma		Immediate	Delayed
Effect when locally applied pressure removed		May stop bleeding	Bleeding recurs
Spontaneous bleeding into skin or mucosa, or from mucosa or gingivae		Common	Uncommon
Bleeding from minor superficial injuries (e.g. needle prick)		Common	Uncommon
Deep haemorrhages or haemarthroses		Rare	Common
Bleeding time		Prolonged	Normal
Tourniquet (Hess) test		Positive	Negative
Platelet count		Often low	Normal
Clotting function		Normal	Abnormal

[a]Purpura is rarely vascular.

factors, especially excessive trauma. By contrast, even patients who know that they have a serious haemorrhagic tendency can keep the fact to themselves unless specifically asked.

It should be stressed again that a history of previous haemorrhagic episodes is the most important feature since screening tests of haemostasis do not always detect mild defects.

Special emphasis must be placed on the following, suggestive of a bleeding disorder:

- deep haemorrhage into muscles, joints or skin – suggests a clotting defect
- bleeding from and into mucosae – suggests purpura (Fig. 8.7).

Females often state that they 'bruise easily', but any such bruises are usually insignificant and small. Excessive menstrual bleeding is also rarely due to a bleeding disorder. Most significant congenital bleeding disorders become apparent in childhood and patients may carry a warning card (Fig. 8.8). However, mild haemophiliacs can escape recognition until adult life if they manage to avoid injury or surgery. A mild haemophiliac can then have oozing from an extraction socket for 2–3 weeks despite local measures such as suturing.

Patients who have had tonsillectomy or dental extractions without trouble are most unlikely to have a severe congenital bleeding disorder. If previous dental bleeding was controlled by local measures, the patient is unlikely to have a serious haemorrhagic disease. On the other hand, admission to hospital, and blood transfusion or comparable measures have obvious implications. Haemorrhagic disease in a blood relative is strongly suggestive of a clotting defect.

Many drugs such as anticoagulants may cause bleeding tendencies, as may hepatic, renal, HIV and other disease. Some herbal products may impair platelet aggregation and prolonging bleeding (Ch. 26).

Laboratory tests must follow consultation with the haematologist to ensure that they are appropriate. All that is needed on the request form is to state: 'History of prolonged bleeding. Would you please investigate haemostatic function?' and to give as much clinical detail as possible. A routine 'blood count' will not identify a clotting defect but may show platelet deficiency. The sample should be adequately labelled and sent immediately for testing together with relevant clinical information.

Essential tests usually include:

- full blood count, film, platelet count
- prothrombin time (PT) and international normalized ratio (INR)
- activated partial thromboplastin time (APTT)
- thrombin time (TT) (citrated sample)
- serum for blood grouping and cross-matching.

To exclude platelet defects, a platelet count and full blood examination are essential, and assays of platelet function may be indicated. Aspirin should be avoided for at least 7 days before assessing platelet function. In the Hess test (tourniquet test), more than a few petechiae appearing on the forearm when a sphygmomanometer cuff is inflated suggests a platelet or vascular defect, but the test is not particularly sensitive and is not specific. A bleeding time is not completely reliable. *In vitro* tests of platelet adhesion and aggregation may be required to demonstrate abnormal function. Platelet aggregation can also be measured using aggregating agents such as ristocetin. Unfortunately such tests are difficult to standardize and do not identify all platelet disorders; the clinical features are more important.

Precise characterization of a congenital clotting defect depends on assay of the individual factors and a wide range of other investigations may be indicated according to the type

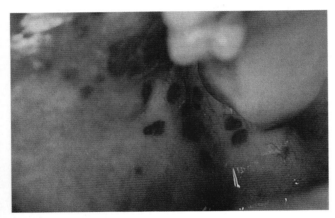

Fig. 8.7 Oral purpura

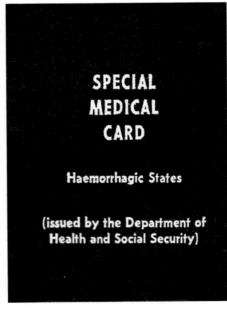

SPECIAL
MEDICAL
CARD

Haemorrhagic States

(issued by the Department of
Health and Social Security)

IN CASE OF INJURY, BLEEDING, OR SERIOUS ILLNESS, THIS PERSON MAY HAVE URGENT NEED OF CARE AT A SPECIAL CENTRE.

IN EMERGENCY, TELEPHONE THE CENTRE NAMED OPPOSITE.

NEITHER INTRA-MUSCULAR INJECTIONS NOR ASPIRIN PREPARATIONS SHOULD BE GIVEN.

A   B

Fig. 8.8 (A) Special medical card that should be carried at all times by patients with haemorrhagic states; (B) special medical card showing warnings inside the cover

of case. For example, the assays usually used in diagnosis of haemophilia A are the APTT and the factor VIII coagulant (FVIIIC) activity. The whole blood clotting time is uninformative and obsolete.

It is important also to investigate patients with a suspected bleeding tendency for anaemia. This is because:

- anaemia is an expected consequence of repeated haemorrhages
- any further bleeding as a result of surgery will worsen the anaemia, or the anaemia may need to be treated before surgery can be carried out
- anaemia may be an essential concomitant of the haemorrhagic tendency – as in leukaemia.

Patients may also need to be screened for liver disease and for bloodborne infections, particularly HIV and hepatitis viruses.

Patients with bleeding disorders may need to be treated with replacement of the missing factor. Earlier, use of blood or blood fractions sometimes resulted in the transmission of blood-borne viruses and other infections. Recombinant factors are therefore preferred. In many countries, blood is now collected from donors under careful precautions, and screened to exclude antibodies to infections such as HIV, hepatitis B, hepatitis C, syphilis or cytomegalovirus.

In the developed countries, all cellular blood products are leukodepleted to limit any possible risk of transmission of prions and some other infections. Leukocytes in erythrocyte and platelet concentrates are now considered as a contaminant since they can cause many other adverse effects, such as the transmission of other cell-associated infectious agents (e.g. herpesviruses, prions and *Toxoplasma*), febrile non-haemolytic reactions, graft-versus-host disease and immunosuppression.

VASCULAR PURPURA

Vascular purpura rarely causes serious bleeding; any bleeding into mucous membranes or skin starts immediately after trauma but stops within 24–48 h.

HEREDITARY HAEMORRHAGIC TELANGIECTASIA (OSLER–RENDU–WEBER SYNDROME)

Hereditary haemorrhagic telangiectasia (HHT) is an autosomal dominant condition characterized by telangiectasia on the skin and mucosae. There may be associated with IgA deficiency or, rarely, von Willebrand disease (see later).

Clinical features

Telangiectasia on the skin or any part of the oral, nasal, gastrointestinal or urogenital mucosa (Fig. 8.9) leads to bleeding and, consequently, often to iron-deficiency anaemia or, rarely, even to cardiac failure.

General management

This is by cryosurgery or argon laser treatment if the telangiectases have bled significantly or are cosmetically unacceptable.

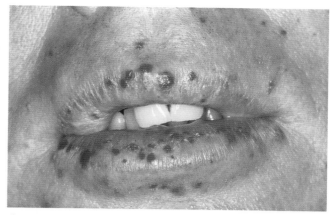

Fig. 8.9 Hereditary haemorrhagic telangiectasia

Dental aspects

Telangiectases may be seen in any part of the mouth and may be conspicuous on the lips. Bleeding from oral surgery is unlikely to be troublesome.

Rarely, brain abscesses or other infections have followed oral procedures that cause bacteraemias but there is no consensus as to the need for antibacterial prophylaxis.

Regional LA should be avoided because of the risk of deep bleeding. Conscious sedation can be given if required. In general anaesthesia (GA), nasal intubation is best avoided and close post-operative observation is advisable.

LOCALIZED ORAL PURPURA ('ANGINA BULLOSA HAEMORRHAGICA')

Blood blisters are occasionally seen, typically in older persons, in the absence of obvious trauma, generalized purpura, any other bleeding tendency or evidence of any systemic disease. These blood blisters are often in the palate and may sometimes be a centimetre or more in diameter and after rupture may leave a sore area for a few days. When a large blood blister of this type is in the pharynx, it can cause an alarming choking sensation and was therefore originally termed 'angina bullosa haemorrhagica'. However, almost any site in the mouth can be affected.

A systemic cause of the blood blisters must be excluded before the diagnosis of localized oral purpura can be made confidently and the patient reassured. Other causes of blood blisters in the mouth include: systemic causes of purpura such as platelet disorders, amyloidosis (causing factor X deficiency), leukaemia, infectious mononucleosis, HIV or rubella; trauma; corticosteroid inhalers; or bleeding into subepithelial blisters such as in mucous membrane pemphigoid (Ch. 11).

PLATELET DISORDERS

Platelets may be lacking because of failed platelet production in rare congenital disorders [thrombocytopenia and absent radii (TAR), Wiskott–Aldrich syndrome, Bernard–Soulier syndrome, trisomy 13 or 18, thrombocytopenia with Robin syndrome, giant haemangiomas (Kasabach–Merritt syndrome), type IIb von Willebrand disease]; because of megakaryocyte depression (drugs, viruses, chemicals); because of general bone marrow failure (e.g. alcoholism, cytotoxic drugs, irradiation, chemicals, drugs, viruses, aplastic anaemia, leukaemia, metastases, megaloblastic anaemia); or because of excessive platelet destruction (Fig. 8.10). This can be autoimmune [idiopathic thrombocytopenic purpura (ITP) or HIV] or due to drugs (e.g. aspirin, cytotoxics, beta-lactam antibiotics and valproate) or diseases (disseminated intravascular coagulation, thrombotic thrombocytopenic purpura, systemic lupus erythematosus, chronic lymphocytic leukaemia and malaria). *Abnormal platelet function* is seen in Glanzmann disease and dysproteinaemias. *Abnormal platelet distribution* is seen in splenomegaly or transfusion of stored blood (Table 8.3).

Platelet numbers or function, if impaired, can cause a bleeding tendency and purpura and changes in results of laboratory investigations (Table 8.4).

Idiopathic thrombocytopenic purpura

Idiopathic thrombocytopenic purpura (ITP), one of the more common causes of thrombocytopenia, is autoimmune and can lead to purpura and prolonged bleeding.

Clinical features

Clinical features include petechiae, ecchymoses and postoperative haemorrhage.

General management

Full blood picture and platelet counts are indicated. Corticosteroids or other immunosuppressives are the main treatments. Splenectomy is sometimes needed.

Dental aspects of platelet disorders

The main danger is haemorrhage but it is rarely as severe as in the clotting disorders. Regional LA block injections can be given if the platelet levels are above $30 \times 10^9/L$. Haemostasis after dentoalveolar surgery is usually adequate if platelet levels are above $50 \times 10^9/L$. Major surgery requires platelet levels above $75 \times 10^9/L$. Conscious sedation can be given but, if by the intravenous route, care must be taken not to damage the vein. GA can be given in hospital but expert intubation is needed to avoid the risk of submucous bleeding into the airway.

Platelets can be replaced or supplemented by platelet transfusions, but sequestration of platelets is very rapid. One

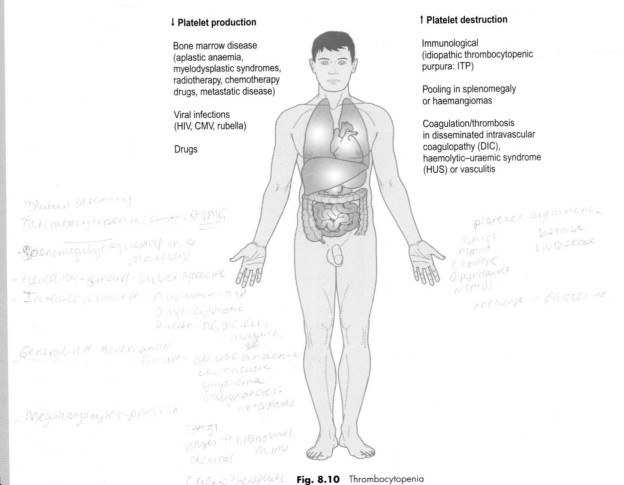

↓ Platelet production

Bone marrow disease
(aplastic anaemia,
myelodysplastic syndromes,
radiotherapy, chemotherapy
drugs, metastatic disease)

Viral infections
(HIV, CMV, rubella)

Drugs

↑ Platelet destruction

Immunological
(idiopathic thrombocytopenic
purpura: ITP)

Pooling in splenomegaly
or haemangiomas

Coagulation/thrombosis
in disseminated intravascular
coagulopathy (DIC),
haemolytic–uraemic syndrome
(HUS) or vasculitis

Fig. 8.10 Thrombocytopenia

Table 8.3 Platelet defects

	Defect	Manifestations	Management
Thrombasthenia (Glanzmann syndrome)	Defective platelet aggregation due to defective membrane protein	Severe bleeding tendency	Platelet infusions needed pre-operatively
Bernard–Soulier syndrome	Giant platelets with defect in platelet glycoprotein which acts as receptor for von Willebrand factor	Heritable disorder resembling von Willebrand disease but considerably more rare	Platelet infusions needed pre-operatively
Storage pool deficiency	Platelets lack capacity to store serotonin and adenine nucleotides and consequently fail to aggregate	Usually congenital with autosomal inheritance. If associated with albinism, is termed Hermansky–Pudliak syndrome	Platelet infusion or cryoprecipitate corrects the bleeding tendency
HIV infection	Purpura is a relatively common feature of HIV infection. May be autoimmune but there appears also to be a platelet defect resulting from the infection; drugs such as zidovudine or some protease inhibitors and bone marrow disease may also contribute	Oral purpura in HIV infection may closely mimic oral lesions of Kaposi sarcoma (Ch. 20)	See Ch. 20
Chronic renal failure	See Ch. 12		
Drugs heparin, dextrans	See Ch. 8		
Dysproteinaemias	See Ch. 8		
Myelodysplastic syndrome	See Ch. 8		

HIV, human immunodeficiency virus.

Table 8.4 Typical findings in platelet disorders

Disorder	Bleeding time	Platelet count	Clot retraction	Platelet aggregation	Platelet FIII activity
Thrombocytopenia	↑	↓	↓	–	–
Thrombasthenia	↑	N	↓	↓	↓
Storage pool deficiency	↑	N	N	N or ↓	↓
Aspirin/von Willebrand disease	↑	N	N	↓ (only with ristocetin)	N
Thrombocythaemia	↑	↑	N or ↓	N or ↓	N or ↓

Arrows indicate a value above ↑ or below ↓ normal (N).
FIII, factor III.

unit of platelets should raise the count by around 10×10^9 platelets/L. Platelet transfusions are therefore best used for controlling already established thrombocytopenic bleeding. When given prophylactically, platelets should be given – half just before surgery to control capillary bleeding and half at the end of the operation to facilitate placement of adequate sutures. Platelets should be used within 6–24 h after collection and suitable preparations include platelet-rich plasma (PRP), which contains about 90% of the platelets from a unit of fresh blood in about half this volume, and platelet-rich concentrate (PRC), which contains about 50% of the platelets from a unit of fresh whole blood in a volume of only 25 ml. PRC is thus the best source of platelets. Platelet infusions carry the risk of isoimmunization, infection with blood-borne agents and, rarely, graft-versus-host disease. Where there is immune destruction of platelets (e.g. in ITP), platelet infusions are less effective.

The need for platelet transfusions can be reduced by local haemostatic measures and use of desmopressin or tranexamic acid or topical administration of platelet concentrates. Absorbable haemostatic agents such as oxidized regenerated cellulose (Surgicel), synthetic collagen (Instat) or microcrystalline collagen (Avitene) may be put in the socket to assist clotting.

Splenectomy predisposes to infections, typically with pneumococci, and especially within the first 2 years. Systemic infection post-splenectomy, involving oral streptococci, is rare and antimicrobial prophylaxis is not therefore generally recommended before invasive dental procedures.

Long-term corticosteroids can cause well-recognized problems (Ch. 6). Drugs such as aspirin and other non-steroidal anti-inflammatory drugs (NSAIDs) which damage platelets should be avoided (Table 8.5). Aspirin's effects are *not* dose dependent: even a single tablet can affect platelet cyclo-oxygenase (COX) irreversibly for about a week. Other NSAIDs

Table 8.5 Some drugs that may impair platelets or their function

Class	Examples
Alcohol	
Antibiotics	Amoxicillin Ampicillin and derivatives Azithromycin Carbenicillin Cephalosporins Gentamicin Methicillin Penicillin G (benzyl penicillin) Rifampicin Sulfonamides Trimethoprim
Analgesics and other platelet inhibitors	Aspirin and other NSAIDs Clopidogrel
Cytotoxic drugs	Many
General anaesthetic agents	Halothane
Psychoactive drugs	Antihistamines (some) Chlorpromazine Diazepam Haloperidol Tricyclic antidepressants Valproate
Diuretics	Acetazolamide Chlorothiazide Furosemide
Antidiabetics	Tolbutamide
Cardiovascular drugs	Digitoxin Quinine Oxprenolol Heparin Methyldopa

NSAIDs, non-steroidal anti-inflammatory drugs.

may have a reversible effect and act for only up to 48 h. COX-2 inhibitors have no such effect on platelets.

Perioperative management is summarized in Table 8.6. Submucous purpura may be conspicuous and sometimes seen as 'blackcurrant jelly' blood blisters.

Thrombocytosis

A raised platelet count (thrombocytosis) may be found in many conditions, and predisposes to arterial thrombosis.

COAGULATION DEFECTS

Coagulation defects are due mainly to genetic defects of clotting factors (von Willebrand disease and haemophilia), to anticoagulant therapy or to a range of diseases, especially liver or kidney diseases (Box 8.1).

Clotting disorders cause a range of changes in results of laboratory investigations (Table 8.7).

Congenital coagulation defects

The most important hereditary bleeding disorder in terms of prevalence and severity is von Willebrand disease, but haemophilia A and B are the other most common coagulopathies. Haemophilia A and B (Christmas disease) are hereditary X-linked recessive disorders characterized by deficiencies in blood clotting factors VIII and IX, respectively. Factor XI deficiency is also important. Less common disorders are summarized in Table 8.8 and Appendix 8.1.

Haemophilia A

Haemophilia

Haemophilia A affects approximately 1 in 5000 males. Carriers of haemophilia rarely manifest a bleeding tendency clinically.

Table 8.6 Thrombocytopenia manifestations and management of surgery

Platelet count (x 10⁹/L)	Severity of thrombocytopenia	Manifestations	MANAGEMENT IN RELATION TO TYPE OF ORAL SURGERY	
			Dentoalveolar	Maxillofacial
100–150	Mild	Mild purpura sometimes. Slightly prolonged post-operative bleeding	No platelet transfusion. Local haemostatic measures.ᵃ Observe	Consider platelet transfusion. Local haemostatic measures.ᵃ Observe
50–100	Moderate	Purpura, post-operative bleeding	Platelets may be needed. Local haemostatic measures.ᵃ Consider post-operative tranexamic acid mouthwash for 3 days	Platelets needed. Local haemostatic measures.ᵃ Post-operative tranexamic acid mouthwash for 3 days
30–50	Severe	Purpura, post-operative bleeding, even from venepuncture	Platelets needed. Local haemostatic measures.ᵃ Post-operative tranexamic acid mouthwash for 3 days	Platelets needed. Local haemostatic measures.ᵃ Avoid surgery where possible. Post-operative tranexamic acid mouthwash for 3 days
< 30	Life-threatening	Purpura, spontaneous bleeding	Platelets needed. Local haemostatic measures.ᵃ Avoid surgery where possible. Post-operative tranexamic acid mouthwash for 3 days	Platelets needed. Local haemostatic measures.ᵃ Avoid surgery where possible. Post-operative tranexamic acid mouthwash for 3 days

ᵃLocal haemostatic measures = compressive packing, sutures, and microfibrillar collagen or oxidized cellulose.

Box 8.1 Main coagulation defects

- Anticoagulants and thrombolytic agents
- Chronic renal failure
- Deficiencies of factors XII and XIII and others
- Disseminated intravascular coagulation
- Dysproteinaemias, especially multiple myeloma
- Haemophilia
- Liver disease, including obstructive jaundice
- Lupus erythematosus
- Von Willebrand disease

Table 8.8 Coagulation factor defects: in descending order of frequency

Factor deficient	Inheritance	Incidence. 1 in
VIII	X-linked	10 000
IX	X-linked	60 000
VII	Autosomal recessive	500 000
V	Autosomal recessive	1 million
X	Autosomal recessive	1 million
XI	Autosomal recessive	1 million
XIII	Autosomal recessive	1 million
Fibrinogen	Autosomal recessive	1 million
Prothrombin	Autosomal recessive	2 million

Table 8.7 Laboratory findings in clotting disorders

Disorder	PT	APTT	TT	FL	FDP
Haemophilia A; haemophilia B; von Willebrand disease; deficiency of factors XI and XII	N	↑	N	N	N
Warfarin or other coumarin therapy; obstructive jaundice, or other causes of vitamin K deficiency; deficiency of factor V or X	↑	↑	N	N	N
Heparin therapy; disseminated intravascular coagulation	↑	↑	N	N	N
Parenchymal liver disease	↑	↑	↑	↓	↑
Deficiency of factor VII	↑	N	N	N	N

APTT, activated partial thromboplastin time (or KPTT); FDP, fibrin degradation products; FL, fibrinogen level; PT, prothrombin time; TT, thrombin time. Arrows indicate a value above ↑ or below ↓ normal (N).

General aspects

Haemophilia A is an X-linked disorder resulting from a deficiency in blood clotting factor VIII, a key component of the coagulation cascade.

Haemophilia A affects males. Sons of carriers have a 50:50 chance of developing haemophilia while daughters of carriers have a 50:50 chance of being carriers. All daughters of an affected male are carriers but sons are normal. Carriers rarely have a clinically manifest bleeding tendency.

Haemophilia A, with a prevalence of about 5 per 100 000 of the population, is about ten times as common as haemophilia B except in some Asians, where frequencies are almost equal. Haemophilia A arises from a variety of mutations: some 150 different point mutations have been characterized. A family history can be obtained in only about 65% of cases.

Clinical features

Haemophilia is characterized by excessive bleeding, particularly after trauma and sometimes spontaneously. Haemorrhage appears to stop immediately after the injury (due to normal vascular and platelet haemostatic responses) but intractable oozing with rapid blood loss soon follows. Haemorrhage is dangerous either because of acute blood loss or due to bleeding into tissues, particularly the brain, larynx, pharynx, joints and muscles (Fig. 8.11). Bleeding into the cranium, or compression of the larynx and pharynx following haematoma formation in the

neck, can be fatal. Abdominal haemorrhage may simulate an 'acute abdomen'. Haemarthroses can cause joint damage and cripple the patient.

Abnormal bleeding after extractions has sometimes led to recognition of haemophilia. Dental extractions lead to prolonged bleeding and, in the past, have been fatal.

The severity of bleeding in haemophilia A correlates with the level of factor VIII:coagulant (VIII:C) activity and degree of trauma (Table 8.9). Normal plasma contains 1 unit of factor VIII per millilitre, a level defined as 100%.

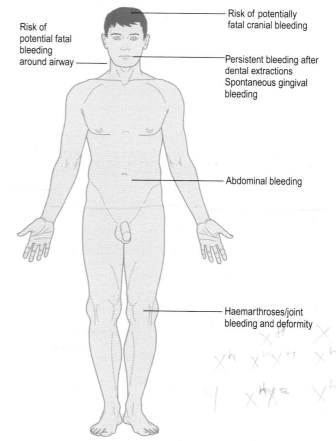

Risk of potentially fatal cranial bleeding

Persistent bleeding after dental extractions Spontaneous gingival bleeding

Risk of potential fatal bleeding around airway

Abdominal bleeding

Haemarthroses/joint bleeding and deformity

Fig. 8.11 Haemophilia

General management

The diagnosis of haemophilias is based upon the clinical presentation, a positive family history, coagulation studies and clotting factor assays. Typical findings are shown in Box 8.2.

Haemophiliacs should be under the care of recognized haemophilia reference centres. Factors VIII or IX must be replaced to adequate levels during episodes of bleeding and ascertained pre-operatively. Synthetic vasopressin (DDAVP) acts to increase factor VIII levels and may be used in very mild haemophilia. 'Gene therapy' and 'gene-delivery systems' raise the possibility of a potential cure for haemophilia in the future.

Rarely, von Willebrand disease may mimic haemophilia, and though the history may help to distinguish them, laboratory testing is essential (see later).

Factor VIII must be replaced to a level adequate to ensure haemostasis if bleeding starts or is expected. In mild haemophilia, desmopressin and antifibrinolytics such as tranexamic acid may be adequate (see later).

Replacement of the missing clotting factor is achieved with porcine factor VIII or recombinant factor VIII. Plasma (fresh or frozen), cryoprecipitate or fractionated human factor concentrates obtained from pooled blood sources have had, and may still occasionally have, the potential to carry blood-borne pathogens. Regular prophylactic replacement of factor VIII is used when possible but necessitates daily injections as the half-life is around 12 h, and its use may be complicated by antibody formation. Desmopressin (deamino-8-D-arginine vasopressin; DDAVP) is a synthetic analogue of vasopressin that induces the release of factor VIIIC, von Willebrand factor and tissue plasminogen activator from storage sites in endothelium. Desmopressin cover just before surgery, and repeated 12-hourly if necessary for up to 4 days, is useful to cover minor surgery in some very mild haemophiliacs, but factor VIII cover may be needed if there is any doubt about haemostasis. Desmopressin can be given as an intranasal spray of 1.5 mg desmopressin per ml with each 0.1 ml pump spray, or as a slow intravenous infusion over 20 min of 0.3–0.5 µg/kg.

Tranexamic acid (Cyklokapron) is a synthetic derivative of the amino acid lysine. It exerts an antifibrinolytic effect through the reversible blockade of lysine binding sites on plasminogen molecules. Tranexamic acid significantly reduces blood loss after surgery in patients with haemophilia and can be used topically or systemically. Systemically, it is given in a dose of 1 g (30 mg/kg) orally, four times daily starting at least 1 h pre-operatively for surgical procedures, or as infusion 10 mg/kg in 20 ml normal saline over 20 min, then 1 g orally three times daily for 5 days (child's dose is 20 mg/kg). However, nausea is a common adverse effect and antifibrinolytics must not be used systemically where residual clots are present (e.g. in the urinary tract or intracranially). Tranexamic acid is not approved for use in the USA by the Food and Drug Administration (FDA), where epsilon-aminocaproic acid is an alternative.

Dental aspects

Many of the coagulation defects present a hazard to surgery and to LA injections, but in general the teeth erupt and exfoliate without problems, and non-invasive dental care is safe.

Table 8.9 Severity of haemophilia

	% factor VIII	Clinical features
Severe	< 1	Spontaneous bleeding, typically from childhood with bleeding into muscles or joints (haemarthroses), easy bruising and prolonged bleeding from minor injuries
Moderate	1–5	Comparatively minor trauma may still lead to significant blood loss
Mild	> 5–25	Comparatively minor trauma may still lead to significant blood loss. Bleeding after dental extractions is sometimes the first or only sign of mild disease
Very mild	> 25	Patient can generally lead a normal life and may remain undiagnosed but there can be prolonged bleeding after trauma or surgery. Some may not bleed excessively even after a simple dental extraction, so that the absence of post-extraction haemorrhage cannot reliably be used to exclude haemophilia. Most will, however, bleed excessively after more traumatic surgery, such as tonsillectomy

Box 8.2 Laboratory findings in haemophilias

- Normal prothrombin time (and INR)
- Normal bleeding time
- Prolonged activated partial thromboplastin time
- Reduced factor VIII:C level (haemophilia A)
- Reduced factor IX level (haemophilia B)
- Normal levels of von Willebrand factor

Close cooperation is needed between the physician and dentist to plan safe, comprehensive dental care.

Haemophiliacs form a priority group to minimize the need for dental operative intervention, which can cause severe, or occasionally fatal, complications. Education of patients or parents, and preventive dentistry, should be started as early as possible in the young child, when the teeth begin to erupt. Caries must be minimized or avoided. The use of fluorides, fissure sealants, dietary advice on the need for sugar restriction and regular dental inspections from an early age are crucial to the preservation of teeth. Prevention of periodontal disease is also imperative. Comprehensive dental assessment is needed at the age of about 12–13, to plan to decide how best to forestall difficulties resulting from overcrowding, or misplaced third molars or other teeth.

Local anaesthesia injections or surgery can be followed by persistent bleeding for days or weeks, the haemorrhage cannot be controlled by pressure alone and the problem may be life-threatening. Management of haemophiliacs should take consideration of the factors listed in Box 8.3.

The bleeding tendency can be aggravated by NSAIDs. It may also be aggravated by other factors such as liver damage after hepatitis, in HIV disease, by thrombocytopenia and the effects of drugs such as protease inhibitors. Paracetamol, codeine and COX-2 inhibitors are safer.

Table 8.10 Topical haemostatic agents

Agent	Main constituent	Source
Avitene	Collagen	Bovine
Beriplast	Fibrin	Various
Colla-Cote	Collagen	Bovine
Cyclokapron	Tranexamic acid	Synthetic
Gelfoam	Gelatin	Bovine
Helistat	Collagen	Bovine
Instat	Collagen	Bovine
Surgicel	Cellulose	Synthetic
Thrombinar	Thrombin	Bovine
Thrombogen	Thrombin	Bovine
Thrombostat	Thrombin	Bovine

Local anaesthesia regional blocks, lingual infiltrations or injections into the floor of the mouth must not be used in the absence of factor VIII replacement because of the risk of haemorrhage hazarding the airway and being life-threatening. Rarely, even submucosal LA infiltrations have caused widespread haematoma formation. If factor VIII replacement therapy has been given, regional LA can be used, providing the factor VIII level is maintained above 30%, but infiltration LA is still preferable. Lingual infiltration should be avoided. Intraligamentary LA injections are safer.

Intramuscular injections of drugs should be avoided unless replacement therapy is being given, as they can cause large haematomas. Oral alternatives are, in any case, usually satisfactory.

In all but severe haemophiliacs, non-surgical dental treatment (taking into consideration the question of LA discussed above) can usually be carried out under antifibrinolytic cover (usually tranexamic acid).

Conservative dentistry treatment of the primary dentition may be carried out without LA. If conservative treatment in the permanent dentition is not feasible without LA, papillary or intraligamentary infiltration is unlikely to cause serious bleeding. Alternative techniques such as electronic dental anaesthesia may be also effective. Soft tissue trauma must be avoided and a matrix band may help prevent gingival laceration. However, care must be taken not to let the matrix band cut the periodontal tissues and start gingival bleeding. A rubber dam is also useful to protect the mucosa from trauma but the clamp must be carefully applied. Cotton rolls may cause mucosal bleeding unless they are wetted before removal. High-speed vacuum aspirators and saliva ejectors can cause haematomas. Trauma from the saliva ejector can be minimized by resting it on a gauze swab in the floor of the mouth.

Endodontic treatment may obviate the need for extractions and can usually be carried out without special precautions other than care to avoid instrumenting through the tooth apex. The use of an electronic endometric instrument will reduce the number of intraoperative radiographs. Topical application of 10% cocaine to the exposed pulp is recommended for vital pulp extirpation. Intracanal injection of LA solution containing epinephrine or topical application (with paper points) of epinephrine 1:1000 may be useful to minimize bleeding. However, in severe haemophilia, bleeding from the pulp and periapical tissues can be persistent and troublesome.

Periodontal surgery necessitates LA and factor VIII replacement to a level of 50–75%. In all but severe haemophiliacs, scaling can be carried out under antifibrinolytic cover. Minor procedures may be carried out with topical anaesthesia.

Orthodontics: there is no contraindication to the movement of teeth in haemophilia. However, there must be no sharp edges to appliances, wires, etc., which might traumatize the mucosa.

Extractions and dentoalveolar surgery should be carefully planned. Ideally all necessary surgery (and other dental treatment) should be performed at one operation. A factor VIII level of 50–75% is required. Panoramic radiographs should be taken for any unsuspected lesion and to assess whether further extractions might prevent future trouble. LA should be given as discussed above. Local measures are important to minimize the risk of post-operative bleeding. Surgery should be carried out with minimal trauma to both bone and soft tissues, and careful mouth toilet post-operatively is essential. Suturing is desirable to stabilize gum flaps and to prevent post-operative disturbance of wounds by eating. A non-traumatic needle must be used, and the number of sutures minimized. Vicryl sutures are preferred and catgut is best avoided. Non-resorbable sutures such as black silk should be removed at 4–7 days. Suturing carries with it the risk, if there is post-operative bleeding, of causing blood to track down towards the mediastinum with danger to the airway due to inadequate pre-operative replacement therapy or factor VIII inhibitors being present.

In the case of difficult extractions, when mucoperiosteal flaps must be raised, the lingual tissues in the lower molar regions should preferably be left undisturbed since trauma may open up planes into which haemorrhage can track and endanger the airway. The buccal approach to lower third molars is safer. Minimal bone should be removed and teeth should be sectioned for removal where possible. Acrylic protective splints are now rarely used, in view of their liability to cause mucosal trauma and to promote sepsis, but they are sometimes useful in sites such as the palate. The packing of extraction sockets is unnecessary if replacement therapy has been adequate but a little oxidized cellulose soaked in tranexamic acid placed into the base of the sockets, or collagen, or cyanoacrylate or fibrin glues (Table 8.10) may be used. Fibrin sealant, which consists mainly of fibrinogen and thrombin, provides rapid haemostasis as well as tissue sealing and adhesion. Liquid fibrin sealant has been used but fibrin glue is unavailable in USA, because of the risk of viral infections: recombinant fibrin glues are becoming available. Local use of fibrin glue and swish and swallow rinses of tranexamic acid before and after the dental extractions is a cost-effective regimen.

Post-operatively, a diet of cold liquid and minced solids should be taken for up to 5–10 days. Care should be taken to watch for haematoma formation which may manifest itself by swelling, dysphagia or hoarseness. The patency of the airway must always be ensured. Infection also appears to induce fibrinolysis, so antimicrobials such as oral penicillin V 250 mg or amoxicillin 500 mg four times daily should be given post-operatively for a full course of 7 days to reduce the risk of secondary haemorrhage. Antibiotic prophylaxis may be indicated for patients with prosthetic joints (Ch. 16). In HIV-infected patients, mild cytopenias are common but severe anaemia, neutropenia and thrombocytopenia that predispose to oral manifestations and surgical complications are rare and post-operative bleeding is uncommon in HIV-infected haemophiliacs.

After trauma to the head and neck in haemophiliacs, factor VIII replacement is essential because of the risk from bleeding into the cranial cavity or into the fascial spaces of the neck. Haemophiliacs should, therefore, be given factor VIII to achieve a level of 100% prophylactically after head or facial trauma. If there are lacerations that need suturing, a minimum level of factor VIII of 50% is required at the time, with further cover for 3 days (see Table 8.11).

Haemophiliacs with inhibitors

The haematologist must always be consulted. Factor VIII inhibitor levels should be checked pre-operatively and, in general, patients with low-titre inhibitors can have dental treatment in the same way as those who have no antibodies.

Those with high-titre inhibitors need special care. In the latter group, traumatic procedures must be avoided unless absolutely essential. Human factor VIII inhibitor bypassing fractions (FEIBA) can often be effective; these are usually either non-activated prothrombin complex concentrates (PCC) or activated prothrombin complex concentrates (APCC), which act by activating factor X, directly bypassing the intrinsic pathway of blood clotting. The danger with these products is of uncontrolled coagulation with thromboses. The real choice lies between either prothrombin-complex concentrates (e.g. FEIBA), or recombinant factor VIIa. In some cases, desmopressin is an effective alternative, and antifibrinolytics may help.

Conscious sedation can be given but, if intravenous, great care must be taken to avoid damaging the vein. If GA is needed, nasal intubation should be avoided.

Haemophilia B

General and clinical aspects

Haemophilia B (Christmas disease; factor IX deficiency) is clinically identical to haemophilia A and inherited in the same way, but is about one-tenth as common as haemophilia A except in some Asians, where frequencies are almost equal. Female carriers of haemophilia B (unlike haemophilia A) often have a mild bleeding tendency.

General management

Replacement therapy is with synthetic factor IX, which is more stable than factor VIII with a half-life of 18 h but often up to 2 days, so that replacement therapy can sometimes be given at longer intervals than in haemophilia A. A dose of 20 units of factor IX per kilogram body weight is given intravenously 1 h pre-operatively.

Dental aspects

Comments on dental management in haemophilia A apply to patients with haemophilia B, apart from using factor IX, and not using desmopressin.

Von Willebrand disease

General aspects

Von Willebrand disease (vWD; pseudohaemophilia) is the most common inherited bleeding disorder and is due to a deficiency of von Willebrand factor (vWF). This is synthesized in endothelium and megakaryocytes, mediates platelet adhesion to damaged endothelium and protects factor VIII from proteolytic degradation. Von Willebrand factor has binding sites for collagen and for platelet glycoprotein (GP) receptors, and thus normally acts in three ways. vWF normally binds to GP Ib and

---

Table 8.11 Outline of management of haemophiliacs requiring surgery

Operation	Factor VIII level required	Pre-operatively give	Post-operative schedule
Dental extraction, dentoalveolar or periodontal surgery	Minimum of 50% at operation	Factor VIII i.v.[a] Tranexamic acid 1 g i.v. (or by mouth starting 24 h pre-operatively)	Local haemostatic measures[c]
Maxillofacial surgery	75–100% at operation; at least 50% for 7 days post-operatively	Factor VIII i.v.[b]	Local haemostatic measures[c] Rest as inpatient for 7 days unless resident close to centre (then 3 days) Soft diet. For 10 days give tranexamic acid 1 g qid and pencillin V 250 mg qid If there is bleeding during this period, give repeat dose of factor VIII[a] Rest inpatient for 10 days Soft diet. Twice daily i.v. factor VIII[a] for 7–10 days

[a]Factor VIII dose in units = weight in kilograms × 25 given 1 h pre-operatively.
[b]Factor VIII dose in units = weight in kilograms × 50 given 1 h pre-operatively.
[c]Local haemostatic measures (see Table 8.10).

Table 8.12 Types of von Willebrand disease (vWD)

Type	% vWD	Defect in von Willebrand factor (vWF)	Factor VIIIC	Features
1	80	Partial lack	May be normal	Autosomal dominant inheritance. Disease is mild and is characterized by bleeding from mucous membranes – nose bleeds, gingival haemorrhage and gastrointestinal blood loss
2A	15	Partial lack but impaired function	Low	
2B	Rare	Partial lack but impaired function	Low	
2M	Rare	Partial lack but impaired function	Low	
2N	Rare	Partial lack but impaired function	Low	
3	5	Complete lack	Low	Bleeding is more severe than in types 1 and 2 but joint and muscle bleeds characteristic of haemophilia are rare

Local haemostatic measures (as Table 8.10 + tranexamic acid mouthwash).

acts as a carrier for factor VIII protecting it from proteolytic degradation. Thus a deficiency leads also to a low factor VIII concentration in the blood. vWF also mediates platelet adhesion to damaged endothelium. vWF mediates platelet aggregation. Thus a deficiency leads to defective platelet adhesion which causes a secondary deficiency in factor VIII. Clinically significant vWD affects approximately 1% of the population and 6% of women with menorrhagia. This is a frequency at least twice that of haemophilia A. Rarely, vWD may be acquired, particularly in patients with autoimmune or lymphoproliferative diseases.

Von Willebrand disease affects females as well as males and usually has an autosomal dominant inheritance, but a severe form of the disease may be inherited as a sex-linked recessive trait like true haemophilia.

Clinical features

The types of von Willebrand disease are shown in Table 8.12.

Von Willebrand disease causes bleeding that has features similar to those caused by platelet dysfunction, but if severe it can resemble haemophilia (Table 8.13). The common pattern is bleeding from, and purpura of, mucous membranes and the skin. Gingival haemorrhage is more common than in haemophilia. Post-operative haemorrhage can be troublesome: excessive haemorrhage may occur after dental treatment and surgery.

Excessive menstrual bleeding is common in females. Haemarthroses are possible but are rare.

The severity also varies from patient to patient and from time to time. Some patients have a clinically insignificant disorder, while others have factor VIII levels low enough to cause severe clotting defects as well as a prolonged bleeding time. However, the severity does not correlate well with the factor VIII level. Pregnancy and the contraceptive pill may cause transient amelioration.

Rarely, hereditary haemorrhagic telangiectasia, IgA deficiency, mitral valve prolapse or factor XII deficiency may be associated.

General management

Von Willebrand disease is characterized by the laboratory findings shown in Box 8.4.

Before surgery, patients with vWD need treatment to reduce the risk of haemorrhage, which may include the administration of factor VIII concentrate and synthetic vasopressin (DDAVP) (Table 8.14).

Table 8.13 Haemophilia A and von Willebrand disease

	Haemophilia A	Von Willebrand disease
Inheritance dominant	Sex-linked recessive	Autosomal
Haemarthroses/deep haematomas	Common	Rare
Epistaxes	Uncommon	Common
Gastrointestinal bleeding	Uncommon	Common
Haematuria	Common	Uncommon
Menorrhagia	None (males)	Common
Post-extraction bleeding	Starts 1–24 h after trauma, lasts 3–40 days and is not controlled by pressure	Starts immediately, lasts 24–48 h and is often controlled by pressure
Bleeding time	Normal	Prolonged
Factor VIII coagulant activity	Low	Low
Factor VIIIR:RCo (plasma factor VIII complex; ristocetin cofactor)	Normal	Low

Note: severe von Willebrand disease is occasionally identical to haemophilia.

Box 8.4 Laboratory findings in von Willebrand disease

- Prolonged bleeding time
- Prolonged activated partial thromboplastin time
- Low levels of von Willebrand factor (factor VIIIR:Ag).
- Low factor VIIIC levels
- Reduced platelet aggregation in the presence of ristocetin

Dental aspects

Desmopressin (DDAVP) is invariably effective in type 1 vWD and is usually given by either intravenous infusion or subcutaneous injection although a nasal spray is also available. DDAVP may be effective in type 2A and it is often helpful to give patients a trial dose to ascertain the response.

Desmopressin (DDAVP) is contraindicated in type 2B vWD because it stimulates release of dysfunctional vWF, which leads in turn to platelet aggregation and severe but transient thrombocytopenia. Clotting factor replacement is needed. Intermediate purity factor VIII, cryoprecipitate and fresh-frozen plasma are effective though pure factor VIII may be ineffective replacement. DDAVP is contraindicated in type 3 vWD where so little vWF is formed that essentially the same management is required as for haemophilia, a. Clotting factor replacement is needed.

In all types, aspirin and NSAIDs should be avoided. Infiltration or intraligamentary LA should generally be used. Conscious sedation can be given, but care must be taken not to damage the vein. GA must be given in hospital where expert attention is available. Intubation is a possible hazard because of the risk of submucosal bleeding in the airway.

Factor XI deficiency ('haemophilia C')

Common in Ashkenazi Jews, factor XI deficiency is inherited as an autosomal disorder with either homozygosity or compound heterozygosity.

Patients with factor XI deficiency cannot activate thrombin-activatable fibrinolytic inhibitor TAFI; this results in rapid fibrinolysis, which is responsible for the bleeding tendency seen in this disorder. Fresh-frozen plasma or factor XI is required.

Factor XII deficiency

Factor XII (the first component of the intrinsic pathway) is more important for the generation of bradykinin and stimulation of fibrinolysis than for initiation of coagulation. Patients with factor XII deficiency rarely show signs of haemorrhage.

Factor XIII deficiency

Factor XIII, the pro-enzyme of plasma transglutaminase, is normally activated by thrombin in the presence of calcium to catalyse the cross-linking of fibrin monomers.

Factor XIII deficiency leads to neonatal umbilical cord bleeding, intracranial haemorrhage and soft tissue haematomas. Primary haemostasis is normal but delayed bleeding is seen.

Fibrinogen disorders

Inherited disorders in fibrinogen are rare (Table 8.15). In contrast, raised plasma fibrinogen levels are found in coronary artery disease, diabetes, hypertension, peripheral artery disease, hyperlipoproteinaemia, hypertriglyceridaemia, pregnancy, menopause, hypercholesterolaemia, use of oral contraceptives and smoking.

Acquired coagulation defects

Acquired haemorrhagic disorders are far more prevalent than congenital diseases but, except in anticoagulant therapy or liver disease, are usually less severe. Important causes include anticoagulant therapy and liver disease, vitamin K deficiency or malabsorption, disseminated intravascular coagulation, fibrinolytic states, amyloidosis (deficiency of factor X) and auto-immune disorders (e.g. acquired haemophilia). Some patients also have clinical bleeding tendencies but no defect detectable by current laboratory methods.

ANTICOAGULANT TREATMENT
GENERAL ASPECTS

Anticoagulants are given to prevent and treat thromboembolic disease but have many uses. They are used to treat atrial fibrillation, cardiac valvular disease, ischaemic heart disease and post-myocardial infarction (sometimes), deep venous thrombosis (DVT), pulmonary embolism, cerebrovascular accident and many other conditions, and are used when there are heart valve replacements or renal dialysis.

Commonly used anticoagulants are the coumarin warfarin for long-term treatment and heparin for short-term treatment.

Table 8.14 Von Willebrand disease: cover for operations[a]		
Von Willebrand disease type	Desmopressin	Factor VIII replacement
1	Typically effective	–
2A	May be effective: check response with trial dose	±
2B	Contraindicated	+
2M	Contraindicated	+
2N	Unlikely to be of value	±
3	Contraindicated	+

[a]Plus local haemostatic measures (Table 8.10).

Table 8.15 Inherited disorders in fibrinogen			
Condition	Definition	Inheritance	Features
Afibrinogenaemia	Complete lack of fibrinogen	Autosomal recessive	Neonatal umbilical cord haemorrhage, ecchymoses, mucosal haemorrhage, internal haemorrhage and recurrent abortion
Hypofibrinogenaemia	Low levels of fibrinogen below 100 mg/dl (normal – 250–350 mg/dl)	Acquired or inherited	Symptoms similar to but less severe than afibrinogenaemia
Dysfibrinogenaemia	Dysfunctional fibrinogen	Inherited	Haemorrhage, spontaneous abortion and thrombo-embolism
Hypoplasminogenaemia	Plasminogen deficient or defective	Inherited	Fibrin deposits with gingival swelling and sometimes ligneous conjunctivitis

Because it takes several days for the maximum effect of warfarin to be realized, heparin is normally given first.

Warfarin, a 4-hydroxycoumarin derivative, is the most commonly used oral anticoagulant. It is a vitamin K antagonist, which acts by inhibiting the post-translational glutamate carboxylation of blood coagulation factors II, VII, IX and X. Warfarin also inhibits glutamate carboxylation of the proteins C and S. The anticoagulant effect of warfarin results predominantly from reduction in factor II.

Warfarin is most frequently prescribed to control and prevent thromboembolic disorders in atrial fibrillation, after cardiac surgery or organ transplants, after cerebrovascular accident, or in DVT or pulmonary embolism.

Warfarin effects begin after 8–12 h, are maximal at 36 h, and persist for 72 h, prolonging the international normalized ratio – the ratio of the patient's prothrombin time to a standardized control. An INR above 1 indicates that clotting will take longer than normal. The management of patients on warfarin should take into consideration the type of dental procedure, the INR value, the underlying condition for which anticoagulation is used and other risk factors (e.g. hepatic disorders or local inflammation). Surgery is the main oral health care hazard to the patient on warfarin and thus the possibility of alternatives (e.g. endodontics) should always be considered. The INR is used as a guideline to care and should be checked on the day of operation or, if that is not possible, within 24 h prior to surgery.

The plasminogen activators such as t-PA (alteplase) or streptokinase also are useful for controlling coagulation, in particular during the short period after myocardial infarction (Ch. 5). Because t-PA is highly selective for the degradation of fibrin in clots, it is extremely useful in restoring the patency of the coronary arteries after thrombosis. Streptokinase (an enzyme from streptococci) is another plasminogen activator useful from a therapeutic standpoint but it is less selective than t-PA, being able to activate circulating plasminogen as well as that bound to a fibrin clot.

Aspirin, by virtue of inhibiting the activity of the cyclo-oxygenase enzyme, depresses the production of thromboxane TXA_2 and prostacyclin (PGI_2), and inhibits platelet aggregation.

DENTAL ASPECTS

Some patients on anticoagulant drugs have a tendency to bleed excessively after trauma or surgery. Dental preventive care is especially important in order to minimize the need for surgical intervention. Alternatives, such as endodontics, should always be considered. Patients must be warned of the risk of intra- and post-operative bleeding and intra/extraoral bruising (Fig. 8.12). Systemic conditions that may aggravate the bleeding tendency include coagulopathies, thrombocytopenias, vascular disorders such as Ehlers–Danlos syndrome, liver disease, renal disease, malignancy and HIV infection. Drugs that might worsen the bleeding tendency (aspirin and other NSAIDs) should be avoided (see later). Intramuscular injections should be avoided. Regional block LA injections may also be a hazard. Bleeding into the fascial spaces of the neck can threaten airway patency. Intraligamentary or intrapapillary injections are safer. Conscious sedation can be given. If intravenous, care must be

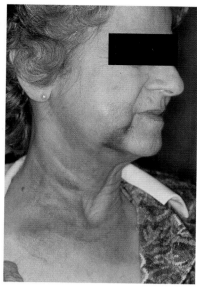

Fig. 8.12 Ecchymosis tracking to mediastinum after oral surgery

taken not to damage the vein. GA requires expert attention in hospital.

In general, anticoagulation should not be stopped except for very good reasons, because it does not necessarily significantly reduce bleeding but, in contrast, may cause hypercoagulability and rebound thrombosis, which has damaged prosthetic cardiac valves and even caused thrombotic deaths in dental patients. Certainly, anticoagulant treatment should not be altered without the agreement of the clinician in charge.

Warfarin does not usually need to be stopped before primary care dental surgical procedures. *Minor dental procedures* such as the administration of infiltration LA, restoration placement, fabrication of fixed and removable prosthetic appliances, and supragingival scaling and polishing do not usually require consideration of the INR, but the prudent dentist will consult with the physician responsible for the patient's warfarin therapy before performing more invasive procedures. Such potentially invasive procedures as the administration of LA via an inferior alveolar nerve block, tooth extractions, periodontal surgery, implant placement, biopsies, subgingival scaling as well as the prescribing of certain medications may need modification. The discussion should include the patient's recent INR values, access to the patient's INR value on the day of surgery, plans to optimize blood pressure control to minimize intraoperative bleeding, and an assurance that the patient is not also receiving antiplatelet agents (such as aspirin and/or clopidogrel). Although it is not uncommon for the physician to concur or support the American Heart Association (AHA) guidelines that permit interruption of anticoagulation for a period of up to 1 week for surgical procedures that carry a risk of bleeding, the dentist should sensitize the physician to the American Dental Association Council on Scientific Affairs (ADA/SCA) guidelines that recognize that, while the AHA guidelines may be relevant for patients undergoing major surgery, they are not applicable for patients having dentoalveolar surgery. Furthermore, they should note that the ADA/SCA and the British Dental Association and the Haemostasis and Thrombosis Task Force of the British Committee for Standards in Hematology, having reviewed the scientific literature, have concluded that warfarin therapy should *not* be discontinued for patients having routine dentoalveolar surgery if the INR = 4. This is because of the difficulty in predicting the drop in the INR value in any given patient and because the risk of experiencing a thromboembolism (which may be fatal) outweighs the risk of experiencing excessive post-operative oral bleeding. These conclusions should be reassuring to the physician, because this level of anticoagulation is far in excess of the 2.0 to 3.0 range (2.5 target) typically prescribed for patients with atrial fibrillation and thus provides an even greater margin of safety. Note however, that there are no studies to date involving significant numbers of patients having more extensive surgeries such as of more than six extractions, removal of impacted teeth, alveolectomies and tori removal. See Appendix 8.4 for guidelines from the National Patient Safety Agency (http://www.bcshguidelines.com/pdf/WarfarinandOralSurgery26407.pdf and http://www.npsa.nhs.uk/nrls/alerts-and-directives/alerts/anticoagulant/).

Previously published studies have identified certain procedures or precautions that may limit intraoperative and post-operative haemorrhage when performing oral surgery for these patients. The administration of LA agents containing vasoconstrictors assists in maintaining a dry surgical field and intraligamentary and intrapapillary injections are preferred over regional blocks if the INR is > 4.0 because of an anecdotal risk of bleeding into the floor of mouth and fascial planes of the neck with consequent obstruction of the airway.

To minimize the risk and extent of post-operative bleeding, the number of teeth to be extracted at any one sitting should be limited and, when required, teeth should be sectioned so as to limit the need for bone removal. When required, subperiosteal tension-free flaps should be raised and minimal bone removed so as to enhance clot stabilization. Resorbable gelatin or oxidized cellulose materials should be placed in the socket; the bony wound should be compressed; soft tissues should be closely apposed; and tight multiple interrupted sutures should be placed. The patient should be requested to bite on saline-soaked gauze compresses for 30 min and advised not to exercise or to rinse their mouth for 24 h or eat anything other than a cold liquid diet for 48 h. Some clinicians augment the above by also asking the patient to rinse their mouth with an antifibrinolytic, such as epsilon-aminocaproic acid (or tranexamic acid), four times per day for 2 min.

When planning more complex and invasive maxillofacial surgical procedures, such as an extraoral open reduction of facial fractures, which is associated with extensive bleeding, for patients without a history of prior stroke, transient ischaemic attack, systemic embolisms or mechanical heart valve, the AHA's guidelines may be applicable. The patient's warfarin therapy should be managed with the patient's physician and the patient's INR must be evaluated on the day of surgery. Older individuals are slower to normalize an elevated INR and may experience warfarin-related bleeding events at lower INRs than do younger individuals. In some instances the physician may prescribe 'bridging anticoagulation' of subcutaneous low-molecular-weight heparin (LMWH) in order to shorten the time that the patient is unprotected from thromboembolism. Typically, the last pre-operative dose of LMWH is

administered 24 h before surgery. The first post-operative dose is given no earlier than 24 h after surgery, and commonly on the second post-operative day when haemostasis has been secured. Warfarin therapy may be reinstituted on the evening of surgery if haemostasis has been assured; if not, then it is started 24 h post-operatively.

Most cases of post-operative bleeding are easily treated with local measures such as packing with a haemostatic dressing, suturing and pressure.

For patients awaiting elective dental procedures who are taking warfarin for a limited period (e.g. 6 months for a DVT), the procedure should be postponed until the warfarin has been stopped.

UK Medicines Information (UKMI) summarises as follows:

- An INR should be measured within 24–72 h of undertaking the procedure.
- The UKMI recommends that no individuals should have a dental procedure in primary care if they have an INR > 4.0; however, the British Committee for Standards in Haematology guidelines recommend that the INR should be no greater than 2 at the time of the procedure.
- The UKMI also recommends that warfarin patients with renal or hepatic disease or those on chemotherapy or cytotoxics should have dental procedures in hospital.

Medication and dietary interactions with warfarin

Warfarin's effect may be changed by several drugs (Table 8.16). Even *topical* miconazole gel has led to bleeding. Aspirin and other NSAIDs can also interfere with platelet function and cause gastric bleeding.

Of greater significance is the increased risk of intracranial haemorrhage from the concurrent administration of warfarin and aspirin.

For post-operative pain management, paracetamol (acetaminophen; an intake of four 500-mg tablets per day for up to 5 days) is recommended as the general analgesic and antipyretic of choice for short-term use in patients on oral anticoagulant therapy. Paracetamol is preferred over NSAIDs because it does not affect platelets, but excessive and prolonged administration can enhance warfarin activity. An intake of fewer than six tablets of 325 mg of paracetamol per week has little effect on INR; however, four tablets a day for a week significantly affects the INR. The concurrent administration of warfarin and paracetamol at a dose of four 325-mg tablets a day for 7 days will raise the INR and risk of haemorrhage because one of the metabolites inhibits a key enzyme in the vitamin K cycle required for the liver's production of coagulation factors. Paracetamol will affect the INR within 18–48 h of administration.

Codeine may be prescribed with the paracetamol to enhance the analgesic effect. COX-2-selective NSAIDs (celecoxib and rofecoxib), which were potential alternatives, are contraindicated because of cardiotoxicity. Tramadol occasionally interferes with warfarin and raises the INR.

Certain other medications when taken over a number of days concurrently with warfarin may increase the patient's INR value and risk of haemorrhage unless the warfarin dosage is adjusted.

Table 8.16 Drug use in patients on warfarin[a]

Drug group	Avoid: warfarin effect is enhanced	Alternatives that can probably be used safely[b]
Analgesics	Aspirin and other NSAIDs Tramadol	Acetaminophen (paracetamol) Celecoxib Codeine
Antibacterials	Ampicillin Amoxicillin Amoxicillin plus clavulanic acid Benzylpenicillin Cephalosporins (2nd, 3rd generation) Clarithromycin Ciprofloxacin Co-trimoxazole (and other sulfonamides) Doxycycline Isoniazid Metronidazole Neomycin Quinolones Tetracyclines	Azithromycin Cephalosporins, (others) Clindamycin Erythromycin Penicillins (others)
Antifungals	Azoles (fluconazole, itraconazole, ketoconazole, miconazole) Griseofulvin	Amphotericin Nystatin
Antivirals	Ritonavir Saquinavir	
Antidepressants	SSRIs (see Ch. 10)	TCAs (see Ch. 10)

[a]Warfarin effect may be enhanced by several drugs but where a single dose of amoxicillin is required there should be no problem. If infection is present, no elective surgery should be done until the patient has been treated with antibiotics and is free from acute infection. In case of emergency, careful haemostatic control should suffice.
[b]Patients should still be advised to be vigilant for excessive bleeding.
NSAIDs, non-steroidal anti-inflammatory drugs; SSRIs, selective serotonin reuptake inhibitors; TCAs, tricyclic antidepressants.

Warfarin's anticoagulation effect is derived as discussed, from its ability to prevent the metabolism of vitamin K to its active form, which is needed in the liver's synthesis of clotting factors II, VII, IX and X. Some antimicrobials (tetracylines, broad-spectrum penicillins – amoxicillin, ampicillin) further decrease available vitamin K because they destroy some of the normal intestinal bacteria which produce it. The INR and risk of haemorrhage may also be increased by antimicrobials such as metronidazole and the macrolides (erythromycin, azithromycin, clarithromycin) because they inhibit the normal metabolism of warfarin. If a full antimicrobial course is indicated, the narrow-spectrum penicillin V (or clindamycin for those allergic to penicillin) is the preferred medication. Azole antifungals, such as ketoconazole, flucanozole, clotrimazole, itraconazole and miconazole, may also increase the INR by inhibiting the hepatic metabolism of warfarin.

Other medications that may adversely interact include dicloxacillin, nafcillin, phenobarbital and chloral hydrate, which can induce enzyme systems to metabolize warfarin rapidly.

Table 8.17 Oral anticoagulant therapy and oral surgery

	Prothrombin time(s)	Thrombotest	INR
Normal level	< 1.3	> 70%	1
Therapeutic range	2–4.5	5–20%	2–5
Levels at which dentoalveolar surgery can be carried out[a]	< 2.5	> 15%	< 4

[a]Uncomplicated forceps extraction of 1–3 teeth.
INR, international normalized ratio.
A normal prothrombin time is around 12 s.

Warfarin's effect can also be influenced by irregular tablet taking; diets high in vitamin K (avocado, beet, broccoli, Brussels sprouts, cabbage, chick peas, green peas, green tea, kale, lettuce, liver, spinach and turnips) can lower the INR; alcohol can inhibit warfarin, but may have the converse effect if there is liver disease; diseases such as diarrhoea, liver disease and malignant disease can raise the INR; and cranberry juice (*Vaccinium macrocarpon*), popularly used to prevent cystitis, may enhance warfarin activity.

Dental aspects

The management of patients on anticoagulants (Table 8.17) should take into consideration: the type of procedure; the INR value, which can be tested approximately if necessary with a bedside machine (Fig. 8.13); the underlying condition for which anticoagulation is used; and other risk factors.

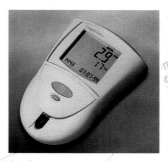

Fig. 8.13 CoaguChek for measuring INR

The INR should be used as a guideline, not a commandment, since stopping warfarin does not necessarily stop bleeding but may cause hypercoagulability. Stopping warfarin before dental surgery has led to rebound thrombosis, which has damaged prosthetic cardiac valves and occasionally been fatal. Unless serious bleeding is anticipated, therefore, warfarin should be continued. In any case, anticoagulant treatment should never be altered without the agreement of the clinician in charge. Generally speaking, dental bleeding due to warfarin is usually easier to control than any thrombotic complications.

The INR should be checked on the day of operation or, if that is not possible, the day before. For patients with a constant INR level of up to 2.5 needing emergency surgery, the authors rely on the last known INR level, provided it was determined within 1 week before surgery. A bedside device, the

CoaguChek (Roche Diagnostics), may be used. It appears that there may be statistically significant INR differences between CoaguChek and the international reference preparations, but these test strips achieve a clinically acceptable level of accuracy.

Medicolegal and other considerations suggest that one should act on the side of caution and fully inform and discuss treatment with the patient, take medical advice in any case of doubt and arrange adjustment of warfarin for patients with INR > 4.0, or > 3 if the procedure is not minor.

Always refer patients to hospital for care in the presence of any of the following conditions: INR > 4; the need for more than simple surgical procedures; the presence of additional bleeding risk factors or logistical difficulties; and drug interactions with warfarin.

If oral surgery is limited, such as the uncomplicated forceps extraction of 1–3 teeth and INR < 4.0 (some suggest 3.5), and no other risk factors are present, local methods of haemostasis should suffice. Resorbable gelatin sponge and multiple sutures, either alone or accompanied by fibrin glue or a mouthwash with tranexamic acid, should give satisfactory haemostasis. If post-operative bleeding starts, in an emergency, an antifibrinolytic agent (tranexamic acid) can be used topically to control it.

If surgery is to be more than simple or minor, or INR > 4.0, or other risk factors are present, the patient should be treated in hospital and consideration given to whether the anticoagulation will need to be modified, possibly changing to heparin during the pre-operative period (Table 8.18). If anticoagulants are to be continued after the operation, vitamin K should be avoided, as it makes subsequent anticoagulation difficult. Usually, it is simply best to discontinue the warfarin for 2 or 3 days pre-operatively. A 2-day suspension appears to be a simple and safe policy for patients with prosthetic heart valves who are anticoagulated. If necessary, low-molecular-weight heparins can be used. To prevent post-operative bleeding, an antifibrinolytic agent (tranexamic acid; see later) can be used topically to control haemorrhage. Warfarin therapy should be restarted simultaneously with heparin unless a contraindication exists or the patient is suspected of having a hypercoagulable state.

Heparin should be stopped once the INR reaches the required therapeutic level. Generally, heparin and warfarin overlap for approximately 4 days. Follow-up INR with the patient's physician should be arranged for 3 days after discharge.

Whenever possible, potentially problematic surgical procedures are best carried out in the morning, allowing more time for haemostasis before nightfall, and early in the week, to avoid problems at the weekend when staffing may be less intense. Unless the patient is also an active cocaine abuser, 2% lidocaine with 1:80 000 or 1:100 000 epinephrine should be used. Epinephrine should then be avoided.

Surgery should be carried out with minimal trauma to both bone and soft tissues. Local measures are important to protect the soft tissues and operation area to minimize the risk of post-operative bleeding. In the case of difficult extractions, when mucoperiosteal flaps must be raised, the lingual tissues in the lower molar regions should preferably be left undisturbed since trauma may open up planes into which haemorrhage can track and endanger the airway. The buccal approach to lower third molar removal is safer. Minimal bone should be removed and the teeth should be sectioned for removal where possible.

Bleeding should be assessed intraoperatively and, if there is concern, an absorbable haemostatic agent such as oxidized regenerated cellulose, resorbable gelatin sponge or collagen (synthetic or microcrystalline or porcine) can be placed in the socket. Cyanoacrylate or fibrin glues provide rapid haemostasis as well as tissue sealing and adhesion. Recombinant fibrin products are preferred.

Suturing is desirable to stabilize flaps and to prevent post-operative disturbance of wounds by eating. Resorbable sutures are preferred since they retain less plaque. Gauze pressure (a gauze soaked with tranexamic acid helps; see later), using 10 min biting on gauze, helps haemostasis. If bleeding is controlled, the patient should be dismissed and given a 7-day follow-up appointment and phone number of the office with instructions to call if bleeding starts. Additional risk factors for bleeding should prompt the treating clinician to be more cautious (i.e. to place more sutures and to prescribe in advance an antifibrinolytic drug such as topical 4.8% tranexamic acid, for up to 7 days).

Post-operatively, the patency of the airway must be ensured. Care should be taken to watch for haematoma formation, often signified by swelling, dysphagia or hoarseness.

Many patients can be managed post-operatively with antifibrinolytic agents given topically as mouthwashes during the first 7–10 days. Systemic tranexamic acid does not result in therapeutic concentrations in saliva. Topical tranexamic acid is effective even when anticoagulant therapy remains unchanged. Controlled studies have shown the efficacy and safety of tranexamic acid mouthwashes, and their lack of unwanted systemic effects. Overall, tranexamic acid reduces bleeding complications to 0–7% from 13–40% in controls. Tranexamic acid is used topically as 10 ml of a 4.8–5% w/v solution used as a mouthwash for 2 min, four times daily for 7 days.

Infection also appears to induce fibrinolysis and therefore antimicrobials, such as oral penicillin V 250–500 mg four times daily or clindamycin, should be given post-operatively for a full course of 7 days if there is risk of secondary haemorrhage. Metronidazole is contraindicated, and amoxicillin and erythromycin

Table 8.18 Protocol for warfarinized patients having oral surgery		
Pre-operatively	**Perioperatively**	**Post-operatively for 24 h**
Check INR within 24 h of operation If INR < 3.5 (some suggest < 3), and no liver disease, do not change warfarin If INR < 3.5, and liver disease, or If INR > 4, consult physician about reducing warfarin No NSAIDs	Minimize trauma Use regional block LA only if essential Local haemostatic measures[a] No NSAIDs	Rest No mouth-rinsing No hot food or drink No chewing No NSAIDs

[a]Local haemostatic measures (see Table 8.10).
INR, international normalized ratio; LA, local analgesia; NSAIDs, non-steroidal anti-inflammatory drugs.

are less appropriate because of possible drug interactions with warfarin, which may enhance bleeding.

For post-operative pain management, paracetamol is the analgesic and antipyretic of choice for *short-term use* in patients on oral anticoagulant therapy. It is preferred over NSAIDs since it does not affect platelets. Codeine is a suitable alternative analgesic. A diet of cool liquid and minced solids should be taken for several days.

Post-operative prolonged bleeding should be controlled by biting on a moist gauze, a gauze pad soaked in tranexamic acid, or a moist tea bag with firm pressure for 30 min. Faced with persistent bleeding, it is important to establish whether the situation is urgent, when the patient will require admission for intravenous fluids, or reversal of anticoagulation. This may be required if the patient is losing large quantities of blood or is hypotensive (hypovolaemic).

To stop oral bleeding, a LA injection containing epinephrine should be given and a sterile gauze pad soaked with tranexamic acid should be pressed over the extraction socket for 10–15 minutes. The socket edges should be approximated by squeezing with the fingers. The socket should then be sutured using black silk sutures to ensure tight closure. A resorbable haemostatic preparation may be placed in the socket before suturing. If the patient continues to bleed, consult the physician about possible use of vitamin K.

HEPARINS

General aspects

Heparin is a natural product, abundant in granules of the mast cells that line the vasculature and is released in response to injury. Heparin is also used as a parenteral anticoagulant given subcutaneously or intravenously, for acute thromboembolic episodes or for hospitalization protocols that include significant surgical procedures, to prevent deep venous thrombosis and pulmonary emboli. Heparin is a sulfated glycosaminoglycan originally obtained from liver (hence *heparin*). Heparin acts immediately on blood coagulation to block the conversion of fibrinogen to fibrin, mainly by inhibiting the thrombin–fibrinogen reaction via its binding to and catalysing antithrombin III, which then inhibits the serine proteases of the coagulation cascade to inactivate thrombin. Heparin also acts on activated factors IX–XII and increases platelet aggregation but inhibits thrombin-induced activation. The anticoagulant effect of standard or unfractionated heparin has an immediate action on blood clotting, which is usually lost within 6 h of stopping it.

The prothrombin, activated partial thromboplastin and thrombin times are prolonged. Most patients are monitored with the APTT and are maintained at 1.5–2.5 times the control value (the therapeutic range). Large doses of heparin can also prolong the INR. Platelet counts should also be monitored if heparin is used for more than 5 days, since it can cause thrombocytopenia. Autoimmune thrombocytopenia is possible within 3–15 days, or sooner if there has been previous heparin exposure.

Heparin is available as standard or unfractionated heparin, or low-molecular-weight heparins (LMWHs). The latter, such as certoparin, interact with factor Xa but do not affect standard blood test results. Low-dose heparin therapy, such as Minihep, is used to reduce the risk of DVT. Some heparins are also being used for other effects, such as immunosuppression.

Low-molecular-weight heparins (LMWHs) have more predictable pharmacokinetic and pharmacodynamic properties than

have largely replaced, unfractionated heparin (UFH). Antifactor Xa monitoring is superior to measurement of APPT, and is prudent in patients with severe obesity or renal insufficiency, and UFH infusion is preferable to LMWH injection in patients with renal failure. Protamine may help reverse bleeding related to LWMH. The synthetic pentasaccharide fondaparinux is a promising new antithrombotic agent.

Dental aspects

For uncomplicated forceps extraction of 1–3 teeth, there is usually no need to interfere with heparin or LMWH anticoagulation.

Before more advanced surgery in a heparin-treated patient, medical advice should be sought. Heparin has an immediate effect on blood clotting but acts for only 4–6 h and no specific treatment is therefore needed to reverse its effect. The effect of heparin is best assessed by the APTT. Withdrawal of heparin is adequate to reverse anticoagulation where this is necessary. In an emergency, this can be reversed by intravenous protamine sulfate given in a dose of 1 mg per 100 IU heparin, but a medical opinion should be sought first. Where heparin has been stopped, any surgery can safely be carried out after 6–8 h. In renal dialysis patients, or patients having cardiopulmonary bypass or other extracorporeal circulation with heparinization, surgery is best carried out on the day after dialysis. The effects of heparinization have then ceased and there is maximum benefit from dialysis.

Low-molecular-weight heparins may have little effect on post-operative bleeding, despite their longer activity (up to 24 h). However, the advice of the haematologist should be sought before surgery.

ASPIRIN

Aspirin irreversibly impairs platelet aggregation and is used long-term in the prevention of cardiovascular events and stroke in patients at risk. In large doses, aspirin may also cause hypoprothrombinaemia. Even small doses of aspirin prolong the bleeding time and impair platelet adhesiveness. Aspirin may worsen bleeding tendencies if there are other anticoagulation medications or other bleeding disorders, such as uraemia.

In patients with no other cause for a bleeding tendency and receiving up to 100 mg aspirin daily, in general, for uncomplicated forceps extraction of 1–3 teeth, there is no need to interfere with aspirin treatment. Suturing and packing the socket with resorbable gelatin sponge, oxidized cellulose or microfibrillar collagen can be carried out if necessary.

In patients with no other cause for a bleeding tendency and receiving doses of aspirin higher than 100 mg daily, if there is concern, the current value of the bleeding time should be established. If it is over 20 min, surgery should be postponed.

In practice, aspirin rarely interferes significantly with dental surgical procedures.

OTHER DRUGS AFFECTING HAEMOSTASIS

Other parenteral agents influencing haemostasis include *heparinoids* such as danaparoid; *hirudins* such as lepirudin and desirudin; *antiplatelet drugs* such as clopidogrel, and glycoprotein

Table 8.19 Other parenteral anticoagulants				
Antiplatelets	**Heparinoids**	**Hirudins**	**Low-molecular-weight heparins**	**Prostacyclin**
Aspirin	Danaparoid	Lepirudin	Certoparin	Epoprostenol
Clopidogrel		Desirudin	Dalteparin	
Dypiridamole			Enoxaparin	
Ticlopidine			Reviparin	
Abciximab			Tinzaparin	
Eptifibatide				
Tirofiban				

IIb/IIIa inhibitors (abciximab, eptifibatide and tirofiban) (Table 8.19). These can have some effect on the APTT and on post-operative bleeding. The physician should be consulted before any major surgical procedure but dentoalveolar surgery is usually uncomplicated.

VITAMIN K DEFICIENCY AND MALABSORPTION

GENERAL ASPECTS

Vitamin K is a fat-soluble vitamin present in the diet and also synthesized by the gut flora. It is absorbed in the small gut, in the presence of bile salts. After transport to the liver, vitamin K is used for the synthesis of factors II (prothrombin), VII, IX and X. Haemorrhagic disease may, therefore, result from interference with vitamin K use by:

- anticoagulants
- malabsorption
- obstructive jaundice
- severe liver disease.

GENERAL MANAGEMENT

In liver disease, many haemostatic functions are severely impaired and vitamin K is of little or no value (Box 8.5).

DENTAL ASPECTS

Dental management in vitamin K deficiency may be complicated by the clotting defect and the underlying disorder, particularly obstructive jaundice (Ch. 9). The latter may be caused by gallstones, viral hepatitis or carcinoma of the head of the pancreas.

The underlying disorder should preferably be corrected but vitamin K can be given if surgery is urgent. Phytomenadione (5–25 mg) is the most potent and rapidly acting form and should preferably be given intravenously. The prothrombin time should be monitored after 48 h and, if the defect has not been corrected by then, this suggests parenchymal liver disease.

Liver disease is an important cause of bleeding disorders related to: impaired vitamin K metabolism; excessive

Box 8.5 Causes of vitamin K deficiency

- Lack of vitamin K synthesis in the gut
- Broad-spectrum antibiotics used for prolonged periods
- In-patients on parenteral feeding
- Poor absorption
- Malabsorption syndromes
- Blind loop
- Obstructive jaundice
- Failure of utilisation
- Oral anticoagulant treatment
- Liver failure
- Responds to parenteral vitamin K

Viral hepatitis also has an obstructive component.

fibrinolysis; failure of synthesis or overconsumption of normal clotting factors; synthesis of abnormal clotting factors; and thrombocytopenia.

Haemorrhage can be severe and difficult to manage because of the complexity of these defects.

Antifibrinolytic treatment and fresh-frozen plasma may sometimes be effective. If there is an obstructive element to the disease, vitamin K may be effective, but only if parenchymal disease is mild (Ch. 9).

FIBRINOLYTIC DRUGS

Fibrinolytic drugs such as streptokinase may cause abnormal bleeding and dental surgery should be deferred where possible.

ACQUIRED HAEMOPHILIA

Acquired haemophilia is a rare disorder due to circulating antibodies to factor VIII, which typically are of unknown origin but may rarely form in autoimmune disorders such as rheumatoid arthritis, drug therapy (especially with penicillin), and in pregnancy or the puerperium. In contrast to congenital haemophilia, females are affected just as frequently as males.

Specialist haematological attention is required before any operative treatment is considered.

OTHER DISORDERS ASSOCIATED WITH BLEEDING TENDENCIES

These may include:

- after massive transfusions
- antibodies to clotting factors
- chronic renal failure (Ch. 12)
- cyanotic congenital heart disease (Ch. 5)
- disseminated intravascular coagulopathy
- Gram-negative shock
- head injuries (Ch. 24)
- hypertension
- myelofibrosis, leukaemia or lymphoma (Ch. 8)
- polycythaemia vera (Ch. 8).

BLOOD TRANSFUSION

Blood can supply a range of products useful in a variety of situations (Fig. 8.14). Perioperative blood loss and anaemia is best dealt with by reducing the amount of blood lost at surgery through minimising trauma, improving mechanical haemostasis, limiting phlebotomy to essential diagnostic tests, using microsample laboratory techniques and using antifibrinolytics such as epsilon-aminocaproic acid or tranexamic acid (or for high-risk procedures, aprotinin). Erythropoeitin can also help where blood has been lost but the replacement of blood by transfusion can be essential after severe haemorrhage and in some other circumstances. Allogeneic blood transfusion may carry hazards of:

- incompatibility
- fluid overload
- transmission of infections (Box 8.6)
- post-transfusion purpura
- transfusion-associated graft-versus-host disease
- transfusion-associated acute lung injury (TRALI).

In the UK, therefore, blood is now screened and leukodepletion also used, as this reduces the risk of infection and also of acute non-haemolytic transfusion reactions and transfusion-associated graft-versus-host disease.

Some medications may be transmitted, and this is especially a concern with pregnant women and prostatic medications such as dutasteride and finasteride (Ch. 25). Allogeneic transfusion may lead to an increased risk of post-operative bacterial infections and multiorgan failure.

Autologous transfusion reduces the need for allogeneic transfusion and is most widely used in elective surgery. The three main techniques are pre-deposit transfusion, intraoperative haemodilution, and intraoperative and post-operative salvage. Autologous transfusion is more cost-effective than allogeneic transfusion and clinical outcomes are improved.

If blood transfusion is needed:

- establish an intravenous line
- take blood for grouping and cross-matching
- seek a surgical opinion and begin a thorough secondary survey
- organize quarter-hourly, or half-hourly, observations of pulse rate, blood pressure, respiratory rate, daily urine output and fluid balance (usually daily).

Blood transfusion is not needed to replace losses of less than 500 ml in an adult, unless there was pre-existing anaemia or deterioration of the general condition warrants transfusion. Blood should therefore never be given unless warranted and in some faiths such as Jehovah's Witnesses is not permissible but their principles are being reconsidered (Fig. 8.15 and Ch. 30), as discussed above.

Box 8.6 Diseases known to be transmitted via allogeneic blood transfusion

- Bacteria (various)
- Chagas disease
- Cytomegalovirus
- Hepatitis A virus
- Hepatitis B virus
- Hepatitis C virus
- Human immunodeficiency viruses (HIV-1 and HIV-2)
- Human T-lymphotropic viruses (HTLV-1 and HTLV-2)
- Malaria
- *Treponema pallidum*
- West Nile virus
- Variant Creutzfeldt–Jakob disease (prions)

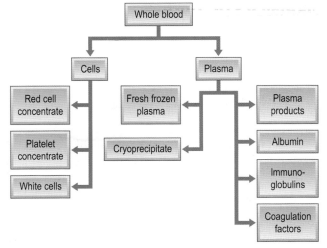

Fig. 8.14 Blood products

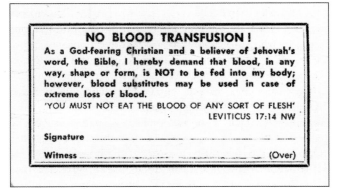

Fig. 8.15 Jehovah's Witness declaration

Table 8.20 Disorders predisposing to thromboses

Factor involved	Genetic forms	Acquired forms	Management
Antithrombin deficiency	AD. Affects ≈ 1 per 2000 of population	Eclampsia, DIC. Nephrotic syndrome	Resistant to heparin anticoagulation – use oral anticoagulants or fresh-frozen plasma
Factor V Leiden	AD. Affects ≈ 5% of population	Liver transplantation	Warfarin
Platelets (thrombocytosis and thrombocythaemia)	–	Exercise; pregnancy; trauma; post-splenectomy; chronic inflammatory disease; malignancy	Treat underlying cause. Pre-operative aspirin, dipyridamole or heparin
Protein C deficiency	AD	Warfarin; Liver disease; Vitamin K deficiency; Sepsis; DIC; thrombosis; asparaginase	Protein C concentrate or anticoagulation
Protein S deficiency	Genetic	Liver disease, DIC	Management takes place in the event of acute venous thromboembolism or in patients with asymptomatic carrier states without a thrombotic event. Heparin therapy and then warfarin

AD, autosomal dominant; DIC, disseminated intravascular coagulopathy.

SUPERFICIAL VEIN THROMBOSIS

Superficial vein thrombosis may complicate intravenous injections, particularly of diazepam, but does not lead to pulmonary embolism. Treatment of acute episodes of thrombosis is by subcutaneous injection or infusion of heparin (for 5–7 days) followed by oral anticoagulant therapy.

✱ DEEP VEIN THROMBOSIS AND THROMBOEMBOLIC DISEASE

Blood contains natural anticoagulants, mainly antithrombin, which inhibits several activated coagulation factors including thrombin, factor IXa and factor Xa, by forming a stable complex with the various factors. Heparin and heparan sulfates increase the activity of antithrombin at least 1000-fold. Other natural anticoagulants include protein S and protein C, which inhibit activated factor V (Table 8.20).

Deep vein thrombosis (DVT) and subsequent pulmonary embolism (PE) are important sequelae and causes of death or significant morbidity, especially in elderly, bed-ridden and post-operative patients as a consequence of immobility, pressure on the calf from prolonged bed rest and increased blood coagulability in pregnancy. It may also follow GA and surgery. Several other factors may contribute, including, sometimes, dehydration or oral contraceptives (Fig. 8.16).

Hypercoagulability is when there is a risk of thrombosis under circumstances that would not cause thrombosis in a normal person. Hypercoagulation is common post-operatively, during long-haul flights ('economy class syndrome') and in obesity. Oestrogen use (e.g. contraceptive pill), malignant and myeloproliferative disease, congestive cardiac failure, homocystinuria and systemic lupus erythematosus (anticardiolipin antibodies) also lead to a hypercoagulable state.

Hypercoagulability (thrombophilia) can be predisposed to by defects of natural anticoagulants (antithrombin or protein C or protein S), because of impaired fibrinolysis or because of Leiden factor (Table 8.21). About 5% of Europeans have abnormal blood clotting factor V (termed factor V Leiden), which cannot be inhibited by protein C.

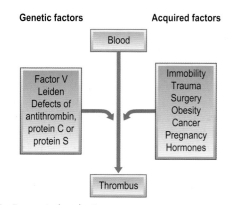

Fig. 8.16 Deep vein thrombosis

Table 8.21 Causes of anaemia

Nature of anaemia	Cause
Increased RBC loss	Menstrual blood loss Gastrointestinal blood loss Haemolysis
Reduced RBC production	Haematinic deficiency Bone marrow infiltration
Increased tissue requirements	Puberty Pregnancy
Decreased tissue requirements	Hypothyroidism

RBC, red blood cell.

Clinical features

Venous thrombosis usually affects the deep calf veins. Pain in the calf, especially on flexing the ankle (Homan sign), is characteristic but the absence of this clinical sign should certainly not be relied upon to exclude the diagnosis.

General management

Prophylaxis against venous thromboembolism is important but not reliably effective. Consideration should be given to stopping the contraceptive pill pre-operatively.

The calves must not rest on hard objects during surgery and stasis may be eliminated by calf contractions stimulated electrically, by use of compression hosiery or by pneumatic compression. Early mobilization and leg movements post-operatively must be encouraged.

A positive D-dimer test is a useful screen to indicate the presence of an abnormally high level of fibrin degradation products, suggesting thrombosis. Doppler ultrasound may be required to confirm the diagnosis.

Heparin anticoagulation is the most effective method of preventing thromboembolism but must be balanced against the risks of haemorrhage. However, low-dose heparin sufficient to provide an INR between 1.5 and 2 protects against DVT without inducing a significant risk of bleeding. Fondaparinux sodium (which blocks factor X) is an alternative.

Treatment of DVT is by heparin, starting with at least 5000 units intravenously, then continuous infusion at 1000 units per hour or 15 000 units subcutaneously each 24 h, with laboratory monitoring of APTT.

PULMONARY EMBOLISM

Pulmonary embolism secondary to venous thrombosis may be fatal as a result of sudden circulatory collapse, may cause minor pulmonary infarcts with haemoptysis or pleurisy, or may gradually cause pulmonary hypertension and right-sided heart failure.

Massive pulmonary embolism with collapse and cardiac arrest requires immediate:

- external cardiac massage, which may break up the embolus
- oxygen
- intravenous heparin
- thrombolytic agent such as streptokinase.

Minor pulmonary embolism usually resolves spontaneously but anticoagulants should be given.

Dental aspects

Venous thrombosis may affect the deep calf veins as a consequence of immobility, pressure on the calf, and increased blood coagulability, which follows GA and surgery (see earlier).

Thrombophilia and hypofibrinolysis may possibly underlie so-called neuralgia-inducing cavitational osteonecrosis (NICO) or Ratner bone cavities, which may cause severe pain. NICO appears due to resistance to activated protein C or to low protein C levels, or low levels of stimulated tissue plasminogen activator.

Bone sites most frequently involved, in decreasing order of prevalence, are mandibular molars, maxillary molars and maxillary canines/lateral incisors. Third molar sites account for 45% of all jawbone involvement. Unlike abscesses, cysts or periapical lesions, the cavities in NICO are often not apparent on radiographs, though thin-slice computed tomography scanning may show the areas. They may be detectable by technetium-99 methylene diphosphonate radioisotope scanning or ultrasonography.

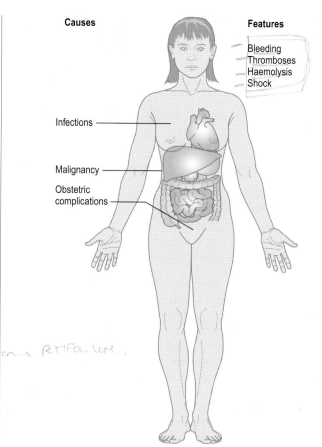

Fig. 8.17 Disseminated intravascular coagulopathy

DISSEMINATED INTRAVASCULAR COAGULATION

Disseminated intravascular coagulation (DIC; consumption coagulopathy or defibrination syndrome) is an uncommon, complex and not fully understood process with potentially fatal activation of the haemostasis-related mechanisms within the circulation. It can lead to bleeding, thrombosis, haemolysis and shock (Fig. 8.17). Haemorrhagic tendencies result from the consumption of platelets and clotting factors internally and from activation of the fibrinolytic system. Purpura and bleeding from sites such as the gastrointestinal tract and gingivae can result. In the case of head injuries, DIC may lead to intracranial haemorrhage. Thrombotic phenomena include clotting in capillaries, which can damage any organ, but the kidneys, liver, adrenals and brain are particularly vulnerable. Red cells become damaged as a result of the changes in the capillaries (microangiopathic haemolysis). Shock may be caused by adrenal damage or obstruction of the pulmonary circulation by fibrin deposition and other factors.

Precipitating causes of DIC include incompatible blood transfusions, severe sepsis, obstetric complications, burns and cancers in various sites or severe trauma. In one series of head injuries some degree of DIC was found in 57%. Brain ischaemia by vascular occlusion may therefore complicate head injury, as a result of DIC.

When there are symptoms suggestive of DIC, such as bleeding from the gingival, nausea, vomiting, muscle and abdominal pain, seizures and oliguria, a D-dimer test, along with PT, APTT, fibrinogen and platelet count help the diagnosis.

Disseminated intravascular coagulation is an acute emergency; the underlying cause and any hypoxia or acidosis should be corrected, and heparinization, replacement of clotting factors and platelets or antifibrinolytic therapy given as appropriate. The management of DIC is controversial and must in any case depend on the cause and pathological changes taking place. No single programme of treatment is effective for all cases.

Dental aspects

The main importance of DIC is in relation to head injuries as discussed earlier. Gingival bleeding may be seen.

PLASMINOGEN DEFICIENCY (HYPOPLASMINOGENAEMIA)

In health, body fluid fibrinolytic activity clears fibrin deposits but does not cause systemic fibrinolysis.

Plasminogen can be activated by tissue plasminogen activator, kallikrein or drugs such as streptokinase. Tissue plasminogen activator is produced by damaged endothelial cells and activates plasminogen to plasmin when it is bound to fibrin. If plasminogen is deficient, this mechanism fails, leading to fibrin deposition.

Some patients develop gingival swelling, corneal involvement and blindness, others may also develop congenital occlusive hydrocephalus. Whether therapy with topical heparin or intravenous purified plasminogen concentrate will effectively control the lesions remains to be established.

Dental aspects

Plasminogen deficiency may rarely underlie ligneous conjunctivitis, an idiopathic form of chronic membranous conjunctivitis associated with fibrin deposits and often with associated lesions in the larynx, nose, cervix and gingivae.

ERYTHROCYTES

Erythrocytes are responsible for oxygen (O_2) carriage from the lungs to the tissues. Erythrocytes are produced (*erythropoiesis*) in the bone marrow from nucleated stem cells (undifferentiated *pluripotent* stem cells), via immature intermediate cells (*reticulocytes*), which retain their organelles, have nuclear remnants and can still divide. Reticulocytes are prematurely released into the blood (reticulocytosis) when demand is high. Erythropoiesis is triggered by *erythropoietin* released from the kidney when low O_2 levels are detected, and this stimulates the pluripotent stem cells. Erythrocytes, when mature, contain only haemoglobin – the molecule responsible for the transport of O_2 and carbon dioxide (CO_2). Haemoglobin (Hb) production requires iron, protoporphyrin and globin chains. Haemoglobin is a heterogeneous group of proteins consisting of four globin chains and four haem groups. In adults, the normal haemoglobins are HbA, HbA_2 and HbF. Effete erythrocytes are broken down largely in the spleen and haemoglobin is degraded to haem and then bilirubin in the liver (Fig. 8.18).

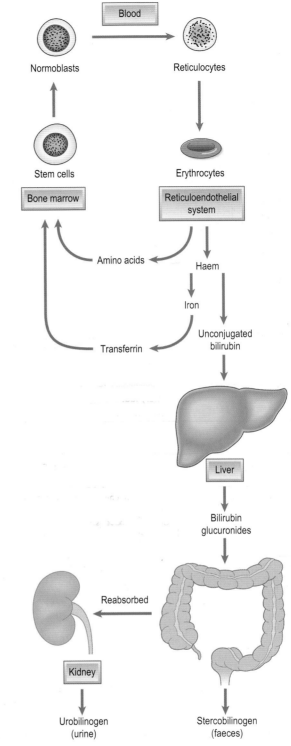

Fig. 8.18 Red cell life history

ANAEMIA

Anaemia is defined as a haemoglobin (Hb) level below the normal for the age, gender and ethnic background of the individual and may be due to insufficient red blood cell (RBC) numbers or Hb content. Up to puberty a haemoglobin level below 11.0 g/dl and, in adult females, below 11.5 g/dl, and

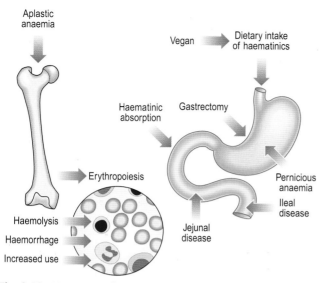

Fig. 8.19 Main causes of anaemia

Table 8.22	Causes of anaemia
Cause	**Examples**
Poor intake of haematinics (uncommon)	Socioeconomic reason Dietary fads Dysphagia
Impaired absorption of haematinics	Diseases of small intestine particularly (e.g. coeliac disease)
Increased demands for haematinics	Pregnancy and haemolysis, especially
Impaired erythropoiesis	Aplastic anaemia and leukaemia Drugs Chronic disease (e.g. rheumatoid arthritis) Viral infections
Haemolytic anaemias	Sickle cell and thalassaemia mainly
Blood loss (most common cause)	Menorrhagia Any gastrointestinal lesion (ulcers or carcinoma) Lesions of the urinary tract Trauma

Macrocytic anaemia (MCV more than 99 fl) is usually caused by vitamin B_{12} or folate deficiency (not infrequently in alcoholics), sometimes because folate and vitamin B_{12} are used up in chronic haemolysis, pregnancy or malignancy, and is sometimes caused by drugs (methotrexate, azathioprine, cytosine or hydroxycarbamide). Macrocytic anaemia may also be caused by liver disease, myxoedema or sometimes aplastic anaemia.

Normocytic anaemia (MCV between 79 and 98 fl) may result from chronic diseases such as leukaemia, chronic inflammatory disease, liver disorders, renal failure, infection, malignancy and sickle cell disease.

Clinical features

Patients with anaemia are commonly symptomless in the early stages or if the onset is slow. However, as the anaemia worsens and the oxygen-carrying capacity of the blood falls, cardiac symptoms and signs develop (tiredness, dyspnoea, palpitations, tachycardia, flow murmurs and eventual cardiac failure). Pallor of the oral mucosa, conjunctiva or palmar creases suggests severe anaemia, but skin colour can be misleading. Anaemia may worsen the symptoms of pre-existing coronary, peripheral and cerebrovascular disease. The different types of anaemia have many clinical features in common (Box 8.7).

General management

Anaemia is diagnosed from the haemoglobin level, but the precise nature and underlying cause must be established. The key to management of anaemia is the establishment and treatment of the underlying cause. Depending on the clinical presentation, the following investigations may be indicated.

- Full blood count – to ascertain the Hb level and RBC indices; it is important to include a reticulocyte count.
- Blood film – this may demonstrate abnormal RBC forms (sickle cells in sickle cell disease and pencil cells in iron-deficiency anaemia; Figs 8.21 and 8.22).
- Erythrocyte sedimentation rate (ESR) or, better, since it changes earlier in disease and is unaffected by drugs, the plasma viscosity (PV).
- Haemoglobin electrophoresis for haemoglobinopathy screening.
- Haematinics – serum vitamin B_{12}, folate and ferritin levels; the ferritin is also an acute-phase reactant and can rise in inflammatory states.
- Endoscopy – to identify sources of gastrointestinal blood loss.
- Bone marrow biopsy – to exclude bone marrow infiltration and disease.

Haematinic deficiency states must be corrected with iron, folic acid and/or vitamin B_{12} supplements. Blood transfusion may be indicated if the onset of anaemia has been rapid so as to prevent worsening of ischaemic symptoms. In end-stage renal failure, the hormone erythropoietin may be administered regularly to encourage haemopoiesis.

in adult males below 13.5 g/dl are the criteria of anaemia. The effect of anaemia is to lower the oxygen-carrying capacity of the blood. Its causes are outlined in Table 8.21 and Fig. 8.19. Although common, anaemia is not a disease in itself: it may be a feature of many diseases (Table 8.22 and Fig. 8.20).

The most common cause of anaemia in developed countries is chronic blood loss and consequent iron deficiency, usually in women from heavy menstruation. Folate and vitamin B_{12} (cobalamin) deficiency are the next most common causes.

Anaemia is classified on the basis of red cell size as microcytic (small), macrocytic (large) or normocytic (normal size erythrocytes; Table 8.23).

Microcytic anaemia is the most common and usually due to iron deficiency, occasionally to thalassaemia or chronic diseases. The mean corpuscular (cell) volume (MCV) falls below 78 fl.

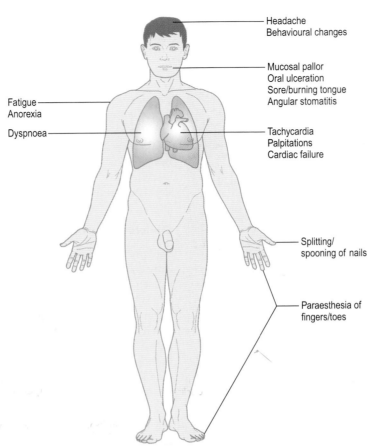

Fig. 8.20 Anaemia-features

Headache
Behavioural changes

Mucosal pallor
Oral ulceration
Sore/burning tongue
Angular stomatitis

Fatigue
Anorexia

Dyspnoea

Tachycardia
Palpitations
Cardiac failure

Splitting/
spooning of nails

Paraesthesia of
fingers/toes

Table 8.23	Main types of anaemia	
Type of anaemia	**Examples**	**Comments**
Microcytic hypochromic	Iron deficiency Thalassaemia	Blood loss from menstruation or occult sources (gastrointestinal or genitourinary) Malabsorption (post-gastrectomy)
Macrocytic	Vitamin B_{12} deficiency Folate deficiency Haemolysis Hypothyroidism Liver disease Aplastic anaemia	Malabsorption (post-gastrectomy)
Normocytic anaemia	Chronic diseases Renal failure Haemolysis Hyothyroidism	

Box 8.7 Clinical features of anaemia

Typically none in the early stages
General lassitude
Cardiorespiratory
- Dyspnoea
- Tachycardia
- Congestive cardiac failure
- Murmurs
- Palpitations
- Angina pectoris

Cutaneous
- Pallor
- Brittle nails
- Koilonychia (spoon-shaped nails – iron deficiency)

Oral
- Sore mouth
- Ulceration
- Angular stomatitis
- Glossitis
- Burning mouth symptoms

Automated examination of blood provides a quick and reliable haemoglobin estimation and count of all the blood cells. It also shows important cytological features of red cells such as red cell distribution width (RDW), MCV and Hb content. The laboratory investigation of the common anaemias is summarized in Figure 8.21. A blood film may also be required, especially as a mixed macro- and microcytic picture may sometimes not be revealed by an automated counter (a mix of large and small cells may produce an average within the normal range) and other abnormalities may be seen. For this purpose, a sample of EDTA-anticoagulated blood should be sent, with as much clinical information as possible, to the haematologist. The terminology used in the description of examination of a stained blood film is shown in Figure 8.22.

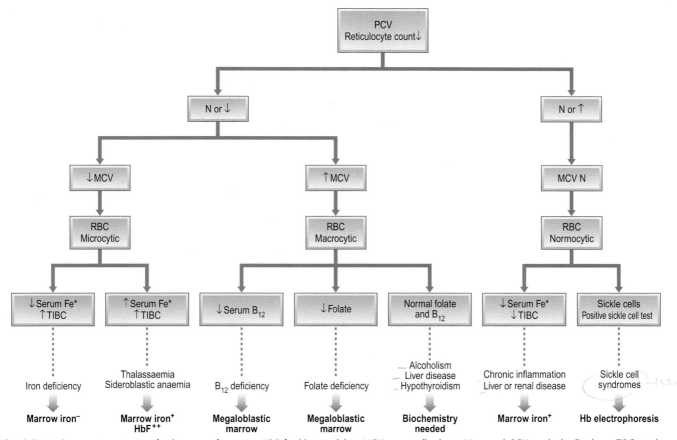

Fig. 8.21 Laboratory investigations for the cause of anaemia. HbF, fetal haemoglobin; MCV, mean cell volume; N, normal; PCV, packed cell volume; TIBC, total iron-binding capacity; *Fe, ferritin.

Special investigations are discussed under the specific diseases.

Haemoglobin can be replaced by blood transfusions, haematinics or occasionally the hormone erythropoietin to encourage natural haemopoiesis. It is better to treat with haematinics such as iron or folic acid. Blood transfusions should be used only when absolutely necessary, when the haemoglobin concentration has fallen to below 7 g/dl, since they may carry the risk of infection, circulatory overload and allergic reactions. Erythropoietin is mainly used in the treatment of anaemia of chronic renal failure or cytotoxic therapy.

Dental aspects

Local anaesthesia is usually satisfactory for pain control. Conscious sedation may be given only if there is supplemental oxygen. Deeper levels of sedation are more likely to lead to hypoxia. Nitrous oxide is theoretically contraindicated in vitamin B$_{12}$ deficiency (see later). When GA is given, it is vital to ensure full oxygenation. Nevertheless, the myocardium may be unable to respond to the demands of anaesthesia. Whenever possible, therefore, the anaemia should be corrected pre-operatively and the haemoglobin level must be raised, if necessary by transfusion. Anaemia of sickle cell disease can make GA especially hazardous (see later). Elective operations under GA should not usually be carried out when the haemoglobin is less than 10 g/dl (male). In an emergency, anaemia can be corrected by whole blood transfusion,

but this should only be given to a young and otherwise fit patient. Packed red cells avoid the risk of fluid overload and can be given in emergency to the older patient or those with incipient congestive cardiac failure. A diuretic given at the same time further reduces the risk of congestive cardiac failure. The patient should be stabilized at least 24 h pre-operatively and it should be noted that haemoglobin estimations are unreliable for 12 h post-transfusion or after acute blood loss.

Some anaemias can also cause oral lesions such as ulcers, glossitis or angular stomatitis (Fig. 8.23).

DEFICIENCY ANAEMIAS

Iron-deficiency anaemia

General aspects

Dietary iron is found mainly as iron salts, partly as haem from the myoglobin and haemoglobin in meat. Dietary iron exists as haem iron only in animal tissues; in plant foods it is present as non-haem iron, which is less easily absorbed. In a mixed omnivorous diet around 25% of dietary iron is non-haem iron. The amount of iron absorbed from various foods ranges from around 1–10% from plant foods to 10–20% from animal foods. Fibre, phytates, oxalates and phosphates present in plant foods, and tannin in tea can inhibit iron absorption. Foods rich in vitamin C, including citrus fruits, green peppers and fresh leafy

Red cell abnormalities		Causes	Red cell abnormalities		Causes
	Microcyte	Iron deficiency, haemoglobinopathy		Spherocyte	Hereditary spherocytosis, autoimmune haemolytic anaemia, septicaemia
	Macrocyte	Liver disease, alcoholism, megaloblastic anaemia		Fragments	DIC, microangiopathy, HUS, TTP, burns, prosthetic valves
	Target cell	Iron deficiency, liver disease, haemoglobinopathies, post-splenectomy		Elliptocyte	Hereditary elliptocytosis
	Stomatocyte	Liver disease, alcoholism		Tear drop poikilocyte	Myelofibrosis, extramedullary haemopoiesis
	Pencil cell	Iron deficiency		Basket cell	Oxidant damage, e.g. G6PD deficiency, unstable haemoglobin
	Ecchinocyte	Liver disease, post-splenectomy		Howell-Jolly body	Hyposplenism, post-splenectomy
	Acanthocyte	Liver disease, abetalipoproteinaemia, renal failure		Basophilic stippling	Haemoglobinopathy, lead poisoning, myelodysplasia, haemolytic anaemia
	Sickle cell	Sickle cell anaemia		Siderotic granules (Pappenheimer bodies)	Disordered iron metabolism, e.g. sideroblastic anaemia, post-splenectomy

Fig. 8.22 Red cell morphological changes. DIC, disseminated intravascular coagulation; G6PD, glucose-6-phosphate dehydrogenase; HUS, haemolytic–uraemic syndrome; TTP, thrombotic thrombocytopenic purpura.

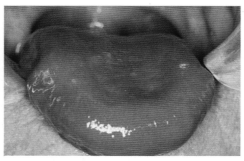

Fig. 8.23 Glossitis in anaemia

green vegetables, promote absorption of non-haem iron. Citric acid, sugars, amino acids and alcohol, as well as meat, poultry, fish and orange juice, also promote intestinal absorption of iron. Good sources of iron for vegetarians include wholegrain cereals and flours, leafy green vegetables, pulses such as lentils and kidney beans, and some dried fruits. Gastric acid is needed for the adequate conversion of iron salts from ferric to ferrous forms for their absorption from the proximal small intestine. Iron is stored in the bone marrow as haemosiderin. The remainder is stored in the liver and spleen, and a small amount is present as myoglobin, which acts as an oxygen store in muscle tissue. Iron is required for synthesis of haem, respiratory cytochromes and myeloperoxidase. Iron also plays a vital role in many metabolic reactions (Fig. 8.24).

The most common causes of anaemia in the West are iron deficiency as a result of nutritional deficiencies or chronic blood loss, and 'in developing countries' malaria and chronic blood loss (Fig. 8.25).

Excessive chronic menstrual or gastrointestinal blood loss is the main cause – women of child-bearing age and older are mainly affected. About 5% of American women may have mild iron-deficiency anaemia and up to 25% may have low iron levels without anaemia. Neonates maintained on a milk diet may become iron deficient. Very many older children are mildly iron deficient because of the high demands for growth, especially during adolescence. By contrast, iron deficiency in an adult male almost invariably indicates blood loss, usually from the gastrointestinal or genitourinary tracts. The same holds true for post-menopausal women.

Clinical features

The important features of iron-deficiency anaemia are summarized in Box 8.8. Impaired exercise capacity, koilonychia (Fig. 8.26) and beeturia (urine appearing red after eating beetroot) may be seen. In childhood, iron deficiency may also predispose to developmental or behavioural disorders. However, symptoms ascribed to iron deficiency do not always respond to iron replacement.

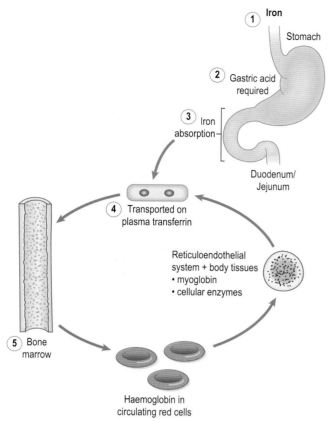

Fig. 8.24 Iron sources and fate

Labels in Fig. 8.24:
1. Iron — Stomach
2. Gastric acid required
3. Iron absorption — Duodenum/Jejunum
4. Transported on plasma transferrin
Reticuloendothelial system + body tissues
• myoglobin
• cellular enzymes
5. Bone marrow
Haemoglobin in circulating red cells

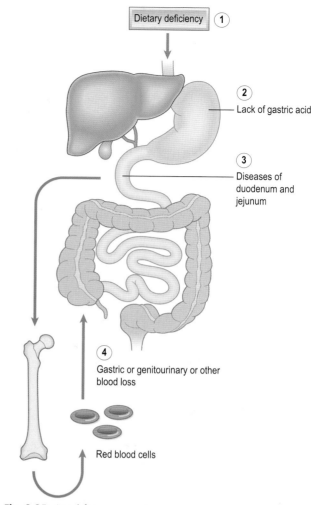

Fig. 8.25 Iron-deficiency anaemia

Labels in Fig. 8.25:
1. Dietary deficiency
2. Lack of gastric acid
3. Diseases of duodenum and jejunum
4. Gastric or genitourinary or other blood loss
Red blood cells

General management

Iron deficiency is the main cause of a microcytic anaemia (Table 8.24). In the early stages, stainable iron is lost from the bone marrow (Table 8.25): deficiency only appears after stores are depleted. Erythrocyte size changes show as an abnormal red cell distribution width on automated red cell sizing, before the transport iron, serum iron and ferritin levels fall.

Falling serum ferritin levels are one of the most sensitive indices of iron deficiency, but this test is not universally available and the level rises in inflammation as ferritin is an acute-phase protein. The serum iron-binding capacity rises and transferrin saturation (total iron binding capacity/serum iron) falls: a value of less than 16% indicates iron deficiency. Declining erythrocyte size (microcytosis and a low MCV) follows, with rising red cell protoporphyrin concentrations. Later there is a fall in haemoglobin and a hypochromic microcytic anaemia. Hypochromic microcytic anaemia with normal marrow iron stores is not caused directly by iron deficiency but is a feature of thalassaemia and sideroblastic anaemia, as discussed later.

The cause of the iron deficiency must be sought and treated. The best treatment for iron deficiency is an iron salt such as ferrous sulfate 200 mg three times daily orally, which is better absorbed than ferric salts. Ferrous gluconate 250 mg/day can be given if ferrous sulfate is not tolerated. Nausea or constipation are fairly common. The stools are black whilst on oral iron therapy and this should not be mistaken for melaena. Oral iron may need to be given for 3 months or more after the haemoglobin has reached normal levels, to replenish marrow iron stores.

Box 8.8 Causes of iron deficiency

- Achlorhydria
- Blood loss
- Dietary ignorance
- Malabsorption
- Old age
- Poor iron intake
- Poverty

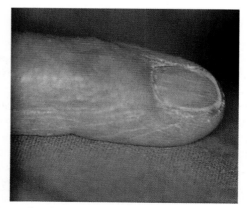

Fig. 8.26 Koilonychia

Parenteral iron does not raise the haemoglobin level more rapidly than oral iron, it must be given intramuscularly, and it may cause reactions including arrhythmias. Parenteral iron only has advantages when, for example, the patient cannot take iron by mouth or when inflammatory bowel disease is aggravated by oral iron.

Dental aspects

Local anaesthesia is satisfactory for pain control. Conscious sedation can be given if full oxygenation is possible. For GA, see earlier.

A sore, physically normal tongue can develop before the haemoglobin falls below the lower limit of normal. Atrophic glossitis – soreness of the tongue with depapillation or colour change – is the best known effect of severe anaemia. It is seen much less frequently than in the past. The Paterson–Brown-Kelly (Plummer–Vinson) syndrome of glossitis and dysphagia with hypochromic (iron deficiency) anaemia is uncommon. Women are mainly affected and the prevalence appears to be highest in northern Europe. There is a substantial risk of carcinoma in the post-cricoid region or in the mouth (Fig. 8.27). Candidosis can be aggravated or precipitated by anaemia and may be the presenting feature. Angular stomatitis is a well-known sign of iron-deficiency anaemia, but it affects only a minority. Nowadays it is more frequently caused by infection, mainly by *Candida albicans*, which may be promoted by the anaemia itself. Occasionally, adequate treatment of anaemia alone, without antifungal treatment, relieves the infection. The

majority of patients with chronic mucocutaneous candidosis, particularly the familial and diffuse types, are also iron deficient and treatment with iron appears to improve the response to antifungal treatment.

Aphthous-like ulceration is sometimes associated with iron deficiency, which, if remedied, can sometimes bring about a cure. Deficiencies should be suspected, especially in patients of middle age or over who develop ulcers.

Staining of the teeth by iron can be prevented in children by using sodium iron edetate as the iron source, as it is also sugar-free and more palatable than ferrous sulfate. Some iron preparations can cause tooth erosion as can chewable vitamin C.

Vitamin B₁₂ (cobalamin) deficiency

General aspects

Vitamin B$_{12}$ is needed by the body to synthesize and break down amino acids, and to synthesize DNA/RNA. This is needed to build new cells, especially blood, skin and mucosal cells. Vitamin B$_{12}$ is found in the diet in meat, especially liver.

Vitamin B$_{12}$ is bound to gastric intrinsic factor secreted by parietal cells, and absorbed in the terminal ileum. Vitamin B$_{12}$ is stored in the liver (Fig. 8.28).

Deficiency of vitamin B$_{12}$ is usually due to a defect in intrinsic factor (as a result of pernicious anaemia or gastrectomy), occasionally ileal disease or resection, or rarely a congenital ileal absorption defect a vegan diet or drugs (Box 8.9 and Fig. 8.29). Nitrous oxide can also interfere with vitamin B$_{12}$ metabolism and with neurological function if administration continues for 12 hours or more, or if it is used as a drug of abuse.

Lack of vitamin B$_{12}$ leads to accumulation of homocysteine (with a possible risk of cardiovascular disease) and methylmalonic acid. Pernicious (Addisonian) anaemia, the most common type of macrocytic anaemia, is caused by a specific defect of absorption of vitamin B$_{12}$, caused by autoantibodies against gastric parietal cells and/or the intrinsic factor. The underlying lesion is an atrophic gastritis causing failure of production of intrinsic factor by parietal cells and of gastric acid (achlorhydria). There may be gastrointestinal symptoms and also a greater risk of stomach cancer. Ultimately there is macrocytic (megaloblastic) anaemia with depressed production of all blood cells. Pernicious anaemia typically affects women in middle age or over, particularly of northern European descent. It is sometimes seen with other autoimmune diseases, especially hypothyroidism, or less often as a feature of the autoimmune polyendocrinopathy syndrome (Ch. 6). Pernicious anaemia

Table 8.24 Differential diagnosis of microcytosis

Index	Iron deficiency	Heterozygous α- or β-thalassaemia trait	Lead poisoning
Haemoglobin	Low	Low	Normal[a]
MCV	Low	Low	Normal[a]
RDW	Raised	Normal	Normal
FEP	Raised	Normal	Raised
Serum iron	Low	Normal	Normal
TIBC	Raised	Normal	Normal
Ferritin	Low	Normal	Normal

[a]May be low if the blood lead concentration is in excess of 100 mg/dl.
FEP, free erythrocyte protoporphyrin; MCV, mean corpuscular volume; RDW, red cell distribution width; TIBC, total iron-binding capacity.

Table 8.25 Laboratory findings during development of iron-deficiency anaemia

	MCV	Hb	MCHC	Serum ferritin	Transferrin saturation[a]	Marrow iron stores
Normal	N	N	N	N	33%	N
Mild anaemia	↓	N or ↓	N	↓	< 16%, < 33%	↓
Moderate anaemia	↓	↓	↓	↓	< 16%	↓
Severe anaemia	↓↓	↓↓	↓↓	↓↓	< 16%	↓↓

Hb, haemoglobin; MCHC, mean corpuscular haemoglobin concentration; MCV, mean corpuscular volume. Arrows indicate a value below normal (N).
[a]It is better to measure ferritin.

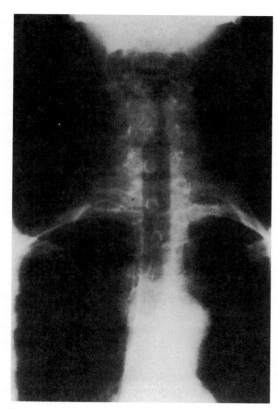

Fig. 8.27 Post-cricoid carcinoma in patient with Paterson–Brown-Kelly (Plummer–Vinson) syndrome

Box 8.9 Causes of vitamin B₁₂ deficiency

Autoimmune (pernicious anaemia)
Poor intake
• Strict vegetarians (vegans and some Hindu Indians)
Malabsorption
• Defective intrinsic factor production
• Congenital
• Gastrectomy
• Ileal disease
• Coeliac disease
• Tropical sprue
• Crohn disease (more frequently folate deficiency)
• Blind loop syndrome
• Resections
• Fish tapeworm (Finland, Asia)
• Transcobalamin II deficiency
Drugs (rarely)
• Colchicine
• Neomycin
• Nitrous oxide
• Omeprazole

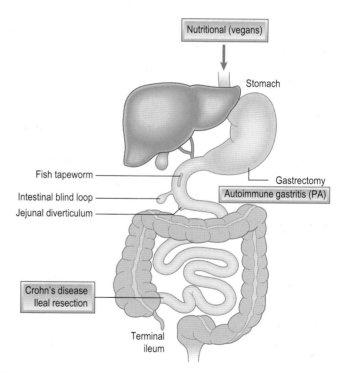

Fig. 8.29 Vitamin B₁₂ deficiency. PA, pernicious anaemia.

affects around 1 in 1000 of the north European population and about 1% of females over age 70.

Clinical features

Deficiency of vitamin B₁₂ develops slowly since liver stores last up to 3 years. In addition to the usual signs and symptoms of anaemia, neurological symptoms – particularly paraesthesiae of the extremities – develop in about 10%. Early signs include loss of toe positional sense and diminished perception of the vibration of a tuning fork. These early neurological changes are reversible with treatment.

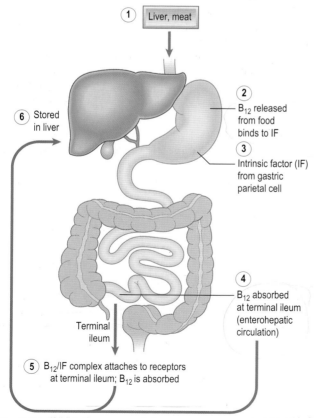

Fig. 8.28 Vitamin B₁₂ source and absorption

In the USA, 5% of persons over 50 appear to have low serum vitamin B_{12} levels. Neurological damage can precede anaemia or even macrocytosis, and lead to subacute combined degeneration of the spinal cord and, ultimately, paraplegia. Absence of macrocytosis is occasionally due to concomitant iron deficiency, but in another study on 70 patients with very low (less than 100 ng/L) serum vitamin B_{12} levels, anaemia was absent in 19% and macrocytosis was absent in 33%. In some of these cases, vitamin B_{12} deficiency was manifested first as cerebral abnormalities and what has been termed 'megaloblastic madness'.

Premature greying of the hair is another well-recognized feature.

General management

The diagnosis of pernicious anaemia depends on the clinical findings and low serum B_{12} levels together with autoantibodies against gastric parietal cells and/or intrinsic factor. Impairment of vitamin B_{12} absorption is shown by the Schilling test, summarized in Box 8.10.

Serum vitamin B_{12} levels may occasionally be low in the absence of an abnormal Schilling test, may be low even though there is no deficiency or may remain normal in patients who are deficient. Measurement of the raised serum levels of methylmalonic acid and homocysteine appears to be more sensitive and specific for deficiency than assay of serum vitamin B_{12} itself, though renal and other disorders may confuse the interpretation.

Pernicious anaemia is treated for life with intramuscular hydroxycobalamin 1 mg five times at 3-day intervals to replete liver stores, and then at about 3-monthly intervals.

Dental aspects

Local anaesthesia is satisfactory. Conscious sedation can be given if the haemoglobin level is only moderately depressed and supplemental oxygen can be given. Nitrous oxide is (theoretically) contraindicated. GA should be postponed until low haemoglobin has been remedied.

A physically normal, sore or burning tongue can be caused by early vitamin B_{12} deficiency, often with normal haemoglobin levels. It is important to have haematological examination of these patients. As discussed earlier, anaemia or macrocytosis may be absent at this stage. It can also, at this early stage, occasionally be associated with neurological disorders. In early B_{12} deficiency, the tongue is sore and may, alternatively, show a pattern of red lines without depapillation or red sore patches

may form. These may come and go, but range from pin-head red spots to circular areas up to a centimetre across, which may resemble erythroplasia clinically and, though they resolve with treatment of the anaemia, may show dysplasia histologically.

Paterson–Brown-Kelly syndrome is rarely associated with a macrocytic anaemia.

Candidosis can be aggravated or precipitated by anaemia and may be the presenting feature. Angular stomatitis is uncommon. Aphthous stomatitis is occasionally the presenting feature and pernicious anaemia should be considered when ulceration starts in middle age or later.

Folate (folic acid) deficiency

General aspects

Folic acid is needed by the body to synthesize and break down amino acids, and to synthesize DNA/RNA, needed to build new cells, especially blood, skin and mucosal cells. Folic acid is found in fresh leafy and other vegetables especially spinach, kale, Brussels sprouts and asparagus. Folic acid is absorbed from the proximal small intestine (Fig. 8.30). There are virtually no body stores of folic acid. Most folic acid deficiency is caused by dietary deficiency (Fig. 8.31). Some is caused by disease of the small intestine, such as coeliac disease, or drugs (Box 8.11), but occasionally no cause can be discovered.

Clinical features

The effects of folate deficiency are very similar to B_{12} deficiency. Both cause megaloblastic changes in the marrow and macrocytic anaemia, defective DNA synthesis, impaired production of blood cells and, ultimately, of many other cells.

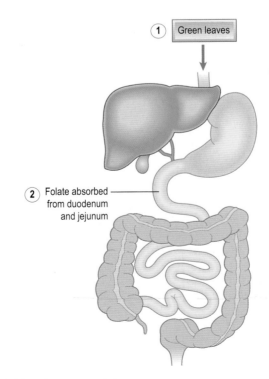

Fig. 8.30 Folate source and absorption

Box 8.10 Schilling test for vitamin B_{12} deficiency

1 Radiolabelled vitamin B_{12} (small dose) given orally
2 Unlabelled vitamin B_{12} (large dose) given i.m. 2 h later
3 Collect urine over 24 h (or whole-body counting)
• Normal: excrete more than 15% of radiolabelled B_{12} in 24 hours
• B_{12} deficiency: excrete less than 15% of radiolabelled B_{12} in 24 hours
4 Repeat with added intrinsic factor
• Pernicious anaemia: excretion of B_{12} increases to normal
• Ileal disease: excretion of B_{12} remains low

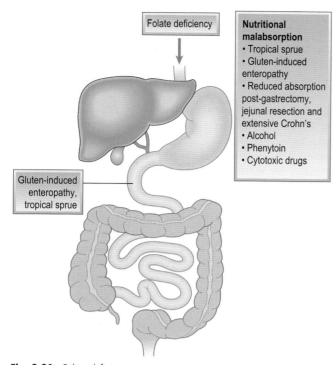

Folate deficiency

Nutritional
malabsorption
• Tropical sprue
• Gluten-induced
  enteropathy
• Reduced absorption
  post-gastrectomy,
  jejunal resection and
  extensive Crohn's
• Alcohol
• Phenytoin
• Cytotoxic drugs

Gluten-induced
enteropathy,
tropical sprue

Fig. 8.31 Folate deficiency

Box 8.11 Causes of folate deficiency

Poor intake
- Poverty
- Dietary ignorance
- Old age
- Alcoholism

Malabsorption
- Coeliac disease
- Crohn disease
- Other malabsorption states

Increased demands
- Infancy
- Pregnancy
- Chronic haemolysis (haemolytic anaemia)
- Malignant disease
- Exfoliative skin lesions
- Chronic dialysis

Drugs
- Alcohol
- Azathioprine
- Barbiturates
- Co-trimoxazole
- Methotrexate
- Oral contraceptives
- Pentamidine
- Phenytoin
- Primidone
- Pyrimethamine
- Sulfasalazine
- Triamterene
- Zidovudine

Folate deficiency in adults leads to anaemia. Folic acid deficiency in pregnancy appears to predispose to neural tube defects or cleft lip–palate in the fetus. Folic acid prophylaxis is thus recommended. Folate deficiency in adults does not lead to subacute combined degeneration of the cord. Folate deficiency in adults predisposes to raised homocysteine levels and possibly ischaemic heart disease.

General management

The red-cell folate levels are low, serum B_{12} normal and the B_{12} absorption (Schilling) test is normal; these tests enable the important distinction to be made from B_{12} deficiency. Red-cell folate levels, when low, are unequivocal evidence of folate deficiency but may remain normal for a time in a few folate-deficient patients until older erythrocytes are replaced. Serum folate assays are considerably less reliable.

Once the cause has been found and rectified, treatment with folic acid (5 mg daily by mouth) rapidly restores the normal blood picture. Treatment is usually given for at least 4 months.

Dental aspects

Local anaesthesia, conscious sedation and GA considerations apply as for pernicious anaemia, but there is no contraindication to nitrous oxide.

Soreness of the tongue without depapillation or colour change can be caused by early deficiencies, often with normal haemoglobin levels.

Atrophic glossitis is the best known effect of severe anaemia but is much less frequently seen than in the past. Angular stomatitis is also a well-known sign, but affects only a minority. Aphthous stomatitis is sometimes associated and, if remedied, can sometimes bring about a cure.

HAEMOLYTIC ANAEMIAS

General aspects

Haemolytic anaemia may result from: inherited abnormalities of haemoglobin formation (the haemoglobinopathies) or erythrocyte structure or function [spherocytosis; glucose-6-phosphate dehydrogenase (G6PD) deficiency], or from damage to erythrocytes (autoimmune, drug-induced or infective). Worldwide, malaria is the most common cause.

Clinical features

Accelerated erythrocyte destruction leads to bilirubin overproduction and sometimes jaundice. The spleen may enlarge and increased red cell turnover raises the reticulocyte count, plasma lactate dehydrogenase (LDH), bilirubin and uric acid levels. This raises the demand for folic acid and may in turn cause macrocytic changes.

General management

The cause should be treated if possible. Folic acid may be required and, in some instances, blood transfusion, but this carries the possibility of iron overload.

Dental aspects

Local anaesthesia is the safest method of pain control. Conscious sedation may be given, with supplemental oxygen if necessary. Any of the haemolytic anaemias may be a contraindication to GA but, in practical terms, sickle cell disease is by far the most important cause of difficulties in dental management.

Haemoglobinopathies

The fetus is normally born with fetal haemoglobin (HbF) as the main haemoglobin and, in infancy, this is replaced with adult haemoglobin (HbA) and a small amount of HbA2. These haemoglobins differ in their peptide chain composition (Table 8.26).

Table 8.26   Normal haemoglobins

Haemoglobin	Alpha chain	Beta chain	Gamma chain	Delta chain
Fetal HbF	2		2	
Adult HbA	2	2		
HbA2	2			2

Haemoglobinopathies are genetically determined disorders of haemoglobin production. Each of the haemoglobin peptide (globin) chains has a unique amino acid sequence, which can be altered as a result of DNA mutations. Qualitative defects in the production of haemoglobin then lead to 'variant haemoglobins'. Quantitative defects in the production of globins lead to the thalassaemias.

Haemoglobinopathies are seen mostly in non-Caucasians. Sickling disorders are common in Afro-Caribbean, Mediterranean, Middle Eastern, Indian, Bangladeshi and Pakistani patients (Fig. 8.32). In the UK, about one in ten Afro-Caribbeans and one in 100 Cypriots and Asians carry the sickle cell trait. Thalassaemias and G6PD deficiency are seen mainly in Mediterranean, Vietnamese, Cambodian, Laotian and Chinese peoples. In the UK, about one in ten from the Indian subcontinent, about one in 30 Chinese and one in 50 Afro-Caribbeans have thalassaemia.

Haemoglobinopathies result in consequences ranging from significant morbidity and mortality in sickle cell disease, to no significant clinical effect as in haemoglobin E disease. Patients may have combinations of more than one haemoglobinopathy. Short stature, abnormal skeletal development and jaundice are often found, in addition to signs and symptoms of anaemia.

The diagnosis of haemoglobinopathy rests on the history, examination and laboratory investigations. A family history is especially important. A full blood picture and red cell indices should be obtained and blood should also be sent for electrophoresis (4 ml of EDTA-anticoagulated blood) and for assay of variant haemoglobins. Special tests such as the Sickledex may also be useful (see later).

The sickling disorders

General aspects

Amino acid substitution in the Hb globin chain results in changes in haemoglobin (HbS), which assumes a propensity to polymerize or precipitate, causing gross distortions in the shape of erythrocytes, with impaired deformability and membrane damage. The erythrocytes cause vascular occlusions in the microcirculation. Integrins on the erythrocyte surface bind to vascular endothelial adhesion molecules, which are upregulated by tumour necrosis factor (TNF) and other pro-inflammatory cytokines, thus obstruction is more common during infections.

Inheritance in the sickling disorders is autosomal. Sickling disorders mainly affect people of African heritage. In West Africa about 2% of the population have sickle cell disease and up to 30% have the trait. Sickle cell trait is many times more common than sickle cell anaemia in Britain and affects some 10% of people of Afro-Caribbean descent, and 20% of African descent. The sickling disorders include the following (see Table 8.27).

Sickle cell *anaemia or disease* (HbSS is present in erythrocytes) is homozygous and usually a serious disease with widespread complications (Box 8.12). It frequently becomes apparent about the third month of life.

Sickle cell *trait* (HbSA is present) is heterozygous and at least ten times as common. Sickle cell trait is frequently asymptomatic, but sickle cell crises can be caused by low O_2 tension (see later; GA, high altitudes or unpressurized aircraft). At times such patients may have renal complications causing haematuria or splenic infarcts. Sickle cell trait may be associated with another haemoglobinopathy.

Clinical features

Sickle cell disease presents six main clinical problems as listed below.

Painful crises, which are usually due to infarction as a result of sickling, are brought on by infection, dehydration, hypoxia, acidosis or cold, and cause severe pain and pyrexia. Infarcts form mainly in the spleen (with eventual auto-splenectomy), bones and joints, brain, kidneys, lungs, retinae and skin. Bone

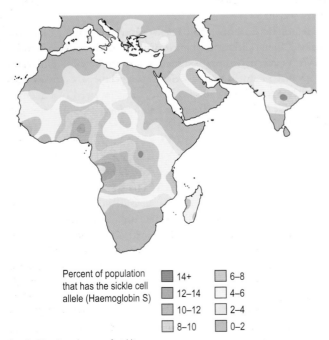

Percent of population that has the sickle cell allele (Haemoglobin S)

14+
12–14
10–12
8–10
6–8
4–6
2–4
0–2

Fig. 8.32 Distribution of sickling

Table 8.27 The sickling disorders

Disorder	Hb type	Origins of predominant ethnic groups affected	Clinical features
Sickle cell anaemia	SS	Africa, West Indies, Mediterranean, India	Severe anaemia
Sickle cell trait	SA	Africa, West Indies, Mediterranean, India	Usually asymptomatic
Sickle cell – HbC disease	SC	West Africa, South-East Asia	Variable anaemia
Sickle cell – HbD disease	SD	Africa, India, Pakistan	Moderately severe anaemia
Sickle cell – HbE disease	SE	South-East Asia	Moderately severe anaemia
Sickle cell – thalassaemia	SAF	Mediterranean, Africa, West Indies	Moderately severe anaemia

Box 8.12 Features of sickle cell anaemia

Anaemia
Crises
- Painful crises
- Aplastic crises
- Dactylitis – painful osteitis in the hands (Fig. 8.33)
- Infarcts of central nervous system, lungs, kidney, spleen, bone
- Skin ulcers
Haemolysis
- Jaundice
- Gallstones
- Reticulocytosis
Impaired growth
Skeletal deformities
Susceptibility to infections

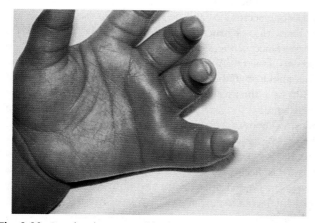

Fig. 8.33 Dactylitis showing painful red swellings

infarcts can cause inflammation and pain, especially in the hands and feet. Pulmonary infarcts cause chest pain and eventually lead to pulmonary hypertension and right-sided cardiac failure. The kidneys may also be affected, causing haematuria and a nephrotic syndrome. Ocular defects or a cerebrovascular accident – often with hemiplegia – are possible. Priapism is a sustained painful erection due to infarction in the corpora cavernosa. Abdominal crises may mimic a surgical emergency.

Haematological crises are caused by parvovirus infection and can be haemolytic, aplastic or sequestration.

Chronic anaemia – with a haemoglobin level often as low as 5–9 g/dl.

Chronic hyperbilirubinaemia predisposes to bile pigment gallstones.

Infections: an immune defect results from splenic infarction and dysfunction. The main cause of death in sickle cell disease is infection, particularly by pneumococci, meningococci, *Haemophilus* and salmonellae. Most patients are kept on prophylactic phenoxymethyl penicillin.

Sequestration syndromes – these include sequestration of sickle cells in:

- the lungs impeding gas exchange (chest syndrome)
- the spleen (septicaemia may result)
- the liver, or 'girdle syndrome' may be associated with bowel dilatation.

Morbidity and early mortality rates are high in sickle cell disease. Most eventually succumb to cardiac failure, renal failure, overwhelming infection or stroke.

General management
Sickling disorders should be suspected in those with a positive family history and in any patient of African, West Indian or (less frequently) Asian or Mediterranean descent. Many already carry warning cards (Fig. 8.34).

In sickle cell *disease*, the haemoglobin level is typically below 9 g/dl. Target cells, reticulocytosis of 5–25%, and sometimes sickled erythrocytes may be seen in a stained blood film. Haemoglobin electrophoresis shows mainly HbS and up to 15% HbF, but no HbA.

In sickle cell *trait*, haematological findings are often normal. Electrophoresis shows 40% HbS and up to 60% HbA.

Sickling may be demonstrated both in sickle cell *disease* and in *trait*, by tests relying on the low solubility of HbS (Sickledex; Fig. 8.35) or by the addition of a reducing agent (such as 10% sodium metabisulfite or dithionite) to a blood sample.

Patients with sickle cell *disease* need regular blood pictures, a comprehensive care programme, folic acid regularly and sometimes blood transfusions for cerebrovascular symptoms in early childhood or recurrent pulmonary thromboses. However, many patients remain with moderate degrees of anaemia for most of their lives. Transfusions can and should usually be minimised, especially because of the risk of hepatitis virus and HIV infection. A growing number of patients with sickle cell disease survive into late middle age. Infections and thromboses are the main causes of death.

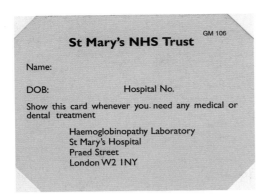

St Mary's NHS Trust

GM 106

Name:

DOB: Hospital No.

Show this card whenever you need any medical or dental treatment

Haemoglobinopathy Laboratory
St Mary's Hospital
Praed Street
London W2 1NY

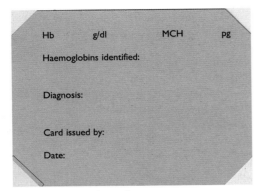

Hb   g/dl   MCH   pg

Haemoglobins identified:

Diagnosis:

Card issued by:

Date:

Fig. 8.34 Haemoglobinopathy card

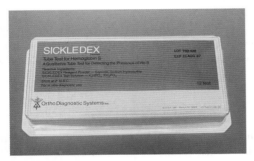

Fig. 8.35 Sickledex test

The main principles in patients with sickle cell *disease* are to prevent trauma, infection, hypoxia, acidosis or dehydration, all of which can precipitate a crisis. Infections must be treated early. Painful crises should be treated promptly with analgesics, such as diamorphine or pethidine, and hydration. Patients with sickle cell anaemia are treated with hydroxycarbamide (hydroxyurea), which raises the levels of HbF and iron-chelating agents (desferrioxamine, deferasirox or deferiprone).

Patients with sickle cell *trait* are less liable to complications from trauma, infection, hypoxia, acidosis or dehydration, but if severe these can precipitate a crisis.

Dental aspects

All those at risk from sickling disorders should be investigated if GA is to be given. Sickle cell anaemia is probable if the haemoglobin is less than 11 g/dl, and presents a hazard for GA. If the sickle cell test is positive, haemoglobin electrophoresis is required to confirm the diagnosis.

Patients with sickle cell *trait* (HbSA) present few problems in management but, if GA is necessary, full oxygenation must be maintained.

For patients with sickle cell *disease* (HbSS) LA is the preferred mode of pain control. It may be preferable to avoid prilocaine which may, in overdose, cause methaemoglobinaemia. Aspirin is best avoided as, in large doses, it may cause acidosis and precipitate a crisis; paracetamol and codeine are effective alternatives. Conscious sedation with relative analgesia can be used safely. At least 30% O_2 is needed and, provided that there is no respiratory depression or obstruction, normal procedures can be used. Benzodiazepines are best avoided.

Elective surgery should be carried out in hospital and during a phase when haemolysis is minimal. Anaemia should be corrected before GA and the haemoglobin brought up to at least 10 g/dl. Exchange transfusion is occasionally required for major surgery but only in selected patients. It carries the risk of red cell alloimmunization in up to 20%. Blood should be available for transfusion. At least 30% O_2 is needed and, provided that there is no respiratory depression or obstruction, normal anaesthetic procedures can be used. If a crisis develops, O_2 is given and bicarbonate infused. A packed red cell transfusion may be required if the haemoglobin falls below 50%.

Prophylactic antimicrobials (penicillin V or clindamycin) should be given for surgical procedures and infections must be treated vigorously, since the patient may be immunocompromised if the spleen is non-functional. As a consequence of multiple transfusions, some patients have become infected with blood-borne viruses. Drugs that can cause respiratory depression, including sedative agents, should not be given. Acidosis and hypotension must also be avoided.

Orofacial manifestations of sickle cell disease include painful infarcts in the jaws (which may be mistaken for toothache) or osteomyelitis. Pulpal symptoms are common in the absence of any obvious dental disease and sometimes pulpal necrosis has resulted. Lesions suggestive of bone infarction (dense radio-opacities) may be seen in the jaws and/or skull. Bone scans using technetium diphosphonate show stronger uptake in these areas. Radiographic findings include a 'stepladder' trabeculae pattern. Some patients have such severe pain during crises that they abuse analgesics and become addicts (Ch. 34). Hypercementosis may be seen. Bone marrow hyperplasia leads to an enlarged haemopoietic maxilla with excessive overjet, and overbite. Skeletal but not dental maturation is delayed. The skull is thickened but osteoporotic with a hair-on-end pattern to the trabeculae. The diploë are thickened, especially in the parietal regions, giving a tower skull appearance. Enamel hypomineralization and calcified pulp canals may be seen. The lamina dura is distinct and dense, and the permanent teeth may be hypomineralized, though neither caries nor periodontal disease is more severe.

The thalassaemias

Thalassaemias are autosomally dominant inherited disorders in which either alpha- or beta-globin chains are synthesized at a low rate, thereby lessening the production of haemoglobin A. The unaffected chains are produced in excess and precipitate within the erythrocytes to cause excessive erythrocyte fragility and haemolysis. Thalassaemias are characterized by a hypochromic microcytic anaemia. Thalassaemias are predominantly found in persons of Mediterranean, Middle Eastern or Asian descent. Thalassaemias may be severe (major; homozygous) or mild (minor; heterozygous) and may affect alpha-chain (alpha-thalassaemias) or beta-chain (beta-thalassaemias) production.

Alpha-thalassaemias

Alpha-thalassaemias result from deficient synthesis of alpha chains and are mainly found in Asians. There are four main subtypes, of varying degrees of severity. In alpha-thalassaemia major, there is no compensatory mechanism for the loss in alpha-chain production, so tetramers of the beta and gamma chains combine to form, respectively, haemoglobin H and Barts, both of which are ineffective O_2 carriers. Thus the condition is lethal *in utero* or infancy.

Beta-thalassaemias

General aspects Beta-thalassaemias (Mediterranean anaemia) result from the depressed production of beta chains. They mainly affect peoples from the Mediterranean littoral, Afro-Caribbeans, South-East Asians and Africans. In the homozygous form they can be life-threatening. A relative increase in delta and gamma chains is associated with raised levels of haemoglobin A_2 and F. Homozygous beta-thalassaemia (Cooley anaemia; thalassaemia major) is characterized by failure to thrive, increasingly severe anaemia, hepatosplenomegaly and skeletal abnormalities. Heterozygotes for beta-thalassaemia may be asymptomatic.

Clinical features Homozygotes for thalassaemia suffer from chronic anaemia, marrow hyperplasia, skeletal deformities, splenomegaly, cirrhosis, gallstones and iron overload. There is no pubertal growth spurt. Affected children are susceptible to folate deficiency (as in other chronic haemolytic states) and also to infection.

Patients with homozygous beta-thalassaemia become overloaded with iron (haemosiderosis) from high gut absorption and from repeated transfusions. The iron damages the heart (cardiac haemosiderosis), causing cardiomyopathy and arrhythmias, which often result in death in early adult life. Iron deposits cause liver and pancreas dysfunction, and deposits in salivary glands can cause a sicca syndrome. Some survive, probably because they have a milder variant, such as beta-thalassaemia with high levels of HbF.

Heterozygous beta-thalassaemia (thalassaemia minor or thalassaemia trait) is common and usually asymptomatic, except for mild hypochromic anaemia. Anaemia may be aggravated by pregnancy or intercurrent illness.

General management Diagnosis of beta-thalassaemia is confirmed by finding severe microcytic hypochromic anaemia with gross aniso- and poikilocytosis, target cells and basophilic stippling of erythrocytes, normal or raised serum iron and ferritin, and normal total iron-binding capacity (TIBC). There is a great increase in HbF and some increase in HbA2.

The main treatment measures in beta-thalassaemia are blood transfusions, folic acid supplements and iron-chelating agents (desferrioxamine, deferasirox or deferiprone) and ascorbic acid. Hydroxycarbamide is now used but the side-effects can be a significant disadvantage. Splenectomy may be required if there is hypersplenism causing greater blood destruction, which leads to accumulation of iron elsewhere and other complications.

Dental aspects Hepatitis B or C, or HIV carriage, may be a complication in repeatedly transfused patients. Since splenectomy results in an immune defect, it may be prudent to cover surgical procedures with prophylactic antimicrobials.

Local anaesthesia is safe. Conscious sedation may be given with oxygen levels not less than 30%. GA induction may be complicated by enlargement of the maxilla, which may cause difficulties in intubation, but in any event, the chronic severe anaemia, and often cardiomyopathy, are contraindications.

Orofacial manifestations include expansion of the diploë of the skull causing a hair-on-end appearance that is frequently conspicuous on lateral skull radiographs. Enlargement of the maxilla is caused by bone marrow expansion (chipmunk facies); there is often spacing of the teeth and forward drift of the maxillary incisors, so that orthodontic treatment may be indicated. Alveolar bone rarefaction produces a chicken-wire appearance on radiography. Pneumatization of the sinuses may be delayed. Less common oral complications include painful swelling of the parotids and xerostomia caused by iron deposition, and a sore or burning tongue related to the folate deficiency.

Sickle cell trait with another haemoglobinopathy

Persons who have sickle cell trait with another haemoglobinopathy, such as thalassaemia, or both sickle cell haemoglobin S and C (SC disease) are usually not as ill as those with isolated sickle cell disease. However, they are at about the same level of risk from GA as are those with sickle cell disease.

Patients with other combined defects should be managed in the same way as those with sickle trait alone.

Other haemoglobin variants

Other haemoglobin variants that can cause haemolytic anaemia, particularly when certain drugs are given, include Hb Zurich (which causes acute haemolytic reactions when sulfonamides are given), and HbH (a relatively common variant in the Far East in which oxidants cause acute haemolysis in homozygotes, similar to that in G6PD deficiency). Various drugs may worsen haemolysis and the physician must be consulted.

ERYTHROCYTE MEMBRANE DEFECTS

General and clinical aspects

Hereditary spherocytosis (acholuric jaundice) is the main form of congenital haemolytic anaemia in Caucasians. It is an autosomal dominant trait characterized by haemolytic anaemia, jaundice, splenomegaly, gallstones, haemochromatosis and skin ulcers. Episodes of haemolysis may be precipitated by infections.

Similar autosomal dominant disorders characterized by chronic haemolytic anaemia are *hereditary elliptocytosis (ovalocytosis)* and *hereditary stomatocytosis.*

General management

Splenectomy and folic acid treatment are almost invariably required.

Dental aspects

Local anaesthesia is safe. Conscious sedation or GA may be given if there is optimal oxygenation.

ERYTHROCYTE METABOLIC DEFECTS

The most common disorder of this type is glucose-6-phosphate dehydrogenase deficiency; various drugs are contraindicated (Table 8.28).

Table 8.28 Drugs in glucose-6-phosphate dehydrogenase (G6PD) deficiency	
Contraindicated	**Drugs with possible risk**
Dapsone Methylene blue (methylthioninium chloride) Nitrofurantoin and quinolones including ciprofloxacin, moxifloxacin, nalidixic acid, norfloxacin and ofloxacin Prilocaine Primaquine – although 30 mg weekly for 8 weeks has been found to be without harmful effects in African and Asian people Sulfonamides, including co-trimoxazole – although some sulfonamides like sulfadiazine are not haemolytic in many with G6PD deficiency Sulfonylureas	Aspirin – although up to 1 g daily is usually harmless Chloroquine, quinidine and quinine Vitamin K analogues (e.g. menadione and water-soluble derivatives like menadiol sodium phosphate)

ACQUIRED HAEMOLYTIC ANAEMIAS

These can be caused by factors such as gross trauma, complement-mediated lysis, toxins and malaria. These may occasionally have dental relevance because of anaemia, corticosteroid treatment or haemorrhagic tendencies.

Microangiopathic haemolytic anaemia (MAHA) is caused by fibrin strands depositing in small vessels and damaging erythrocytes. Causes include: pre-eclampsia; disseminated intravascular coagulopathy; malignant hypertension; thrombotic thrombocytopenic purpura – usually caused by a defect in breakdown of von Willebrand factor; and haemolytic–uraemic syndrome (HUS), which is usually caused by *Escherichia coli* with a verotoxin, or a defect in factor H – the complement regulatory protein.

OTHER ANAEMIAS

Aplastic anaemia

General aspects

Aplastic anaemia is pancytopenia with a non-functioning bone marrow. It is a rare disease causing leukopenia, thrombocytopenia and refractory anaemia.

Chemicals such as benzene, drugs, hepatitis viruses, irradiation and graft-versus-host disease (GVHD) are important causes (Box 8.13), but many cases are idiopathic, though probably immunologically mediated.

Clinical features

The clinical manifestations are those of anaemia (normochromic, normocytic or macrocytic) together with abnormal susceptibility to infection and bleeding. Purpura is often the first manifestation.

General management

The principles of management include removal of the cause (even when this is discoverable, as in the case of drugs such as chloramphenicol, marrow damage may still be irreversible); isolation and antibiotics to control infection; bone marrow transplantation [BMT; haemopoietic stem cell transplantation; HSCT (Ch. 35)] after intense immunosuppression [this in turn may cause GVHD, which is often fatal (Ch. 35)]; androgenic (anabolic) steroids may be of some value (corticosteroids are of questionable benefit); blood transfusion – but this carries risks from iron overload or infection.

The prognosis is poor and 50% of patients die within 6 months, usually from haemorrhage or infection. Iron overload may result from repeated blood transfusions.

Dental aspects

Treatment modification needs to take into consideration:

- anaemia
- haemorrhagic tendencies

Box 8.13 Causes of aplastic anaemia
Genetic
• Fanconi anaemia
• Dyskeratosis congenita
Immunological
• Autoimmune
• Graft-versus-host disease
Drugs
• NSAIDs
• Antithyroids
• Allopurinol
• Phenylbutazone
• Chloramphenicol
• Sulfonamides
• Gold
• Penicillamine
• Anticonvulsants
• Cytotoxic agents
Chemicals
• Benzene
• Toluene
• Heavy metals
• Glue-sniffing
Viruses
• Hepatitis
Irradiation

NSAIDs, non-steroidal anti-inflammatory drugs.

- susceptibility to infections
- effects of corticosteroid therapy (Ch. 6)
- hepatitis B and other viral infections (Ch. 9).

Local anaesthesia is satisfactory. Conscious sedation and GA should be avoided because of the anaemia.

Oral manifestations of aplastic anaemia, and management, are somewhat similar to those of leukaemia, viz. ulceration, haemorrhagic tendencies, and susceptibility to infections. Oral lichenoid lesions, or a Sjögren-like syndrome, may develop if there is GVHD following marrow transplantation to relieve the anaemia (see later and Ch. 35). Gingival swelling may develop if ciclosporin is used.

Fanconi anaemia

Fanconi anaemia is a rare autosomal dominant disorder with bone marrow failure, absent radii and predisposition to malignant disease, including oral cancer.

Pure red cell aplasia

Pure red cell aplasia is a rare disease which may be congenital or acquired. The latter is often associated with a thymoma and sometimes chronic mucocutaneous candidosis. These patients need regular blood transfusions and are therefore at risk from hepatitis viruses and HIV infection.

Anaemia caused by bone marrow infiltration

Bone marrow infiltration by abnormal cells (metastases, leukaemias, myeloma or myelofibrosis) causes normocytic anaemia and often leukopenia or thrombocytopenia with a leukoerythroblastic peripheral blood picture. There may be extramedullary haemopoiesis in other organs. Dental care may be complicated by susceptibility to infections, haemorrhage (as in aplastic anaemia) or the underlying disease.

Anaemia associated with systemic disease

Anaemia of various types may be associated with chronic systemic disorders which include chronic inflammation (infections, or connective tissue disease such as rheumatoid arthritis); neoplasms, particularly leukaemia; liver disease (Ch. 9); uraemia (Ch. 12); HIV infection (Ch. 20); or, rarely, endocrinopathies (hypothyroidism, hypopituitarism or hypoadrenocorticism (Ch. 6).

WHITE BLOOD CELLS

Several types of leukocyte (white blood cells) exist, but all are produced and derived from a multipotent bone marrow stem cell. Leukocytes are found throughout the body and are discussed in Ch. 20.

LEUKOPENIA (SEE CH. 20)

MALIGNANT DISEASE

Malignant diseases involving lymphoid cells (lymphoreticular malignancies – leukaemias and lymphomas) are potentially fatal. Lymphoid tissue is widely spread throughout the body, and thus lymphoreticular malignancies have wide effects.

In most forms of malignant disease, some form of staging is used to assist treatment planning and in making a possible prognosis. Staging aims to determine the spread of the malignant neoplasm from its original site. Staging is based on history, physical examination and investigations, such as blood tests, biopsies (e.g. of lesions; lymph nodes; bone marrow), and imaging – radiography, computed tomography (CT) and magnetic resonance imaging (MRI) scans or ultrasound.

Treatment of malignant disease can be with surgery, radiotherapy, cytotoxic drugs singly or in combination, stem cell transplantation, immunotherapy (monoclonal antibodies and, on the horizon, vaccines) and gene therapy.

Quality of life is as, or more, important than simply extending survival.

LEUKAEMIAS

General aspects

Leukaemias are potentially fatal diseases in which there is neoplastic proliferation of bone marrow white blood stem cells associated with specific gene mutations, deletions or translocations. The aetiology is unknown in most cases but may include a genetic predisposition (e.g. patients with Down syndrome) and exposure to ionizing radiation, chemicals such as benzene, or viruses.

Leukaemias are classified by:

- cell of origin (lymphoblast or non-lymphoblast)
- cell maturity – immature (acute) versus mature (chronic).

The classification allows a patient's prognosis to be assessed and has implications for treatment. The acute leukaemias are characterized by primitive blast cells in the blood and bone marrow. They account for nearly 50% of all malignant disease in children and are the most common cause of non-accidental death. A total of 85% of leukaemia in children is acute lymphoblastic leukaemia.

Chronic leukaemias are characterized by an excess of mature leukocytes in blood and bone marrow, and are mainly diseases of adult life. They are chronic disorders but may progress to acute leukaemia. In acute leukaemias, primitive blast leukocytes are released into the blood, whereas in chronic leukaemias the abnormal cells retain most of the morphological features of their normal counterparts.

Clinical features

Many of the manifestations of leukaemia arise from the crowding out of normal blood cells from the marrow by the leukaemic cells, leading to:

- anaemia (fatigue, pallor, etc.)
- thrombocytopenia (purpura and a bleeding tendency)

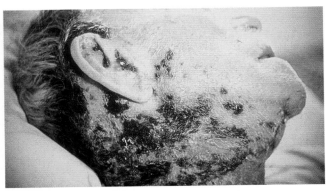

Fig. 8.36 Herpes zoster (shingles) of the upper cervical nerves in a patient dying from leukaemia

Table 8.29 Clinical features of leukaemia

Site of disease	Clinical manifestation
Bone marrow failure	
Anaemia	Pallor, lethargy, dyspnoea
Neutropenia	Recurrent infection
Thrombocytopenia	Mucosal bleeding and bruising
Tissue infiltration	
Lymphatics	Lymphadenopathy
Liver and spleen	Hepatosplenomegaly
Mediastinum	Hilar lymphadenopathy
Gingiva and skin	Gingival and skin deposits
Meninges and brain	Meningitis-like syndrome
Bone	Bone pain and pathological fractures

- liability to infections (Fig. 8.36)
- lymphadenopathy, especially in lymphatic leukaemias.

The different types of acute leukaemia are not reliably distinguishable clinically.

The clinical features of leukaemia are variable but broadly reflect the degree of tissue infiltration by the leukaemic cells and the extent of bone marrow failure (Table 8.29).

General management

Diagnosis and prognosis are established by haematological examination (especially a raised white cell count and blood film examination showing immature blast forms). This is supplemented by bone marrow biopsy, chest radiography, CT and MRI scans, and lumbar puncture. There is an excess of circulating white blood cells but there may be phases when few are released from the bone marrow (aleukaemic leukaemia). Cytochemistry, analysis of membrane markers and immunophenotyping are required for categorization of the cell type. Detection of chromosomal abnormalities may guide treatment and prognosis.

The treatment of leukaemia is dependent upon the accurate diagnosis and staging of the disease. It generally involves combination chemotherapy with a variety of cytotoxic agents such

Table 8.30 Examples of possible chemotherapy regimes for lymphoproliferative disorders

Disease		Agents
Acute leukaemias	ALL	Vincristine, prednisolone, asparaginase, daunorubicin
	AML	Daunorubicin and cytosine arabinoside
Chronic leukaemias	CLL	Sometimes chlorambucil
	CML	Hydroxycarbamide
Lymphomas	Hodgkin disease	ABVD or MOPP
	Non-Hodgkin lymphomas	CHOP

ABVD, Adriamycin, bleomycin, vinblastine, dacarbazine; ALL, acute lymphoblastic leukaemia; AML, acute myeloblastic leukaemia; CHOP, cyclophosphamide, doxorubicin hydrochloride, Oncovin, prednisolone; CLL, chronic lymphocytic leukaemia; CML, chronic myeloid leukaemia; MOPP, mustine, Oncovin (vincristine), procarbazine, prednisolone.

as shown in Table 8.30, and includes induction of remission with cytotoxic drugs singly or in combination and, increasingly, bone marrow transplantation (haemopoietic stem cell transplantation; Ch. 35). Post-remission treatment (consolidation) and, in some instances, maintenance therapy are indicated.

Newer treatments include retinoids, monoclonal antibodies, T-cell infusions, peptide vaccines and cytokines, such as granulocyte colony-stimulating factor (G-CSF). Minimal residual disease (MRD) may remain, and this guides further care. Prognosis of most leukaemias in the absence of treatment is very poor; few patients survive more than a year after diagnosis.

Cytotoxic chemotherapeutic drugs may need to be given by intravenous, oral, intramuscular, or intrathecal routes. Cytotoxic drugs damage all proliferating cells including epithelium, bone marrow and reproductive tissues. Their toxic nature causes nausea and vomiting, impaired immunity, alopecia and mucositis. They are also teratogenic. Patients are highly susceptible to infection at this time and may need to be isolated during the induction of remission. Supportive care includes control of nausea, infections, haemorrhagic tendencies, anaemia, hyperuricaemia (gout) and renal malfunction. Nausea may be controllable with phenothiazines (prochlorperazine) or domperidone or, if severe, by 5-hydroxytryptamine (5HT) antagonists such as granisetron.

Dental aspects

Orofacial manifestations include mucositis, ulcers or gingival swelling and bleeding.

Dental management can often be complicated by bleeding tendencies and susceptibility to infection. Septicaemias may spread from oral infections in these patients, as in other immunocompromised persons (Ch. 20).

Cytotoxic drugs are potentially hazardous to staff, who should only handle them wearing medical gloves and protective eyewear, should dispose of waste and sharps carefully, and should not handle them while pregnant.

Oral health care principles are summarized in Table 8.31.

Table 8.31 Synopsis of principles of oral health care in leukaemia

Pre-chemotherapy	During induction chemotherapy	During remission	Long term
Assessment Treatment planning Remove unsaveable teeth Treat caries Dietary advice Start fluoride prophylaxis Oral hygiene advice Start chlorhexidine prophylaxis	Continue preventive oral health care Antifungal prophylaxis (nystatin) Antiviral prophylaxis (aciclovir)	Continue preventive oral health care	Continue preventive oral health care Monitor craniofacial and dental development

Table 8.32 Acute leukaemia: typical features

General features	Features due to leukaemic infiltration of bone marrow	Features due to leukaemic infiltration of lymphoreticular system
Weight loss	Anaemia (pallor)	Lymphadenopathy
Weakness	Bone pain	Splenomegaly
Anorexia	Ineffective leukocytes (infections)	Thrombocytopenia (purpura and bleeding from mucous membranes)

Box 8.14 Considerations in the care of acute lymphoblastic leukaemia

- Abnormal susceptibility to infection – patient may be kept in isolation, such as in a laminar flow room, when strict asepsis is indicated. Antimicrobial cover is needed for surgery, particularly for those with indwelling atrial catheters
- Anaemia
- Bleeding tendencies
- Complications of bone marrow transplantation (haemopoietic stem cell transplantation; Ch. 35)
- Corticosteroid treatment (Ch. 6)
- Disseminated intravascular coagulopathy
- Hepatitis B or C (Ch. 9) and human immunodeficiency virus (HIV) infection (Ch. 21; pre-operative precautions include screening for hepatitis B and HIV in blood transfusions)
- Interaction between methotrexate and nitrous oxide (largely theoretical)

Acute lymphoblastic leukaemia (ALL)

General aspects

Acute lymphoblastic leukaemia (ALL) is the most common childhood leukaemia; it has a peak incidence at 2–4 years but can affect any age group. Aetiological factors may include ionizing radiation and exposure to benzene. Electromagnetic radiation from power lines has little observable effect.

Acute lymphoblastic leukaemia is usually a B-lymphocyte neoplasm. Malignant lymphoblasts proliferate and infiltrate the bone marrow (causing granulocytopenia, anaemia and thrombocytopenia), viscera, skin and nervous system.

Clinical features

Anaemia, lymphadenopathy, splenomegaly, infections, fever, bruising and bleeding tendencies are the main features. Central nervous system (CNS) involvement is not uncommon. ALL is clinically indistinguishable from non-lymphoblastic (myeloblastic) leukaemia (Table 8.32).

General management

Treatment is initially with cytotoxic drugs including vincristine and prednisolone plus an anthracycline (daunorubicin or idarubicin). Intravenous plus intrathecal methotrexate may be used to combat CNS involvement. Over 90% of children have a remission within 6 weeks. During induction of remission, the child may need to be kept in isolation, such as in a laminar flow room, because of the high susceptibility to infection. Strict asepsis is indicated, live vaccines must not be given and infected persons should be kept away.

The risk of relapse is greatest in the first 18 months and maintenance therapy is usually continued for 2–3 years. Relapse is higher in males, partly because of occult testicular or CNS disease. Methotrexate weekly and vincristine and steroids monthly form a common regimen. Craniospinal irradiation is no longer routine in low-risk ALL patients but intrathecal methotrexate may be given. Bone marrow transplantation (haemopoietic stem cell transplantation; Ch. 35) may give better control if chemotherapy fails to prevent relapse. The 5-year survival rate is over 50%.

Dental aspects

Dental treatment should only be carried out after consultation with the physician, as it may be affected by various aspects of management and the probable life expectancy.

Preventive oral health care is essential and, where indicated, conservative dental treatment may be possible. Surgery should be deferred (except for emergencies such as fractures, haemorrhage, potential airways obstruction or dangerous sepsis) until a remission phase.

The main dental management problems to consider in ALL are listed in Box 8.14.

Regional LA injections may be contraindicated if there is a severe haemorrhagic tendency. Conscious sedation is usually possible. Anaemia may be a contraindication to GA – intravenous sedation or relative analgesia may be used as alternatives. However, nitrous oxide, which interferes with vitamin B_{12} and hence folate metabolism, is possibly contraindicated if the patient is being treated with methotrexate. The toxic effects of the latter may be exacerbated.

Because of the dangers of haemorrhage and infections such as osteomyelitis or septicaemia, desmopressin or platelet infusions or blood may be needed pre-operatively, and antibiotics given until the wound has healed. Penicillin is the antibiotic of choice; intramuscular injections should be avoided as a haematoma may result. Sockets should not be packed, as this appears to predispose to infection. Operative procedures must be performed with strict asepsis and with the least trauma. Absorbable polyglycolic acid sutures are preferred.

Aspirin and other NSAIDs should not be given, since they can aggravate bleeding.

Oropharyngeal lesions can be the presenting complaint in over 10% of cases of acute leukaemia. Oral bleeding and petechiae are typical manifestations, together with mucosal pallor and sometimes gingival swelling (localized or generalized), mucosal or gingival ulceration, pericoronitis and cervical lymphadenopathy. Severe bleeding from the mouth, particularly from the gingival margins, may result from the thrombocytopenia. It needs treatment with desmopressin or even platelet transfusion. Gentle oral hygiene measures should control gingivitis which, otherwise, aggravates the bleeding.

Herpetic oral and perioral infection is common and troublesome, as are varicella-zoster infections. They should be treated vigorously, usually with aciclovir. Varicella-zoster (VZV) and measles viruses can also cause encephalitis or pneumonia. Prophylactic aciclovir has greatly reduced the incidence, morbidity and mortality from VZV infections, including those secondary to bone marrow transplants.

Candidosis is particularly common in the oral cavity and the paranasal sinuses, and usually caused by *Candida albicans*. Prophylactic antifungal therapy, such as nystatin mouthwashes or pastilles, or amphotericin lozenges, is therefore indicated. Fluconazole-resistant candidal species and a rising number of cases of infection with *Candida krusei* are seen.

Aspergillosis or mucormycosis can involve the maxillary antrum and be invasive.

Bacterial infections with Gram-negative species occasionally cause oral lesions, which can be a major source of septicaemia or metastatic infections in leukaemic patients. Lesions tend to become infected with bacteria such as *Pseudomonas* or *Escherichia*, or with *Candida* or *Aspergillus*. In severely immunosuppressed patients, over 50% of systemic infections result from oropharyngeal micro-organisms. Microbiological investigations with care to obtain specimens for anaerobic culture are essential to enable appropriate antimicrobial therapy to be given. Meticulous oral hygiene should be carefully maintained, with regular frequent warm 0.2% aqueous chlorhexidine mouth rinses and the use of a soft nylon toothbrush.

Gram-negative bacteria can sometimes form a white adherent plaque on the tongue.

Other oral findings include tonsillar swelling, paraesthesiae (particularly of the lower lip), extrusion of teeth, and painful swellings over the mandible and of the parotid (Mikulicz syndrome).

Bone changes seen on radiography may include destruction of the crypts of developing teeth, thinning or disappearance of the lamina dura, especially in the premolar and molar regions, and loss of the alveolar crestal bone. Bone destruction near the apices of mandibular posterior teeth may also be seen. These bone changes may be reversible with chemotherapy.

Many of the cytotoxic drugs can precipitate mucositis, with oral ulceration.

Adult acute lymphoblastic leukaemia

Adult acute lymphoblastic leukaemia has a worse prognosis than childhood ALL, but treatment schedules are similar.

Acute non-lymphoblastic (myeloblastic) leukaemia (ANLL)

General aspects

Acute non-lymphoblastic (myeloblastic) leukaemia (ANLL) is less common than ALL in children. Acute myeloblastic leukaemia (AML) is the most common of the seven subtypes described, and is the most common acute leukaemia of adults. Acute promyelocytic leukaemia is seen particularly in Hispanic peoples in the USA.

Clinical features

Anaemia, lymphadenopathy, splenomegaly, infections, fever, bruising and bleeding tendencies are the main features. CNS involvement is rare, though the disease occasionally causes cranial nerve palsies.

General management

Combination chemotherapy has greatly improved the prognosis in AML but is less successful than in childhood ALL. High-dose cytarabine (Ara-C) with an anthracycline, and sometimes with thioguanine or etoposide, is often used. Allopurinol is also needed for hyperuricaemia. Remission can be obtained in up to 85% of patients but is rarely maintained. Whenever possible, bone marrow transplantation (haemopoietic stem cell transplantation; Ch. 35) is employed and 5-year survival rates of up to 60% are then reported.

Some patients with AML have been treated with the monoclonal antibody gemtuzumab, or antibody linked to a chemical toxin, calicheamicin.

Acute promyelocytic leukaemia is frequently successfully treated with the vitamin A analogue, all-trans retinoic acid (ATRA). Arsenic trioxide, a recently introduced agent, may also be used to treat this subtype of acute leukemia.

Dental aspects

Treatment modifications are as provided earlier for ALL. Orofacial manifestations develop in 65–90% of cases (Box 8.15).

Oral bleeding and petechiae are typical manifestations, together with mucosal pallor and sometimes gingival swelling (localized or generalized), mucosal or gingival ulceration, pericoronitis and cervical lymphadenopathy. Acute myeloblastic leukaemia particularly may cause gingival swelling in 20–30% of patients. Gingival swelling results from an abnormal response to dental plaque, causing the tissues to be distended by dysfunctional white cells. Improvement in oral hygiene, aided by chlorhexidine, for example, can greatly ameliorate or abolish the swelling. ATRA, used in the treatment of acute promyelocytic leukaemia, may also cause gingival swelling.

Box 8.15 Oral and perioral manifestations of leukaemia

Lymph node enlargement
Pallor
Purpura, and bleeding from gingivae
Infections
- Candidosis and other fungal infections
- Herpesvirus infections

Oral ulceration
- Caused by herpesviruses, drugs and other factors

Gingival swelling
- Caused by leukaemic infiltrate

Drug side-effects
- Mucositis and ulceration (many of the cytotoxics)
- Dry mouth [doxorubicin (Adriamycin)]
- Pigmentation (busulfan)
- Candidosis (antimicrobials)

Chronic lymphocytic leukaemia

General aspects

Chronic lymphocytic leukaemia (CLL) is the most common type of leukaemia. In 10% there is a positive family history of the disease. Men are particularly affected; CLL is rare in Asians. CLL is almost invariably a B-cell neoplasm but there are several variants (Table 8.33).

Table 8.33 Chronic lymphoid leukaemias[a]

Disorder	Particular features
Chronic lymphocytic leukaemia	Splenomegaly, skin lesions
	Prolonged survival possible
Sézary syndrome	Generalized lymph node enlargement; pruritus; exfoliating erythroderma, sometimes oral deposits
	Chemotherapy relatively ineffective
Hairy cell leukaemia	Splenomegaly; may be associated with HTLV-1 infection; predisposes to mycobacterial infection
	Relatively long survival
	Responds to interferon-alpha
Prolymphocytic leukaemia	Splenomegaly; resistant to chemotherapy and radiotherapy
Adult T-cell leukaemia–lymphoma	Resembles lymphocytic leukaemia
	Poor prognosis

[a]Except for T-cell leukaemia and Sézary syndrome, which involve T cells, most involve B cells.
HTLV-1, human T-lymphotropic virus 1.

Clinical features

Many patients with CLL are asymptomatic, some 60% of cases are detected coincidentally during a blood screen for an unrelated reason, and life expectancy may not be affected.

In others, CLL is insidiously progressive, with fatigue, fever, weight loss, anorexia, lymphadenopathy, haemorrhage and infections. Lymph nodes enlarge early, whereas the liver and spleen enlarge later. Other effects are anaemia and thrombocytopenia. Leukaemic infiltration of the skin is more common than in chronic myeloid leukaemia and may be a major manifestation. In some, autoimmune disorders, such as haemolytic anaemia or thrombocytopenia, or both (Evan syndrome), may develop.

About 15% of patients with CLL undergo transformation to a more rapidly progressive form of leukaemia, or lymphoma (Richter syndrome).

General management

Asymptomatic patients may not need treatment. Those patients who are symptomatic can be treated with radiotherapy and cytotoxic drugs, usually:

- CHOP – cyclophosphamide, doxorubicin, vincristine (Oncovin) and prednisolone
- CAP – cyclophosphamide, doxorubicin (Adriamycin) and prednisolone
- CVP – cyclophosphamide, vincristine and prednisolone.

Fludarabine and other purine analogues (pentostatin; cladribine) are second-line drugs, which are effective but predispose to infections. Chlorambucil is particularly effective, though it predisposes to epithelial cancers. It may be used with steroids or cyclophosphamide. The monoclonal antibody alemtuzumab has helped some patients who are refractory to chemotherapy. Splenectomy may be needed. The 5-year survival is over 50%. Interferon, 2-deoxycoformycin and cladribine are used for hairy cell leukaemia.

Dental aspects

The prognosis of chronic leukaemia is better than for acute leukaemia and routine dental treatment is more likely to be required. Close cooperation with the haematologist is needed since there may be:

- bleeding tendencies
- liability to infection
- anaemia
- susceptibility to hepatitis B, C and HIV infection.

In addition, ampicillin and amoxicillin may cause irritating rashes similar to those seen in infectious mononucleosis and unrelated to penicillin allergy. Gingival bleeding, oral petechiae or oral ulceration may also be features. Ulceration may be aggravated by cytotoxic therapy. Herpes simplex or zoster, and candidosis, are common. Gingival swelling is less frequent than in the acute leukaemias. Palatal swelling (submucosal leukaemic nodules) may develop. Drug treatment of chronic leukaemia can also cause oral complications.

Local anaesthesia is satisfactory. Conscious sedation can be given if required. GA must be carried out in hospital.

Chronic myeloid leukaemia

General aspects

Chronic myeloid leukaemia (CML) is characterized by proliferation of myeloid cells in the bone marrow, peripheral blood and other tissues. A total of 90% of patients with CML have the Philadelphia chromosome and the BCR-ABL gene, which can aid diagnosis and treatment monitoring. Most patients with CML suffer from chronic granulocytic leukaemia (CGL) and are over 40 years of age, but there are several rare subgroups (Table 8.34).

Table 8.34 Chronic myeloid leukaemia

Disorder	Particular features
Chronic granulocytic leukaemia	Splenomegaly
	Positive for Philadelphia chromosome
	Fairly responsive to chemotherapy
Atypical chronic granu-locytic leukaemia	Negative for Philadelphia chromosome
	Less responsive to chemotherapy
Juvenile	Mainly young children; lymphadenopathy. Poor response to chemotherapy
Chronic myelomonocytic leukaemia	Little response to chemotherapy
Chronic neutrophilic leukaemia	Difficult to differentiate from a benign leukocytosis
Eosinophilic leukaemia	Eventual cardiac damage

Clinical features

Anaemia, weight loss, joint pains, splenomegaly and hepatomegaly are common but lymphadenopathy is rare.

Chronic myeloid leukaemia, after about a 4–5-year phase, transforms to an acute phase similar to AML (blast crisis). Fever, haemorrhage or bone pain are then common.

General management

Treatment choices for CML include interferon-alpha alone or with other drugs, or a donor or autologous stem cell transplant. Imatinib mesylate has recently been shown to normalize blood cell counts in nearly all patients with CML and is advocated where the response to interferon is poor. It acts by blocking the BCR-ABL gene-encoded protein. Radiotherapy may be useful later.

The prognosis of CML is variable, but sooner or later there is transformation to a blast crisis. In blast transformation, the same treatment is given as for AML, but the acute phase is usually refractory and the patient may die within a few months.

Dental aspects

The prognosis of chronic leukaemia is better than for acute leukaemia and routine dental treatment is more likely to be required. Close cooperation with the haematologist is needed since there may be:

- bleeding tendencies
- liability to infection
- anaemia
- susceptibility to hepatitis B, C and HIV infection.

Side-effects of treatment include pulmonary fibrosis as a result of busulfan. Ampicillin and amoxicillin may cause irritating rashes. These are similar to those seen in infectious mononucleosis and unrelated to penicillin allergy. Interferon-alpha can disturb taste and cause xerostomia.

In CML, oral haemorrhage may result from platelet deficiency. Leukaemic infiltration can cause swelling of lacrimal and salivary glands (Mikulicz syndrome). Granulocytic sarcoma is a rare tumour-like proliferation of leukaemic cells, which can affect the jaws or soft tissues and may rarely precede other manifestations or herald a blast crisis.

Drug treatment of chronic leukaemia can also cause oral complications.

MYELODYSPLASTIC (PRE-LEUKAEMIC) SYNDROMES

General aspects

The myelodysplastic syndromes (MDSs; Box 8.16) are a group of diseases found especially in the elderly that originate in a bone marrow stem cell. Though the bone marrow is initially active, erythrodyspoiesis and dysplastic changes develop later.

There is a tendency to transform to acute myeloid leukaemia. The poor quality of the blood cells means that a significant number of them are destroyed, leading to pancytopenia.

Box 8.16 The myelodysplastic syndromes

- Refractory anaemia alone (RA)
- Refractory anaemia with ring sideroblasts (RAS)
- Refractory anaemia with excess blasts (RAEB)
- Refractory anaemia with blasts in transformation (RABT)
- Chronic myelomonocytic leukaemia (CML)

Clinical features

Myelodysplastic syndromes mainly affect males over the age of 60 who have neutropenia, macrocytic anaemia and/or thrombocytopenia.

The usual signs and symptoms are therefore excessive tiredness on exertion, breathlessness, bleeding, easy bruising, infection and enlargement of spleen or liver. Some patients succumb to marrow failure.

General management

Diagnosis is from examination of blood and bone marrow. There is usually a monocytosis.

Treatment of MDSs is mainly supportive, since the majority of patients with these syndromes are too old to be eligible for a bone marrow transplant. This treatment includes erythrocyte and platelet transfusions, erythropoietin, G-CSF or granulocyte–macrophage colony-stimulating factor (GM-CSF), antibiotics, folic acid and vitamin B_6, and systemic corticosteroids.

Dental aspects

Dental management may be complicated by:

- bleeding tendencies due to thrombocytopenia
- anaemia
- neutropenia and a liability to infection, including hepatitis B and HIV (Ch. 20)

Table 8.35 Important findings in myeloproliferative diseases

	RBC count	WBC count	Platelet count	Alkaline phosphatase	Marrow fibrosis	Splenomegaly
Polycythaemia rubra vera	↑	↑	↑	↑	−	+
Agnogenic myeloid metaplasia	↓	↑	N or ↑	↑	+	++
Essential thrombocythaemia	N	N	↑↑↑	N	−	+

RBC, red blood cell; WBC, white blood cell. Arrows indicate a value above (↑) or below (↓) normal (N).

- corticosteroids (Ch. 6)
- gingival infiltration and oral ulceration may develop in CML but not in the other myelodysplastic syndromes.

HYPEREOSINOPHILIC SYNDROME

Hypereosinophilic syndrome (HES) is an uncommon disorder in which there is hypereosinophilia in the absence of allergic disease. T-cell proliferation or parasitic infestation, together with disease of various organs, especially cardiomyopathy, and various rashes are typical. Mucosal erosions and ulcers may be an early feature. HES is sometimes pre-lymphomatous.

Management is with systemic corticosteroids and usually hydroxycarbamide, or interferon.

MYELOPROLIFERATIVE DISORDERS

Myeloproliferative disorders, characterized by proliferation of bone marrow cells other than leukocyte stem cells, are regarded as separate entities from leukaemias but may progress to acute leukaemia. They have several common features, and transition between them is common (Table 8.35). All are rare. Chronic granulocytic leukaemia is sometimes also included in this group.

Polycythaemia rubra vera

General aspects

Polycythaemia is an expansion mainly in the red cell population. It may be primary and idiopathic and associated with normal erythropoietin levels. Polycythaemia rubra vera (PRV; Fig. 8.37) is mainly a disease of the elderly, of smokers, has a slight male predominance and also causes proliferation of other blood cells.

Clinical features

Red cell overproduction leads to hyperviscosity syndrome (see later) and the risk of thromboses because of changes in platelets and clotting mechanisms. Stroke, myocardial infarction or less serious consequences can follow.

Granulocyte overproduction and excessive cell turnover may lead to hyperuricaemia, gout and renal damage. Platelet overproduction with platelet dysfunction leads to haemostatic defects, bruising or bleeding. Bone marrow replacement by erythropoietic tissue causes bone pain and there may eventually be myelofibrosis, and myeloid metaplasia in the liver and spleen.

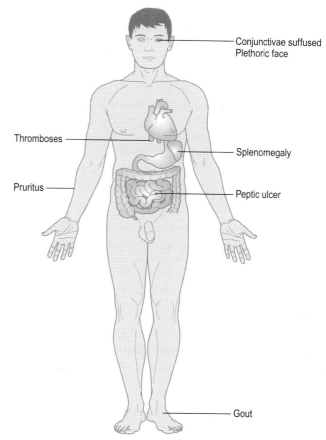

Fig. 8.37 Polycythaemia

General management

In the absence of treatment, few patients with PRV survive more than 2 years.

Repeated venesection shrinks the red cell mass and extends survival to more than 10 years. Phosphorus-32 is also a simple and effective method of depressing erythropoiesis but may increase the risk of leukaemia. Cytotoxic agents (busulfan, chlorambucil or melphalan) may be given to suppress marrow activity, especially if there is thrombocytosis, but they also raise the risk of neoplasia. Cyproheptadine to control pruritus and allopurinol for gout may also be needed.

Dental aspects

The main dental management problems are susceptibility to thrombosis and haemorrhage. Venesection is especially important, if surgery is indicated, since post-operative morbidity and mortality are greatly increased by thrombotic complications.

Local anaesthesia regional blocks should be avoided. Conscious sedation can be given. GA is a matter for expert attention in hospital.

There may be oral complications from cytotoxic chemotherapy.

Agnogenic myeloid metaplasia and myelofibrosis

General aspects

Myelofibrosis may be primary (agnogenic myeloid metaplasia) or it may be secondary to PRV, carcinomatosis or tuberculosis. Most patients are elderly.

Clinical features

Fibrosis of the bone marrow gradually depresses cell proliferation and extends throughout the reticuloendothelial system. There may be loss of weight, anaemia, thrombocytopenia purpura and bleeding tendencies, weakness, bone pain, splenomegaly, hepatomegaly, and gout.

General management

Most patients need correction of anaemia and thrombocytopenia by transfusion. Bone pains and hyperuricaemia also need to be controlled. Corticosteroids are used occasionally. The median survival time is about 5 years, but less in myelofibrosis secondary to carcinomatosis or polycythaemia.

Dental aspects

Management problems may result from:

- anaemia
- haemorrhage
- possible hepatitis B and C or HIV carriage
- corticosteroid treatment.

Essential thrombocythaemia

General aspects

Thrombocythaemia may be an isolated abnormality or associated with other myeloproliferative disorders.

Clinical features

The common effects are thromboses or haemorrhages. There is usually gross thrombocytosis with functionally defective, giant platelets.

General management

Radioactive phosphorus is the treatment of choice. If this fails, cytotoxic drugs are used. Aspirin and dipyridamole are useful for preventing thrombosis, but heparin may be required.

Dental aspects

Surgery must be avoided until the disease is controlled, particularly because of the haemorrhagic tendencies.

CRYOGLOBULINAEMIA

Cryoglobulinaemia is a condition where cryoglobulins – immunoglobulins that precipitate when cooled below the normal body temperature – are formed.

Cryoglobulins are of three main types as follows.

- Type I is monoclonal, and a typical feature of lymphoproliferative and related diseases.
- Types II and III are typically associated with connective tissue diseases and infections, where the effects may result from immune complex formation.

Cryoglobulins can occasionally cause effects as a result of their physical properties, particularly Raynaud phenomenon. Occasionally they cause peripheral thromboses and obstruction of small vessels. Purpura or bleeding tendencies may also result. Plasmapheresis may be beneficial.

LYMPHOMAS

Lymphomas are solid tumours that originate in lymph nodes or extranodal lymphoid tissue in any part of the body, from any type of lymphocyte. Lymphocytic lymphoma may be associated with lymphocytic leukaemia.

Lymphomas comprise Hodgkin and non-Hodgkin types (Table 8.37). They are not reliably distinguishable clinically.

Most lymphomas are non-Hodgkin lymphomas (NHL). About 10% of all lymphomas are Hodgkin disease, which can affect any age group but particularly males in their thirties.

Classification of lymphomas has been confusing; the European Organization for Research and Treatment of Cancer (EORTC) classification (1997) and the World Health Organization (WHO) classification of haematological malignancies (2000) – the Revised European–American Lymphoma (REAL) modification – are usually used (Table 8.36).

Microscopic appearance, immunological characterization of the cell lineage and the clinical extent of the disease (staging) determine the treatment and prognosis (Table 8.37). The higher the stage, the worse the prognosis.

Treatment often includes chemotherapy given under various acronyms (Table 8.38) and irradiation.

Dental management may be complicated by anaemia, liability to infection and radiation, corticosteroid or cytotoxic therapy.

Hodgkin disease

General aspects

Hodgkin disease appears to originate in a cell of the monocyte-histiocyte series, and is defined by the presence of the Reed–Sternberg cell. It is usually classified using the REAL/WHO classification.

Hodgkin disease may be related to Epstein–Barr virus (EBV) infection, and the prevalence is greater in persons who are immunocompromised.

Table 8.36 Revised European–American Lymphoma (REAL)/World Health Organisation (WHO) classification of lymphomas

Classical Hodgkin disease	
Lymphocyte rich	
Nodular sclerosing	
Mixed cellularity	
Lymphocyte depleted	
Nodular lymphocyte predominant (some suggest this is NHL)	
Non-Hodgkin lymphoma (NHL)	
Nodular	**Indolent course usually**
Poorly differentiated lymphocytic	Most frequent; disseminated
Mixed cellular (lymphocytic and histiocytic)	Good response to chemotherapy
Histiocytic	Aggressive; behaves like diffuse
Diffuse	**Aggressive course usually**
Lymphocytic	Chronic if well differentiated
	Others disseminated
Mixed cellular	Disseminated
Histiocytic	Formerly called reticulum cell sarcoma
Lymphoblastic	50% develop acute lymphoblastic leukaemia
Burkitt lymphoma	Good response to chemotherapy

Table 8.37 Staging and treatment in lymphomas

Stage[a]	Definition	Treatment
I	Involvement of a single lymph node or group of nodes	Radiotherapy
II	Involvement of two or more groups of lymph nodes on one side of diaphragm, or localized involvement of an extralymphatic organ or site and of one or more lymph nodes on the same side of diaphragm	Radiotherapy
III	Involvement of lymph nodes on both sides of diaphragm ± splenic or other sites	Radiotherapy (IIIA) or quadruple therapy (IIIB)[b]
IV	Diffuse or disseminated disease of one or more extralymphatic organs or tissues ± associated lymph node involvement	Quadruple therapy[b]

[a]Stage is also qualified by a suffix A or B. B, presence of fever, night sweats or weight loss; A, absence of such systemic symptoms.
[b]Quadruple therapy is combined chemotherapy, either MOPP or ABVD (Table 8.39).

Table 8.38 Chemotherapeutic regimens

Acronym	Regimen
ABVD	Adriamycin, Bleomycin, Vinblastine, Dacarbazine
CHOP	Cyclophosphamide, Adriamycin, Oncovin, Prednisolone
M-BACOD	Methotrexate, Bleomycin, Adriamycin, cyclophosphamide, Oncovin, Decadron
m-BACOD	Methotrexate, Bleomycin, Adriamycin, Cyclophosphamide, Oncovin, Decadron
MOPP	Mechlorethamine, Oncovin, Procarbazine, Prednisone
Pro-MACE-MOPP	Prednisone, Methotrexate, Adriamycin, Cyclophosphamide, Etoposide followed by MOPP
Pro-MACE-CytaBOM	Prednisone, Methotrexate, Adriamycin, Cyclophosphamide, Etoposide, Cytarabine, Bleomycin, Oncovin, Methotrexate
MACOP-B	Methotrexate, Adriamycin, Cyclophosphamide, Oncovin, Prednisone, Bleomycin
PACEBOM	Prednisone, Adriamycin, Cyclophosphamide, Etoposide, Bleomycin, Oncovin, Methotrexate
COPP	Cyclophosphamide, Oncovin, Procarbazine, Prednisone
BEACOPP	Bleomycin, Etoposide, Adriamycin, plus COPP

Clinical features

There is progressive involvement of lymphoid tissue, often beginning in the neck (Fig. 8.38). The lymph nodes become enlarged, discrete and rubbery, and can cause symptoms by pressure on other organs or ducts. Alcoholic drinks may cause pain in affected lymph nodes in nodular sclerosing Hodgkin disease.

Systemic symptoms, which indicate a poor prognosis, include pain, remittent fever, night sweats, weight loss, malaise, bone pain and pruritus. Anaemia is common late in the disease.

Cellular immunity is impaired so that fungal and viral infections are common and may disseminate.

General management

Treatment of Hodgkin disease includes chemotherapy and radiotherapy depending on the staging of the disease (Ann Arbor staging). ABVD was the commonly used chemotherapeutic regimen. However, it can damage heart and lungs. BEACOPP is more effective (Table 8.37).

Radiotherapy, especially mantle radiotherapy, may be required. This can lead to radiation damage to lungs (pneumonitis), heart (pericarditis) and thyroid (hypothyroidism), and predisposes to acute leukaemia.

With such management, the 5-year survival in the earlier stages approaches 100% and is over 60% even in more advanced Hodgkin disease. Those who relapse usually do so within the first 2 years.

Hodgkin disease pursues a more aggressive course in HIV disease.

Dental aspects

The main problems from lymphomas that may influence oral health care are:

- anaemia
- corticosteroid therapy
- bleeding tendencies

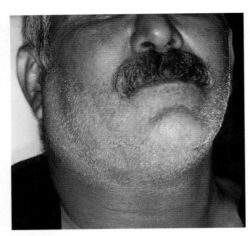

Fig. 8.38 Lymphoma

- impaired respiratory function (pulmonary fibrosis due to irradiation)
- mediastinal irradiation – may impair lung function or cause cardiac disease
- acute leukaemia (7% of treated patients).

Local anaesthesia regional blocks should be avoided if there is any haemorrhagic tendency. Conscious sedation may be given if required. GA is a matter for expert attention in hospital. Orofacial manifestations are as follows.

- Painless enlarged cervical lymph nodes are the initial complaint in 50%.
- Hodgkin disease very rarely affects the mouth. When it does, it is not clinically distinguishable from NHL.
- Oral infections, especially with viruses and fungi.
- Mucositis and oral ulceration caused by cytotoxic drugs.
- Xerostomia (from irradiation involving salivary glands).
- Herpes zoster, herpetic stomatitis and oral candidosis, especially in those on cytotoxic or radiation therapy. Zoster, secondary to immunodeficiency, may be the first sign of the disease.
- Hodgkin disease of salivary glands is exceptionally rare and usually involves juxtaglandular lymphoid tissue.

Non-Hodgkin lymphomas

General aspects

Non-Hodgkin lymphomas (NHL) are more common than Hodgkin disease and have a variable but generally poor prognosis. European types of NHL (seen in Europe, USA and Australia) are seen mainly in older persons, differ in age profile from NHL in other areas and are growing in frequency.

Most NHLs are of B-cell origin. NHLs are more frequent in association with immune defects such as HIV infection, in which NHL may be EBV-related and is second only to Kaposi sarcoma in frequency. Chronic immunosuppression or cytotoxic chemotherapy also predispose to the condition. Post-transplantation lymphoproliferative disease is often NHL.

NHLs are more frequent in association with connective tissue diseases and may sometimes have a recognized microbial aetiology, such as Epstein–Barr virus, hepatitis C virus, HTLV-1, or *Helicobacter pylori*.

A further strong risk factor is a family history of NHL, which entails a 3–4-fold greater risk to relatives. Weaker factors are occupational exposure, especially to pesticides and herbicides, and a weak, inconsistent association with hair dye use.

Clinical features

Non-Hodgkin lymphomas have a predilection for sites such as the gastrointestinal tract and CNS. They frequently involve the mesenteric lymph nodes and bone marrow, but often enlargement of cervical lymph nodes is the first sign.

General management

Non-Hodgkin lymphomas are broadly classified as either indolent (usually follicular types) or aggressive (usually diffuse). NHL is staged along the same lines as Hodgkin disease. In general, NHL is treated by multiple chemotherapy, since early dissemination is common. CHOP is the standard treatment. Chlorambucil or fludarabine may be used for indolent NHL. Treatment of B-cell lymphomas using rituximab, an antibody directed at the CD20 antigen on follicular lymphoma cells, has become important.

Dental aspects

The main problems from lymphomas that may influence oral health care are:

- oral infections, especially with viruses and fungi
- mucositis or oral ulceration caused by cytotoxic drugs
- anaemia
- corticosteroid therapy
- bleeding tendencies
- impaired respiratory function (pulmonary fibrosis due to irradiation)
- acute leukaemia (7% of treated patients)
- painless enlarged cervical lymph nodes are the initial complaint in 50% of cases.

Local anaesthesia regional blocks should be avoided if there is any bleeding tendency. Conscious sedation can be given if required. GA should be given in hospital.

Lymphomas rarely form in the oral cavity or oropharynx, but more frequently in HIV infection. Involvement of Waldeyer's ring is more common in NHL than in Hodgkin disease. Lesions appear as erythematous swellings, often with surface ulceration as a result of trauma. The jaws are rarely involved.

Herpes zoster, herpetic stomatitis and oral candidosis may be seen, especially in those receiving cytotoxic or radiation therapy.

Non-Hodgkin lymphoma is one of the most common types of non-epithelial tumour of salivary glands in adults, but accounts for only about 5% of salivary gland tumours. Its diagnosis causes difficulties in this site because of possible confusion with benign lymphoepithelial lesion and Sjögren syndrome, and the fact that these may progress to lymphoma in about 20% of cases.

Other lymphomas

African Burkitt lymphoma is often EBV-related, and is seen particularly in children, presenting mainly with jaw swellings but also frequently involving abdominal viscera. It responds well to chemotherapy.

T-cell lymphomas are rare but the cause of midline granuloma syndrome. The mouth may be involved by spread from the nasal cavity.

Nasopharyngeal (peripheral) T-cell lymphomas

Nasopharyngeal (peripheral) T-cell lymphomas can be clinically indistinguishable from Wegener granulomatosis in their early stages. If allowed to progress, they can cause mid-facial destruction, which if neglected can be so severe as to open the cranial cavity to the exterior. In such cases, death from intercurrent infection was common.

Downward spread of the disease from the nasal cavity can lead to palatal necrosis and ulceration. In such cases, superimposed infection from the oral cavity can seriously confuse the microscopic picture and make diagnosis even more difficult. In uncomplicated cases, the microscopic picture is highly pleomorphic but typically characterized by angiocentric and angiodestructive changes, which mimic vasculitis.

T-cell lymphomas can have a highly variable course, sometimes with prolonged survival or even apparently spontaneous remissions. Wide dissemination follows sooner or later.

The optimal form of treatment is therefore uncertain, but radiotherapy and cytotoxic chemotherapy may be effective if the disease is not too far advanced.

Midline granuloma syndromes (fatal midline granuloma)

This group of diseases starts in the nasal or paranasal tissues and can cause mid-facial destruction, sometimes of hideously disfiguring degree (so-called Stewart-type granuloma) and often with a fatal systemic involvement (Table 8.39).

These 'idiopathic' diseases mainly affect adults between 40 and 50 years of age, males more than females, and are usually nasopharyngeal T-cell lymphomas (the so-called Stewart-type granuloma) or Wegener granulomatosis diseases, which are not reliably distinguishable clinically (Box 8.17).

The most common upper respiratory tract symptoms are nasal stuffiness and crusting, and often discharge, which can be bloody.

PLASMA CELL DISEASES

Plasma cells derive from B lymphocytes. Plasma cell diseases are uncommon disorders, sometimes termed paraproteinaemias or monoclonal gammopathies, characterized by overproduction of a specific immunoglobulin detectable on electrophoresis, and often dominating other proteins (Box 8.18).

These homogeneous immunoglobulins (monoclonal immunoglobulins) are defective (leading to immunodeficiency), and the rates of production of immunoglobulin light or heavy chains may be unbalanced, leading to overproduction of light chains appearing in urine (Bence Jones protein) or heavy chains detectable in the serum and urine (Table 8.40).

Table 8.39 Features of the main types of idiopathic midline granuloma syndrome

	Wegener granulomatosis	Peripheral T-cell lymphomas
Destruction of facial skeleton and soft tissues	±	+++
Systemic involvement	Pulmonary cavitation Glomerulonephritis	Predominantly lymphatic spread. Liver, kidneys or other viscera may become involved
Biopsy findings	Necrotizing vasculitis, fibrinoid necrosis, multiple giant cells, ill-formed granulomas	Highly pleomorphic cellular picture, T cells recognizable by immunocytochemistry. Angiocentric and angiodestructive changes
Suggested treatment	Cyclophosphamide or azathioprine + prednisolone[a]	Radiotherapy + cytotoxic chemotherapy

[a]Or co-trimoxazole.

Box 8.17 Important causes of midline granuloma syndromes

- Idiopathic
- Wegener granulomatosis
- Peripheral T-cell lymphomas[a]
- B-cell lymphomas (rarely)
- Infections
- Tuberculosis[b]
- Syphilis[b]
- Deep mycoses

[a]Previously called lymphomatoid granulomatosis, polymorphic reticulosis, midline malignant reticulosis, Stewart-type granuloma, etc.
[b]Unlikely to be seen as a cause of this syndrome now.

Box 8.18 Plasma cell diseases (dyscrasias)

- Multiple myeloma
- Solitary myeloma
- Waldenstrom macroglobulinaemia
- Heavy-chain disease
- Idiopathic monoclonal gammopathy

Multiple myeloma (myelomatosis: Kahler disease)

General aspects

Multiple myeloma is a disseminated plasma cell neoplasm, predominantly causing bone lesions. The malignant plasma cells produce defective immunoglobulins and release osteoclast-activating factors, which cause bone resorption and pain.

Multiple myeloma is a disease mainly of the middle-aged and elderly. It has a slight predilection for males and is occasionally related to exposure to ionizing radiation or petroleum products.

Clinical features

Abnormal serum immunoglobulins form early and are occasionally detectable by chance during routine haematological examination, by a raised ESR, rouleaux formation or high

Table 8.40 Paraproteins found in the serum and urine in plasma cell diseases

	Serum	Bence Jones proteinuria
Heavy-chain disease	Alpha chain (or gamma or mu)	–
Idiopathic monoclonal gammopathy	IgG (or IgA or IgM)	–
Multiple myeloma	IgG (50%)	+
	IgA (25%)	
	IgD or IgE rarely	
Waldenstrom macroglobulinaemia	IgM	Rarely

Ig, immunoglobulin.

Box 8.19 Multiple myeloma: clinical findings

- Bone infiltration and destruction
- Bone pain (especially spinal)
- Pathological fractures
- Hyperviscosity syndrome
- Weakness
- Visual disturbances
- Bleeding tendencies
- Renal failure
- Anaemia
- Susceptibility to infections
- Neurological lesions
- Paraesthesiae
- Weakness

Box 8.20 Multiple myeloma: investigational findings

Radiological osteolytic lesions
Biochemical
- Hypergammaglobulinaemia
- Bence Jones proteinuria
- Monoclonal IgG (less often IgA, rarely IgD or IgE) on electrophoresis of serum or urine (IgG in 55%, IgA in 25% and only light chains in 20%)
- Plasma cell proliferation on marrow biopsy
- Uraemia (in renal disease)
- Hypercalcaemia
- Hyperuricaemia (after treatment)

Haematological
- Normochromic anaemia
- Leukopenia
- Thrombocytopenia
- ESR very high

Skeletal radiographs or bone scanning
- Osteolytic lesions

ESR, erythrocyte sedimentation rate; Ig, immunoglobulin.

plasma viscosity, or serum protein investigations. Many years may elapse before symptoms appear.

Neoplastic proliferation of plasma cells in the bone marrow and their release of cytokines, such as interleukin-1, ultimately cause pain, osteolysis and bone destruction, hypercalcaemia, suppression of haemopoiesis, and other secondary effects. Circumscribed areas of bone destruction are typically seen in the vault of the skull. The defective immunoglobulins may lead to plasma hyperviscosity with a clotting or bleeding tendency, renal failure, liability to infections and neurological sequelae (Box 8.19).

General management

Diagnostic findings include those listed in Box 8.20.

Symptomatic patients, or those with progressive bone lesions or worsening paraproteinaemia, are treated by chemotherapy with melphalan, cyclophosphamide or chlorambucil plus corticosteroids. More complicated chemotherapeutic regimens have not been shown to be consistently superior, though relapses are probably best treated with vincristine, Adriamycin (doxorubicin) and dexamethasone (VAD). New treatments include interferon, thalidomide, revlimid, lenalidomide, bortezomib, bone marrow transplantation (haemopoietic stem cell transplantation; Ch. 35) and haemopoietic growth factors. Bisphosphonates, such as pamidronate, help prevent pathological fractures.

The prognosis is variable, but the survival of treated symptomatic patients averages 3 years. Anaemia, chronic renal failure, low serum albumin and high levels of serum beta2-microglobulin in the absence of renal disease, indicate a poor prognosis. A few patients treated with cytotoxic chemotherapy develop acute myelomonocytic leukaemia.

A growing number of asymptomatic patients are found to have myelomatosis by electrophoretic evidence of hypergammaglobulinaemia. Such patients must be followed and treatment started when appropriate.

Dental aspects

Dental treatment may be complicated by anaemia, infections, haemorrhagic tendencies, renal failure or corticosteroid therapy.

The skull, especially the calvarium, is ultimately affected with rounded, discrete (punched-out) osteolytic lesions in about 70%. Jaw lesions are seen less frequently but can be the first sign. Small, punched-out, osteolytic lesions involving the posterior mandible are typical. Root resorption, loosening of teeth, mental anaesthesia and, rarely, pathological fractures are other possible effects. Rare complications are gingival bleeding, oral petechiae, cranial nerve palsies and herpes simplex or zoster infections. Amyloid may be deposited in the oral soft tissues causing local or more widespread swellings, such as macroglossia, the nature of which can be confirmed by biopsy.

Melphalan can cause severe mucositis. Biphosphonates may cause osteonecrosis.

Solitary plasmacytoma

Solitary plasmacytomas (localized myeloma) occasionally form in the jaws or soft tissues nearby, and are more likely than bone lesions to remain localized for a time. There is usually no abnormal immunoglobulin production but, even when present, levels are low.

Local radiotherapy may be useful, but cytotoxic chemotherapy is contraindicated. Patients should be kept under observation as multiple myeloma develops in many, even after 20 years.

Waldenstrom macroglobulinaemia (primary macroglobulinaemia)

General aspects

Macroglobulinaemia is a rare disease in which B lymphocytes produce excessive amounts of monoclonal IgM.

Clinical features

The large monoclonal IgM molecules increase blood viscosity and cause hyperviscosity syndrome (see later).

There is usually also anaemia, recurrent infections and haemorrhagic tendencies and a wide variety of other possible manifestations, particularly lymphadenopathy and splenomegaly. In contrast to myeloma, foci of bone destruction and hypercalcaemia are not features, and renal involvement is uncommon.

The prognosis of macroglobulinaemia is slightly better than that of myeloma, but it may progress to lymphoma and a more rapid termination.

General management

The clinical course is very variable, nearly 25% of patients need no treatment for long periods and there is a median survival of over 3 years.

Dental aspects

The major problems of dental treatment are bleeding tendencies, corticosteroid therapy (Ch. 6) or anaemia. Local anaesthesia regional blocks should be avoided if there is a bleeding tendency. Conscious sedation can be given if required. GA must be given in hospital.

Haemorrhagic tendencies may cause spontaneous gingival bleeding or post-extraction haemorrhage. Deep punched-out ulcers of the tongue, buccal mucosa or palate may form, but are rare.

HEAVY-CHAIN DISEASES

Heavy-chain diseases are rare disorders in which gamma, alpha or mu immunoglobulin heavy chains appear in serum and urine. Gamma-chain disease (Franklin disease) may cause palatal swelling due to lymphoid proliferation in Waldeyer's ring.

Benign monoclonal gammopathy

Benign monoclonal gammopathy or monoclonal gammopathy of undetermined significance (MGUS) is when excessive amounts of monoclonal immunoglobulins are found in the serum of elderly patients who otherwise appear healthy. Investigations are needed to rule out myeloma (Table 8.41).

Benign is only a relative term. Prolonged follow-up is essential since 20% ultimately develop myeloma and some others die from amyloid renal disease. However, it is essential not to interpret this finding as necessarily indicating myeloma.

Amyloid deposition in the tongue may cause macroglossia.

Table 8.41 Differentiation of myeloma from monoclonal gammopathy

	Myeloma	Benign monoclonal gammopathy
Plasma paraprotein level at presentation	High	Low
Plasma paraprotein levels observed over months and years	Rise	Stable
Other plasma immunoglobulin levels	Depressed	Normal
Imaging	Bone lesions	No evidence of lesions

Secondary macroglobulinaemia

Large amounts of serum IgM, which is often polyclonal and not a precursor to myeloma or macroglobulinaemia, can be an incidental finding on blood examination. It can be secondary to chronic disorders such as connective tissue diseases, liver disease or lymphocytic leukaemia.

Hyperviscosity syndrome

General aspects

Hyperviscosity syndrome is caused by excessive amounts of high-molecular-weight plasma proteins, which adsorb to platelets and erythrocytes causing excessive platelet adhesiveness and erythrocyte rouleaux formation.

Polycythaemia, Waldenstrom macroglobulinaemia or myeloma account for most cases.

Clinical features

Hyperviscosity syndrome is characterized by slowing of the peripheral circulation. The large protein molecules also activate clotting factors and complement, causing local thrombosis and inflammation.

General management

Venesection may be tried. Plasmapheresis reduces the viscosity, but treatment should be aimed at the primary condition. Penicillamine is useful for a short period only, since the side-effects can be severe.

Dental aspects

Gingival or post-extraction haemorrhage, or taste loss and oral ulceration due to penicillamine, may be features.

LANGERHANS CELL HISTIOCYTOSIS (SOLITARY AND MULTIFOCAL EOSINOPHILIC GRANULOMA)

Langerhans cell histiocytosis is a group of tumours or tumour-like lesions of Langerhans cells, antigen-presenting counterparts of macrophages. This cell is recognizable on electron microscopy by the presence of rod-shaped Birbeck granules and by immunohistochemistry. The three main types of Langerhans cell histiocytosis are shown in Table 8.42.

Solitary eosinophilic granuloma

General aspects

Eosinophilic granuloma is an osteolytic lesion of bone with a predilection for the mandible.

Clinical features

Adults mainly are affected. Typical symptoms are pain, tenderness, swelling or bone destruction.

General management

Radiographs show a tumour-like area of rarefaction. A bone scan should be carried out to ensure that the disease is not multifocal. Diagnosis is confirmed by biopsy typically showing foamy histiocytes and eosinophils with ill-defined, somewhat fibrillar background and areas of necrosis.

Eosinophilic granuloma is relatively benign and sometimes resolves spontaneously. Otherwise it responds to curettage or, if recurrent, to modest doses of irradiation, or chemotherapy.

Dental aspects

Eosinophilic granuloma is an osteolytic lesion of bone with a predilection for the mandible. It can produce a characteristic form of periodontal destruction with gross gingival recession and alveolar bone loss, typically involving a small group of teeth and often exposing the roots of the teeth, with a 'teeth floating in air' appearance on radiography.

Eosinophilic granuloma can also affect the oral soft tissues, but less frequently than the mandible. However, a histologically somewhat similar lesion (eosinophilic granuloma or ulcer) can be traumatic in origin or reactionary without any history of trauma and there is some doubt about the nature of eosinophilic granulomas of soft tissues reported in the past. 'Traumatic' eosinophilic granuloma eventually resolves spontaneously, though it may need to be excised for cosmetic reasons. Alternatively, the lesion may be excised because of its clinical resemblance to a tumour.

Multifocal eosinophilic granuloma and Hand–Schuller–Christian disease

General aspects

These lesions are the same histologically as the solitary eosinophilic granuloma and are sometimes referred to indifferently as Hand–Schuller–Christian disease.

Clinical features

Multifocal eosinophilic granuloma most frequently develops before the age of 5 years.

Hand–Schuller–Christian disease, strictly speaking, comprises osteolytic lesions of the skull, exophthalmos and diabetes insipidus; it is a variant of multifocal eosinophilic granuloma but develops in only 25%.

Flat bones, including the mandible, are the main sites. Soft tissues also become involved. Lymphadenopathy and hepatosplenomegaly may develop in up to 50%. Malaise, fever and infections of the ear, mastoid and respiratory tract are common.

General management

Diagnosis is by biopsy, which shows essentially the same features as solitary eosinophilic granuloma. Skeletal radiography or bone scans show the extent of the disease.

In approximately 50%, the lesions gradually resolve spontaneously over the course of years but can leave residual disabilities as a result of limb lesions or diabetes insipidus. To reduce such complications, or in refractory cases, chemotherapy in relatively modest doses may be given as for solitary lesions. The mortality may be 25–30%. The younger the patient and the more widespread the disease, the worse the prognosis.

Dental aspects

Complications can arise from radiotherapy to the oral or para-oral regions, or chemotherapy with corticosteroids or cytotoxic agents.

Table 8.42 Langerhans cell histiocytoses

	Age of onset	Bone lesions	Skin or mucosal lesions	Visceral lesions	Pituitary lesions	Treatment	Prognosis
Solitary eosinophilic granuloma	> 10 years	+	+/−	−	−	Surgery local radiotherapy	Good
Multifocal eosinophilic granuloma (Hand–Schuller–Christian disease)	< 5 years	+	+	±	+	Chemotherapy	Variable
Letterer–Siwe disease	Infancy	+	+	+	+	Chemotherapy Steroids	Often fatal

Multifocal eosinophilic granuloma of childhood or Hand–Schuller–Christian disease rarely has initial manifestations in the jaws. However, it can produce a characteristic form of periodontal destruction like that seen in solitary eosinophilic granuloma.

Letterer–Siwe disease

General aspects

Letterer–Siwe disease typically affects children between the ages of 2 and 3 years.

Clinical features

The main features of Letterer–Siwe disease are lymphadenopathy, hepatosplenomegaly, and bone and skin lesions. Fever, infections and bleeding tendencies are secondary to pancytopenia, which results from marrow displacement by the histiocyte-like cells.

It sometimes follows a rapidly fatal course. Rarely death follows within a week of diagnosis.

General management

Diagnosis is by biopsy, showing infiltration of the tissues by proliferating histiocyte-like cells. Treatment is with radiotherapy, corticosteroids and cytotoxic drugs, and may be successful. Occasionally the course of the disease is less acute and recoveries are possible.

Dental aspects

In view of the age group mainly affected and the rapidity of the course, patients are unlikely to be seen by dentists. In the few older patients with a more chronic form of the disease, the features relevant to dentistry are essentially those of severe types of multifocal eosinophilic granuloma. Corticosteroid or cytotoxic treatment may complicate dental management.

MASTOCYTOSIS

Proliferation of mast cells with release of their mediators may result in urticaria pigmentosa, pruritus, flushing, diarrhoea, bone pain and neuropsychiatric problems. The condition is treated with steroids and antihistamines. Trauma, stress, extremes of temperature and various drugs (NSAIDs, codeine, opiates, radiographic media and some GA agents) may precipitate exacerbations.

TRANSFUSION-ASSOCIATED GRAFT-VERSUS-HOST DISEASE

Transfusion-associated graft-versus-host disease is a rare but serious complication of blood transfusion. People at risk include those who have:

- received blood transfusions from HLA-matched donors, including family members
- had a stem cell transplant
- inherited immune defects
- acquired immune defects such as Hodgkin disease
- been treated with purine analogues, such as fludarabine, cladribine or deoxycoformycin.

Transfusion-associated graft-versus-host disease results from transfused leukocytes; gamma irradiation of the transfused blood will obviate the reaction.

Patients should be pre-warned and carry a warning card (Fig. 8.39).

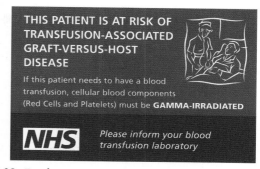

Fig. 8.39 Transfusion-associated graft-versus-host disease warning card

BONE MARROW TRANSPLANTATION (HAEMOPOIETIC STEM CELL TRANSPLANT; SEE CH. 35)

GRAFT-VERSUS-HOST DISEASE (SEE CH. 35)

USEFUL WEBSITES

http://www.merck.com/mmpe/index.html.
http://www.nlm.nih.gov/medlineplus/encyclopaedia.html
http://www.leukemia-lymphoma.org/all_page?item_id=4689
http://www.cancer.gov/cancertopics
http://www.leukemia.org/hm_lls/
http://www.rialto.com/g6pd/

FURTHER READING

Aframian, D.J., Lalla, R.N., Peterson, D.E., 2007. Management of dental patients taking common hemostasis-altering medications. Oral Surg Oral Pathol Oral Radiol Endod 103 (Suppl), S45.e1–e11.

Al-Mubarak, S., Rass, M.A., Alsuwyed, A., Alabdulaaly, A., Cianico, S., 2006. Thromboembolic risk and bleeding in patients maintaining or stopping oral anticoagulant therapy during dental extraction. J Thromb Haemost 4, 689–691.

Ansell, J., Hirsh, J., Dalen, J., et al., 2001. Managing oral anticoagulant therapy. Chest 119 (1 Suppl), 22S–38S.

Ardekian, L., Gaspar, R., Peled, M., Brener, B., Laufer, D., 2000. Does low-dose aspirin therapy complicate oral surgical procedures? J Am Dent Assoc 131 (3), 331–335.

Baker, R.I., Coughlin, P.B., Gallus, A.S., Harper, P.L., Salem, H.H., Wood, E.M., 2004. Warfarin Reversal Consensus Group. Warfarin reversal: consensus guidelines, on behalf of the Australasian Society of Thrombosis and Haemostasis. Med J Aust 181, 492–497.

British Committee for Standards in Haematology. Guidelines for the management of patients on oral anticoagulants requiring dental surgery, 2007.

Chugani, V., 2004. Management of dental patients on warfarin therapy in a primary care setting. Dent Update 31, 379–382, 384.

De Araujo, M.R., Ribas, M.O., Koubik, A.C.G.A., Mattioli, T., de Lima, A.A.S., Franca, B.H.S., 2007. Fanconi's anaemia; clinical and radiographic oral manifestations. Oral Dis 13, 291–295.

Delaney, J.A., Opatrny, L., Brophy, J.M., Suissa, S., 2007. Drug interactions between antithrombotic medications and the risk of gastrointestinal bleeding. CMAJ 177, 347–351.

Diz Dios, P., Fernández Feijoo, J., 2001. Tooth removal in patients receiving oral anticoagulants. Oral Surg Oral Med Oral Pathol Oral Radiol Endod 92, 248–249.

Douketis, J.D., 2002. Perioperative anticoagulation management in patients who are receiving oral anticoagulant therapy: a practical guide for clinicians. Thromb Res 108, 3–13.

Evans, I.L., Sayers, M.S., Gibbons, A.J., Price, G., Snooks, H., Sugar, A.W., 2002. Can warfarin be continued during dental extraction? Results of a randomized controlled trial. Br J Oral Maxilliofac Surg 40, 248–252.

Fang, M.C., Go, A.S., Chang, Y., et al., 2007. Death and disability from warfarin-associated intracranial and extracranial hemorrhages. Am J Med 120, 700–705.

Ferrieri, G.B., Castiglioni, S., Carmagnala, D., Cargnel, M., Strohmenger, L., Abati, S., 2007. Oral surgery in patients on anticoagulant therapy without treatment interruption. J Oral Maxillofac Surg 65, 1149–1154.

Gómez-Moreno, G., Cutando, A., Arana, C., Scully, C. 2005. Hereditary blood coagulation disorders. Management and dental treatment. Journal of Dental Research 84, 978–985.

Garfunkel, A.A., Haze, C., Eldor, A., 2000. A suggested protocol for oral surgery patients on anticoagulant medications. J Isr Dent Assoc 17, 22–23.

Herman, W.W., Konzelman, J.L., Sutley, S.H., 1997. Current perspectives on dental patients receiving coumarin anticoagulant therapy. JADA 128 (3), 327–335.

Holbrook, A.M., Pereira, J.A., Labiris, R., et al., 2005. Systematic overview of warfarin and its drug and food interactions. Arch Intern Med 165, 1095–1106.

Jaffer, A.K., 2006. Anticoagulant management strategies for patients on warfarin who need surgery. Cleve Clin J Med 73 (Suppl 1), S100–S105.

Jafri, S.M., 2004. Periprocedural thromboprophylaxis in patients receiving chronic anticoagulation therapy. Am Heart J 147, 3–15.

Jeske, A.H., Suchko, G.D., 2003. Lack of scientific basis for routine discontinuation of oral anticoagulation therapy before dental treatment. J AM Dent Assoc 134, 1492–1497.

Juurlink, D.N., 2007. Drug interactions with warfarin: what clinicians need to know. CMAJ 177, 369–371.

Little, J.W., Miller, C.S., Henry, R.G., McIntosh, B.A., 2002. Antithrombotic agents; implications in dentistry. Oral Surg 93, 544–551.

Mask Jr., A.G., 2000. Medical management of the patient with cardiovascular disease. Periodontology 23, 136–141.

Mehra, P., Cottrell, D.A., Bestgen, S.C., Booth, D.F., 2000. Management of heparin therapy in the high-risk, chronically anticoagulated, oral surgery patient: a review and a proposed nomogram. J Oral Maxillofac Surg 58 (2), 198–202.

Nash, M.J., Cohen, H., 2004. Management of Jehovah's Witness patients with haematological problems. Blood Rev 18, 211–217.

Nelson, L.P., Savilli-Castillo, I., 2002. Dental management of a pediatric patient with mastocytocsis. Pediatr Dent 24, 343–346.

Perry, D.J., Noakes, T.J., Helliwell, P.S., 2007. Guidelines for the management of patients on oral anticoagulants requiring dental surgery. Br Dent J 203, 389–393.

Randall, C., 2005. Surgical management of the primary care dental patient on warfarin. Dent Update 32, 414–426.

Rice, P.J., Perry, R.J., Afzal, Z., Stockley, I.H., 2003. Antibacterial prescribing and warfarin: a review. Br Dent J 194, 411–415.

Russo, G., Corso, L.D., Biasiolo, A., Berengo, M., Pengo, V., 2000. Simple and safe method to prepare patients with prosthetic heart valves for surgical procedures. Clin Appl Thromb Hemost 6, 90–93.

Sacco, R., Sacco, M., Carpenedo, M., Moia, M., 2006. Oral surgery in patients on oral anticoagulant therapy: a randomized comparison of different INR targets. J Thromb Haemost 4, 688–689.

Salam, S., Yusuf, H., Milosevic, A., 2003. Bleeding after dental extractions in patients taking warfarin. Br J Oral Maxillofac Surg 45, 463–466.

Schardt-Sacco, D., 2000. Update on coagulopathies. Oral Surg Oral Med Oral Pathol Oral Radiol Endod 90, 559–563.

Scully, C., Chaudhry, S., 2007. Aspects of Human Disease 16. Chronic renal failure (CRF). Dental Update 43, 597.

Scully, C., Chaudhry, S., 2007. Aspects of Human Disease 17. Anaemia. Dental Update 43, 661.

Scully, C., Chaudhry, S., 2008. Aspects of Human Disease 18. Von Willebrand's disease (vWD). Dental Update 35, 69.

Scully, C., Chaudhry, S., 2008. Aspects of Human Disease 19. Haemophilia. Dental Update 35, 69.

Scully, C., Chaudhry, S., 2008. Aspects of Human Disease 20. Leukaemia. Dental Update 35, 141.

Scully, C., Diz Dios, P., Giangrande, P., Lee, C., 2002. Oral health care in hemophilia and other bleeding tendencies. World Federation on Hemophilia Treatment of Hemophilia Monograph Series No. 27.

Scully, C., Diz Dios, P., Shotts, R., 2004. Oral health care in patients with the most important medically compromising conditions; 1. platelet disorders. CPD Dentistry 5, 3–7.

Scully, C., Diz Dios, P., Shotts, R., 2004. Oral health care in patients with the most important medically compromising conditions; 2. congenital coagulation disorders. CPD Dentistry 5, 8–11.

Scully, C., Diz Dios, P., Shotts, R., 2004. Oral health care in patients with the most important medically compromising conditions; 3. anticoagulated patients. CPD Dentistry 5, 47–49.

Scully, C., Diz Dios, P., Shotts, R., 2004. Oral health care in patients with the most important medically compromising conditions; 4. patients with cardiovascular problems. CPD Dentistry 5, 50–55.

Scully, C., Diz Dios, P., Shotts, R., 2004. Oral health care in patients with the most important medically compromising conditions; 5. patients at risk for endocarditis. CPD Dentistry 5, 75–79.

Scully, C., Gokbuget, A., Kurtulus, I., 2007. Hypoplasminogenaemia, gingival swelling and ulceration. Oral Diseases 13, 515–518.

Scully, C., Watt-Smith, P., Dios, P., Giangrande, P.L.F., 2002. Complications in HIV-infected and non-HIV-infected hemophiliacs and other patients after oral surgery. Int J Oral Maxillofac Surg 31, 634–640.

Scully, C., Wolff, A., 2002. Oral surgery in patients on anticoagulant therapy. Oral Surg Oral Med Oral Pathol Oral Radiol Endod 94, 57–64.

Silingardi, M., Ghirarduzzi, A., Tincani, E., Iorio, A., Iori, I., 2000. Miconazole oral gel potentiates warfarin anticoagulant activity. Thromb Haemost 83, 794–795.

Stubbs, M., Lloyd, J.A., 2001. Protocol for the dental management of von Willebrand's disease, haemophilia A and haemophilia B.. Aust Dent J 46, 37–40.

Thijssen, H.H., Soute, B.A., Vervort, L.M., Classens, J.G., 2004. Paracetamol (acetaminophen) warfarin interaction: NAPQI, the toxic metabolite of paracetamol, is an inhibitor of enzymes in the vitamin K cycle. Thromb Haemost 92, 797–802.

Vanderlinde, E.S., Heal, J.M., Blumberg, N., 2002. Autologous transfusion. BMJ 324, 772–775.

Vassilopoulos, P., Palcanis, K., 2000. Bleeding disorders and periodontology. Periodontology 2007, 44, 211–223.

Wahl, M.J., 2000. Myths of dental surgery in patients receiving anticoagulant therapy. J Am Dent Assoc 131, 77–81.

Ward, B.B., Smith, M.H., 2007. Dentoalveolar procedures for the anticoagulated patient: literature recommendations versus current practice. J Oral Maxillofac Surg 65, 1454–1460.

Zanon, E., Martinelli, F., Bacci, C., Zerbinati, P., Girolami, A., 2000. Proposal of a standard approach to dental extraction in haemophilia patients. A case-control study with good results. Haemophilia 6, 533–536.

Appendix 8.1   Rare coagulation-related factor defects

Coagulation factor defect	Bleeding tendency	APTT	PT	Basic defect
V	+	−	−	Genetic: AR, streptomycin, liver disease, others
VII	+	−	−	Genetic: AR, liver disease, anticoagulants, many others
X Stuart–Prower factor	+ usually	−	−	Genetic: AR, primary amyloid, others
XI Plasma thromboplastin antecedent	+	−	−	Genetic: high frequency in Ashkenazi Jews
XII Hageman factor	−	−	−	Genetic: AR, liver disease
XIII Fibrin stabilizing factor	+	−[a]	−[a]	Genetic: AR
α-Antiplasmin (Miyasato disease)	+	−	−	Genetic: AR, many others
Fibrinogen	+	−	−	Genetic: AR
Prekallikrein (Fletcher factor)	−	−	−	Genetic: AR, nephritic syndrome, liver disease

APTT, activated partial thromboplastin time; AR, autosomal recessive; PT, prothrombin time.
Assay by α-antiplasmin function.
[a]Assay by clot solubility.

Life is impossible without the liver. The liver (hepar) consists of hepatocytes, organized for optimal contact with sinusoids (blood vessels) and bile ducts, and makes and breaks down sugar, proteins, and fats; stores nutrients; produces bile and removes metabolic products and other toxins from the blood. Bile drains to the gall bladder and via the bile duct to the small intestine, at which point it is intimately associated with the head of the pancreas, swelling of which may cause biliary obstruction and jaundice (Fig. 9.1).

The liver turns glucose into glycogen (stored in the liver). This is converted back into glucose when required, maintaining stable blood glucose levels. Excess carbohydrates and protein are converted to fat.

The liver makes many proteins – blood proteins (e.g. most blood-clotting factors using vitamin K metabolites), and albumin, hormones, transporter proteins and complement. The liver also forms bile acids, which are essential for fat digestion and absorption of fat-soluble vitamins (A, D, E and K), and produces or stores these vitamins folate and vitamin B_{12}, and stores minerals (e.g. copper and iron). Bile (gall) is made up of water, cholesterol, phospholipids, bicarbonate, bile pigments and bile salts. It is a bitter yellow or green fluid secreted by hepatocytes, stored in the gall bladder between meals, and upon eating is discharged into the duodenum where it is required for the absorption of fats and fat-soluble vitamins. The bile salts sodium glycocholate and sodium taurocholate are produced by the liver from cholesterol, and they help emulsify fats for their absorption and facilitate the activity of pancreatic lipase.

The breakdown of haemoglobin, cholesterol, proteins, sex steroids and many drugs occurs at least partly in the liver. The enzyme haem oxygenase acts on haem to form biliverdin, which in turn is converted into bilirubin. Biliverdin and bilirubin are termed bile pigments. Bilirubin is not water-soluble (unconjugated bilirubin) and needs a carrier (albumin) to be transported. In the liver, bilirubin is conjugated by combining with glucuronic acid and becomes water-soluble *conjugated* bilirubin. This then enters the bile, and flows into the bile duct and finally the intestine.

In the intestine, conjugated bilirubin can be excreted in the stool after being changed into urobilinoids. Alternatively, the process of conjugation can be reversed by beta-glucuronidase, which converts the conjugated bilirubin back into unconjugated bilirubin. Unlike conjugated bilirubin, unconjugated bilirubin can be reabsorbed from the intestine back into the blood (enterohepatic recirculation). Conjugated bilirubin can also be excreted in the urine, which it darkens. Increased levels of bilirubin in the blood can cause the body, especially the sclerae of the eyes, to appear yellow (jaundice).

Water-soluble toxins and waste products can be eliminated via the kidneys in the urine, but non-water-soluble toxins need to be chemically modified by the liver to allow this process to occur. Digested proteins in the form of amino acids are broken down further in the liver, a process known as deamination. Nitrogenous products such as ornithine and arginine are converted to urea, which is excreted into the urine by the kidneys. Sex steroids, such as the masculinizing hormone testosterone and the feminizing hormone oestrogen, are inactivated in the liver.

Most drugs, including alcohol, are metabolized/excreted via the liver (Table 9.1). In particular, oral drugs are absorbed by the gut and transported via the portal circulation to the liver. In the liver, drugs may undergo first-pass metabolism, in which they are modified, activated or inactivated before they enter the systemic circulation. Drugs (e.g. alcohol and barbiturates), which can induce the cytochrome P450 system, can lead to diminished effects of drugs such as the contraceptive pill, phenytoin or warfarin. By contrast, some drugs (e.g. cimetidine, omeprazole, sulfonamides or valproate) impair P450 activity causing enhanced activity of drugs, such as carbamazepine, ciclosporin, phenytoin or warfarin.

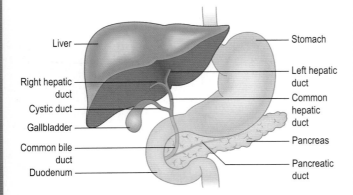

Fig. 9.1 Liver anatomy

Liver — Stomach
Right hepatic duct
Cystic duct
Gallbladder
Common bile duct
Duodenum
Left hepatic duct
Common hepatic duct
Pancreas
Pancreatic duct

Table 9.1 Some drugs metabolized by the liver

Local anaesthetics	Bupivacaine, lidocaine, mepivacaine, prilocaine, articaine
Analgesics	Acetaminophen, aspirin, codeine, ibuprofen, meperidine
Antimicrobials	Ampicillin, metronidazole, tetracyclines, vancomycin
Sedatives	Diazepam

LIVER DISEASE

GENERAL ASPECTS

The liver has some powers of regeneration but this capacity can be exceeded by repeated or extensive damage by infective agents, alcohol, drugs or poisons. Alcohol abuse is a major cause of liver disease. Chronic liver disease includes chronic hepatitis, and cirrhosis. Chronic hepatitis is the term for hepatitis that persists longer than 6 months: it may follow acute hepatitis (or appear without warning) and may progress to cirrhosis. The most important causes of chronic hepatitis are hepatitis C virus, alcohol, drugs or autoimmune hepatitis (Table 9.2).

Excessive alcohol intake, viral hepatitis and drugs also account for the majority of cases of cirrhosis (Box 9.1).

Cirrhosis is characterized by liver cell necrosis and inflammation followed by replacement of normal functioning liver with fibrotic tissue and regenerating nodules of hepatocytes and vascular derangement. Liver function deteriorates and the blood flow through it becomes obstructed.

Box 9.1 Causes of chronic liver disease

- Alcoholic and drug-induced liver disease
- Gaucher disease
- Haemochromatosis
- Portal hypertension
- Primary biliary cirrhosis
- Primary sclerosing cholangitis
- Sarcoidosis
- Viral hepatitis
- Wilson disease
- Zellweger syndrome (cerebrohepatorenal syndrome; a rare congenital leukodystrophy)

CLINICAL FEATURES

Liver diseases can have many effects according to the degree of liver damage – including jaundice, a bleeding tendency, and impaired drug and metabolite degradative and excretory activities (Table 9.3). Many patients with liver disease are asymptomatic and the problem frequently remains subclinical for years or decades. Malaise, anorexia and fatigue are common, sometimes with low-grade fever and upper abdominal discomfort.

Bilirubin ester is normally excreted in bile and is one of the factors that colour the faeces. If bilirubin is not conjugated (enzyme defect or parenchymal liver disease) or excreted (biliary obstruction), it accumulates in the body and colours the skin and mucous membranes (jaundice) and the whites of the eyes (icterus), detectable clinically at levels > 40 µmol/L, and the urine darkens.

Jaundice is often caused by liver disease but may also result from haemolysis. The main causes of jaundice are abuse of alcohol or other drugs, and infection (Table 9.4).

Pale, fatty faeces and malabsorption result from failure of bile salts to reach the intestine (obstructive diseases), causing malabsorption of fats, and of the fat-soluble vitamins (e.g. vitamin K) needed for clotting factor synthesis. Bile salts accumulating in the blood may cause itching, nausea, anorexia and vomiting.

A bleeding tendency results from depressed synthesis of blood-clotting factors and excess fibrinolysins. Prothrombin time (PT), the international normalized ratio (INR) and activated partial thromboplastin time (APTT) are all increased. Chronic bleeding may cause anaemia.

Cirrhosis chiefly affects the middle-aged or elderly, and is frequently asymptomatic in its earlier stages. Anorexia, malaise and weight loss are common, but effects can be widespread (Box 9.2; Fig. 9.2).

Cirrhosis is a potentially fatal disorder. Obstruction to the portal circulation can lead to portal hypertension, oesophageal varices and the risk of vomiting of blood (haematemesis), which can cause anaemia or fatal gastrointestinal haemorrhage. Thrombocytopenia from splenomegaly, and low blood clotting factor levels, leads to a bleeding tendency which can worsen the haemorrhage from oesophageal varices. Anaemia may also result. Portal obstruction can also lead to portal-systemic (hepatic) encephalopathy and tremor (liver flap or asterexis), due to failure to detoxify normal metabolites, and this can be exacerbated by drugs, gastrointestinal haemorrhage or a high-protein diet and can lead to coma. Metabolism is disturbed, and sex-steroid accumulation can lead to gynaecomastia and testicular atrophy.

Spontaneous bacterial peritonitis is a potential and serious problem. Diabetes mellitus, peptic ulceration, renal dysfunction, gallstones, immune dysfunction and hepatoma are other potential complications.

The patient may develop finger-clubbing, opaque nails (leukonychia), palmar erythema, asterixis, spider naevi (angiomata), scratch marks, purpura, gynaecomastia, scant body hair, testicular atrophy, hepatomegaly, splenomegaly, distended abdominal veins in which flow is away from the umbilicus (caput medusae), ascites (fluid in the peritoneal cavity) (Fig. 9.3) and ankle oedema.

Table 9.2 Causes of chronic hepatitis

Hepatitis	Drugs	Autoimmune	Inflammatory bowel disease	Metabolic
Hepatitis B or C virus	Acetaminophen (paracetamol) Alcohol Aspirin Cytotoxics Halothane Isoniazid Methyldopa Nitrofurantoin			Alpha$_1$-antitrypsin deficiency Wilson disease

Table 9.3 Manifestations of liver diseases

Impaired	Main causes	Consequences	Clinical features
Bilirubin metabolism	Congenital hyperbilirubinaemia	Hyperbilirubinaemia	Jaundice
Bilirubin excretion	Hepatocellular disease Extrahepatic obstruction	Hyperbilirubinaemia Bilirubinuria	Jaundice Dark urine Pale stools
Excretion of bile salts	Extrahepatic obstruction Hepatocellular disease	Rise in serum alkaline phosphatase and 5'-nucleotidase Malabsorption of fats and fat-soluble vitamins (especially vitamin K) causing prolonged prothrombin time	Pruritus Fatty stools Bleeding tendencies
Liver cell function	Hepatocellular disease	Impaired clotting factor synthesis and prolonged prothrombin time Impaired albumin synthesis Impaired drug metabolism Rise in serum transaminases Portal venous hypertension Disorganized liver structure Cirrhosis	Bleeding tendencies Oedema Coma or neurological disorders Bleeding from oesophageal varices

Table 9.4 Causes of jaundice

CONGENITAL	ACQUIRED		
	Hepatocellular disease (parenchymal liver disease)	Extrahepatic biliary obstruction	Haemolysis
Haemolysis, such as in rhesus incompatibility	Viral hepatitis	Gallstones	Malaria
Prematurity	Drug-induced hepatitis	Carcinoma of pancreas	Yellow fever
Gilbert syndrome (Table 9.14)	Cirrhosis (often alcoholic)	Biliary atresia	Sickle cell diseases
Various rare syndromes (Table 9.14)	Primary biliary cirrhosis	Others	Incompatible transfusion
Others	Chronic hepatitis		
	Others		

Box 9.2 Cirrhosis: clinical features

- Jaundice
- Oedema
- Ascites
- Swollen ankles
- Gastrointestinal haemorrhage
- Mental confusion
- Hepatomegaly
- Splenomegaly
- Finger-clubbing
- Skin manifestations
- Spider naevi
- Palmar erythema
- Opaque nails
- Sparse hair

Other occasional manifestations

- Parotid swelling (sialosis)
- Gynaecomastia
- Bleeding (liver failure)
- Portal hypertension and varices

Alcoholic cirrhosis may have associated parotid swelling (sialosis) (Fig. 9.4), Dupuytren contracture (Fig. 9.5), gastric ulceration or pancreatitis.

GENERAL MANAGEMENT

The diagnosis depends on the history, physical examination, evaluation of liver function tests (Table 9.5) and other studies.

In chronic hepatitis, clinical and laboratory features are diagnostically helpful. Liver enzymes, especially aminotransferases, are raised. Values of bilirubin and alkaline phosphatase are variable. Serological markers are common in autoimmune hepatitis and include immunoglobulin G (IgG) elevations, antinuclear antibody, smooth muscle (anti-actin) antibody, LE cells, rheumatoid factor, and antibodies directed against liver and kidney microsomes. Liver biopsy is essential for definitive diagnosis.

Autoimmune hepatitis generally improves substantially with treatment with corticosteroids, with or without azathioprine. Treatment for chronic hepatitis B virus (HBV) and HCV

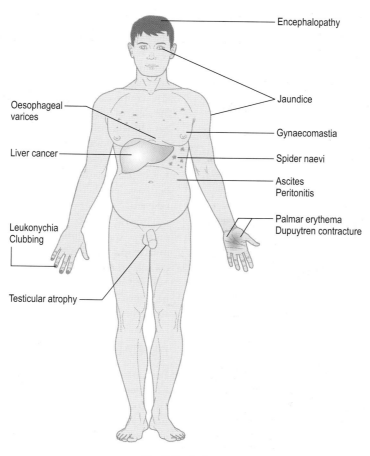

Fig. 9.2 Cirrhosis

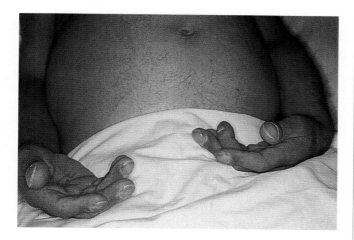

Fig. 9.3 Ascites and finger-clubbing in chronic liver disease

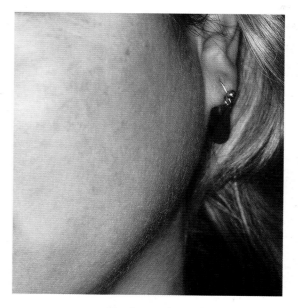

Fig. 9.4 Sialosis

is with interferon-alpha to suppress viral replication. Treatment of chronic HBV infection with lamivudine gives results comparable to interferon and is well tolerated, but treatment for 1–3 years is usually needed and a mutant strain of the virus often emerges. Treatment with defovir dipivoxil is another choice. Chronic HCV is treated with a combination of ribavirin plus interferon-alpha or pegylated interferon.

Prognosis is highly variable and patients with chronic hepatitis usually survive several years or decades, but hepatocellular failure, cirrhosis, or both, often follow eventually. Liver transplantation is fairly successful for HCV-related hepatitis.

Although HCV infection universally persists, the clinical course is generally indolent, and long-term survival rates are relatively high. Transplantation has not generally been effective for HBV end-stage liver disease, because of aggressive disease recurrence in the graft, but treatment with lamivudine can now help ameliorate it.

In cirrhosis, laboratory tests for haemochromatosis or Wilson disease are specific but many others are non-specific. Serum albumin is often low but bilirubin, immunoglobulins, transaminases and alkaline phosphatase may be raised. Haematological abnormalities include a prolonged prothrombin time, thrombocytopenia, anaemia, macrocytosis and sometimes leukocytosis.

Computed tomography (CT), ultrasound or other imaging may be indicated, as may liver biopsy.

Treatments that can stop or delay further progression and complications include treatment of any viral cause, and interferon to inhibit activation of hepatic stellate cells and degradation of the collagenous matrix by metalloproteinases, activated by TIMP (tissue inhibitor of metalloproteinases). Adequate nutrition should be maintained and management is mainly directed towards prevention and treatment of complications. For example, for ascites and oedema, a low-sodium diet or the use of diuretics, may help. For portal hypertension, a beta-blocker may be needed. Varices are managed by ligation, beta-blockers and possibly transjugular intrahepatic portosystemic shunting. Encephalopathy can be managed with a low-protein diet supplemented with ornithine, aspartate, benzoate or phenylacetate. Lactulose plus neomycin may also be used.

The molecular absorbent recirculating system (MARS) removes water-soluble and protein-bound toxins, which accumulate in liver failure, based on an albumin-filled circuit recirculating through a charcoal and cholestyramine column.

Liver transplantation is necessary when complications cannot be controlled or when the liver becomes so damaged that it stops functioning completely.

DENTAL ASPECTS

Patients with acute or chronic liver disease can present serious bleeding problems if surgery is needed. There may be a risk from transmission of infection. Impaired drug metabolism causes central nervous system (CNS) depressants, such as sedatives, analgesics and general anaesthesia (GA) in particular, to be potentiated and can cause coma. The maximum

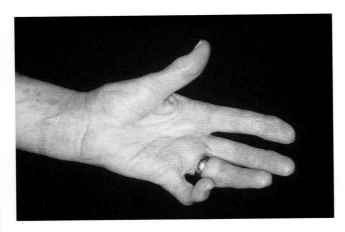

Fig. 9.5 Dupuytren contractures involve the fifth and fourth fingers in alcoholic liver disease

Table 9.5	**Liver function tests[a]**
Serum Test	**Comments**
Bilirubin	Positive in urine in most patients with jaundice except unconjugated hyperbilirubinaemia. Bilirubin rises in serum because of overproduction or obstruction. In liver disease, the total serum bilirubin may rise (hyperbilirubinaemia). The total bilirubin includes that which has undergone conjugation (the direct or conjugated bilirubin) plus the portion of bilirubin that has not been metabolized (unconjugated bilirubin). When the direct bilirubin fraction is elevated, the cause is typically gallstones. If the direct bilirubin is low, while the total bilirubin is high, this reflects liver cell damage or bile duct damage within the liver itself
Hyaluronic acid (HA)	Raised serum levels in liver fibrosis; marker of pre-cirrhosis
Alanine aminotransferase (ALT)	Leaks from damaged liver. Most sensitive marker of any form of hepatocyte damage. Also known as serum glutamic–pyruvic transaminase (SGPT)
Aspartate aminotransferase (AST)	Leaks from damaged liver, heart or muscle. Rises in liver, heart or muscle damage. Also known as serum glutamic–oxaloacetic transaminase (SGOT)
5′-Nucleotidase	Found in liver, thyroid and bone. Rises in biliary obstruction
Gamma-glutamyl transpeptidase (GGT or GGTP)	Found in liver, kidneys, pancreas, prostate. Rises in obesity, alcoholism, most liver diseases, pancreatitis, diabetes, myocardial infarct and with some drugs. Medications commonly cause GGT to be elevated but alcohol is the main drug cause of an increase in the GGT.
Alkaline phosphatase	Found in biliary canaliculi, osteoblasts, intestinal mucosa and placenta. Rises in pregnancy, liver disease, gallstones and bone disease Renal or intestinal damage can also cause the alkaline phosphatase to rise. One way to assess the aetiology of a raised level is to examine isoenzymes
Albumin	Low albumin (hypoalbuminaemia) may indicate that the synthetic function of the liver has been markedly diminished, such as in cirrhosis. Falls in malnutrition, nephrotic syndrome and gastrointestinal disease
Prothrombin time (and INR)	Prolonged in liver disease, malnutrition (decreased vitamin K ingestion)

[a]Statins and other drugs can disturb liver function tests.
INR, international normalized ratio.

safe dose of local anaesthesia (LA) is also lower than in healthy persons.

The hepatologist or haematologist should be consulted if surgery, GA or drug therapy is needed. Surgery is hazardous also because of possible HCV or HBV carriage, or infection, diabetes, anaemia, drug therapy, poor wound healing and a liability to peritonitis. A clotting screen and prothrombin time may be indicated. If the prothrombin time is prolonged, vitamin K_1 10 mg parenterally (phytomenadione) should be given daily for several days pre-operatively to improve haemostatic function. If there is an inadequate response as shown by the prothrombin time, a transfusion of fresh blood or plasma may be required. Repeated gastrointestinal bleeding may cause anaemia (Ch. 8) or be fatal.

Routine dental treatment can usually be carried out without any particular problem, though alcoholism may influence treatment planning and procedures (Ch. 34).

Because drug metabolism can be impaired, and protein synthesis depressed, care must be taken when considering using drugs, particularly such as some analgesics, antimicrobials and CNS-active drugs (Table 9.6). Impaired drug detoxification and excretion mean that the effects of drugs are not entirely predictable: age, gender, the type and severity of the liver disease, hypoalbuminaemia (depressed protein-binding of drugs) and the possible induction of hepatic drug-metabolizing enzymes by previous medication may influence the outcomes of drug use. Drugs that are hepatotoxic should obviously be avoided.

Local anaesthesia is safe given in normal doses, but prilocaine or articaine are preferred to lidocaine. Drugs liable to cause respiratory depression are dangerous and coma can be precipitated by sedatives, hypnotics or opioids. The doses of midazolam used for conscious sedation should be reduced. Inhalational sedation is preferable to intravenous sedation with a benzodiazepine. Nitrous oxide with pethidine or phenoperidine appears to be suitable for GA but it is essential to avoid hypoxia; isoflurane or sevoflurane are preferable to halothane (see later: *halothane hepatitis*). Desflurane should be used in lower than normal doses. Suxamethonium is best avoided because of impaired cholinesterase activity.

Aspirin and most other non-steroidal anti-inflammatory drugs (NSAIDs), such as indometacin, should be avoided because of the risk of gastric haemorrhage in those with portal hypertension or peptic ulcers. Analgesia is best achieved with acetaminophen or codeine used in lower than normal doses.

Anticoagulants can cause uncontrollable haemorrhage and broad-spectrum antibiotics (at least in theory) may further reduce vitamin K availability by destroying the gut flora. Antimicrobials that can usually safely be used in normal doses include penicillin, cefalexin, cefazolin and imipenem.

If a jaundiced patient must undergo major surgery, aggressive treatment with intravenous fluids and diuresis with mannitol are indicated to avoid acute renal failure, which may complicate hepatic failure (hepatorenal syndrome; Ch. 12). There may also be considerations related to alcoholism (Ch. 34), autoimmune disease, hepatitis B, C or D antigen carriage or diabetes (Ch. 6).

Spontaneous bacterial peritonitis is a potential problem in cirrhosis with ascites. Though most infections are with normal

Table 9.6 Drugs contraindicated and alternatives in liver disease

Type of drug	Drugs contraindicated	Alternatives to use
Analgesics	Aspirin Codeine Dextropropoxyphene Indometacin Mefenamic acid Meperidine[a] NSAIDs Opioids Pentazocine	Acetaminophen/ paracetamol[a] Oxycodone
Antimicrobials	Aminoglycosides Azithromycin Azole antifungals (miconazole, ketoconazole, itraconazole) Clarithromycin[a] Clindamycin[a] Co-amoxiclav* Co-trimoxazole Doxycycline Erythromycin estolate Flucloxacillin Metronidazole[a] Minocycline Moxifloxacin Roxithromycin Talampicillin Tetracyclines	Amoxicillin Ampicillin, cephalosporins Nystatin, fluconazole Erythromycin stearate Imipenem Penicillin Nystatin Penicillin Tetracycline Penicillin
Corticosteroids	Prednisone	Prednisolone
Antidepressants	Monoamine oxidase inhibitors Tricyclicsal	SSRIs
Muscle relaxants	Suxamethonium	Atracurium, cisatracurium, pancuronium, vecuronium
Local anaesthetics	Lidocaine[a]	Articaine, prilocaine
General anaesthetics	Halothane Methohexitone Propofol[a] Thiopental	Desflurane Isoflurane Sevoflurane
Anxiolytics/sedatives	Barbiturates Diazepam[a] Midazolam[a] (and flumazenil) Phenothiazines Promethazine	Lorazepam[a] Oxazepam[a] Pethidine[a]
Anticonvulsants	Carbamazepine Lamotrigine Phenytoin	
Others	Anticoagulants Biguanides Diuretics Etretinate Liquid paraffin Lomotil Methyldopa Oral contraceptives Pilocarpine Sumatriptan	

[a]Or given in lower doses than normal.

NSAIDs, non-steroidal anti-inflammatory drugs; SSRIs, selective serotonin reuptake inhibitors.

gut aerobic bacteria or Gram-positive bacteria, invasive dental or oral surgical procedures may increase the risk and, since the mortality approaches 30%, antibiotic prophylaxis must be considered. Amoxicillin orally 2–3 g with metronidazole 1 h preoperatively or intravenous imipenem are recommended.

Some patients have sialosis, or tooth erosion from gastric regurgitation.

There is an association between liver cirrhosis and oral carcinoma.

HEPATITIS

'Hepatitis' is the term for liver inflammation, which can result from many insults, including drugs, poisons and, particularly, various infections.

VIRAL HEPATITIS

Viral hepatitis is especially important since the agents can be transmitted in body fluids in health care and other settings. Many viruses causing hepatitis have been identified (Table 9.7), but hepatitis B and C are the most relevant to health care.

Jaundice during childhood is often caused by hepatitis A and is of little consequence. Jaundice in the teenager or young adult may be due to viral hepatitis A, B, C, D or E. Several of these viruses, particularly hepatitis A and E, are transmitted faeco-orally. Some, especially hepatitis A and B, and probably C, can be spread sexually. Hepatitis A and E are more of a problem for travellers, since they are seen mainly in the developing world and transmitted faeco-orally; hepatitis E is more severe among pregnant women, especially in the third trimester. The term 'viral hepatitis' used in health care usually refers to infection by hepatitis B, D or C viruses, which are transmitted parenterally (Table 9.8). Hepatitis B has been of greatest importance, but, in the absence of a vaccine, hepatitis C has become a more serious problem. These viruses can also be transmitted in health care facilities and they constitute a cross-infection risk in dentistry. Universal (standard) precautions against transmission of infection must always be employed since these viruses, particularly HBV, HCV and hepatitis D virus (HDV) can be transmitted in blood and blood products and other body fluids including by practices where infection control is lacking, particularly in intravenous drug use where there is needle or syringe sharing. Any practice where there is a skin breach, such as body-piercing or tattooing (Fig. 9.6), can also constitute a risk. Co-infection with other blood-borne agents, such as human immunodeficiency virus (HIV), is common, particularly in intravenous drug users.

All hepatitis viruses can cause acute, or short-term, illness, and jaundice is common (Fig. 9.7). Some hepatitis viruses, particularly HCV and HBV, also have a small acute mortality. HBV, HCV and HDV can also cause chronic hepatitis, in which the infection is prolonged, sometimes lifelong, and may be associated with virus carriage, chronic liver disease and liver cancer (hepatoma) or can be responsible for aplastic anaemia and other extrahepatic manifestations. The clinical and laboratory features of viral hepatitis are summarized in Table 9.9.

Table 9.7   Viral causes of hepatitis

Hepatitis viruses	Herpesviruses	Others
Hepatitis A virus	Cytomegalovirus	Coxsackie B virus
Hepatitis B virus	Epstein–Barr virus	Yellow fever
Hepatitis C virus	Herpes simplex virus	
Hepatitis D virus		
Hepatitis E virus		
Hepatitis G virus		
SEN viruses		
Transfusion transmitted virus (torque teno virus; TTV)		

Hepatitis A ('infectious hepatitis')

General aspects

Hepatitis A is caused by the hepatitis A virus (HAV) and is rarely a serious disease. Hepatitis A is endemic throughout the world, is seen particularly where socioeconomic and living conditions are poor and, in those areas, infection (and consequent immunity) is common in childhood (Fig. 9.8). In the developed world, many people reach adulthood without infection and have no immunity, and are therefore are at risk from infection if they travel to endemic areas.

Spread of hepatitis A is largely faecol-oral by consumption of contaminated water or food, particularly raw shellfish. For example, nearly 300 000 persons were infected in one outbreak in Shanghai, originating from contaminated clams. Hepatitis A can also be transmitted sexually and by close person-to-person contact, and in body fluids including saliva. Persons in the armed forces, food handlers, health care workers, sewage workers, travellers to areas of high endemicity, children and employees at day care centres, promiscuous individuals who do not practise safe sex, and injecting drug users are at greatest risk.

Clinical features

The incubation period is 2–6 weeks. The disease is frequently subclinical or anicteric, but clinical features are similar to those of other forms of viral hepatitis (though muscle pains, rashes and arthralgia are rare), and include fatigue, nausea and vomiting, abdominal pain or discomfort, loss of appetite, low-grade fever, jaundice and itching.

Recovery is usually uneventful. Blood and faeces become non-infective during or shortly after the acute illness. There is no evidence of either a carrier state or progression to chronic liver disease. About 15% have relapses over a 6–9-month period, but the mortality is less than 0.1%. Hepatitis A gives long-lasting immunity.

General management

The diagnosis of hepatitis A can be confirmed if necessary by demonstrating serum antibodies to the virus (HAAb).

No specific treatment is usually needed; normal human immunoglobulin may prevent or attenuate the clinical illness and is used mainly in sporadic outbreaks. HAV vaccine

Table 9.8 Comparative features of more common forms of viral hepatitis

	Hepatitis virus					
	A	**B**	**C**	**D**	**E**	**G**
Alternative terminology	Infectious	Serum	Non-A non-B	Delta agent	Non-A non-B[a]	Non-A non-B[a]
Prevalence in developed world	Common	Uncommon; about 5–10%	Uncommon; about 1–5%	In countries with low prevalence of chronic HBV infection, HDV prevalence is low among both HBV carriers (< 10%) and patients with chronic hepatitis (< 25%)	Rare except in endemic areas in far East	Uncommon; about 1–2% of general population Associated with some cases of acute or chronic non-A, non-B, non-C, non-D, non-E hepatitis
Type of virus	Picornaviridae (RNA)	Hepadnaviridae (DNA)	Flaviviridae (RNA)	Circular RNA similar to plant viroid Delta virus	Similar to calcivirus (RNA)	Flaviviridae (RNA)
Incubation	2–6 weeks	2–6 months	2–22 weeks	3 weeks–2 months	2–9 weeks	?
Main route of transmission	Faecal–oral	Parenteral	Parenteral	Parenteral	Faecal–oral	Parenteral
Severity	Mild	May be severe	Moderate	Severe	May be severe	No consequences known
Carrier states	–	+	+	+	–	–
Complications	Rare Acute mortality 0.1%	Chronic liver disease in 10–20% Hepatoma Polyarteritis nodosa Chronic glomerulonephritis Acute mortality 1–2%	Many Chronic liver disease in > 70% Hepatoma	Can cause fulminant hepatitis	Rare except in pregnancy	–
Vaccine available	+	+	–	–	–	–

[a]Several forms of enteric non-A non-B (NANB) exist (E, G).

is available especially for prophylaxis in travellers to high-risk endemic areas such as Asia, South America and Africa. A combined vaccine against HAV and HBV is also available.

Dental aspects

Patients are unlikely to seek dental treatment during the acute phase. There appears to be no risk of transmission of hepatitis A during dentistry conducted properly.

Hepatitis B (serum hepatitis; homologous serum jaundice)

General aspects

Hepatitis B is caused by the hepatitis B virus and is a serious disease. It can cause lifelong infection, cirrhosis (scarring) of the liver, liver cancer, liver failure and occasionally fulminant hepatitis and death.

Hepatitis B infection is endemic throughout the world, especially in institutions such as for custodial care, in cities and in poor socioeconomic conditions. It is especially common in the developing world where prevalence exceeds

8%: sub-Saharan Africa, the Pacific Basin, south-East Asia, Central Asia, parts of the Middle East, South America's Amazon Basin and some Eastern European countries are the areas of highest endemicity. Over 75% of some populations such as Australian aboriginals (hence the older term 'Australia antigen') are carriers. In parts of sub-Saharan Africa, Asia and the Pacific, nearly all children are infected. The prevalence is low (under 2%) in north-western Europe, North America and the Antipodes. Intermediate levels (2–8%) are found in Mediterranean countries, the Middle East, the Indian sub-continent and Japan.

Spread of hepatitis B is mainly parenteral (via unscreened blood or blood products, particularly by intravenous drug abuse, and by tattooing/body-piercing), sexually (especially among promiscuous individuals who do not practise safe sex) and perinatally. HBV is a robust virus, surviving for a week or more in dried blood on surfaces. Hepatitis B virus has been transmitted to patients and staff in health care facilities and has been transmitted between patients in a dental setting. Health care workers in the past were not infrequently infected; however, adherence to standard infection control procedures, and immunization, have resulted in a decline in infections over the past two decades.

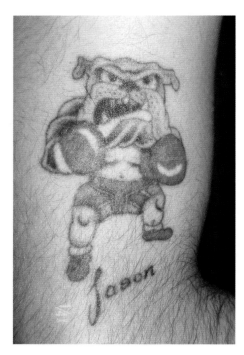

Fig. 9.6 Tattoo; safe if done under aseptic conditions, but can otherwise transmit blood-borne infections such as hepatitis viruses or human immunodeficiency virus

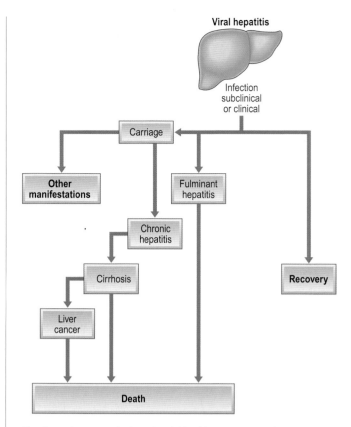

Fig. 9.7 Outcomes of infection with blood-borne viruses such as hepatitis B, C or D virus

Nevertheless, in USA, 91 health care workers were known to have transmitted HBV to patients in the health care setting over the decade to 2006. Apart from health care workers, those in the armed forces, missionaries and aid workers, and persons travelling to the developing world are at risk (Box 9.3).

Clinical features

The incubation period for HBV is 2–6 months, and the acute mortality rate is less than 2%. However, rarely, where there has been co-infection with HDV, the death rate has been as high as 30%.

About 30% have no signs or symptoms, and most patients with clinical hepatitis recover completely with no untoward effect, apart perhaps from some persistent malaise. The effects of HBV infection, therefore, range from subclinical infections without jaundice (anicteric hepatitis) to fulminating hepatitis, acute hepatic failure and death.

The prodromal period of 1–2 weeks is characterized by anorexia, malaise and nausea. Hepatitis B viraemia usually precedes the clinical illness by weeks or months and lasts for some weeks before clearing completely.

As jaundice becomes clinically evident, the stools become pale and the urine dark due to bilirubinuria. The liver is enlarged and tender, and pruritus may be troublesome (Table 9.9). Muscle pains, arthralgia and rashes are more common in hepatitis B than hepatitis A, and there is often fever.

Complications of hepatitis B include a carrier state, chronic infection, cirrhosis, liver cancer, polyarteritis nodosa or death. A carrier state, in which HBV persists within the body for more than 6 months, develops in 5–10%. It is more frequent in anicteric infections or those contracted early in life. Although 5–10% of carriers lose the hepatitis antigen each year, carriage may persist for up to 20 years and may be asymptomatic. Some patients, especially those who have received blood products, those infected with HDV and those who have immune defects, are 'high risk', and predisposed to the carrier state. Most carriers are healthy but others, especially those with persistently abnormal liver function tests, develop chronic liver disease (see later), 15–25% of whom die from it.

Table 9.9 Acute viral hepatitis: clinical and biochemical features					
Stage	Clinical features	Serum bilirubin	AST	ALT	Alkaline phosphatase
Prodrome	Anorexia, lassitude, nausea, abdominal pain	N or ↑	↑	↑↑	N or ↑
Clinical hepatitis	As above plus jaundice, pale stools, dark urine, pruritus, fever, hepatomegaly	↑	↑	↑↑↑	N or ↑

Arrows indicate a value above normal (N).

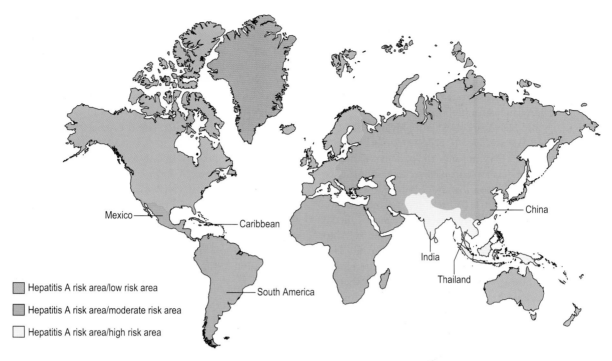

Fig. 9.8 Hepatitis A is seen worldwide

Mexico · Caribbean · South America · China · India · Thailand

☐ Hepatitis A risk area/low risk area

☐ Hepatitis A risk area/moderate risk area

☐ Hepatitis A risk area/high risk area

Box 9.3 Viral hepatitis – high-risk groups for hepatitis B

- Patients (e.g. haemophiliacs, thalassaemics) who have received unscreened blood products or multiple plasma or blood transfusions, especially in the Far East or Africa
- Patients receiving haemodialysis for end-stage renal disease
- Immunosuppressed or immunodeficient patients (e.g. HIV-infected, post-transplantation or due to malignant disease)
- Residents and staff of long-stay institutions, particularly prisons
- Persons in occupations that involve exposure to human blood – health care and laboratory personnel (especially surgeons)
- Intravenous drug abusers
- Sexually active individuals, especially promiscuous individuals who do not practise safe sex
- Patients from the developing world, especially Africa and Asia
- Tattooing and acupuncture, especially in the Far East
- Individuals travelling to regions with high infection rates of HBV, such as sub-Saharan Africa, South-East Asia, the Amazon Basin, the Pacific Islands and the Middle East
- People with certain other disorders (e.g. Down syndrome, polyarteritis nodosa)
- Consorts of patients with hepatitis or any of the above groups
- Patients with some chronic liver diseases
- Household contacts of someone who has a chronic HBV infection
- Newborns whose mothers are infected with HBV are also at high risk. The same is true of infants and children whose parents were born in areas where HBV infection is widespread

HBV, hepatitis B virus; HIV, human immunodeficiency virus.

Infection with HBV confers immunity. Active immunity can therefore be acquired naturally. In the past, a high proportion of health care staff working in developing countries or in institutions were not immunized and developed antibody to hepatitis B despite a low incidence of overt hepatitis.

General management

Serum enzyme estimations are useful in the diagnosis of hepatitis: aspartate transaminase (AST) and alanine transaminase (ALT) are raised in proportion to the severity of acute hepatitis. Alkaline phosphatase, alpha-fetoprotein and serum bilirubin levels are also raised.

Electron microscopy of serum from HBV-infected patients shows three types of particle: the Dane particle, which probably represents intact HBV, and consists of an inner core containing DNA and core antigens (HBcAg), and an outer envelope of surface antigen (HBsAg); and smaller spherical forms and the tubular forms, which represent excess HBsAg.

Diagnosis and prognosis depend, however, on serological markers. HBsAg (Australia antigen, hepatitis-associated antigen, hepatitis B antigen) is a non-infectious protein found transiently in those with acute hepatitis B, and persists in the serum in carriers and in some who are non-infectious. In a typical case, HBsAg develops 20–100 days after exposure, is detectable in the serum for 1–120 days and then disappears. The serum becomes negative for HBsAg about 6 weeks after the onset of clinical jaundice. Persistence of HBsAg beyond 13 weeks of the clinical illness often implies that a carrier state is developing. Hepatitis B surface *antibody* (anti-HBs) develops after infection or vaccination and, in the absence of HBsAg, implies immunity.

HBcAg is found in liver biopsies in acute hepatitis B. Hepatitis B core *antibody* is a sensitive marker of viral replication indicating either current or recent infection. Anti-HBc associated with anti-HBs appears to indicate recovery and immunity to hepatitis. However, if anti-HBs is absent, anti-HBc suggests the carrier state or chronic hepatitis.

Hepatitis B e antigen (HBeAg) and its antibody, anti-HBe, are useful markers to determine the likelihood of spread of HBV (transmissibility) by persons affected with chronic hepatitis B viral infection: the presence of HBeAg means ongoing viral activity and the ability to infect others, whereas the presence of anti-HBe signifies a more inactive state of the virus and less risk of transmission. HBeAg indicates high infectivity and is found only in serum that is also HBsAg-positive, but only in about 25% of those who are HBsAg-positive. If HBeAg persists beyond about 4 weeks of the onset of symptoms, the patient will probably remain infectious and develop chronic liver disease. Absence of HBeAg has usually indicated low infectivity. However, in some individuals infected with HBV, the genetic material for the virus has undergone a particular structural change, called a pre-core mutation, which results in an inability of the HBV to produce HBeAg, even though it is actively reproducing. This means that, even though no HBeAg is detected in the blood, HBV is still active in these persons and they can infect others.

Anti-HBe usually indicates complete recovery and loss of infectivity, provided HBeAg is lost. Asymptomatic HBsAg carriers often possess anti-HBe, and are usually at lower infective risk than those with HBeAg and DNA polymerase (supercarriers). The most specific marker of HBV reproduction is the measurement of HBV DNA in the blood; the polymerase chain reaction (PCR) is the most sensitive assay (Table 9.10).

Acute hepatitis B will resolve on its own in most symptomatic individuals and so management usually includes a high carbohydrate diet and avoiding hepatotoxins (e.g. alcohol). Antiviral therapy is not warranted.

Chronic HBV infection, however, can be effectively treated with interferon-alpha 2b (intron A). This is given for 4–6 months but can have a number of adverse reactions. Lamivudine is used for those who fail to respond to interferon and is usually better tolerated, but treatment for 1–3 years is usually needed and a variant mutant virus strain YMDD eventually emerges in 50% of treated patients. Adefovir dipivoxil is also available.

Prevention is best achieved by hepatitis B vaccination and by avoiding contact with the virus (Box 9.4). Infection from contact with hepatitis B can also be minimized by giving HBIG (hepatitis B immune globulin) and vaccine within 12 h after birth, to infants born to HBV-infected mothers.

Vaccination is recommended for all clinical students and staff, and for people working with high-risk groups, and those travelling to high prevalence areas. The vaccine is a recombinant vaccine of HBsAg. After vaccination, anti-HBs develops and confers 90% protection for many years and possibly for life but may not protect against pre-core variants. Vaccination also protects indirectly against hepatitis D. Hepatitis B vaccine rarely causes any significant adverse effects. Concerns that giving hepatitis B vaccine to infants might contribute to sudden infant death syndrome (SIDS), or that the vaccine may trigger autoimmune diseases, especially multiple sclerosis (MS) or lichen planus, proved unfounded.

After routine vaccination of most infants, children, adolescents or adults, post-vaccination testing for adequate antibody response is not necessary. For health care workers with normal immune status who have demonstrated an anti-HBs response following vaccination, booster doses of vaccine are not recommended nor periodic anti-HBs testing (Fig. 9.9). Post-vaccination testing is recommended for persons who:

- are immunocompromised (e.g. haemodialysis patients)
- received the vaccine in the buttock
- are infants born to HBsAg-positive mothers
- are health care workers who have contact with blood
- are sex partners of persons with chronic hepatitis B virus infection.

Post-vaccination testing in these groups should be completed 1–2 months after the third vaccine dose for results to be meaningful. A protective antibody response is ≥ 10 mIU/ml).

Combined hepatitis A and hepatitis B vaccine is available for some travellers, injecting drug users, promiscuous individuals who do not practise safe sex, and persons with clotting factor disorders who receive therapeutic blood products. It is indicated for vaccination of persons aged > 18 years in these groups. Hepatitis B vaccine is recommended for travellers to areas of high or intermediate hepatitis B endemicity who plan to stay for > 6 months and have frequent close contact with the local population.

Dental aspects

Drugs should be used with caution (Tables 9.1 and 9.6).

Patients with normal platelet counts and normal prothrombin times (and INR) can undergo dental intervention safely.

Table 9.10 Hepatitis B serum markers in relation to disease progress

Marker	HBsAg	Anti-HBs	Anti-HBc (total)	Anti-HBc IgM	HBeAg	Anti-HBe	HBV DNA
Acute infection – early phase	+	–	+	+	+	+	+
Acute infection – mid phase	+	–	+	+	–	+	–
Acute infection – later phase	–	–	+	+	–	+	–
Recovery and immunity	–	+	+	–	–	–	–
Successful vaccination	–	+	–	–	–	–	–
Chronic infection with active reproduction	+	–	+	–	+ or –	–	+
Chronic infection in the inactive phase	+	–	+	–	–	+	–
Recovery, false positive or chronic infection	–	–	+	–	–	+ or –	–

Box 9.4 Prevention of viral hepatitis

- Always following routine barrier precautions and safely handling needles and other sharps
- Drug addicts never sharing needles, syringes, or water for injection
- Not sharing personal care items that might have blood on them (razors, toothbrushes)
- Avoiding having a tattoo or body piercing, unless the piercer follows strict health practices
- Using condoms: hepatitis B virus (HBV) can be spread by sex as can hepatitis C virus (HCV)
- Not donating blood, organs, or tissue if HBV- or HCV-positive
- Not inhaling cocaine through contaminated straws!

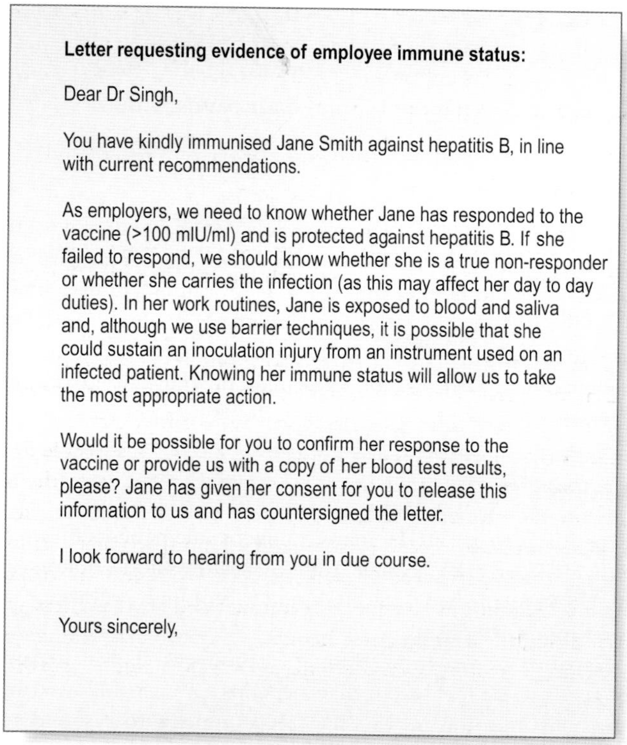

Letter requesting evidence of employee immune status:

Dear Dr Singh,

You have kindly immunised Jane Smith against hepatitis B, in line with current recommendations.

As employers, we need to know whether Jane has responded to the vaccine (>100 mIU/ml) and is protected against hepatitis B. If she failed to respond, we should know whether she is a true non-responder or whether she carries the infection (as this may affect her day to day duties). In her work routines, Jane is exposed to blood and saliva and, although we use barrier techniques, it is possible that she could sustain an inoculation injury from an instrument used on an infected patient. Knowing her immune status will allow us to take the most appropriate action.

Would it be possible for you to confirm her response to the vaccine or provide us with a copy of her blood test results, please? Jane has given her consent for you to release this information to us and has countersigned the letter.

I look forward to hearing from you in due course.

Yours sincerely,

Fig. 9.9 Request for hepatitis B virus immune status

However, there may be a bleeding tendency if the platelet count is low (Ch. 8), or if the prothrombin time (INR) is prolonged.

Although pure parotid saliva does not contain HBsAg, saliva collected from the oral cavity may contain HBV (presumably derived from serum via gingival exudate) and may be a source for non-parenteral transmission. However, the risk of transmission by this route appears to be low except where there is very close contact, as in families or children's nurseries or sexual contact. HBV can also be transmitted by human bites. Blood, plasma or serum can be infectious. As little as 0.0000001 ml of HBsAg-positive serum can transmit hepatitis B.

The main danger is from needlestick injuries; some 25% may transmit HBV infection. There is a higher risk for oral surgeons and periodontologists, and for those working with high-risk patients, probably because of needlestick injuries. However, if adequate precautions are taken, the dental surgery is no longer a significant source of transmission. In the past, HBsAg carriage was found in about 1% of dental practitioners and up to 20%

of oral surgeons, who occasionally transmitted the infection to their patients. Now the risk appears to be fairly low, since universal infection control precautions are usually taken and dental staff have been immunized against HBV. Only about 1 in 1000 of the UK population are HBsAg carriers and even among high-risk patients attending dental hospitals fewer than 10% are HBsAg carriers, and 75% of them are HBeAg-negative and probably non-infectious.

Practitioners who are ill with hepatitis should stop dental practice until fully recovered. Testing for HBeAg may indicate those individuals likely to spread hepatitis B. HBeAg-positive dental surgeons and those who are HBeAg-negative but have greater than 1000 HBV viral particles per millilitre of blood should discontinue practice involving exposure-prone procedures.

Needlestick injuries involving HBV can transmit the virus: post-exposure prophylaxis (PEP) with HBIG and/or hepatitis B vaccine series should be considered for occupational exposures after evaluation of the HBsAg status of the source and the vaccination and vaccine-response status of the exposed person within 24 hours of contact.

Hepatitis C

General aspects

Hepatitis C virus (HCV) infection was identified from what was formerly known as post-transfusion non-A non-B hepatitis (NANBH). HCV now ranks second only to alcoholism as a cause of liver disease in the developed world and is responsible for much sporadic viral hepatitis, particularly in intravenous drug abusers, among whom its prevalence is rising. By contrast, transfusion-associated hepatitis C is declining and should decline rapidly now that blood is routinely tested for HCV. The virus can also be transmitted between health care workers and patients. Persons at special risk for hepatitis C include those who have: received blood from a donor who later tested positive for hepatitis C; have ever injected illegal drugs; received a blood transfusion or solid organ transplant before about 1992; received a blood product for clotting disorders produced before about 1987; ever been on long-term renal dialysis; or have evidence of liver disease (e.g. persistently abnormal ALT levels).

Six major HCV genotypes are recognized with varying geographical distributions; genotype 1 accounts for most cases.

Clinical features

Hepatitis C has a similar incubation period to hepatitis B (usually less than 60 but up to 150 days) but most HCV-infected persons develop no signs or symptoms. Clinical hepatitis C is also usually a less severe and shorter illness than hepatitis B (Table 9.8), but a greater proportion (25–80%) of patients have persisting abnormal liver function tests, many develop chronic liver disease (up to 85%), and some develop liver cancer, or die (< 3%). There are associations of HCV in some populations with sicca syndrome, lichen planus, lymphoma, cryoglobulinaemia and other extrahepatic manifestations.

About 15% of patients infected with HCV are co-infected with hepatitis G virus (HGV). Co-infection with HBV and SEN (see below) is also common.

General management

Diagnosis is from the detection of HCV RNA and anti-HCV antibody in the blood, but anti-HCV IgG is usually not detectable until 1–3 months after the acute infection.

Acute HCV infection resolves spontaneously in 50% of patients; both interferon-alpha or pegylated interferon, with or without ribavirin, have been used with some success, but they can have significant adverse effects. Chronic HCV is treated with a combination of ribavirin plus interferon-alpha or pegylated interferon.

There is as yet no vaccine against hepatitis C. Hepatitis C prevention is shown in Box 9.4.

Dental aspects

Hepatitis C virus has been transmitted to patients and staff in health care facilities. There has been a raised prevalence of HCV infection in some dental populations studied. HCV has been found in saliva and infection has followed a human bite. HCV is transmitted in about 10% of needlestick injuries. For HCV post-exposure management, the HCV status of the source and the exposed person should be determined, and for health care personnel exposed to an HCV-positive source, follow-up HCV testing should be performed to determine if infection develops. Immune globulin and antiviral agents (e.g. interferon with or without ribavirin) are not recommended for post-exposure prophylaxis of hepatitis C.

Staff infected with HCV should not perform exposure-prone procedures (Appendix 9.1).

Hepatitis C virus may be associated with oral features – sicca syndrome, non-Hodgkin lymphoma and, in some populations (mainly patients originating from the Mediterranean basin or Japan), with lichen planus. Chronic hepatitis C infection and sicca syndrome have an association with HLA DQB1*02.

Hepatitis D

General aspects

Hepatitis D virus (HDV or delta agent) is an incomplete virus carried within the hepatitis B particle and will only replicate in the presence of HBsAg. Therefore, there is no HDV without HBV infection. HDV spreads parenterally, mainly by shared hypodermic needles. Risk groups are as for HBV (Box 9.3). HDV has been transmitted to patients and staff in health care facilities.

Hepatitis D virus is endemic, especially in the Mediterranean littoral and among intravenous drug abusers, and is found worldwide. It is not endemic in northern Europe or the USA, but some haemophiliacs and others have acquired the infection and the prevalence is rising.

Clinical features

HDV infection may coincide with hepatitis B or superinfect patients with chronic hepatitis B. Infection may produce a biphasic pattern with double rises in liver enzymes, and bilirubin. The incubation period of hepatitis D is unknown; 90% of infections are asymptomatic and HDV infection does not necessarily differ clinically from hepatitis B but can cause fulminant disease with a high mortality. About 70–80% of HBV carriers with HDV superinfection develop chronic liver disease with cirrhosis, compared with 15–30% with chronic HBV infection alone.

General management

Hepatitis D virus antigen indicates recent infection; delta antibody indicates chronic hepatitis or recovery. Vaccination against HBV protects indirectly against HDV.

Drug treatment with interferon-alpha is effective.

Dental aspects

The same considerations apply as for hepatitis B.

Hepatitis E

Hepatitis E virus (HEV) spreads mainly via the faecal–oral route and causes large epidemics in India, South-East Asia, parts of the CIS (the old USSR) and Africa. HEV causes a disease similar to hepatitis A, but in pregnant women has a high mortality rate (up to 40%).

Hepatitis E virus is not known to be transmitted during dentistry.

Hepatitis G

Hepatitis G virus (HGV) may co-infect some patients infected with HCV or HBV. About 1.5% of healthy blood donors in the USA are infected with HGV and it is of high prevalence in intravenous drug users.

Hepatitis G virus infection, if it produces clinical hepatitis, tends to be less severe than hepatitis C but is followed by persistent infection in 15–30%. HGV appears to respond to interferon-alpha.

HGV is not known to be transmitted during dentistry. GB virus C is related to HGV.

Transfusion transmitted virus (torque teno virus)

Transfusion transmitted virus (TTV) has a single strand only of DNA and there is an extraordinarily high prevalence of chronic viraemia in apparently healthy people (up to nearly 100% in some countries). Like HGV, the pathogenicity of TTV has not been proven, it has not yet been aetiologically linked to any other disease and the virus is not known to be transmitted during dentistry.

SEN viruses

SEN is named after the initials of the patient from whom the virus was isolated. SEN V-D and SEN V-H are DNA viruses which are transmitted parenterally and can cause post-transfusion hepatitis. These viruses are otherwise of unknown pathogenicity and not known to be transmitted during dentistry.

LEPTOSPIROSIS

The bacteria *Leptospira icterohaemorrhagiae*, which is associated with rats and *Leptospira hardjo*, found in cattle, can be transmitted to humans by contact with the urine of rats, foxes or cattle, usually via contaminated water or soil. Leptospirosis is an occupational hazard for sewer workers, people who work outdoors or with animals (e.g. farmers and vets) and is a recreational hazard for those who participate in water sports and for campers. There is usually a flu-like illness with severe headaches. It may respond to penicillin or tetracycline.

The severe form (Weil disease), which affects only about 10–15%, causes liver damage and jaundice and has a death rate between 4% and 40%.

ALCOHOLIC HEPATITIS

Alcohol is the major and increasing cause of hepatitis in developed countries. It injures the liver by blocking the metabolism of protein, fats and carbohydrates, and causes fatty change (alcoholic steatosis); in response there is inflammation (alcoholic hepatitis), which is probably initially reversible. The amount of alcohol that can injure the liver varies greatly from person to person: in women, as few as two to three units per day may be responsible, and in men, as few as three to four units per day.

Exposure to alcohol over long periods may cause liver fibrosis, which, in itself, is largely asymptomatic but, as it progresses, can turn into cirrhosis, where the fibrosis alters the architecture and impairs liver function. If cirrhosis progresses, the liver may fail.

Non-alcoholic steatohepatitis (NASH; macrovesicular steatosis; non-alcoholic fatty liver disease or NAFLD) may be caused by obesity, diabetes, protein malnutrition, coronary artery disease or corticosteroid treatment. The prevalence in the developed world may reach 30% and, in about 15% of cases, it may progress to cirrhosis.

DRUG-INDUCED HEPATITIS

Apart from alcohol, halothane, some NSAIDs, some herbs and nutritional supplements, paracetamol/acetaminophen in overdose, and many other drugs can cause hepatitis (Box 9.5). With some drugs, liver damage is a predictable dose-related effect, while with others the damage is unpredictable and may be immunologically mediated (Table 9.11).

Dental aspects

Aspirin ingestion by children, during and after a viral illness (e.g. chickenpox, influenza or other respiratory tract illness), significantly increases the chance of developing Reye syndrome – liver damage with encephalopathy and abnormal accumulations of fat in the liver and other organs, along with a severe rise in intracranial pressure. Reye syndrome can follow several days (1–14 days) after aspirin use, usually in a viral infection, and generally progresses through two stages. The first includes persistent or continuous vomiting, severe tiredness, belligerence due

---

Box 9.5 Hepatotoxic drugs apart from alcohol

- Acetaminophen
- Allopurinol
- Amitriptyline
- Amiodarone
- Atomoxetine
- Azathioprine
- Erythromycin estolate
- Flucloxacillin
- Halothane
- Ibuprofen
- Indometacin
- Isoniazid (INH)
- Ketoconazole
- Loratadine
- Methotrexate
- Methyldopa
- Minocycline
- Nifedipine
- Nitrofurantoin
- Oral contraceptives
- Phenytoin
- Pyrazinamide
- Rifampicin
- Sulfonamides
- Tetracyclines
- Valproic acid
- Zidovudine

Table 9.11 Drug and chemically related liver damage

Dose-related liver damage	Non-dose-related liver damage
Acetaminophen (paracetamol)	Antithyroid drugs
Alcohol	Erythromycin estolate
Anabolic steroids	Flucloxacillin
Isoniazid	Halothane
Ketoconazole	Nitrofurantoin
Methyldopa	Phenylbutazone, phenothiazines, vinyl chloride and carbon tetrachloride
Methyltestosterone	Phenytoin
Tetracyclines	Sulfonamides

---

to illness (moodiness), nausea and loss of energy. The second stage follows with personality changes, bizarre mental and physical behaviour (confusion, restlessness and irrational behaviour), lethargy or inactivity and, sometimes, coma and convulsions. There is a 90% chance of recovery for those diagnosed early but only 10% are likely to recover if diagnosed late. Treatment is typically provided in an intensive care unit for monitoring of fluids, electrolytes, blood gases, intracranial pressure and nutrition. About 90% of cases of Reye syndrome develop in the first 15 years of life, so aspirin or other salicylates are contraindicated for children under 16, except for certain specific diseases. Many over-the-counter medications including mouth ulcer preparations may contain salicylates and these must be avoided. Acetaminophen/paracetamol in moderate dosage is now the preferred analgesic and antipyretic for children below the age of 16.

Antimicrobials may sometimes cause liver problems. Tetracyclines in massive doses can cause liver damage and the danger of hepatotoxicity is greater if there is impaired urinary excretion. Erythromycin estolate is potentially hepatotoxic but the effect is reversible when the drug is stopped (erythromycin stearate is not hepatotoxic). Flucloxacillin can be cholestatic.

Halothane can cause hepatitis, which may follow a single exposure in 1 in 35 000 cases. It is more common when anaesthetics are given repeatedly at intervals of less than 3 months, in middle-aged females, and in the obese. Transient impairment of liver function appears after halothane as after other anaesthetics. The reaction may be some form of hypersensitivity, but the precise mechanism is uncertain and pre-existing liver disease does not appear to be contributory. There also appears to be a genetic susceptibility. Clinically, halothane hepatitis causes pyrexia developing after a week post-operatively. Malaise, anorexia and jaundice may then appear, and if jaundice is severe the prognosis is very poor. Unfortunately, there are no dependable criteria or laboratory tests to indicate when halothane is truly contraindicated. Serum antibodies reacting with halothane-altered liver membrane determinants have been reported in about 75% of patients but, as with antibodies to penicillin, few of these patients have a reaction on a further exposure. Halothane should never be given repeatedly, or within a period of 3 months, and never to any patient who has had malaise, pyrexia or jaundice after exposure to it. Fortunately, newer halogenated anaesthetic agents, such as enflurane, isoflurane, desflurane and sevoflurane, do not induce hepatitis in those who have had an episode of halothane hepatitis. In many hospitals, these agents have, despite their cost, replaced halothane, particularly to carry out several operations on the same patient at short intervals. Flucloxacillin can also cause hepatitis.

AUTOIMMUNE HEPATITIS

Autoimmune hepatitis (autoimmune liver disease; autoimmune chronic active hepatitis) is associated with various autoantibodies and the complement allele C4AQO and with the HLA haplotypes B8, B14, DR3, DR4 and Dw3, and often progresses to cirrhosis. Several types are recognized (Table 9.12). In autoimmune hepatitis, multisystem manifestations are common, especially in young women, and can include acne, arthralgia, amenorrhoea, haemolytic anaemia, nephritis, pulmonary fibrosis, thyroiditis and ulcerative colitis.

Autoimmune hepatitis is typically responsive to immunosuppressants.

PRIMARY BILIARY CIRRHOSIS
GENERAL ASPECTS

Primary biliary cirrhosis (PBC) is an uncommon, progressive, autoimmune disorder with antibodies directed against mitochondrial pyruvate dehydrogenase complex, affecting small intrahepatic bile ducts, seen mainly in middle-aged women. It begins with non-suppurative destructive cholangitis and jaundice, and culminates in cirrhosis.

CLINICAL FEATURES

Patients with PBC may be asymptomatic for many years but, eventually, complaints of weakness, lethargy, weight loss, pale stools and dark urine, jaundice and pruritus emerge. Complications include xanthomas and skin pigmentation, or the complications of any chronic liver disease. Osteoporosis and connective tissue diseases, particularly systemic sclerosis (scleroderma) or Sjögren syndrome, may occur.

GENERAL MANAGEMENT

Primary biliary cirrhosis must be distinguished from other conditions with similar symptoms, such as *autoimmune hepatitis* or *primary sclerosing cholangitis*.

The biochemical features of PBC resemble those of obstructive jaundice with raised serum alkaline phosphatase and elevated AST, ALT and gamma-glutamyl transpeptidase levels. Antibodies against mitochondria are found in about 90%. Approximately 50% have antinuclear antibodies, sometimes against proteins specific to nuclear components; the M2-*IgG* antimitochondrial antibody is the most specific test.

Antinuclear antibodies appear to be prognostic agents in PBC; a*nti-glycoprotein-210 antibodies*, and to a lesser degree *anti-p62 antibodies*, correlate with progression toward end-stage liver failure. *Anticentromere antibodies* correlate with developing portal hypertension.

Table 9.12 Autoimmune hepatitis			
Clinical features	**Type 1**	**Type 2**	**Type 3**
Diagnostic autoantibodies	SMA ANA Anti-actin	Anti-LKM P450 IID6 Synthetic core motif peptides 254–271	Soluble liver–kidney antigen Cytokeratins 8 and 18
Age mainly affected	Any	Children	Adults
Concurrent autoimmune disease (%)	41	34	58
IgG raised	+++	+	++
HLA associations	B8, DR3, DR4	B14, Dr3, C4AQO	Uncertain
Progression to cirrhosis (%)	45	82	75

ANA, antinuclear antibodies; SMA, smooth muscle antibodies.

Abdominal ultrasound or a CT scan is usually performed to rule out blockage to the bile ducts. Previously, most suspected sufferers underwent a liver biopsy, and – if uncertainty remained – endoscopic retrograde cholangiopancreatography (ERCP, an endoscopic investigation of the bile duct). Now most patients are diagnosed without invasive investigation since the combination of antimitochondrial antibodies and typical (cholestatic) liver function tests are considered diagnostic. However, a liver biopsy is still necessary to determine the stage of disease.

Medical treatment includes cholestyramine to relieve pruritus, vitamins and calcium to help prevent osteoporosis (loss of bone), and oral medium-chain triglycerides to improve nutrition. Ursodeoxycholic acid may help improve laboratory values but the effect on prognosis is unclear. Colchicine may play a role in inhibiting liver fibrosis and improves laboratory values but not signs or symptoms.

Orthotopic liver transplantation is highly successful for end-stage liver disease resulting from PBC.

If left untreated, the prognosis is poor, as with other forms of cirrhosis (see later).

Dental aspects

Patients with PBC may present similar management problems to those with other parenchymal liver diseases. Sjögren syndrome complicates 70% or more cases of PBC. Telangiectasias may be seen, and oral lichen planus is an occasional complication. Penicillamine, once used for treatment, occasionally caused thrombocytopenia, polymyositis, pemphigus or myasthenia, and also cause lichenoid lesions, oral ulceration and loss of taste.

PRIMARY SCLEROSING CHOLANGITIS

Primary sclerosing cholangitis (PSC) is an autoimmune form of cholangitis that leads to accumulation of bile, which damages the liver, leading to jaundice and liver failure.

LIVER CANCER
GENERAL ASPECTS

Cancer of the hepatocytes is termed hepatocellular carcinoma or malignant hepatoma. It is common in Africa, South-East Asia, Japan and some Mediterranean countries (mainly areas of high endemicity for HBV and HCV) but uncommon in the USA and the UK, where metastatic cancer to the liver from the colon, lungs, breasts, uterus or other parts of the body is far more common.

Risk factors for hepatocellular carcinoma include male gender, old age, a positive family history, chronic HCV or HBV, oral contraceptive use and cirrhosis. Aflatoxin, a mould that forms on peanuts, corn and other nuts and grains, is an important cause in Asia and Africa.

CLINICAL FEATURES

Liver cancer in the early stages often causes no symptoms. Later, manifestations may include wasting, jaundice, pain or swelling in the abdomen, anorexia and fever.

GENERAL MANAGEMENT

High alpha-fetoprotein serum levels can be a feature of liver cancer. Ultrasound, isotope and magnetic resonance imaging scans, and biopsy are often needed for the diagnosis.

Treatment usually consists of surgical resection (partial hepatectomy) but the prognosis is invariably poor. Liver transplantation may be required.

DENTAL ASPECTS

There appear to be no significant dental considerations other than those applying to other types of severe liver disease.

EXTRAHEPATIC BILIARY OBSTRUCTION
GENERAL ASPECTS

The main causes of extrahepatic biliary obstruction are gallstones and carci noma of the pancreas (Ch. 7). Gallstones are common with advancing age, particularly in females. Around 10–20% of adults have gallstones, but most are symptomless. About 80% are cholesterol-containing stones, others are bile pigment stones. The aetiology of cholesterol stones is usually unclear but some patients with Crohn disease or on clofibrate, oral contraceptives or oestrogens appear to be susceptible. Pigment gallstones may complicate chronic haemolytic anaemias (hereditary spherocytosis, thalassaemia or sickle cell anaemia).

CLINICAL FEATURES

Gallstones are often asymptomatic but passage of the stones into the bile ducts can precipitate pain because of biliary colic, acute cholecystitis or acute pancreatitis. Extrahepatic biliary obstruction causes jaundice, pruritus, dark urine and pale stools with impaired absorption of fats and of vitamin K.

GENERAL MANAGEMENT

There is usually a rise in serum bilirubin esters, alkaline phosphatase, 5'-nucleotidase, gamma-glutamyl transpeptidase and transaminases.

Diagnosis may be by ultrasound and endoscopic retrograde cholangiopancreatography (ERCP). Lithotripsy and medical treatment with chenodeoxycholic acid or ursodeoxycholic acid have a place in the treatment of asymptomatic stones. Cholecystectomy is usually indicated if obstructive jaundice develops.

DENTAL ASPECTS

The main danger in surgery is excessive bleeding resulting from vitamin K malabsorption. Surgical intervention should therefore be deferred wherever possible in the presence of jaundice until haemostatic function returns to normal. If surgery is essential, vitamin K_1 should be given parenterally at a dose of 10 mg daily for several days in an attempt to correct the bleeding tendency (Ch. 8).

General anaesthesia in a severely jaundiced patient can lead to renal failure (hepatorenal syndrome).

POST-OPERATIVE JAUNDICE

Post-operative jaundice is discussed in Ch. 3 (Table 9.13).

Table 9.13 Causes of post-operative jaundice		
Excessive bilirubin load	**Hepatocellular disease**	**Others**
Haemolysis due to haemolytic anaemia or incompatible transfusions	Gilbert syndrome Viral hepatitis	Shock Sepsis Obstructive jaundice Bile duct damage
Resorption of blood from large haematoma	Halothane and other drug-induced hepatitis	Gallstone disease Pancreatitis

CONGENITAL JAUNDICE

GENERAL AND CLINICAL ASPECTS

Transient neonatal jaundice is common, usually due to the normal breakdown of haemoglobin around birth, and is of little consequence.

Severe neonatal jaundice can be caused by prematurity, haemolysis such as in rhesus incompatibility, biliary atresia or hepatic disease, and can lead to kernicterus (damage to the basal ganglia of the brain), which can be fatal, or cause epilepsy or choreoathetosis (with or without learning disability) and deafness.

DENTAL ASPECTS

Disorders associated with an early rise in serum levels of conjugated bilirubin (mainly biliary atresia and haemolysis such as in rhesus disease) can cause a greenish discoloration of the teeth and dental hypoplasia.

Familial liver enzyme disorders that can cause jaundice are shown in Table 9.14.

Table 9.14 Syndromes with congenital hyperbilirubinaemia				
	Gilbert	**Crigler–Najjar**	**Dubin–Johnson**	**Rotor**
Prevalence	Common	Rare		
Prognosis	Usually benign	May be fatal	Benign	
Bilirubinaemia	Unconjugated	Unconjugated	Conjugated	
Pigment in urine	–	–	+	
Associated problems	–	Kernicterus	–	
Comments	May become jaundiced after GA but no other clinical problems	Serious disease	No clinical problems Liver pigmented	Liver not pigmented

LIVER TRANSPLANTATION

GENERAL ASPECTS

Liver transplantation is provided for treatment of end-stage liver disease such as from biliary atresia, metabolic disease, cirrhosis or malignancy. Usually the liver is obtained from a cadaveric or brain-dead donor.

The 1-year survival of liver transplantation is around 80% and, of survivors, 90% survive 5 years and 85% for 10 years. Graft-versus-host disease can follow liver transplantation (Ch. 35).

GENERAL MANAGEMENT

All liver transplant recipients require lifelong immunosuppression to prevent a T-cell, alloimmune rejection response.

Liver transplant recipients may be susceptible to recurrence of their original disease and may develop recurrence of hepatitis B or C, alcoholic liver disease, or one of the autoimmune hepatitides. The severity of recurrence varies from mild to development of progressive allograft failure. HCV recurrence after transplantation is almost universal but the extent of the graft damage is variable. The survival in the short term is not significantly affected, but concerns exist regarding long-term recurrence because the rate of developing cirrhosis at 5 years can be as high as 8–25%.

DENTAL ASPECTS

Dental aspects in addition to those discussed in Ch. 35 are:

- liver failure (bleeding tendencies, impaired drug metabolism)
- children needing liver transplants may have retarded tooth eruption and discoloured and hypoplastic teeth
- gingival swelling may be seen in patients on ciclosporin or some other drugs.

USEFUL WEBSITES

http://www.nhs.uk/conditionspages/bodymap.aspx
http://en.wikipedia.org/wiki/Hepatitis
http://en.wikipedia.org/wiki/Cirrhosis
http://www.nlm.nih.gov/medlineplus/hepatitis.html
http://www.cancerbackup.org.uk/Cancertype/Liver/Primarylivercancer

FURTHER READING

Aimetti, M., Romano, F., Marsico, A., Navone, R., 2008. Non-surgical periodontal treatment of cyclosporin A-induced gingival overgrowth: immunohistochemical results. Oral Dis 14, 244–250.

Carrozzo, M., 2008. Oral diseases associated with hepatitis C virus infection. Part 1. Sialadenitis and salivary glands lymphoma. Oral Dis 14, 123–130.

Ferreiro, MC., Diz Dios, P., Scully, C., 2005. Trasmission of hepatitis C virus by saliva? Oral Diseases 11, 230–235.

Golecka, M., Mierzwinska-Nastalska, E., Oldakowska-Jedynak, U., 2007. Influence of oral hygiene habits on prosthetic stomatitis complicated by mucosal infection after organ transplantation. Transplant Proc 39, 2875–2878.

Guggenheimer, J., Eghtesad, B., Close, J.M., Shay, C., Fung, J.J., 2007. Dental health status of liver transplant candidates. Liver Transpl 13, 280–286.

Kajiya, T., Uemura, T., Kajiya, M., et al., 2008. Pyogenic liver abscess related to dental disease in an immunocompetent host. Intern Med 47, 675–678.

Lodi, G., Bez, C., Porter, S.R., Scully, C., Epstein, J.B., 2002. Infectious hepatitis C, hepatitis G, and TT virus: review and implications for dentists. Special Care Dent 22, 53–58.

Lodi, G., Carrozzo, M., Harris, K., et al., 2000. Hepatitis G virus-associated oral lichen planus; no influence from hepatitis G virus co-infection. J Oral Pathol Med 29, 39–42.

Modi, A.A., Liang, T.J., 2008. Hepatitis C, a clinical review. Oral Dis 14, 10–14.

Naudi, A.B., Ammari, A.B., Fung, D.E., 2008. A report of 2 cases of green pigmentation in the primary dentition associated with cholestasis caused by sepsis. J Dent Child (Chic) 75, 91–94.

Perry, J.L., Pearson, R.D., Jagger, J., 2006. Infected health care workers and patient safety: a double standard. Am J Infect Control 34, 313–319.

Redd, J.T., Baumbach, J., Kohn, W., Nainen, O., Khristova, M., Williams, I., 2007. Patient-to-patient transmission of hepatitis B virus associated with oral surgery. J Infect Dis 195, 1311–1314.

Rustemeyer, J., Bremerich, A., 2007. Necessity of surgical dental foci treatment prior to organ transplantation and heart valve replacement. Clin Oral Invest 11, 171–174.

Scully, C., Chaudhry, S., 2007. Aspects of human disease 15 Chronic liver disease. Dental Update 43, 525.

Scully, C., Chaudhry, S.I., 2007. Aspects of human disease. Dent. Update 34, 525.

Valerin, M.A., Napeñas, J.J., Brennan, M.T., Fox, P.C., Lockhart, P.B., 2007. Modified Child–Pugh score as a marker for postoperative bleeding from invasive dental procedures. Oral Surg Oral Med Oral Pathol Oral Radiol Endod 104, 56–60.

Appendix 9.1 Health Protection Agency Guidance UK Advisory Panel for Healthcare Workers Infected with Bloodborne Viruses (UKAP)

http://www.hpa.org.uk/webw/HPAweb&Page&HPAweb AutoListName/Page/1203496960618?p=1203496960618

The Panel is available for consultation:

- when advice is needed regarding restricting the practice of health care workers infected with blood-borne viruses
- when a lookback exercise may be needed as a result of exposure-prone procedures being undertaken on patients by a health care worker infected with a blood-borne virus
- for general advice concerning the categorization of clinical procedures as exposure prone.

The Panel works within the framework of government guidance concerning health care workers and blood-borne viruses, and aims to interpret the guidance in relation to individual cases on a consistent basis.

UK DEPARTMENT OF HEALTH GUIDANCE

HEPATITIS B INFECTED HEALTHCARE WORKERS AND ANTIVIRAL THERAPY (2007)

http://www.dh.gov.uk/en/publicationsandstatistics/ publications/publicationspolicyandguidance/dh_073164

HEALTH CLEARANCE FOR TUBERCULOSIS, HEPATITIS B, HEPATITIS C AND HIV: NEW HEALTHCARE WORKERS (2007)

http://www.dh.gov.uk/en/publicationsandstatistics/ publications/publicationspolicyandguidance/dh_073132

MEDICAL AND DENTAL STUDENTS: HEALTH CLEARANCE FOR HEPATITIS B, HEPATITIS C, HIV AND TUBERCULOSIS. MEDICAL SCHOOLS COUNCIL (FEBRUARY 2008)

http://www.chms.ac.uk/documents/bbvsguidance-feb2008_000.pdf

HEALTH SERVICE CIRCULAR HSC 2000/020: HEPATITIS B INFECTED HEALTH CARE WORKERS

http://www.dh.gov.uk/en/publicationsandstatistics/ publications/publicationspolicyandguidance/dh_4008156

Guidance extended the previous restrictions placed upon hepatitis B-infected health care workers. Both those who carry the e antigen (i.e. are HBeAg positive) and those who are e-antigen negative with a viral load (HBV DNA level) that exceeds 10^3 genome equivalents per millilitre are restricted from performing exposure-prone procedures. The guidance names two dedicated laboratories in the UK where tests for HBV DNA are to be carried out using a specified assay and standardized controls.

Hepatitis B-infected health care workers who are HBeAg negative and do not have an HBV DNA level exceeding 10^3 are not restricted from performing exposure-prone procedures but are subject to exposure-prone procedures.

PROTECTING HEALTH CARE WORKERS AND PATIENTS FROM HEPATITIS B

The guidance recommends that carriers of the hepatitis B virus who are known to be e-antigen positive must not carry out procedures where there is a risk that injury to themselves will result in their blood contaminating a patient's open tissues. Such procedures are termed 'exposure-prone procedures'.

- Addendum to HSG(93)40: Protecting health care workers and patients from hepatitis B (April 2004)
- Addendum to HSG(93)40: Protecting health care workers and patients from hepatitis B (26 September 1996)
- Protecting health care workers and patients from hepatitis B [HSG(93)40]
- Protecting health care workers and patients from hepatitis B (Olive Book).

HEALTH SERVICE CIRCULAR HSC 2002/010: HEPATITIS C INFECTED HEALTH CARE WORKERS

Guidance recommends that health care workers known to be infected with hepatitis C and who are viraemic (i.e. HCV RNA positive) should not perform exposure-prone procedures. The guidelines also recommend that health care workers intending to embark upon careers that rely upon the performance of exposure-prone procedures should be tested for hepatitis C (antibodies and, if positive, HCV RNA). This would mean prospective dental students before entry into dental schools. This is intended to apply to prospective students for undergraduate training, and not to those already qualified seeking post-graduate training. As in the HIV guidance, there is also a section about those at risk coming forward for testing for hepatitis C.

GUIDANCE FOR CLINICAL HEALTH CARE WORKERS: PROTECTION AGAINST INFECTION WITH BLOOD-BORNE VIRUSES (HSC 1998/063)

http://www.dh.gov.uk/en/publicationsandstatistics/publications/publicationspolicyandguidance/dh_4002766

This booklet contains guidance on measures to protect clinical health care workers against occupational infection with blood-borne viruses. It is based on the recommendations of the Expert Advisory Group on AIDS and the Advisory Group on Hepatitis. It draws also on work done by the Advisory Committee on Dangerous Pathogens and the Microbiology Advisory Committee.

MENTAL HEALTH

Mental health problems include mental illness; medically unexplained symptoms (MUS – formerly termed psychogenic problems); dementia, discussed in Ch. 13; and learning impairment discussed in Ch. 28.

Mental health is often affected by social, psychological, biological, genetic and environmental factors and changes in the brain neurotransmitters in the central nervous system (CNS) (Table 10.1).

Emotion is not a function of any specific brain area but of a circuit that involves interconnected basic structures, the hypothalamus, the anterior thalamic nucleus, the cingulate gyrus, the hippocampus: the prefrontal area, the parahippocampal gyrus and subcortical groupings like the amygdala, the medial thalamic nucleus, the septal area, the basal nuclei and a few brainstem formations (Table 10.2)

BRAIN NEUROTRANSMITTERS

Brain neurotransmitters include monoamines, acetylcholine, amino acids, gamma-aminobutyric acid, peptides, substance P and opioids (Table 10.3).

Monoamines include catecholamines (norepinephrine, epinephrine and dopamine), serotonin (5-hydroxytryptamine or 5HT) and histamine. Norepinephrine (noradrenaline) is released by post-ganglionic neurons of the sympathetic branch of the autonomic nervous system. Acetylcholine (ACh) mediates transmission at brain synapses involved in the acquisition of short-term memory. Amino acids such as glutamic acid (Glu) are involved in transmission at excitatory synapses and are essential for long-term potentiation (LTP), a form of memory. Gamma-aminobutyric acid (GABA) is released at inhibitory synapses to hyperpolarize the post-synaptic membrane, resulting in an inhibitory post-synaptic potential (IPSP). Peptides not only serve as brain neurotransmitters but some are also hormones, such as vasopressin (antidiuretic hormone; ADH), oxytocin, gonadotropin-releasing hormone (GnRH), angiotensin II and cholecystokinin (CCK). Other transmitters include substance P, which transmits pain impulses and opioids – a term used for all enkephalins, endorphins and morphine-like peptide chemicals, including dynorphin.

Enkephalins (from the Greek *kephale* meaning head) are pentapeptides. One enkephalin, leu-enkephalin, terminates in a leucine; the other, met-enkephalin, terminates in a methionine. Enkephalins are released at synapses on neurons involved in transmitting pain signals to the brain and act as an intrinsic pain-suppressing system, hyperpolarizing the post-synaptic membrane and thus inhibiting pain signals.

Endorphins are small-chain peptides that activate opiate receptors, producing feelings of well-being, as well as tolerance to pain. These compounds are hundreds or even thousands of times more potent than morphine. Four groups of endorphins – alpha, beta, gamma, and sigma – have been identified.

Table 10.1 Main parts and functions of the brain

Main part of brain (Fig 10.1)		Neurological functions	Mental and other functions
Supratentorial	Cerebrum	Initiation of movement, coordination of movement, temperature, touch, vision, hearing,	Higher functions, memory, judgment, ideas, reasoning, problem solving, emotions, learning. Skillful intellectual tasks (e.g. Reading, writing mathematical calculations). Limbic system contains several nuclei of grey matter around the brain stem. This commands certain behaviours necessary for survival (allow the person to distinguish between the agreeable and the disagreeable: affective functions are developed, such as the one that induces the females to nurse and protect their toddlers, or the one which induces playful moods). Emotions and feelings, like wrath, fright, passion, love, hate, joy and sadness, originate in the limbic system. This system is also responsible for aspects of personal identity and important functions related to memory.
	Brainstem, includes midbrain, pons, and medulla	Movement of eyes and mouth, relaying sensory messages (i.e., hot, pain, loud), hunger, respiration, consciousness, cardiac function, body temperature, involuntary muscle movements, sneezing, coughing, vomiting, and swallowing	Self preservation. Mechanisms of aggression and repetitive behaviour. Instinctive reactions of the so-called reflex arcs and the commands which allow some involuntary actions and the control of visceral functions (cardiac, pulmonary, intestinal, etc),
Infratentorial	Cerebellum	Coordinates voluntary muscle movements and maintains posture, balance, and equilibrium	-

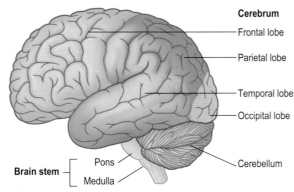

Fig. 10.1 Brain Structure

Dynorphins are other brain opioid peptides.

Factors that influence the production of enkephalins, endorphins and dynorphins include prolonged strenuous activity, transcutaneous electrical nerve stimulation (TENS), acupuncture and placebos. Enkephalins and endorphins bind to neuroreceptors in the brain to give relief from pain. This effect appears to be responsible for the so-called runner's high, the temporary loss of pain after severe injury, and the analgesic effects that acupuncture and chiropractic adjustments of the spine can offer.

Enkephalins are found especially in the thalamus and in parts of the spinal cord that transmit pain impulses and the adrenal medulla. Enkephalins act as analgesics and sedatives and appear to affect mood and motivation. Blood levels rise after exercise and sexual activity, and may explain how someone severely wounded can continue to function. Endorphins may act to prevent the release of substance P, which may account for the sedating effects of endogenous endorphins and of opioids given therapeutically. Endorphins also have anti-ageing effects by removing superoxide, anti-stress activity, pain-relieving effects and memory-improving activity. Endorphins may link the emotional state of well-being and the health of the immune system.

Once any neurotransmitter has acted, it must be removed from the synaptic cleft, usually by reuptake or breakdown, to prepare the synapse for the arrival of the next action potential. All the neurotransmitters except ACh do this via reuptake. ACh is removed from the synapse by enzymatic breakdown by acetylcholinesterase into inactive fragments.

Other factors that affect mental health include the following.

- *Antidepressant drugs:* monoamine oxidase inhibitors block the breakdown of monoamines, such as noradrenaline and serotonin. Selective serotonin reuptake inhibitors (SSRIs) block the reuptake only of serotonin, but tricyclics interfere with noradrenaline and serotonin reuptake from synapses and thus enhance the action.
- *Amino acids* such as tyrosine, phenylalanine, methionine, tryptophan and GABA are essential for the production of neurotransmitters and are, therefore, natural antidepressants. Organic sulfur in the form of methylsulfonylmethane (MSM) is needed for their production and utilization. Dietary supplementation with MSM may improve alertness and elevate mood.
- *Hormones:* act indirectly via control of blood sugar, calcium, and sodium balance, and they affect behaviour in general – anger, love, anxiety, panic attacks and agitation.

Table 10.2   Main parts and functions of the brain involved wiht emotion and mood

Brain area	Emotions/moods
Amygdala	Mediates and controls major affective activities like friendship, love and affection, expressions of mood and fear, rage and aggression
Cingulate gyrus	Coordinates smells and sights with pleasant memories of previous emotions and participates in the emotional reaction to pain and in the regulation of aggressive behaviour
Hippocampus	Responsible for long-term memory
Hypothalamus	Connects wiht other proscencephalic areas and the mesencephalus.Involved with several vegetative functions and some so-called motivated behaviours, like thermal regulations, sexuality, combativeness, hunger and thirst. Also play a role in emotion, with pleasure and rage, aversion, and laughing.
Nucleus accumbens	Responsible for pleasurable sensations, some of them similar to orgasm.
Septal region	Associated with different kinds of pleasant sensations, mainly those related to sexual experiences. Anterior frontal lobe is important in the genesis and expressoin of affection, joy, sadness, hope or despair as well as the capacity for concentration, problem-solving and abstraction.
Thalamus	Associated with emotional/reactivity due to connections with other limbic system structures. The medical dorsal nucleus connects with the frontal area and hypothalamus. The anterior nuclei connect with the mamilary bodies, and through them, via fornix, with the hippocampus and the cingulate gyrus

Hypoglycaemia can cause agitation, depression and poor mental concentration. Hypothyroidism can cause impotence and depression. Hyperthyroidism can cause agitation, irritability and lack of sleep. Addison disease can cause severe depression, while those treated with high corticosteroid doses can become euphoric or have hallucinations and psychoses. Sex steroids such as testosterone clearly affect mood and behaviour. The mood swings associated with premenstrual stress and menopause may be reduced with natural progesterone cream derived from wild yam – all sex steroids were originally produced from wild (elephant foot) yam. Melatonin may ease depression.

- *Drugs that bind to the GABA receptor* to enhance the inhibitory effect of GABA in the CNS. These include sedatives such as phenobarbital, alcohol, and anxiolytics such as benzodiazepines.
- *Drugs such as chlorpromazine and haloperidol bind to dopamine receptor* leading to greater synthesis of dopamine at the synapse easing some of the symptoms of schizophrenia.
- *Naloxone binds to the opioid kappa receptor,* and blocks both enkephalin-degrading enzyme inhibitors (enkephalinase inhibitors) and kappa antagonist.

Table 10.3 Some neurotransmitters, functions and associated disorders

Neurotransmitter	Functions	Associated disorders
Acetylcholine (ACh)	Alertness, memory Muscle tone, learning, primitive drives, emotions, release of vasopressin, which is involved in learning and in regulation of urine output. ACh-releasing neurons in the pons are active in rapid eye movement (REM) sleep (dreaming) ACh is also related to sexual performance and arousal – helps control blood flow to genitals, heart rate, and blood pressure during sexual intercourse	Alzheimer disease is associated with 90% loss of ACh in the forebrain and hippocampus
Dopamine	Produces feelings of bliss ('the pleasure chemical'). Regulates information flow into the frontal lobe from other areas of brain. More dopamine in the frontal lobe lessens pain and increases pleasure. Affects voluntary movement, learning, memory, emotion	Parkinson disease is brought on when dopamine fails to reach the basal ganglia Dopamine is also related to attention deficit hyperactivity disorder (ADHD) Schizophrenia is associated with the inability of dopamine to reach the frontal lobe Excess dopamine in the limbic system and not enough in the cortex may produce paranoia or inhibit social interaction. A shortage of dopamine in the frontal lobes may cause poor memory Cocaine, opiates and alcohol produce effects in part via dopamine release
Endorphins and enkephalins	Involved in pain reduction, pleasure (enhance release of dopamine) and hibernation as well as a number of other behaviours. Endorphins block pain at receptor sites. Endorphins also facilitate the dopamine pathway that feeds into the frontal lobe, thereby replacing pain with pleasure. Also produced by the pituitary gland and released as hormones	Opiates (natural and synthetic) bind to endorphin and enkephalin brain receptors and alter behaviour
Epinephrine (adrenaline)	Physiological expressions of fear and anxiety (fright, fight and flight)	Epinephrine in excess is seen in anxiety disorders
Gamma-aminobutyric acid (GABA)	Major inhibitory neurotransmitter lessening anxiety. Brain produces substances which enhance anxiety (beta-carbolines) as well as substances which lower anxiety (e.g. allopregnanolone). All modify GABA brain receptors to produce effects	Anxiolytic drugs, such as benzodiazepines, act by enhancing effects of GABA at synapses
Glutamate	Glutamate is the main brain excitatory neurotransmitter, with actions mediated at NMDA and AMPA receptors involved in memory formation	Glutamate is involved in a 'suicidal' response when the brain is damaged, as in stroke. Excess glutamate is neurotoxic and neurons are damaged by the excessive calcium that enters the cell due to glutamate binding. Glutamate is produced excessively in ALS.
Neuropeptide Y/ polypeptide YY (NPY/PPYY)	Affect hypothalamus and bring about excessive food intake and fat storage	Linked with eating disorders
Norepinephrine (noradrenaline)	Stimulant to the body and mind. Norepinephrine causes some of the physiological expressions of fear and anxiety (fright, fight and flight response). Modulates heart rate, blood pressure, learning, memory, waking, emotion	Most forms of depression are associated with a deficiency of norepinephrine. High levels of norepinephrine can cause aggression. Stress in children can create permanently high levels of norepinephrine, creating the potential for violent behaviour. Raised levels of norepinephrine mixed with dopamine and phenylethylamine produce feelings of infatuation
Oxytocin	Raised levels of oxytocin give mothers an impulse to cuddle their newborns	High oxytocin levels contribute to multiple orgasms in women
Phenylethylamine	Phenylethylamine in the limbic system gives feelings of bliss	A natural ingredient in chocolate
Serotonin (5-hydroxytryptamine)	Serotonin is the 'feelgood' hormone that enables us to relax and enjoy life. Serotonin is synthesized from the amino acid L-tryptophan. Serotonin also serves as a precursor for the pineal hormone melatonin, which regulates the body clock: sleep, appetite, sensory perception, temperature regulation, pain suppression and mood	Most forms of depression are associated with a deficiency of serotonin at functionally important serotonergic receptors
Substance P	Substance P is a neurotransmitter that mediates pain. It is found throughout the pain pathway and its release can be blocked by enkephalins and endorphins	–

ALS, amyotrophic lateral sclerosis; AMPA, alpha-amino-3-hydroxyl-5-methyl-4-isoxazole-propionate; NMDA, N-methyl-D-aspartate.

ENVIRONMENTAL FACTORS

Life stresses such as bereavement and divorce can play a significant role in mental health. Lifestyles can also influence mental health: brisk exercise can, by stimulating release of norepinephrine and endorphins, lift depression and create a sense of euphoria. Sunlight stimulates the pineal gland to release serotonin and improve mood. This is one reason why more people tend to be depressed during the darker winter months – SAD (seasonal affective disorder).

GENETIC FACTORS

Genetics plays a role in shaping our personality and consequently our psychological status. The interactions of genetic and environmental factors are believed to cause a number of mental health problems from autism to bipolar disorder.

NEUROIMMUNOLOGICAL MECHANISMS

There appears to be a relationship between mental health and the immune system, which can be both overactive or suppressed, leading to associated diseases. There is growing evidence that such neuroimmunological mechanisms might influence immunological and inflammatory disorders and defence against infection. It has, for example, been suggested that stress might underlie some periodontal and other oral diseases. The major route identified for neuroimmunomodulation is via the neuroendocrine system.

In addition to recognizable neurotransmitters, the nervous system contains significant levels of cytokines and their receptors. Thus the possibility of a two-way exchange of information is clearly present. Immune cells possess a host of receptor profiles for modulatory substances and many of these are common to the nervous system. Two different pathways and effects of immediate stress can be demonstrated as follows.

- The endocrine path, in which the CNS is central to the control of release of glucocorticosteroids such as cortisol, which have an immunosuppressive effect and have temporary adverse effects on cognitive functions, such as learning and memory.
- The second, direct neural pathway to the adrenal medulla, releases other transmitters, particularly catecholamines, which depress chemotaxis and phagocytosis, and beta-adrenergic agonists, which have general effects on white blood cells.

In severe long-term stress, natural opioids are released–the adrenals release met-enkephalin and the hypothalamus releases β-endorphin, which leads to enhanced antitumour activity of NK cells and proliferative response of lymphocytes.

Inflammatory cytokines-interleukin (IL)-1b, IL-6 and tumour necrosis factor (TNF) α-activate the hypothalamo–pituitary–adrenal (HPA) axis. IL-1 modulates brain catecholamine activity: depletion of central catecholamines potentiates severity of inflammation and also affects the release of corticotropin-releasing hormone (CRH) and adrenocorticotropic hormone (ACTH). IL-1, IL-6 and nitric oxide modulate brain serotonin activity, depletion of which enhances inflammatory response.

Under stress conditions, if immune activity is not controlled, it may reach a state of activation in which host injury and tissue destruction can take place (autoimmunity).

MENTAL HEALTH AND DISEASE

Good mental health is not just the absence of diagnosable mental health problems, but is characterised by the ability to:

- learn
- feel, express and manage a range of positive and negative emotions
- form and maintain good relationships with others
- cope with and manage change and uncertainty.

When a person experiences severe and or enduring mental health problems they are sometimes described as mentally ill, but there is no universally agreed cut-off point at which behaviour becomes abnormal enough to be termed mental illness and, in any event, the term mental illness can imply that all such problems are solely caused by medical or biological factors, whereas most seen to result from complex interactions of medical, biological, social and/or psychological factors.

Mental health problems traditionally have been classified as *Organic* (identifiable brain disease) or *Functional* (no obvious brain structural abnormality); or as *Neuroses* (severe forms of normal experiences such a low mood, anxiety with insight retained) or *Psychoses* (severe distortion of a person's perception of reality with loss of insight). Neuroses covers those symptoms which can be regarded as severe forms of 'normal' emotional experiences such as depression, anxiety or panic; are now more often termed "common mental health problems" and include problems such as anxiety, depression, phobias, obsessive compulsive and panic disorders. Psychoses are less common and manifest with symptoms which interfere with a person's perception of reality; may include hallucinations such as seeing, hearing, smelling or feeling things that no-one else can and include severe and enduring mental health problems such as schizophrenia and bipolar affective disorder (manic depression).

Personality disorder is defined as 'an enduring pattern of inner experience and behaviours that deviates markedly from the expectation of the individual's culture, is pervasive and inflexible, has an onset in adolescence or early adulthood, is stable over time and leads to distress or impairment'.

Several diagnostic and classification frameworks have been developed to help identify mental health problems. The main two are the ICD (International Statistical Classification of Diseases and Related Health Problems) of the WHO (ICD-10 is version 10) and the DSM (Diagnostic and Statistical Manual of Mental Disorders) of the American Psychiatric Association (DSM-IV-TR is version 4 revised) classify mental health problems in a series of families or categories (Box 10.1).

DENTAL ASPECTS

Preventive dentistry is crucial in patients with mental health problems. The patient may neglect oral hygiene, dental appointments and instructions unless a caregiver or family member is also involved. Dental staff must use great tact, patience and a sympathetic, unpatronizing manner in handling patients with mental health problems. To avoid causing adverse drug interactions, take special precautions when administering certain antibiotics, analgesics and sedatives. The treatment should be in the morning, when cooperation tends to be best, with the usual carertakers present and in a familiar environment, and allowing time to explain every procedure before it is carried out. The patient should be treated while sitting upright in the dental chair or slightly reclined, to avoid aspiration and postural hypotension (Ch. 5).

PERSONALITY DISORDERS

In mental health, the word 'personality' refers to the collection of characteristics or traits that makes each of us an individual, including the ways that we think, feel and behave.

Personality may develop in a way that makes it difficult for us to live with ourselves and/or other people – traits or disorders usually noticeable from childhood or early teens. Personality disorders are chronic abnormalities of character or maladjustment to life that shade into neuroses or psychoses and may make it difficult to make or keep relationships, get on with friends and family or with people at work, keep out of trouble or control feelings or behaviour. However, insight is retained and most patients manage to pursue a relatively normal life. Personality disorders are shown in Table 10.4.

Causes include upbringing (neglect, physical or sexual abuse, violence in the family, parents who drink too much alcohol), early problems (childhood severe aggression, disobedience and temper tantrums) or brain problems (these remain to be defined). Personality disorders may be aggravated by drugs or alcohol, interpersonal conflicts, financial problems or other mental health problems.

People with personality disorders are often made unhappy by poor relationships or frequent conflicts and severe antisocial

Table 10.4 Types of personality disorder

Personality disorder	Features
Cluster A	**Paranoid**
Paranoid	Suspicious, distrustful, litigious, lacking humour, blames others Feel that other people are being unpleasant (even when evidence shows this isn't true), sensitive to rejection, tend to hold grudges
Schizoid	Socially distant, detached, secretive, isolated, lack friends Emotionally 'cold', don't like contact with other people, prefer own company; have a rich fantasy world
Schizotypal	Odd, eccentric, difficulties with thinking, lack of emotion, or inappropriate emotional reactions, can see or hear strange things, related to schizophrenia
Cluster B	**Emotional and impulsive**
Antisocial or dissocial	Impulsive, aggressive, manipulative, selfish, callous, disloyal, in conflict with everyone and everything, don't care about the feelings of others, easily frustrated Tend to be aggressive, commit crimes, find it difficult to make intimate relationships, don't feel guilty, don't learn from unpleasant experiences
Borderline	Impulsive, self-destructive, unstable, find it hard to control emotions Feel bad about self, often self-harm, feel 'empty', make relationships quickly, but easily lose them, can feel paranoid or depressed, when stressed, may hear noises or voices
Histrionic	Emotional, dramatic, theatrical, immature, manipulative, attention-seeking, shallow interpersonal relationships, overdramatize events, self-centred Show strong emotions, but which change quickly and don't last long Can be suggestible, worry a lot about appearance, crave new things and excitement, can be seductive
Narcissistic	Boastful, egotistical, 'superiority complex', strong sense of own self-importance Dream of unlimited success, power and intellectual brilliance, crave attention, but show few warm feelings in return, exploit others, ask for favours not then returned
Cluster C	**Anxious**
Avoidant	Shy, timid, ('inferiority complex'), very anxious and tense, worry a lot Feel insecure and inferior, have to be liked and accepted Extremely sensitive to criticism
Dependent	Dependent, submissive, clinging, passive, rely on others to make their own decisions, find it hard to cope with daily chores, feel hopeless and incompetent Easily feel abandoned by others
Obsessive–compulsive (anankastic)	Perfectionistic, rigid, controlling, chronically worried about standards and self-image; unable to relax and are often depressed Rigid; cautious, preoccupied with detail, worry about doing the wrong thing, find it hard to adapt; often have high moral standards Judgemental; sensitive to criticism; can have obsessional thoughts and images (although these are not as bad as those in obsessive–compulsive disorder)

personality disorders can lead to criminal behaviour. Dangerous and severe personality disorders are the subject of a recent review of the Mental Health Act; these patients may be detained under the Act regardless of the absence of treatable disease.

Handling patients with personality disorders requires enormous patience and tolerance, and the exercise of tact and skills. These skills only come with appreciation of the existence of these disorders and with experience, but are difficult to acquire. Even with such skills, little progress may still be possible. Antipsychotics, antidepressant or mood-stabilizing drug therapy may be helpful.

BORDERLINE PERSONALITY DISORDER

General aspects

Borderline personality disorder (BPD) is characterized by pervasive instability of mood, interpersonal relationships, self-image and behaviour. It frequently disrupts family and work, long-term planning, and the individual's sense of self-identity. BPD affects 2% of adults, mostly young women.

Brain imaging studies in BPD show that individual differences in the ability to activate regions of the prefrontal cerebral cortex thought to be involved in inhibitory activity, predict the ability to suppress negative emotion.

Clinical features

A person with BPD may experience intense bouts of anger, depression and anxiety that may last only hours, or at most a day, while a person with depression or bipolar disorder (see below) typically endures the same types of mood for weeks. Bouts of BPD may be associated with episodes of impulsive aggression, self-injury, and drug or alcohol abuse. People with BPD may exhibit other impulsive behaviours, such as excessive spending, binge eating or risky sex. Distortions in cognition and sense of self can lead to frequent changes in long-term goals, career plans, jobs, friendships, gender identity and values.

Borderline personality disorder is often associated with other psychiatric problems, particularly bipolar disorder, depression, anxiety disorders, substance abuse and other personality disorders. Thus BPD often causes highly unstable patterns of social relationships.

General management

Dialectical behaviour therapy, developed specifically to treat BPD, involves four primary modes of treatment: individual therapy, group skills training, telephone contact and therapist consultation. Antidepressants and antipsychotic drugs may also be used.

Dental aspects

Persons with personality disorders may make unreliable patients. They are unlikely to have any conscience about missing appointments or to pay much attention to oral health care instructions. Treatment plans may be argued about or frankly refused. Payment may be withheld and litigation threatened.

Dental staff may also have personality disorders and find themselves in conflict with others, including colleagues – often to the dental staff's disadvantage – and may find it difficult not to antagonize patients and colleagues.

ANXIETY AND STRESS

Stress may play a greater role in health and disease than formerly supposed. Humans are sensitive to stressors (e.g. operations) and even visits for health care can activate the HPA system. Anxiety generated by such ordeals as dental or medical appointments, or by public speaking, solo musical performances, examinations or interviews is normal. Stress is also fairly common in dental students and staff. Work stressors may include examinations, fear of failure, difficulties with accommodation or study facilities, inadequate holidays or relaxation time, financial difficulties, criticism, and time and scheduling demands. Stress can lead to reactions affecting a wide range of functions (Table 10.5).

Fear, an emotion that deals with danger, causes an automatic, rapid protective response in many body systems, coordinated by the amygdala. Emotional memories stored in the central amygdala may play a role in disorders involving very distinct fears, such as phobias, while different parts may be involved in other forms of anxiety.

The hippocampus – an area of the brain critical to memory and emotion – is involved in intrusive memories and flashbacks typical of post-traumatic stress disorder, and results in raised levels of stress hormones – cortisol, epinephrine and norepinephrine.

Table 10.5 Some possible effects of acute and chronic stress

	Mild stress	Acute stress	Chronic stress
Central nervous system	Mood change	Improved concentration and clarity of thought	Anxiety, loss of sense of humour, depression, fatigue, headaches, migraines, tremor
Cardiovascular	Rise in pulse rate and blood pressure	Tachycardia, arrhythmias	Hypertension, chest pain Ischaemic heart disease
Respiratory	Raised respiratory rate	Hyperventilation	Cough and asthma
Mouth	Slight dryness	Dry mouth	Dry mouth, ulcers
Gastrointestinal	Raised bowel activity	Impaired digestion	Peptic ulceration Irritable bowel syndrome
Sexual	Male impotence and female irregular menstruation	Male impotence and female irregular menstruation	Male impotence and female amenorrhoea

Danger induces high levels of enkephalins and endorphins, natural opioids, which can temporarily mask pain, and in some anxiety states higher levels persist even after the danger has passed.

Cortisol is the major steroid hormone produced in the adrenal glands and is essential for the body to cope with stress. Cortisol levels exhibit a natural rise in the morning and fall at night. If this rhythm is disturbed, mineral balance, blood sugar control and stress responses are affected. Lack of cortisol can lead to fatigue, allergies and arthritis, while excess cortisol can have an even greater negative effect on the body. While short-term elevations of cortisol are important for dealing with the stress of life-threatening issues, illness and wound healing, chronically elevated levels of cortisol can result in tiredness, depression and accelerated ageing with hypertension muscle loss, bone destruction, obesity and diabetes. Prolonged stress or prolonged exposure to glucocorticoids can also have adverse effects on the hippocampus to cause atrophy, and memory deficits such as have been demonstrated in Cushing syndrome, depression and post-traumatic stress disorder.

Dehydroepiandrosterone (DHEA), the most abundant steroid hormone in the body, appears to counter the effects of high levels of cortisol and improves the ability to cope with stress. Low levels of DHEA have been associated with impaired immunity, cardiovascular disease, Alzheimer disease, hypothyroidism and diabetes.

Anxious or stressed patients may require drugs to control the anxiety but they respond better to beta-blocking agents (such as propranolol) than to benzodiazepines, and with less impairment of performance. Stress may lead to substance abuse (Ch. 34). Anxiety may be caused or aggravated by using caffeine or street drugs like amphetamines, LSD or Ecstasy.

CLINICAL FEATURES

Anxiety can cause several physical effects as a result of overwhelming autonomic activity. Sympathetic activity via the release of catecholamines causes apprehension, tachycardia, hyperventilation, hypertension, sweating, tremor and dilated pupils. Parasympathetic activity may lead to involuntary defaecation and urinary incontinence. These changes may be recognized by features as in Table 10.6.

DIAGNOSIS

Pathological anxiety may be difficult to diagnose and requires careful consideration of an individual's personal history and presenting clinical features. A thorough history and perhaps psychiatric assessment may be appropriate, but underlying organic causes such as hyperthyroidism and mitral valve prolapse should be excluded first. Anxiety can be classified into the following diagnostic categories:

- panic disorder – discrete attacks with no external stimulus
- phobias – discrete attacks with stimuli
- generalized anxiety disorder – a generalized persistent state of anxiety
- anxiety as a manifestation of other psychiatric disease such as depression.

MANAGEMENT

Treatment of anxiety and stress may require:

- appropriate management of any underlying organic disease
- lifestyle changes to reduce stressors and avoid precipitating factors
- behavioural techniques
- pharmacotherapy (anxiolytics and beta-blockers)
- psychotherapy – this may be used to aid adjustment of lifestyle (supportive) or to explore patient conflicts and secondary gain (psychodynamic).

Psychotherapy involves talking with a mental health professional, such as a psychiatrist, psychologist, social worker or counsellor, to learn how to deal with problems. Cognitive behavioural therapy (CBT) and behavioural therapy are effective for several anxiety disorders, particularly panic disorder and social phobia. There are two components – the cognitive component helps to change thinking patterns that keep them from overcoming their fears, and the behavioural component seeks to change reactions to anxiety-provoking situations. A key element of this component is exposure, in which people have to confront the things they fear. Behavioural therapy alone, without a strong cognitive component, has been used effectively to treat specific phobias. Here, persons are gradually exposed to the objects or situations that are feared. Often the therapist will accompany them to provide support and guidance. After treatment, the beneficial effects of CBT may last longer than those of medication for people with panic disorder; the same may be true for obsessive–compulsive disorder (OCD), post-traumatic stress disorder and social phobia.

Drugs can play a part in the treatment of some people with anxiety or phobias. Medications used include anxiolytics, such as benzodiazepines (BZPs), which relieve symptoms quickly with few side-effects, except often for some drowsiness. Benzodiazepines include clonazepam, which is used for social phobia and generalized anxiety disorder (GAD), and alprazolam, which is helpful for panic disorder and GAD; and lorazepam, which is also useful for panic disorder. BZPs should be prescribed for short periods of time because of development of tolerance (rising doses to get the same effect) and dependence. Panic disorder is an exception, for which BZPs may be used for 6 months to a year. Those who abuse drugs or alcohol are not usually good candidates for BZPs because they can become dependent. Withdrawal symptoms, and in certain instances rebound anxiety, can follow after stopping BZPs. Benzodiazepines should not be given to children, the elderly, alcoholics (except to treat withdrawal), or pregnant or lactating women. Temazepam is particularly prone to become abused and is a controlled drug.

Table 10.6	Features suggesting anxiety		
	FEATURES		
	Physiological	Behavioural	Cognitive
Child	Pallor Increased pulse rate Tension Hyperventilation	Crying Uncooperative, restless or disruptive Silent or sullen	Scared Anxious Negative thoughts
Adult	Dry mouth	Verbal abuse Excessive talking Cancelling appointments, arriving late or not at all	Negative thoughts

Table 10.7 Modified dental anxiety scale (modified from Humphris et al., 2000)					
	Not anxious	Slightly anxious	Fairly anxious	Very anxious	Extremely anxious
If you went to your dentist for treatment tomorrow, how would you feel?					
If you were sitting in the waiting room (waiting for treatment), how would you feel?					
If you were about to have a tooth drilled, how would you feel?					
If you were about to have your teeth scaled and polished, how would you feel?					
If you were about to have a local anaesthetic injection, how would you feel?					

Beta-blockers, such as propanolol, are helpful in certain anxiety disorders, particularly social phobia. Antidepressants can help to relieve anxiety.

DENTAL ASPECTS

Anxiety can be generated by dental or medical appointments, even amongst normal patients and is a perfectly natural reaction to an unpleasant experience. A total of 65% of patients report some level of fear of dental treatment. It is essential, therefore, not to dismiss patients who will not accept a proposed treatment as being 'phobic' or 'uncooperative', though a small number of patients will require psychological or even psychiatric assessment and/or treatment. Younger patients have significantly more fear of treatment than older patients. Among fearful patients, changes in pulse rate (> 10 beats/min) and changes in blood pressure are detectable.

Quantification of anxiety levels can be achieved using a modified dental anxiety scale (Table 10.7). Other scales and a range of techniques to manage such patients are outlined by Rafique et al. (2008).

Dental 'phobia' is more extreme than straightforward anxiety, and previous frightening dental experiences are often cited as the major factor in their development. Patients fear the noise and vibration of the drill (56%), the sight of the injection needle (47%) and sitting at the treatment chair (42%) especially. Effects include muscle tension (64%), faster heartbeat (59%), accelerated breathing (37%), sweating (32%) and stomach cramps (28%). Patients with a true phobic neurosis about dental treatment are uncommon but, when seen, demand great patience. Phobic patients, who may genuinely want dental care but be unable to cooperate, are often unaware of their anxiety and, as a consequence, may be hostile in their responses or behaviour. Some patients are difficult or even impossible to manage because of anxiety, phobia or personality disorders.

Patients who apply for treatment at a dental fear clinic are not just dentally anxious; they often show a wide range of other complaints. Persons with clinically significant fear tend to have poorer perceived dental health, a longer interval since their last dental appointment, a higher frequency of past fear behaviours, more physical symptoms during dental injections, and higher percentage of symptoms of anxiety and depression. They may chatter incessantly, have a history of failed appointments, and appear tense and agitated ('white knuckle syndrome').

Dental treatment in anxiety states is usually straightforward. Early morning appointments, with pre-medication and no waiting, can help. The main aids are careful, painlessly performed dental procedures, psychological approaches, confident reassurance, patience and, sometimes, the use of pharmacological agents, for example anxiolytics such as oral diazepam, supplemented if necessary with intravenous, transmucosal or inhalational sedation during dental treatment. General techniques to help overcome anxiety include relaxation techniques (e.g. deep breathing), distraction (e.g. watching TV), control strategies (e.g. 'put your hand up if you wish me to stop') and positive reinforcement (e.g. praise). Other techniques include systematic desensitization, biofeedback, modelling and hypnosis, and may need support from a psychologist.

Symptoms such as agitation, slight tachycardia and dry mouth, mainly caused by sympathetic overactivity, are usually controllable by reassurance and possibly a very mild anxiolytic or sedative, such as a low dose of a beta-blocker or a short-acting (temazepam) or moderate-acting (lorazepam or diazepam) benzodiazepine, provided the patient is not pregnant and does not drive, operate dangerous machinery or make important decisions for the following 24 h. Temazepam 10 mg orally on the night before and 1 h before dental treatment can be used to supplement gentle sympathetic handling and reassurance of the anxious patient. Intravenous or intranasal sedation with midazolam, or relative analgesia using nitrous oxide and oxygen, is also useful. Benzodiazepine metabolism is impaired by azole antifungals, and by macrolide antibiotics such as erythromycin and clarithromycin. Alcohol, antihistamines and barbiturates have additive sedative effects with benzodiazepines. The analgesic dextropropoxyphene should be avoided in patients taking alprazolam as it may cause toxicity.

Difficulties may also result from alcoholism or drug dependence, or drug treatment with major tranquillizers, monoamine oxidase inhibitors or tricyclic antidepressants. Oral manifestations, such as facial arthromyalgia, dry mouth, lip-chewing or bruxism may be complaints in chronically anxious people. Cancer phobia is also an indication of an anxiety.

STRESS IN DENTAL STAFF

Dentistry can be a stressful occupation both for dentist and ancillary staff. There appears to be a significant level of dissatisfaction amongst dental nurses and hygienists in general practice, in terms of working conditions, relations with other staff and management skills of the dentist.

Increasingly, dentists in general practice appear concerned about the business aspects of practice, and seem to experience more physical and mental ill-health compared with other health professionals. In contrast, community dentists may be more worried about clinical matters, such as treating medical emergencies or difficult patients.

OBSESSIVE–COMPULSIVE DISORDER (OCD)

General aspects

Obsessional personality traits are common, especially amongst dental and medical personnel, and often salutary. Many healthy people have features of OCD and secondary ritualistic behaviours such as checking that the door is locked several times before or after leaving the house. In true OCD, the urge to do or think certain things repeatedly can dominate life unhelpfully, with obsessive activities consuming at least 1 h a day, causing significant disruption of normal life. For example, one dental surgeon felt compelled to telephone his patients late at night because he was obsessed with the notion that, having prepared the cavity, he might have forgotten to place the restoration. The basal ganglia and striatum appear to be involved in OCD. OCD strikes males slightly more commonly and usually starts in childhood, adolescence or early adulthood.

OCD is the fourth most common mental disorder, affecting 1–2% of the population and it appears to be increasing.

Clinical features

OCD is comprised of thoughts (obsessions) that create anxiety, and things the patient does to reduce the anxiety (compulsions). Obsessional patients are often intelligent, many are unmarried and many have a pre-morbid state, such as an uncertain and vacillating, or alternatively a stubborn, rigid, morose and irritable, personality. Obsessional thoughts are those that come repeatedly into consciousness against the patient's will, are usually unpleasant, but always recognized as the patient's own thoughts. Typical obsessions are the repeated checking, questioning of decisions, hoarding, counting, religious compulsions, the fear of harm or harming, or the fear of dirtiness or contamination.

However, the thoughts are not accepted by the patients as harmless or inevitable and an internal struggle against them leads to secondary ritualistic thought or behaviour patterns (compulsions). The compulsions may include rituals, checking, avoidance, hoarding and reassurance. A prominent example was the millionaire Howard Hughes who was so severely affected that he eventually ended up sitting naked in the middle of his hotel room obsessed with concerns about 'contamination' with six aides 'cleaning' him.

The obsessional thoughts may also in turn generate depression or other anxiety disorders, and some people with OCD also have eating disorders. Obsessional features can also be associated with disorders such as depression, schizophrenia or, rarely, organic brain disease.

The course of OCD is variable. Symptoms may come and go, may ease over time or they can grow progressively worse.

General management

Treatment is often difficult, though OCD may respond to psychotherapy, or medication with antidepressants, especially SSRIs, clomipramine, and the tricyclic antidepressants, which are useful when there is also depression. The benzodiazepines may be useful when anxiety is predominant.

Dental aspects

It is questionable whether true obsessions often become centred on the mouth but they may, for example, result in compulsive toothbrushing or excessive use of antiseptic mouthwashes. Occasional patients become obsessed with the possibility of infections or cancer in the mouth (as, for example, a patient who was obsessed with the idea that his Fordyce spots were thrush) and refuse to be reassured. Some patients become obsessed with the notion that they have oral malodour.

POST-TRAUMATIC STRESS DISORDER

General aspects

Post-traumatic stress disorder (PTSD) is an anxiety state that can follow exposure to a terrifying event where victims can see danger, where life is threatened, or they see other people dying or being injured. Traumatic events that can trigger PTSD include personal assaults, such as rape or mugging, disasters, accidents or military combat.

Many people with PTSD repeatedly re-experience the ordeal in the form of flashback episodes, memories, nightmares or frightening thoughts, or being 'on guard', especially when exposed to events or objects reminiscent of the trauma. Anniversaries of the event can also trigger symptoms. Most people with PTSD thus try to avoid any reminders or thoughts of the ordeal (avoidance and numbing).

Clinical features

Post-traumatic stress disorder symptoms typically begin within 3 months of the traumatic event, but occasionally not until years later. Headaches, gastrointestinal complaints, dizziness, chest pain or discomfort elsewhere can be disabling. Emotional numbness and sleep disturbance, depression, anxiety, irritability or outbursts of anger and feelings of intense guilt are common.

Associated depression, alcohol or other substance abuse, or another anxiety disorder are also common.

General management

Cognitive behavioural therapy, group therapy, eye movement desensitization and reprocessing (EMDR) and exposure therapy, in which patients gradually and repeatedly relive the frightening experiences under controlled conditions to help them work through the trauma, can be effective. Medications, particularly SSRIs, are frequently prescribed (tricyclic antidepressants are as effective), and help to ease associated symptoms of depression and anxiety and to promote sleep.

Dental aspects

Frightening though dentistry may be, it is not known to have precipitated PTSD. However, patients who are suffering from PTSD may present with a variety of unexplained pain problems.

GENERALIZED ANXIETY DISORDER

General aspects

Generalized anxiety disorder differs from normal anxiety in that it is chronic and fills the day with exaggerated and unfounded worry and tension. GAD is twice as common in women as in men.

Clinical features

People with GAD are always anticipating disaster, often worrying excessively about health, money, family, or work and may have physical symptoms, such as fatigue, headaches, muscle tension, muscle aches, difficulty in swallowing, trembling, twitching, irritability, sweating and hot flushes, and trouble falling or staying asleep. Unlike other anxiety disorders, people with GAD do not characteristically avoid certain situations. GAD is often accompanied by other conditions associated with stress, such as irritable bowel syndrome. GAD may be accompanied by another anxiety disorder, depression or substance abuse.

General management

Generalized anxiety disorder is diagnosed when someone spends at least 6 months worrying excessively about everyday problems. GAD is commonly treated with CBT and benzodiazepines such as clonazepam or alprazolam. Venlafaxine, a drug closely related to the SSRIs, is also useful. Buspirone, an azipirone, is also used: it must be taken consistently for at least 2 weeks to achieve effect; possible side-effects include dizziness, headaches and nausea.

PANIC DISORDER

General aspects

Panic disorder is the term given to recurrent unpredictable attacks of severe anxiety with physical symptoms such as palpitations, chest pain, dyspnoea, paraesthesiae and sweating ('panic attacks'). There are associations with mitral valve prolapse in 50%.

Clinical features

Panic attacks can come at any time, even during sleep. In a panic attack, there are features of catecholamine release – the heart pounds and the patient may feel sweaty, weak, faint or dizzy. The hands may tingle or feel numb, and there may be nausea, chest pain, a sense of unreality or fear of impending doom.

Many or most of the symptoms may result from hyperventilation. An attack generally peaks within 10 min, but some symptoms may last much longer.

Many suffer intense anxiety between episodes, worrying when and where the next attack will strike.

Panic disorder is often accompanied by other conditions such as depression, drug abuse or alcoholism and may lead to a pattern of avoidance of places or situations where panic attacks have struck.

General management

Panic disorder is one of the most readily treatable disorders and usually responds to psychotherapy or medication with alprazolam or lorazepam. Fluoxetine or other SSRIs are prescribed frequently, but tricyclic antidepressants are as effective. Hyperventilation is effectively treated by rebreathing into a paper bag.

SOCIAL PHOBIA (SOCIAL ANXIETY DISORDER)

General aspects

Social phobia involves overwhelming anxiety and excessive self-consciousness in normal social situations, resulting in a persistent, intense and chronic fear of being watched and judged by others and being embarrassed or humiliated by their own actions. Women and men are equally likely to develop social phobia, usually beginning in childhood or early adolescence.

Clinical features

Accompanying physical symptoms may include blushing, profuse sweating, trembling, nausea and difficulty in talking. Anxiety disorders or depression are common and substance abuse may develop.

General management

Social phobia can usually be treated successfully with psychotherapy or medications. Beta-blockers, such as propanolol or clonazepam, are helpful. Fluoxetine or other SSRIs are frequently prescribed but tricyclic antidepressants are as effective.

SPECIFIC PHOBIAS (PHOBIC NEUROSES)

General aspects

A phobia is a morbid fear or anxiety out of all proportion to the threat, an intense irrational fear of something that poses little or no actual danger. Twice as common in women as in men, phobias usually appear first during childhood or adolescence and tend to persist into adulthood.

Clinical features

Phobic neuroses differ from anxiety neuroses in that the phobic anxiety arises only in specific circumstances, whereas patients with anxiety neuroses are *generally* anxious. Claustrophobia (fear of closed spaces) is probably the most common phobic disorder. Magnetic resonance imaging is sometimes impossible to carry out because of claustrophobia.

Some of the other more common specific phobias are centred around heights, tunnels, driving, water, flying, insects, dogs and injuries involving blood. When phobias are centred on threats such as flying, anaesthetics or dental treatment, normal life is possible if such threats are avoided. Phobias may also be a minor part of a more severe disorder, such as depression, obsessive neurosis, anxiety state, personality disorder or schizophrenia.

General management

Specific phobias are highly treatable with carefully targeted psychotherapy. Behaviour therapy aims at desensitization by slow and gradual exposure to the frightening situation. Implosion is a technique where patients are asked to imagine a persistently frightening situation for 1 or 2 h. Phobias can sometimes be controlled by anxiolytic drugs. Buspirone is particularly useful, since it lacks the psychomotor impairment, dependence and some other effects of benzodiazepine use. Antidepressants, especially tricyclic antidepressants, are used if there is a significant depressive component.

CHILDHOOD DISORDERS

These include attention-deficit/hyperactivity disorder, conduct disorder (the antisocial personality disorder of childhood) and oppositional defiant disorder (not only in children).

ATTENTION-DEFICIT/HYPERACTIVITY DISORDER

General aspects

Mischievous children are not abnormal. Overactivity or hyperactivity applies to gross misbehaviour such as reckless escapes from parents while on public transport. Hyperactive children always seem to be in motion and seem unable to curb their immediate reactions or think before they act. Although parents not infrequently describe their badly behaved child as 'overactive', the term should be limited to those who demonstrate gross behavioural abnormalities, including uncontrolled activity, impulsiveness, impaired concentration, motor restlessness and extreme fidgeting. These activities are seen particularly when orderliness is required, for example in the dental waiting room or surgery. Deficit in attention and motor control and perception may be a variant.

Attention-deficit/hyperactivity disorder (ADHD), once called *hyperkinesis* or *minimal brain dysfunction*, is characterized by inattention and hyperactivity and/or impulsivity, which are excessive, long-term and pervasive. ADHD is one of the most common of childhood mental disorders, affecting 3–5% of children; it is twice as common in boys as in girls and often continues into adolescence and adulthood.

Commonly associated disorders may include:

- oppositional defiant disorders affect nearly half of all children with ADHD, overreacting or lashing out when they resent anything
- developmental language disorders
- motor and coordination difficulties
- specific learning disabilities
- Tourette syndrome.

Overactivity can be caused by minor head injuries or undetectable brain damage, or refined sugar and food additives. It also be caused by factors affecting parents, or the child or the child–parent relationship, or external factors (Table 10.8).

Table 10.8 Causes of hyperactivity in a child

Child	Parental	External
Hyperkinetic syndrome	Child–parent relationship	Institutionalization
Brain damage	Rejection or overprotection	Excessive demands at school
Low intelligence	Inconsistent discipline	
Tartrazine sensitivity	Lack of parental love	
Anxiety states	Marital disharmony	
Drug abuse	Depression	

Clinical features

To make a diagnosis of ADHD, the abnormal behaviours above must be severe and appear before age 7 years, and continue for at least 6 months. Signs of inattention include becoming easily distracted by irrelevant sights and sounds, failing to pay attention to details and making careless mistakes, rarely following instructions carefully and completely, or losing or forgetting things such as toys, or pencils, books and tools needed for a task.

Signs of hyperactivity and impulsivity include feeling restless, often fidgeting with hands or feet, or squirming, running, climbing, or leaving a seat, in situations where sitting or quiet behaviour is expected, blurting out answers before hearing the whole question, having difficulty waiting in a queue or for a turn.

General management

Behavioural therapy, emotional counselling and practical support are required. Sedatives and tranquillizers should be avoided as they may impair learning ability or cause paradoxical reactions – such as aggressive behaviour. Stimulants surprisingly seem to be the most effective treatment in both children and adults, and include methylphenidate, atomoxetine and dextroamfetamine (dexamfetamine), or, in the USA, Adderall – a 'cocktail' mixture of four different amfetamine salts.

Dental aspects

- Overactive children can often be almost impossible to manage in the dental surgery and frequently succeed in frustrating all concerned.
- 'Tell-show-do' may be of value.
- Tranquillizers such as diazepam should be avoided as they usually exacerbate rather than depress overactivity.
- Dental treatment may not be possible without conscious sedation or GA. Such patients are, therefore, often referred to hospital for dental care. The drug treatment may create resistance to conscious sedation. LA containing adrenaline may interact with atomoxetine to increase blood pressure.

SOMATIZATION DISORDERS

GENERAL ASPECTS

Many people suffer inner anxieties and some are prone to turn these into symptoms; these are termed 'somatizers'. They typically develop inappropriate health-seeking behaviours, with multiple consultations and investigations, use of many conventional and alternative therapies, and may accumulate huge medical records ('fat folder syndrome'). *Somatic disorders* are those that are thought to be initiated or aggravated by psychological factors and that persist for over 2 years. Typical examples are unexplained breathlessness, chest pain, fatigue, dizziness, paraesthesiae or chronic facial pain. Allergies, migraine, anorexia nervosa, psychogenic vomiting and, sometimes, obesity may also have a psychogenic basis. In addition psychological factors may contribute to factitious injuries.

Features that may suggest that symptoms are related to somatization, but not necessarily depressive, may include any of the following.

- Absence of organic cause or physical signs. The affected area typically appears normal and if, for example, a putatively diseased tooth is extracted, symptoms are unaffected. The symptoms cause real enough suffering to the patient and this must be acknowledged while emotional factors are explored.
- Persistence of symptoms for very long periods, sometimes for years. Clearly, after such periods any organic cause would have become apparent.
- The symptoms may be bizarre, such as 'drawing' or 'gripping' sensations or apparently exaggerated 'unbearable' pain in spite of normal physical health or often sleep.
- The site of the symptom is often somewhat vague, the distribution of pain, for example, may not follow an anatomical pattern, and the patient may be unable to put a finger precisely upon the painful area.
- Symptoms are usually not provoked by recognizable stimuli such as hot or cold foods, or mastication.
- Patients may have several chronic physical complaints at the same time.

In contrast to patients with severe organic disease who typically reach for medication, many patients with chronic pain make little attempt to get relief from them. Frequently drugs, after a brief trial, are said to be totally ineffective.

Patients' personality and manner are highly variable. Some appear obviously neurotic but few are overtly depressed. Indeed the organic symptoms can be regarded as more acceptable substitutes ('depressive equivalents') for more typical manifestations of depression. These varied clinical pictures are discussed more fully below.

Sometimes the patients bring notes (Fig. 10.2) or drawings (Fig. 10.3) to illustrate their problems. These may reflect genuine disease, or may indicate the emotional nature of the complaint(s) (*la maladie du petit papier*). However, increasingly, informed patients who have no mental health problems bring notes or computer print-outs to consultations.

In some patients the response to antidepressant drugs is dramatic, with relief of symptoms and striking general improvement in mood, sometimes before the drug has had time to produce true antidepressant effect. However, effective dosage varies widely and, in the case of tricyclic antidepressants, the response is generally related to the plasma levels achieved. Thus doses may sometimes have to be very high before an effect is evident.

Psoriasis from head to inbetween toes
Perpetual scream in left ear
Spasmodic pressure above left ear
Constant ulcers in mouth and on tongue
Asthma, bronchitis, severe bouts of indigestion
Sore mouth due to grinding of bottom right molar
Severe pain under crutch after any exertion
Constant irritation around back passage
Spasmodic bleeding piles

Medicines taken internally
Predisalone
Ventolin
Asilone suspension
Bronchipax

Fig. 10.2 Note as presented by a patient. Such histories vary in length, detail and imagination and sometimes suggest that the patient is disturbed (*maladie du petit papier*)

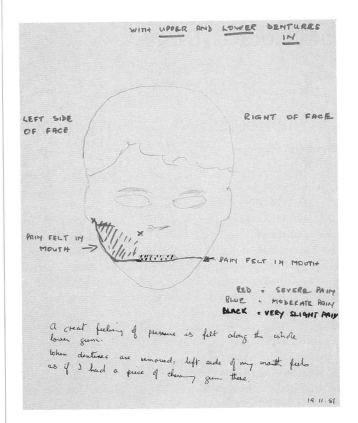

Fig. 10.3 Drawing produced by a patient

Many patients over the course of years go from specialist to specialist (doctor-shopping) with negative results from innumerable investigations or response to any form of treatment. Indeed, the patient persistently refuses to accept advice or reassurance, and may even seem to take a sort of perverse pride in the resistance of the pain to the challenge of medical science.

Conflict between patient and carer is not uncommon, and patients may believe they are not receiving proper care.

Chronic physical symptoms can generally be regarded as a plea for help or attention. This occasionally becomes distressingly apparent in a patient who, at the start, appears well-balanced and self-controlled – even occasionally joking about symptoms – but after a little while is crying uncontrollably. At the other extreme, many patients reject the possibility of mental illness and aggressively assert that 'It's not my nerves' (even if no such suggestion has been made) and typically also reject the idea of psychiatric help, however obliquely and sympathetically suggested.

Examples of these varied clinical pictures therefore include the following.

- The patient may be overtly depressed and cries readily or is obviously having difficulty in restraining tears. Alternatively, initial self-control is followed by unrestrained crying.
- The patient may complain (in effect) of depression by saying that the pain or other symptom makes them miserable.
- Some, when allowed to discuss their symptoms, relate them to 'stress' or trouble with the family or at work.
- A few are already having, or have had, antidepressant drugs but the symptoms have not been controlled.
- A few have associated bizarre (delusional) symptoms such as 'powder' or 'slime' coming out of the painful area as mentioned earlier.
- A few, given the chance of a sympathetic hearing, gratefully expand on their problems and welcome the suggestion of help.
- The most difficult and relatively common group is the 'rejectors', who refuse to accept the idea of mental disturbance, refuse to have the possibility investigated and refuse to accept that any drugs (which they equate with drugs of dependence) may be helpful

It should not need to be emphasized that, where psychological problems are suspected, discussion with the patient must be conducted patiently, gently and sympathetically. Surprisingly, this may perhaps be the first opportunity that patients have had to unburden themselves. Listening, tolerance, empathy and compassion are required. Unfortunately, some doctors are at least as intolerant of such 'neurotic' patients as some members of the public. This is not to suggest that the dentist should attempt to be an amateur psychiatrist but an effort must be made understand the nature of the symptoms. It is probably unnecessary to enquire into full details of family relationships or broken homes. If a patient is depressed, the cause is often as much the patient's susceptibility to depression as the so-called life situation. In any case, improvement in the life situation is unlikely to be feasible, and it is only too common for those so affected to be unable to overcome their difficulties without help from drugs or other sources. It is important to stress to the patient that we now understand that damage to the periphery, perhaps from unnecessary dental treatment, causes wind up and central sensitization so that the brain becomes hypervigilant. Such an explanation allows both doctor and patient to understand how the pain changes and moves around; the problem is not some localized pathology but a disorder of pain signalling requiring both pharmacological and cognitive help.

The key feature is that the presenting complaint cannot be explained by any known medical condition and there appears to be unconscious/involuntary symptom production; these are sometimes termed medically unexplained symptoms (MUS).

Careful investigation is therefore essential to exclude possible organic causes; however, the dentist must be careful not to overinvestigate the patient as this has been shown to make problems more difficult to treat. It is important to achieve a shared understanding and management plan; try diaries to record the problems; avoid manipulation by the patient; and minimize involvement of other health care professionals ('doctor shopping').

The concurrence of emotional and physical disease is one of the most common problems in medicine requiring a mature clinical understanding.

Types of disorder previously termed "Psychosomatic" include those shown in Box 10.2.

> **Box 10.2 Types of somatization disorder**
>
> - Somatization disorder
> - Hypochondriasis
> - Conversion disorder
> - Somatoform pain disorder
> - Body dysmorphic syndrome
> - Malingering
> - Factitious disorders
> - Hysterical states

SOMATIZATION DISORDER

This consists of complaints of multiple unexplained symptoms, which rarely remit completely but are presented in colourful exaggerated terms.

Patients are rarely men but inconsistent historians with depressed mood and anxiety symptoms. Diagnostic criteria include:

- four pain symptoms, plus
- two gastrointestinal symptoms, plus
- one sexual/reproductive symptom, plus
- one pseudoneurological symptom
- if within a medical condition, excessive symptoms
- laboratory abnormalities are absent
- cannot be intentionally feigned or produced.

HYPOCHONDRIASIS

Minor degrees of hypochondriasis are common, especially among the elderly, particularly (and quite understandably) if they are living alone. Hypochondriacal neurosis is a morbid preoccupation with physical symptoms or bodily functions, in which minute details are related incessantly; there is excessive preoccupation with fear of disease or strong belief in having disease due to false interpretation of a trivial symptom and it may be graphically described as 'illness as a way of life'. Features include:

- the medical history being presented in excessive detail
- absence of organic disease or physiological disturbance
- unwarranted fears or ideas persisting despite reassurances
- clinically significant distress
- complaints not restricted to appearance or delusional intensity
- negative physical examination and laboratory results.

General management

Organic disease should always be excluded, as should schizo-phrenia. Most patients with hypochondriasis are depressed and some are deluded.

Reassurance and supportive care are then needed, and anti-depressant drugs may be helpful. Unnecessary interventions must also be avoided.

Dental aspects

The common oral symptoms are dry or burning mouth, dis-turbed taste and oral or facial pain.

Other syndromes related to dentistry include the so-called chronic candidosis ('candidiasis') syndromes and mercury allergy syndrome.

CONVERSION DISORDER ('HYSTERIA')

In conversion disorder, the patient complains of isolated symp-toms that appear to be motivated to achieve a gain of some sort and have no physical cause (e.g. blindness, deafness, stocking anaesthesia and features that do not conform to known ana-tomical pathways or physiological mechanisms).

Diagnostic criteria include:

- symptoms are preceded by stress
- no neurological, medical, substance abuse or cultural explanation
- severe distress
- significant laboratory findings are absent or insufficient.

Nevertheless, in 10–50% of these patients, a physical disease process will ultimately become apparent.

SOMAT1SATION PAN DISORDER (BRIQUET'S SYNDROME)

Somatisation disorder is characterized by physical symptoms that mimic disease or injury for which there is no identifiable physical cause but are not the result of conscious malingering of factitious disorders (Ch. 13).

BODY DYSMORPHIC DISORDER (BDD; DYSMORPHOPHOBIA)

In BDD, the affected person is excessively concerned and preoc-cupied by a perceived defect in their physical features, causing psychological distress that impairs occupational and/or social functioning, sometimes to the point of depression, anxiety, or social withdrawal. BDD affects men and women equally, with the onset of symptoms generally in adolescence or early adult-hood. BDD is characterized by an unusually exaggerated degree of worry or concern about a specific part of the face or body, rather than the general size or shape of the body, The most com-mon areas of focus is the face (size, shape, or lack of symmetry).

BDD is distinguished from anorexia nervosa and bulimia nervosa, as those patients are generally preoccupied with their overall weight and body shape. About 50% of patients with BDD however, also meet the criteria for a delusional disorder,

which is characterized by beliefs that are not based in reality. The defect in BDD exists only in the eyes of the beholder, and others can rarely agree that anything is defective. Thus the patient may adopt compulsive behaviour which can include:

- Compulsive checking in mirrors, windows and other reflective surfaces.
- Attempts to camouflage the imagined defect
- Excessive grooming
- Compulsive skin-touching
- Reassurance-seeking
- Compulsive information seeking
- Obsession with cosmetic procedures such as orthognathic or plastic surgery, with little satisfactory results for the patient. With the number of elective cosmetic dentistry procedures being performed, dentists may be the first health care provider to notice BDD.

Patients with BDD may well be unrealistically dissatisfied with results of treatments and procedures or unable to verbal-ize expectations. BDD has a high rate of comorbidity, most commonly with major depression, social phobia, or obsessive-compulsive disorder (OCD), BDD patients can also be self-destructive, including performing surgery on themselves (e.g. sawing down teeth or removing facial scars with sandpaper) and attempted or completed suicide. There is a completed-suicide rate double that of major depression. So it is a major risk factor for suicide. CBT and SSRIs are indicated.

MALINGERING

Malingering is the deliberate simulation or exaggeration of symptoms for obvious and understandable gain. The gain can be monetary (e.g. compensation or incapacity benefit), or to avoid work or other unpleasant tasks (e.g. service in the armed forces) or criminal prosecution. True malingering is rare. Diag-nosis can be difficult but a key is whether the symptoms persist when the patient believes they are not being watched.

FACTITIOUS INJURIES

Factitious (self-induced) disorders are distinguished from somatoform disorders by the voluntary production of symp-toms, and distinguished from malingering by the lack of external incentive. Physical or psychological symptoms are intentionally produced to assume a sick role. It is more com-mon in men than women, and seen most frequently in health care workers, who intentionally produce signs of medical and/ or mental disorders.

Serious deliberate self-inflicted lesions in the mouth are con-siderably less common than on the skin. This may be due to an underlying need or desire for attention and oral lesions are insufficiently obvious.

Factitious disorders are not uncommon in depressed patients, and in those with schizophrenia and learning disability. Exam-ples include self-induced cigarette burns (Fig. 10.4) or cuts. Rare causes of self-injury also include any cause of sensory loss, pain insensitivity, such as in the Riley–Day syndrome, Lesch–Nyhan syndrome (Ch. 23), and Gilles de la Tourette syndrome – multiple tics and coprolalia (involuntary uttering of obscenities).

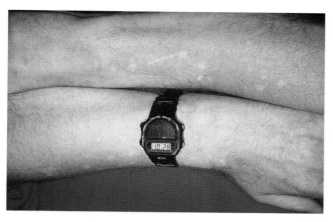

Fig. 10.4 Self-induced burns from cigarettes as an attention-seeking device

Clinical features

Minor, subconsciously self-induced oral lesions are common, the classic examples being bruxism and cheek-biting (morsicatio buccarum). Other lesions may be accidentally self-inflicted when the oral mucosa is anaesthetized, after a local anaesthetic, surgery or damage to the trigeminal nerve.

The most commonly reported type of self-inflicted oral injuries has been so-called self-extraction of teeth. Soft-tissue lesions can be produced, typically by picking at the gingivae with the fingernails. In adults injuries may be produced by the use of the pointed end of a nail file, often also at the gingival margins.

Other types of injury include the application of caustic substances to the lips or injuries from attempts at suicide.

General management

Self-inflicted lesions should be suspected when the lesions do not correspond with those of any recognized disease; are of bizarre configuration with sharp outlines and in an otherwise healthy patient; are in sites accessible only to the patient; or if the patient shows signs that suggest emotional disturbance, is under stress, is known to be under psychiatric treatment, or has a learning impairment.

Few patients will admit to injuring themselves. More frequently the diagnosis can be confirmed only by discreet observation after admission of the patient to hospital. However, even when seen to cause the injuries, the patient may still deny having made them. Once the diagnosis has been made, the family doctor or specialist psychiatrist should see the patient.

HYSTERICAL STATES

Hysterical personality disorders, neuroses and acute psychoses are recognized.

Hysterical neuroses

Hysterical neuroses mainly affect females – sometimes those working in medical or paramedical occupations – as conversion neurosis or as a dissociative state. Hysterical conversion neurosis is characterized by physical complaints that have no demonstrable organic basis, such as pain, anaesthesia, dysphagia, fainting, fits, paralysis or tremor, but frequently result in patients submitting to repeated operations and may as a result have multiple scars (see later; Munchausen syndrome). Dissociative states are characterized by disturbances of consciousness or identity (but no physical symptoms) in the absence of demonstrable organic disease. Amnesia, states of fugue (when the patient wanders aimlessly away), or (rarely) multiple personalities, are examples.

It is often difficult to establish that the patient is gaining something by the illness, although in compensation neurosis the nature of the potential gain is easily recognized.

Dental aspects

Patients who aggressively insist on their symptoms and demand surgery for undetectable lesions are fortunately rare.

Munchausen syndrome

Munchausen syndrome is a disorder in which patients go to considerable length to fabricate histories and simulate symptoms without an external incentive (cf. malingering) but apparently for the sake of undergoing operations. This may be done repeatedly, even occasionally by assuming false names and travelling to many hospitals scattered about the country. Patients are often intelligent and resourceful. Common complaints are of acute abdominal pain; fever; haematuria; or infected wounds. Ultimately the patient may become extensively scarred and develop complications from the repeated operations.

Munchausen syndrome-by-proxy is the term given to a parent or other carer who invents symptoms in, and demands unnecessary medical or surgical treatment for, a child.

Treatment is difficult and often fails; the main aims should be to avoid unnecessary drug use (especially opiates) and surgery.

Compensation neurosis

Compensation neurosis usually follows an accident (especially a head injury) or operation, and is characterized by paralysis, chronic pain (often headache) or other symptoms of obscure origin and of no obvious organic cause. Men and women are equally susceptible, there is no previous history, and the lack of insight is less convincing than in hysteria.

Settlement of the claim for compensation typically results in rapid disappearance of the symptoms.

PSYCHIATRIC DISORDERS

Psychiatric disorders are common; perhaps one third of the population suffer at some time during their life. They are often underdiagnosed, and what may appear simply to be unusual behaviour may actually be a manifestation. Psychiatric illnesses cause significant incapacity, but, equally, organic illness can cause major behavioural changes and sometimes precipitate psychiatric disease (Box 10.3).

Box 10.3 Some possible behavioural reactions to organic disease

- Denial
- Anger
- Frustration
- Aggression
- Anxiety
- Fear
- Withdrawal
- Apathy
- Dependency
- Depression

Box 10.4 Axis I

- Disorders first diagnosed in infancy
- Delirium, dementia, and amnestic and other cognitive disorders
- Mental disorders caused by a general medical condition
- Substance-related disorders
- Schizophrenia and other psychotic disorders
- Mood disorders
- Anxiety disorders
- Somatoform disorders
- Factitious disorders
- Dissociative disorders
- Sexual and gender identity disorders
- Eating disorders
- Sleep disorders
- Psychological factors affecting medical conditions
- Impulse control disorders not classified elsewhere
- Adjustment disorders
- Other conditions that may be the focus of medical attention

Table 10.9 Classification of psychosocial health

Axis	Description
I	Clinical disorders (Box 10.4)
II	Personality disorders
III	General medical conditions
IV	Psychosocial and environmental problems
V	Global assessment of functioning

Table 10.10 The most common mental disorders

Condition	Anxiety disorders	Depression	Schizophrenia
Prevalence (approximate)	1 in 10 people	1 in 10 people	1 in 100 people

Diagnostic criteria for the most common mental disorders are outlined in *Diagnostic and statistical manual of mental disorders*, 4th edition (DSM-IV), the American Psychiatric Association, Washington, DC, 1994 (revised 2000; Table 10.9). The most significant psychiatric disorders are shown in Table 10.10.

Some mental disorders have defined organic causes. Mental disorders underlie many complaints and extend the recovery time from many others.

Mental disorders frequently coexist with diverse other illnesses. Depression, for example, may be associated with a high prevalence (around 65%) of common chronic medical conditions such as hypertension, coronary artery disease, diabetes, arthritis and chronic lung disorders. About 15% of people with a mental disorder also indulge in substance abuse.

DENTAL ASPECTS

Mental disorders can significantly influence oral health care, not least because of behavioural disorders or interpersonal difficulties. Patients with mental disease may be unable to cooperate. Drug misuse may explain abnormal behaviour in some patients.

- Compliance with appointments or treatment is often poor.
- There may be difficulties in gaining informed consent to treatment.
- There may also be oral neglect with a high prevalence of caries and periodontal disease, difficulties coping with dental prostheses, and self-induced lesions or other oral symptoms caused by the psychiatric illness or its treatment.
- Some of the more severely ill or neglected patients with mental disorders are at high risk from diseases of deprivation and lifestyle, such as tuberculosis.
- Drugs such as antidepressants, phenothiazines, lithium or barbiturates can cause xerostomia or other orofacial disorders, or otherwise influence dental care.

MOOD DISORDERS

DEPRESSION

Depression is a common emotion which all of us experience at some time. It becomes a disorder of emotion when it is characterized by a persistent lowering of mood and negative patterns of thinking and may impact significantly on an individual's quality of life. Depression is also often a feature of a medical problem but is sometimes so severe and enduring that it becomes an illness in itself.

Depression as an illness, involves mood and thoughts, and affects the way persons eat and sleep, feel about themselves and think about things. Although depression alone may be seen (unipolar disorder), about one in ten people who suffer from serious depression will also have periods when they are too happy and overactive (bipolar disorder – which used to be called manic depression).

The lifetime risk for depression is approximately 10%, with rates being doubled in women; hormonal factors may contribute, particularly menstrual cycle changes, pregnancy, miscarriage, the post-partum period, pre-menopause and the menopause. Depression may be genetic and can often run in families; onset may be at any stage from childhood onwards. Episodes can be triggered by adverse life events, such as a serious loss, difficult relationships, financial problems or any stressful (unwelcome or even desired) change in life patterns.

Some cases are precipitated by serious medical illnesses such as stroke, a heart attack, cancer, Parkinson disease, hormonal disorders, or illnesses that are long and uncomfortable or painful, such as arthritis or bronchitis. Some people become depressed after viral infections, like influenza or glandular fever.

The main effects of depression appear to relate to changes in hypothalamic centres that govern food intake, libido and circadian rhythms: various hormones, particularly serotonin, dopamine and norepinephrine, are implicated and hypercortisolism is common. Antidepressants increase concentrations of these chemicals at brain nerve endings and so seem to boost the function of those parts of the brain that use serotonin and noradrenaline.

The danger in depression is of suicide; death from suicide in men is four times that of women, though more women attempt it.

Clinical features

Features of major depression include (Box 10.5): a persistently sad, anxious or 'empty' mood; feelings of hopelessness and pessimism, of guilt, worthlessness and helplessness; loss of interest or pleasure in hobbies and activities that were once enjoyed, including sex; lack of energy, fatigue and a feeling of being 'slowed down'; difficulty concentrating, remembering, making decisions; insomnia, early-morning awakening or oversleeping; appetite and/or weight loss, or overeating/weight gain; restlessness and irritability. A depressive episode is diagnosed if five or more of these symptoms last most of the day, nearly every day, for a period of 2 weeks or longer:

- feel unhappy most of the time (but may feel a little better in the evenings)
- lose interest in life and can't enjoy anything
- find it harder to make decisions
- can't cope with things that you used to
- feel utterly tired
- feel restless and agitated
- lose appetite and weight (some people find they do the reverse and put on weight)
- take 1–2 h to get off to sleep, and then wake up earlier than usual
- lose interest in sex
- lose your self-confidence
- feel useless, inadequate and hopeless
- avoid other people
- feel irritable
- feel worse at a particular time each day, usually in the morning
- think of suicide.

Patients may exhibit: lack of energy, fatigue, reduced concentration, insomnia, early-morning awakening, oversleeping, loss of appetite and weight loss or gain. Depression may also

---

Box 10.5 Features of depression

- Sadness
- Hopelessness
- Pessimism
- Lack of pleasure
- Irritability
- Fatigue
- Sleep disturbance
- Loss of libido and appetite

---

manifest as chronic pain: 50% of patients who are depressed have pain as their presenting complaint.

Chronic pain or other persistent bodily symptoms that are not caused by physical illness or injury are common. Men are less likely to admit to depression, and doctors are less likely to suspect it. It is often masked by manifesting in men, not as feeling hopeless and helpless, but as being irritable, angry and discouraged. Alternatively it may be suppressed by alcohol or drugs, or by the socially acceptable habit of working excessively long hours.

There may be thoughts of death or suicide, and suicide attempts. Warning signs include: talking about feeling suicidal or wanting to die; feeling hopeless, that nothing will ever change or get better; feeling helpless, that nothing they do makes any difference; feeling a burden to family and friends; abusing alcohol or drugs; putting affairs in order (e.g. organizing finances or giving away possessions to prepare for death); writing a suicide note; putting themselves in harm's way, or in situations where there is a danger of being killed. Risks for suicide appear to be higher earlier in the course of the illness.

Dysthymic disorder is a chronic, less intense form of depression but may progress to major depression. It involves long-term, chronic symptoms that do not disable, but keep patients from functioning well or from feeling happy. Many dysthymics also experience major depressive episodes at some time.

Seasonal affective disorder (SAD) is a chronic cyclical form of depression that appears as daylight hours shorten, related to melatonin production. Its features also include winter somnolence and craving for carbohydrates.

Involutional melancholia is characterized by severe anxiety and hypochondriasis, beginning in later life and mainly affecting women.

Bipolar disorder is the term given to depression alternating with mania, which may amount to a psychosis. The various mood states in bipolar disorder may be regarded as a spectrum with severe depression at one end and mania at the other. Bipolar 1 disorder consists of alternating depression and mania; bipolar 2 disorder is alternating depression with hypomania; while mixed bipolar disorder is when depression and mania occur concurrently – usually as aggression plus depression.

General management

Diagnosis of depression is dependent upon identifying:

- a persistent lowering of mood
- alterations of biological function (as outlined above)
- altered thought content. Negative pessimistic thoughts about themselves, the world and the future (Beck cognitive triad).

It is important to remember that depressed patients often present with other symptoms, such as pain, and questionnaires to screen for thought and biological disturbances are therefore useful diagnostically.

Anyone thinking about committing suicide needs immediate attention, preferably from a psychiatrist. Important measures, if there is an attempt, are to call a doctor or emergency services to get immediate help; ensure the suicidal person is not left alone and that there is no access to medications, weapons or other items that could be used for self-harm.

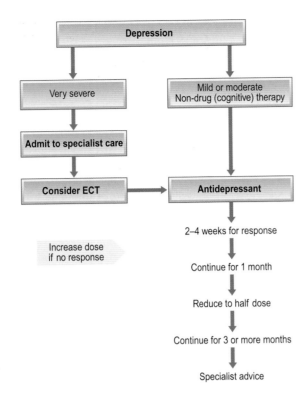

Fig. 10.5 Depression, tricyclic antidepressants and electroconvulsive therapy (ECT)

Treatment of depression is by psychotherapy and medication. (Fig. 10.5) Psychotherapy involves talking with a mental health professional, such as a psychiatrist, psychologist, social worker or counsellor, to learn how to deal with problems.

The majority of patients with depression can be managed in the primary health care setting by using the following.

- Appropriate risk assessment for suicide, self-neglect and danger to others. Psychiatric referral is needed if suicide risk is high or the depression is severe and unresponsive to initial treatment. Following the recent review of the Mental Health Act 2008 in UK, all doctors are required to be able to judge a patient's capacity to make decisions; psychiatrists are further required to assess dangerousness.
- Psychological techniques (cognitive behavioural and supportive therapy).
- Pharmacotherapy (Tables 10.11 and 10.17).
- Electroconvulsive therapy (ECT) – for very severe cases, where significant physical retardation or delusions (fixed unshakeable false beliefs) are present.

Antidepressants

Antidepressant drugs raise brain levels of serotonin and norepinephrine. None of them is perfect and all suffer from at least one of the following drawbacks:

- delayed onset of action from 7 to 28 days – although some improvements may be seen in the first few weeks, most antidepressant medications must be taken regularly for 3–4 weeks (in some cases, as many as 8 weeks) before the full therapeutic effect starts

Table 10.11 Classification of antidepressants (see Table 10.15)

Class	Examples
Tricyclic antidepressant (TCA)	Amitriptyline
Serotonin norepinephrine reuptake inhibitor (SNRI)	Venlafaxine
Selective serotonin reuptake inhibitor (SSRI)	Fluoxetine
Norepinephrine reuptake inhibitor (NRI)	Reboxetine
Norepinephrine and specific serotonergic agonist	Mirtazapine
Serotonin reuptake inhibitor (SRI)	Nefazodone
Reversible inhibitor of monoamine oxidase A (RIMA)	Moclobemide
Monoamine oxidase inhibitor (MAOI)	Phenelzine

Table 10.12 Monoamine oxidase inhibitors (MAOIs)

MAOI	Special comments
Isocarboxazid	Contraindicated in liver or CVS disease
Phenelzine	Contraindicated in liver or CVS disease
Tranylcypromine	The most dangerous MAOI
Moclobemide	Less reactive with foods or drugs

CVS, cardiovascular system.

- anticholinergic effects
- sedation
- agitation
- cardiotoxicity
- weight gain.

Patients often are tempted to stop medication too soon but they should continue the medication for at least 4–9 months to prevent recurrence.

Monoamine oxidase inhibitors

Monoamine oxidase inhibitors (MAOIs) were the first effective antidepressants but are now rarely prescribed (Table 10.12) because of their adverse effects. Dry mouth and hypotension are common side-effects of MAOIs. The most serious adverse effects of the earlier and non-selective irreversible MAOIs, such as phenelzine, isoniazid and tranylcypromine, are drug or food interactions. Hypertensive crises have resulted from interaction of these MAOIs with foods containing tyramine, particularly cheese, and also with yeast products, chocolate, bananas, broad beans, some red wines and beer, pickled herring or caviar. However, the frequency of such reactions has been greatly overestimated. Selective MAOIs, such as selegiline, used mainly in Parkinsonism rather than depression, contrary to earlier beliefs can also provoke similar reactions. Interactions of MAOIs with pethidine and other opioids are the most dangerous reactions and have sometimes been fatal (Table 10.13). Interactions with tricyclic antidepressants are also dangerous. Ephedrine and similar drugs, which are often present in nasal decongestants or cold remedies, may cause severe hypertension.

The most commonly used MAOIs are phenelzine and isocarboxazid; phenelzine, for example, is helpful for people with panic disorder and social phobia.

Table 10.13 Monoamine oxidase inhibitors: possible adverse effects and interactions

Possible adverse effects	Possible interactions
Xerostomia	Hypertensive reactions with norepinephrine, ephedrine or phenylephrine, or tyramine-containing foods
Hypotension	Epinephrine can safely be used
Anorexia	Enhanced action of respiratory depressants such as general anaesthetic agents, sedatives, antihistamines, opioids
Nausea	With tramadol, there is a risk of seizures
Constipation	
Sexual dysfunction	

Table 10.14 Some possible adverse effects and interactions of tricyclic antidepressants

	Possible adverse reactions	Possible interactions
Cardiovascular	Postural hypotension Cardiotoxic Arrhythmias Tachycardias	Hypertensive reaction with norepinephrine
Neurological	Seizures Dizziness Ataxia Tremor Insomnia Agitation Drowsiness	Potentiation of central nervous system depressants With tramadol, there is a risk of seizures
Liver	Jaundice	
Blood	Leukopenia	
Others	Dry mouth Sexual dysfunction Nausea Constipation Urinary retention Blurred vision	

Tricyclic antidepressants

Tricyclic antidepressants (TCAs) are probably the most effective antidepressants, which have stood the test of time, despite their undesirable adverse effects (Table 10.14); they are useful when there is associated anxiety. Their most common adverse effects, and ways to deal with some of them, are:

- dry mouth – it is helpful to drink sips of water, chew sugarless gum and clean teeth daily
- constipation – bran, prunes, fruit and vegetables should be in the diet
- bladder difficulties – emptying the bladder may be troublesome, and the urine stream may be weak
- sexual difficulties – sexual function may deteriorate
- blurred vision
- dizziness – rising from the bed or chair slowly is helpful
- drowsiness as a daytime problem (Table 10.12). The more sedating antidepressants are generally taken at bedtime to help sleep and minimize daytime drowsiness. A person feeling drowsy or sedated should not drive or operate dangerous equipment.

The onset of action of TCAs is slow and they may take 4 weeks to exert their full effect. The action is dose-dependent and lack of effect is often the result of failure to achieve adequate plasma levels. Tricyclics are contraindicated in patients with cardiac disorders (recent myocardial infarct, arrhythmias, heart block, cardiac failure), epilepsy, liver dysfunction, blood dyscrasias, glaucoma and urinary obstruction (e.g. prostatic hypertrophy). Tricyclics should only be given after a full blood count, liver function tests and, if the patient is over 45, an ECG is indicated. TCAs should not be used within 2 weeks of the use of MAOIs.

The most commonly used TCAs are amitriptyline, dothiepin (dosulepin) and imipramine. Sedation is a common side-effect, particularly with amitriptyline, but this may be an advantage if the patient is agitated (Table 10.15). Side-effects of the tricyclics are more serious in older people. Various other tricyclics have particular advantages: imipramine, for example, is mildly stimulating and clomipramine appears to be useful where there are obsessional or phobic problems. Lofepramine has fewer

Table 10.15 Tricyclic and related antidepressants

Drug	Special comments[a]
Amitriptyline	More cardiotoxic, sedative and antimuscarinic than many tricyclic antidepressants (TCAs) Caution with general anaesthesia
Amoxapine	May cause tardive dyskinesia
Clomipramine	Possibly low sedative activity
Dothiepin/dosulepin	Sedative
Doxepin	Sedative: fewer cardiac effects
Imipramine	Less sedative than most but more antimuscarinic and cardiac effects
Lofepramine	Avoid in renal or hepatic disease
Nortriptyline	Possibly low antimuscarinic effects
Trimipramine	Photosensitive rashes
Related drugs	
Maprotiline	Less antimuscarinic but more epileptogenic than TCAs
Mianserin	Possible hepatic and haematological reactions
Trazodone	Fewer antimuscarinic and cardiac effects

[a]Up to 4 weeks are required before symptom control can be expected. Reduce doses in the elderly. Arrhythmias and heart block may be seen as well as drowsiness, dry mouth, urinary retention and constipation (antimuscarinic actions). Contraindicated after myocardial infarction. Cardiotoxic in overdose.

antimuscarinic effects than some others and is less dangerous in overdose. Doxepin (similar to imipramine) is the drug of choice if there is cardiovascular disease. Clomipramine is the only tricyclic prescribed for OCD, while imipramine may be given for panic disorder and GAD.

Table 10.16 Selective serotonin reuptake inhibitors: possible adverse effects and drug interactions

Possible adverse effects	Possible interactions with effects	
Xerostomia	Carbamazepine	Serotonin syndrome
Arrhythmias	Lithium	Serotonin syndrome
Gastrointestinal upsets	Monoamine oxidase inhibitors	Serotonin syndrome
	Terfenadine	Arrhythmias
	Tramadol	Risk of seizures
	Tricyclics	Serotonin syndrome

Table 10.17 Antidepressants[a] (see Table 10.9)

Class	Acronym	Actions	Examples
Monoamine oxidase inhibitors	MAOI	Inhibit monoamine oxidase A (MAO-A)	Moclobemide
Noradrenergic and specific serotonergic antidepressants	NASSA	Block norepinephrine, $5HT_2$ and $5HT_3$ reuptake	Mirtazapine
Noradrenaline reuptake inhibitors	NARI	Block norepinephrine reuptake	Reboxetine
Selective serotonin reuptake inhibitors	SSRI	Block 5HT (serotonin) reuptake	Citalopram Fluoxetine Fluvoxamine Paroxetine Sertraline
Serotonin norepinephrine reuptake inhibitors	SNRI	Block norepinephrine and 5HT reuptake	Duloxetine Venlafaxine
Serotonin reuptake inhibitors	SRI	5HT antagonists	Nefazodone
Tricyclic antidepressants	TCAs	Block norepinephrine and 5HT (serotonin) reuptake	Amitriptyline Dosulepin Doxepin Lomipramine Lofepramine Nortriptyline Protriptyline

[a]For adverse effects, see Tables 10.12–10.16.
5HT, 5-hydroxytryptamine.

Selective serotonin reuptake inhibitors

Selective serotonin reuptake inhibitors are newer antidepressants, and have the advantage over older antidepressants of less severe antimuscarinic activity, weight gain or cardiac conduction effects. SSRIs do not interact with alcohol and are thus often preferred by both patients and practitioners; however, gastrointestinal effects are common.

Adverse effects of SSRIs include anorexia, nausea, anxiety, diarrhoea and sexual dysfunction, and rarely mania, paranoia or extrapyramidal features (Table 10.16). Fluoxetine (Prozac) has been hailed as a valuable antidepressant (makes you feel 'better than well!'), but in the USA has allegedly been associated with aggressive behaviour, including murders. More recently the same allegations have been made against paroxetine.

Selective serotonin reuptake inhibitors may interact with TCAs or neuroleptics to cause a rise in plasma concentration and exaggerated effects of these drugs. SSRIs may interact with MAOIs, TCAs, carbamazepine or lithium to produce the serotonin syndrome (Table 10.16), which comprises CNS irritability, hyperreflexia and myoclonus, and is occasionally fatal. SSRIs should not therefore be used with TCAs, or within 2 weeks of MAOIs. They are also contraindicated in epilepsy, cardiac disease, diabetes, glaucoma, bleeding tendencies, pregnancy, liver or renal disease.

They may have other adverse effects:

* arrhythmias if the patient is using terfenadine
* headache
* nausea
* nervousness and insomnia (trouble falling asleep or waking often during the night); dosage reductions or time will usually resolve these complaints
* agitation
* xerostomia.

Selective serotonin reuptake inhibitors such as fluoxetine or sertraline are commonly prescribed for panic disorder, OCD, PTSD and social phobia, and may be preferred for anxiety disorders. SSRIs can inhibit cytochrome P450 enzymes and thus inhibit the metabolism of benzodiazepines, carbamazepine, codeine and erythromycin.

Summary

The SSRIs and other newer antidepressants that affect neurotransmitters, such as dopamine or norepinephrine, generally have fewer adverse effects than TCAs, and both SSRIs and TCAs are overall safer than MAOIs, which can interact, even fatally, with some foods and drugs (Table 10.17).

Herbal therapy

St John's wort (*Hypericum perforatum*) has been shown to be effective in mild depression but it may interact with SSRIs to produce the serotonin syndrome. It also stimulates cytochrome P450, and thus impairs the activity of drugs such as chemotherapeutic drugs (e.g. irinotecan, the vinca alkaloids, etoposide, teniposide, anthracycline, paclitaxel, docetaxel and tamoxifen), ciclosporin, digoxin, warfarin, indinavir (HIV protease inhibitor), oral contraceptives, opioids and general anaesthetic agents.

Electroconvulsive therapy

Electroconvulsive therapy (ECT) is sometimes given for severe depression, where drugs have been ineffective or where there is a strong risk of suicide. A muscle relaxant is given before treatment, which is given under general anaesthesia (GA). Electrodes are placed at precise locations on the head to deliver electrical impulses. The stimulation causes a brief (about 30s) seizure. The patient does not consciously experience the electrical stimulus. Amnesia is the main side-effect.

Dental aspects of depression

The features aiding recognition of depression have been suggested above. Dental staff should be alert to this possibility, particularly where the patient appears withdrawn, difficult or aggressive, or where there are oral complaints of the types described earlier. Great tact, patience and a sympathetic, friendly manner are needed. Dental treatment is preferably deferred until depression is under control but preventive programmes should be instituted at an early stage.

In patients taking TCAs, epinephrine in local anaesthetics has not been shown clinically (despite statements to the contrary) to cause hypertension. However, severe hypertension has resulted from high concentrations (1:20 000) of norepinephrine in local anaesthesia (LA) agents, whether or not the patient was receiving antidepressants. Norepinephrine has no advantages as a vasoconstrictor and norepinephrine preparations have been withdrawn.

Acetaminophen (paracetamol) can inhibit the metabolism of TCAs, and atropinics are potentiated by TCAs.

Patients on MAOIs are at risk from GA, since prolonged respiratory depression may result. Any CNS depressant, especially opioids and phenothiazines, given to patients on MAOIs (or within 21 days of their withdrawal) may precipitate coma. Pethidine is particularly dangerous.

Indirectly acting sympathomimetic agents, such as ephedrine or cocaine, can interact with MAOIs to cause hypertension, and must therefore not be used. There is no evidence of any danger to patients on MAOI from epinephrine in LA solutions.

Tricyclics and MAOIs can cause postural hypotension. Dental patients using these drugs should not be stood immediately upright if they have been recumbent during treatment and the chair should be brought upright slowly. Some depressed patients resort to drug misuse, and this must be considered (Ch. 34).

Benzodiazepines, carbamazepine, codeine and erythromycin may be potentiated by SSRIs.

The most common oral complaint of depressed patients under treatment is of a dry mouth, especially as a result of the use of TCAs, MAOIs or lithium. This may even predispose to oral candidosis and accelerated caries. Taste sensation may also be disturbed and patients tend to eat more sugar. The effect of xerostomia can occasionally result in ascending suppurative parotitis. The most effective treatment is to change the antidepressant to another that has little anticholinergic activity. If this is not acceptable, the dry mouth should be managed as in Sjögren syndrome (Ch. 16). Smoking, and other drugs which may add to the xerostomia, such as antihistamines, hyoscine or other atropine-like drugs, or SSRIs, should therefore be avoided. Both MAOIs and TCAs have also been reported occasionally to cause facial dyskinesias and prolonged use of flupentixol can lead to intractable tardive dyskinesia.

Bodily complaints, often related to the mouth, are common in depression and the dental surgeon should appreciate the possibility of a psychological basis for such oral complaints. Depression is associated especially with the following painful disorders of the orofacial region:

- chronic facial pain
- burning mouth or sore tongue (oral dysaesthesia)
- occasionally temporomandibular pain dysfunction syndrome

- other oral complaints may be delusional and include discharges (of fluid, slime or powder coming into the mouth) dry mouth or sialorrhoea despite normal salivary flow spots or lumps halitosis disturbed taste sensation.

Depression may also accompany: other mental diseases, such as schizophrenia; viral infections (e.g. influenza, hepatitis or infectious mononucleosis); drugs (particularly reserpine, methyldopa, fenfluramine and corticosteroids) or their withdrawal (e.g. of amfetamines, benzodiazepines or antidepressants); and serious medical disorders – such as Parkinsonism or stroke, myocardial infarction, malignant diseases or endocrinopathies, such as diabetes.

CHRONIC FATIGUE SYNDROME (ME; MYALGIC ENCEPHALITIS; MYALGIC ENCEPHALOMYOPATHY)

General aspects

Chronic fatigue syndrome (CFS) is a disorder characterized by lack of energy, tiredness, or muscle and joint pains after minimal effort, emotional lability, poor concentration and memory and often other symptoms. This clinical picture was described in 1867 and termed 'neurasthenia'. CFS is underdiagnosed in more than 80% of the people who have it; at the same time, it is often misdiagnosed as depression.

Chronic fatigue syndrome often begins after an infection such as influenza or infectious mononucleosis, or after a period of high stress. Since the symptoms may resemble those of the recovery phase of a viral infection, the complaint is termed 'post-viral fatigue syndrome', but claims for Epstein–Barr virus, herpes virus 6 and Coxsackie B having a causative role have not been substantiated. Parvovirus has been implicated in some patients.

Genetic, immunological, infectious, metabolic and neurological aetiologies have been suggested to explain CFS. Several mechanisms have been suggested such as excessive oxidative stress following exertion, immune imbalance characterized by decreased natural killer cell and macrophage activity, immunoglobulin G subclass deficiencies (IgG_1, IgG_3) and decreased serum concentrations of complement component. Autoantibodies have also been suggested as a possible factor: recent studies indicate that antiserotonin, anti-microtubule-associated protein 2 and antimuscarinic cholinergic receptor 1 antibodies may play a role. It has been demonstrated that impairment in vasoactive neuropeptide metabolism may explain the symptoms of CFS. Genes for haematological disease and function, immunological disease and function, cancer, cell death, immune response and infection have altered expression. Increases in elastase activity and protein kinase and RNase L enzymes support the clinical importance of these immune dysfunctions in CFS.

Clinical features

Unlike most post-viral symptoms, which usually abate in a few days or weeks, CFS symptoms, particularly fatigue, either persist or fluctuate, frequently for more than 6 months. CFS also has eight other possible primary symptoms, which include: loss of memory or concentration, sore throat, painful and mildly enlarged lymph nodes in the neck or axilla, myalgia, polyarthralgia without swelling or redness, headache of a new type, pattern or severity, sleep disturbance or extreme exhaustion after normal exercise or exertion. A person meets the diagnostic criteria of CFS when unexplained fatigue persists for 6 months or more with at least four of the above eight primary symptoms also present.

General management

Tests showing any disorders of muscle function or any other organic lesion have not been substantiated. By contrast, those with organic neuromuscular diseases do not have the mental symptoms characteristic of 'ME'.

Management of CFS aims to relieve symptoms by using gradual but steady exercise and treatment of symptoms. CFS may respond to antidepressant drugs.

Dental aspects

Unexpectedly perhaps, atypical (idiopathic) facial pain has not been reported as a feature of CFS. The only oral symptom reported has been dry mouth.

PSYCHOSES

Psychoses are serious disorders in which insight is often lacking (Table 10.18).

Table 10.18 Psychoses: features

Bipolar disorder (manic depression)	Mainly severe depression but may be manic episodes for weeks, months or years
Schizophrenia	Severe disorder of thought, behaviour and affect, with hallucinations, delusions and illusions
Korsakoff syndrome	Recent amnesia and confabulation
Brief psychotic disorder	Short non-recurrent psychosis
Delusional disorder	One or more fixed belief
Shared psychotic disorder	"Folie a deux"–a delusional disorder shared by two people

BIPOLAR DISORDER

General aspects

Bipolar disorder is characterized by cycling mood changes of severe highs (mania) and lows (depression). Hypomania with major depression is termed bipolar I disorder (Table 10.19). Sometimes the mood switches are dramatic and rapid, but most often they are gradual.

About one in every 100 adults has bipolar disorder. Men and women are affected equally. It usually starts in late adolescence or early adulthood. It is unusual for it to start after the age of 40. However, symptoms may sometimes start during childhood, or alternatively in later in life when they may indicate organic disease such as a neoplasm, or an effect of drugs, such as corticosteroids, alcohol or another drug of dependence.

Table 10.19 Bipolar disorders

Terminology	Comments
Bipolar I	At least one high, or manic episode, lasting longer than 1 week. Some people with bipolar I will have only manic episodes, although most will also have periods of depression Untreated, manic episodes generally last 3–6 months Depressive episodes last rather longer – 6–12 months without treatment
Bipolar II	More than one episode of severe depression, but only mild manic episodes – 'hypomania'
Cyclothymia	Mood swings not as severe as in full bipolar disorder, but can be longer. May develop into full bipolar disorder
Rapid cycling	More than four mood swings in a 12-month period

When in the manic cycle, the person may be overactive, over-talkative and have excessive energy. In the depressed cycle, any or all of the symptoms of a depressive disorder are prominent.

Mania

Mania, left untreated, may worsen to a psychotic state. It is characterized by:

- abnormal or excessive elation, 'high', excessively euphoric mood
- unusual irritability
- less need for sleep
- grandiose notions and unrealistic beliefs in abilities and powers
- excessive talking
- racing thoughts, jumping from one idea to another (butterfly mind)
- distractibility
- excessive sexual desire
- greatly increased energy and provocative, intrusive or aggressive behaviour
- poor judgement
- inappropriate social behaviour
- spending sprees
- abuse of drugs, particularly cocaine, alcohol and sleeping medications
- denial that anything is wrong.

A manic episode is diagnosed if elevated mood comes with three or more of the other symptoms for most of the day, nearly every day, for 1 week or longer.

Mania often affects thinking, judgement and social behaviour in ways that can cause serious problems and embarrassment. The individual in a manic phase may feel elated, full of grand schemes that might range from unwise business decisions to romantic sprees. Frequently, therefore, the family rather than the patient feel the ill-effects and complain accordingly.

A mild to moderate level of mania is called hypomania and it may be enjoyed by the patient, and may even be associated with good functioning and enhanced productivity. Thus, even when family and friends learn to recognize the mood swings as possible bipolar disorder, the person may deny that anything is wrong. Alternation between mild mania and depression is termed cyclothymia.

Sometimes, severe episodes of mania or depression include psychotic symptoms, such as hallucinations (hearing, seeing or otherwise sensing the presence of things not actually there) and delusions (false, strongly held beliefs not influenced by logical reasoning or explained by a person's usual cultural concepts). Psychotic symptoms in bipolar disorder tend to reflect the extreme mood state at the time. For example, delusions of grandiosity, such as believing one is the President or has special powers or wealth, may be experienced during mania. Delusions of guilt or worthlessness, such as believing that one is ruined and penniless or has committed some terrible crime, may appear during depression. People with bipolar disorder who have these symptoms are sometimes incorrectly diagnosed as having schizophrenia.

General management of mania

Cognitive behavioural therapy may be effective. Psychoeducation involves teaching people with bipolar disorder about the illness and its treatment, and how to recognize signs of relapse so that early intervention can be instituted before a full-blown episode. Lithium, carbamazepine and valproate are the main mood-stabilizing drugs. 'Atypical' antipsychotic medications (such as olanzapine) may help.

Lithium can have several adverse effects. It affects thyroid function and the ECG, and can produce nephrogenic diabetes insipidus. It is also a teratogen. It must only be used where blood levels can be monitored, as overdose can cause tremor, ataxia, convulsions and renal damage. Patients with cardiovascular, renal or thyroid disorders are at risk. Side-effects include thirst and dry mouth, and nausea. Povidone–iodine is contraindicated.

Carbamazepine has fewer adverse effects than lithium and is given when the latter is not tolerated. An important adverse effect is ataxia.

Valproate may lead to adverse effects. It depresses platelet numbers and function to produce a bleeding tendency. Valproate may lead to adverse hormone changes in teenage girls and polycystic ovary syndrome in women who start taking the medication before age 20, so young female patients taking it should be monitored carefully by a physician. NSAIDs, erythromycin and benzodiazepines are also contraindicated.

Newer anticonvulsant medications, including lamotrigine, gabapentin and topiramate, are being studied for their effect in stabilizing mood. Atypical antipsychotic medications, including clozapine, olanzapine, risperidone and ziprasidone, are also possible treatments.

If insomnia is a problem, a high-potency benzodiazepine, such as clonazepam or lorazepam, may help. These medications may be habit-forming and should be prescribed short term only, and therefore other types of sedative medication, such as zolpidem, are sometimes used instead.

Treatments of unproven worth in mania include St John's wort (*Hypericum perforatum*) and omega-3 fatty acids found in fish oil.

Table 10.20 Potential drug interactions with lithium

Drug interacting with lithium	Consequences
Carbamazepine	Lithium toxicity
Diazepam	Hypothermia
Droperidol and other neuroleptics	Facial dyskinesias
Non-steroidal anti-inflammatory analgesics (NSAIDs)	Lithium toxicity
Metronidazole	Lithium toxicity
Phenytoin	Lithium toxicity
Selective serotonin reuptake inhibitors (SSRIs)	Serotonin syndrome
Suxamethonium and other muscle relaxants	Prolonged muscle relaxation
Tetracyclines	Lithium toxicity

Dental aspects

An excited manic patient can be difficult to manage and treatment may have to be delayed until after stabilization. Lithium treatment should be monitored by regular assay of plasma levels. Arrhythmias may be precipitated, particularly during GA. Lithium can interact with many drugs, and it may be advisable to stop lithium treatment 2–3 days before GA (Table 10.20).

Most NSAIDs and metronidazole should be avoided as they can induce toxicity, but aspirin, acetaminophen and codeine are safe to use.

Manic-depressive patients may be treated with lithium and also antidepressant drugs – with oral side-effects such as xerostomia.

SCHIZOPHRENIA

The term 'schizophrenia' covers a number of chronic conditions of complex aetiology characterized by dopamine overactivity in the mesolimbic pathways of the brain. It is a disabling condition and has a lifetime prevalence of approximately 1%, although in recent years prevalence figures are falling for reasons which are not clear.

There is a significant genetic component in the aetiology, probably related to chromosomes 13 and 6. Schizophrenia appears to be due to some imbalance of the complex interrelated chemical systems of the brain, involving dopamine and glutamate; many studies have found abnormalities in brain structure, and suggest it may be a developmental disorder leading to neurons forming inappropriate connections during fetal development. Marijuana use may precipitate schizophrenia and abuse of PCP, crack cocaine, LSD and amphetamines can cause a similar picture (Ch. 34). There is a high prevalence in the socially deprived and in penal institutions. It may also be common in some people of African heritage.

Clinical features

Acute schizophrenia typically presents in young individuals with positive symptoms (hallucinations, delusions and thought disorder). The person generally lacks insight and concern is initially raised by a friend or relative. Acute schizophrenia may develop in previously normal individuals, is often precipitated by organic disorders or external stress, and affective symptoms such as depression may be associated. Chronic schizophrenia is more common and characterized by inappropriate affect, disordered thought processes, delusions and hallucinations. Some patients are strikingly paranoid, others have mainly motor symptoms (catatonia), a bizarre mixture of emotional, behavioural and thought disturbances, or neuroses. Chronic schizophrenia may present insidiously with negative symptoms (apathy, loss of affect and social withdrawal) and thus be misdiagnosed.

Intelligence is unimpaired and insight may even be retained. Occasionally, as a result, patients may be aware that their behaviour is bizarre and even of the consternation that such behaviour creates in others.

Mood, thoughts and behaviour are disorganized and appear irrational and exaggerated. Disorders of perception (hallucinations) and thought (delusions) are common. Disintegration of the individual's personality results in social isolation and withdrawal. Some patients are strikingly paranoid whilst others exhibit motor impairment (catatonia) or a mixture of emotional, behavioural and thought disturbances (hebephrenia). Thoughts and behaviour can be totally inappropriate and incomprehensible.

The first signs of schizophrenia often appear as confusing, or even shocking, changes in behaviour. Schizophrenics often suffer terrifying symptoms such as hearing internal voices not heard by others, or believing that other people are reading their minds, controlling their thoughts, or plotting to harm them – such symptoms may leave them fearful and withdrawn.

Schizophrenics often suffer a severely impaired emotional expressiveness – a 'blunted' or 'flat' affect (mood). Signs of normal emotion are diminished or missing, the voice monotonous, facial expressions mask-like and the person may appear apathetic. Schizophrenics may withdraw socially, avoiding contact with others and, when forced to interact, may have nothing to say ('impoverished thought').

Disordered thinking is common. Schizophrenics may not be able to sort out what is relevant and what is not relevant to a situation. Thoughts may come and go rapidly. The patient may not be able to concentrate on one thought for very long and may be easily distracted, unable to focus attention. Schizophrenic thought disorder causes loss of cohesion between logical thought sequences, with thoughts becoming disorganized and fragmented. Speech and behaviour can be so disorganized as to be incomprehensible or frightening to others. Speech may include non-existent words (neologisms) or be inconsequential ('word salad'). There may be disruption of the stream of speech (thought-blocking), which can make conversation very difficult.

If people cannot make sense of what an individual with schizophrenia is saying, they are likely to become uncomfortable and tend to leave that person alone, and this, together with inappropriate affect (mood) and withdrawal from social contact, leads to isolation. Motivation can thus be greatly weakened, as can interest in or enjoyment of life. In some severe cases, a person can spend entire days doing nothing at all, even neglecting basic hygiene. These problems with emotional expression and motivation may be extremely troubling to family members and friends, but are symptoms of schizophrenia, not character flaws or personal weaknesses.

Hallucinations and delusions have no connection to an appropriate source and can involve any sensory form – auditory, visual, tactile, gustatory and olfactory. However, hearing voices that other people do not hear is the most common type of hallucination. Such voices may describe the patient's activities, carry on a conversation, warn of impending dangers or even issue orders. Schizophrenics live in a world distorted by hallucinations and delusions, and may feel frightened, anxious and confused, and may behave very differently at various times. Sometimes they may seem distant, detached or preoccupied, and may even sit as rigidly as a stone, not moving for hours or uttering a sound. Other times they may move about constantly – always occupied, appearing wide awake and alert. The bizarre nature of the disorder may be made obvious when they shout back at the unheard voices.

Delusions, on the other hand, describe a sensory stimulus that is present but is incorrectly interpreted by the individual. Delusions are false personal beliefs not subject to reason or contradictory evidence and are not explained by a person's usual cultural concepts. Delusions may take on different themes. For example, patients suffering from paranoid-type symptoms – roughly one-third of schizophrenics – often have delusions that they, or a member of the family or someone close to them, are the focus of persecution. Alternatively, they may have false and irrational beliefs that they are being cheated, harassed, poisoned or conspired against. Delusions of grandeur, in which the individual believes that he or she is a famous or important figure, are common. The best known schizophrenic delusion, in the past, was that of being Napoleon! Sometimes the delusions are quite bizarre; for instance, believing that a neighbour is controlling their behaviour with magnetic waves; that people on television are directing special messages to them, or that their thoughts are being broadcast aloud to others. Murderous attacks on others are sometimes ordered by the illusory inner voices.

Paranoia is a projection of the patient's internal disturbance, which, as a consequence, is believed to be the result of the hostility of others, such as neighbours, secret agents or foreign powers, who may be projecting mysterious rays to achieve their malign objectives, for example.

Catatonia with abnormalities of movement, posture and speech, negativism, echolalia, mannerisms and stereotypia may also be features.

General management

Diagnosis is not easy at times, since even normal individuals may feel, think or act in ways that resemble schizophrenia. At the same time, people with schizophrenia do not always act abnormally. Indeed, some people with the illness can appear completely normal and be perfectly responsible, even while they experience hallucinations or delusions. An individual's behaviour may change over time, seeming close to normal when receiving appropriate treatment, but becoming bizarre when medication is stopped.

The diagnosis should thus only be made by an experienced psychiatrist. The diagnostic criteria for schizophrenia vary but include the recognition of Schneider's first-rank symptoms:

- auditory hallucinations – thought echo or voices talking about the patient in the third person

- passivity – the feeling of being controlled by external forces
- thought insertion or withdrawal
- thought broadcasting
- delusions
- hallucinations.

Some people with symptoms of schizophrenia exhibit prolonged extremes of elated or depressed mood, mimicking a manic-depressive (or bipolar) disorder or major depressive disorder. When such symptoms cannot be clearly categorized, a diagnosis a 'schizoaffective disorder' is sometimes made.

It is important to rule out other illnesses, as sometimes similar symptoms are due to undetected underlying medical conditions or drug abuse and, for this reason, a medical history should be taken and a physical examination and laboratory tests should be done to rule out other possible causes.

Coping with the symptoms of schizophrenia can be especially difficult for family members who remember how involved or vivacious a person was before they became ill.

Treatment of schizophrenia includes:

- early active intervention before the illness becomes chronic
- assessment of a patient's risk to themselves or others (individuals may require acute psychiatric admission under the Mental Health Act)
- family therapy
- cognitive behavioural therapy
- long-term psychotherapy and antipsychotic drug therapy (Table 10.21)
- supportive therapy via community psychiatric services.

Table 10.21 Antipsychotic drugs used to treat schizophrenia

Class	Examples
Atypical antipsychotics	Clozapine
Piperazine phenothiazines	Prochlorperazine
Phenothiazines	Chlorpromazine
Butyrophenones	Haloperidol
Thioxanthines	Flupentixol
Diphenylbutylpiperidines	Pimozide

A person with schizophrenia can be more sensitive to stress, so it is best to avoid arguments and keep calm.

Treatment with individual psychotherapy is of questionable value. Rehabilitation, family education and self-help groups can help. Treatment usually includes drugs, which can be the older (typical) antipsychotics that work by reducing brain dopamine but can cause side-effects such as stiffness and shakiness and feeling slow, restlessness, sexual difficulties and unwanted movements, mainly of the mouth and tongue. Some of these antipsychotic medications, including haloperidol, fluphenazine, perphenazine and others, are available in long-acting injectable forms that eliminate the need to take pills every day. The newer (atypical) antipsychotics are less likely to produce unwanted movements but can cause weight gain, diabetes, tiredness and sexual problems (Table 10.22).

Antipsychotic medications alter the dopamine/cholinergic balance in the basal ganglia so that extrapyramidal and anticholinergic effects are common and can be disabling. The long-term side-effects of antipsychotic drugs, especially drowsiness, hypotension, xerostomia, interference with temperature regulation and extrapyramidal symptoms may pose particularly serious problems. Extrapyramidal features from medication are most common with the piperazine phenothiazines, butyrophenones and depot preparations, and include:

- dystonia and dyskinesia (abnormal movements)
- akathisia (restlessness)
- parkinsonism; anti-parkinsonian drugs such as benztropine or orphenadrine are required to control extrapyramidal symptoms, which sometimes develop after only a few doses. Levodopa is contraindicated.

Maintenance therapy is conveniently carried out with long-acting preparations such as fluphenazine or flupentixol, but these can cause intractable tardive dyskinesia. Phenothiazines can also cause the neuroleptic malignant syndrome, dose-related impaired temperature regulation, obstructive jaundice, leukopenia or ECG changes.

Most schizophrenic patients need and show substantial improvement with antipsychotic drugs but there have been sudden deaths in asthmatics. Some people have only one such psychotic episode; others have many episodes during a lifetime, but lead relatively normal lives during the interim periods; but those with 'chronic' schizophrenia, or a continuous or recurring pattern of illness, typically require long-term treatment. Schizophrenia can be remarkably disturbing for patients and for those in contact with them; hospitalization may therefore be necessary in severe cases. Overall, about 10% remain hospitalized and a further 30% remain seriously handicapped.

Electroconvulsive therapy may be given if there is poor response to medication or if there is catatonia.

Tardive dyskinesia

Tardive dyskinesia (TD), characterized by involuntary movements, most often affecting the mouth, lips and tongue, and sometimes the trunk or other parts of the body, such as arms and legs, affects about 15–20% of patients who have been receiving phenothiazines for many years, but sometimes only for short periods. The symptoms of TD are usually mild so that the patient may be unaware of the movements. TD does not respond to withdrawal of the causative drug or to any other medication.

Neuroleptic malignant syndrome

Neuroleptic malignant syndrome (NMS) is a rare but potentially life-threatening drug-induced disorder associated with the use of antipsychotic medications. It is characterized by disturbances in mental status, hyperpyrexia, and disturbed autonomic and extrapyramidal functions. Laboratory findings include leukocytosis, raised creatine phosphokinase and metabolic acidosis. Treatment of NMS consists primarily of early recognition, discontinuation of triggering drugs, management of fluid balance, cooling and monitoring for complications. Use of dopamine

Table 10.22 Important drugs used to treat schizophrenia

	Examples	Features
Phenothiazines with pronounced sedative effects, but moderate antimuscarinic and extrapyramidal effects	Chlorpromazine, methotrimeprazine or promazine	If there is considerable anxiety or hyperactivity, chlorpromazine is most commonly used but parenteral fluphenazine enanthate or decanoate, pipothiazine palmitate or zuclopenthixol decanoate by biweekly injection overcomes compliance difficulties
Phenothiazines with low extrapyramidal effects, moderate sedative and antimuscarinic effects	Pericyazine, pipotiazine or thioridazine	Fewer extrapyramidal effects than other phenothiazines Thioridazine may be cardiotoxic
Piperazine phenothiazines, with low sedative and antimuscarinic activity	Fluphenazine, perphenazine, prochlorperazine or trifluoperazine	If no sedation is needed piperazine phenothiazines may be given but may have pronounced extrapyramidal effects and may worsen depression
Butyrophenones	Benperidol, droperidol or haloperidol	Useful mainly for violent patients
Thioxanthines	Flupentixol and zuclopenthixol	Extrapyramidal effects common
Atypical antipsychotics	Clozapine, amisulpride, olanzapine, quetiapine, risperidone, sertindole, zotepine	All apart from clozapine are first-line treatment for newly diagnosed schizophrenia. Clozapine is used for resistant cases; it does not cause tardive dyskinesia but has significant antimuscarinic effects and can cause agranulocytosis
Diphenylbutylpiperidines	Fluspirilene and pimozide	Danger of sudden unexplained, probably cardiac, death

agonists or dantrolene, or both, should be considered and may be indicated in more severe, prolonged or refractory cases.

Dental aspects

Mild schizophrenic features (which are often unrecognized) include loss of social contact, flatness of mood or inappropriate social behaviour, which may appear at first as mere tactlessness or stupidity. Thus the patient, when asked to sit down in the surgery, may sit in the operator's rather than the dental chair. Attempts at communication are met by a response that indicates a failure to get through or are interrupted by totally irrelevant remarks. Such patients may have delusional oral symptoms, the treatment of which is beyond the expertise of dental staff, and then psychiatric help must be sought.

Phenothiazines can cause epinephrine reversal in patients given a LA: there is vasodilatation instead of the anticipated vasoconstriction, because of phenothiazines' alpha-adrenergic blocking activity. Any practical importance of this in relation to LA is unclear.

- Conscious sedation is safe.
- With tramadol, there is a risk of seizures.
- Haloperidol and phenothiazines may cause orthostatic hypotension. Patients should be raised slowly and carefully assisted from the dental chair.
- Haloperidol and droperidol reportedly block the vasoconstrictor activity of epinephrine.
- General anaesthesia, especially with intravenous barbiturates, can lead to severe hypotension and should therefore be avoided if possible.
- The long-term use of neuroleptics can lead to xerostomia (with susceptibility to candidosis and caries, and, occasionally, ascending parotitis), oral pigmentation and severe extrapyramidal symptoms.
- Muscular rigidity or tonic spasms (facial dyskinesias; frequently involve the bulbar or neck muscles, with

subsequent difficulties in speech or swallowing. Alternatively, there may be uncontrollable facial grimacing (orofacial dystonia), which may start after only a few doses. This may be controlled by stopping the neuroleptic and giving anti-parkinsonian antimuscarinic drugs.
- Haloperidol and clozapine can cause hypersalivation.

KORSAKOFF PSYCHOSIS

Korsakoff psychosis is characterized by amnesia for recent events, impaired ability to learn new facts and fabricated descriptions of recent events (confabulation). Nevertheless the patient is alert, responsible and behaves in an otherwise normal manner.

The disease results from a symmetrical lesion in the periaqueductal area, thalamus, mammillary bodies and cerebellar vermis; chronic alcoholism associated with thiamine deficiency is an important cause, though relatively few alcoholics develop the syndrome. Other possible causes include cerebrovascular disease, tumours or degenerative disorders.

OTHER PSYCHOSES

Psychoses can complicate various endocrine disturbances, the puerperium, or drugs such as alcohol, amfetamine or psychotomimetics (see Table 10.23).

SYSTEMIC DISEASE CAUSING MENTAL DISORDERS

Many endocrine diseases can be complicated by mental disturbances, as may alcoholism, drug abuse or drug treatment. Major trauma, surgery or severe life-threatening disease can also frequently cause emotional reactions, such as anxiety or depression, or conditions such as compensation neurosis.

Table 10.23 Some drug-induced mental states

Mental State	DRUGS SOMETIMES RESPONSIBLE	
	Used in medicine mainly	Used in dentistry also
Confusion	Antihypertensives Antihistamines Tricyclic antidepressants	Benzodiazepines
Aggressive behaviour	Dopa derivatives	Benzodiazepines (in children)
Nightmares or hallucinations	Some antihypertensives	Pentazocine or ketamine
Mania	Levodopa	Corticosteroids
Depression	Antihypertensives Contraceptive pill	Pentazocine Corticosteroids
Delirium	Antihypertensives Antitubercular drugs Anticonvulsants Oral hypoglycaemics	Procaine penicillin Sulfonamides
Paranoia	Antihypertensives Anticonvulsants Amphetamines	Ephedrine Corticosteroids

LEGISLATION

Legislation and policy decisions affect individuals' rights and in particular their rights to health care provision, including oral health care. Legislation in the UK has evolved significantly over recent years to protect the rights of the individual, and a summary is presented below.

MENTAL HEALTH ACT 1983

This Act is primarily concerned with the care and treatment of people with a mental health problem which requires that they be detained or treated in the interests of their own health and safety or with a view to protecting other people. This Act is now over 20 years old and new legislation has been passed through parliament in the form of the Mental Health Act 2007.

MENTAL CAPACITY ACT 2005

This Act applies to everyone involved in the care, treatment or support of people aged 16 years and over in England and Wales, and who lack capacity to make all or some decisions for themselves. This Act also applies to situations where a person may lack capacity to make a decision at a particular time due to illness or drugs or alcohol. Assessments of capacity should be time and decision specific.

The Act clarifies the term 'mental capacity' and 'lack of mental capacity' and says that a person is unable to make a particular decision if they cannot do one or more of the following:

- understand information given to them
- retain that information long enough to be able to make the decision
- weigh up the information available to make the decision

- communicate their decision; this could be done, for example, by talking, using sign language or even simple muscle movements, such as blinking an eye or squeezing a hand.

A new criminal offence of ill-treatment or wilful neglect of people who lack capacity also came into force in 2007. Within the law, 'helping with personal hygiene' (that would include toothbrushing) will attract protection from liability as long as the individual has complied with the Act by assessing a person's capacity and acting in their best interests. 'Best interest' decisions made on behalf of people who lack capacity should be the least restrictive of their basis rights and freedoms.

Further changes within the Act include the introduction of *lasting powers of attorney* (LPA) which extend to health and welfare decisions. When a health professional has a significant concern relating to decisions taken under the authority of an LPA about serious medical treatment, the case can be referred for adjudication to the Court of Protection, which is ultimately responsible for the proper functioning of the legislation. The Act also creates a new Public Guardian which will have responsibility for the registration and supervision of both LPAs and Court-appointed deputies. Furthermore, independent mental capacity advocates have been introduced to support particularly vulnerable incapacitated adults – most often those who lack any other forms of external support – in making certain decisions.

USEFUL WEBSITES

http://www.mssm.edu/msjournal/65/05_miy.pdf
http://www.nimh.nih.gov/publications/index.shtml
http://www.abess.com/glossary.html
http://www.rcpsych.ac.uk/
http://www.depressionalliance.org/
http://www.samaritans.org
http://www.nice.org.uk/guidance/index.jsp
http://www.anxietyuk.org.uk
http://www.ccbt.co.uk
http://www.uktrauma.org.uk
http://www.ncptsd.va.gov/ncmain/information
http://www.trauma-pages.com
http://bmj.com/cgi/content/full/316/7138/1105
http://bmj.com/cgi/content/full/320/7226/26
http://med.annualreviews.org/cgi/content/full/50/1/453
http://www.merck.com/mmpe/index.html

FURTHER READING

Abrahamsson, K.H., Berggren, U., Carlsson, S.G., 2000. Psychosocial aspects of dental and general fears in dental phobic patients. Acta Odontol Scand 58, 37–43.

Adshead, G., 2000. Psychological therapies for post-traumatic stress disorder. Br J Psychiatry 177, 144–148.

American Psychiatric Association (APA), 1994. Diagnostic and statistical manual of mental disorders, 4th edn. (DSM-IV). APA, Washington, DC.

Barskey, A.J., 2001. The patient with hypochondriasis. N Engl J Med 345, 1395–1399.

Bassi, N., Amital, D., Amital, H., Doria, A., Shoenfeld, Y., 2008. Chronic fatigue syndrome: characteristics and possible causes for its pathogenesis. Isr Med Assoc J 10, 79–82.

Bateman, A., Tyrer, P., 2004. Psychological treatment for personality disorders. Adv Psychiatr Treat 10, 378–388.

Bateman, A., Tyrer, P., 2004. Services for personality disorder: organisation for inclusion. Adv Psychiatr Treat 10, 425–433.

Blenkiron, P., 2001. Treatment of obsessive compulsive disorder (review). Cont Prof Dev Bull Psychiatry 2, 68–72.

British Medical Association and Law Society, 2004. Assessment of mental capacity: guidance for doctors and lawyers. BMJ, London.

Coid, J., 2003. Epidemiology, public health and the problem of personality disorder. Br J Psychiatry 182 (Suppl 44), s3–s10.

Coid, J., Yang, M., Tyrer, P., Roberts, A., Ullrich, S., 2006. Prevalence and correlates of personality disorder in Great Britain. Br J Psychiatry 188, 423–431.

Core interventions in the treatment of obsessive-compulsive disorder and body dysmorphic disorder. Clinical guidelines 31 (Quick reference guide), National Institute for Health and Clinical Excellence, November 2005.

Foa, E., Keane, T., Friedman, M. (eds), 2000. Effective treatments for PTSD: guidelines from the International Society of Traumatic Stress Studies. Guilford Press, New York.

Freeman, R., 2000. The psychology of dental patient care; a common sense approach. BDJ Books, Basingstoke.

Friedlander, A.H., Norman, D.C., 2002. Late-life depression: psychopathology, medical interventions and dental implications. Oral Surg 94, 404–412.

Geddes, J., 2003. Bipolar disorder. Evid Based Ment Health 6, 101–102.

General Medical Council. Consent: patients and doctors making decisions together 2008. General Medical Council 51. http://www.gmc-uk.org/guidance/ethical_guidance/consent_guidance/index.asp.

Glaros, A.G., 2000-01. Emotional factors in temporomandibular joint disorders. J Indiana Dent Assoc 79 (4), 20–23.

Goodwin, G.M., 2003. Evidence-based guidelines for treating bipolar disorder: recommendations from The British Association for Psychopharmacology. J Psychopharmacol 17, 149–173.

Griffith, J.P., Zarrouf, F.A., 2008. A systematic review of chronic fatigue syndrome: don't assume it's depression. Prim Care Companion J Clin Psychiatry 10, 120–128.

Hagglin, C., Hakeberg, M., Hallstrom, T., et al., 2001. Dental anxiety in relation to mental health and personality factors. A longitudinal study of middle-aged and elderly women. Eur J Oral Sci 109, 27–33.

Hill, J., 2003. Early identification of individuals at risk for antisocial personality disorder. Br J Psychiatry 182 (Suppl 44), s11–s14.

Hull, A.M., Alexander, D.A., Klein, S., 2002. Survivors of the Piper Alpha oil platform disaster: long-term follow-up study. Br J Psychiatry 181, 433–438.

Humphris, G.M., Freeman, R., Campbell, J., Tuuti, H., D'Sousza, V., 2000. Further evidence for the reliability and validity of the Modified Dental Anxiety Scale. Int Dent J 50, 367–370.

Kendell, R., 2002. The distinction between personality disorder and mental illness. Br J Psychiatry 180, 110–115.

Kerr, J.R., Petty, R., Burke, B., et al., 2008. Gene expression subtypes in patients with chronic fatigue syndrome/myalgic encephalomyelitis. J Infect Dis 197, 1171–1184.

Lab, D., Santos, I., de Zulueta, F., 2008. Treating post-traumatic stress disorder in the 'real world': evaluation of a specialist trauma service and adaptations to standard treatment approaches. Psychiatr Bull 32, 8–12.

Lebowitz, B.D., Pearson, J.L., Schneider, L.S., et al., 1997. Diagnosis and treatment of depression in late life: consensus statement update. JAMA 278, 1186–1190.

Locker, D., Thomson, W.M., Poulton, R., 2001. Psychological disorder, conditioning experiences, and the onset of dental anxiety in early adulthood. J Dent Res 80, 1588–1592.

Mellor, A., 2007. Management of the anxious patient: what treatments are available? Dent Update 34, 108–114.

Mental Capacity Act 2005. s2(1) Department of Constitutional Affairs. Mental Capacity Act 2005, summary, P. 1.

Morriss, R., 2004. The early warning symptom intervention for patients with bipolar affective disorder. Adv Psychiatr Treat 10, 18–26.

NICE clinical guideline 26: Post-traumatic stress disorder: the management of PTSD in adults and children in primary and secondary care. http://www.nice.org.uk/Guidance/CG26.

NICE clinical guideline 28, September 2005. The treatment of depression in children and young people. National Institute for Clinical Excellence, London.

NICE clinical guideline 38, 2006. Bipolar disorder: the management of bipolar disorder in adults, children and adolescents, in primary and secondary care. National Collaborating Centre for Mental Health, London.

Rafique, S., Banerjee, A., Fiske, J., 2008. Management of the petrified dental patient. Dent Update 35, 196–198 201–2, 204 passim.

Rey, J.M., Tennant, C.C., 2002. Cannabis and mental health. BMJ 325, 1183.

Scully, C., Diz Dios, P., Kumar, N., 2007. Special care in dentistry. handbook of oral healthcare. Churchill Livingstone, Edinburgh.

Scully, C., Chaudhry, S., 2008. Aspects of Human Disease 21. Anxiety, stress and depression Dental Update 35, 213.

Scully, C., Chaudhry, S., 2008. Aspects of Human Disease 22. Schizophrenia, Dental Update 35, 285.

Seishima, M., Mizutani, Y., Shibuya, Y., Arakawa, C., 2008. Chronic fatigue syndrome after human parvovirus B19 infection without persistent viremia. Dermatology 216, 341–346.

Talis, F., 1992. Understanding obsessions and compulsions. Sheldon Press, London a self-help manual.

Tate, P., 2007. The doctor's communication handbook. Radcliffe Publishing, Oxford.

Tyrer, P. (ed.), 2002. Personality disorders, psychiatry 2002, The Medicine Publishing Company, Oxford.

Tyrer, P., Bateman, A., 2004. Drug treatment for personality disorders. Adv Psychiatr Treat 10, 389–398.

Tyrer, P., Coombs, N., Ibrahimi, F., et al., 2007. Critical developments in the assessment of personality disorder. Br J Psychiatry 190 (Suppl 49), s51–s59.

Understanding NICE guidance: information for people with OCD or body dysmorphic disorder, their families and carers, and the public. Printed copies from NHS response line; downloadable from: http://www.nice.org.uk/guidance/index.jsp?action=byID&o=10976.

US Department of Health and Human Services, 1999. Mental health: a report of the Surgeon General. US Department of Health and Human Services, Substance Abuse and Mental Health Services Administration, Center for Mental Health Services. National Institutes of Health, National Institute of Mental Health, Rockville, MD.

Veale D, Willson R. Overcoming obsessive-compulsive disorder: a self-help book using cognitive-behavioural techniques. Constable and Robinson, London.

Yehuda, R. (ed.), 2002. Treating trauma, survivors with PTSD. American Publishing, Washington, DC.

MUCOSAL, ORAL AND CUTANEOUS DISORDERS

SKIN DISEASES

The common skin diseases are discussed here.

ECZEMA

General aspects

Eczema is a term describing a range of persistent skin conditions that include dryness and recurring rashes characterized by redness, itching, crusting, flaking, blistering, cracking, oozing or bleeding.

Clinical features

Common types of eczema include the following.

- *Atopic eczema* is believed to have a hereditary component (often runs in families whose members also have asthma and/or hay fever). It is particularly noticeable on face and scalp, neck, inside of elbows, behind knees and buttocks.
- *Contact dermatitis* is irritant (resulting from direct reaction to a solvent) or allergic.
- *Seborrhoeic dermatitis* causes dry or greasy scaling of scalp and eyebrows, scaly pimples and red patches.

General management

Patch-testing, raised serum immunoglobulin E (IgE), eosinophilia, radioallergosorbent test (RAST) or paper radioimmunosorbent test (PRIST; Chs 17) may be diagnostically helpful. There is no known cure; treatments, which aim to control symptoms, reduce inflammation and relieve itching, include topical emollients, corticosteroids, or calcineurin inhibitors. Ciclosporin, azathioprine or methotrexate may rarely be needed.

ACNE

General aspects

Acne is a common skin disorder in which hair follicles become blocked with oil and hypertrophied epithelium, and is characterized by clogged pores and pimples. More than four out of five people, particularly adolescent males, develop acne. Several factors – including hormones, bacteria, medications such as corticosteroids, heredity and stress – play a role. Many adult women experience mild to moderate acne due to hormonal changes associated with menstrual cycles, starting or stopping oral contraceptives or pregnancy.

Clinical features

Pimples appear as hair follicles, become plugged with oil and dead skin cells, causing the follicle wall to bulge and produce a 'whitehead'. If the pore stays open and traps dirt, the plug surface oxidises and darkens, causing a 'blackhead'. Blockages and inflammation deep inside hair follicles can produce scarring and cysts. Acne is rarely serious, but it often causes emotional distress.

General management

Effective lotions generally contain benzoyl peroxide or azeleic acid. Topical erythromycin and clindamycin are effective treatments for inflamed lesions. Systemic acne treatment should start with antimicrobials (tetracyclines or erythromycin). Options for scarring cystic acne or acne that fails to respond to other treatments are, in women, cyproterone acetate or isotretinoin (vitamin A analogue, only prescribable by consultant dermatologists). For men, only isotretinoin is available. Oral contraceptives, including a combination of norgestimate and ethinylestradiol, can improve acne in women. Maternal use of vitamin A congeners must be avoided since birth defects similar to those in Di George syndrome can result – the *fetal isotretinoin syndrome*.

Dermabrasion (removing the top skin layers with a rapidly rotating wire brush) may help more severe scarring. Laser resurfacing can achieve the same effect.

PSORIASIS

General aspects

Psoriasis is a common chronic skin disease characterized by scaling and inflammation. Psoriasis has a strong genetic background with HLA-Cw6 and HLA-DR7. T cells trigger inflammation, and excessive skin cell reproduction underlies the pathogenesis. There are sometimes associations with stress and alcoholism.

Clinical features

Psoriasis causes thick pruritic erythematous plaques covered with silvery scales (Fig. 11.1) predominantly on scalp, elbows and knees, lower back, face, palms, and soles of feet, and 'ice-pick' pitting or onycholysis of fingernails and toenails (Fig. 11.2). About 15% have joint inflammation (psoriatic arthropathy).

General management

Treatment of psoriasis initially is with topical agents – corticosteroids, vitamin D_3, vitamin A analogues (retinoids), coal tar or anthralin. Failing this, light (phototherapy) is used. Sunlight often helps but more controlled artificial light treatment may be used in mild psoriasis (ultraviolet B phototherapy), or psoralen and ultraviolet A (PUVA) therapy in more severe or extensive psoriasis.

Severe cases of psoriasis may need systemic treatment with methotrexate, ciclosporin or retinoids.

Dental aspects

Local anaesthesia (LA) is safe. Conscious sedation can be given if required.

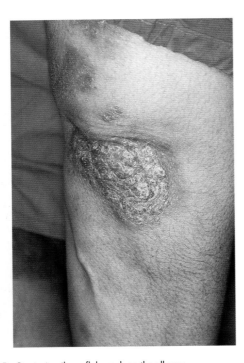

Fig. 11.1 Psoriasis; silvery flaky rash on the elbows

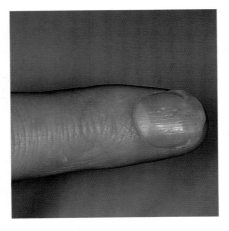

Fig. 11.2 Psoriasis affecting nails

Oral lesions such as white or reddish mucosal plaques are rare. There may be a higher prevalence of erythema migrans and fissured tongue, particularly in pustular psoriasis. The temporomandibular joint is involved in up to 60% of patients with psoriatic arthropathy.

Oral complications of the treatment of psoriasis, such as gingival swelling from ciclosporin, or ulceration from methotrexate, may be seen.

SKIN CANCER

General aspects

The three major types of skin cancer, all on the increase, are (see also ch. 22):

- basal cell carcinoma (BCC; rodent ulcer)
- squamous cell carcinoma (SCC)
- melanoma.

Nearly half of all men over 65 years will develop a skin cancer. Risk factors are shown in Box 11.1.

Box 11.1 Risk factors for skin cancer

- Fair skin; patients with blond or red hair, light-coloured eyes, and who freckle or sunburn easily, are 20–30 times more prone
- Sunburn increases the risk. People who live in areas of strong sunshine are at greatest risk; immigrants to Australia and southern USA, or at high elevations, are frequent victims. Severe sunburn as a child or teenager is a particular risk. Overuse of sun-beds for tanning is another cause
- Moles; people who have > 20 naevi are at greater risk of skin cancer
- Pre-cancerous skin lesions (e.g. actinic keratoses) can increase the risk of developing skin cancer
- A family history of skin cancer
- A personal history of skin cancer
- An immune defect
- Exposure to environmental hazards, such as chemicals (including some herbicides) or psoriasis treatments, increases the risk of skin cancer

---

Clinical features and management

Skin cancer develops mainly on areas of sun-exposed skin: the scalp, face, lips, ears, neck, chest, arms and hands, and on the legs in women. BCC is superficial and highly treatable, especially if found early. It appears as a pearly or waxy lump on the face, ears or neck or a flat, flesh-coloured or brown scarlike lesion on the chest or back, typically in persons after middle age, but responds to excision. In Gorlin syndrome, BCC can start to form in childhood.

Squamous cell carcinoma is superficial, slow-growing and is highly treatable, especially if found early. It presents as a firm, red nodule on the face, lip, ears, neck, hands or arms or a flat lesion with a scaly, crusted surface on the face, ears, neck, hands or arms. It usually responds to wide excision.

Melanoma has the greatest potential to spread and is potentially fatal. It typically appears as: a large brownish spot with darker speckles, anywhere; a simple mole anywhere that changes in colour or size or consistency, or that bleeds or exhibits new growth; a small lesion with an irregular border and red, white, blue or blue–black spots on the trunk or limbs; shiny, firm, dome-shaped nodules anywhere; dark lesions on palms, soles, tips of fingers and toes, or on mucous membranes; or a red flat lesion (amelanotic melanoma). Malignant melanomas can also form in the retina or rarely, even in areas protected from sunlight such as the mouth.

Treatment of melanoma is usually excision, and if the tumour is superficial (Breslow depth < 1.5 mm) the prognosis is excellent at 90% 5-year survival. The prognosis of malignant melanoma is usually poor as a consequence of late diagnosis and rapid spread: survival averages only 2 years.

Dental aspects

Dentists are a risk group for skin cancers (from excess vacational sun exposure!).

MUCOCUTANEOUS DISORDERS

Several mucocutaneous diseases can involve the mouth or may influence dental treatment. The most common is lichen planus. The most serious are pemphigus (which is potentially fatal), erythema multiforme and mucous membrane pemphigoid (which may involve other mucosae). Oral lesions herald some mucocutaneous diseases or may be the main manifestation. Immunostaining can often help the diagnosis (Table 11.1).

Many of the mucocutaneous diseases are treated with corticosteroids (topically or systemically), which may, if used for prolonged periods, cause adrenocortical suppression (Ch. 6).

ACQUIRED DISORDERS

This section discusses mainly those mucocutaneous diseases that are acquired, as these are most common, though many have at least some genetic background.

Lichen planus

General aspects

Lichen planus (LP) is a common skin and mucosal disease. The immunopathogenesis includes a dense T-lymphocyte infiltrate, to an unidentified provoking antigen.

Lesions clinically and histologically similar or identical to lichen planus (lichenoid lesions) can be related to dental restorations, particularly amalgam and drugs, particularly to non-steroidal anti-inflammatory drugs (NSAIDs), gold, antimalarials, and beta-blockers. Reported associations of oral LP with diabetes mellitus and hypertension have not been confirmed, and the so-called Grinspan syndrome of LP, diabetes mellitus and hypertension is probably related to drug treatment. Similar lesions may be to chemicals, such as photographic developing solutions, graft-versus-host disease (Ch. 35), chronic liver disease and virus infections, and hepatitis C or human immunodeficiency virus (HIV).

Approximately 1% of cases of oral LP may develop malignant change after 10 years.

Clinical features

Skin lesions are usually small polygonal purplish or violaceous itchy papules particularly affecting the flexor surfaces of the wrist (Fig. 11.3), and also elsewhere such as the shins (Fig. 11.4) or periumbilically, but rarely, if ever, on the face. Examination with a lens may show a fine lacy white network of striae (Wickham striae) on these papules (Fig. 11.5). Mouth and genital lesions in LP include white striae, papules, plaques, or red atrophic areas or erosions (Fig. 11.6). The nails or hair may be affected (Fig. 11.7).

Table 11.1 Immunostaining in skin and oral mucosal diseases

Disease	Direct immunofluorescence	Epithelial location	Indirect immunofluorescence	Type of antibody[a]	Main epithelial antigen
Pemphigus vulgaris	Yes	Intercellular	Yes	IgG	Desmoglein
Paraneoplastic pemphigus	Yes	Intercellular[b]	Yes	IgG	Desmoplakin
IgA pemphigus	Yes	Intercellular	Yes	IgA	?Desmocollin
Bullous pemphigoid	Yes	Basement membrane area	Yes	IgG	BP1
Mucous membrane pemphigoid	Yes	Basement membrane area	Rarely	IgG	BP2
Angina bullosa haemorrhagica	No	–	No	–	–
Dermatitis herpetiformis	Yes	Basement membrane area	No	IgA	Transglutaminase
Linear IgA disease	Yes	Basement membrane area	No	IgA	Laminin
Systemic lupus erythematosus	Yes	Basement membrane area	Yes	ANA	NR
Chronic discoid lupus erythematosus	Yes	Basement membrane area	No	ANA	NR
Lichen planus	Often	Basement membrane area	No	(Usually fibrin)	?
Chronic ulcerative stomatitis	Yes	Basal cell layer	No	IgG/ANA	?

[a]Usually with complement deposits.
[b]Transitional epithelium.
ANA, antinuclear antibody; BP, bullous pemphigoid; Ig, immunoglobulin; NR, not relevant;

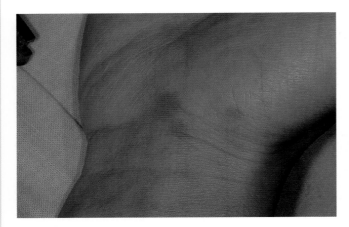

Fig. 11.3 Lichen planus rash

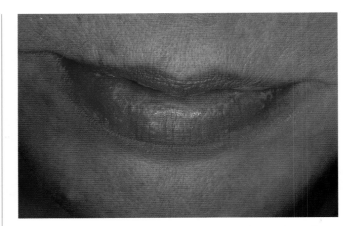

Fig. 11.6 Lichen planus on lips

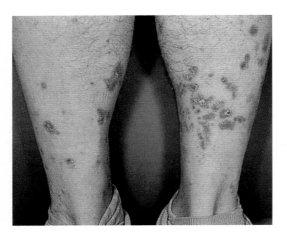

Fig. 11.4 Lichen planus rash

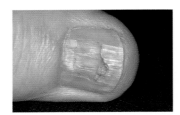

Fig. 11.7 Lichen planus affecting nails

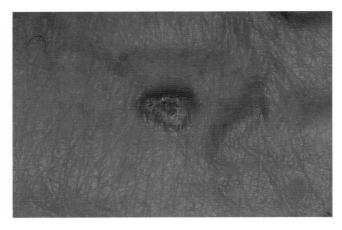

Fig. 11.5 Wickham striae in lichen planus

General management

A drug history should be taken in order to exclude possible reactions. If there is any doubt about the diagnosis, a biopsy is needed, particularly to differentiate LP from lupus erythema-

tosus, chronic ulcerative stomatitis or keratoses. Topical corticosteroids or tacrolimus can be useful to control symptomatic LP, especially severe erosive lesions. Aloe vera reportedly gives effective symptomatic relief.

Exceptionally severe LP sometimes responds only to systemic corticosteroids. Other drugs such as vitamin A analogues (etretinate), dapsone, ciclosporin or alefacept are used only rarely.

Dental aspects

Local anaesthesia is safe. Conscious sedation can be given if required.

Oral lesions in LP can persist for years, although the skin lesions frequently resolve within a few months. Oral lesions characteristically are bilateral and sometimes strikingly symmetrical; they affect particularly the posterior buccal mucosa but may also involve the tongue, gingivae or other sites. Gingival lesions are usually atrophic and red ('desquamative gingivitis').

Replacement of amalgam with non-metallic alternatives may sometimes cause lesions to resolve, but relapse is possible.

PEMPHIGUS

Pemphigus is a potentially fatal autoimmune reaction against proteins, usually within the stratified squamous epithelium, characterized by widespread formation of skin vesicles and bullae. The mouth is frequently the first site of attack. Variants include those listed in Table 11.2.

Table 11.2 Pemphigus variants

Pemphigus variant	Desmosomal antigens	Serum antibodies	Oral lesions	Comments
Pemphigus vulgaris localized to mucosae (mucosal)	Desmoglein 3	IgG	Common	Fatal
Pemphigus vulgaris also involving skin/other mucosae (mucocutaneous)	Desmoglein 3 Desmoglein 1	IgG	Common	Fatal
Pemphigus vegtans	Desmoglein 1	IgG	Uncommon	Variant of vulgaris
Pemphigus foliaceus	Desmoglein 1	IgG	Uncommon	–
Pemphigus erythematosus	Desmoglein 1	IgG	Uncommon	Variant of foliaceous
Drug-induced pemphigus	Desmoglein 3	IgG	Common	–
Paraneoplastic pemphigus	Desmoplakin 1 Desmoplakin 2	IgG or IgA	Common	Rare. Associated with lymphoproliferative disorders
IgA pemphigus	Desmocollin 1 Desmocollin 2 Desmoglein 3	IgA	Common	Rare

Ig, immunoglobulin.

PEMPHIGUS VULGARIS

General aspects

Pemphigus vulgaris is an uncommon disease, which mainly affects middle-aged women. Pemphigus may occasionally be associated with other autoimmune diseases, such as lupus erythematosus, inflammatory bowel disease, or thymoma and myasthenia gravis. Rarely, it is induced by a drug such as rifampicin, penicillamine or captopril. The main immunological finding is circulating antibodies to desmoglein 3 of intercellular attachments (desmosomes) of epithelial cells of stratified squamous epithelia. These IgG antibodies, and complement components, are deposited (and can also be localized by immunostaining) around the epithelial cells, and result in loss of adherence of the cells to one another (acantholysis). Pemphigus is characterized by widespread formation of intraepithelial vesicles and bullae.

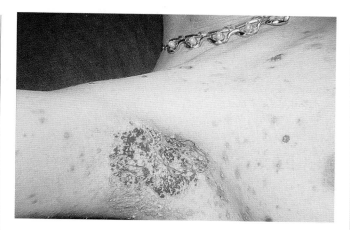

Fig. 11.8 Pemphigus

Clinical features

Pemphigus vulgaris is characterized by thin-roofed vesicles or bullae, followed by ulceration (Fig. 11.8), and is usually fatal in the absence of treatment. It frequently first appears in the mouth. Stroking the skin or mucosa with a finger may induce vesicle formation in an apparently unaffected area or cause a bulla to extend (Nikolsky sign). If untreated, pemphigus vulgaris is usually fatal, as a result of extensive skin and mucosal damage leading to fluid and electrolyte loss, and often infection.

General management

Rapid and precise diagnosis of pemphigus vulgaris is essential since acute cases need immediate immunosuppressive treatment. Diagnosis is confirmed by biopsy. The specimen should be halved to enable both light and immunofluorescent microscopy to be carried out. Light microscopy on a paraffin section is usually distinctive and shows suprabasal cleft formation and intraepithelial vesicles containing free-floating acantholytic cells. Immunofluorescence examination shows IgG and C3 deposits intercellularly. It can be carried out by the direct method using fluorescein-conjugated anti-human IgG and anti-complement (C3) sera on the frozen specimen or on exfoliated cells. In the indirect method, the patient's serum is incubated with normal animal mucosa, which is then labelled with fluorescein-conjugated antihuman globulin (Table 11.1).

The usual treatment of pemphigus vulgaris is with high doses of systemic corticosteroids plus a steroid-sparing agent such as azathioprine. Gold may sometimes be used. Cyclophosphamide, methotrexate or mycophenolate mofetil also appear to be effective. With current methods of treatment, the mortality may be reduced to about 8% but is often a complication of immunosuppressive treatment. Long-term remission has been reported but many require prolonged therapy.

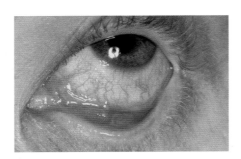

Fig. 11.9 Pemphigoid affecting conjunctiva

Dental aspects

Local anaesthesia and conscious sedation can be given as required. Orofacial manifestations are as described above. However, blisters are so fragile as rarely to be seen intact in the mouth. They leave painful erosions.

MUCOUS MEMBRANE PEMPHIGOID

General aspects

Mucous membrane pemphigoid is a group of subepithelial immune blistering diseases with autoantibodies directed to different epithelial basement membrane proteins. Oral pemphigoid-like lesions have occasionally been reported in association with internal cancers or the use of certain drugs, such as penicillamine. Autoantibodies against basement membrane proteins cause loss of attachment of the epithelium to the connective tissue and blister formation. The common variant of mucous membrane pemphigoid has antibodies against bullous pemphigoid antigen 2 (BP2) but the types that mainly affect the mouth have antibodies against integrin or epiligrin. Serum autoantibodies are demonstrable by conventional techniques in relatively few patients.

Clinical features

Mucous membrane pemphigoid predominantly affects women between 50 and 70 years of age. Intact vesicles or bullae are frequently visible. Sometimes the blisters fill with blood and then must be distinguished from generalized or localized oral purpura. The gingivae may be particularly affected and pemphigoid is an important cause of so-called 'desquamative gingivitis'. Progress is typically indolent and lesions may remain restricted to one site, such as the mouth, for several years or possibly never develop elsewhere, depending on the type.

Scarring after healing of the bullae is a serious complication in sites such as the eyes, larynx, oesophagus or genitalia. Ocular involvement is the most common dangerous manifestation since it can impair or destroy sight (Fig. 11.9). Laryngeal or oesophageal stenosis secondary to scarring is also possible.

General management

The diagnosis of pemphigoid must be confirmed by biopsy. The section should be halved and a frozen section tested for localization of immunoglobulins or complement components along the basement membrane (see Table 11.1). It may be difficult otherwise to differentiate pemphigoid from other mucosal blistering diseases. Paraffin sections show separation of the epithelium from the underlying connective tissue, which is infiltrated by inflammatory cells, often with many eosinophils. Localization of immunoglobulins (IgG) along the line of the epithelial basement membrane can be shown in fewer than 50% but complement components may be demonstrable in about 80%. If there is any suspicion of ocular involvement, referral to an ophthalmologist is essential. The danger of ocular involvement is regarded as an indication for giving systemic corticosteroids. Other lesions can often be adequately controlled by potent topical corticosteroids. Dapsone or systemic corticosteroids may be needed for more severe cases.

Dental aspects

Local anaesthesia is safe and conscious sedation can be given if required. Orofacial manifestations are as described above.

BULLOUS PEMPHIGOID

Bullous pemphigoid is essentially a skin disease which rarely affects the mouth but histologically or immunologically does not appear to differ from mucous membrane pemphigoid. There are associations with diabetes or psoriasis.

DERMATITIS HERPETIFORMIS

Dermatitis herpetiformis is an uncommon chronic skin disease related to coeliac disease.

Clinical features

Dermatitis herpetiformis usually affects males past middle age, and causes an itchy papulovesicular eruption, usually on the extensor surfaces of the upper limbs and trunk. It leaves pigmented areas on healing. The coeliac disease is milder than in isolated coeliac disease. There may be associations with thyroid disease, gastric achlorhydria and pernicious anaemia, and lymphoma.

General management

Diagnosis of dermatitis herpetiformis is by demonstrating deposits of IgA in the papillae at the epithelial basement membrane zone (BMZ), with papillary tip microabscesses and a subepithelial split. The biopsy should be from uninvolved skin. Anti-endomysial and anti-transglutaminase antibodies may be detectable. Serum immune complexes are often detectable, but decline if the patient is put on a gluten-free diet, which may be of considerable benefit (see Ch. 7). Patients are usually treated with dapsone, or sulfapyridine or sulfamethoxypyridazine.

Dental aspects

Indometacin may exacerbate the condition and should be avoided. Oral lesions are usually innocuous but may be erythematous, vesicular, purpuric or sometimes erosive. They may be confused with pemphigoid. Coeliac-type enamel defects may rarely be seen.

Drug reactions may be seen. Dapsone rarely causes a lichenoid eruption; sulfapyridine or other sulfonamides may cause erythema multiforme.

LINEAR IgA DISEASE

General aspects

Linear IgA disease (LAD) is a rare variant of dermatitis herpetiformis, in which the IgA deposits are linear at the BMZ, but coeliac disease is absent. LAD may occasionally be induced by vancomycin.

Clinical features

Similar oral manifestations to dermatitis herpetiformis may be seen and LAD is most likely to be confused with pemphigoid. A variant seen in childhood is termed chronic bullous dermatosis of childhood. There may be an association with lymphoma.

General management

The diagnosis and treatment are as for dermatitis herpetiformis but a gluten-free diet is not required.

Dental aspects

Oral lesions are clinically indistinguishable from those in dermatitis herpetiformis.

ERYTHEMA MULTIFORME

General aspects

Erythema multiforme (EM) primarily affects young males and is characterized by recurrent mucosal and/or cutaneous lesions including virtually any type of rash. The aetiology is uncertain but it may be an immune complex disorder in which the antigens can be various micro-organisms or drugs (Table 11.3). Herpes simplex may be involved in most cases limited to the mouth.

Severe cases with multiple mucosal involvement and fever are termed toxic epidermal necrolysis (TEN), or Stevens–Johnson syndrome. TEN is the term often used when there is very extensive skin detachment and involvement of mucosae and the condition is drug induced. It has of up to 40% mortality.

Stevens–Johnson syndrome is a less severe form than TEN, also affecting several sites.

Clinical features

Skin, and ocular, genital or oral mucous membranes may be involved together or in isolation. The typical skin lesion is the target or iris lesion (Fig. 11.10) in which there are concentric erythematous rings affecting particularly the hands and feet. Vesicles or bullae may also be seen. Typical oral features are grossly swollen, crusted and blood-stained lips, and widespread superficial oral ulceration with ill-defined margins (Fig. 11.11).

General management

When typical mucosal lesions are associated with dermal lesions, the diagnosis can usually be made largely on clinical grounds. Diagnosis can be difficult when the disease is limited to mucosae. Other suggestive features are recent use of drugs (particularly sulfonamides), or recent infections, particularly by herpes simplex or *Mycoplasma pneumoniae*. Biopsy can be useful to exclude other more serious diseases, such as early-onset pemphigus. An ophthalmological opinion should be obtained if the conjunctivae are involved. Oral lesions can

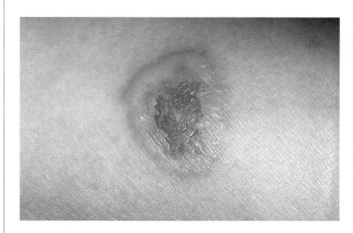

Fig. 11.10   Erythema multiforme target lesion

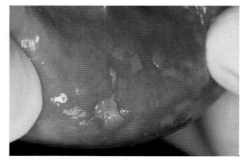

Fig. 11.11   Erythema multiforme on lips

Table 11.3 Erythema multiforme: possible causes		
Micro-organisms	**Drugs**[b]	**Others**
Herpes simplex virus[a] Mycoplasma	Barbiturates Carbamazepine Chlorpropamide Codeine Hydantoins Penicillins Phenylbutazone Salicylates Sulfonamides Tetracyclines Thiazides	Pregnancy Irradiation Internal malignancy

[a]Most common cause of recurrent erythema multiforme.
[b]Most drugs have at some time been implicated in erythema multiforme.

Box 11.2 Causes of desquamative gingivitis

- Lichen planus
- Pemphigoid
- Chronic ulcerative stomatitis
- Dermatitis herpetiformis
- Linear IgA disease
- Pemphigus
- Erythema multiforme
- Pyostomatitis vegetans

Box 11.3 Behçet disease: clinical features and possible complications

Oral
- Aphthous-like stomatitis

Ocular
- Uveitis and hypopyon
- Retinal vasculitis
- Optic atrophy
- Blindness

Genital
- Ulcers

Cutaneous
- Pustules
- Erythema nodosum

Joints
- Arthralgia (large joints)

Vascular
- Aneurysms
- Thromboses of vena cava

Renal
- Proteinuria
- Haematuria

Neuropsychiatric
- Syndromes resembling multiple sclerosis
- Syndromes resembling pseudobulbar palsy
- Benign intracranial hypertension
- Brainstem lesions
- Depression

---

be symptomatically managed with topical corticosteroids, chlorhexidine or lidocaine gel to ease the pain. Healing usually takes 10–14 days.

Severe erythema multiforme and TEN may necessitate hospital admission as feeding may be difficult; systemic corticosteroids are frequently given but may not give anything more than symptomatic relief. Aciclovir is indicated for prophylaxis of recurrent EM, since herpes simplex virus (HSV) is often involved.

Dental aspects

Local anaesthesia is safe. Conscious sedation can be given if required. Orofacial manifestations are as described above.

DESQUAMATIVE GINGIVITIS

Desquamative gingivitis is the term given to the clinical description of chronically red and occasionally sore gingivae. It is caused mainly by pemphigoid or lichen planus, and sometimes other mucocutaneous disorders (Box 11.2).

BEHÇET DISEASE

General aspects

Behçet disease is a clinical triad of oral and genital ulceration, and uveitis, tending particularly to strike people with 'Silk Road' bloodlines, especially those from Turkey and Japan. Behçet disease mainly affects young adult males, and there is an association with HLA-B5 and HLA-B51(B5101). Features such as arthralgia and leukocytoclastic vasculitis suggest an immune complex-mediated basis. The immunological changes seen mimic those seen in patients with recurrent aphthous stomatitis (RAS), with various T-lymphocyte abnormalities (especially T-suppressor cell dysfunction), changes in serum complement, and increased polymorphonuclear leukocyte motility. There is also evidence that mononuclear cells may initiate antibody-dependent cellular cytotoxicity to oral epithelial cells, and evidence of disturbance of natural killer cell activity.

Clinical features

Behçet disease is a multisystem disease with a wide variety of manifestations. Oral ulceration is the most constant feature of Behçet disease and is indistinguishable from the common types of aphthous-like stomatitis. Ocular and genital lesions are common, as are rashes, arthritis, thrombophlebitis, cardiovascular disease and central nervous system involvement (Box 11.3).

MAGIC syndrome (Mouth And Genital ulcers and Interstitial Chondritis) is a recognized variant of Behçet disease.

General management

A clinical diagnosis of Behçet disease is usually made on the presence of any two of oral, genital and ocular features, but similar oral ulceration may also develop in other diseases that have multisystem involvement and these must be excluded when making the diagnosis. Behçet disease must enter into the differential diagnosis of recurrent aphthae but the diagnosis may be difficult to confirm for reasons given earlier. Oral and genital ulceration may also result from folate deficiency, when other features characteristic of Behçet syndrome are lacking. Recurrent oral, ocular and genital lesions may also be seen in erythema multiforme and sometimes in ulcerative colitis and other conditions. According to the *international criteria for classification of Behçet's disease*, the primary features of Behçet disease are as follows.

- Recurrent oral ulceration (painful aphthous-like ulcers, testing negative for herpes) in almost 100% of patients.
- Plus any two of the following four:
  recurrent genital ulcerations

eye inflammation (uveitis, or retinal vasculitis)

skin lesions (erythema nodosum, pseudofolliculitis, papulopustular lesions or acneiform nodules)

a positive pathergy test (a skinprick test using a sterile needle and sterile saline solution).

However, UK or US patients rarely test positive, even during disease activity.

Other manifestations that may be useful in diagnosis, but are not considered part of the international Behçet criteria, include:

- subcutaneous thrombophlebitis, deep vein thrombosis
- epididymitis, arterial occlusion and/or aneurysm
- central nervous system involvement (including difficulties in movement or speech or memory loss)
- severe headaches with stiff neck, joint pain or non-destructive arthritis
- gastrointestinal tract involvement (bloating, cramping, diarrhoea, bloody stools)
- renal involvement
- pulmonary vascular inflammation and pleuritis.

Reliable diagnostic tests for Behçet disease are not available but there are many immunological findings including: circulating autoantibodies (e.g. against intermediate filaments, cardiolipin and neutrophil cytoplasm); circulating immune complexes and abnormal levels of complement; immunoglobulins and complement deposition within and around blood vessel walls; depressed T-helper (CD4):T-suppressor (CD8) ratio. Behçet disease is thus diagnosed mainly on clinical grounds alone though findings of HLAB5101 and pathergy are supportive, as are antibodies to cardiolipin and neutrophil cytoplasm. Activity of the disease may be assessed by serum levels of acute-phase proteins or antibodies to intermediate filaments, both raised in active Behçet disease.

Medical and ophthalmological opinions should be obtained since ocular involvement often culminates in impaired sight.

Available treatments include mainly colchicine, systemic corticosteroids, azathioprine and thalidomide. However, the multiplicity of other medications, including levamisole, cyclophosphamide, dapsone and ciclosporin or chlorambucil confirms their overall low level of success.

Dental aspects

Oral lesions can be managed symptomatically like common aphthae. Topical tetracycline mouthwash is the topical drug of choice for controlling the ulcers. Topical corticosteroids and LA may help. Colchicine may be of value and thalidomide may be the most effective treatment for otherwise intractable oral ulceration.

SWEET SYNDROME

Sweet syndrome, or acute neutrophilic dermatosis, is rare but consists of persistent high fever, raised erythrocyte sedimentation rate and neutrophilia, and a rash. Some cases are associated with malignancy (especially acute myeloid leukaemia), and

some have followed infections – especially upper respiratory tract infections.

The rash consists of dull red skin nodules or plaques on the neck and forearms especially; these may become pustular. Sweet syndrome may also include oral ulceration, conjunctivitis, episcleritis and arthralgia. Treatment is with systemic corticosteroids.

GENETIC DISORDERS

ECTODERMAL DYSPLASIA

General aspects

Ectodermal dysplasia is a relatively common genodermatosis characterized by hypoplasia or agenesis of many skin appendages. There are many variants. The skin is fragile and nails may be defective. The teeth and salivary glands may also be defective or fail to form. Sweat glands may fail to form and heat control is then defective (hypohidrotic ectodermal dysplasia).

Clinical features

There may be frontal bossing and a depressed nasal bridge. The hair is fine, blond and scanty (hypotrichosis), especially in the tonsural region, and the eyelashes and eyebrows may be absent. If the teeth are absent, there may be a prematurely senile (nutcracker) profile with protuberant lips.

Dental aspects

Ectodermal dysplasia rarely causes management problems apart from those related to its oral manifestations. LA is safe. Conscious sedation is safe. GA, as with other dental patients, must be given in hospital. Especial care is indicated in intubation in hypohidrotic forms. Teeth are often few in number (hypodontia or oligodontia), and those present may be of simple conical form. The enamel is thin. Either, or in extreme cases both, the deciduous and permanent dentition may fail to form (anodontia), causing hypoplasia of the jaws. Salivary glands may fail to form, which causes xerostomia. Preventive dental care is therefore particularly important.

EPIDERMOLYSIS BULLOSA

General aspects

Epidermolysis bullosa is an uncommon bullous disease affecting mainly skin and mucosae. There are several forms that show different patterns of inheritance and vary greatly in severity. The severe form appears soon after birth; milder forms may not become evident until adolescence or later (Table 11.4).

An acquired form, with antibodies against collagen VII, is also recognized.

Clinical features

Vesicles and bullae form in response to mild or insignificant trauma and may lead to disabling scarring.

Table 11.4 The main types of epidermolysis bullosa

Type	Onset	Main site of lesions[a]	Oral mucosal lesions	Dental defects	Nail defects	Scarring	Inheritance
I. Non-scarring types							
Simplex[b]	Neonatal onwards	Hands, feet and elbows	Rarely	No	No	No	AD
Letalis[c]	Birth	Widespread	Yes[d]	Yes	Severe	No	AR
II. Scarring types							
Dermolytic dominant (dystrophic)[e]	Childhood	Extremities	Uncommon	No	Yes	Yes. Soft scars	AD
Dermolytic recessive (polydysplastic)[g]	Birth or infancy	Widespread	Yes. Severe, mutilating	No	Destruction	Mutilating[f]	AR

[a]Usually also any site of trauma.
[b]May improve by puberty: commonest type.
[c]Usually fatal in neonatal period or childhood. Also known as Herlitz disease.
[d]Vermilion border of lips spared: lesions are perioral and perinasal. May be corneal lesions.
[e]A cemental defect has been reported, but destruction and loss of teeth from caries and periodontal care is a typical result of inability to brush the teeth.
[f]Typically leads to destruction of hands and feet. Oesophageal stricture may lead to aspiration into airway.
[g]Rare and fatal.
AD, autosomal dominant; AR, autosomal recessive.

General management

Corticosteroids may help prevent blister formation and some success has been claimed for vitamin E and phenytoin.

Dental aspects

Early dietary advice and preventive dental care is overwhelmingly important; since even 'normal' toothbrushing can cause ulceration. Adequate oral hygiene is difficult to achieve, and dental diseases such as caries and periodontal disease are common. Oral scarring and severe microstomia may restrict access. Blistering, erosions and aggravation of scarring following dental treatment (however carefully carried out) may possibly be reduced by applying KY jelly or silicone oil to the mucosa. A short pre-operative course of corticosteroids an hour before treatment, again on the following day, and then tapering the dose off over the next 3 days, may possibly help.

Intramuscular injections can cause sloughing and adhesive tapes easily traumatize the epidermis and thus should be avoided. Antimicrobials to cover surgery may possibly be helpful.

General anaesthesia should be avoided where possible. Bullae may form on the face or in the airway if intubation is attempted. If it must be used, the face should be protected with petroleum jelly gauze and intubation should be oral rather than nasal. Iron deficiency anaemia is common and may need correction before GA (Ch. 5). Intravenous ketamine has proved a useful anaesthetic in these patients. Atropinics are often needed to control excessive salivation.

Rarely, squamous cell carcinoma can complicate the oral lesions. Rare cases are associated with poikiloderma congenitale and may present with early-onset periodontitis or desquamative gingivitis.

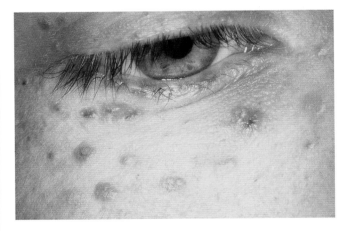

Fig. 11.12 Basal carcinomas in Gorlin–Goltz syndrome

MULTIPLE BASAL CELL NAEVI SYNDROME (GORLIN–GOLTZ SYNDROME)

General aspects

The multiple basal cell naevi syndrome consists of multiple basal cell carcinomas of early onset, keratocystic odontogenic tumors, anomalies of the vertebrae and ribs and many other abnormalities. It is an autosomal dominant trait with poor penetrance.

Clinical features

Skin lesions appear in childhood or adolescence. Multiple naevoid basal cell carcinomas over the nose, eyelids, cheeks and elsewhere are often an early sign (Fig. 11.12).

There is frontal and temporoparietal bossing, a broad nasal root, prominent supraorbital ridges and a degree of mandibular prognathism. Multiple jaw cysts develop. Short fourth meta-carpals are common. There may also be pitting of the palms or soles.

Many other problems may be associated, including learning impairment or cerebral tumours. Pseudohypoparathyroidism has been described in some patients and there is also a slightly greater incidence of diabetes mellitus. Cardiac lesions may be present and cerebral tumours can be fatal.

General management

Radiography may reveal bifid ribs, vertebral defects with kyphoscoliosis and calcification of the falx cerebri.

Dental aspects

Local anaesthesia is safe. Conscious sedation can be given. GA must be given in hospital for treatment of the jaw cysts.

GARDNER SYNDROME (FAMILIAL ADENOMATOUS POLYPOSIS COLI)

General aspects

Gardner syndrome is the association of multiple osteomas, skin fibromas and epidermoid cysts, and pigmented ocular fundus lesions with colonic polyposis.

It is an autosomal dominant trait of variable penetrance.

Clinical features

Multiple osteomas characteristically involve the jaws, facial skeleton or frontal bone and appear in adolescence. Fibromas, desmoid tumours, epidermoid cysts or lipomas affect any site. Multiple colonic polyps invariably undergo malignant change. Thyroid, adrenal and biliary carcinomas may also develop.

General management

Colonic resection is usually required. Desmoid tumours often arise in the abdominal wall scar.

Dental aspects

Local anaesthesia is safe. Conscious sedation can be given if required. Multiple osteomas, particularly on the alveolar margins, should suggest the presence of Gardner syndrome. Compound odontomes and dental anomalies may be associated.

COWDEN SYNDROME

This is an autosomal dominant condition of multiple hamartomas, with a predisposition to carcinomas of the breast, thyroid or colon. Skin and mucosal papules precede the onset of malignant disease. Other lesions include keratoses on the palms and soles, and sometimes learning impairment.

Oral mucosal papillomatosis may suggest the diagnosis. When associated with cerebellar hypertrophy, the syndrome is known as Cowden–L'Hermitte syndrome.

THE PHAKOMATOSES

The phakomatoses (neurodermatoses) are hereditary hamartomatous autosomal dominant disorders affecting the skin and nervous system. They include neurofibromatosis, tuberous sclerosis and Sturge–Weber syndrome. Sporadic cases are not uncommon. The fourth member of this group, cerebroretinal angiomatosis, is not discussed here.

NEUROFIBROMATOSIS, TYPE I (VON RECKLINGHAUSEN DISEASE)

General aspects

Neurofibromatosis type I is a simple autosomal dominant condition in which there are multiple neurofibromas or, less often, neurilemmomas.

Clinical features

Neurofibromas sometimes form in vast numbers. These may be disfiguring but are often asymptomatic unless pressure effects develop, for example on the spinal nerve roots with compression of the spinal cord. Patches of skin hyperpigmentation (café-au-lait spots) are common. Sarcomatous change may develop in about 10% of severely affected patients. There is also a greater frequency of cerebral gliomas.

Complications may include learning impairment and epilepsy in a minority. Multiple neuroendocrine adenoma syndrome may be associated (Ch. 6).

Dental aspects

Local anaesthesia can be given safely. Conscious sedation can be given if required. GA must as always be given in hospital.

Oral mucosal neurofibromas are uncommon and more typically associated with endocrine disorders (MEA type III; see Ch. 6). Neurofibromatosis type II is characterized by bilateral acoustic neuromas, which can cause deafness and any of the symptoms of cerebellopontine angle lesions but the skin lesions of type I are lacking.

TUBEROUS SCLEROSIS (BOURNEVILLE DISEASE; EPILOIA)

General aspects

Tuberous sclerosis is characterized by adenoma sebaceum and leaf-shaped depigmented naevi of the skin, epilepsy and sometimes learning disability.

It is a simple autosomal dominant trait linked to chromosome 9 or 16.

Clinical features

The skin adenoma sebaceum are angiofibromas typically distributed in a butterfly pattern across the cheeks, nasolabial folds, bridge of the nose, forehead and chin. Epilepsy, learning impairment and cardiac or renal involvement, or endocrinopathies, particularly diabetes mellitus, may be features.

Dental aspects

Dental management may be complicated by cardiac or renal involvement, or diabetes mellitus, in addition to epilepsy and sometimes learning impairment. LA with or without conscious sedation can be given unless there is severe cardiac or renal involvement. GA must, as always, be given in hospital.

The facial 'adenomas' may be conspicuous and suggest the diagnosis. Oral lesions include hyperplastic gingivitis and pit-shaped dental defects in both dentitions.

STURGE–WEBER SYNDROME

General aspects

Sturge–Weber syndrome (encephalotrigeminal angiomatosis) is characterized by an angiomatous defect (hamartoma), which is usually on the upper part of the face and also within the skull.

Clinical features

The angioma is often large, usually in the upper part of the face, and may appear to occupy the area of a division of the trigeminal nerve, extending into the mouth. The occipital lobe of the brain is usually involved, but the parietal and frontal lobes may be affected if the lower face is involved by the angioma.

Clinically, there are often convulsions, hemiplegia and learning impairment.

Dental aspects

Dental surgery in the area affected by the haemangioma may be complicated by profuse haemorrhage and should therefore only be attempted in hospital. When the vascular naevus involves the face, it usually extends to the underlying oral mucosa and gingivae, which are red and sometimes hyperplastic, and also to the alveolar bone.

Local anaesthesia is safe. Conscious sedation can usually be given if required.

PSEUDOXANTHOMA ELASTICUM

Pseudoxanthoma elasticum is a rare autosomal recessive disorder of connective tissue characterized by yellow papular or reticular skin lesions, visual impairment and cardiovascular abnormalities. The skin is hyperextensible and there may be blue sclerae and loose-jointedness. Abnormalities in the eyes include streaks beneath the retina (angioid streaks) and often haemorrhages and scarring.

Cardiovascular involvement includes calcification of elastic tissue in vessel walls leading to poor blood flow causing ischaemic heart disease and intermittent claudication. Hypertension is common. Some patients have a normal lifespan but others succumb to haemorrhage, cardiac disease or cerebrovascular accidents. Some patients develop hypothyroidism; others bleed from the upper gastrointestinal tract, uterus, renal or respiratory tracts.

Dental management may be complicated particularly by cardiovascular disease.

Lesions may be seen around the face and mouth, and there may be nodules in the lips or rarely in the mouth.

ORAL MUCOSAL DISORDERS

Mouth ulcers are generally caused by local factors but some are recurrent aphthae; others are due to malignant disease (Ch. 22), drugs or systemic disease (diseases of blood, infections, gastrointestinal disease, or skin diseases: Chs. 5,7,21).

RECURRENT APHTHAE (RECURRENT APHTHOUS STOMATITIS)

General aspects

Recurrent aphthae (recurrent aphthous stomatitis; RAS) typically appear as round or ovoid ulcers, with onset usually in childhood or adolescence, and recurrences at intervals. RAS is common and may affect up to 25% of the population. The cause is usually unclear and most patients are otherwise healthy but there are occasional associations with a familial basis, no tobacco use, menstrual cycle, haematinic deficiency (iron, folate or vitamin B_{12}), trauma, stress and particular foods.

Aphthous-like ulcers may be seen in relations to a number of conditions (Box 11.4).

Box 11.4 Aphthous-like ulcers: related conditions

- Intestinal diseases, notably coeliac or Crohn disease, or ulcerative colitis
- Behçet syndrome, when there is usually genital ulceration, uveitis and other lesions
- Human immunodeficiency virus infection: major aphthae may be the presenting feature
- Cyclic neutropenia: typically (but rarely) causes recurrent infections, fever, malaise and enlarged cervical lymph nodes. Oral ulceration may appear at 21-day intervals, coincident with the falls in circulating neutrophils, and may be the main manifestation of the disease. In others, severe periodontal disease may develop
- Autoinflammatory syndromes such as periodic fever, aphthous stomatitis, pharyngitis and cervical adenitis (PFAPA)
- Drugs: cytotoxics, NSAIDS, nicorandil

Clinical features

The onset is usually in childhood or adolescence. Ulcers are typically round or ovoid and recur at intervals. Three different clinical patterns are recognized (Table 11.5).

General management

In addition to a careful history, patients with aphthous-like ulcers should be screened haematologically, particularly if the history suggests a systemic disorder or if the ulcers develop or worsen in middle age or later. A full screen includes haemoglobin and blood indices, serum ferritin (or iron and iron-binding capacity), vitamin B_{12} levels, corrected whole blood or red cell folate levels, and transglutaminase and anti-endomysial antibodies (to exclude coeliac disease). There are no useful laboratory diagnostic tests for RAS. Systemic conditions such as Behçet disease and HIV infection should be excluded if the history is suggestive.

There is no specific or reliably effective treatment; topical corticosteroids are often used. For severe or intractable RAS, systemic

Table 11.5 Clinical variants of aphthae

Minor aphthae	Major aphthae	Herpetiform aphthae
Common Usually round or ovoid discrete ulcers Not on attached gingiva or hard palate and rarely on dorsum of tongue Most are 2–4 mm in diameter Heal within 10 days without scarring	Uncommon Usually round or ovoid discrete ulcers Ulcers may be one to several centimetres in diameter Persist for months before healing with scarring	Uncommon Ulcers initially 1–3 mm across but later coalesce to form ragged ulcers Ulcers form in crops of 10–100 with widespread erythema

corticosteroids or other immunosuppressants may be given, but overall thalidomide appears to be most effective. In patients with HIV infection, aphthous-like ulcers may respond to antiretroviral therapy (ART) or highly active antiretroviral therapy (HAART), granulocyte–macrophage colony-stimulating factor or thalidomide.

PERIODIC FEVER, APHTHOUS STOMATITIS, PHARYNGITIS AND CERVICAL ADENITIS (PFAPA; SEE CH. 19)

CHRONIC ULCERATIVE STOMATITIS

General aspects

Chronic ulcerative stomatitis (CUS) is a rare disease with an appearance similar to erosive lichen planus, which mainly affects the oral mucosa. CUS is associated with unusual antinuclear antibodies reacting exclusively with squamous epithelia (squamous epithelium-specific antinuclear antibodies; SES-ANA). Sera from CUS patients bind a keratinocyte protein KET, which is closely related to the p53 tumour suppressor gene. The *KET* gene is expressed exclusively in epithelia and thymus and thus may play a role in keratinocyte cell cycle control. This might explain the specificity of SES-ANA for keratinocytes. However, the antibodies persist after clearance of mucosal lesions, are fixed *in vivo* and also in uninvolved skin and other mucosa, and may appear in patients without CUS. Thus their pathogenic potential remains to be established.

Clinical features

Chronic ulcerative stomatitis mainly affects older females. The clinical appearances are similar to erosive lichen planus (see later) and it seems likely that many cases of CUS have been misdiagnosed clinically as lichen planus.

General management

Antimalarials are initially highly effective. Relapses respond usually only to combined therapy with chloroquine and small doses of corticosteroids.

FREY SYNDROME (GUSTATORY SWEATING)

General and clinical aspects

Parotidectomy or trauma to the parotid region is sometimes followed by sweating and flushing of the pre-auricular skin on that side, in response to stimulation of salivation. Similar conditions may follow surgery to other salivary glands.

Gustatory sweating is due to the joining of the damaged post-ganglionic parasympathetic nerve fibres with the sympathetic nerve endings, so that sweating and flushing occur rather than salivation.

General management

Antiperspirants such as 20% aluminium chloride hexahydrate may be effective in controlling the sweating.

INFLAMMATORY DENTAL DISEASE

Increasing evidence supports, but does not prove, an association between periodontal infection and atherosclerotic cardiovascular disease or its sequelae, and possibly other conditions. The possible mechanisms behind these associations ultimately include increased systemic inflammation due to periodontal diseases and/or dissemination of bacteria and direct damage on endothelium and other target organs. There is some evidence supporting links with pre-eclampsia, pre-term and low birthweight babies, endometriosis, ischaemic heart disease, cerebrovascular disease, aspiration pneumonia, diabetes mellitus, metabolic syndrome, chronic kidney disease, osteoporosis, Alzheimer disease, pancreatic cancer, kidney cancer, haematological cancers and even oral cancer. It is possible that endodontic infections have similar associations, as chronic inflammatory lesions following carious lesions could both trigger a systemic inflammatory state as well as induce short-lived bacteraemias.

ORAL CANCER (Ch.22)
SALIVARY NEOPLASMS (Ch.14)

USEFUL WEBSITES

http://www.nlm.nih.gov/medlineplus/oralcancer.html
http://www.tambcd.edu/outreach/lichen/
http://www.aad.org/pamphlets/lichen.html
http://www.pemphigus.org/
http://www.niams.nih.gov/Health-Info/default.asp
http://www.nhsdirect.nhs.uk/condition/Behcets-disease

FURTHER READING

Aoki, T., Tanaka, T., Akifuji, Y., et al., 2000. Beneficial effects of interferon-alpha in a case with Behçet's disease. Intern Med 39, 667–669.
Awano, S., Ansai, T., Takata, Y., et al., 2008. Oral health and mortality risk from pneumonia in the elderly. J Dent Res 87, 334–339.

Baioni, C.S., de Souza, C.M., Ribeiro Braosi, A.P., et al., 2008. Analysis of the association of polymorphism in the osteoprotegerin gene with susceptibility to chronic kidney disease and periodontitis. J Periodontal Res 43, 578–584.

Bagan, J., Lo Muzic, L., Scully, C., 2005. Mucous membrane pemphigoid Oral Diseases 11, 197–218.

Bassani, D.G., Olinto, M.T., Kreiger, N., 2007. Periodontal disease and perinatal outcomes: a case-control study. J Clin Periodontol 34, 31–39.

Beck, J.D., Offenbacher, S., 2005. Systemic effects of periodontitis: epidemiology of periodontal disease and cardiovascular disease. J Periodontol 76 (11 Suppl), 2089–2100.

Behle, J.H., Papapanou, P.N., 2006. Periodontal infections and atherosclerotic vascular disease: an update. Int Dent J 56 (4 Suppl 1), 256–262.

Bez, C., Hallet, R., Carrozzo, M., et al., 2001. Lack of association between hepatotropic transfusion transmitted virus infection and oral lichen planus in British and Italian populations. Br J Dermatol 145, 990–993

Black, M., Mignogna, M., Scully, C., 2005. Pemphigus Oral Diseases 11, 119–130.

Bobetsis, Y.A., Barros, S.P., Offenbacher, S., 2006. Exploring the relationship between periodontal disease and pregnancy complications. J Am Dent Assoc 137 (Suppl), 7S–13S. Erratum in J Am Dent Assoc 2008;139(3):252.

Calabrese, L., Fleischer, A.B., 2000. Thalidomide: current and potential clinical applications. Am J Med 108, 487–495.

Caplan, D.J., Chasen, J.B., Krall, E.A., et al., 2006. Lesions of endodontic origin and risk of coronary heart disease. J Dent Res 85, 996–1000.

Challacombe, S.J., Setterfield, J., Shirlaw, P., Harman, K., Scully, C., Black, M.M., 2001. Immunodiagnosis of pemphigus and mucous membrane pemphigoid. Acta Odontol Scand 59, 226–234.

Chen, M.C., Feng, I.J., Lu, C.H., eta al., 2008. The incidence and risk of second primary cancers in patients with nasopharyngeal carcinoma: a population-based study in Taiwan over a 25-year period (1979–2003). Ann Oncol 19, 1180–1186.

Choonhakarn, C., Busaracome, P., Sripanidkulchai, B., Sarakarn, P., 2008. The efficacy of aloe vera gel in the treatment of oral lichen planus:. a randomized controlled trial. Br J Dermatol 158, 573–577.

Cota, L.O., Guimarães, A.N., Costa, J.E., Lorentz, T.C., Costa, F.O., 2006. Association between maternal periodontitis and an increased risk of pre-eclampsia. J Periodontol 77, 2063–2069.

Craig, R.G., 2008. Interactions between chronic renal disease and periodontal disease. Oral Dis 14, 1–7.

Craig, R.G., Kotanko, P., Kamer, A.R., Levin, N.W., 2007. Periodontal diseases – a modifiable source of systemic inflammation for the end-stage renal disease patient on haemodialysis therapy?. Nephrol Dial Transplant 22, 312–315.

Dahn, K.A., Glode, M.P., Chan, K.H., 2000. Periodic fever and pharyngitis in young children: a new disease for the otolaryngologist?. Arch Otolaryngol Head Neck Surg 126, 1146–1149.

D'Aiuto, F., Graziani, F., Tetè, S., Gabriele, M., Tonetti, M.S., 2005. Periodontitis: from local infection to systemic diseases. Int J Immunopathol Pharmacol 18 (3 Suppl), 1–11.

Dave, S., Batista Jr., E.L., Van Dyke, T.E., 2004. Cardiovascular disease and periodontal diseases: commonality and causation. Compend Contin Educ Dent 25 (7 Suppl 1), 26–37.

Davè, S., Van Dyke, T., 2008. The link between periodontal disease and cardiovascular disease is probably inflammation. Oral Dis 14, 95–101.

Farrell, S., Ide, M., Wilson, R.F., 2006. The relationship between maternal periodontitis, adverse pregnancy outcome and miscarriage in never smokers. J Clin Periodontol 33, 115–120

Farthing, P., Bagan, J., Scully, C., 2005. Erythema multiforme Oral Disease 11, 261–267.

Feder Jr., H.M., 2000. Periodic fever, aphthous stomatitis, pharyngitis, adenitis: a clinical review of a new syndrome. Curr Opin Pediatr 12, 253–256.

Femiano, F., Gombos, F., Scully, C., 2002. Pemphigus vulgaris with oral involvement; evaluation of two different systemic corticosteroid therapeutic protocols. J Eur Acad Dermatol Venereol 16, 353–356.

Franek, E., Blaschyk, R., Kolonko, A., et al., 2006. Chronic periodontitis in hemodialysis patients with chronic kidney disease is associated with elevated serum C-reactive protein concentration and greater intima-media thickness of the carotid artery. J Nephrol 19, 346–351

Gcnzatez-Moles, M.A., Scully, C., Gil-Montoya, J.A., 2008. Oral lichen planus:controversies surrounding malignant transformation. Oral Diseases 14, 229–243, Feb 22; [Epub ahead of print].

Hajishengallis, G., Sharma, A., Russell, M.W., Genco, R.J., 2002. Interactions of oral pathogens with toll-like receptors: possible role in atherosclerosis. Ann Periodontol 7, 72–78.

Herranz, P., Arribas, J.R., Navarro, A., et al., 2000. Successful treatment of aphthous ulcerations in AIDS patients using topical granulocyte–macrophage colony-stimulating factor. Br J Dermatol 142, 171–176.

Hingorani, A.D., Vallance, P., Deanfield, J., 2007. Treatment of periodontitis and endothelial function. N Engl J Med 356, 911–920.

Irwin, C., Mullally, B., Ziada, H., Byrne, P.J., Allen, E., 2008. Periodontics: 9. Periodontitis and systemic conditions – is there a link?. Dent Update 35, 92–94, 97–98, 100–101.

Kamer, A.R., Craig, R.G., Dasanayake, A.P., Brys, M., Glodzik-Sobanska, L., de Leon, M.J., 2008. Inflammation and Alzheimer's disease possible role of periodontal diseases. Alzheimers Dement 4, 242–250.

Kamer, A.R., Dasanayake, A.P., Craig, R.G., Glodzik-Sobanska, L., Bry, M., de Leon, M.J., 2008. Alzheimer's disease and peripheral infections: the possible contribution from periodontal infections, model and hypothesis. J Alzheimers Dis 13, 437–449.

Katsura, K., Sasai, K., Sato, K., Saito, M., Hoshina, H., Hayashi, T., 2008. Relationship between oral health status and development of osteoradionecrosis of the mandible: a retrospective longitudinal study. Oral Surg Oral Med Oral Pathol Oral Radiol Endod 105, 731–738.

Kavoussi, S.K., West, B.T., Taylor, G.W., Lebovic, D.I., 2009. Periodontal disease and endometriosis: analysis of the National Health and Nutrition Examination Survey. Fertil Steril 91, 335–342.

Lindy, O., Suomalainen, K., Mäkelä, M., Lindy, S., 2008. Statin use is associated with fewer periodontal lesions: a retrospective study. BMC Oral Health 8, 16.

Lodi, G., Carrozzo, M., Harris, K., et al., 2000. Hepatitis G virus-associated oral lichen planus; no influence from hepatitis G virus co-infection. J Oral Pathol Med 29, 39–42.

López, N.J., Da Silva, I., Ipinza, J., Gutiérrez, J., 2005. Periodontal therapy reduces the rate of preterm low birth weight in women with pregnancy-associated gingivitis. J Periodontol 76 (11 Suppl), 2144–2153.

López, R., 2008. Periodontal disease and adverse pregnancy outcomes. Evid Based Dent 9, 48.

McBride, D.R., 2000. Management of aphthous ulcers. Am Fam Physician 62, 149–154, 160.

Mealey, B.L., Rose, L.F., 2008. Diabetes mellitus and inflammatory periodontal diseases. Curr Opin Endocrinol Diabetes Obes 15, 135–141.

Meyer, M.S., Joshipura, K., Giovannucci, E., Michaud, D.S., 2008. A review of the relationship between tooth loss, periodontal disease, and cancer. Cancer Causes Control 19, 895–907.

Michaud, D.S., Liu, Y., Meyer, M., Giovannucci, E., Joshipura, K., 2008. Periodontal disease, tooth loss, and cancer risk in male health professionals: a prospective cohort study. Lancet Oncol 9, 550–558.

Niedzielska, I., Janic, T., Cierpka, S., Swietochowska, E., 2008. The effect of chronic periodontitis on the development of atherosclerosis: review of the literature. Med Sci Monit 14, RA103–RA106.

Porter, S.R., Hegarty, A., Kaliakatsou, F., Hodgson, T.A., Scully, C., 2000. Recurrent aphthous stomatitis. Clin Dermatol 18, 569–578.

Porter, S.R., Scully, C., 2000. Aphthous ulcers: recurrent. Clin Evid 5, 606–612; 2001;6:1037–41; and 2002;7:1232–8; and Clin Evid Concise 2002;7:234.

Pussinen, P.J., Alfthan, G., Jousilahti, P., Paju, S., Tuomilehto, J., 2007. Systemic exposure to Porphyromonas gingivalis predicts incident stroke. Atherosclerosis 193, 222–228.

Schara, R., Medvescek, M., Skaleric, U., 2006. Periodontal disease and diabetes metabolic control: a full-mouth disinfection approach. J Int Acad Periodontol 8, 61–66.

Scully, C., 2001. The mouth in dermatological disorders. Practitioner 245, 942–952.

Scully, C., Carrozzo, M., Gandolfo, S., Puiatti, P., Monteil, R., 1999. Update on mucous membrane pemphigoid (an immune mediated sub-epithelial blistering disease); a heterogeneous entity. Oral Surg Oral Med Oral Pathol 88, 56–68.

Scully, C., Challacombe, S.J., 2002. Pemphigus vulgaris: update on etiopathogenesis, oral manifestations and management. Crit Rev Oral Biol Med 13, 397–408.

Scully, C., Eisen, D., Carrozzo, M., 2000. Management of oral lichen planus. Am J Clin Dermatol 1, 287–306.

Scully, C., Gorsky, M., Lozada-Nur, F., 2002. Aphthous ulcerations. In: Camisa, C. (ed.), Diagnosis and treatment of oral lesions, Dermatologic Therapy, 15, pp. 185–205.

Scully, C., Carrozzo, M., 2008. Oral mucosal diseases: Lichen planus. British Journal of Oral and Maxillofacial Surgery 46, 15–21, 2007, Sep 4; [Epub ahead of print]

Scully, C., Bagan, J.V., 2008. Oral mucosal diseases: Erythema multiforme. British Journal of Oral and Maxillofacial Surgery 46, 90–95, 2007 Sep 1; [Epub ahead of print]

Scully, C., Lo Muzio, L., 2008. Oral mucosal diseases: Pemphigoid. British Journal of Oral and Maxillofacial Surgery 46, 358–366, 2007 Sep 3; [Epub ahead of print]

Scully, C., Mignogna, M., 2008. Oral mucosal diseases: Pemphigus. British Journal of Oral and Maxillofacial Surgery 46, 272–277, 2007 Sep 14; [Epub ahead of print].

Scully, C., Porter, S., 2008. Oral mucosal diseases: Recurrent aphthous stomatitis. British Journal of Oral and Maxillofacial Surgery 46, 198–206, 2007 Sep 10; [Epub ahead of print].

Shimazaki, Y., Saito, T., Yonemoto, K., Kiyohara, Y., Iida, M., Yamashita, Y., 2007. Relationship of metabolic syndrome to periodontal disease in Japanese women: the Hisayama Study. J Dent Res 86, 271–275.

Ship, J.A., 2003. Diabetes and oral health: an overview. J Am Dent Assoc 134 (Sp. No), 4S–10S.

Shotts, R., Scully, C., 2002. How to identify and deal with tongue problems. Pulse 62, 73–76.

Skamagas, M., Breen, T.L., LeRoith, D., 2008. Update on diabetes mellitus: prevention, treatment, and association with oral diseases. Oral Dis 14, 105–114.

Tezal, M., Sullivan, M.A., Reid, M.E., et al., 2007. Chronic periodontitis and the risk of tongue cancer. Arch Otolaryngol Head Neck Surg 133, 450–454.

Tucker, R., 2006. Periodontitis and pregnancy. J R Soc Health 126, 24–27.

Williams, R.C., Barnett, A.H., Claffey, N., et al. 2008. The potential impact of periodontal disease on general health: a consensus view. Curr Med Res Opin 24, 1635–1643.

Appendix 11.1 Congenital oral and intestinal disorders

Syndrome	Cutaneous and other extraintestinal features	Gastrointestinal lesions
Cowden syndrome	Skin nodules Breast malignancy	Polyps
Gardner syndrome (familial adenomatous polyposis coli)	Osteomas of jaws (especially mandible), epidermal cysts, sebaceous cysts, lipomas, fibroma, dental anomalies	Colon polyps, adenocarcinomas, biliary neoplasia
MEA III	See Ch. 6	Mucosal neuromas
Peutz–Jeghers syndrome	Pigmented macules of mouth, lips and digits. Risk of neoplasia	Small intestine polyps and carcinoma rarely
Tylosis	Hyperkeratosis of palms and soles	Oral leukoplakia Oesophageal carcinoma

Renal function is required to maintain normal body fluid volumes and composition including acid–base balance, to excrete many metabolites and drugs, and to synthesize vitamin D and erythropoietin. The nephron makes urine by filtering small molecules and ions from the blood and then reclaiming useful materials such as glucose (Fig. 12.1). The nephron consists of a Bowman's capsule, glomerulus (a capillary network within Bowman's capsule), and proximal convoluted tubule, loop of Henle, and distal convoluted and collecting tubules (Table 12.1).

The kidneys constantly pass urine through the ureters to the bladder, where it is stored in the bladder to be passed from time to time via the urethra (Fig. 12.2). Nearly a quarter of the blood volume perfuses the kidneys each minute. The glomerular filtration rate (GFR) can be calculated from creatinine clearance, inulin clearance, or clearance of isotopes, such as ^{125}I-iothalamate, ^{51}Cr-EDTA (ethylenediamine tetra-acetic acid) or ^{99m}Tc-DPTA (diethylenetriamine penta-acetic acid), or plasma creatinine levels; it is increasingly expressed as an estimate calculated by using the Modification of Diet in Renal Disease (MDRD) Study equation, which takes into account patient age, gender and serum creatinine level. In health, the GFR is around 120 ml/min per 1.73 m² for women and 130 ml/min per 1.73 m² for men. In population terms, this declines by 1–2 ml/min per year over the age of 20 years. The kidneys also act in the excretion of drugs and hormones and as endocrine organs for the synthesis of hydroxycholecalciferol (active vitamin D), erythropoietin, renin and prostaglandins, and are target organs for parathyroid hormone and aldosterone.

RENAL DISEASE

Nephrology deals with many different kidney disorders including acid–base disorders, electrolyte disorders, nephrolithiasis, hypertension, acute kidney disease and end-stage renal disease.

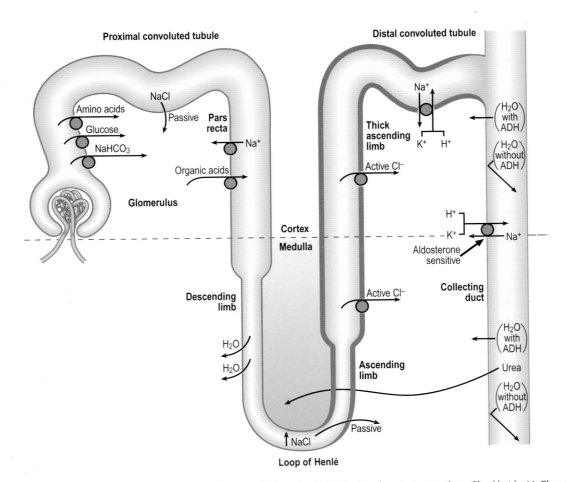

Fig. 12.1 Diagram of renal tubular structure. ADH, antidiuretic hormone; H₂O, water; NaHCO₃, bicarbonate; Na⁺, sodium; Cl⁻, chloride; NaCl, sodium chloride; H⁺, hydrogen; K⁺, potassium

Table 12.1 The kidney: constituents and functions

	Proximal convoluted tubule	Loop of Henle	Distal convoluted tubule	Collecting tubule
Functions	Actively reabsorbs glucose, amino acids, uric acid and inorganic salts	Water continues to leave by osmosis	More Na⁺ is reclaimed by active transport, and still more water follows by osmosis	Final adjustment of body Na⁺ and water content
	Active transport out of Na⁺ controlled by angiotensin II			Surplus or waste ions and molecules flow out as urine
	Active transport of phosphate (PO_4^{3-}) suppressed by parathyroid hormone			
	Water follows by osmosis			

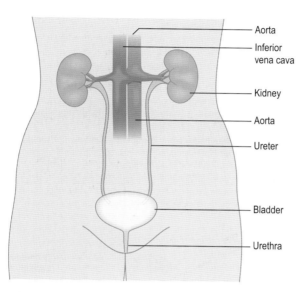

Fig. 12.2 Genitourinary anatomy

Historically, chronic kidney disease has been classified according to the part of the renal anatomy that is involved, as follows.

- Vascular, which includes disease of large vessels (e.g. bilateral renal artery stenosis) or small vessels (e.g. ischaemic nephropathy, haemolytic–uraemic syndrome and vasculitis).
- Glomerular, a diverse group subclassified into disease that is primary (e.g. focal segmental glomerulosclerosis and immunoglobulin A nephritis) or secondary (e.g. diabetic nephropathy and lupus nephritis).
- Tubulointerstitial, which includes polycystic kidney disease, drug- and toxin-induced chronic tubulointerstitial nephritis and reflux nephropathy.
- Obstructive, as with renal or bladder stones and prostate diseases.

Renal failure can come on suddenly (acute renal failure), as after surgery or severe injuries, or when renal blood vessels become obstructed, but more usually develops slowly (chronic renal failure; CRF). Renal failure results in fluid retention, acidosis, accumulation of metabolites and drugs, damage to platelets (leading to a bleeding tendency), hypertension, anaemia and endocrine effects.

ACUTE RENAL FAILURE

Acute renal failure (ARF) can be caused by pre-renal, renal or post-renal factors.

- *Pre-renal factors* (55%), such as hypotension (haemorrhage or severe burns), renal thrombosis, sepsis, heat stroke or drugs causing renal shutdown, for example non-steroidal anti-inflammatory drugs (NSAIDs) and angiotensin-converting enzyme (ACE) inhibitors.
- *Renal factors* (15%), such as: interstitial nephritis; toxic acute tubular necrosis; complicated surgery or trauma (myoglobin blocks tubular function); drugs [contrast dyes used in arteriography, antibiotics (especially streptomycin or gentamicin or amphotericin), aspirin and other NSAIDs, acetaminophen (paracetamol) overdose]; toxins (betel, heavy metals, solvents); multiple organ failure, in which the heart, lungs, liver, brain and kidneys totally or partially shut down (most often the result of major trauma or sepsis); the haemolytic–uraemic syndrome, which is caused in children by *Escherichia coli* O157:H7 (which expresses verotoxin – also called Shiga toxin) and in adults by human immunodeficiency virus (HIV), antiphospholipid syndrome, post-partum renal failure, malignant hypertension, scleroderma or cancer chemotherapy.
- *Post-renal factors*, such as obstructed urine flow.

Acute renal failure is a medical emergency, which may lead to confusion, seizures and coma. Management is often by dialysis.

CHRONIC KIDNEY DISEASE (CHRONIC RENAL DISEASE)

GENERAL ASPECTS

Chronic kidney disease (CKD) is defined as the presence of kidney damage, or a reduction in the GFR, for 3 or more months. All individuals with a GFR < 90 ml/min per 1.73 m² for 3 months are classified as having CKD, if there is also proteinuria or haematuria. They are at increased risk of loss of kidney function and development of cardiovascular disease (Table 12.2) CKD is not a specific disease, the most common causes (75% of all adult cases) are diabetes, hypertension and glomerulonephritis. Renal diseases (e.g. chronic glomerulonephritis, polycystic renal disease, renal artery stenosis), systemic diseases

Table 12.2 Stages of chronic kidney disease

Stages[a]	Renal health	GFR ml/min/1.73 m²	Features
–	Normal	130	–
1	Diminished renal reserve (early CRF)	> 90	Abnormalities in blood or urine tests or imaging studies but few overt symptoms
2	Mild CRF (azotaemia)	60–89	Abnormalities in blood or urine tests or imaging studies
3	Moderately severe	30–59	Abnormalities in blood or urine tests or imaging studies
4	Severe CRF	15–29	Uraemic symptoms
5	End-stage renal failure (ESRF), also called end-stage renal disease (ESRD), chronic kidney failure (CKF) or chronic renal failure (CRF).	< 15	Life-threatening and requires some form of renal replacement therapy

[a]Stages are based on estimated GFR (eGFR): National Kidney Foundation. Am J Kidney Dis 2002;39(2 Suppl 1):S1–S266.
CRF, chronic renal failure; GFR, glomerular filtration rate.

(lupus erythematosus, myeloma, amyloid), poisoning (e.g. lead or betel) and drugs (e.g. long-term use of aspirin or other NSAIDs, or large amounts of acetaminophen) are other causes. CKD leads to a progressive loss of renal function through five stages defined by the National Kidney Foundation. CKD can be compensated by structural and functional hypertrophy of surviving nephrons, to a point at which around 50% of renal function remains, when chronic renal insufficiency ensues. This inevitably progresses to end-stage renal disease (ESRD).

CLINICAL FEATURES

Chronic kidney disease is symptomless at first and only when kidney function has fallen to less than 25% of normal do nocturia and anorexia appear, and serum levels of nitrogenous compounds (urea) become raised (azotaemia or uraemia). Advanced CKD causes significant impairment of all renal functions, affects virtually all body systems and causes changes in urea and electrolytes and other blood constituents (Table 12.3; Fig. 12.3). CKD can result in a range of clinical manifestations (Table 12.4).

Hypertension is common. Anaemia is common and caused by toxic suppression of the bone marrow, lack of renal production of erythropoietin and/or iron deficiency, from blood loss in the gut. Purpura and a bleeding tendency may appear from abnormal platelet production, diminished platelet factor 3 (thromboxane), which impairs conversion of prothrombin to thrombin; raised prostacyclin (prostaglandin I); leading to vasodilatation and poor platelet aggregation; and defective von Willebrand factor. A liability to infection arises because of defective phagocyte function, which results from reduced interleukin-2 (IL-2), but rises in pro-inflammatory cytokines (IL-1, IL-6, tumour necrosis factor).

Renal osteodystrophy is common: phosphate retention leads to depression of plasma calcium levels and subsequently raised parathyroid activity (secondary hyperparathyroidism). There is also deficiency of renal production of 1,25-dihydroxycholecalciferol (vitamin D₃) and calcium absorption is thereby impaired. Parathyroid hyperplasia may eventually become adenomatous and irreversible (tertiary hyperparathyroidism).

Table 12.3 Laboratory features of chronic kidney disease

Urea	Creatinine	Potassium	Phosphate	Calcium	Haemoglobin
Raised	Raised	Normal or Raised	Raised	Low	Low

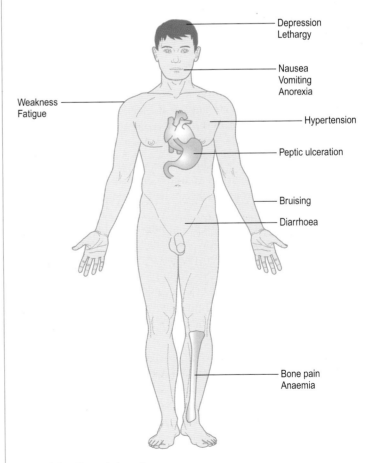

Depression
Lethargy

Nausea
Vomiting
Anorexia

Weakness
Fatigue

Hypertension

Peptic ulceration

Bruising

Diarrhoea

Bone pain
Anaemia

Fig. 12.3 Chronic kidney disease

Table 12.4 Chronic kidney disease: clinical features

Blood and immune	Cardiovascular	Gastrointestinal	Neuromuscular	Metabolic and endocrine	Skin
Bleeding Anaemia Lymphopenia Liability to infections	Hypertension Congestive cardiac failure Pericarditis Cardiomyopathy Atheroma, peripheral vascular disease	Anorexia Nausea and vomiting Hiccoughs Peptic ulcer and gastrointestinal bleeding	Weakness and lassitude Drowsiness leading to coma Headaches, confusion Disturbances of vision Sensory disturbances Tremor	Nocturia and polyuria Thirst Glycosuria Raised urea, creatinine, lipids and uric acid Electrolyte disturbances Secondary hyperparathyroidism renal osteodystrophy Impotence, amenorrhoea, infertility	Pruritus Bruising Hyperpigmentation Infections

GENERAL MANAGEMENT

Chronic renal failure is diagnosed by clinical history and presentation; rising plasma urea and creatinine levels and a falling GFR, which is increasingly expressed as an estimate (eGFR; calculated by using the MDRD equation, which takes into account patient age, gender, serum creatinine level). There is also a correction that can be applied for those of Afro-Caribbean background.

The decline in eGFR can be plotted over time, allowing accurate prognosis of events (such as timing of requirement for dialysis, creation of arteriovenous fistulae, etc.). It also allows for demonstration of effects of therapy, the most important of which is blood pressure (BP) control – by using angiotensin-converting enzyme inhibitors (ACEi) and angiotensin-II blockers (ARBs). Underlying causes of CKD should be treated where possible and any stress, infection or urinary tract obstruction should be treated, as this may precipitate symptoms. The treatment goal is to slow down or halt the progression of CKD to stage 5, measured by a falling eGFR and rising plasma urea (in the USA, blood urea nitrogen; BUN) and rising creatinine levels, and aimed at reducing cardiovascular risk, which is the main cause of mortality. A normal diet (low-protein diets are now rarely advocated); potassium restriction; and salt or water control are used. Because cardiovascular risk is high in patients with low GFR, management includes statins, aspirin, smoking cessation, etc (Ch. 5).

Symptoms and complications such as hiccough, vomiting, fits and calcium loss are treated. Iron stores are replenished using iron and epoietin (recombinant erythropoietin) or darbepoietin, which has a longer half-life. Calcium carbonate, vitamin D_3 or its synthetic analogue, a low-phosphate diet or intravenous clodronate help inhibit bone resorption. Cinacalcet, which reduces parathyroid hormone, may be used. Parathyroidectomy may be necessary in cases of tertiary hyperparathyroidism (Ch. 06). A bisphosphonate may be needed for the management of renal osteodystrophy.

Drug therapy requires certain cautions: dosages of drugs cleared renally, such as penicillins, cephalosporins and erythromycin, should be reduced based on renal function (Table 12.5). The least nephrotoxic agents should be used (NSAIDs or tetracyclines should be avoided), and alternative medications should be prescribed if necessary to avoid potential drug interactions. Clinicians should be aware of drugs with active metabolites that can exaggerate pharmacological effects in patients with CKD. Patients with CKD should also be asked about over-the-counter and herbal medicine use.

RENAL REPLACEMENT THERAPY

When the patient reaches stage 5 CKD, renal replacement therapy is required.

Dialysis

Renal dialysis is used to remove metabolites (e.g. urea, potassium) and excess water, by exposing the patient's blood across a semi-permeable membrane to a hypotonic solution to allow the diffusion and osmosis of solutes and fluid from the body. The dialysis solution has levels of minerals like potassium and calcium that are similar to their natural concentration in healthy blood. For another solute, bicarbonate, dialysis solution level is set slightly higher than that in normal blood, to encourage diffusion of bicarbonate into the body, to neutralize the metabolic acidosis often present. There are two primary types of dialysis.

Peritoneal dialysis (PD) works on the principle that the peritoneal membrane can act as a natural semi-permeable membrane and, though less efficient than haemodialysis, it is as beneficial overall, since it is done more frequently. Dialysis fluid is instilled via a catheter into the patient's abdominal cavity (often a Tenckhoff catheter) placed near the umbilicus (Fig. 12.4) or tunnelled under the skin from near the sternum (called a pre-sternal catheter). PD has other advantages since it is relatively easy to learn, fluid balance is usually easier than on haemodialysis, it is usually done at home and it is relatively easy to travel with (bags of dialysis solution can be transported to the holiday destination). Continuous ambulatory peritoneal dialysis (CAPD) has around 4–5 manual changes daily, while with continuous cyclic peritoneal dialysis (CCPD) a machine does the exchanges at night. Intermittent peritoneal dialysis (IPD) uses the same type of machine as CCPD; if done overnight it is called nocturnal intermittent peritoneal dialysis (NIPD).

Haemodialysis (HD) is often carried out at home or as an outpatient. Optimal effects are from 5–7 dialysis sessions of 6–8 h each per week, but most patients have two or three 3–6-hourly sessions per week. An arteriovenous fistula is usually created surgically above the wrist to facilitate the introduction of infusion lines (Fig. 12.5); alternatively, a Gortex or

Table 12.5 Drug modification in patients with chronic kidney disease[a]

	Usually safe (no dosage change usually required)	Fairly safe (dosage change only in severe renal failure)	Less safe (dosage reduction indicated[b] even in mild renal failure)	Avoid (best avoided in any patient with renal failure)
Antimicrobials	Azithromycin Cloxacillin Doxycycline Flucloxacillin Fucidin Minocycline Rifampicin	Ampicillin Amoxicillin Benzylpenicillin Clindamycin Co-trimoxazole Erythromycin Ketoconazole Lincomycin Metronidazole Phenoxymethyl penicillin	Aciclovir[c] Cephalosporins[d] Ciprofloxacin Etafloxacin Fluconazole Levofloxacin Ofloxacin Vancomycin	Aminoglycosides Carbenicillin Cefadroxil Cefalexin Cefixime Cephalothin Gentamicin Imipenem/cilastatin Itraconazole Sulfonamides Tetracyclines[e] Valaciclovir
Anaesthetics	Lidocaine	Prilocaine, articaine	–	–
Analgesics	Paracetamol/ acetaminophen	Codeine	Aspirin NSAIDs	Dextropropoxyphene opioids Meperidine, morphine Pethidine Tramadol
Anticonvulsants			Carbamazepine Gabapentin Lamotrigine	
Sedatives	Diazepam Midazolam			

[a]Many other drugs unlikely to be used in dentistry may be contraindicated: check the formulary. Gadolinium-containing contrast agents are contraindicated as they may cause nephrogenic system fibrosis.
[b]Severe renal failure – glomerular filtration rate (GFR) < 10 ml/min; moderately severe renal failure – GFR < 25 ml/min; mild renal failure – GFR < 50 ml/min.
[c]Systemic aciclovir.
[d]Except cephaloridine and cefalothin, which are contraindicated.
[e]Except doxycycline and minocycline.
NSAIDs, non-steroidal anti-inflammatory drugs.

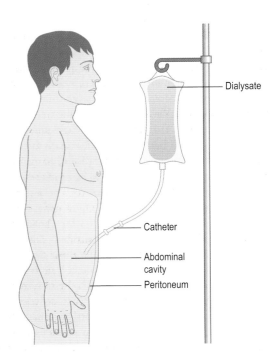

Fig. 12.4 Peritoneal dialysis

Dialysate

Catheter

Abdominal cavity

Peritoneum

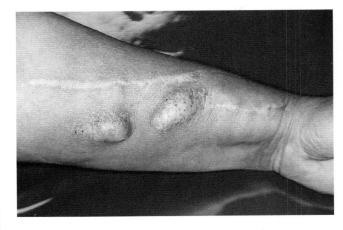

Fig. 12.5 Arteriovenous anastomosis (shunt) for haemodialysis

polytetrafluoroethylene (PTFE) graft is placed, or an indwelling tunnelled cuffed catheter used. The patient is heparinized during dialysis to keep both the infusion lines and the dialysis machine tubing patent and the patient's blood is circulated through an extracorporeal circulation (Fig. 12.6).

Dialysis can totally rehabilitate up to 20% of patients, but cannot prevent all complications and is itself associated with

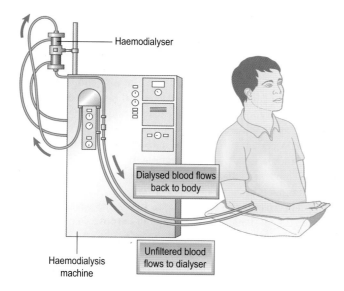

Haemodialyser

Dialysed blood flows back to body

Unfiltered blood flows to dialyser

Haemodialysis machine

Fig. 12.6 Haemodialysis

some adverse effects (sometimes collectively referred to as dialysis 'hangover' or 'washout'). These symptoms are caused by removing fluid too rapidly or to excess, and include low BP, fatigue, chest pains, leg cramps, nausea and headaches. Other and longer term adverse effects include worsened ischaemic heart disease, cardiac valve calcification (especially affecting the aortic valve), dialysis-related amyloidosis and neuropathies.

Cardiovascular disease and infection are the leading causes of death. Control of infection is of paramount importance, since PD also carries the risk of peritonitis (as well as fluid leaks into the tissues and hernias). Infections of the PD catheter's exit site or 'tunnel' however, are less serious. HD grafts and catheters may also be at risk of infection, and bacterial endocarditis, osteomyelitis and blood-borne virus infections (mainly hepatitis or HIV), and tuberculosis, were common in the past. Inflammatory periodontal disease may also contribute to the infective load and it is possible that therapy may decrease systemic levels of C-reactive protein. In addition, haemodialysis may mechanically damage platelets creating an additional bleeding tendency.

Haemofiltration

In haemofiltration, the blood is pumped through a 'haemofilter' as in dialysis but, rather than a dialysate being used, a pressure gradient is applied. Water thus moves across the very permeable membrane rapidly, facilitating the removal of metabolites, importantly those with large molecular weights that are cleared less well by haemodialysis. The salts and water lost from the blood during haemofiltration are replaced with a 'substitution fluid' infused into the extracorporeal circuit during the treatment. Haemodiafiltration combines haemodialysis and haemofiltration in one process.

Renal transplantation

Transplantation is now strongly recommended for all patients with end-stage renal disease who are medically suitable, since a successful transplant offers enhanced quality and duration of life and is more effective (medically and economically) than chronic dialysis. Transplantation is the renal replacement modality of choice for child patients and patients with diabetic nephropathy.

Outcomes are improved by 'pre-emptive' live donor transplantation, meaning using a kidney from an unaffected relative and performing the transplant before the patient needs to have dialysis. Transplants can be from cadaveric or living donors with graft survival as high as 90% at 1 year, about 70% survival at 5 years, and with an overall mortality of less than 5%.

The transplanted kidney is usually sited in the right iliac fossa of the abdomen. All kidney transplant recipients require lifelong immunosuppression to prevent a T-cell alloimmune rejection response. Induction therapy is a short course of intensive treatment with intravenous antilymphocyte antibody. Patients then need to be immunosuppressed, traditionally with a corticosteroid plus a steroid-sparing drug, such as azathioprine, but now more commonly ciclosporin or tacrolimus or sirolimus, or mycophenolate mofetil. Basiliximab or daclizumab are increasingly used, with a calcineurin inhibitor.

Complications of transplantation include transplant rejection, increased risk of atheroma and ischaemic heart disease, ciclosporin-induced nephropathy and immunosuppression-induced infection or malignancy (Ch. 35).

DENTAL ASPECTS OF CHRONIC KIDNEY DISEASE

The haematologist should first be consulted; dental treatment is usually best carried out on the day after dialysis, when there has been maximal benefit from the dialysis and the effect of the heparin has worn off. Careful haemostasis should be ensured if surgical procedures are necessary (Ch. 8). Should bleeding be prolonged, desmopressin (DDAVP) may provide haemostasis for up to 4 h. If this fails, cryoprecipitate may be effective, has a peak effect at 4–12 h and lasts up to 36 h. Conjugated oestrogens may aid haemostasis: the effect takes 2–5 days to develop but persists for 30 days.

Infections are poorly controlled by the patient with CKD, especially if immunosuppressed, and may spread locally as well as giving rise to septicaemia. They also accelerate tissue catabolism causing clinical deterioration and there is some evidence that periodontitis can perpetuate inflammation in CKD. Tuberculosis is also more frequent, but is usually extrapulmonary and therefore does not constitute a risk to dental staff. Infections can be difficult to recognize as signs of inflammation are masked. Haemodialysis predisposes to blood-borne viral infections such as hepatitis virus. Odontogenic infections should be treated vigorously (Table 12.5). Erythromycin, flucloxacillin, and fucidin can be given in standard dosage. Penicillins (other than phenoxymethyl penicillin and flucloxacillin) and metronidazole, however, should be given in lower doses, since very high serum levels can be toxic to the central nervous system. Benzylpenicillin has significant potassium content and may also be neurotoxic and may therefore be contraindicated. Tetracyclines can worsen nitrogen retention and acidosis and are best avoided, though doxycycline or minocycline may be given.

Patients with CKD before having dental extractions, scaling or periodontal surgery should be considered for antimicrobial prophylaxis, especially those with renal transplants (Ch. 35), those with polycystic kidneys (who may also have mitral valve prolapse), those on PD or those on HD with prosthetic bridge grafts of PTFE or tunnelled cuffed catheters. An alternative is to give 400 mg teicoplanin intravenously during dialysis, which gives cover for at least a day. Vascular access infections are usually caused by skin organisms such as *Staphylococcus aureus* and only rarely by oral micro-organisms; thus patients with most arteriovenous fistulas are not considered at risk from infection during dental treatment. Patients with indwelling intraperitoneal catheters are not considered to require antimicrobial prophylaxis.

Drugs excreted mainly by the kidney may have undesirably enhanced or prolonged activity, if doses are not lowered. Drug therapy may need to be adjusted, depending on the degree of renal failure, the patient's dialysis schedule or the presence of a transplant. Except in emergency, such drugs should be prescribed only after consultation with the renal physician. Drugs which are directly nephrotoxic must be avoided (Table 12.5).

Aspirin (75 mg dose will often already be being given as prophylaxis against cardiovascular disease) and other NSAIDs should be avoided, since they aggravate gastrointestinal irritation and bleeding associated with CKD. Their excretion may also be delayed and they may be nephrotoxic, especially in the older patient or where there is renal damage or cardiac failure. Some patients have peptic ulceration – a further contraindication to aspirin. Even cyclo-oxygenase (COX)-2 inhibitors may be nephrotoxic and are best avoided. Use of NSAIDs is linked to a risk for acute renal failure, nephrotic syndrome with interstitial nephritis and chronic renal failure. Sodium excretion is reduced and can lead to peripheral oedema, elevated blood pressure and exacerbation of heart failure. Antihypertensive effects of beta-blockers, ACEi or ARBs can be decreased. Short-term NSAID use is well tolerated if the patient is well hydrated and has good renal function and no heart failure, diabetes or hypertension. Serum creatinine should be checked every 2–4 weeks in early treatment.

Antihistamines or drugs with anti-muscarinic side-effects may cause dry mouth or urinary retention.

Systemic fluorides should not be given, because of doubt about fluoride excretion by damaged kidneys. Fluorides can usually safely be used topically for caries prophylaxis. Antacids containing magnesium salts should not be given as there may be magnesium retention. Antacids containing calcium or aluminium bases may impair absorption of penicillin V and sulfonamides. Cholestyramine, sometimes used in CKD, may also interfere with the absorption of penicillins.

Consideration must also be given to the effect on dental care of underlying diseases, such as hypertension (Ch. 5), diabetes (Ch. 6), systemic lupus erythematosus (Ch. 16), polyarteritis nodosa (Ch. 5), myelomatosis (Ch. 8) and amyloidosis (Ch. 8), or complications such as peptic ulceration (Ch. 7). Major surgical procedures may be complicated by hyperkalaemia as a result of tissue damage, acidaemia and blood transfusion, which predisposes to arrhythmias and may cause cardiac arrest. Dialysis is deferred post-operatively if possible since heparinization is required.

Local anaesthesia is safe unless there is a severe bleeding tendency. For conscious sedation, relative analgesia is preferred since the veins of the forearms and the saphenous veins are lifelines for patients on regular haemodialysis. If it is necessary to give intravenous sedation, or take blood, other veins such as those at or above the elbow should be used because of the risk of consequent fistula infection or thrombophlebitis. Never put a cannula into the arteriovenous fistula arm. Midazolam is preferable to diazepam because of the lower risk of thrombophlebitis.

General anaesthesia is contraindicated if the haemoglobin is below 10 g/dl. Patients are also highly sensitive to the myocardial depressant effects of anaesthetic agents, and may develop hypotension at moderate levels of anaesthesia. Myocardial depression and cardiac arrhythmias are especially likely in those with poorly controlled metabolic acidosis and hyperkalaemia. Enflurane is metabolized to potentially nephrotoxic organic fluoride ions and therefore should be avoided if other nephrotoxic agents are used concurrently. Isoflurane and sevoflurane are probably safer. Induction with thiopental followed by very light GA with nitrous oxide is generally the technique of choice.

Although data are conflicting, most studies show that dental health of CKD patients is comparable with controls, but there is more periodontal disease. Secondary hyperparathyroidism does not have an appreciable effect on periodontal indices and radiographic bone height. Osseous lesions include loss of the lamina dura, osteoporosis and osteolytic areas (renal osteodystrophy). Secondary hyperparathyroidism may lead to giant cell lesions. There may be abnormal bone repair after extractions, with socket sclerosis. Patients with renal disease should therefore be screened carefully for bone disease before implant placement. Dry mouth, halitosis and a metallic taste, and insidious oral bleeding and purpura can also be conspicuous. The salivary glands may swell, salivary flow is reduced, there are protein and electrolyte changes and there is calculus accumulation. In children with CRF, jaw growth is usually retarded and tooth eruption may be delayed. There may be malocclusion and enamel hypoplasia with brownish discoloration, but tetracycline staining of the teeth should no longer be seen. A lower caries rate and less periodontal disease have been reported in children with CKD. A variety of mucosal lesions may be seen. The oral mucosa may be pale because of anaemia and there may be oral ulceration.

DENTAL ASPECTS OF RENAL TRANSPLANTATION IN ADDITION TO THOSE DISCUSSED ABOVE AND IN CH. 35

Any oral sign of infection must be examined immediately and treated aggressively in an immunosuppressed transplant recipient.

Consideration should also be given to haematological abnormalities, such as anaemia and platelet–haemostatic dysfunction; viral hepatitis B and C; and cardiovascular disorders such as hypertension, atherosclerotic heart disease with myocardial infarction, congestive heart failure, and left ventricular hypertrophy. Bone and joint disease is common because of low calcium levels, high phosphorus concentrations and elevated serum parathyroid hormone. Dental pulp narrowing has been noted – apparently a corticosteroid effect.

THE NEPHROTIC SYNDROME

GENERAL ASPECTS

The nephrotic syndrome is a non-specific condition in which glomerular damage (usually because of minimal change disease, diabetic nephropathy or systemic lupus erythematosus) leads to massive proteinuria with hypoalbuminaemia and oedema.

CLINICAL FEATURES

Oedema affects especially the face, genitals and lower limbs, and there are transudates in serous cavities (especially the peritoneal cavity – ascites). Loss of immunoglobulins (especially IgG) in the urine predisposes to infections with encapsulated bacteria such as *Haemophilus influenzae* and *Streptococcus pneumonia*. Loss of antithrombin III with raised factor VIII, fibrinogen and other clotting factors, leads to hypercoagulability – predisposing to thromboses. Loss of cholecalciferol-binding protein leads to vitamin D deficiency, secondary hyperparathyroidism and bone disease. In response to albumin loss, the liver synthesizes more of its proteins and levels of large proteins (such as alpha$_2$-macroglobulin and lipoproteins) increase. Patients also develop hypercholesterolaemia and become susceptible to atheroma and ischaemic heart disease.

GENERAL MANAGEMENT

Treatment aims to reduce proteinuria, control infections and prevent thromboembolism, and to remove or treat the basic cause of nephrosis. Many of the considerations in the management of the patient with CKD are also applicable to the nephrotic patient. Corticosteroids, a low-salt but high-protein diet, warfarin and prophylactic antimicrobials may be given.

DENTAL ASPECTS

Long-term corticosteroid therapy is the main problem (Ch. 6). Prophylactic antimicrobials may be indicated for procedures likely to cause a bacteraemia. Cardiovascular and haematological disorders and anticoagulation may complicate care (Ch. 8).

RENAL STONES (NEPHROLITHIASIS)

Renal stones (calculi) are not uncommon, may cause symptoms of renal colic or secondary renal damage and 90% can be seen on radiography. Systemic disease is rarely identified as underlying renal stones, but they may complicate gout, hyperparathyroidism, hyperoxaluria, cystinosis or renal tubular acidosis. A recent outbreak in China was related to melamine contamination of milk. There is no known predisposition to salivary calculi or dental calculus formation in patients who develop renal stones Renal calculi are treated by lithotripsy or surgical removal.

RENAL CANCER

Most kidney cancers (90%) are adenocarcinomas – renal cell cancers. Transitional cell cancer is rare. It is rare for people under 40 to have renal cancer, but the rare Wilms tumour (nephroblastoma) affects very young children. Renal cancer affects more men than women. Risk factors are shown in Box 12.1.

> **Box 12.1 Risk factors for renal cancer**
> - Cigarette smoking
> - Dialysis
> - Heredity: von Hippel–Lindau disease
> - Hypertension
> - Obesity
> - Occupation (working in the steel and coal industries with blast furnaces or coke-ovens, or exposure to cadmium, lead or asbestos)

CLINICAL FEATURES

Renal cancer may be symptomless but blood in the urine is the most common feature, and may induce pain. A lump or pain in the area of the kidney, or persistent fevers, night sweats, tiredness and weight loss may also be seen.

GENERAL MANAGEMENT

Diagnosis is confirmed by cystoscopy, ultrasound, computed tomography/magnetic resonance imaging, intravenous urography and biopsy. The main treatment is surgery, usually nephrectomy. Other treatments may include biological treatments (interferon-alpha or the IL-2 analogue aldesleukin) or targeted treatments [the multikinase inhibitors sorafenib, sunitinib, or bevacizumab or temsirolimus]. Occasionally radiotherapy or chemotherapy is used, or hormones.

DENTAL ASPECTS

Renal cancer occasionally metastasizes to the jaws or mouth.

USEFUL WEBSITES

http://www.niddk.nih.gov/health
http://www.uihealthcare.com/topics/index.html
http://www.nci.nih.gov/dictionary
http://www.cancerbackup.org.uk/Cancertype/Kidney
http://www.kidney.org.uk/Medical-Infopublished
http://www.sign.ac.uk/guidelines/index.html

FURTHER READING

Bansal, N., Hsu, C.Y., 2008. Long-term outcomes of patients with chronic kidney disease. Nat Clin Pract Nephrol 4, 532–533.

Bayraktar, G., Kazancioglu, R., Bozfakioglu, S., Yildiz, A., Ark, E., 2004. Evaluation of salivary parameters and dental status in adult hemodialysis patients. Clin Nephrol 62, 380–383.

Bayraktar, G., Kurtulus, I., Duraduryan, A., et al., 2007. Dental and periodontal findings in hemodialysis patients. Oral Dis 13, 393–397.

Bayraktar, G., Kurtulus, I., Kazancioglu, R., et al., 2008. Evaluation of periodontal parameters in patients undergoing peritoneal dialysis or hemodialysis. Oral Dis 14, 185–189.

Chou, C.Y., Cheng, S.Y., Liu, et al., J.H., et al., 2008. Association between betel-nut chewing and chronic kidney disease in men. Public Health Nutr 23, 1–5.

Crawford, P.W., Lerma, E.V., 2008. Treatment options for end stage renal disease. Prim Care 35, 407–432.

Criag, R.G., 2008. Interactions between chronic renal disease and periodontal disease. Oral Dis 14, 1–7.

Cunha, F.L., Tagliaferro, E.P., Pereira, A.C., Meneghim, M.C., Hebling, E., 2007. Oral health of a Brazilian population on renal dialysis. Spec Care Dentist 27, 227–231.

Frankenthal, S., Nakhoul, F., Machtei, E.E., et al., 2002. The effect of secondary hyperparathyroidism and hemodialysis therapy on alveolar bone and periodontium. J Clin Periodontol 29, 479–483.

Kerr, A.R., 2001. Update on renal disease for the dental practitioner. Oral Surg 92, 9–16.

Kotano, P., 2008. Chronic inflammation in dialysis patients – periodontal disease, the new kid on the block. Oral Dis 14, 8–9.

Moghaddam, S.M., Alavian, S.M., Kermani, N.A., 2008. Hepatitis C and renal transplantation: a review on historical aspects and current issues. Rev Med Virol 18, 375–386.

Munar, M.Y., Singh, H., 2007. Guidelines for drug dosing regimens in chronic kidney disease. Am Fam Physician 75, 1487–1496.

NEUROLOGY

KEY POINTS

- Neurological disorders often lead to significant disability
- Headaches are common and usually inconsequential but can signify life-threatening disease
- Stroke is a common cause of collapse, disability and death

The central nervous system (CNS) via electrical impulses that pass from the nervous system to muscles and glands is, together with the endocrine system, responsible for coordination of body cellular activities. The CNS consists of the brain and spinal cord. The brain contains the cerebral motor and sensory cortices essential for life: other specific areas have specialized functions (Tables 10.1 and 13.1; Figs. 10.1, 13.1 and 13.2.). Brain damage can lead to motor and/or sensory defects, disability, loss of consciousness and/or death.

The CNS controls the peripheral nervous system (PNS), which consists of the somatic (SNS) and (ANS) autonomic nervous systems, and extends to the limbs and organs (Fig. 13.2). The somatic nervous system is under conscious control and is responsible for receiving external stimuli and for coordinating movement. The autonomic nervous system consists of the sympathetic, parasympathetic and enteric nervous systems. The sympathetic system responds to danger or stress by release of adrenaline – increasing anxiety, cardiac rate and output, and other physiological changes. The parasympathetic system is responsible for slowing the heart, dilating blood vessels, and stimulating the digestive and genitourinary systems. The enteric nervous system controls digestion throughout the gastrointestinal tract.

The core components of the nervous system are neurons. Action potentials travel down the neuronal axon to open calcium (Ca^{++}) channels in the plasma membrane, triggering the exocytosis of vesicles containing neurotransmitters, which affect a receiving cell. The main neurotransmitters are acetylcholine (ACh) and noradrenaline. However, there are many other neurotransmitters (see Table 10.1).

Neurotransmitters such as ACh at excitatory synapses depolarize the post-synaptic membrane, causing an excitatory post-synaptic potential and an action potential in the post-synaptic cell. ACh is released at the terminals of all motor

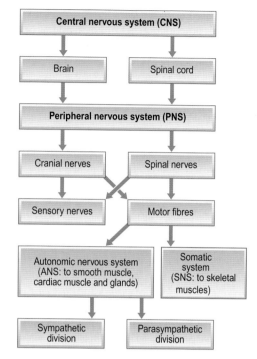

Fig. 13.1 Nervous system

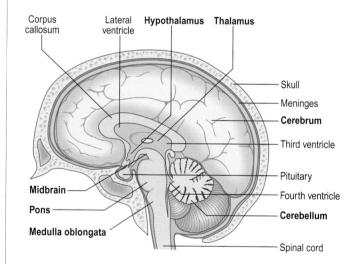

Fig. 13.2 Brain

Table 13.1	Location of the main functions in the cerebral cortex				
Cortex	Frontal	Pre-central gyrus	Post-central gyrus	Superior temporal	Occipital
Functions	Olfactory	Motor	Sensory (somatosensory)	Hearing	Vision
	Language (on dominant side) and speech (Broca's area)			Word comprehension (Wernicke's area)	

neurons activating skeletal muscle, all pre-ganglionic neurons of the autonomic nervous system and the post-ganglionic neurons of the parasympathetic system. ACh also mediates transmission at brain synapses involved in acquisition of short-term memory. Amino acids such as glutamic acid are involved in transmission at excitatory synapses in the CNS and are essential for long-term potentiation, a form of memory. Neurotransmitters such as GABA at inhibitory synapses hyperpolarize the post-synaptic membrane, causing an inhibitory post-synaptic potential because they counteract any excitatory signals that may arrive at that neuron.

NEUROLOGICAL DISEASE

The most common neurological complaints are shown in Box 13.1.

Patients whose symptoms have a neurological basis are relatively common and dental professionals may well be involved in their care, especially of people with the most important brain disorders, such as cerebral palsy, epilepsy, cerebrovascular accidents (CVAs; strokes) and facial palsy. Patients with head or maxillofacial injuries may have brain damage with impaired ocular movements or pupil reactions and loss of the sense of smell (anosmia). Orofacial pain is common and may have a neurological cause. Dental professionals should therefore be able to examine and recognize gross neurological abnormalities,

---

Box 13.1 The 12 most common neurological complaints

- Cerebrovascular accidents
- Compressive neuropathies (e.g. carpal tunnel syndrome)
- Diabetic neuropathy
- Epilepsy
- Headaches
- Meningitis
- Multiple sclerosis
- Parkinsonism
- Tremors
- Trigeminal neuralgia
- Tumours
- Zoster

---

and especially problems involving the cranial nerves, particularly the trigeminal, facial, glossopharyngeal, vagal and hypoglossal nerves.

NEUROLOGICAL EVALUATION

The nervous system may need to be evaluated as in Table 13.2.

If cognitive functions appear normal and there is no related complaint, and the patient appears, behaves and answers a history normally, formal cognitive evaluation is not required. Mental status can be assessed using a standard screening test such as mini-mental state examination (MMSE) or Folstein test (simple questions and problems in a number of areas: the time

---

Table 13.2	**Neurological evaluation**	
Aspects	**Details**	**Assessment**
Speech	Dysarthria may be detected	
Mental state or higher mental function	Table 13.3	
Level of consciousness	Ch. 24	Glasgow coma scale is widely used
Cognition	Table 13.3	
Sensory system	Sensory nerves carry information from the body to the brain about such things as touch, pain, heat, cold, vibration, position of body parts, and the shape of objects	Test using a pin and a blunt object to see if the patient can distinguish. Test person's ability to feel light touch, heat and vibration. Test position sense – move finger or toe up or down and ask the person to describe its position without looking. Dermatomes are shown in Fig. 13.3
Motor system	Muscle weakness or paralysis may indicate damage to the muscle, motor nerve or synapse, brain, or spinal cord A reflex is an automatic response to a stimulus. Those most commonly tested are the knee jerk, and elbow, ankle and plantar reflexes. The knee jerk tests the pathway consisting of the sensory nerve to the spinal cord, the spinal cord connections, and the motor nerves back to the muscle	Muscle size change (increased size or wasting or atrophy); involuntary movements or twitching; strength; and tone changes – increase (spasticity, rigidity) or decrease (flaccidity). The plantar reflex, tested by firmly stroking the outer border of the sole of foot with an object that causes minor discomfort, normally causes toes to curl downward: if the big toe goes upward and other toes spread out, this suggests a brain or spinal cord lesion (except in infants < 6 months). The extent of brain injury in a comatose person is tested by noting whether pupils constrict when light is shined on them (pupillary light reflex). Facial sensation and movement are determined by whether eyes blink when the cornea is touched (corneal reflex)
Cerebrum and cerebellum	Gait, coordination, and balance testing: require integration of signals from sensory and motor nerves by brain and spinal cord	Gait tested by asking the patient to walk in a straight line, placing one foot in front of the other; walk on heels, on toes, then hop on each foot. Coordination is tested by asking the patient to use the forefinger to reach out and touch an object, and then the person's own nose, and then to repeat actions rapidly and then with eyes closed. Balance is tested by the Romberg test: the patient stands still with feet together and eyes closed. In health, balance should be retained
Autonomic nervous system (ANS)		Tested by determining whether blood pressure changes when the person lies, sits or stands (orthostatic hypotension), or if there is a reduction or absence of sweating
Cranial nerves	Table 13.12	

Table 13.3 Testing mental status	
Test	**Test indicates**
Give today's date State the place you are Name specific people	Orientation in time, place and person
Name the last three Prime Ministers	Knowledge
Describe an event that happened yesterday	Recent memory
Describe events from schooldays	Remote memory
Interpret a proverb (e.g. 'there is many a slip between cup and lip')	Abstract thinking
Do simple arithmetic	Ability to calculate numbers
Repeat a short list of objects	Attention
Recall the short list of objects after 5 minutes	Immediate recall
Describe feelings and opinions about your illness	Insight
Explain how you feel today	Mood
Comb your hair	Ability to perform action
Name simple objects and body parts	Ability to use language
Identify, without seeing them, small objects held in the hand, and discriminate between being touched in two places	Ability of brain to process and interpret complex information from the hand
Follow simple command involving different body parts on different sides (such as 'put your right thumb in your left ear and stick out your tongue')	Language comprehension
Draw a clock, cube or house	Ability to understand spatial relationships

and place of the test, repeating lists of words, arithmetic, language use and comprehension, and basic motor skills). Testing can also be achieved as shown in Table 13.3.

HEADACHES AND OROFACIAL PAIN

Headache and orofacial pain are the most common neurological complaints, often chronic and mainly caused by local disease, psychogenic disorders, neurological disorders or vascular disease (see also Table 13.4 and Box 13.2). The pain receptors can be stimulated by stress, muscular tension, dilated blood vessels and other triggers.

Headaches can also signal serious disorders such as brain tumour, infection or bleeding (Box 13.3). Features suggesting serious or life-threatening headaches are shown in Box 13.4.

Some headaches are less serious and have quite specific and obvious precipitating factors (Table 13.5). Foods such as alcohol, caffeine, chocolate, cheeses and nuts can cause headaches in some people and, in some, trigger migraine.

Virtually *all other* types of headache, at least to some extent, depend on emotional factors and individual personalities. About 50% of patients seen in headache clinics are thought to suffer from muscle contraction (tension) headaches, which appear to involve the tightening or tensing of facial and neck muscles because of stress (see below).

LOCAL CAUSES OF OROFACIAL PAIN

The mouth

Oral causes of facial pain (e.g. pulpitis, apical periodontitis, periodontal abscesses, pericoronitis and various intraosseous lesions) are discussed in other texts.

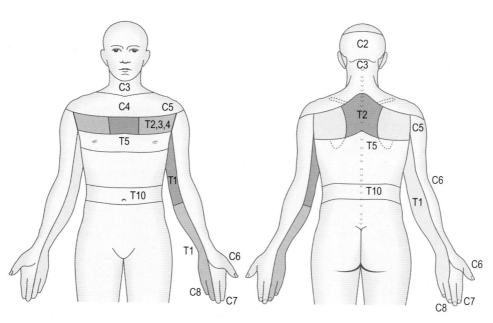

Fig. 13.3 Cervical and thoracic dermatomes

Table 13.4 Causes of headache and orofacial pain

Cause	Diseases
Local	Dental or oral disease Infections or tumours of paranasal sinuses and nasopharynx Neck lesions Ocular lesions
Psychogenic	Tension headaches Atypical (idiopathic) facial pain Temporomandibular pain-dysfunction syndrome Oral dysaesthesia
Neurological	Trigeminal neuralgia Glossopharyngeal neuralgia Herpetic neuralgia Raeder neuralgia Intracranial disease
Vascular	Migraine Migrainous neuralgia Temporal arteritis
Other	Referred pain (e.g. heart or chest) Raised intracranial pressure Meningeal irritation Diseases of the skull Medical diseases (e.g. severe hypertension) Trauma Drugs (e.g. vinca alkaloids, nitrites, dapsone, some analgesics)

The sinuses and nasopharynx

Sinusitis causes localized pain. In acute maxillary or frontal sinusitis, local pain and tenderness (but not swelling), and radio-opacity of the affected sinuses, usually follow a cold (Ch. 14).

Tumours of sinuses or nasopharynx can also cause facial pain. These are rare, usually carcinomas, and involve trigeminal nerve branches and may cause pain simulating pain-dysfunction syndrome. They can remain undetected until late.

Eagle syndrome, due to calcification of the stylohyoid ligament, may be a rare cause of pain on chewing, swallowing or turning the head. The elongated styloid process may be visualized radiographically, and palpation of it in the wall of the pharynx causes intense pain. The stylohyoid process can be shortened surgically, but regrowth and relapse are common.

The eyes

Glaucoma (raised intraocular pressure) may cause pain in and around the orbit. Disorders of refraction can cause frontal headaches. Retrobulbar neuritis (e.g. in multiple sclerosis) can cause pain in and around the orbit.

The ears

Pharyngeal or middle ear disease may cause headaches. Oral disease can rarely cause pain referred to the ear: the classic picture is that of the older man with tongue cancer whose complaint is earache.

Box 13.2 International Headache Society classification of headache

1. Migraine
1.1 Migraine without aura
1.2 Migraine with aura
1.3 Ophthalmoplegic migraine
1.4 Retinal migraine
1.5 Childhood periodic syndromes that may be precursors to or associated with migraine
1.6 Complications of migraine
1.7 Migrainous disorder not fulfilling above criteria
2. Tension-type headache
2.1 Episodic tension-type headache
2.2 Chronic tension-type headache
2.3 Tension-type headache not fulfilling above criteria
3. Cluster headache and chronic paroxysmal hemicrania
3.1 Cluster headache
3.2 Chronic paroxysmal hemicrania
3.3 Cluster headache-like disorder not fulfilling above criteria
4. Miscellaneous headaches not associated with structural lesion
4.1 Idiopathic stabbing headache
4.2 External compression headache
4.3 Cold stimulus headache
4.4 Benign cough headache
4.5 Benign exertional headache
4.6 Headache associated with sexual activity
5. Headache associated with head trauma
5.1 Acute post-traumatic headache
5.2 Chronic post-traumatic headache
6. Headache associated with vascular disorders
6.1 Acute ischaemic cerebrovascular disorder
6.2 Intracranial haematoma
6.3 Subarachnoid haemorrhage

6.4 Unruptured vascular malformation
6.5 Arteritis
6.6 Carotid or vertebral artery pain
6.7 Venous thrombosis
6.8 Arterial hypertension
6.9 Headache associated with other vascular disorder
7. Headache associated with non-vascular intracranial disorder
7.1 High CSF pressure
7.2 Low CSF pressure
7.3 Intracranial infection
7.4 Intracranial sarcoidosis and other non-infectious inflammatory diseases
7.5 Headache related to intrathecal injections
7.6 Intracranial neoplasm
7.7 Headache associated with other intracranial disorder
8. Headache associated with substances or their withdrawal
8.1 Headache induced by acute substance use or exposure
8.2 Headache induced by chronic substance use or exposure
8.3 Headache from substance withdrawal (acute use)
8.4 Headache from substance withdrawal (chronic use)
8.5 Headache associated with substances but with uncertain mechanism
9. Headache associated with non-cephalic infection
9.1 Viral infection
9.2 Bacterial infection
9.3 Headache related to other infection
10. Headache associated with metabolic disorder
10.1 Hypoxia
10.2 Hypercapnia
10.3 Mixed hypoxia and hypercapnia
10.4 Hypoglycaemia
10.5 Dialysis
10.6 Headache related to other metabolic abnormality

Box 13.2 International Headache Society classification of headache—cont'd

11. Headache or facial pain associated with disorder of cranium, neck, eyes, ears, nose, sinuses, teeth, mouth, or other facial or cranial structures

11.1 Cranial bone
11.2 Neck
11.3 Eyes
11.4 Ears
11.5 Nose and sinuses
11.6 Teeth, jaws and related structures
11.7 Temporomandibular joint disease

12. Cranial neuralgias, nerve trunk pain and deafferentation pain

12.1 Persistent (in contrast to tic-like) pain of cranial nerve origin
12.2 Trigeminal neuralgia
12.3 Glossopharyngeal neuralgia
12.4 Nervous intermedius neuralgia
12.5 Superior laryngeal neuralgia
12.6 Occipital neuralgia
12.7 Central causes of head and facial pain other than tic douloureux
12.8 Facial pain not fulfilling criteria in groups 11 or 12

13. Headache not classifiable

Headache Classification Committee of International Headache Society. Classification and diagnostic criteria for headache disorders, cranial neuralgias and facial pain. Cephalalgia 1988; 8 (Suppl 7): 1–96.

CSF, cerebrospinal fluid.

Box 13.3 Serious causes of headache

- Acute glaucoma
- Acute hypertension
- Acute lesions affecting the carotid vessels
- Brain tumours
- Giant cell arteritis
- Meningitis
- Subarachnoid haemorrhage
- Subdural or epidural haemorrhage

Box 13.4 Indicators of seriousness in headache

- Abrupt, severe 'thunderclap' or bilateral headache
- After a recent sore throat or respiratory infection
- Confusion, loss of consciousness, convulsions, fever, stiff neck, rash, mental confusion, seizures, diplopia, weakness, numbness, pain in the eye or ear, or dysarthria
- Disrupting normal life
- New headache pain after age 55
- Persistent in a person who was previously headache-free
- Preceded by head trauma
- Recurring in children
- Severe headache
- Worse after coughing, exertion, straining or a sudden movement

---

Table 13.5 Some less serious causes of headache

	Causes
Chinese restaurant syndrome	Monosodium glutamate
Hangover headache	Acetaldehyde
Hot dog headache	Nitrites/nitrates
Post-coital headache	Intercourse
Vitamin A-induced headache	Vitamin A

The neck

Cervical vertebral disease occasionally causes headache or pain referred to the face and may aggravate tension headaches. Nerve block with local anaesthesia (LA) may temporarily relieve this pain. Carotidynia is unilateral pain arising from the cervical carotid artery that radiates to the ipsilateral face and ear, and sometimes to the head. Carotid artery tenderness and overlying soft tissue swelling are the signs. It is responsive to corticosteroids.

PSYCHOGENIC CAUSES OF HEADACHE OR OROFACIAL PAIN (See Ch.10)

Tension headaches

Tension headaches are common, especially in young adults, particularly in emotionally tense, aggressive, frustrated and anxious individuals. They may be caused by sustained contraction of the head and neck muscles and vasoconstriction of nutrient arterioles. Patients are frequently adamant that they suffer from migraine and sometimes the two conditions do coexist. The possibility of associated depression should also be considered.

Clinical features

The pain is experienced more than 15 days monthly to be classified as tension headache. Pain affects the frontal, occipital or temporal muscles, and is felt as a constant ache or band-like pressure, of mild or moderate intensity, bilateral in location, lasting from 30 min to 7 days. The pain onset often is associated with emotional conflict but does not worsen with routine physical activity. Nausea is absent, but photophobia or phonophobia may be present. Pain can often be elicited by palpation of the trapezius or pericranial muscles, is often worse in the evening and at night, but does not waken the patient.

General management

Hypertension and hyperthyroidism should be excluded, as must drug-associated headaches (e.g. analgesics, antihistamines, anticonvulsants, ergotamine, steroids and antibiotics). The pain may be treated by rest, simple analgesics or with combination drugs with biofeedback, and particularly with counselling. Reassurance may be effective and may be helped by a short course of diazepam, which is both an anxiolytic and muscle relaxant. Failing this, amitriptyline is usually effective. Even acupuncture may offer relief.

ORAL DYSAESTHESIAS

A complaint of a burning tongue or mouth is the common type of oral dysaesthesia. Dry mouth, disturbed taste sensations or delusions of halitosis are other dysaesthesias. These are often manifestations of monosymptomatic hypochondriasis, somatization pain disorder or a depressive neurosis. There is sometimes cancer phobia, or anxiety about the possibility, for example, of venereal disease or human immunodeficiency virus (HIV).

Burning mouth syndrome (glossopyrosis; glossodynia)

General aspects

Burning mouth 'syndrome' (BMS) is a common chronic complaint seen especially in middle-aged or elderly females. Organic causes of burning mouth include:

- glossitis
- erythema migrans (geographic tongue)
- candidosis
- lichen planus
- dry mouth
- drugs (such as angiotensin-converting enzyme inhibitors)
- habits and denture difficulties
- diabetes.

Burning mouth syndrome is the term usually used when symptoms persist in the absence of identifiable organic aetiological factors. Many of these cases appear related to psychogenic factors such as cancer phobia, depression or anxiety. Sometimes, factors such as restricted tongue space from poor denture construction, or parafunction, such as tongue-thrusting, may be at play. Denture allergy is probably never responsible. Systemic disorders such as a haematological deficiency state are found in some (Table 13.6).

Table 13.6   Organic causes of burning mouth

	Examples	Comments/examples
Local causes	Candidosis	Sometimes associated with xerostomia
	Denture problems	–
	Erythema migrans (geographical tongue)	–
	Lichen planus	–
Systemic causes	Deficiency of:	B vitamins, especially B_{12}
		Folate
		Iron
	Diabetes	–
	Drugs	–
	Dry mouth	–
	Psychogenic	Anxiety states
		Cancerophobia
		Depression
		Hypochondriasis

Clinical features

The symptoms are of a burning sensation that starts after waking and grows in intensity during the day. It may sometimes be relieved by chewing or drinking. By contrast, pain caused by organic lesions is typically made worse by eating.

Burning mouth syndrome most frequently affects the tongue but may also affect the palate, or less commonly the lips or lower alveolus. There are often multiple oral and/or other psychogenic related complaints, such as dry mouth, bad taste, headaches, chronic back pain, irritable bowel syndrome or dysmenorrhoea.

Patients are often high users of health care services: there have often already been multiple consultations and attempts at treatment. There are no clinically detectable signs of mucosal disease, no tenderness or swelling of tongue or affected areas, a total lack of objective signs and all investigations are negative. Patients use analgesics only uncommonly.

Three types have been described on the basis of the pattern of symptoms of burning sensation (Table 13.7).

Table 13.7   Types of burning mouth syndrome

Type	Symptom pattern	Frequency	Other features
1	No symptoms on waking, but increasing during the day	–	Unremitting
2	Symptoms on waking and through the day	Most common	Unremitting
3	No regular pattern of symptoms	Least common	May remit

General management

Laboratory screening may be indicated to rule out anaemia, vitamin or iron deficiency (blood tests), diabetes (blood and urine analyses), xerostomia (salivary flow rates) and candidosis (smear or ruse). Pontine infarction should be excluded or ruse (see below).

Few patients with BMS have spontaneous remission and thus treatment is indicated, including attention to any local factors such as dentures, psychogenic assessment and occasionally psychiatric care, but many refuse this. Psychological screening using, for example, the hospital anxiety and depression (HAD) scale may be helpful. Treatment may include topical agents such as capsaicin or antidepressants, such as amitriptyline, doxepine, dosulepine, trazodone, prothiadine or fluoxetine.

ATYPICAL FACIAL PAIN (IDIOPATHIC OR PSYCHOGENIC FACIAL PAIN)

General aspects

The International Headache Society (IHS) defines this as 'facial pain not fulfilling other criteria' or

> persistent facial pain that does not have the characteristics of the cranial neuralgias and is not associated with physical signs or demonstrable organic causes. It is present daily and persists for most or all of the day. It is confined at onset to a limited area on one side of the face and may spread to the upper and lower jaws or other areas of the face or neck. It is deep and poorly

localized. The pain is not associated with sensory loss or other physical signs. Laboratory investigations including radiographs of face and jaws do not demonstrate relevant abnormalities.

A few patients with similar symptomatology eventually prove to have organic disorders such as an adenocystic carcinoma that has invaded perineurally but in others it may be a somatization pain disorder (Ch.10).

Clinical features

Pain is continuous, often of a dull boring or burning type and ill-defined location, but particularly in the maxilla. The pain may waken the patient in the early morning. The pain has no obvious precipitating factors, although it may be attributed to dental disease or treatment, and is rarely completely relieved by analgesics. There are often multiple oral and/or other psychogenic related complaints. There have often been multiple consultations and treatment attempts.

General management

Idiopathic facial pain is a clinical diagnosis by careful examination of the mouth, perioral structures and cranial nerves. Imaging with computed tomography (CT) or magnetic resonance imaging (MRI) scan to exclude organic disease is important.

Cognitive therapy is indicated but, since many of these patients have already rejected the idea of mental illness, it may be difficult to persuade them of the need for this help. Sometimes it is helpful to make it clear that depression is both common and is an illness like any other and, like other illnesses, can also cause physical symptoms. Sometimes the pain may appear as a hysterical conversion neurosis and many patients have obsessional personality traits.

Antidepressants that can be useful include amitriptyline, dothiepin (dosulepin), nortriptyline or fluoxetine.

Idiopathic odontalgia is a variant characterized by the complaint of severe throbbing pain in one or several teeth, which are hypersensitive to any stimulus. Extractions typically lead to transference of the symptoms to adjacent teeth.

TEMPOROMANDIBULAR PAIN-DYSFUNCTION SYNDROME (FACIAL PAIN-DYSFUNCTION, MYOFASCIAL PAIN-DYSFUNCTION, TMJ PAIN-DYSFUNCTION OR FACIAL ARTHROMYALGIA)

General aspects

Temporomandibular joint (TMJ) pain-dysfunction is a common problem predominantly affecting young women. The TMJ shows no pathology in contrast to internal derangement of the TMJ, which may also cause pain. The cause is unclear but there have been many hypotheses from trauma to malocclusion and even psychogenic causes.

Some occupations or hobbies, such as scuba-diving, may predispose to abnormal habits and TMJ pain-dysfunction.

There may be a greater frequency of migraine, rhinitis, peptic ulcer and irritable bowel syndrome associated, leading some to believe that depression may be contributory. A psychiatric basis

for the syndrome however is controversial, but it may be seen particularly in ambitious obsessional personalities, in anxiety states or in agitated depression.

Clinical features

There is typically dull pain, usually in front of the TMJ, which tends to radiate over the masseter and temporalis muscles and sometimes occipitally or cervically. There is typically tenderness in the masticatory muscles including the pterygoids.

There may be an audible click or palpable crepitus in the joint, the mandible often deviates towards the affected side on opening and there may be restricted mouth opening, or 'locking'. There is sometimes faceting on the teeth, ridging of the tongue margins and buccal mucosa at the occlusal line, and sometimes signs of lip-chewing if patients frequently grind or clench their teeth or develop various (parafunctional) habits, such as pencil chewing.

General management

Radiography shows no significant abnormality but, nevertheless, organic disease must be excluded. In any case, symptoms eventually resolve spontaneously. Degenerative joint disease is not usually a consequence. Treatment consists of reassurance. A bite-raising appliance to provide a free, sliding occlusion may help. Mild anxiolytics such as diazepam, which is also a muscle relaxant, may help but should only be given for a limited period and may need to be supplemented with analgesics or peri-articular injection of benzocaine. If there is real evidence of depression, tricyclic antidepressants may be more useful.

Dental aspects

Limited mouth-opening may interfere with dental treatment. Attrition may require special restorative care. Dental treatment may be blamed for the onset of symptoms.

NEUROLOGICAL CAUSES OF FACIAL PAIN

Sensory innervation of the face and scalp is carried by the trigeminal nerve. Lesions of the trigeminal at any stage from its nuclei along its course from the pons can cause facial pain or sensory loss, sometimes with serious implications.

Idiopathic trigeminal neuralgia

General aspects

Trigeminal neuralgia (TN) has been described by the IHS as 'a painful, unilateral affliction of the face, characterized by brief electric-shock, lightning-like (lancinating) pains limited to the distribution of one or more divisions of the trigeminal nerve.' TN usually afflicts patients over the age of 50. The incidence is less than 0.2% in those under 40 years but rises to 25% in those over 70.

About 15% of cases have structural causes: about 5% are produced by posterior fossa tumours (meningiomas, acoustic neurinomas or carcinomas) that are not suspected before operation and a slightly smaller percentage have multiple sclerosis.

The cause of *idiopathic* trigeminal neuralgia is unclear but it may be caused by demyelination caused by a tortuous arteriosclerotic blood vessel in the posterior cranial fossa pressing on the trigeminal (the disease predominantly affects older people, many of whom have hypertension or arteriosclerosis).

Clinical features

The pain of trigeminal neuralgia has the following characteristics.

- It is confined to the trigeminal area of one side, usually the maxillary or mandibular division or occasionally both. Infraorbital or lower lip/lower jaw pain is common, and supraorbital pain uncommon.
- It is severe and sharply stabbing (lancinating), of only a few seconds' duration, but paroxysms may follow in quick succession. The pain is typically remarkably severe and a patient seen crying with pain during an attack is not easily forgotten.
- Triggers are mild stimuli, which, applied to trigger zones within the trigeminal area, typically provoke an attack, and include

  shaving
  stroking or touching the face
  eating
  drinking a hot or cold liquid
  brushing teeth
  talking
  putting on cosmetics
  encountering a cold breeze
  walking into an air-conditioned room.

Idiopathic trigeminal neuralgia is likely when there is an intact corneal reflex, no abnormal neurological signs, no objective sensory loss in the area and no other defined neurological deficit.

Secondary trigeminal neuralgia is more likely if the patient's pain started when younger than 40 years, if there is predominant forehead and/or orbit pain (i.e. first division of the trigeminal nerve), if the pain is bilateral, if there are abnormal trigeminal reflexes, or if there are physical signs such as facial sensory or motor impairment. The latter can result from posterior cerebral fossa lesions, particularly tumours or aneurysms (the combination of neuralgia with hemifacial spasm also suggests a posterior cranial fossa lesion), multiple sclerosis, brainstem ischaemia or infarction in cerebrovascular disease, neurosyphilis or other lesions.

Atypical trigeminal neuralgia is a syndrome that overlaps TN and trigeminal neuropathy, and affects up to 5% after facial surgery or significant trauma, and in up to 1% after the removal of impacted teeth. It includes unusual symptoms, such as more continuous rather than lightning attacks of pain, or triggering by warmth rather than cold, and may result from lesions or injuries of the trigeminal nerve root distal to the root entry zone but with even greater compression than found in the idiopathic form of TN. Attacks consist of constant pain that episodically intensifies and produces both lancinating triggered pain and a baseline, constant, dull and throbbing discomfort.

General management

The diagnosis and clinical.

The diagnosis is cliniceal Organic disease must be excluded by neurological examination to confirm normal corneal reflexes, sensory appreciation, masseter muscle bulk and strength. Loss of the corneal reflex excludes the diagnosis of idiopathic trigeminal neuralgia, unless a previous trigeminal nerve section procedure has been performed. The other main differential diagnoses are from glossopharyngeal neuralgia (the two can coexist), atypical facial pain, Raeder paratrigeminal syndrome and Frey syndrome.

Investigations, required especially if there are any neurological features, may include skull radiographs, MRI or CT brain scans, and occasionally CSF examination, or neurophysiological tests (e.g. trigeminal evoked potentials and corneal reflex latency). Many now advocate MRI as a routine.

A few patients with mild symptoms recover spontaneously but most require treatment. This is initially with anticonvulsants, particularly carbamazepine, which change GABA levels in the central pain-inhibiting systems. Spontaneous remissions of a month or two are relatively common and may make the assessment of treatment difficult. Carbamazepine is indicated first, if only because its use may constitute a therapeutic challenge to the correct diagnosis. If, for example, a patient presumed to have TN does not respond to carbamazepine in 24–48 h, then the physician may wish to reconsider the initial diagnosis. Carbamazepine is not an analgesic and, if given when an attack starts, will not relieve the pain. If used prophylactically, it may control up to 90% of cases over the first few months, but this falls to about 25% by 1 year.

Carbamazepine absorption is slow, and its antineuralgic activity depends on its metabolites, and therefore it must be given continuously for long periods until symptoms are controlled or adverse effects become excessive. Though about 80% obtain pain relief within 24 h, about 20 days are required before the full effect is noted. Carbamazepine can cause severe ataxia but the many other possible toxic effects are uncommon. Ataxia and drowsiness are dose-related, may interfere with driving and can be dose-limiting.

Carbamazepine is contraindicated in HLA-B1502-positive Asians from China and Thailand (may develop Stevens–Johnson syndrome), in pregnancy and porphyria, and should be used with caution in persons with hepatic, renal, cardiac (especially atrioventricular conduction defects) or bone marrow disease. Monitoring of blood carbamazepine levels and, for adverse reactions, by regular assessment of blood pressure, blood urea and electrolytes, liver function, platelet and white cell counts is helpful.

Carbamazepine may predispose to liver damage from acetaminophen and may interfere with the effectiveness of the contraceptive pill, though most patients are beyond the age of concern in that respect. Drugs such as erythromycin, cimetidine and isoniazid can raise serum carbamazepine levels.

Should carbamazepine in maximum dosage fail to control neuralgia, oxcarbazine or gabapentin appears to be the most satisfactory alternative. Additional therapeutic agents that may be added or replace carbamazepine include baclofen or lamotrigine, or phenytoin.

Surgery may be indicated if medical therapy fails (25–50% of patients eventually fail to respond to drugs) or adverse effects are intolerable. Surgery (surgical division, cryosurgery, injections of alcohol or phenol) to the trigeminal nerve branches involved is usually carried out under open operation under LA. Cryosurgery can bring pain relief without permanent anaesthesia. However, the benefit of all peripheral nerve procedures may only be temporary, with relapse common within 2 years. If these treatments fail, intracranial neurosurgery is available. All destructive surgical procedures result in a sensory deficit in up to 20% of patients, relapse is common beyond 2 years and the more peripheral the procedure, the greater the risk of recurrence.

Percutaneous radiofrequency trigeminal (retrogasserian) rhizotomy (PRTR) is the most widely used technique and is minimally invasive involving inserting a needle but has morbidity and some mortality. Trigeminal-innervated muscle weakness is a significant early side-effect and anaesthesia also results, causing danger of damage to the cornea.

Percutaneous trigeminal ganglion compression (rhizotomy) is minimally invasive and uses a Fogarty balloon. This may be effective. Over 50% of patients have mild to moderate post-operative numbness, but no corneal numbness, and 16% have ipsilateral masseter/pterygoid weakness. The overall recurrence rate is 26% but 60% of patients are pain-free 8 years after surgery.

Microvascular decompression (MVD) is an invasive procedure via a suboccipital craniotomy. This may be effective but occasionally results in damage to the VIIth or VIIIth cranial nerves and also carries a small mortality.

Gamma knife radiosurgery (GKR) is non-invasive. It involves delivering high doses of radiation to the trigeminal nerve root without any need for injection or skin incision. It can be successful in eliminating pain in up to 80% but pain recurs in more than half the cases.

Neurosurgical techniques can occasionally be followed by continuous facial pain (anaesthesia dolorosa) that responds very poorly to treatment.

Dental aspects

Patients may be reluctant to brush their teeth or attend for dental treatment.

Glossopharyngeal (vagoglossopharyngeal) neuralgia

Glossopharyngeal neuralgia is rare and usually idiopathic, possibly caused by an abnormal intracranial blood vessel, as in trigeminal neuralgia. The pain is similar to that of TN (rarely, the two coexist), but affects the throat, especially the tonsillar region and is typically triggered by swallowing or coughing. Pain may also be felt in the ipsilateral ear (Vago–Collet–Sicard syndrome) and this may simulate neuralgia of the nervus intermedius (Hunt neuralgia). There are no sensory or motor defects but, in 10%, there is associated bradycardia and fall in blood pressure, sometimes with syncope, especially when the neuralgia is secondary to a throat tumour. During longer attacks, asystole may occur and long severe attacks may be marked by protracted

cardiac arrest, absence of pulse, pallor, mental confusion, syncope or convulsions.

The mechanism usually proposed has been spillover of impulses from the glossopharyngeal nerve via the tractus solitarius to the dorsal motor nucleus of the vagus nerve, resulting in reflex bradycardia, heart block or asystole.

Unlike TN, glossopharyngeal neuralgia rarely appears to be associated with intracranial tumours and even more rarely with multiple sclerosis. Tumours in the posterior cranial fossa or jugular foramen (jugular foramen syndrome) can rarely cause similar pain together with lesions of the vagus (X) and accessory (XI) nerves (see Appendix 13.2). Hoarseness, dysphagia, palatal deviation to the intact side, anaesthesia of the posterior pharyngeal wall, and weakness of the sternomastoid and upper trapezius are then seen.

A 10% cocaine or other anaesthetic throat spray will cause temporary pain relief which is diagnostic. Therapy is as for TN, but carbamazepine is usually less effective and gabapentin is probably better. If drugs fail to give adequate relief, neurosurgery is indicated but is more difficult than for TN and has a higher morbidity and mortality.

Raeder paratrigeminal neuralgia

Raeder paratrigeminal neuralgia is severe, persistent pain in and around the eye, with associated Horner syndrome, often caused by a lesion at the skull base requiring neurological attention.

Herpetic and post-herpetic facial neuralgia

Herpes zoster (shingles) is often preceded, usually accompanied and sometimes followed by neuralgia in up to 70% of cases. It mainly affects older people, but antivirals may help prevent it (Ch. 21).

Post-herpetic neuralgia is defined as pain persisting a month after the eruption of zoster, causing continuous burning pain, worse with movement and thermal change, and sometimes sensory changes in the affected area. Treatment is difficult, and pain may be so intolerable that suicide can become a risk. However, spontaneous improvement may sometimes follow after about 18 months.

Non-steroidal anti-inflammatory drugs are generally ineffective but topical lidocaine or capsaicin as a cream may help. Tricyclic antidepressants, particularly desipramine or amitriptyline, may relieve the pain better than valproate or carbamazepine. Transcutaneous electrical nerve stimulation or neurosurgery may sometimes help.

Pontine infarction

Pontine ischaemia may be due to bilateral ventral pontine infarction. Lateral medullary infarction may cause a similar but unilateral effect. Burning orofacial pain may be an early symptom.

Bilateral ventral pontine infarction causes the syndrome of quadriplegia, lower cranial nerve palsies but preservation of movement of the upper eyelids and vertical gaze (termed the ' locked-in syndrome' because the patient, though able to understand what is being said and happening, is imprisoned by their inability to speak or move anything apart from their eyes). The prognosis is poor.

Cerebellopontine angle tumours

Lesions in the posterior cranial fossa (e.g. cerebellopontine angle tumours) can cause facial pain associated with an absent corneal reflex (Vth nerve), deafness, tinnitus and vertigo (from involvement of the VIIIth nerve), facial palsy (VIIth nerve involvement), ataxia, intention tremor and nystagmus (cerebellar involvement) and spasticity of the leg (pyramidal tract involvement). Acoustic neuromas and meningiomas are usually operable.

Middle cranial fossa lesions

Middle cranial fossa lesions can involve the Vth and VIth nerves, and also cause lateral rectus palsy. Carotid aneurysms, especially those in the cavernous sinus, or cavernous sinus thrombosis, may also cause facial pain and associated cranial nerve lesions (IIIrd, IVth and VIth nerves; Fig. 6.3).

Cavernous sinus thrombosis

Cavernous sinus thrombosis is a life-threatening complication that may rarely result from infection spreading back through the emissary veins from the maxillary or nasal region, or upper teeth, or from infected thrombi in the anterior facial vein or less commonly the pterygoid plexus. Infection can reach the cavernous sinus via either the ophthalmic veins or the foramen ovale.

Clinically, cavernous sinus thrombosis causes gross eyelid oedema, ipsilateral pulsatile exophthalmos, cyanosis due to venous obstruction, rigors and high swinging pyrexia. The superior orbital fissure syndrome (proptosis, fixed dilated pupil and limitation of eye movements) rapidly develops.

There is a mortality of up to 50% and a further 50% of those that survive are likely to lose the sight of one or both eyes. Vigorous and early use of anticoagulants, antibiotics, drainage and elimination of infection are essential.

Bell palsy

Bell (facial) palsy is preceded or accompanied by pain in the region of the ear, spreading down the jaw in about half the cases. However, the appearance of the typical facial paralysis leaves little doubt as to the diagnosis (see below).

Facial pain caused by extracranial lesions

Branches of the trigeminal nerve may be affected by inflammatory, traumatic or neoplastic lesions causing pain or sensory loss in their distribution.

VASCULAR CAUSES OF FACIAL PAIN

Vasomotor states are responsible for certain headaches, but either widening or narrowing of extracranial and intracranial arteries may produce pain. Both vasodilatation and neurogenic

inflammation are under the influence of serotonin (5HT): the $5HT_{1B}$ receptor controls vasodilatation, whereas $5HT_{1D}$ regulates neurogenic inflammation. Serotonin agonists such as ergotamine and triptans can prevent neurogenic inflammation.

Migraine

General aspects

Migraine is a recurrent headache combined with autonomic disturbances, affecting over 14% of women and 7% of men. The prodrome is usually accompanied by diminished cerebral blood flow, possibly the result of a neuronal trigger mechanism in the trigeminovascular nucleus, but the headache is usually associated with increased cerebral and extracranial blood flow possibly caused by serotonin adsorbed to blood vessel walls, since platelet serotonin rises before a migraine headache. This may cause the trigeminal nerve to release neuropeptides, and the combination of serotonin and bradykinin may cause blood vessels to become dilated and inflamed.

Clinical features

Migraine attacks may be precipitated by foods containing tyramine or nitrites (Table 13.8). The highest levels of tyramine are in aged cheeses, spoiled meats, aged and cured meats, Marmite yeast extract, sauerkraut, fermented soybean products, broad (fava) bean pods, and draft (tap) beer, but there is little or no tyramine in beverages, breads, fats, cottage cheese, ricotta, cream cheese, soft farmer's cheese, mozzarella cheese, processed cheese slices, sour cream, yogurt, milk, eggs, oranges, tomatoes, fresh meat, poultry, fish, shellfish and soy milk.

There is some evidence that large quantities of nuts (peanuts, coconuts and brazil nuts) may trigger hypertensive reactions and headaches, but not via tyramine.

Other foods precipitating migraine include alcohol (especially beer and red wine), nitroglycerin, aspartame and monosodium glutamate (a flavour-enhancing ingredient in some Asian foods, certain seasonings, and in many tinned and processed foods). Other precipitants include the menstrual cycle, pregnancy, contraceptive pill or stress and environmental factors (noise, smoke, etc.). The fact that attacks are more frequent at weekends, for example, should not be interpreted as excluding stress, as there is no doubt that some find the company and demands of their families more stressful than their work. Going away on holiday (Freud's *reise fieber* – 'travel fever') is also highly stressful for many. Changes in the weather, season, altitude level, time zone or sleep patterns; bright lights; drugs, including cimetidine, fenfluramine, nifedipine and theophylline; low blood sugar, changes in mealtimes, skipped meals or fasting; intense physical exertion, including sexual activity; and tobacco, including passive smoking, are other factors.

Several types of migraine are recognized (Table 13.9); migraine without aura is the most frequent type, presenting with unilateral headache, but migraine with aura is the most readily recognizable type. Another recognized variant is an aura without headache.

Classical migraine presents with an aura (warning symptoms), which may last about 15 min and consists of visual,

Table 13.8 Tyramine in foods

Tyramine-containing	Low tyramine	Not usually tyramine-containing
All tap beer and ale, Chianti, port, sherry and vermouth, red wine, white wine	Domestic bottled beers	Non-alcoholic beverages
Most aged cheeses	Cream cheese and cottage cheese	Regular cheese of the kind typically used on bread and pizza
Banana skin, figs, grapes, oranges, pineapples, plums, prunes, raisins, overripe avocados	Avocados – provided not overripe	Chocolate
Broad beans, eggplant		Tomatoes
Processed foods; Marmite, Vegemite, sauerkraut, and shrimp paste		Processed cheese
Processed meats, cured or pickled meats, and meat by-products and broths. Game birds and wild animals if hung; old liver and meat		Fresh liver, meat, poultry and fish and shellfish
All soy products; soybeans; soy sauce, tofu, miso and teriyaki sauce		Soy milk

Table 13.9 Migraine variants

Type	Subtype	Clinical features
Migraine	Classic	Unilateral headache preceded by an aura[a]
	Hemiplegic	Often familial; hemiparesis may outlast headache by several days; may rarely cause facial palsy
	Ophthalmoplegic	Affects children (boys) mainly; pain around eye with impaired eye movement
	Vertebrobasilar	Affects adolescent girls mainly. Aura associated with ataxia, vertigo, diplopia; headache usually occipital; may be loss of consciousness at the onset
	Complicated	Any form of migraine complicated by residual neurological defect after attack
Migrainous neuralgia	Classic	Pain typically around the eye, often with visible effects of vasodilatation
	Facial migraine	Affects lower face (lower-half migraine)

[a]Migraine frequently lacks the 'classic' features and may not be strictly unilateral or there may be no aura. It is then difficult to distinguish from non-migrainous headache.

sensory, motor or speech disturbances. Visual phenomena are typically of zigzag flickering light (fortification spectra) or other transient visual defects. Sensory phenomena include paraesthesia or anaesthesia – usually of the contralateral upper limb, or face and mouth. Motor symptoms are mainly weakness – again of the contralateral upper limb. Epilepsy is slightly more common in migraine sufferers than in the general population. Obvious vascular phenomena may be associated but are variable in character, and range from facial flushing and oedema on the affected side to temporary hemiplegia. Unilateral headache (hemicrania), which is usually severe, often becomes throbbing and generalized and may be associated with facial pallor, can last for hours or days. Photophobia and sometimes phonophobia, nausea and sometimes vomiting may be seen. The number, frequency, intensity and duration of migraine attacks vary widely, but they tend to diminish in frequency and intensity with increasing age.

General management

The diagnosis of migraine is clinical.

Migraine is usually managed with drugs and avoidance of precipitating factors but there is also a significant placebo factor in the relief of migraine. Spontaneous remissions are not uncommon and migraine tends to improve during pregnancy. In acute attacks, patients usually prefer to lie in a quiet dark room. Analgesics such as aspirin, acetaminophen or ibuprofen can be effective. Intranasal lidocaine can give early relief within 5 min in over half those suffering from migraine, but the pain returns after about an hour in half of the responders. Triptans, serotonin ($5HT_1$) receptor agonists, such as sumatriptan, are effective in up to 80% if given within 1 h. Possible adverse effects include nausea, dizziness, muscle weakness and, rarely, stroke or myocardial infarction. Triptans are contraindicated for patients taking monoamine oxidase inhibitors (MAOIs). Sumatriptan may cause coronary spasm and angina, or permanent neurological damage if given in hemiplegic migraine or with ergotamine.

If triptans are not effective, ergotamine given orally may abort an attack but, in many cases, absorption by mouth is too slow to be effective and a better alternative is to use it by inhalation from a Medihaler. Even so, ergotamine must not be used within 6 h of sumatriptan. The maximum permissible dose of ergotamine is 4 mg in 24 h; this must not be exceeded and treatment must not be repeated at intervals of less than 4 days. Ergotamine can cause peripheral vasospasm and gangrene, abdominal pain, nausea and vomiting. Ergotamine can also be given with caffeine, or as a suppository, which overcomes the problem of poor absorption if the patient is vomiting.

Antiemetics, such as metoclopramide, domperidone or buclizine, should be given orally early to overcome the autonomic dysfunction preventing gastric emptying. In severe cases of vomiting, an antiemetic such as metoclopramide or prochlorperazine by suppository may also be required.

If attacks of migraine are more frequent than two a month, the treatment of choice is prophylaxis with propranolol or another beta-blocker, but sometimes a serotonin antagonist (pizotifen or cyproheptadine) or amitriptyline is used. Pizotifen can cause drowsiness, and should be used with caution in renal disease, pregnancy, glaucoma or urinary retention. Low-dose aspirin may reduce attacks by 20%, probably by blocking prostaglandin production in response to stimulation of a 5HT (serotonin) receptor. Calcium-channel blockers, such as verapamil or nifedipine, may be useful alternatives. Methysergide may help but has dangerous toxic effects (retroperitoneal fibrosis and fibrosis of heart valves and pleura) and is therefore given only for refractory cases under specialist supervision.

Dental aspects

Dental procedures, such as tooth extraction, amalgam removal or the use of occlusal splints, are of no proven value in the management of true migraine.

Migrainous neuralgia (periodic migrainous neuralgia, cluster headaches, Horton neuralgia, superficial petrosal neuralgia, histamine cephalgia, Sluder headaches)

General aspects

Migrainous neuralgia is less common than migraine. It is a pain in the head and face, defined by the IHS as

unilateral excruciatingly severe attacks of pain principally in the ocular, frontal and temporal areas, recurring in separate bouts with daily or almost daily attacks for weeks or months, usually with ipsilateral lacrimation, conjunctival injection, photophobia and nasal stuffiness and/or rhinorrhoea.

Males are mainly affected and attacks often begin in middle age.

Occasionally, pain mimicking migrainous neuralgia is due to organic disease, such as ocular disease, lesions of the trigeminal, brainstem or in the middle cranial fossa near the midline, such as lesions involving the cavernous sinus, circle of Willis or pituitary. Presentation is then atypical.

Clinical features

Attacks of migrainous neuralgia are sometimes precipitated by factors shown in Box 13.5. Typical features are the onset of severe pain at night (classically at around 02.00), and clustering of attacks at the same time, for several weeks.

Migrainous neuralgia causes unilateral pain localized usually around the maxillary premolars, eye, forehead, cheek and temple (Table 13.10). Pain may occasionally be occipital, cervical

---

Box 13.5 Precipitants of migrainous neuralgia

- Alcohol
- Cocaine
- Exercise
- High altitude
- Histamine
- Hot baths
- Hypoxaemia
- Nitroglycerin

Table 13.10 Differentiation between migraine and migrainous neuralgia

	Migraine	Migrainous neuralgia
Sex mainly affected	Females	Males
Family history positive	Often	Rarely
Pain unilateral	Usually	Always
Frequency of attacks	<3 per week	May be daily
Time of attacks	Usually daytime	Often at night
Duration of attacks	Hours to days	Minutes to hours
Other features	May be aura, nausea and vomiting	May be nasal congestion and lacrimation

---

or scapular. Episodes, which commence and often terminate suddenly, last less than 1 h (often 30–45 min), and may recur from one to eight times daily. Autonomic features include flushing and/or sweating of the affected side of the face and features such as lacrimation, conjunctival injection and nasal congestion, and sometimes Horner syndrome.

General management

Migrainous neuralgia should be differentiated from migraine and other headaches (Table 13.10).

Diagnosis is clinical but, as similar symptoms may be related to tumours around the cavernous sinus and craniospinal junction, CT/MRI is indicated.

Precipitants should be avoided and oxygen inhalations help (pain relief from these is sometimes regarded as diagnostic). Other therapies include ipsilaterally applied intranasal lidocaine; triptans [usually sumatriptan (an antagonist of 5HT receptors), where there is neither hypertension nor coronary artery disease; zolmitriptan, rizatriptan, eletriptan or naratriptan are also available; ergotamine; butorphanol tartate nasal spray; capsaicin and pizotifen. Preventive (prophylactic) medications include ergotamine, propranolol, amitriptyline, cyproheptadine, diltiazem, lithium carbonate, prednisolone and verapamil. Neurosurgery may be required for those with intractable cluster headaches.

Dental aspects

Migrainous neuralgia must be distinguished from dental pain by the characteristic history and confirmation of the absence of a dental cause.

Short-lasting unilateral neuralgia with conjunctival injection and tearing

The short-lasting unilateral neuralgia with conjunctival injection and tearing (SUNCT) syndrome is seen mainly in males who have short-lasting unilateral attacks of pain in the periocular region accompanied by various autonomic disturbances, such as conjunctival injection, lacrimation, nasal stuffiness and rhinorrhoea, and subclinical forehead sweating. SUNCT is therefore similar to migrainous neuralgia but may occur in daytime. Only lamotrigine and gabapentin have been reported to prevent SUNCT.

Idiopathic stabbing headache (ice-pick pains)

Idiopathic stabbing headache is pain confined to the head and exclusively or predominantly felt unilaterally in the distribution of the first division of the trigeminal nerve (orbit, temple and parietal area), mostly in the orbital region. It often recurs in the same place, but may move to other places on the same side of the head or, less commonly, to the opposite side. Pain forms a single stab or a series of stabs; each stab lasts for seconds only and episodes recur at irregular intervals of hours to days.

Diagnosis depends upon the exclusion of structural changes at the site of pain and in the distribution of the affected cranial nerve. Indometacin is the only drug known to relieve idiopathic stabbing headache.

Chronic paroxysmal hemicrania

Chronic paroxysmal hemicrania is similar to migrainous neuralgia, but only sometimes comes at night and is rarely triggered by alcohol. In 20% it follows head injury or whiplash injury, and invariably it responds well to indometacin.

Cranial arteritis (temporal or giant cell arteritis)

General aspects

Cranial arteritis is an immunologically mediated vasculitis closely related to polymyalgia rheumatica, causing inflammation of the walls of medium-sized arteries with prominent giant cells, and obliteration of the vessel lumen and ischaemia of the part supplied. Women are predominantly affected, usually after the age of 55.

Clinical features

The most common complaint is severe unilateral throbbing headache, mainly in the temporal region. Associated features may be malaise, proximal muscle stiffness, weight loss and fever. The superficial temporal artery is typically prominent, tortuous and tender.

The most severe complication of cranial arteritis is ischaemia of the optic nerve causing blindness in up to 30%. Hemiplegia or myocardial infarction are also possible. Pain on mastication (misnamed jaw claudication) is seen in about 20% of cases and occasionally there is limitation of opening the mouth.

General management

Cranial arteritis should be suspected in an older patient who suddenly experiences headache associated with a warm, tender scalp vessel. There is no diagnostic serological test but erythrocyte sedimentation rate (ESR) is usually greatly raised. Serum levels of interleukin-6 and alkaline phosphatase may also be raised. Temporal artery biopsy is the one confirmatory diagnostic measure and even this may be negative as lesions are patchily distributed.

Because of the risk of eye involvement, it is obligatory to give systemic corticosteroids (60 mg prednisolone daily, reducing as the ESR returns to normal) as soon as the diagnosis is made to prevent this complication. The clinical response to the drug is rapid.

Dental aspects

Ischaemic pain in the muscles of mastication can cause severe pain when eating and has been reported in 20% of patients. A rare manifestation is ischaemic necrosis and gangrene of the tongue or lip.

OTHER CAUSES OF HEADACHE AND OROFACIAL PAIN (SEE TABLE 13.4)

Orofacial pain may be referred from the chest, particularly in ischaemic heart disease but occasionally in lung cancer. Headache can be a feature of many systemic diseases, such as any fever, hypertension, chronic obstructive airways disease or some endocrinopathies, and head injuries.

Head injuries

Headaches after head injuries, though common, do not normally persist. If they do, neurological advice must be sought to exclude intracranial haemorrhage. In the absence of neurological complications, persistent post-traumatic headaches may be due to compensation neurosis (Chs 10).

Raised intracranial pressure

Raised intracranial pressure is one of the most serious but also the least common cause of headache. It may be caused by malignant hypertension, a tumour, abscess or haematoma. The headache is severe and often worse on waking, but improves during the day. Nausea and vomiting are common and the headache is aggravated by straining, coughing, sneezing or lying down. Neurological attention is essential.

Skull disease

Headache is occasionally the presenting feature of diseases of the skull such as bony metastases or Paget disease (Ch. 16).

Meningeal irritation

Meningeal irritation, seen in meningitis or subarachnoid haemorrhage, provokes severe headache with nausea, vomiting, neck pain or stiffness (inability to kiss the knees) or pain on raising the straightened legs (Kernig sign). Urgent neurological attention is needed.

New daily persistent headache

Epstein–Barr virus appears to be associated with these headaches in young adults that recur daily but resolve spontaneously within a year.

Drugs

Facial pain may occasionally be induced by drugs (e.g. nitrites, vinca alkaloids, phenothiazines or even analgesics).

GENERAL MANAGEMENT OF HEADACHE AND OROFACIAL PAIN

Features of pain that need to be ascertained are previous episodes, duration, onset, site, nature, duration, moderating factors, referral and severity. Patients with headache should be evaluated initially by history supplemented by physical examination, including examination of the cranium, sinuses, ears and eyes, and mental and neurological status. Some differentiating features are shown in Table 13.11.

Investigations may need to include a full blood picture, basic blood chemistry and possibly endocrinological examination, as well as urinalysis, imaging (CT or MRI) and sometimes lumbar puncture, electroencephalography, electrocardiography or arteriography.

CRANIAL NERVE LESIONS

Cranial nerves can be damaged by trauma, infections, tumours, drugs or chronic diseases (e.g. diabetes, connective tissue diseases, leukaemia, sarcoidosis, midline granulomas, Behçet disease or demyelinating diseases; Table 13.12).

History and full neurological and physical examinations are essential aspects of assessment, including of people with cranial nerve lesions. Investigations that may be useful include: blood tests (full blood count, electrolytes, liver, kidney or endocrine function tests); CSF examination – lumbar puncture; electrophysiological studies (electroencephalography; EEG); imaging [plain radiography, CT, MRI and positron emission tomography (PET) – allows cerebral functional studies and opened the way for advances, such as single-photon emission computed tomography; SPECT].

OLFACTORY (IST CRANIAL) NERVE

The olfactory nerve permits the smelling of odours. Unilateral anosmia is often unnoticed but bilateral anosmia causes loss of ability to smell odours though, in practice, the patient may complain of loss of taste rather than of smell. Anosmia is common in upper respiratory infections and after head injuries, as the nerves may be torn as they pass through the cribriform plate and is experienced especially in Le Fort III fractures of the middle third of the facial skeleton. Olfactory neuroblastoma is a rare tumour linked tentatively to dental staff. An olfactory lesion is confirmed by inability to smell substances, such as orange, soap, coffee, and cloves or peppermint oil. Each nostril is tested separately. Ammoniacal solutions must not be used, as they stimulate the trigeminal rather than the olfactory nerve.

OPTIC (IIND CRANIAL) NERVE

The optic nerve is central to vision (Fig. 13.4) and can be damaged by trauma, glaucoma, raised intracranial pressure, neoplasms, radiation, toxins or drugs, resulting in impaired vision. Visual ability is tested by asking the person to read an eye chart. Peripheral vision is tested by asking the person to detect objects or movement from the corners of the eyes. The ability to detect light is tested in a darkened room by shining a bright light (as from a flashlight) into each pupil.

OCULOMOTOR (IIIRD CRANIAL) NERVE

Extraocular (orbital) muscles are complex but responsible for moving the globe. The medial rectus (supplied by the IIIrd nerve) moves the eye medially (adducts). The adducted eye is depressed by the superior oblique muscle (IVth nerve) and

Table 13.11 Differentiation of headaches and orofacial pain of different cause				
	TMJ pain-dysfunction	Psychogenic	Idiopathic trigeminal neuralgia	Migraine
Age (years)	20–30	35–60	50+	Any
Sex	F > M	F > M	F > M	F > M
Site	Temple, ear, jaws, teeth Usually unilateral	Diffuse, deep, sometimes across midline	Mandible or maxilla Unilateral	Any
Associated features	Click in TMJ, trismus	Life events, back pain, etc. Stress, fatigue	± Trigger area	± Photophobia Nausea Vomiting
Character	Dull, continuous	Dull, boring, continuous	Lancinating	Throbbing
Duration of episode	Weeks to years	Weeks to years	Brief (seconds)	Hours (or usually days)

TMJ, temporomandibular joint.

Table 13.12   Cranial nerves: main features, causes of lesions and testing

Number	Name	Main functions	How to test the nerve	Main lesion features	Main causes
I	Olfactory	Olfaction	With an odorous substance	Anosmia or hyposmia	Trauma Infection Neoplasm
II	Optic	Vision	Vision chart. Ask patient to stare at your face from about 12 in away and (with both eyes open and with each eye shut in turn) report if any part of your face is missing	Visual defect or blindness	Trauma Infection Neoplasm CVA Multiple sclerosis
III	Oculomotor	Most eye muscles	'Follow the moving finger' in a 'rugby post' configuration	Ptosis Dilated pupil Diplopia Eye points 'down and out'	Diabetes Trauma
IV	Trochlear	Superior oblique eye muscle	Look down at the tip of the nose	Diplopia Unable to look down when looking medially	Trauma
V	Trigeminal	Facial sensation, muscles of mastication	Touch the face, clench the teeth	Anaesthesia or hypo-aesthesia	Trauma Infection Neoplasm Multiple sclerosis Connective tissue disease
VI	Abducens	Lateral rectus eye muscle	Look to each side	Diplopia Unable to look laterally to the affected side	Trauma Neoplasm CVA Raised intracranial pressure
VII	Facial	Facial expression, taste	Smile, raise the eyebrows Test taste for sugar and salt	Facial palsy	Trauma Infection Neoplasm CVA Multiple sclerosis Connective tissue disease
VIII	Auditory/vestibular	Hearing and balance	Tuning fork	Impaired hearing or balance	Trauma Infection Neoplasm CVA Bone disease
IX	Glossopharyngeal	Pharynx sensation	Test gag reflex	Impaired gag reflex	Trauma Neoplasm
X	Vagus	Pharynx and larynx muscles, parasympathetic	Check for hoarseness, open wide and say 'Ah'	Voice changes Impaired gag reflex	Trauma Neoplasm CVA
XI	Accessory	Sternomastoid and trapezius	Test turning the head or shrugging shoulders	Weakness	CVA Trauma Infection (polio)
XII	Hypoglossal	Tongue muscles	Protrude tongue	Tongue deviation to affected side, and sometimes wasting	Trauma Neoplasm

CVA, cerebrovascular accident

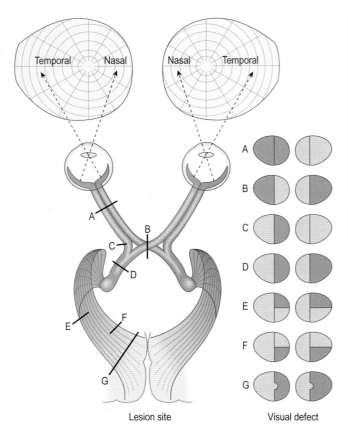

Fig. 13.4 Optic nerve lesions, site of lesion and resultant visual defects

Lesion site

Visual defect

elevated by the inferior oblique (IIIrd nerve). The lateral rectus (VIth nerve) abducts the eye. The abducted eye is depressed by the inferior rectus (IIIrd nerve) and elevated by the superior rectus (IIIrd nerve).

The oculomotor nerve thus supplies most of the orbital muscles (not the lateral rectus and superior oblique), as well as the ciliary muscle, the constrictor of the pupil, and the muscle that raises the upper eyelid. Disruption of the IIIrd nerve can be caused by extracranial causes (trauma, arteriosclerosis, diabetes, orbital apex disease, cavernous sinus disease, aneurysm of the posterior communicating artery) or supratentorial (raised intracranial pressure with uncal herniation). Disruption of the IIIrd nerve causes the following.

- Paralysis of internal, upward and downward movement of the eye. Lateral movement is retained.
- Double vision (diplopia) and a divergent squint with the affected eye pointing downwards and laterally – 'down and out' in all directions except when looking towards the affected side.
- Ptosis (drooping upper eyelid).
- A dilated pupil, which fails to constrict on accommodation or when light is shone either on to the affected eye (negative direct light reaction) or into the unaffected eye (negative consensual light reaction), i.e. a fixed pupil.

The upper eyelid is checked for drooping (ptosis). The pupils' response to light is checked by shining a bright light (as from a flashlight) into each pupil in a darkened room. The ability

to move each eye up, down and inward is tested by asking the person to follow a target moved by the examiner.

TROCHLEAR (IVTH CRANIAL) NERVE

The trochlear nerve supplies only the superior oblique muscle, which moves the eye downwards and medially towards the nose. Damage may be caused by vascular disease, diabetes, cavernous sinus syndrome, trauma or orbital apex syndrome. A trochlear lesion is characterized by:

- the head tilted away from the affected side
- diplopia, maximal on looking downwards and inwards, and causes difficulty descending stairs, or reading
- normal pupils.

The ability to move each eye down and inward is tested by asking the person to follow a target moved by the examiner. There is often damage to the IIIrd and VIth nerves as well.

TRIGEMINAL (VTH CRANIAL) NERVE

The trigeminal (= three twins) nerve supplies sensation over the face (apart from the angle of the jaw), scalp (back to a line drawn across the vertex, between the ears) and most of the mucosae of the oral cavity, conjunctivae, nose, tympanic membrane and paranasal sinuses (Fig. 13.5). Taste fibres from the anterior two-thirds of tongue are carried in the trigeminal nerve. The motor division of the trigeminal nerve supplies the muscles of mastication. Secretomotor fibres to submandibular and sublingual salivary glands and lacrimal glands are also carried in trigeminal branches Damage to the trigeminal can be extracranial [trauma (e.g. surgical, fractures), bone disease, drugs, multiple sclerosis, diabetes or tumours] or intracranial [trauma (e.g. surgical, fractures), inflammatory (infections, sarcoidosis, connective tissue disorders), tumours, cerebrovascular disease, syringobulbia, diabetes, bone disease, drugs or multiple sclerosis].

Trigeminal sensory loss (Table 13.13)

Normal facial sensation, mediated by the trigeminal, is important to protect the skin, mucosae and especially the cornea from damage. Loss of facial sensory awareness, which can be caused by lesions of a sensory branch of the trigeminal nerve or the central connections, may be completely lost (*anaesthesia*) or partially lost (*hypoaesthesia*). *Paraesthesia* does not mean loss of sensation; rather it means abnormal sensation, often 'pins and needles' or similar discomfort.

Extracranial causes of facial sensory loss are most common and include damage to the trigeminal from trauma, which is the usual cause – especially by inferior alveolar local analgesic injections, fractures or surgery (particularly lower third molar removal, osteotomies or jaw resections), mainly after orthognathic or cancer surgery. Rarely, endodontics or implants may be responsible. Ipsilateral lower labial hypoaesthesia or anaesthesia usually results. The lingual nerve may be damaged, especially during removal of lower third molars, particularly when the lingual split technique is used. Ipsilateral lingual hypoaesthesia or anaesthesia usually results. Occasionally the mental foramen is

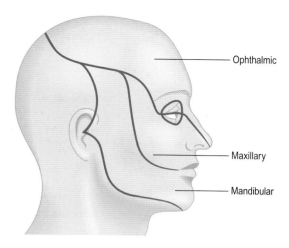

Ophthalmic

Maxillary

Mandibular

Fig. 13.5 Distribution of sensory divisions of the trigeminal nerve

Table 13.13	Causes of sensory loss in the trigeminal area	
Intracranial		
Congenital	Syringobulbia	
Acquired	Inflammatory	Multiple sclerosis
		Neurosyphilis
		Sarcoidosis
		Tuberculosis
		Connective tissue disease
		HIV/AIDS
	Neoplastic	Cerebral tumours
	Vascular	Cerebrovascular disease
		Aneurysms
	Drugs	Stilbamidine
	Occupational	Trilene (dry cleaning)
	Idiopathic	Benign trigeminal neuropathy
		Paget disease
Extracranial		
Acquired	Trauma	To infraorbital, inferior dental, lingual or mental nerves or middle cranial fossa fracture
	Inflammatory	Osteomyelitis
	Neoplastic	Carcinoma of antrum or nasopharynx
		Oral carcinoma
		Metastatic tumours
		Leukaemic deposits

AIDS, acquired immune deficiency syndrome; HIV, human immunodeficiency virus.

close beneath a lower denture and there is anaesthesia of the lower lip on the affected side, as a result of pressure from the denture. Damage to branches of the maxillary division may be caused by the following.

- Trauma (usually middle-third facial fractures).
- Bone disease (osteomyelitis in the mandible may affect the inferior alveolar nerve to cause labial anaesthesia). Paget disease is a rare cause of sensory loss.
- Malignant disease (oral carcinomas may invade the jaws to cause anaesthesia. Jaw metastases or malignant disease in the bone marrow may damage the nerve supply. Tumours such as carcinoma of the maxillary antrum may cause ipsilateral upper labial hypoaesthesia or anaesthesia. Nasopharyngeal carcinomas may invade the pharyngeal wall to infiltrate the mandibular division of the trigeminal nerve, causing pain and sensory loss and, by occluding the Eustachian tube, deafness (Trotter syndrome). Tumours around the skull base may also involve the trigeminal nerve. Numbness that spreads is a possible indicator of malignancy.
- Neuropathies (multiple sclerosis, diabetes, sarcoidosis, toxin).
- Drug-induced (e.g. mefloquine), infections [e.g. HIV, herpes simplex virus (HSV), syphilis, leprosy], amyloidosis or sickle cell disease.

Intracranial lesions affecting the trigeminal or connections are uncommon but serious, and include inflammatory disorders (multiple sclerosis, sarcoidosis, connective tissue disorders), infections (e.g. HIV, HSV, syphilis, leprosy), neoplasms (tumours around the Gasserian ganglion or posterior cranial fossa may involve the trigeminal nerve; numbness that spreads is a possible indicator of malignancy), syringobulbia or drugs.

Since other cranial nerves are anatomically close, there may be neurological deficits associated with intracranial causes of facial sensory loss. In posterior cranial fossa lesions, for example, there may be cerebellar features such as ataxia. In middle cranial fossa lesions, there may be associated neurological deficits affecting cranial nerve VI and thus mediolateral eye movements.

Benign trigeminal neuropathy is a transient sensory loss in one or more divisions of the trigeminal nerve that seldom occurs until the second decade or affects the corneal reflex. The aetiology is unknown, though some patients prove to have connective tissue disorder. *Psychogenic causes of facial sensory loss* include hysteria, and particularly hyperventilation syndrome. Facial sensation is mediated through the trigeminal nerve but the skin over the angle of the mandible is supplied by cervical nerves.

Trigeminal neuropathy or post-traumatic trigeminal neuropathy may develop after irreparable damage to the trigeminal nerve, most commonly after destructive procedures, such as rhizotomies used for treatment of trigeminal neuralgia, but also after craniofacial trauma (road traffic accidents), or dental or sinus trauma (e.g. Caldwell–Luc procedures).

Other causes of neuropathic pain can be metabolic (diabetes), inflammatory, infective (post-herpetic neuralgias), neoplastic and, rarely, after local analgesic injections.

Hypoaesthesia or anaesthesia may become associated with abnormal sensations or pain, related to excessive firing of pain-mediating nerve cells (phantom or deafferentation pain), which can start immediately or days to years later. Neuropathic pain may be burning, stabbing, stinging, or like an electric shock. Trigeminal neuropathic pain often presents as a constant, unilateral, often mild facial pain with prominent sensory loss, spontaneous and unremitting. In the most extreme form (anaesthesia dolorosa), there is continuous severe pain in areas of complete numbness.

Analgesics are rarely effective. The first-line treatment is with a tricyclic antidepressant, such as amitriptyline; gabapentin is the best alternative. Topical capsaicin, which appears to deplete substance P, may also be effective. Trigeminal nerve stimulation procedures may offer relief. More invasive procedures, such as brain surface (pre-motor cortex) stimulation or tractotomy, may be needed.

The blink reflex is tested by touching the cornea of the eye with a cotton wisp. Facial sensation is tested using a pin and a wisp of cotton. Strength and movement of muscles that control the jaw are tested by asking the person to clench the teeth and open the jaw against resistance.

Damage to a sensory branch of the trigeminal causes hypoaesthesia in its area of distribution, initially result in a diminishing skin response to pinprick and, later, complete anaesthesia. Lesions involving the ophthalmic division cause corneal anaesthesia: gently touching the cornea with a wisp of cotton wool (which the patient must not see), twisted to a point (corneal reflex), normally causes a blink, but not if the cornea is anaesthetic, or the facial nerve is damaged.

It is important, with patients complaining of facial anaesthesia, to test all areas but particularly the corneal reflex, and the reaction to pinprick over the angle of the mandible. If, however, the patient complains of complete facial or hemifacial anaesthesia, but the corneal reflex is retained or there is anaesthesia over the angle of the mandible, the symptoms are probably functional rather than organic.

Damage to taste can be tested with sweet, salt, sour or bitter substances carefully applied to the dorsum of the tongue.

Trigeminal motor neuropathy

Trigeminal motor neuropathy may occasionally be seen in isolation – possibly related to a viral infection. Trigeminal motor neuropathy is more frequently associated with trigeminal sensory neuropathy or due to lesions affecting the motor division of the trigeminal nerve when there are usually other cranial nerve deficits, sometimes caused by an intracranial tumour. Weakness may develop sometimes with masseter and temporalis wasting. Damage to the motor part of the trigeminal can be difficult to detect, is usually asymptomatic if unilateral but the jaw may deviate towards the affected side on opening. It is easier to detect motor weakness by asking the patient to open the jaw against resistance, rather than by trying to test the strength of closure.

ABDUCENS (VITH CRANIAL) NERVE

The abducens nerve supplies only the lateral rectus muscle. Damage to this nerve may be caused by vascular disease, cavernous sinus syndrome, trauma, orbital apex syndrome or raised intracranial pressure. Lesions can be surprisingly disabling, presenting with (Fig.13.6):

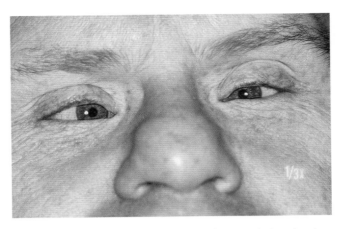

Fig. 13.6 Lesions of the abducens nerve. With the patient looking directly ahead, the affected left eye deviates medially as its lateral rectus muscle is functionless

- paralysis of abduction of the eye
- deviation of the affected eye towards the nose, and convergent squint – the diplopia is maximal on looking laterally towards the affected side
- normal pupils.

The ability to move each eye outward beyond the midline is tested by asking the person to look to the side.

FACIAL (VIITH CRANIAL) NERVE

The facial nerve is the motor supply to the muscles of facial expression (Fig. 13.7), but it also carries taste sensation from the anterior two-thirds of the tongue (via the chorda tympani), secretomotor fibres to the submandibular and sublingual salivary glands and lacrimal glands, and branches to the stapedius muscle.

Causes of damage to the facial nerve include, especially, stroke, trauma and infection but are shown in Table 13.14.

The motor neurons supplying the lower face receive upper motor neurons (UMNs) from the contralateral motor cortex, whereas the neurons to the upper face receive bilateral UMN innervation. Thus an UMN lesion (e.g. stroke) causes

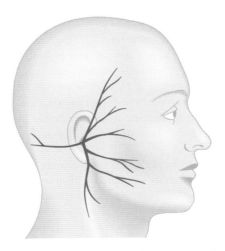

Fig. 13.7 Motor branches of the facial nerve to muscles of facial expression

unilateral facial palsy with some sparing of the frontalis and orbicularis oculi muscles (because of the bilateral cortical representation) and, although voluntary facial movements are impaired, the face may still move with emotional responses (e.g. laughing). Paresis of the ipsilateral arm (monoparesis), or arm and leg (hemiparesis), or dysphasia, may also be associated because of more extensive cerebrocortical damage.

In contrast, lower motor neuron (LMN) facial palsy (e.g. Bell palsy) is characterized by unilateral paralysis of all muscles of facial expression – for both voluntary and emotional responses.

In facial palsy, the forehead is unfurrowed, the patient unable to close the eye on that side and attempted closure causes the eye to roll upwards (Bell sign). Lacrimation is diminished in an VIIth nerve lesion but, because of the weakness, tears tend to overflow on to the cheek (epiphora), the nasolabial fold is obliterated, and the corner of the mouth droops and saliva may dribble from it and cause angular stomatitis. On the affected side, food collects in the vestibule and plaque accumulates on teeth. Other defects such as loss of taste or hyperacusis may be associated.

Facial weakness is demonstrated by asking patients to smile, to close their eyes against resistance, to raise the eyebrows, to whistle or to raise the lips to show their teeth. The Schirmer test, carried out by gently placing a strip of filter paper on the lower conjunctival sac and comparing the wetting of the paper with that on the other side, may show reduced lacrimation. Taste is tested by applying sugar, salt, sour lemon juice or vinegar and bitter (aspirin, quinine, or aloes) on the tongue and asking the patient to identify each.

Bell palsy

Bell palsy is facial paralysis where no local or systemic cause can be identified, though it is now recognized to be a lower motor neuron palsy and mainly due to infection with herpes simplex virus. There appears to be inflammation of the facial nerve in the stylomastoid canal, sometimes with demyelination.

Similar features may occasionally be seen after other herpesvirus infections [e.g. varicella zoster virus (VZV), cytomegalovirus (CMV) and Epstein–Barr virus (EBV)], influenza viruses, retroviruses (e.g. HIV and HTLV-1), and other infections such as Lyme disease (*Borellia burgdorferi*). There are occasional associations with hypertension, lymphoma, Melkersson–Rosenthal syndrome, sarcoidosis, Crohn disease, connective tissue disorders, acoustic neuroma, Guillain–Barré syndrome, multiple sclerosis and a variety of other disorders (Table 13.14). Bell palsy is more common in pregnancy, diabetes, influenza, a cold or another respiratory illness.

Clinical features

There is acute unilateral facial paralysis (with no other paralyses) over a few hours, maximal within 48 h (Fig. 13.8). Pain in the region of the ear or in the jaw may precede the paralysis

Table 13.14 Localization of site of lesion in, and causes of, unilateral facial palsy

Muscles paralysed	Lacrimation	Hyperocusis	Sense of taste	Other features	Probable site of lesion	Type of lesion
Lower face	N	–	N	Emotional movement retained ± monoparesis or hemiparesis ± aphasia	Upper motor neuron (UMN)	Stroke Brain tumour Trauma HIV infection
All facial muscles	↓	+	↓	± VIth nerve damage	Lower motor neuron (LMN) Facial nucleus	Multiple sclerosis
All facial muscles	↓	+	↓	± VIIIth nerve damage	Between nucleus and geniculate ganglion	Fractured base of skull Posterior cranial fossa tumours Sarcoidosis
All facial muscles	N	±	N or ↓	–	Between geniculate ganglion and stylomastoid canal	Otitis media Cholesteatoma
All facial muscles	N	–	N	–	In stylomastoid canal or extracranially	Bell palsy Trauma Local analgesia (e.g. misplaced inferior dental block) Parotid malignant neoplasm Guillain–Barré syndrome Herpes simplex virus Lyme disease HIV infection Granulomatous disorders
Isolated facial muscles	N	–	N	–	Branch of facial nerve extracranially	Trauma Local analgesia

N, normal; +, present; ↓, reduced.

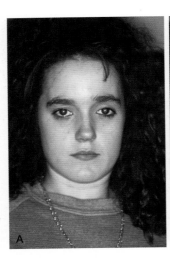
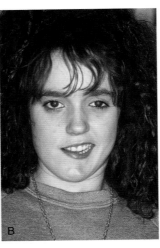

Fig. 13.8 Bell palsy: the right side of the face is completely paralysed, as demonstrated when the patient tries to smile (B)

by a day or two. Occasionally hyperacusis (oversensitivity to sound, due to loss of function of nerve to stapedius), or loss of taste (chorda tympani) on the anterior tongue, or changes in salivation/lacrimation are associated (Table 13. 14). Patients may complain of facial numbness, but sensation is intact on testing.

General management

Lower motor neuron palsy must be distinguished from upper motor neuron palsy (Table 13.15).

Electromyography (EMG) can confirm nerve damage and its severity. If paralysis is progressive, imaging of the internal acoustic canal, cerebellopontine angle and mastoid may be needed to exclude an organic lesion. Most patients with Bell palsy, however, are otherwise healthy, present no management difficulties and totally recover spontaneously within weeks. Nevertheless, active treatment is indicated and includes anti-inflammatory medication (short course of prednisolone may result in 80–90% complete recovery compared with about 50–60% in the absence of such treatment); antiviral medication (aciclovir or famciclovir); and facial massage (may help prevent permanent contractures of the paralysed muscles

during the acute phase; the cornea should be protected with an eye pad). Where paralysis is complete, only 50% recover completely within 1 week, but another 25% recover over 2 weeks or so. Few who have not recovered by 2 weeks will do so. Favourable prognostic signs are incomplete paralysis in the first week and persistence of the stapedial reflex, measured by electroneurography. Bad prognostic signs are hyperacusis, severe taste impairment and/or diminished lacrimation or salivation, especially in older, diabetic or hypertensive patients. Although many patients recover spontaneously, the after-effects in the remaining 10–20% can be severe and distressing, when surgical decompression of the nerve in the stylomastoid canal may be attempted. If paralysis persists and function remains incomplete, the palpebral fissure may narrow, the nasolabial fold deepens and facial spasm may develop. Rare complications, apparently caused by anomalous regeneration of the facial nerve, include irregular or anomalous lacrimation (crocodile tears) when the facial muscles are used, for example, during eating, retraction of the commissure when the eye is closed, or hemifacial spasm.

Dental aspects

In chronic palsy, construction of a splint to support the angle of the mouth may improve aesthetics to some degree, as may a facial graft or other manoeuvres such as facial–hypoglossal nerve anastomosis, but results are not always entirely satisfactory.

Ramsay–Hunt syndrome

Severe facial paralysis with vesicles in the ipsilateral pharynx and external auditory canal (Ramsay–Hunt syndrome) may be due to VZV of the facial nerve geniculate ganglion.

Bilateral facial paralysis

Bilateral facial paralysis is rare but may result from acute idiopathic polyneuritis (Guillain–Barré syndrome, Ch 37); sarcoidosis (Heerfordt syndrome, Ch. 37), arachnoiditis or posterior cranial fossa tumours.

Other causes of facial weakness

An apparent facial palsy may be caused by myasthenia gravis, some myopathies or Romberg syndrome.

VESTIBULOCOCHLEAR (VIIITH CRANIAL OR AUDITORY) NERVE

This nerve has two components, the vestibular (concerned with appreciation of the movements and position of the head) and the cochlear (hearing).

Damage to the auditory nerve can be caused by loud noise (explosions, music or occupations where loud sounds are produced), ageing, infections of inner ear and brain, drugs (e.g. aminoglycosides), trauma, stroke or multiple sclerosis. Damage to the vestibular component may be caused by infections (vestibular neuritis and labyrinthitis).

Table 13.15 Differentiation of upper (UMN) from lower motor neuron (LMN) lesions of the facial nerve

Action	UMN lesion	LMN lesion
Emotional movements of the face	Retained	Lost
Blink reflex	Retained	Lost
Ability to wrinkle forehead	Retained	Lost
Drooling from commissure	Uncommon	Common
Lacrimation, taste and hearing	Unaffected	May be affected
Tongue protrusion	Normal	Deviates to unaffected side

Lesions of the auditory nerve may cause loss of hearing, vertigo or ringing in the ears (tinnitus). An otological opinion should be obtained, as special tests are needed for diagnosis. Hearing is tested with a tuning fork or with headphones that play tones of different frequencies (pitches) and loudness (audiometry). Balance is tested by asking the person to walk a straight line.

GLOSSOPHARYNGEAL (IXTH CRANIAL) NERVE

The glossopharyngeal nerve supplies to the posterior third of tongue and the pharynx, and carries taste sensation from the posterior third of tongue, motor supply to stylopharyngeus and secretomotor fibres to the parotid. The glossopharyngeal can be damaged by infections, trauma, tumours or surgery in the cerebellopontine angle, pharynx or parapharyngeal space, and lesions are usually associated with lesions of vagus, accessory and hypoglossal nerves (bulbar palsy) and usually cause impaired pharyngeal sensation – so that the gag reflex may be weakened. Bulbar palsy is the term given to weakness or paralysis of muscles supplied by the medulla (tongue, pharynx, larynx, sternomastoid and upper trapezius; cranial nerves IX–XII inclusive). Acute bulbar palsy can be caused by poliomyelitis or diphtheria, chronic, progressive bulbar palsy by tumours or aneurysms of the posterior cranial fossa or nasopharynx, or strokes. Various other syndromes, some of which are rare, are tabulated in Appendix 13.2. Because the IXth and Xth cranial nerves control similar functions, they are tested together. The person is asked to swallow; to say 'aah' (to check movement of the palate and uvula); and the back of the throat may be touched with a tongue blade, which evokes the gag reflex in healthy people. The person is asked to speak to determine whether the voice sounds nasal.

VAGUS (XTH CRANIAL) NERVE

The vagus has a wide parasympathetic distribution to the thoracic and upper abdominal viscera and the motor supply to some soft palate, pharyngeal and laryngeal muscles. The vagus can be damaged particularly by trauma including neck surgery, in particular carotid artery surgery or thyroid surgery. Lesions of one vagus are rare in isolation but can cause impaired gag reflex, hoarse voice and bovine cough and, if the patient is asked to say 'aah', the soft palate moves towards the unaffected side.

ACCESSORY (XITH CRANIAL) NERVE

The accessory nerve gives the motor supply to sternomastoid and trapezius muscles. It can be damaged iatrogenically, surgically in neck resections or occasionally in lymph node biopsy or excision. Accessory nerve lesions are often associated with damage to the IXth and Xth nerves and cause ipsilateral sternomastoid weakness (on turning the head away from the affected side) and weakness of the trapezius on shrugging the shoulders. There may be an asymmetric neckline, a drooping shoulder, weakness of forward elevation of the shoulder, and a winged scapula – exaggerated on arm abduction.

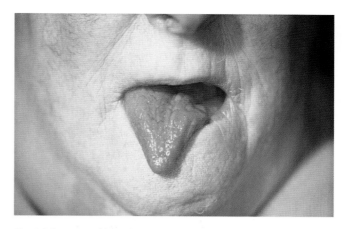

Fig. 13.9 Lesion of hypoglossal nerve with wasting of the left side of the tongue (lower motor neuron lesion)

Testing this nerve is also useful in differentiating patients with genuine palsies from those with functional complaints since, in an accessory nerve lesion, there is weakness on turning the head away from the affected side but those shamming paralysis often simulate weakness when turning the head towards the 'affected' side.

HYPOGLOSSAL NERVE (XIITH CRANIAL) NERVE

The hypoglossal nerve is the motor supply to the tongue muscles and may be damaged in its intracranial or extracranial course. A tumour or bone disease at the skull base, stroke, infection of the brainstem, or an injury to the neck, such as during endarterectomy, or amyotrophic lateral sclerosis, can damage the nerve. Intracranial lesions typically cause bulbar palsy (see later). Disease in the condylar canals, such as Paget disease or bone tumours, and peripheral lesions, such as glomus jugulare, carotid body or other tumours, trauma or radiation damage, can cause an isolated hypoglossal nerve deficit. In an upper motor neuron lesion the tongue is spastic but not wasted; in a lower motor neuron lesion there is wasting and fibrillation of the affected side (Fig. 13.9).

Hypoglossal lesions cause dysarthria (difficulty in speaking), particularly for lingual sounds, and deviation of the tongue towards the affected side on protrusion.

DISORDERS OF TASTE

The complex process of tasting begins when molecules stimulate special sensory (gustatory or taste) cells in the nose, mouth or throat. Another chemosensory mechanism, the common chemical sense, contributes to appreciation of food flavour, especially to sensations like the sting of ammonia, the coolness of menthol and the irritation of chilli peppers.

Humans can commonly identify at least five different taste sensations: sweet, sour, bitter, salty and umami (the taste elicited by glutamate, found in chicken broth, meat extracts and some cheeses). Flavours are recognized mainly through the sense of smell. Taste buds are present on the tongue mainly, but

Table 13.16 Causes of taste loss or change

Cause	Examples
Ageing	
Local causes	Xerostomia Irradiation of the oral cavity or salivary glands
Drugs	Antihistamines Antihypertensives Antidepressants Cytotoxic agents Protease inhibitors
Neurological disorders	Alzheimer disease Chorda tympani damage Facial palsy Head trauma Multiple sclerosis Parkinson disease Riley–Day syndrome Temporal lobe epilepsy
Nutritional defects	Cancer Vitamin B deficiency Zinc deficiency
Endocrinopathies	Addison disease Diabetes Cushing syndrome Hypopituitarism Hypothyroidism
Metabolic disorders	Chronic renal failure Hepatic disease
Viral infections	Various

also on the soft palate, uvula, epiglottis, pharynx, larynx and oesophagus. Taste perception can be tested with salt (sodium chloride), sweet (saccharin), acidic (citrus) and bitter (quinine) or by electrogustometry. Disorders of taste (dysguesia) are fairly common and have a wide range of causes (Table 13.16), similar to those causing halitosis.

Perceived loss of taste usually reflects a smell loss, which is often confused with a taste loss. The sense of taste can also be temporarily disturbed by the use of chemicals such as chlorhexidine.

Rarely there is complete lack of perception to taste sweet, sour, bitter, salty and umami (ageusia). More commonly, testing may demonstrate a weakened ability to taste (hypogeusia). In other disorders of the chemical senses, the system may misread and/or distort an odour, a taste, or a flavour. The most common taste complaint is of phantom taste perceptions. Alternatively, a person may detect a foul taste from a substance that is normally pleasant tasting.

Loss of taste can be due to medical disorders, or anaesthesia of the nerves involved, particularly surgery with lingual nerve damage (e.g. resections or third molar extraction); damage to the chorda tympani (from middle ear surgery, herpes zoster oticus, otitis media, mastoiditis or cholesteatoma); upper respiratory infections; head injury; radiation therapy; diabetes; hypertension; malnutrition; chemicals such as insecticides; some drugs (gymnemic acid abolishes the perception of sweet tastes while amiloride abolishes salt perception); or degenerative neurological diseases (Parkinson disease, Alzheimer disease and Korsakoff psychosis).

CEREBROVASCULAR ACCIDENTS, STROKES AND TRANSIENT ISCHAEMIC ATTACKS

GENERAL ASPECTS

The blood enters the brain from the two carotid and two vertebral arteries, which branch to supply each specific area of brain. If blood flow from these arteries is interrupted for more than a few seconds, brain cells can die, causing infarction and damage, resulting in loss of function – a stroke or cerebrovascular accident (CVA) – the syndrome of rapidly developing clinical signs and symptoms of focal and, at times, global disturbance of cerebral function lasting greater than 24 h (or death within that time).

Strokes are a common cause of death (the third leading cause of death, accounting for one out of every 15 deaths in the developed world) and disability, especially in older people. The high mortality relates not only to the acute brain damage but also to complications (thrombosis and infection, especially respiratory). A stroke may be preceded by a transient ischaemic attack (TIA) which, by definition, is characterized by a focal neurological deficit, which lasts less than 60 min and resolves completely within 24 h. Patients who have had a TIA are at high risk of a stroke and require prompt evaluation. A reversible ischaemic neurological deficit (RIND) is similar but persists for > 24 h; again, it is a predictor of a stroke.

The most common cause of CVA is carotid or intracerebral artery atheroma, in which plaque rupture results in arterial occlusion or thrombosis. An embolism from the left side of the heart (a potential complication of atrial fibrillation) may also obstruct cerebral blood flow and intracerebral or subarachnoid haemorrhages account for the other 20% of strokes. TIAs are typically embolic and cause focal cerebral and neurological deficits. Risk factors for CVA include increasing age, hypertension, atrial fibrillation, ischaemic or valvular heart disease, preceding CVA, diabetes, hypercholesterolaemia, smoking, alcohol, obesity, hyperviscosity syndromes, prothrombotic and haemorrhagic states. Emboli may also reach the cerebral vessels from fibrillating atria. Rarely, CVAs are secondary to carotid stenosis or dissection; cocaine use; fibromuscular dysplasia; or syphilis. Prevention involves controlling risk factors and taking more exercise.

CLINICAL FEATURES

The clinical manifestations vary according to the duration, severity and pattern of cerebral ischaemia. Typical features include sudden visual deterioration (monocular or homonymous), speech disturbance (expressive or receptive dysphasia) and hemiplegia (loss of voluntary movement of the opposite side of the body to the cerebral lesion). Most patients who sustain an ischaemic or haemorrhagic stoke remain conscious but, if the ischaemia, oedema or haemorrhage is extensive, raised intracranial pressure may impair consciousness – progressing to coma and/or death. Approximately 45% of people with a stroke die within a month; 50% of those who survive 6 months may survive another 7 years. Of survivors, 40% have mild disability, 40% require special care, 10% recover completely and 10% require long-term hospitalization. Prognosis is better in young patients and if there is incomplete paralysis of a limb, no loss of consciousness at onset or later, and no confusion.

Transient ischaemic attacks are typically embolic and may cause focal cerebral deficits such as facial numbness, hemiplegia or dysarthria, and about 30% progress to stroke. *Reversible ischaemic neurological deficit* is similar to TIA but persists for > 24 h.

Stroke-in-evolution is when such a cerebral deficit persists and worsens. Common symptoms include changes in vision, speech and comprehension, weakness, vertigo, loss of sensation in part of the body, or changes in conscious level.

Typical features of *full stroke* (Table 13.17) include: sudden unconsciousness often going on to coma or death; hemiplegia (loss of voluntary movement of the opposite side of the body to the brain lesion); changes in speech [slurred, thick, difficult speech or inability to speak (aphasia)] often with loss of the ability to write (both the result of a left-sided brain lesion); and visual loss or deterioration, especially in one eye. Other symptoms depend on the area of brain affected, the extent of damage, and the cause, but may include numbness, paraesthesia or other sensation changes, or recognizing or identifying

sensory stimuli (agnosia) resulting in 'neglect' of one side of the body; difficulty in understanding speech, reading or writing; vertigo; swallowing difficulties; personality or emotional changes, including depression or apathy; loss of bladder or bowel control; cognitive decline, dementia, easily distracted, impaired judgement and limited attention.

The four main types of stroke (Table 13.18) are as follows.

- *Cerebral arterial thrombosis*, the most common cause, follows atherosclerosis; it tends to be the least rapid in development and has lowish acute mortality (30%).
- *Intracerebral haemorrhage* mainly affects individuals past middle age and is the most lethal type with mortality of 80%. Bleeding into the brain destroys and tears apart the tissue and acts as an expanding lesion, distorting the brain and causing gross cerebral oedema. Predisposing factors are hypertension and atherosclerosis.
- *Subarachnoid haemorrhage* accounts for only about 10% of strokes, originates from a ruptured congenital aneurysm (berry aneurysm) on the arterial circle of Willis (more common in polycystic kidney disease, Ehlers–Danlos syndrome, fibromuscular dysplasia with renal artery stenosis, polyarteritis nodosa and coarctation of the aorta). Hypertension, atherosclerosis, trauma, cocaine or amphetamine abuse, and acute physical or emotional stress may be contributory. Clinically, subarachnoid haemorrhage is characterized by sudden, excruciatingly severe headache, which is quickly followed by coma; unlike other types of stroke, localizing signs, such as hemiplegia, are typically absent. In some cases slow aneurysm leakage causes headache or minor neurological dysfunction preceding the acute attack. The prognosis is poor: about 30% of patients die from the initial haemorrhage and only 50% survive.
- *Cerebral embolism* is relatively uncommon and usually originates from a fibrillating atrium or intracardiac thrombosis secondary to a myocardial infarct, rarely from endocarditis or a thrombosed prosthetic heart valve. Embolic strokes are *not* associated with activity levels, can occur at any time, and are typically dramatically sudden and may affect a younger person.

Table 13.17 Disability following stroke (see Table 3.22)

	Right-sided brain lesion	Left-sided brain lesion
Side paralysed	Left	Right
Other deficits	Thought, perception	Language, speech
Other problems	Memory Problems performing tasks and using mirrors	Memory Problems in organization

Table 13.18 Clinical features of different types of stroke

	HAEMORRHAGE		THROMBOSIS	EMBOLISM
	Intracerebral	Subarachnoid		
Prodrome	–	±	Transient ischaemic attacks (TIAs)	–
Onset	Rapid	Rapid	Gradual	Sudden
First symptom	Headache	Intense headache	Ill-defined	Headache
Progression	Hemiplegia and aphasia	Coma	Gradual and intermittent	Immediate
Underlying diseases	Hypertension Atherosclerosis	Aneurysm	Hypertension Atherosclerosis	Atrial fibrillation, etc.
Prognosis	High mortality	High mortality	From minimal dysfunction to death in a week	80% recur

GENERAL MANAGEMENT

Diagnosis of a CVA is essentially clinical, based upon a history and clinical features. Specific neurological, motor and sensory deficits often correspond closely to the brain damage location. Neck stiffness, Brudzinski sign (flexing the neck causes patient to flex knees and hips), and Kernig sign (flexing the hip 90° and straightening knee causes pain) become positive in subarachnoid haemorrhage. Examination may also show changes in vision or visual fields, abnormal eye movements, muscle weakness, impaired sensation and other changes. A 'bruit' may be heard over the carotid arteries in the neck. There may be signs of atrial fibrillation. It is also important to assess risk factors including co-morbid medical conditions. MRI or CT may localize the site and assess the degree of cerebral damage. However, MRI is not always possible and CT may be normal in the early stages of ischaemic stroke or in patients with minor symptoms. Cardiac investigations (electrocardiogram and echocardiogram) help in arrhythmias and valvular heart disease. Carotid duplex scans assess carotid artery stenosis and arterial blood flow to the brain.

Cerebral arteriography can identify a source of haemorrhage. Brainstem evoked response audiometry and clotting, thrombophilia and vasculitic screens may help. Blood biomarkers of stroke, such as S-100b (a marker of astrocytic activation), B-type neurotrophic growth factor, von Willebrand factor, matrix metalloproteinase-9 and monocyte chemotactic protein-1 have yet to be proved superior to conventional investigations.

Virtually all stroke victims or those with developing stroke should be admitted early to hospital for assessment and management, the goal being to prevent a stroke or prevent its spread, and to maximize the patient's ability to function. The time of the stroke, progression and conscious level (using the Glasgow coma scale; Ch. 24) should be recorded. Early treatment in a dedicated stroke unit lowers mortality and morbidity. Supportive care includes protection of the airway including appropriate ventilatory support; speech and language assessment; if swallowing is impaired, the patient should be kept nil by mouth and a nasogastric tube placed to reduce the risk of an aspiration pneumonia; pressure sensitive nursing to avoid the development of bed sores; urinary catheterization and incontinence pads if urethral and anal sphincteric reflexes are impaired; physiotherapy to reduce muscle wasting and disuse atrophy; and occupational therapy for long-term rehabilitation. The airway must be protected during the acute phase and, for virtually all strokes, hospitalization is required, possibly including intensive care and life support, and oxygen.

It is essential to establish the type of stroke since patients under good care have mortality reduced by 25% and recurrence by a similar amount. The degree of disability can be assessed according to one of several scales (e.g. the Barthel Index, Glasgow Outcome Scale, Hunt and Hess Classification of Subarachnoid Hemorrhage, Modified Rankin Scale or NIH Stroke Scale). Anticoagulation may help if it is certain that the stroke is thrombotic or embolic. Alteplase is recommended for ischaemic stroke. Recombinant tissue plasminogen activator (RTPA) lyses clots and potentially restores blood flow to the affected area to prevent further cell death and permanent damage, but there are strict criteria because of the risk of serious bleeding for those who can receive it. The most important is that the stroke victim be evaluated and treated by a specialized stroke team within 3 h of onset of symptoms. Aspirin and other antiplatelet drugs are also used to prevent non-haemorrhagic strokes.

Antihypertensive medication is frequently indicated. Control of atrial fibrillation is needed to prevent recurrent strokes. Analgesics are required to control severe headache. Nimodipine (a calcium antagonist) helps reduce intracranial vasospasm.

Surgical treatment may include emergency neurosurgery or interventional neuroradiology to clip or glue a leaking aneurysm, or evacuate a large intracerebral bleed. Carotid endarterectomy facilitates removal of atheroma to improve blood flow to the cerebral arteries.

Precautions must be taken in the later care of the comatose patient, to prevent pressure sores and sometimes urinary catheterization or bladder/bowel control programmes to control incontinence. If the person has swallowing difficulties, nutrients and fluids may be given through an intravenous line or via a nasogastric or gastrostomy tube. Longer term care involves rehabilitation, based on the symptoms, and prevention of future strokes. Recovery is possible as other areas of the brain take over functioning for the damaged areas. Depression and other symptoms should be treated. People should stay active within their physical limitations but safety must be considered, since some stroke victims appear to have no awareness of their surroundings on the affected side. Friends and family members should repeatedly reinforce important cues, like name, age, date, time and where they live, to help reduce disorientation. Communication may require pictures, demonstration, verbal cues or other strategies, depending on the type and extent of language deficit. In-home care, nursing homes, adult day care or convalescent homes may be required to provide a safe environment, control aggressive or agitated behaviour, and meet physiological needs. Visiting nurses or aides, volunteer services, homemakers, adult protective services and other community resources may be helpful. Speech therapy, occupational therapy, physical therapy, positioning, range of motion exercises, and other therapies may prevent complications and promote maximum recovery of function. Legal action may make it easier to make ethical decisions regarding the care of the person with organic brain syndromes such as stroke.

For TIAs or RIND, aspirin reduces the chance of progression to full stroke. Antihypertensive medication is frequently indicated. Otherwise, the investigations are as above for stroke.

DENTAL ASPECTS

Many patients with a stroke initially suffer confusion and emotional lability; therefore, encouragement is an extremely important motivating factor. Access, mobility and communication may be impaired in many, since they may have cognitive and visual defects as well as dysarthria, aphasia, confusion, memory loss and emotional distress and depression. Support with preventive care is critical; oral hygiene tends to deteriorate on the paralysed side, and impaired manual dexterity may interfere with toothbrushing. Use of an electric toothbrush or adapted holders may help.

Dentists should defer for 3–6 months elective and invasive dental care. It is important to communicate clearly with the patient by not wearing a mask, by facing the patient and by speaking slowly, clearly and using language that is not complex. Short treatment sessions in mid-morning are desirable for these patients, who are best treated in the upright position, with extra care taken to avoid foreign bodies from entering the pharynx. The practitioner needs to monitor blood pressure and anticoagulation status before beginning any dental treatment.

Dental management modifications in a patient with a stroke may also include consideration of problems of loss of protective reflexes, such as swallowing and gag reflexes in brainstem lesions. Patients are best treated sitting upright and extra care must be taken to avoid foreign bodies entering the pharynx. Good suction must be at hand.

Subarachnoid or cerebral haemorrhage can be precipitated by acute hypertension and, in the past, has resulted from the use of norepinephrine in LA. Cerebral haemorrhage can also result from hypertension caused by interactions of monoamine oxidase inhibitors with other drugs, particularly pethidine. Opioids are best avoided in strokes as they may cause severe hypotension. It is thus important to have short stress-free treatment sessions in mid-morning and to monitor blood pressure; use the minimal amount of epinephrine in LA; avoid the use of epinephrine-containing gingival retraction cords; and possibly avoid electronic dental analgesia.

Multidisciplinary care is required for modifications related to anticoagulation, hypertension, cardiovascular disease, diabetes mellitus or old age.

Patients after a stroke may have unilateral (upper motor neuron) facial palsy. Oral hygiene tends to deteriorate on the paralysed side and impaired manual dexterity may interfere with toothbrushing. An electric toothbrush may help. Oropharyngeal dysphagia post-stroke in around 50% of patients has a significant contribution to morbidity and mortality, since it predisposes to respiratory infection, malnutrition and weight loss.

Strokes are a possible cause of sudden loss of consciousness in the dental surgery and should be recognizable, especially by the sudden loss of consciousness and, usually, signs of one-sided paralysis as already described. Protection of the airway and a call for an ambulance are the only useful immediate measure (Ch. 1).

Calcified atherosclerotic plaques may sometimes be detected on dental panoramic radiographs.

LOCKED-IN SYNDROME

Locked-in syndrome is a condition in which a patient is aware and awake, but cannot move or communicate due to complete paralysis of nearly all voluntary muscles. It is usually due to a brainstem lesion, such as a stroke, trauma, infection or tumour, but higher centres remain intact. Some patients can move certain facial muscles, most often some extraocular eye muscles. There is a 90% early mortality. Of survivors, most do not regain motor control, but assistive computer interface technologies may help patients to communicate.

MOVEMENT DISORDERS

Muscles may move without the person meaning them to. For example, tiny muscle twitches (fasciculations) may indicate nerve damage to that muscle. Other possible involuntary movements are rhythmic movements of a body part (tremor), twitches (tics), sudden flinging of a limb (hemiballismus), quick fidgety movements (chorea) or snake-like writhing (athetosis), all of which suggest motor incoordination due to basal ganglia disease. Muscle tone that is evenly increased (rigidity) may be due to Parkinson disease. Muscle tone is severely reduced (flaccid) immediately and temporarily after a spinal cord injury produces paralysis. Muscle tone that is uneven and suddenly increased (spasticity) may be due to a stroke or spinal cord injury.

One of the most common involuntary movements is a tremor, which may have many causes – essential tremor, Parkinson disease, Huntington chorea and cerebellar disease (Table 13.19).

PARKINSON DISEASE (PARALYSIS AGITANS)

General aspects

Parkinson disease (PD) is a common serious brain disorder causing trembling, muscle rigidity, difficulty in walking, and problems with balance and coordination, whose prevalence

Table 13.19 Motor abnormalities; terms, features and main causes

Disorder	Features	Main causes
Akathisia	Restlessness	Neuroleptic drugs
Akinesia	Lack of movement	Parkinsonism
Athetosis	Dystonia of limbs	Athetoid cerebral palsy
Chorea	Continual flow of jerky movements	Huntington and Sydenham chorea (rheumatic fever)
Clonus	Rhythmic contractions	UMN (upper motor neuron) lesions
Dyskinesia	Involuntary chewing or grinding	Phenothiazines
Dystonia	Sustained spasms causing abnormal posture	Phenothiazines
Fasciculation	Spontaneous contractions of muscle fibres	LMN (lower motor neuron) lesions
Hemiballismus	Chorea affecting half of the body	Subthalamic lesion
Rigidity	Limbs resist passive movement	Parkinsonism
Spasticity	Excess tone in arm flexors, leg extensors	Cerebral palsy; UMN lesion
Tremor	Rhythmic movements of a part at rest	Parkinsonism, anxiety, drugs, thyrotoxicosis, benign, or brain lesion. Worse with anxiety; better with alcohol, benzodiazepines or beta-blockers
	On intention to move	Cerebellar disease

increases with age. Parkinson disease affects mainly the basal ganglia with degeneration of the substantia nigra pigmented cells that normally release dopamine – the neurotransmitter between the substantia nigra and corpus striatum, which enables muscles to make smooth controlled movements.

Most PD is idiopathic and people who have an affected first-degree relative are at three times greater risk of developing it themselves. *PINK1* mutations tend to be diagnosed as the early-onset autosomal recessive form of PD. Parkinsonism may also be caused by cerebrovascular disease, head injury (particularly in boxers), drugs [particularly phenothiazines and butyrophenones (dopamine receptor blockers), valproate, metoclopramide and prochlorperazine], and (rarely) encephalitis lethargica (von Economo disease). Severe parkinsonism has followed the use of an illicitly manufactured opioid (MPTP; methyl phenyl tetrahydropyridine), and this led to the suggestion that many cases of apparently idiopathic disease are due to environmental toxins, such as pesticides, herbicides, manganese, heavy metals or carbon monoxide. PD is more common in people engaged in farming, living in rural areas or who drink well water. Lower oestrogen levels may also raise the risk of PD: menopausal women who receive little or no hormone replacement therapy (HRT) and those who have had hysterectomies may be at higher risk, while menopausal women using HRT appear to have a decreased risk.

Clinical features

The earliest features of PD can be as subtle as an arm that does not swing when walking, a mild tremor in the fingers, or soft or mumbling speech difficult to understand. The main features of established PD are shown in Box 13.6 and Fig. 13.10.

Many people with PD develop voices which become monotonous and very soft, a special problem for older adults because the voice may not be audible to a partner with poor hearing. Even the digestive tract functioning may slow down, causing problems with swallowing, digestion and elimination, and constipation is often a major problem. PD may cause either urinary incontinence or urine retention, and anticholinergic drugs used to treat the disease make it hard to urinate. Bradykinesia may progress to akinesia and total rigidity.

Complications of PD may include subtle psychiatric disorders, deformities of the hands and feet, ocular abnormalities, urinary and gastrointestinal disturbances and autonomic

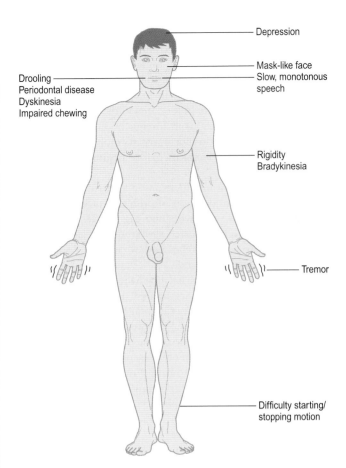

Fig. 13.10 Parkinsonism

dysfunction (which may cause mild postural hypotension, disordered respiratory control and hypersalivation that, with the movement defect, may result in drooling). The face in PD is often expressionless and there is a loss of the blink reflex as a response to gentle tapping of the bridge of the nose. Oculogyric crises may be seen in drug-induced or post-encephalitic disease.

General management

Supportive care is required. Treatment aims to enhance brain dopamine – but treatment with dopamine itself is impossible, since it fails to cross the blood–brain barrier. Drug treatment aims to increase dopamine by increasing L-dopa; by inhibiting dopamine breakdown; or with agonists of dopamine (Table 13.20). Dopaminergic drugs may cause daytime sleepiness. Anticholinergics also reduce tremor and they [or selegiline or catechol-*O*-methyl transferase (COMT) inhibitors) may be given together with levodopa in severe cases. Adenosine A(2A) receptor antagonists may prove useful in the future.

Deep brain stimulation (DBS), which involves implanting a brain stimulator, similar to a heart pacemaker, within the subthalamic nucleus, may control symptoms so well that medications can be reduced. The device can also be placed in the thalamus for tremor control or the globus pallidus to produce effects similar to pallidotomy.

Box 13.6 Features of parkinsonism

- Tremor – mainly affecting the hands (pill-rolling) and arms, and worst at rest. Tremors also may develop in the head, lips or feet
- Rigidity – the arms are flexed and held stiffly at the sides. Limb movement has a so-called cog-wheel rigidity
- Abnormal posture – the neck and shoulders are rigid, causing a stooping posture
- Restlessness (akathisia) is typical
- Slowness (bradykinesia) – slowness in the initiation and execution of movements and poverty of spontaneous movements. The patient may be slow at starting to walk but then runs forwards (festinant gait) or shuffles with slow short steps. This can make performing the simplest tasks difficult and time-consuming. Speech may be affected

Table 13.20   Drug treatment in Parkinson disease

Drug examples	Action	Comments
Levodopa (L-dopa); usually given with inhibitor of degradative enzyme dopa decarboxylase, e.g. carbidopa (co-careldopa) or benserazide (co-beneldopa)	Replaces dopamine	L-dopa is converted into dopamine in the brain, and may improve akinesia and imbalance. Adverse effects include involuntary movements (dyskinesia), nausea, arrhythmias, liver dysfunction, depression, psychoses and hallucinations. L-dopa is contraindicated in glaucoma
Bromocriptine Pergolide Lysuride Ropinirole Cabergoline Pramipexole Apomorphine (injection)	Dopamine agonists	Useful when L-dopa cannot be tolerated, but can cause hypotension or serious neuropsychiatric adverse effects, and pulmonary, retroperitoneal and pericardial fibrosis
Amantadine	Acts like dopamine agonist	An antiviral
Monoamine oxidase B (MAO-B) inhibitor (selegiline)	Inhibits monoamine oxidase B (MAO-B) and thus dopamine breakdown	Toxic reactions have occurred in some patients who took selegiline with the narcotic meperidine
Catechol-O-methyl transferase (COMT) inhibitors block the liver enzyme that breaks down dopamine	Inhibit dopamine and dopa breakdown	Tolcapone has been linked to liver damage and liver failure. Entacapone may help manage fluctuations in the response to levodopa in people with Parkinson disease
Benzhexol Benztropine Orphenadrine Procyclidine	Anticholinergics (block ACh)	Effective at reducing the tremor at rest.

Neurosurgery may reduce tremor but carries a number of risks, including slurred speech, disabling weakness and vision problems, especially when performed bilaterally. Thalamotomy, the destruction of small amounts of tissue in the thalamus, is useful to reduce tremor. Pallidotomy, use of an electric current to destroy a small amount of tissue in the pallidum (globus pallidus), may improve tremors, rigidity and slowed movement but benefits do not always persist.

Experimentally, brain grafts of fetal substantia nigral tissue have been given, but its value is as yet unclear, and one large study reported that as many as 15% of recipients developed severe dyskinesias as a result of *excess* dopamine.

Dental aspects

It is essential in patients with PD not to let the blankness of expression and apparent unresponsiveness be mistaken for lack of reaction or intelligence. Sympathetic handling is particularly important, as anxiety increases tremor, which may affect the tongue and/or lips. Patients should be raised upright only cautiously and carefully assisted out of the dental chair, since parkinsonism, L-dopa and some other agents may cause hypotension. The movements, drooling and head positioning associated with PD can make the use of sharp and rotating instruments hazardous and may compromise restorative care. Levodopa in combination with a dopa-decarboxylase inhibitor may interact with epinephrine to cause tachycardia, arrhythmias and hypertension. Epinephrine may interact with COMT inhibitors (tolcapone, entacapone) to cause tachycardia, arrhythmias and hypertension; therefore, LA without epinephrine should be used in these patients. Erythromycin and other macrolides may increase levels of bromocriptine or cabergoline. Pergolide may rarely induce cardiac valvulopathy; pramipexole may cause sudden onset of sleepiness.

Conscious sedation should be safe. Pethidine should be avoided in patients receiving selegeline or other MAOIs, since a serious interaction is possible. Selegeline differs from other MAOIs in that it should not cause acute hypertensive episodes with most other drugs.

Drooling of saliva may be troublesome: injection of botulinum toxoid into salivary glands significantly decreases saliva production, which may be beneficial. Orofacial involuntary movements (dyskinesia), such as 'flycatcher tongue' and lip pursing, are side-effects of levodopa and bromocriptine and may make the use of rotating dental instruments more hazardous.

Levodopa may cause taste disturbances and reddish saliva. Antimuscarinic drugs may produce dry mouth.

HUNTINGTON CHOREA

General aspects

Huntington chorea is an autosomal dominant condition related to a gene on chromosome 4 and the protein *huntingtin*. It is due to atrophy of the caudate nucleus of the basal ganglia, characterized by involuntary movements (chorea), emotional disturbances and progressive dementia, and currently is incurable.

Clinical features

The name *chorea* comes from the Greek for 'dance' and refers to the characteristic and incessant quick, jerky and involuntary movements.

Signs and symptoms usually appear in early to middle age (30–50 years) and may include: involuntary jerky movements of fingers, feet, arms, neck, trunk and face; hesitant, halting or slurred speech; clumsiness or poor balance; wide, prancing gait; and personality changes (moodiness, paranoia) and deterioration in cognitive function (memory, attention, decision-making).

Progress of disease is slow, often leading to difficulty walking so that patients become chair-bound. Life is often ended by intercurrent infection, or sometimes suicide, since patients are usually aware of the family history and poor prognosis.

General management

There is no satisfactory treatment available to stop or reverse Huntington disease and thus genetic counselling, though available, is not always taken up. A high-calorie diet may be advised as the involuntary movements can burn up considerable calories. Medications may help. Some signs and symptoms may be controlled by neuroleptics (e.g. clonazepam). Antipsychotics (e.g. haloperidol and clozapine) help control movements, violent outbursts and hallucinations. Speech therapy can help. Lithium can help control extreme emotions and mood swings. Fluoxetine, sertraline and nortriptyline can help control depression and the obsessive–compulsive rituals that some people with Huntington disease develop. Most people who have Huntington disease eventually become physically and mentally disabled, and therefore may require short-term psychiatric hospitalization and, as the disease progresses, long-term nursing care.

Dental aspects

Patients can often understand what they are being told but may be unable to respond; this can give a false impression of the degree of dementia.

There may be darting movements of the head and tongue that subside somewhat if physical control is applied. The chorea can make operative dentistry or the construction and wearing of prostheses difficult or nigh impossible; GA or conscious sedation may then help but with especial care to protect the airway at all times. Oral hygiene may be impaired through impaired manual dexterity and a predilection to caries and periodontal disease is worsened by medications that cause xerostomia or by a high-calorie diet unless thought is given to avoiding cariogenicity. Orofacial trauma may occur.

NEURAL TUBE DEFECTS (SPINA BIFIDA) (SEE CH. 28)

POLIOMYELITIS

General aspects

Anterior poliomyelitis (polio) is an enteroviral infection, spread faeco-orally, that may damage the lower motor neurons and sometimes motor cranial nerves. Rare in the developed world since the introduction of an effective vaccine, it is still common in the developing world, and appears in the

developed world in some immigrants, or where vaccine uptake is poor.

Clinical features

Typically causing wasting and paralysis of a lower limb, polio may affect other areas including the medulla oblongata when it can cause bulbar palsy and respiratory paralysis.

General management

Patients with respiratory paralysis must be permanently artificially ventilated (on an 'iron lung').

Dental aspects

Patients with bulbar palsy or a high-level spinal lesion may also have impaired gag and cough reflexes, and thus their airway must be carefully protected. Good suction must be used. Patients with quadriplegia may benefit from the dentist constructing a mouthstick or bitestick appliance with which they can perform manual functions or operate a computer, telephone and other means of communication. Those with paraplegia require care similar to persons with spina bifida (see Ch. 28).

SPINAL CORD DAMAGE AND PARAPLEGIA (SEE CH. 28)

ABNORMAL FACIAL MOVEMENTS
DYSTONIAS

Dystonias are a group of uncommon basal ganglia diseases characterized by abnormal movements associated with muscle spasm, and are focal or generalized. An example of focal dystonia is torticollis. Most dystonias are primary (a neurological disorder cannot be identified). Dystonias that result from defined organic diseases affecting the brain are known as secondary dystonias.

Oromandibular dystonia refers to recurrent spasmodic episodes of lip movement, tongue protrusion and retraction, and jaw clenching or opening. This may be associated with blepharospasm, and respiratory muscles and speech may be impaired. Over one-third of patients may suffer from depression. Treatment is difficult but benzodiazepines may be helpful.

Acute oromandibular dystonia (drug-induced parkinsonism) can appear within a short time (hours or days) of starting treatment with neuroleptics, such as phenothiazines and butyrophenones. It may resolve after withdrawal of the drug or be improved with antimuscarinics such as benztropine. However, it is made worse by levodopa, which can itself also cause involuntary spasmodic movements if the dose is too great.

TORTICOLLIS

Torticollis (from the Latin *torti* – twisted, and *collis* – neck) refers to the neck being held in a twisted or bent position. It can be congenital or acquired.

Infants born with torticollis appear healthy at delivery, but over days to weeks develop soft-tissue swelling over an injured sternocleidomastoid due to birth trauma or intrauterine mal-positioning. This mass, which may be confused with a branchial cleft cyst, regresses and leaves a fibrous band in place of the muscle, causing contracture of the neck.

Acquired torticollis or idiopathic spasmodic torticollis is a focal dystonia known as acute wry-neck; it is the type most frequently encountered, and develops overnight in young and middle-aged adults. Symptoms usually resolve spontaneously within 2 weeks with use of heat, massage, supportive cervical collar, muscle relaxants and analgesics. Torticollis may be associated with other forms of focal dystonia, such as blepharospasm, writer's cramp, spasmodic dysphonia or orobuccal dystonia.

DYSKINESIAS

Dyskinesias are abnormal movements of the tongue or facial muscles, sometimes with abnormal jaw movements, bruxism or dysphagia.

Common dyskinesias are involuntary tongue protrusion and retraction, and facial grimacing. Tardive dyskinesia is usually a late (hence tardive) complication of long-term treatment with neuroleptics. It is somewhat similar to oromandibular dystonia. It rarely responds to withdrawal of the offending drug, is usually made worse by giving antimuscarinics and may be resistant to treatment.

FACIAL TICS

Most facial tics are benign spasms (habit spasms) and usually affect children. Common tics are blinking, grimacing, shaking the head, clearing the throat, coughing or shrugging. Emotion or fatigue intensify tics but the natural history is of spontaneous remission. If persistent, haloperidol may be helpful.

GILLES DE LA TOURETTE SYNDROME

Tics and compulsive behavioural rituals sometimes including coprolalia (utterance of obscenities).

HEMIFACIAL SPASM AND BLEPHAROSPASM

Hemifacial spasm (clonic facial spasm) mainly affects adults, particularly older people with a spasm that affects especially the angle of mouth or the eyelid and worsens towards evening. Many cases of hemifacial spasm are idiopathic, but some herald a cerebellopontine angle lesion or other lesion and some follow facial palsy. Occasionally facial paralysis or trigeminal neuralgia follow.

Blepharospasm is a spasm of both eyelids that may be seen in the elderly in isolation, or with hemifacial spasm.

Local injections of botulinum toxin into the affected muscles may give relief for up to 3 months but must be given with extreme care, as there is a hazard of corneal exposure and glaucoma.

FACIAL MYOKYMIA

Facial myokymia is a rare but serious condition in which there are continuous fine, worm-like contractions of one or more facial muscles, especially the perioral or periorbital muscles. Facial myokymia must be distinguished from facial hemispasm, facial tics or blepharospasm (which involves several muscles synchronously), and from benign fasciculation and myokymia of the lower eyelid, which are quite innocuous.

Facial myokymia starts suddenly, lasts for variable periods and is unaffected by voluntary movements; it is frequently associated with multiple sclerosis, brainstem or posterior cranial fossa tumours or other neurological disorders. Neurological assessment is crucial.

MYOCLONUS

Myoclonus refers to a quick, abnormal, involuntary muscle jerk, that usually comes infrequently or many times a minute. In severe cases, it can distort movement and limit the ability to walk, talk and eat. Jerking leg movements while the person is at rest, used to be called myoclonus, but they are now referred to as periodic leg movements (restless legs syndrome). Myoclonus can be normal if it only affects persons as they fall asleep (hypnic jerks). However, it can also be a sign of drug adverse effects (e.g. amitriptyline); metabolic disorders, such as hepatic or renal failure or hyponatraemia; or CNS disorders, such as infection, viral encephalitis or Creutzfeldt–Jakob disease, brain damage (trauma or stroke), multiple sclerosis, epilepsy, Parkinson disease or Alzheimer disease.

Treatment of myoclonus usually is with anticonvulsants.

BOTULINUM TOXIN

Botulinum toxins are increasingly used, especially in cosmetic surgery, but they are neurotoxins and severe, life-threatening, respiratory muscle problems and death have occasionally occurred when the toxin has spread through the body.

Botulinum toxin type A is one of seven distinct neurotoxins produced by *Clostridium botulinum*. It has high specificity and potency, and *small* doses of purified, sterilized toxin may be injected to block the release of acetylcholine and thus temporarily paralyse muscles. It is widely used to paralyse facial muscles to improve the appearance of moderate to severe frown lines between the eyebrows (glabellar lines) or other wrinkles for up to 120 days.

Botulinum toxin type A [Botox (Allergan): BTX; Dysport (Ipsen); Xeomin (Merz Pharma)] has been used for an extensive range of conditions but the most evidence is that it can be useful to treat blepharospasm, hemifacial spasm and cervical dystonia. It also acts on cholinergic synapses in the autonomic nervous system, and injection into salivary glands significantly decreases saliva production, which may be beneficial for patients with sialorrhoea, such as in Parkinson disease or amyotrophic lateral sclerosis. There are no randomized controlled trials of botulinum toxoid in a range of applications (orofacial pain syndromes, cluster headache, chronic paroxysmal hemicrania, trigeminal neuralgia) and only a few small-sized trials in others (cervicogenic headache, chronic neck pain, temporomandibular disorders).

Botox should be injected no more frequently than once every 3 months, and the lowest effective dose should be used. Botulinum toxin type A is contraindicated for use in pregnancy and neuromuscular disorders. Air travel should be avoided for 72 h as decrease in pressure may affect distribution of the toxin. The most common adverse events following injection of Botox are generally temporary, but can last several months and include headache, respiratory infection, flu syndrome, blepharoptosis (droopy eyelids) and nausea. In less than 3%, adverse reactions may include pain in the face, redness at the injection site and muscle weakness. Botulinum toxin type A has occasionally caused severe, life-threatening breathing problems and death. These symptoms occurred as soon as one day and as late as several weeks after botulinum toxin type A injections were given.

Botulinum toxin type B (BoNTB; Myobloc) acts at a slightly different site from toxin A, and is used to treat cervical dystonia. It may cause severe xerostomia and many of the adverse effects seen with botulinum toxin type A. Botulinum toxin type B has occasionally caused severe, life-threatening breathing problems and death as soon as one day and as late as several weeks after injections were given.

DEMYELINATING AND DEGENERATIVE DISEASES

MULTIPLE (DISSEMINATED) SCLEROSIS

General aspects

Multiple sclerosis (MS) is the most common disease of young adults, especially women. There is a high prevalence in northern Europe and North America, and there may be a familial predisposition. MS is thought to be an autoimmune disease in genetically susceptible individuals, perhaps of viral aetiology, possibly due to human herpes virus 6 (HHV-6), with autoantibodies directed against myelin sheath proteins. It is a chronic relapsing disorder, characterized by formation of 'plaques' (areas of demyelination) throughout the CNS. Inflammation and damage to the myelin sheath with multiple areas of scarring (sclerosis) impairs muscle coordination, visual sensation and other nerve signals.

Clinical features

The hallmark of MS is a series of neurological deficits distributed in time and space not explained by any other causes. Up to 35% of cases are subclinical. Clinical features depend on the area of CNS affected and may include fatigue, dizziness, numbness, weakness or paralysis in a limb, brief pain, tingling or electric-shock sensations, tremor, lack of coordination or unsteady gait, visual disturbances causing diplopia or a moving field of vision and pain on eye movement (optic neuritis), urinary incontinence, constipation and sexual dysfunction, or cognitive changes (memory loss and impaired concentration). Nystagmus, ataxia, jerky (scanning) speech, tremors and loss of muscular coordination develop as a result of cerebellar involvement. Occasionally, mental changes, such as forgetfulness or confusion, occur. MS varies in severity and speed of evolution, ranging from a mild illness to one which results in permanent disability (Table 13.21). As the disease progresses, muscle spasms, vision loss, problems with bladder, bowel or sexual function, and paralysis may develop and, ultimately, there can be widespread paralysis and loss of sphincter control and urinary incontinence.

Table 13.21 Multiple sclerosis (MS) subtypes

Subtype	Frequency	Features
Relapsing–remitting	80%+	Short acute attacks about once each year
Primary progressive	10%	Progressive deterioration from outset
Secondary progressive	Uncommon	Progressive deterioration in patients with relapsing–remitting MS, after ≈10 years
Progressive–relapsing	Rare	Relapses in patients with primary progressive MS

General management

Diagnosis is assisted by MRI to identify demyelinating disease (T2-weighted MRI shows demyelinating plaques and gadolinium-enhancing lesions); delayed visual evoked response potentials (VEPs) and CSF examination may demonstrate a slightly raised white cell count, increased protein concentration and oligoclonal bands indicating intrathecal immunoglobulin synthesis.

Management requires a multidisciplinary team. Symptomatic care may include physical and occupational therapy, counselling and drugs.

There is no specific reliably effective treatment for MS, but acute episodes may be ameliorated by disease-modifying agents (DMAs) beta-interferons (interferon-beta-1b and -beta-1a) and glatiramer – an immunomodulator that shifts pro-inflammatory T helper 1 (Th1) cells to regulatory Th2 cells that suppress the inflammatory response. Neither interferon nor glatiramer is recommended by the National Institute for Health and Clinical Excellence (NICE) for the treatment of MS in England and Wales. Other potent anti-inflammatory agents like natalizumab (a monoclonal antibody that inhibits leukocyte migration in the CNS) and alemtuzumab are increasingly used, particularly in patients with breakthrough disease activity. Mitoxantrone – a topoisomerase inhibitor – may help in severe attacks. Intravenous immunoglobulin has a positive effect in relapsing and advanced MS. Corticosteroids promote remission in acute episodes but do not influence long-term prognosis. Low-dose methotrexate is also used. Oral fumarate appears to significantly reduce disease activity in relapsing–remitting MS. Experimental approaches include plasma exchange. Muscle relaxants (baclofen, tizanidine, dantrolene and benzodiazepine) may reduce pain from spastic muscle paralysis. Antidepressants (e.g. fluoxetine), the antiviral amantadine or modafinil (a medication used for narcolepsy) may reduce fatigue.

Dental aspects

There are no specific oral manifestations of MS but this diagnosis should always be considered in a young patient presenting with trigeminal neuralgia, particularly if bilateral, or if there have been other neurological disturbances, or if the pain lasts minutes or hours. It may respond to carbamazepine. Other presentations may include cerebellar tremor; abnormal speech;

abnormal perioral sensation, such as extreme hypersensitivity or anaesthesia; or facial palsy, myokymia or hemispasm. Atropinics used in treatment of bladder dysfunction may cause dry mouth, as may tizanidine. Glatiramer may cause facial oedema.

Dental preventive care and treatment are important since oral hygiene may be poor. Limited mobility and psychological disorders may interfere with routine dental treatment. Patients with severe MS are best not treated fully supine, as respiration may be embarrassed. Treatment is best carried out under LA if possible. Nitrous oxide is probably best avoided since it may theoretically cause demyelination. Some patients are on corticosteroids, with attendant complications (Ch. 6).

GUILLAIN–BARRÉ SYNDROME (INFECTIVE OR IDIOPATHIC POLYNEURITIS)

General aspects

Guillain–Barré syndrome (GBS) appears to be an immunologically mediated disorder mainly of peripheral nerves, which may follow bacterial infections (campylobacteriosis, from eating undercooked food, especially poultry); viral infections (approximately two-thirds of people affected by GBS have had an infection, such as sore throat, diarrhoea, cold or influenza, EBV or CMV infections within 4 weeks before the onset); or operations (5–10% of all cases).

Clinical features

Guillain–Barré syndrome can be devastating because of its sudden onset: signs and symptoms usually appear rapidly over the course of a single day, and may include weakness, paraesthesia or loss of sensation in legs and feet, or in arms or upper body, with hypaesthesia, paraesthesia or moderate pain throughout the body. Difficulty in breathing, eye and facial movement, speaking, chewing or swallowing, and paralysis of legs and arms may follow. There may be bradycardia, hypotension and difficulty with bladder or intestinal control. Generally, GBS progresses quickly, with most patients experiencing the most profound weakness in the legs, arms, chest and other areas within 3 weeks. In some cases, GBS may progress very rapidly with complete paralysis of legs, arms and respiration over a few hours. Recovery may take as little as a few weeks or as long as a few years, and up to 30% have some residual weakness after 3 years.

Miller Fisher syndrome is a rare variant of GBS, characterized by ataxia, ophthalmoplegia and areflexia.

General management

Diagnosis is confirmed by lumbar puncture and EMG. Hospitalization is required and treatment approaches include plasmapheresis, intravenous immunoglobulin and physiotherapy.

MOTOR NEURON DISEASE

General aspects

Motor neuron disease (MND) comprises a group of uncommon fatal neurodegenerative diseases affecting males, especially in old age, and causing damage to motor neurons (especially anterior horn cells; Fig. 13.11). The aetiology is unclear but may be viral; 90% of cases of the most common type are sporadic; a few others are due to a defect in the gene for superoxide dismutase, which normally protects against free radical damage.

Clinical features

There are three subtypes of MND. *Amyotrophic lateral sclerosis* (ALS) is the most common subtype and has an intermediate prognosis. It affects the anterior horn and pyramidal tract, begins in the hands, feet and limbs, then spreads to the trunk. UMN and LMN damage cause hand wasting and weakness and leg spasticity. Early signs and symptoms include cramps and twitching in arms, shoulders and tongue (the hypoglossal nerve may be affected); slow loss of strength and coordination in one or more limbs; weakness in feet and ankles, resulting in a stiff and clumsy gait and in dragging feet. ALS eventually affects bulbar functions such as chewing, swallowing, speaking and breathing but, even in the late stages, sensory, bowel, bladder and cognitive functions are spared. Involvement of the brainstem may lead to pseudobulbar palsy – bulbar palsy with emotional lability (involuntary weeping or laughing). ALS is relentless with respiratory paralysis and death within 5 years.

Progressive bulbar palsy affects brainstem anterior horn cells and thus cranial nerve motor neurons arising in the medulla (IX–XII inclusive), and has the worse prognosis, characterized by wasting, weakness and fasciculation of the muscles of the pharynx, tongue, palate, sternomastoid and trapezius.

Progressive muscular atrophy has the best prognosis, affecting anterior horn below the foramen magnum, causing LMN lesions with wasting and weakness starting in small muscles of the hands and spreading proximally.

General management

Diagnosis is clinical, based on the history and findings of muscle fasciculation, weakness, wasting, spastic dysarthria and exaggerated reflexes. Nerve conduction studies and EMG are confirmatory. Riluzole (an anti-glutamate) may slow the progress of ALS. Physical and occupational therapy, speech therapy, nutritional support and, eventually, breathing assistance are needed. Morphine or pethidine are frequently needed for terminal care.

Dental aspects

Oral hygiene may be impaired as in other conditions with disability. Weakness or paralysis in the neck and head can lead to dysphagia and drooling. Protection of the airway may also be impaired. Botulinum toxoid injection into salivary glands significantly decreases saliva production.

SYRINGOMYELIA

General aspects

Syringomyelia is cavitation of the spinal cord, of unknown aetiology, causing disruption of pain and temperature neurons of the anterior commissure. Syringobulbia is the term used if it affects the brainstem (usually the medulla).

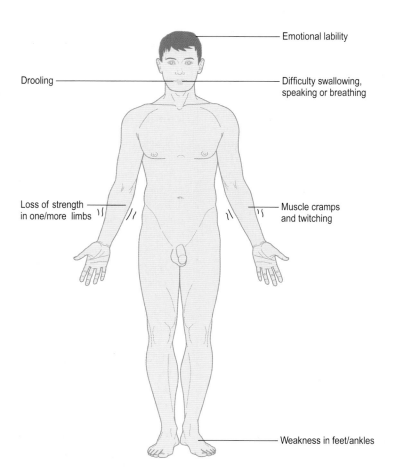

Emotional lability

Drooling

Difficulty swallowing,
speaking or breathing

Loss of strength
in one/more limbs

Muscle cramps
and twitching

Weakness in feet/ankles

Fig. 13.11 *Motor neuron disease*

Clinical features

Symptoms begin in adolescence or adult life and progress errat-
ically. Syringomyelia lead to segmental loss of pain and temperature but preservation of touch senses, leading to painless
ulcers, injuries or burns and deranged (Charcot) joints. Damage to sympathetic neurons in the intermediolateral column of
the spinal cord can cause Horner syndrome. Later, the pyramidal tracts may be involved, causing leg spasticity. Kyphoscoliosis
develops at an early stage.

Syringobulbia may also cause facial or oral sensory changes
or paralyses, but medullary damage rarely significantly affects
the respiratory or cardiovascular centres.

General management

There is no effective treatment. Patients should be protected
from injuries, especially from heat.

Dental aspects

Syringobulbia can cause facial sensory loss with unilateral palatal and vocal cord palsies, nystagmus, weakness and atrophy of
the tongue, dysphagia and dysarthria.

PATIENTS WITH RESPIRATORY PARALYSIS

Spinal cord trauma, infarction, haemorrhage, myelitis or
tumours, or poliomyelitis may cause severe and permanent
disablement, but the type of disability depends largely on the
level and extent of the lesion within the spinal cord. High-level
lesions can be fatal, or cause respiratory paralysis and quadriplegia. Lower level lesions may cause paraplegia and many of
the problems that afflict persons with spina bifida (Ch. 28).

ORGANIC BRAIN DISORDERS

Damage to focal areas of brain from trauma, stroke, tumours or
infections may lead to a range of defined neurological defects
(Table 13.22) and epilepsy, whilst damage that is more gross
may also cause coma or death.

More diffuse cortical damage can lead to acute or chronic
organic brain disease (dementia) and widespread brain dysfunction. *Acute organic brain disease* can have many causes (Table
13.23). Characterized by disorientation, anxiety, fear, hallucinations, delusions and impaired consciousness, patients with acute

Table 13.22	Defects resulting from brain cortex damage
Area damaged	**Examples of resulting defects**
Frontal	Anosmia, abnormal affect, difficulty in motivation/ planning, aphasia, perseveration, personality changes
Occipital	Cortical blindness, homonymous hemianopia, visual agnosia, impaired visual perception
Parietal	Astereognosis (failure to recognize common objects by feel), disorders of learned movements such as writing
Temporal	Memory impairment, cortical deafness, auditory agnosia, impaired musical perception

Table 13.24	Causes of dementia
Common causes	**Uncommon causes**
Alcoholism	Brain-occupying lesion
Alzheimer disease	Chronic traumatic encephalopathy
Hydrocephalus	Creutzfeldt–Jakob disease
Lewy body dementia	HIV infection/AIDS
Multi-infarct dementia	Hypothyroidism
Tumours	Huntington chorea
	Pick disease (frontal lobar atrophy)
	Syphilis
	Vitamin B_{12} deficiency
	Wernicke–Korsakoff syndrome

Table 13.23	Possible causes of acute organic brain disorders
Causes	**Mental complications that may result**
Chemicals	Various
Drugs	Various
Endocrine disease	
Acromegaly	Emotional lability
Addison disease	Apathy, mild recent amnesia
Corticosteroid therapy,	Euphoria
Cushing syndrome and disease	Euphoria or depression. Psychoses with delusions or hallucinations
Hypoglycaemia (in treated diabetes mellitus)	Confusion, dementia
Hypothyroidism	Impaired concentration, amnesia, depression, paranoia, acute confusion
Hyperparathyroidism with hypercalcaemia	Apathy, depression
Thyrotoxicosis	Anxiety and agitation, depression
Infections	See text
Trauma	See Ch. 24
Tumours	See text

Table 13.25	Diagnostic features of dementia		
Development of multiple cognitive defects	Cognitive disturbances	Language (aphasia) Motor activities (apraxia) Recognition (agnosia) Planning Organizing	
Memory impairment			

organic brain disease must be handled carefully with tact and reassurance, and may need sedation and psychiatric help (Ch. 10).

Chronic organic brain disease (dementia) is more common than acute, and probably affects 1% of those aged 60 years, doubling every 5 years thereafter so that, by age 85 years, up to 50% are affected. Dementia is not a feature of old age *per se* but has many causes; almost two-thirds is Alzheimer disease and one-quarter is multi-infarct (vascular) dementia (Table 13.24).

Everyone has occasional lapses in memory, especially with advancing age, and it is often quite normal to forget the names of people whom you rarely see, but it is not a normal part of ageing to forget the names of familiar people and objects.

Dementia is an acquired progressive loss of cognitive functions, intellectual and social abilities, severe enough to interfere with daily functioning, and characterized by amnesia (especially for recent events), inability to concentrate, disorientation in time, place or person, and intellectual impairment (including loss of normal social awareness; Table 13.25). Other less

specific symptoms include mood changes or paranoia. Anxiety, fear, hallucinations and delusions can be features.

Dementia is often accompanied by disruptive behaviour, and may be mimicked by acute organic brain disease, confusional states, drug-induced disorders and psychiatric disease.

Informed consent is a fraught issue in patients with dementia. They themselves are rarely able to give informed consent and, in many countries, relatives and staff have no legal right to give such consent on the patient's behalf. If a person is not capable of giving or refusing consent, and has not validly refused such care in advance, treatment may still be given lawfully if it is deemed to be in the patient's best interests. However, this should happen only after full consideration of its potential benefits and unwanted effects, and consultation with the carer(s), relatives and other people close to the patient.

ALZHEIMER DISEASE (ALZHEIMER DEMENTIA)

General aspects

Alzheimer disease (AD) is the most common form of dementia. It may affect 10–15% of those over 65 and 20% of those over 80 years of age.

Alzheimer disease is a neurodegenerative disease in which, according to the 'amyloid cascade hypothesis', there is abnormal processing of beta-amyloid precursor protein (betaAPP) into toxic amyloid-beta (Abeta) peptides. The hallmarks on histology are neurofibrillary tangles and argentophile plaques consisting of dying neurons clustered close to amyloid deposits. Tangles are threads of *tau* protein, normally responsible for the internal support structure for brain neurons. Plaques are made up of the normally harmless amyloid-beta. The brain degenerates, with reduced neurotransmitter levels, creating signalling problems and a progressive decline in memory and mental abilities. Similar brain changes can be seen in Down syndrome; both have a defect on chromosome 21, where the amyloid precursor protein (*APP*) gene is located. Mutations in this *APP* gene, or the presenilins PS-1 or PS-2, or inheritance of the apoplipoprotein E allele, are responsible for some cases of AD.

Clinical features

Alzheimer disease may manifest with slight memory loss and confusion and an inability to perform previously simple tasks, but eventually leads to decreasing cognitive skills and severe, irreversible mental impairment that destroys a person's ability to remember, reason, learn and imagine (Box 13.7).

Box 13.7 Changes in cognition (mental ability)

- Dementia (dysfunction of multiple cognitive functions)
- Difficulty performing common motor skills, such as combing one's hair, despite normal strength (apraxia)
- Difficulty in understanding or using language to speak or write (aphasia)
- Failing memory
- Inability recognizing familiar objects (agnosia)
- Inability performing simple arithmetic (acalculia)
- Inability sustaining concentration when performing a task
- Inability distinguishing right from left
- Poor visual–spatial comprehension (e.g. getting lost driving in a familiar area)

Features of anxiety and depression may also be present, often contributing to social difficulties and self-neglect. In advanced dementia, individuals may be disoriented in time, place and person. The ability to recognize family or friends, or carry out the simplest, once-routine tasks that require sequential steps, such as combing the hair or toothbrushing, decreases. There are also general deteriorations in motor skills and difficulties with abstract thinking, decision-making and finding the right word. People with AD may initially have trouble balancing their cheque book, a problem that progresses to trouble understanding and recognizing numbers. Eventually, reading and writing are also affected and inability to solve everyday problems, such as knowing what to do if food on the stove is burning, makes independent living impossible. Ultimately there can be disorientation and grossly inappropriate or bizarre behaviour, in which loss of a sense of time and dates, personality changes, delusions, mood swings or depression and disordered behaviour of many kinds may be associated. Patients may express distrust in others, show increased stubbornness and withdraw socially. Restlessness is also a common sign and eventually patients may even wander from home.

General management

The diagnosis depends on evidence of a progressive decline in cognitive function in the absence of focal neurological deficits and the exclusion of other organic disease such as hypothyroidism and vitamin B_{12} deficiency. Investigations include full blood count, renal and liver profiles, serum vitamin B_{12} and folate levels, syphilis serology, septic screen and MRI. Alzheimer disease differs from multi-infarct dementia as shown in Table 13.26.

Table 13.26 Comparison of Alzheimer disease and multi-infarct dementia

	Alzheimer disease	Multi-infarct dementia
Gender	F > M	M > F
Age at onset	70–90 years	60–80 years
Aetiopathogenesis	? possibly environmental/familial	TIA or stroke
Hypertension and ischaemic heart disease	±	+++
Onset	Slow, progressive deterioration	Acute and stepwise deterioration
Main symptoms	Cognitive loss	Emotional disturbance
Cognitive loss	Global	Patchy
Insight	Lost	Preserved
Personality	Lost	Preserved
Focal signs	±	+++

TIA, transient ischaemic attack.

Patients with dementia should be managed in the community if possible, although a detailed assessment by a psychogeriatrician is often needed. Treatment may involve management of concurrent problems, which may make dementia worse (e.g. respiratory or urinary tract infections); social services (supportive interventions for both patients and carers – long-term residential or nursing home care may become necessary); and drugs. Acetylcholinesterase inhibitors (donepezil, rivastigmine, galantamine) may slow intellectual deterioration. Tacrine is also effective but has liver complications. Gingka biloba may have some benefit. Selective Abeta-peptide-lowering agents (SALA) are being developed to counter the Abeta-initiated neurodegenerative pathology. Memantine use is controversial. An unexpected benefit of statins (HMG-CoA inhibitors) has been their effect on enzymes that generate Abeta-peptides. Glutamatergic agonist and Abeta-peptide immunization, however, have had little impact. Methylene blue is an innovation, promising in early clinical trials. Sedatives and antidepressants may help manage associated anxiety and depression.

In advanced AD, the inability of patients to care for themselves leads to: difficulty eating, incontinence and health problems, such as pneumonia and other infections; urinary incontinence which may require catheterization, and raises the risk of infections; and falls and their complications. Prolonged immobilization, which may be necessary to recover from injuries related to a fall, raises the risk of deep vein thrombosis and pulmonary embolism.

Dental aspects

Up to 75% of patients with AD require dental attention, but the chief problems are behavioural. It is crucial to anticipate future decline in oral hygiene. Carers must be involved. Attention to diet, oral hygiene and preventive care are important but after a time may no longer be practicable. Dental treatment should be planned with the knowledge that the patient may sooner or later become unmanageable for treatment under LA. In the early stages, dental appointments and instructions are forgotten. Later, there is progressive neglect of oral health as a result of forgetting the need, or even how, to brush the teeth or clean dentures. Dentures are also frequently lost or broken or cannot be tolerated. Deterioration of dental care together with hyposalivation can lead to destruction of the dentition by caries and periodontal disease and increase the problems of management because of difficulty in eating and halitosis. Periodontitis has even been suggested as an aetiological factor in AD. Injuries are also common in demented patients. Drugs, such as phenothiazines used to manage behavioural problems, may aggravate xerostomia and may cause dyskinesias. Loss of taste is common. Salivary substitutes may give some symptomatic relief.

Treatment should, as far as possible, be carried out in the morning, when cooperation tends to be best, and with the usual carers present in a familiar environment with care to explain every procedure before it is carried out and to avoid discomfort. Time-consuming and complex treatments should be avoided.

Access can be a serious handicap. Pre-operative sedation with a short-acting benzodiazepine or haloperidol may be required.

BRAIN TUMOURS

Brain (cerebral) tumours are second only to cerebrovascular lesions as a cause of neurological disease. Most are metastatic from carcinomas of the lung, breast, gastrointestinal tract and kidney, but primary cerebral tumours are also usually malignant. A possible relationship between brain tumours and dental radiography has been reported but not as yet confirmed. Intracranial lymphomas are a well-recognized feature of HIV disease and are rising in prevalence. In children, brain tumours account for approximately 2% of all cancer deaths but are second only to leukaemia as a cause of death.

Epileptiform fits developing for the first time in an adult are strongly suggestive of a cerebral tumour. Typical features of a tumour are localizing signs dependent on the site (e.g. convulsions or paralysis), and signs of raised intracranial pressure (headache, vomiting, papilloedema, lapsing consciousness, rising blood pressure and slowing pulse). Cerebral tumours, even those that are histologically benign, have a poor prognosis if not amenable to surgery.

ACOUSTIC NEUROMA (NEUROFIBROMA)

Acoustic neuroma is usually a benign tumour that arises from the neural axon or sheath of the vestibular part of the VIIIth cranial nerve, where it leaves the brainstem in the posterior cranial fossa. Bilateral acoustic neuromas are characteristic of neurofibromatosis type II. Clinically, it causes tinnitus (ringing in the ears), deafness and rotational vertigo (a sensation of spinning) and then postauricular pain, disturbance of balance, facial twitching or weakness and paraesthesia and, as the trigeminal, facial, glossopharyngeal and vagus nerves become stretched over the tumour, difficulty in speaking and swallowing – a

highly characteristic picture. The neuroma can be completely removed surgically in about 60% of cases.

PITUITARY TUMOURS

Adenomas are the most common pituitary tumours. Their endocrine effects dominate the clinical picture (Ch. 6) but they may compress the gland and cause hypopituitarism, or produce signs common to other cerebral tumours.

The craniopharyngioma arises from Rathke's pouch, an upgrowth from the primitive stomatodeum, may resemble an ameloblastoma or calcifying odontogenic cyst microscopically, and most manifest in childhood with headache, vomiting and papilloedema and visual defects. Short stature, delayed sexual development and diabetes insipidus may be associated. Suprasellar calcification may be seen, especially on CT.

Pituitary tumours can be removed, often through a transsphenoidal approach.

CENTRAL NERVOUS SYSTEM INFECTIONS
MENINGITIS

Meningitis is infection of the membranes (meninges) that surround the brain and spinal cord, and has a number of possible causes and sequelae (Table 13.27; and Ch. 21). Viral meningitis is usually fairly inconsequential and self-limiting. However, high fever, severe and persistent headache, stiff neck, nausea and vomiting may appear suddenly and require prompt medical attention since some forms, notably bacterial meningitis, are potentially fatal.

Bacterial (suppurative) meningitis
General aspects

A number of bacteria may cause meningitis, notably *Neisseria meningitidis* (meningococcus), *Streptococcus pneumoniae* (pneumococcus) and *Haemophilus influenzae* B (Hib; Table 13.27). *N. meningitidis* (12 serotypes are known) is carried in the nasopharynx and sometimes causes meningitis epidemics, mainly in children or adolescents. Most cases are caused by serogroups A, B and C, less commonly by serogroups W-135 and Y. Recent outbreaks have been of group B and C. Group B, type 15 meningococcus in particular, causes a severe form of the disease. Spread of bacteria to the meninges is by the bloodstream or occasionally as a result of a maxillofacial fracture involving the ethmoid cribriform plate (Ch. 24).

Clinical features

Meningitis is characterized by severe headache, nausea or vomiting, pain and stiffness of the neck, drowsiness, photophobia, fever, stupor or coma and, occasionally, convulsions. A purpuric rash is characteristic of meningococcal septicaemia, which, as a result of bleeding into the adrenal cortex, can go on to adrenocortical failure with vasomotor collapse, shock and death (Waterhouse–Friedreichsen syndrome).

Table 13.27 Causes and sequelae of meningitis

Causes			Comments
Infective	Viral	Enteroviruses: Coxsackie viruses, ECHO viruses and mumps	Thousands of cases occur each year, mostly affecting babies and children. Most common and usually self-limited to 10 days or less and a mild disease. Although most recover fully, some remain with serious and debilitating after-effects. Specific treatment rarely available
	Bacterial	*Neisseria meningitidis* (meningococcus)	Most cases in babies and young children. Uncommon. Around 7% die and 15% left with severe disability. Meningococcal disease describes meningitis and septicaemia, which can occur alone or more commonly together. Treat urgently with antimicrobials (benzylpenicillin or cefotaxime)
		Streptococcus pneumoniae (pneumococcus)	Most cases in babies and young children under 18 months of age. Increasingly important in adult life, particularly in those with impaired resistance (e.g. alcoholism or sickle cell disease). A life-threatening infection; 20% die and 25% left with severe and disabling after-effects. Intravenous ceftriaxone or cefotaxime (often penicillin-resistant), or if cause is unclear. Vaccine is available
		Haemophilus influenzae	Usually in babies and children under the age of 4. Hib vaccine significantly reduced cases. Treat with cefotaxime
		Listeria monocytogenes	Treat with amoxicillin plus gentamicin
		Mycobacterium tuberculosis	Usually originated from lungs, but in about 2% is haematogenous. Develops slowly. Difficult to diagnose and treat
		Group B streptococcus (*Streptococcus agalactiae*) and *Escherichia coli*	The most common causes in newborn babies. Risks higher for premature babies. Fatality rates as high as 20%
		Staphylococcus aureus	May complicate neurosurgical procedures
		Listeria monocytogenes	Associated with malnutrition and alcoholism
	Fungal	*Cryptococcus neoformans, Candida albicans*	Rare. Typically seen in immunocompromised people. Often develop slowly. Difficult to diagnose and treat
Non-infective	Physical injury Cancer Drugs Systemic lupus erythematosus		

General management

Diagnosis is confirmed with a Gram-stained smear, culturing and examining for meningococci by the polymerase chain reaction (PCR) from throat, lumbar puncture (CSF) specimen and blood. Antibiotic treatment should start immediately, even before microbiology results are available (Table 13. 00). If treatment is prompt, the overall mortality is low, but about 20% suffer permanent neurological damage (e.g. cranial neuropathies – blindness, deafness or palsies – epilepsy or learning impairment).

Patients with middle third maxillofacial injuries should be given prophylactic antimicrobials because of the danger of meningitis (Ch. 24). Family contacts of patients with contagious meningitis require chemoprophylaxis with rifampicin or ciprofloxacin. ACWY Vax is a meningitis quadrivalent vaccine that contains inactivated polysaccharide extracts of meningococci types A, C, W135 and Y.

BRAIN ABSCESS

General aspects

Brain abscesses usually arise secondary to middle ear, sinus or pulmonary infections, head trauma or infective endocarditis. Bacteria from periodontal pockets, particularly anaerobes, or periapical periodontitis are also a recognized focus for cerebral abscess; inhalation of a tooth fragment or materials used in dentistry can cause a lung abscess, which can metastasize to the brain with serious consequences. Patients with congenital heart disease, particularly those with right-to-left shunts, and those with hereditary haemorrhagic telangiectasia, are also at risk of brain abscess.

In immunocompetent persons, frontal lobe abscesses often result from sinusitis and contain a heavy growth of *Streptococcus milleri*. Sphenoidal sinusitis is notorious in this respect and can be difficult to diagnose. Post-traumatic or post-operative brain abscesses are often related to *Staphylococcus aureus*.

Temporal lobe abscesses often arise from middle ear mixed bacterial infections, with large numbers of anaerobes. In immunocompromised persons, brain abscesses may also be fungal (mainly *Candida*, *Aspergillus* or *Cryptococcus*) or protozoal (*Toxoplasma*).

Clinical features

Cerebral abscess causes signs and symptoms similar to other space-occupying lesions of the brain (i.e. headache, nausea, vomiting, diminished level of consciousness, hypertension, bradycardia and respiratory changes).

General management

Computed tomography and MRI are valuable in the diagnosis. Treatment is by immediate high doses of antibiotics (usually penicillin or metronidazole, or both) followed, where necessary, by aspiration or drainage. The mortality is still between 10% and 20%.

ENCEPHALITIS

Encephalitis (inflammation of the brain) is usually caused by viral infection. Symptoms include sudden fever, headache, vomiting, photophobia (abnormal visual sensitivity to light), stiff neck and back, confusion, drowsiness, clumsiness, unsteady gait and irritability.

Some cases are mild, short and relatively benign and patients have full recovery; others are severe, and permanent impairment or death is possible. The acute phase of encephalitis may last for 1–2 weeks, with gradual or sudden resolution of fever and neurological symptoms. Neurological symptoms may require many months before full recovery. No specific treatment is available unless it is caused by herpes simplex virus.

HERPETIC SIMPLEX ENCEPHALITIS

Herpetic simplex encephalitis is rare, although still the most frequent cause of encephalitis in temperate climates. Evidence as to whether it is a primary or reactivation infection is conflicting. Clinical effects are highly variable from early symptoms, such as disorientation, personality changes, hallucinations and ataxia, which can be mistaken for drunkenness or psychosis, to stupor, fits, paralyses and sensory loss. Coma is often pre-terminal.

Herpetic simplex encephalitis has often been fatal, particularly because confirmation of the diagnosis has had to be by brain biopsy, but the prognosis has improved greatly as a result of treatment with aciclovir and related antiviral drugs, which are frequently given on suspicion. The incidence of neurological damage among survivors has also declined.

NEUROSYPHILIS (SEE CH. 32)

HIV-ASSOCIATED NEUROLOGICAL DISEASE (SEE CH. 21)

PRION DISEASE (TRANSMISSIBLE SPONGIFORM ENCEPHALOPATHIES)

Transmissible spongiform encephalopathies (TSEs) are a group of fatal degenerative brain diseases (encephalopathies) characterized by the appearance of microscopic vacuoles in the brain grey matter, giving a sponge-like (spongiform) appearance. TSEs were originally termed slow virus infections – though no virus has ever been associated and current evidence points to the specific association with an abnormal form of a host-encoded protein termed a prion (proteinaceous infectious particle).

Prions are composed of a cell-surface glycoprotein PrP and accumulation in the brain of a protease-resistant isoform (PrP^{sc}) is the common mechanism of pathogenesis of TSEs. PrP^{sc} is remarkably resistant to inactivation by sterilization methods, and this presents significant infection control problems when patients with TSEs undergo health interventions.

All TSEs have prolonged incubation periods of months to years, gradually leading to death over months or years, with varying amounts of PrP^{sc} accumulating in the CNS.

There are several animal TSEs, including bovine spongiform encephalopathy (BSE; also known as 'mad cow disease') in cattle, and scrapie in sheep and goats. The classic example of a human TSE is Creutzfeldt–Jakob disease (CJD). Incubation periods in humans, after peripheral or oral exposure, range from at least 4 years to 40 years, with a mean of 10–15 years.

Infectivity in TSEs is highest in brain tissue, but also present in some peripheral tissues, not in most body fluids, including saliva. Animal studies show prions in the trigeminal nerve, tooth pulp, gingiva and salivary glands and the potential for prion transmission via the dental route. Prions do not evoke a protective immune response or detectable diagnostic antibodies. Nevertheless, attempts at vaccine production are under way.

Human TSE types are inherited, acquired or sporadic (Table 13.28), but are frequently referred to collectively as CJD. The acquired forms include kuru, iatrogenic and variant CJD. Overall, CJD affects approximately 1 per 1 000 000 of the population per annum across the world.

Table 13.28   Types of Creutzfeldt–Jakob disease (CJD)

Type	Abbreviation	Comments
Sporadic	sCJD	–
Familial	fCJD	Autosomal dominant
Kuru	–	Ritualistic cannibalism
Iatrogenic	iCJD	Contaminated surgical instruments; dura mater grafts or pituitary hormones
Variant	vCJD; sometimes termed nvCJD^a	Consumption of BSE-infected material

^{a}New-variant CJD
BSE, bovine spongiform encephalopathy.

Sporadic CJD (sCJD) accounts for about 85% of all cases of CJD. The underlying cause is unknown but it commonly develops in middle to late life as a rapidly progressive multifocal dementia. Up to a third of patients have non-specific prodromal symptoms, such as insomnia, fatigue, depression, weight loss, headache, malaise and pain. Over weeks there is rapid progression to akinetic mutism, with mental deterioration, myoclonus, extrapyramidal and pyramidal signs, cerebellar ataxia and cortical blindness. EEG shows characteristic changes.

Familial CJD (fCJD), which accounts for around 10% of cases, includes rare autosomal dominant disorders that manifest in early to middle adult life. *Fatal familial insomnia* is characterized by progressive insomnia, dysautonomia, disruption of circadian rhythms, motor dysfunction and deterioration in cognition. *Gerstmann–Straussler–Scheinker syndrome* is distinct, with many PrP^{sc}-positive plaques throughout the brain.

Kuru, first described in the 1950s, was endemic among the Fore ethnic group in the eastern highlands of Papua New Guinea and spread by cannibalism. Most cases were in children and women, who ritually consumed brains from deceased relatives. Typically there was progressive cerebellar ataxia but, unlike in CJD, dementia was not common.

Iatrogenic CJD (iCJD) can be transmitted mainly by exposure to cadaver-derived growth hormone, pituitary gonadotropins, dura mater homografting, corneal grafts or inadequately sterilized neurosurgical equipment. There is no evidence to suggest that any patients who have received dura mater allografts for the management of maxillofacial defects have developed iCJD. Concerns exist about the theoretical risk of the use of non-human animal-derived graft materials and heterologous human graft materials in oral or periodontal surgery.

Variant Creutzfeld–Jacob disease (vCJD)

General aspects

Bovine spongiform encephalopathy was first recognized in UK cattle in 1986, and it was eventually recognized that the infective agent was spread by the use of meat and bonemeal in cattle food. Then, in 1990, TSE appeared in domestic cats in the UK, suggesting transmission of TSE in pet foods, and that the causative agent was by no means species-specific. In 1996, a variant of sporadic CJD (variant or vCJD) was first observed in humans in the UK, and linked with the consumption of infected bovine offal. Pathological examination of the CNS revealed plaques of PrP^{sc} and a specific genetic predisposition, with all vCJD patients analysed being homozygous for methionine at codon 129 of the PrP gene. CNS, posterior orbit and (unusually for prion diseases) lymphoreticular tissue are, in descending order of risk, the tissues most likely to be infective. Transfusions of blood or blood derivatives can also transmit the prion, and plasma products were banned in 1998 and all donor blood has been leukodepleted since 1999. To avoid the possibility of transmission via infected brain tissue, recipients of human growth hormone were excluded from blood donation in 1989, and recipients of other human-derived pituitary hormones have been excluded since 1993. There may also be other potential but unproven sources of infection, such as products produced from cell lines grown in the presence of fetal bovine serum, some vaccines, and bovine products such as collagen.

Clinical features

Persons with vCJD have prominent early psychiatric symptoms (severe depression and behavioural manifestations) together with paraesthesias and dysaesthesias, followed by dementia, cerebellar and other neurological signs, myoclonus or other involuntary movements and, finally, akinetic mutism.

General management

The clinical course of vCJD is much longer than that of sCJD and affected patients do not have the same typical EEG changes. Tests and investigations that can contribute to a diagnosis include MRI, which shows characteristic bilateral symmetrical high signals in the thalamic pulvinar nuclei ('the pulvinar sign'). Other tests include blood tests for the genetic mutations, EEG, psychometric tests, CSF analyses to show a rise in the specific CSF proteins 14-3-3 and to exclude other infections. Tonsillar biopsy may help confirm a diagnosis of CJD.

There is no effective treatment for vCJD or other prion diseases. *In vitro*, some success has been achieved with quinacrine and chlorpromazine.

Dental aspects

Conventional dental treatment has no proven association with transmission of any form of CJD. However, PrP^{sc} is remarkably resistant to inactivation with heat, most disinfectants, ionizing, ultraviolet and microwave radiations. Concentrated bleach does appear to achieve inactivation and 20 000 ppm available chlorine of sodium hypochlorite for 1 h or 2M sodium hydroxide for 1 h are considered effective (Box 13.8) as is an enzyme (prionzyme).

Box 13.8 Recommended methods of inactivation of human and TSE agents

- 20 000 ppm available chlorine of sodium hypochlorite for 1 h
- 2M sodium hydroxide for 1 h
- Non-porous load steam sterilizer 134–137°C for a single cycle of 18 min, or six successive cycles of 3 min each[a]

[a]But known not to be completely effective.
TSE, transmissible spongiform encephalopathy.

Effective cleaning to remove adherent tissue, coupled with autoclaving significantly reduces infectivity levels on contaminated instruments if a non-porous load steam sterilizer is used at 134–137°C for a single cycle of 18 min or six successive cycles of 3 min each.

For the management of patients with TSEs, it is useful to divide them into three main groups, as follows.

- Confirmed cases of CJD – all instruments used for invasive procedures should be destroyed after use.
- Suspected cases of CJD (patients who present with a clinical history that is suggestive of CJD but a confirmed diagnosis is unavailable) – the instruments used for invasive procedures should be quarantined pending a confirmation of diagnosis.
- Cases 'at-risk' of CJD who are clinically well, include those 'at risk' by virtue of an inheritable defect in the prion protein gene producing familial CJD, and those who have been exposed to infectious material through the use of human cadaveric derived pituitary hormones, dural and corneal homografts (iatrogenic CJD).

Most guidelines recommend that surgical instruments used to operate on 'high-risk ' tissues (CNS, spinal cord and eye) in patients 'at-risk' of CJD should be disposed of by incineration. For interventions such as routine dental treatment, which do not involve 'high-risk' tissues, some national guidelines recommend the use of stringent instrument decontamination.

Dental health care staff infected or potentially infected with prion disease should not practise invasive clinical procedures in view of the risk of motor and cognitive dysfunction. Orofacial manifestations of human TSEs comprise dysphagia and dysarthia (due to pseudobulbar palsy) and, in vCJD patients, there may be orofacial dysaesthesia or paraesthesia or abnormal taste sensation.

BRAIN DAMAGE

Trauma, hypoxia, infections and hypoglycaemia are the main causes of brain damage.

CEREBRAL PALSY (SEE CH. 28)

HYPOXIC ENCEPHALOPATHY

Acute cerebral hypoxia is particularly important as it can readily cause brain damage: some patients can die and others suffer damage leading, depending on the age, duration and degree of hypoxia, to cerebral palsy, to epilepsy or to a persistent vegetative state.

Hypoxia can follow head injuries, airway obstruction, severe hypotension (e.g. cardiac arrest, shock syndrome, severe bradycardia, stroke) or impaired oxygenation (e.g. respiratory failure or during GA, when the anaesthetic agent can depress respiration, but there may also be partial, often unnoticed, respiratory obstruction). Cerebral hypoxia can remain unrecognized if the patient is already unconscious.

Cerebral hypoxia causes loss of consciousness in less than a minute but, if the blood circulation and oxygenation are restored within about 3 min, recovery should be complete. Hypoxia for longer than about 3 min causes brain damage and coma, with dilated pupils unresponsive to light, inert or rigid limbs, unresponsiveness to all stimuli, abolition of brainstem reflexes and ultimately no electrical activity on electroencephalography (brain death). *The most vigilant supervision of all patients with head injuries, and other patients undergoing or recovering from GA or sedation, is, therefore, essential.* Special care must be taken to ensure that the patient is respiring effectively, that oxygen supplies are adequate and maintained, and that no hypoxia, however slight, develops.

PERSISTENT VEGETATIVE STATE

'Persistent vegetative state' (PVS) is a term that describes the condition of patients with severe brain damage. Patients with PVS have no cerebral cortical function (they are unconscious and unaware), but exhibit irregular circadian sleep–wake cycles with either full or partial hypothalamic and brainstem autonomic functions, and persisting reflexes. PET scan studies have shown ≈50% decreased metabolic activity in the cerebral cortex and cerebellum of patients in PVS.

Patients in a PVS may be aroused by certain stimuli, opening their eyes if they are closed, changing their facial expressions, or even moving their limbs, and they may grind their teeth, swallow, smile, shed tears, grunt, moan or scream without reason. They may move their eyes, but this is merely reflexive and not indicating awareness if they neither fixate on a visual object nor track a moving target with their eyes. Nevertheless, despite no evidence of awareness, their heads and eyes can follow a moving object or move towards a loud sound. PVS is considered permanent when a diagnosis of irreversibility can be established based on the fact that the chances that the patient will regain consciousness are exceedingly small.

Patients with PVS need close medical and nursing support, similar to that for stroke victims, including attention to oral health.

EPILEPSY

Epilepsy is a predisposition for *recurrent* seizures, affects approximately 1% of the adult population and may reflect underlying brain pathology (injury, tumours or infections). A total of 10% of the population suffer at least one seizure in their lifetime, but mainly in childhood when it may be caused by febrile convulsions.

A seizure (fit) is a convulsion or transient disturbance in consciousness, caused by abnormal cerebral cortical electrical activity. Different causes prevail at different ages (Table 13.29).

Table 13.29	Causes of fits at different ages of onset
Age at onset	**More common causes**
Young child	Birth trauma, fevers, metabolic disease, congenital disease or idiopathic
Adolescent	Idiopathic or traumatic
Young adult	Traumatic, neoplastic, idiopathic, alcoholism or barbiturate abuse, acquired immune deficiency syndrome (AIDS)
Middle age	Neoplastic, traumatic, cerebrovascular disease, AIDS or drug abuse
Older	Cerebrovascular disease or neoplasm

Epilepsy is occasionally secondary (symptomatic epilepsy) to cerebral hypoxia; metabolic disturbances (hypoglycaemia or hyperglycaemia) and drugs (alcohol, amphetamines, anticonvulsants, barbiturates, benzodiazepines, cocaine and opioids) may predispose to epilepsy. Many cases, however, have no detectable structural or metabolic cause and are known as idiopathic – when it is likely there is a positive family history and a genetic predisposition (Box 13.9).

Epilepsy is more prevalent in the young and in the mentally or physically impaired. Most cases begin between the ages of 5 and 20 years.

Many seizures in epileptic people have no clear trigger but, in some instances, food and sleep deprivation, hormonal changes (e.g. pregnancy or menstruation), concurrent illness, metabolic disturbances, sensory stimuli (flashing lights, sounds and touch – even, very rarely, an electric toothbrush) and prescribed or illicit drugs (alcohol, chlorpromazine, enflurane, flumazenil, fluoxetine, ketamine, methohexitone, tramadol, tricyclic antidepressants) or their withdrawal may be implicated.

Box 13.9 Causes of epilepsy

Metabolic abnormalities
- Diabetes mellitus or hypoglycaemia
- Electrolyte imbalances
- Renal failure
- Nutritional deficiencies
- Inborn errors of metabolism e.g. Phenylketonuria (PKU)
- Use of, or intoxication from, or withdrawal from alcohol
- Use of, or intoxication from, or withdrawal from illicit drugs, especially cocaine and amphetamines; also alcohol, anticonvulsants, barbiturates, benzodiazepines, ecstasy, opioids

Brain trauma
- May affect any age, highest incidence in young adults
- Most likely if the brain membranes are damaged
- Seizures usually begin within 2 years after the injury
- Early seizures (within 2 weeks of injury) – do not necessarily indicate that chronic seizures (epilepsy) will develop

Brain tumours and other space-occupying brain lesions (such as haematomas)
- May affect any age, more common after age 30
- Partial (focal) seizures most common initially
- May progress to generalized tonic–clonic seizures

Cerebrovascular disease
- Most common cause of seizures after age 60

Degenerative disorders (senile dementia, Alzheimer disease or similar organic brain syndromes) mostly affect older people

Drugs

Infections, which may affect all ages
- Meningitis
- Encephalitis
- Brain abscess
- Acute severe systemic infections
- Chronic infections (e.g. neurosyphilis)
- HIV/AIDS or other immune disorders

Table 13.30 Classification and features of generalized and focal/partial epilepsy

Type	Subtype	Clinical features
Generalized seizures	Tonic–clonic (grand mal)	Loss of consciousness, tonic phase, clonic phase, tongue-biting, incontinence. Seizure lasts < 5 min
	Absence seizure (petit mal)	Brief period of unresponsiveness Duration of absences < 30 s
Partial seizures	Simple (Jacksonian epilepsy)	No impairment of consciousness Motor, sensory and autonomic features
	Complex (temporal lobe epilepsy)	Impaired consciousness Automatic repetitive acts

CLINICAL ASPECTS

The International League Against Epilepsy (ILAE) Classification of Epileptic Seizures (ILAE 1981), and ILEA 1989 are the two systems of classification in use. ILAE 1981 classifies seizures as:

- partial (seizures involving only part of the brain)
- generalized (seizures involving both sides of the brain) and
- unclassifiable.

A problem presented by this simple classification is that the same patient may have more than one type of seizure, either together or in sequence. ILEA 1989 is meant to supplement the 1981 classification, and classifies epilepsies as:

- localization-related (involves one or more distinct parts of the brain)
- generalized (involves both sides of the brain at the same time)
- undetermined whether localized or generalized
- special syndromes (Table 13.30).

In addition to seizures, there may be other features, such as headache, changes in mood or energy level, confusion and memory loss.

The main types of epilepsy are generalized seizures [grand mal (tonic–clonic)], when consciousness is typically lost, and partial seizures, which include simple seizures during which the person remains alert, along with abnormal movements or sensations. Generalized seizures are the most dramatic but partial seizures are the most common.

GENERALIZED: GRAND MAL (TONIC–CLONIC) EPILEPSY

Grand-mal epilepsy usually begins in childhood, or sometimes at about puberty. There is a warning (aura), followed by loss of consciousness, tonic and the clonic convulsions and, finally, a variably prolonged recovery. The aura may consist of a mood change, irritability, brief hallucination or headache. The attack then begins suddenly with total body tonic spasm and loss of consciousness. The sufferer falls to the ground and is in danger of injury. Initially the face becomes pale and the pupils dilate, the head and spine are thrown into extension (opisthotonos), and glottic and respiratory muscle spasm may cause an initial brief cry and cyanosis. There may also be incontinence and biting of the tongue or lips. The tonic phase passes, after less than a minute, into the clonic phase, when there are repetitive jerking movements of trunk, limbs, tongue and lips. Salivation is profuse with bruxism, sometimes tongue-biting and, occasionally, vomiting. There may be urinary or faecal incontinence, and autonomic phenomena such as tachycardia, hypertension and flushing. Clonus is followed by a state of flaccid semi-coma for a further 10–15 min. Confusion and headaches are common afterwards and the patient may sleep for up to 12 h or more before full recovery. The attack may occasionally be followed by a transient residual paralysis (Todd palsy) or by automatic or aggressive behaviour. This full sequence is not always completed.

Complications of major convulsions can be trauma (Fig. 13.12), respiratory embarrassment or brain damage, or progress to status epilepticus, but most seizures end without mishap. A major fit is so dramatic that it seems to be of longer duration than is in fact the case but, if it lasts more than 5 min (by the clock) or starts again after apparently ceasing, the patient must be regarded as being in *status epilepticus*, which is particularly dangerous – the mortality rate can be up to 20%. Brain damage may result from cerebral hypoxia, when tonic and clonic phases

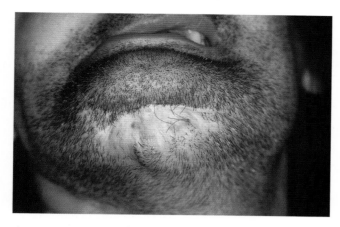

Fig. 13.12 Results of trauma in a person with epilepsy

alternate repeatedly without consciousness being regained and there can also be inhalation of vomit and saliva. *Status epilepticus is a medical emergency by causing severe hypoxia, and is potentially fatal.*

PARTIAL SEIZURES

Petit-mal seizures come most often during childhood and are characterized by minimal or no movements (except for eye-blinking) and an apparently blank stare; brief sudden loss of awareness or of conscious activity that may only last seconds; recur many times and involve learning difficulties (child often thought to be daydreaming). Most patients who have petit mal also have grand-mal attacks.

Simple partial (focal) seizures can be motor, sensory or behavioural, typically remain confined to one area, and include muscle contractions of a specific body part [focal motor epilepsy, which may take the form of clonic movements of a limb or group of muscles, usually in the face, arm or leg though the clonus may spread (march) to adjacent muscles on the same side of the body (Jacksonian epilepsy)]; abnormal sensations; sometimes nausea, sweating, skin flushing, and dilated pupils; sometimes other focal (localized) symptoms.

Partial complex seizures, or temporal lobe epilepsy (psychomotor epilepsy), are characterized by automatism (automatic performance of complex behaviours) such as lip-smacking and chewing movements, or facial grimacing; recalled or inappropriate emotions; changes in personality or alertness; sometimes disorientation, confusion and amnesia, or loss of consciousness; sometimes olfactory (smell) or gustatory (taste) hallucinations or impairments.

GENERAL MANAGEMENT

Disorders that may show features resembling seizures include transient ischaemic attacks, rage or panic attacks, and any disorder that causes loss of consciousness, tremors or tics. Witness accounts are invaluable. A physical examination, including a detailed neurological examination is indicated and may show focal neurological deficits but often is normal. CT and MRI are used to screen for cerebral pathology. An EEG records brain electrical activity and may aid in the diagnosis, usually confirming the seizures and may, in some cases, indicate the location of a lesion. It displays 3-Hz spike and wave activity in primary generalized absence seizures. However, a normal EEG does not completely rule out a seizure disorder. Tests for the cause may also include full blood picture, blood glucose, liver function tests, renal function tests, inflammatory markers (ESR, C-reactive protein), and CSF analysis to exclude infection.

Management of epilepsy includes patient education; identification and avoidance of precipitating or trigger factors; treatment of any identifiable predisposing pathology or disease; and prophylactic anticonvulsants. Anticonvulsants (Table 13.31) are of two broad groups – GABA or receptor potentiators, and neuronal inhibitors. Therapy is typically started with a single drug, raising doses until the disorder is controlled. A second-line drug is then substituted and some 50% will eventually be able to relinquish medication. However, most patients with major epilepsy having more than one attack in a year need to be maintained on anticonvulsants.

Table 13.31 Anticonvulsant treatment of epilepsy

Type of epilepsy	Drugs	Adverse effects[a]
Tonic–clonic seizure	Carbamazepine Phenytoin Sodium valproate Gabapentin	Skin rashes Blood dyscrasias Liver impairment
Absence seizure	Sodium valproate Ethosuximide	Sleep disturbance
Partial seizures	Carbamazepine Sodium valproate	As above

[a]Sodium valproate is best avoided in women of child-bearing age because of significant risk (5–7%) of fetal malformation.

A second drug should only be given *additionally* if a single agent in maximal dosage fails to control fits or causes undesirable toxic effects. Plasma anticonvulsant levels may sometimes need to be monitored, particularly with phenytoin where small changes in dosage can cause disproportionately large changes in plasma levels and toxic effects. Since treatment of major epilepsy is often lifelong, adverse effects can be a problem (Box 13.10).

Box 13.10 Possible adverse effects of phenytoin

- In large doses, nystagmus, ataxia and, possibly, cerebellar damage
- Gingival swelling, thickening of the facial features, hypertrichosis
- Folic acid deficiency and, occasionally, megaloblastic anaemia
- Enhanced catabolism of vitamin D, causing steomalacia, usually subclinical
- Lymphadenopathy with lymphoma-like changes histologically
- Slightly enhanced risk of lymphoma
- Allergy – rashes or lupus erythematosus-like reactions

Patients with epilepsy who are drowsy from medication should not operate unguarded machinery or drive. Epileptics may not drive a motor vehicle until they have been seizure-free for more than 1 year, or over a 3-year period have only had sleep attacks.

Anticonvulsants may interact with other drugs: some interfere with the oral contraceptives. Anticonvulsants in pregnancy, particularly phenytoin, are potentially teratogenic, but there is a greater risk to the fetus from uncontrolled epilepsy. Phenytoin (Epanutin), carbamazepine (Tegretol) and sodium valproate (Epilim) are all known to be teratogenic and can cause fetal anticonvulsant syndrome (FACS), which affects up to 10% of babies born to women taking anticonvulsants during pregnancy. Folic acid can reduce the risk of some of the congenital problems seen. Anomalies reported in FACS include spina bifida, cleft palate, and heart, kidney and limb malformations. The children also usually have distinctive facial features (prominent forehead, broad flattened nasal bridge, thin upper lip, medial deficiency of the eyebrows and infraorbital grooves), which may be particularly apparent in pre-school children but change towards normal as they mature. Anticonvulsant medication is also a risk factor for the development of an autistic spectrum disorder.

Valproate depresses platelet numbers and function to produce a bleeding tendency. Valproate may lead to adverse hormone changes in teenage girls and polycystic ovary syndrome in women who start taking the medication before age 20, so young female patients taking it should be monitored carefully by a physician. Non-steroidal anti-inflammatory drugs, erythromycin and benzodiazepines are also contraindicated.

Antiepileptic drugs should be continued during breast-feeding. Drug treatment should follow the same principles as for non-pregnant patients but plasma levels need to be monitored as they may fall during the later stages.

DENTAL ASPECTS

Dental treatment should be carried out in a good phase of epilepsy, when attacks are infrequent. Various factors can precipitate attacks (Box 13.11).

Box 13.11 Factors sometimes precipitating fits in susceptible subjects

- Withdrawal of anticonvulsant medication
- Epileptogenic drugs (Box 13.12)
- Fatigue, starvation or stress
- Infection
- Menstruation
- Flickering lights (television; strobe lights)

Those who have infrequent seizures or who depend on others (such as those with a learning impairment) may fail to take regular medication and thus be poorly controlled. When carrying out dental treatment in a known epileptic, a strong mouth prop should be kept in position and the oral cavity kept as free as possible of debris. As much apparatus as possible should be kept away from the area around the patient. Drugs can be epileptogenic or interfere with anticonvulsants, or can themselves be changed by anticonvulsant therapy and may, therefore, be contraindicated (Tables 13.32 and 13.33 and Box 13.12).

In the past, particularly, gingival swelling due to phenytoin required treatment by gingival surgery. Carbamazepine or gabapentin obviate this problem.

Table 13.32 Drugs used in dentistry that can increase anticonvulsant activity, leading to overdose

Aspirin	Can increase the bleeding tendency induced by valproate
Azole antifungals	Can interfere with phenytoin Can increase the bleeding tendency induced by valproate Can interfere with carbamazepine
Metronidazole	Can interfere with phenytoin Can increase the bleeding tendency induced by valproate
Propoxyphene	Can interfere with carbamazepine

Table 13.33 Drugs used in dentistry whose activity can be altered by anticonvulsants

| Acetaminophen | Hepatotoxicity may be increased by anticonvulsants |
| Doxycycline | Metabolism may be increased by carbamazepine |

Box 13.12 Drugs contraindicated in epilepsy

- Alcohol
- Chlorpromazine
- Enflurane
- Flumazenil
- Fluoxetine
- Ketamine
- Lidocaine (large doses)
- Metronidazole
- Quinolones
- Tramadol
- Tricyclic antidepressants

Aspirin, azoles and metronidazole can interfere with phenytoin. Propoxyphene and erythromycin can interfere with carbamazepine.

Large doses of lidocaine given intravenously for severe arrhythmias may occasionally cause convulsions. An overenthusiastic casualty officer may therefore blame a dental LA for causing a fit. There is no evidence that this can happen, especially as intravenous lidocaine has also been advocated for the control of status epilepticus.

Conscious sedation in epilepsy should be safe. Stress reduction should reduce the chance of a fit. Benzodiazepines are anti-epileptogenic, but occasionally fits have been recorded in epileptics undergoing intravenous sedation with midazolam. Flumazenil, however, can be epileptogenic. Nitrous oxide can increase the CNS depression in patients on anticonvulsants. It is probably best to avoid electronic dental analgesia.

Temporal lobe (psychomotor) epilepsy in particular is associated with paranoid and schizophrenic features. Antisocial and psychopathic behaviour may then make dental management difficult.

Acrylic is probably better used for prostheses than porcelain, as it is more resilient.

Convulsions may have craniofacial sequelae, especially lacerations, haematomas and fractures. Trauma frequently results from a grand-mal attack when the patient falls unconscious or from the muscle spasm, and a range of injuries can result [e.g. fractures of the vertebrae or limbs, dislocations, periorbital subcutaneous haematomas in the absence of facial fractures, injuries to the face from falling (lacerations, haematomas, fractures of the facial skeleton), fractures, devitalization, subluxation or loss of teeth (a chest radiograph may be required), TMJ subluxation, or lacerations or scarring of the tongue, lips or buccal mucosa].

FEBRILE CONVULSIONS

Febrile convulsions are more common than epilepsy, usually affect children and result from a rise in body temperature commonly caused by infection. Children who develop high fevers (above 38°C) should therefore be put in a cool environment, and bathed with tepid water and given acetaminophen elixir (*not* aspirin). Children under 18 months should be admitted to hospital since the fit may be due to meningitis. Severe febrile convulsions can cause brain damage and about 3% of children with febrile convulsions go on in later life to develop epilepsy; most do not.

PERIPHERAL NEUROPATHIES

Mononeuropathies are commonly caused by nerve compression (e.g. carpal tunnel syndrome) or by vascular disease. Polyneuropathies have a wide range of causes as seen in Box 13.13.

AUTONOMIC DYSFUNCTION

Many disorders can be associated with autonomic dysfunction, most importantly ageing, alcoholism, amyloidosis, diabetes, familial dysautonomia, liver failure, parkinsonism, porphyria and renal failure. Autonomic dysfunction manifests with: abnormal sweating (sometimes gustatory sweating), bladder dysfunction, dry mouth and eyes, gastrointestinal dysfunction, impotence and orthostatic (postural) hypotension. Autonomic dysfunction may also underlie sialosis.

Patients with autonomic dysfunction are sensitive to any agent causing hypotension, such as GA agents, and to being raised quickly from the supine position. Some have mitral valve prolapse.

HORNER SYNDROME

Horner syndrome comprises unilateral:

- miosis (constricted pupil), unreactive to mydriatics
- ptosis (drooping eyelid)
- loss of sweating of the face
- apparent enophthalmos (because of ptosis).

Box 13.13 Peripheral neuropathies

- Abuse of nitrous oxide
- Alcoholism
- Bell palsy
- Diabetes
- Vitamin B$_{12}$ deficiency
- Other, less common causes (see Appendix 13.1).

Horner syndrome is usually caused by interruption of sympathetic nerve fibres post-ganglionically, or at the cervical sympathetic trunk or in the spinal cord or brainstem. It may result, for example, from surgery or trauma to the neck, or bronchogenic or metastatic breast carcinoma infiltrating the sympathetic supply from the superior cervical sympathetic ganglion.

CHOLINERGIC DYSAUTONOMIA

Post-ganglionic cholinergic autonomic dysfunction may be autoimmune, characterized by impaired lacrimation and salivation, mydriasis, decreased gastrointestinal motility, bladder atony, sweating and taste disturbance.

RILEY–DAY SYNDROME (FAMILIAL DYSAUTONOMIA)

Familial dysautonomia, a rare autosomal recessive disorder found almost exclusively in Ashkenazi Jews, is characterized by selective damage to the sensory, motor and autonomic peripheral nervous system.

The main features are depressed pain sensation and impaired regulation of temperature and blood pressure. Aspiration pneumonias and episodes of acute abdominal pain are common.

Orthostatic hypotension can occur, so patients should be raised upright only cautiously. The other most important dental aspect is self-mutilation of hard and/or soft tissues. Splints may be used to protect the soft tissues.

Hypersalivation may be seen, the lingual fungiform papillae and taste sensation are diminished, and oral hygiene may be poor.

DISORDERS OF NEUROMUSCULAR TRANSMISSION

MYASTHENIA GRAVIS (SEE CH. 16)

SLEEP

Sleep affects daily functioning and physical and mental health. Sleep and wakefulness are controlled by neurotransmitters: brainstem serotonin and norepinephrine keep parts of the brain active during wakefulness, other neurons at the base of the brain begin signalling during sleep and 'switch off' signals that maintain wakefulness. Adenosine accumulates throughout waking hours, causing drowsiness, but gradually breaks down during sleep.

Sleep passes through stages 1, 2, 3, 4 and *REM* (rapid eye movement) sleep, then the cycle starts over again with stage 1. A complete sleep cycle takes 90–110 min on average, the first REM period usually occurring about 70–90 min after falling asleep, manifesting with breathing becoming more rapid, irregular, and shallow, eyes jerking rapidly, limb muscles becoming temporarily paralysed and the heart rate increasing; blood pressure rises and males can develop erections. REM sleep stimulates the brain regions used in learning, which may be important for normal brain development, which would explain why infants spend much more time in REM sleep than adults. The first sleep cycles each night contain relatively short REM periods and long periods of deep sleep and, as the night progresses, REM sleep periods lengthen while deep sleep decreases so that, by morning, most people spend nearly all their sleep time in stages 1, 2 and REM.

In stage 1, light sleep, the person can be awakened easily, eyes move slowly and muscle activity slows. In stage 2 sleep, eye movements stop and brain electrical activity subsides, with occasional bursts of rapid waves called *sleep spindles*. In stage 3, extremely slow brain waves called *delta waves* begin to appear, interspersed with smaller, faster waves. By stage 4, the brain produces delta waves almost exclusively. Stages 3 and 4, are called *deep sleep* and this is typified by lack of eye movement and muscle activity, and people awakened during deep sleep do not adjust immediately and often feel disoriented for several minutes after they awaken. Some children experience bedwetting, night terrors or sleepwalking during deep sleep. Deep sleep coincides with growth hormone release in children and young adults and increased production and reduced breakdown of proteins. Activity in parts of the brain that control emotions, decision-making processes, and social interactions is drastically reduced during deep sleep, suggesting this type of sleep may help people maintain optimal emotional and social functioning while awake.

Circadian rhythms are regular changes in mental and physical characteristics that occur in the course of a day (from Latin for 'around a day'), controlled usually by the body's biological 'clock' – the hypothalamic suprachiasmatic nucleus (SCN). The SCN receives information about the amount of light or darkness, and connects with the pineal gland, which produces melatonin. Tryptophan is converted to serotonin (5-hydroxytryptamine) and finally converted to the hormone melatonin (N-acetyl-5-methoxytryptamine). The less light there is, the more melatonin is released and nocturnal melatonin secretion may be involved in physiological sleep onset. At sunset, light cessation triggers the pineal to begin releasing melatonin and this rises, peaking around 2 am (3 am for the elderly), after which it steadily declines to minimal levels by morning. The melatonin regulates many neuroendocrine functions. The SCN has melatonin receptors and melatonin may have a direct action on the SCN to influence 'circadian' rhythms. The SCN also governs functions synchronized with the sleep/wake cycle, including temperature, hormone secretion, urine production and changes in blood pressure.

SLEEP DISORDERS

The amount of sleep each person needs depends on many factors, including age. Children generally require about 12 h a day, teenagers need about 9 h and most adults 7–8 h. Women in the first 3 months of pregnancy often need more. The amount of sleep needed also increases if a person has been deprived of sleep previously – a dangerous situation when operating machinery or driving. Too little sleep causes drowsiness and inability to concentrate, impaired memory and physical performance and reduced ability to carry out calculations. If it continues, hallucinations and mood swings may develop.

Foods can change neurotransmitters and affect sleep, as can drugs (e.g. alcohol, amphetamines, antidepressants, caffeine, cocaine, decongestants, dopaminergic drugs, ecstasy, hypnotics, pramipexole, sedatives, statins and valproate). Antidepressants may suppress REM sleep. Heavy smokers often sleep lightly, have reduced amounts of REM sleep and tend to wake after 3–4 hours due to nicotine withdrawal.

The ability to thermoregulate is lost during REM, so abnormally hot or cold environmental temperatures can disrupt sleep.

Sleep and sleep-related problems play a role in a large number of disorders (Table 13.34).

Insomnia

The best measure of the amount of sleep needed is how the person feels: if they awaken feeling refreshed, they are getting enough. Insomnia can affect almost everyone occasionally because of stress, jet lag, diet or many other factors, and insomnia tends to increase with age. It affects about 40% of women, 30% of men and over 50% of older people. Insomnia is a key symptom of depression and often the major disabling symptom of an underlying medical disorder (Table 13.35).

Insomnia can be a chronic and persistent difficulty in either: (1) falling asleep (initial insomnia); (2) remaining asleep through the night (middle insomnia); or (3) waking up too early (terminal insomnia). Insomnia almost always affects well-being and job performance the next day. Those who have insomnia frequently or for extended periods of time can develop even more serious sleep deficits.

Mild insomnia often can be prevented or cured by practising good sleep hygiene (habits; Box 13.14). For short-term insomnia, hypnotics may help. Counselling may be helpful for psychological disorders that lead to insomnia; antidepressants such as amitriptyline or trazodone can often help. Antihistamines, long-acting or high-dose sedatives can increase daytime drowsiness, over time making the problem worse, not better.

Table 13.34	Effects of disease on sleep
Disorder	**Sleep-related problems**
Depression	Often causes early morning wakening. Extreme sleep deprivation can lead to a seemingly psychotic state of paranoia and hallucinations in otherwise healthy people and disrupted sleep can trigger episodes of mania (agitation and hyperactivity) in people with manic depression
Epilepsy	REM (rapid eye movement) sleep seems to help prevent seizures, while deep sleep may promote the spread of these seizures. Sleep deprivation may trigger seizures
Infectious diseases	Cytokines are powerfully sleep-inducing
Pain	Hospital routines may disrupt sleep, and patients who are unable to sleep also notice pain more
Sleep apnoea	See Ch. 15
Stroke and asthma	Attacks tend to occur more frequently during the night and early morning, perhaps due to changes in hormones and heart rate

Table 13.35 Causes of insomnia (see Table 13.34)	
Causes	**Detail**
Disrupted waking hours	Jet lag, shift work, wake–sleep pattern disturbances, excessive sleep during day
Disturbance of sleep	Bed or bedroom not conducive to sleep, noise, interference with sleep by diseases, including prostate hypertrophy (men), cystitis (women), COPD, arthritis, heartburn and cardiorespiratory problems
Drugs	Nicotine, alcohol, caffeine, food or stimulants at bedtime, medications or illicit 'street drugs' (e.g. excessive thyroxine, amphetamines, caffeine-containing beverages, cocaine, ephedrine, phenylpropanolamine, theophylline), withdrawal of medications (such as sedatives or hypnotics), alcoholism or abrupt alcohol cessation
Endocrine	Hyperthyroidism
Light exposure	Inadequate bright-light exposure during waking hours
Others	Ageing, restless legs syndrome (see later)
Psychological factors	Depression, grief, anxiety, stress, exhilaration or excitement, excessive physical or intellectual stimulation at bedtime

COPD, chronic obstructive pulmonary disease.

Box 13.14 Sleep hygiene

- Having a routine
- Going to the toilet before retiring
- Taking a warm bath
- Going to bed at a reasonable time
- Ensuring the bed is comfortable, warm and in a quiet place
- Avoiding stimulants

See http://www.umm.edu/sleep/sleep_hyg.htm

Jet lag

Jet lag is the result of long-distance travel east/west crossing time zones at a rapid rate, and consists of symptoms such as sleep disturbance, loss of appetite, reduced psychomotor efficiency and general malaise. Circadian rhythms need about 1 day to adapt for each time zone crossed: people adapt more easily after a flight westward because there is a longer day. Melatonin will almost certainly have a role in the treatment but the exact dose regime still requires to be worked out. Benzodiazepines are the current treatments; they appear to suppress melatonin secretion.

Delayed sleep phase syndrome

This is the condition when people are only able to fall asleep late into the night or early in the morning. It is quite common among adolescents.

Somnambulism (sleepwalking)

This disorder falls under the parasomnia group – undesirable motor, verbal or experiential events that occur during sleep. Sleepwalking occurs most commonly in middle childhood and pre-adolescence, with a peak incidence around puberty. There are no specific diagnostic tests. Reassurance usually suffices. Parents may need to lock windows and doors, remove obstacles, and add alarms (if necessary) to decrease the likelihood of injury. Benzodiazepines or tricyclic antidepressants may be useful if necessary.

Seasonal affective disorder (SAD; winter depression)

This is depression occurring in the winter months, associated with hypersomnia, weight gain and carbohydrate craving. Environmental magnetic fields have diminished strength during the winter months and there may be desynchronization of the circadian rhythm. SAD improves with bright light treatment.

Narcolepsy

Narcolepsy is a disorder of sleep regulation which manifests with 'sleep attacks' lasting from several seconds to more than 30 min, at various times, even after a normal night's sleep. Narcolepsy is usually hereditary, linked to HLA-DR2 and the hypocretin receptor 2 gene, but is occasionally caused by brain damage from a head injury or neurological disease. People with narcolepsy also may experience cataplexy (sudden onset of falling or collapse), hallucinations whilst falling asleep, temporary paralysis when they awaken and disrupted night-time sleep. Nearly 50% of patients develop a personality or major affective disorder.

Restless legs syndrome

This is one of the most common sleep disorders, especially among older people. A familial disorder causing unpleasant crawling, prickling or tingling sensations in legs and feet and an urge to move them for relief, it may sometimes be linked to anaemia, pregnancy, or diabetes. Many restless legs syndrome (RLS) patients also have a disorder known as *periodic limb movement disorder* (PLMD), which causes repetitive jerking movements of the limbs, especially the legs. These movements occur every 20–40 s and cause severely fragmented sleep. RLS and PLMD often can be relieved by drugs that affect dopamine.

Snoring

Snoring is caused by the vibration of the uvula and soft palate during breathing whilst asleep. Snoring is at the lower end of a spectrum of sleep-disordered breathing (SDB), which may be related to weak activity of tongue, palate and pharynx muscles. SDB has at its minimal level simple snoring, then upper airways resistance syndrome (UARS) and, finally, obstructive sleep apnoea syndrome (OSAS). SDB has been associated with insulin resistance and glucose intolerance, and is frequently found in people with type 2 diabetes.

At least 30% of adults snore, more as age increases. Snorers tend to have a higher body mass index and snoring is usually due to nasal or pharyngeal obstruction or weakness. Snoring is usually a minor problem, but complications may include inter-personal difficulties from annoyance to others, mouth-breathing and dryness, headache and daytime tiredness. Almost all treatments for snoring are based on ensuring upper airway patency. Advice includes sleeping on the side, losing weight and stopping smoking. Rarely, single-dose injection snoreplasty with sodium tetradecyl sulfate or surgery (or radiofrequency uvulopalatopharyngoplasty or laser-assisted palatoplasty) are indicated.

Central sleep apnoea is a CNS disorder.

Obstructive sleep apnoea syndrome (see Ch. 15)

INTRACRANIAL HYPERTENSION

Raised intracranial pressure is a dangerous condition, usually related to space-occupying lesions such as intracranial haemorrhage or tumours, but is occasionally drug-induced (e.g. tetracyclines).

USEFUL WEBSITES

http://www.cjd.ed.ac.uk
http://www.dh.gov.uk/en/index.htm
http://www.epilepsy.org.uk/
http://www. epilepsy.society.org.uk/
http://www.epilepsy.com/
http://www.brainandspine.org.uk
http://www.mssociety.org.uk/
http://www.stroke.org.uk/
http://www.ninds.nih.gov/disorders/disorder_index.htm
http://www.sleeping.org.uk/
http://www.meningitis-trust.org/
http://www.aesnet.org/
http://www.stroke-site.org/
http://facial-neuralgia.org
http://imigraine.net
http://www.fpasupport.org/

FURTHER READING

Al-Jassim, A.H., Lesser, T.H., 2008. Single dose injection snoreplasty: investigation or treatment? J Laryngol Otol 122, 1190–1193.

Bacigaluppi, M., Hermann, D.M., 2008. New targets of neuroprotection in ischemic stroke. Scientific World J 8, 698–712.

Bakheit, A.M., 2006. The possible adverse effects of intramuscular botulinum toxin injections and their management. Curr Drug Saf 1, 271–279.

Blanchet, P.J., Rompre, P.H., Lavigne, G.J., Lamarche, C., 2005. Oral dyskinesia; a clinical overview. Int J Prosthodont 18, 10–19.

Boyle, C.A., Frölander, C., Manley, G., 2008. Providing dental care for patients with Huntington's disease. Dent Update 35, 333–336.

Chemaly, D., Lefrancois, A., Perusse, R., 2000. Oral and maxillofacial manifestations of multiple sclerosis. J Can Dent Assoc 66, 600–605.

Combarros, O., Sanchez-Juan, P., Berciano, J., De Pablos, C., 2000. Hemiageusia from an ipsilateral multiple sclerosis plaque at the midpontine tegmentum. J Neurol Neurosurg Psychiatry 68, 796.

Costa, M.M., Afonso, R.L., Ruviére, D.B., Aguiar, S.M., 2008. Prevalence of dental trauma in patients with cerebral palsy. Spec Care Dentist 28, 61–64.

Cruccu, G., Gronseth, G., Alksne, J., et al., 2008. AAN-EFNS guidelines on trigeminal neuralgia management. Eur J Neurol 15, 1013–1028.

Dave, S.J., 2008. Pilocarpine for the treatment of refractory dry mouth (xerostomia) associated with botulinum toxin type B. Am J Phys Med Rehabil 87, 684–686.

Fedok, F.G., 2008. Advances in minimally invasive facial rejuvenation. Curr Opin Otolaryngol Head Neck Surg 16, 359–368.

Fiske, J., Boyle, C., 2002. Epilepsy and oral care. Dent Update 29, 180–187.

Hankey, G.J., 2008. Review: statins prevent stroke and reduce mortality. Evid Based Med 13, 113.

Haytac, M.C., Aslan, K., Ozcelik, O., Bozdemir, H., 2008. Epileptic seizures triggered by the use of a powered toothbrush. Seizure 17, 288–291.

Holland, J.N., Weiner, G.M., 2004. Recent developments in Bell's palsy. Br Med J 329, 553–557.

Hupp, W.S., 2001. Seizure disorders. Oral Surg 92, 593–596.

Jacobsen, P.L., Eden, O., 2008. Epilepsy and the dental management of the epileptic patient. J Contemp Dent Pract 9, 54–62.

Jagoda, A., Chan, Y.F., 2008. Transient ischemic attack overview: defining the challenges for improving outcomes. Ann Emerg Med 52, S3–S6.

Kang, Y.K., Lee, E.H., Hwang, M., 2000. Pure trigeminal motor neuropathy: a case report. Arch Phys Med Rehabil 81, 995–998.

Katsara, M., Matsoukas, J., Deraos, G., Apostolopoulos, V., 2008. Towards immunotherapeutic drugs and vaccines against multiple sclerosis. Acta Biochim Biophys Sin (Shanghai) 40, 636–642.

Kocaelli, H., Yaltirik, M., Yargic, I., Ozbas, H., 2002. Alzheimer's disease and dental management. Oral Surg 93, 521–524.

Kumazawa, R., Tomiyama, H., Li, Y., et al., 2008. Mutation analysis of the PINK1 gene in 391 patients with Parkinson disease. Arch Neurol 65, 802–808.

Lamonte, M.P., 2008. Ensuring emergency medicine performance standards for stroke and transient ischemic attack care. Emerg Med Clin North Am 26, 703–713.

Lobbezzoo, F., Naeije, M., 2007. Dental implications of some common movement disorders. Arch Oral Biol 52, 395–398.

Lumley, J.S.P., 2004. Creutzfeld–Jakob disease (CJD) in surgical practice. Ann R Coll Surg Eng 86, 86–88.

Meeks, S.L., Buatti, J.M., Foote, K.D., Friedman, W.A., Bova, F.J., 2000. Calculation of cranial nerve complication probability for acoustic neuroma radiosurgery. Int J Radiat Oncol Biol Phys 47 (3), 597–602.

Moore, P., Naumann, M., 2003. Handbook of botulinum treatment, 2nd edn. Blackwell, Oxford.

Penarrocha, M., Bagan, J.V., Alfaro, A., Penarrocha, M., 2001. Acyclovir treatment in 2 patients with benign trigeminal sensory neuropathy. J Oral Maxillofac Surg 59, 453–456.

Penarrocha, M., Cervello, M.A., Marti, E., Bagan, J.V., 2007. Trigeminal neuropathy. Oral Dis 13, 141–150.

Ramagopal, M., Scharf, S.M., Roberts, D.W., Blaisdell, C.J., 2008. Obstructive sleep apnea and history of asthma in snoring children. Sleep Breath 12, 381–392.

Schulte-Mattler, W.J., 2008. Use of botulinum toxin a in adult neurological disorders: efficacy, tolerability and safety. CNS Drugs 22, 725–738.

Scully C., Chaudhry S., 2008. Aspects of Human Disease 23. Cerebrovascular accident (CVA) Dental Update 35; 357.

Scully C., Chaudhry S., 2008. Aspects of Human Disease 24. Dementia Update 35; 428.

Scully C., Chaudhry S., 2008. Aspects of Human Disease 25. Epilepsy Dental Update 35; 501.

Scully C., Chaudhry S., 2008. Aspects of Human Disease 26. Multiple sclerosis Dental Update 35; 581.

Scully C., Chaudhry S., 2008. Aspects of Human Disease 27. Migraine Dental Update 35; 645 (2008).

Scully, C., Diz Dios, P., 2000. Oral dyskinesias and palsies. In: Alio Sanz, J.J. (ed.), Rapport XV Congress of International Association of Disability and Oral Health, Aula Medica, Madrid, 306–329.

Scully, C., Shotts, R., 2001. The mouth in neurological disorders. Practitioner 245, 539–549.

Shaw, J.E., Punjabi, N.M., Wilding, J.P., Alberti, K.G., Zimmet, P.Z., 2008. International Diabetes Federation Taskforce on Epidemiology and Prevention. Sleep-disordered breathing and type 2 diabetes: a report from the International Diabetes Federation Taskforce on Epidemiology and Prevention. Diabetes Res Clin Pract 81, 2–12.

Simola, N., Morelli, M., Pinna, A., 2008. Adenosine A2A receptor antagonists and Parkinson's disease: state of the art and future directions. Curr Pharm Des 14, 1475–1489.

Smith, A.J., Bagg, J., Ironside, J.W., Will, R.G., Scully, C., 2003. Prions and the oral cavity. J Dent Res 82, 769–775.

Stone, C.A., O'Leary, N., 2008. Systematic review of the effectiveness of botulinum toxin or radiotherapy for sialorrhea in patients with amyotrophic lateral sclerosis. J Pain Symptom Manage 37, 246–258.

Sullivan, F.M., Swan, I.R., Donnan, P.T., et al., 2007. Early treatment with prednisolone or acyclovir in Bell's palsy. N Engl J Med 357, 1598–1607.

Suryadevara, A.C., 2008. Update on perioral cosmetic enhancement. Curr Opin Otolaryngol Head Neck Surg 16, 347–351.

Swope, D., Barbano, R., 2008. Treatment recommendations and practical applications of botulinum toxin treatment of cervical dystonia. Neurol Clin 26 (Suppl 1), 54–65.

Toulouse, A., Sullivan, A.M., 2008. Progress in Parkinson's disease: where do we stand? Prog Neurobiol 85, 376–392.

Vorkas, C.K., Gopinathan, M.K., Singh, A., Devinsky, O., Lin, L.M., Rosenberg, P.A., 2008. Epilepsy and dental procedures. A review. N Y State Dent J 74, 39–43.

Voss, N.F., Vrionis, F.D., Heilman, C.B., Robertson, J.H., 2000. Meningiomas of the cerebellopontine angle. Surg Neurol 53, 439–446.

Welsby, P.D., 2004. The 12, 24, or is it 26 cranial nerves?. Postgrad Med J 80, 602–606.

Xue Ming, Brimacombe, M., Chaaban, J., Zimmerman-Bier, B., Wagner, G.C., 2008. Autism spectrum disorders: concurrent clinical disorders. J Child Neurol 23, 6–13.

Zivadinov, R., Reder, A.T., Filippi, M., et al., 2008. Mechanisms of action of disease-modifying agents and brain volume changes in multiple sclerosis. Neurology 71, 136–144.

Appendix 13.1 Peripheral neuropathies

Hereditary

- Charcot–Marie–Tooth disease
- Refsum disease
- Dejerine–Sottas disease

Acquired

Infective

- Herpes zoster
- Guillain–Barré syndrome
- Leprosy
- Diphtheria
- Lyme disease
- HIV
- HTLV-1 (human T-lymphotropic virus 1)

Neoplasms

- Various

Trauma

Metabolic

- Diabetes mellitus
- Vitamin deficiencies, especially B_{12}

Toxic

- Alcohol
- Heavy metals
- Gold
- Nitrous oxide abuse

Idiopathic

- Bell palsy

Appendix 13.2 Cranial nerve syndromes

Syndrome	Cranial nerves involved	Site of lesion	Other features
Avellis	X	Medulla	Hemiplegia Horner syndrome
Benedikt	III	Midbrain	Cerebellar ataxia Tremor Hemiplegia
Cerebellopontine angle	V, VII, VIII and sometimes IX	Posterior cranial fossa	Cerebellar ataxia
Claude	III	Midbrain	Cerebellar ataxia Tremor
Collet–Sicard	IX, X, XI, XII	Retroparotid space	Paralysed palate, pharynx, tongue
Foix	III, IV, V (ophthalmic), VI	Cavernous sinus	Proptosis
Gradenigo	V, VI	Petrous temporal	Pain
Jackson	X, XII	Medulla	Hemiplegia Horner syndrome
Jacob	II, III, IV, V, VI	Middle cranial fossa	–
Millard–Gubler	VII, VI	Pons	Hemiplegia
Moebins	VI, VII	Pons	Lack of facial expression
Nothnagel	III	Midbrain	Cerebellar ataxia
Parinaud	III, IV, VI	Midbrain	Abormal eye movements with pupil dysfunction
Sphenoid fissure (superior orbital fissure)	III, IV, V (ophthalmic), VI and sometimes II	Superior orbital fissure	Proptosis
Vernet	IX, X, XI	Jugular foramen Nasopharynx	Paralysed soft palate, pharynx and vocal cords
Villaret	IX, X, XI, XII	Retroparotid space	Horner syndrome
Wallenberg (posterior inferior cerebellar artery, PICA; lateral medullary)	V, IX, X, XI	Medulla	Ipsilateral cerebellar ataxia and Horner syndrome, and loss of pain and temperature sense on face, and paralysis of palate/pharynx/larynx. Contralateral loss of pain and temperature sense elsewhere. Vertigo, nystagmus
Weber	III	Midbrain	Hemiplegia

Appendix 13.3 Anticonvulsant drugs: uses and adverse effects

Drug	Use	Systemic adverse effects	Oral adverse effects
Carbamazepine	TLE GM	Ataxia Drowsiness Leukopenia Lupoid syndrome SIADH (Ch. 6)	Dry mouth Erythema multiforme Dyskinesias
Valproate	GM PM	Drowsiness Bleeding diathesis	Purpura
Phenytoin	GM TLE	Cerebellar damage Hirsutes Nephrotic syndrome Hyperglycaemia	Gingival swelling Dental anomalies Erythema multiforme Lupoid syndrome or ulcers Cervical lymphadenopathy
Ethosuximide	PM	Lupoid syndrome Renal damage Eosinophilia	
Primidone	GM TLE PM	Drowsiness Ataxia Oculomotor palsy	Megaloblastic anaemia causing ulcers
Gabapentin	GM PM	Dizziness Drowsiness	Dry mouth
Topiramate	GM PM	Allergic reactions Various others	Dry mouth oedema

GM, grand mal; PM, petit mal; SIADH, syndrome of inappropriate antidiuretic hormone secretion; TLE, temporal lobe epilepsy.

OTORHINOLARYNGOLOGY

KEY POINTS

- Upper respiratory infections are ubiquitous
- Voice changes may herald laryngeal cancer

The upper respiratory tract (URT) includes the nose paranasal sinus, pharynx and larynx but the salivary glands and oral cavity are closely adjacent. Salivary disorders are discussed mainly in Chs. 14, 18 and 22, oral disorders in Chs 11 and 22. The URT may become damaged by pollutants such as smoke, soot, dust and chemicals or infected with micro-organisms from the inspired air. Pain from sinus or aural problems may radiate or be referred to the mouth; equally, oral problems may cause pain in the sinus or ear.

UPPER RESPIRATORY TRACT INFECTIONS

A wide variety of respiratory pathogens may cause a single clinical syndrome and, vice versa, any one pathogen may cause a range of clinical diseases. Most diseaes are viral.

The URT is colonized by normal bacterial flora, which rarely cause disease, but may under certain circumstances cause upper or lower respiratory tract (LRT) disease or even systemic or transmissible infections. For example, the normal nasal bacterial flora may include *Staphylococcus aureus* and *S. epidermidis* and aerobic corynebacteria ('diphtheroids'). Some people carry meticillin-resistant *Staphylococcus aureus* (MRSA) in their nose, which can cause disease. Bacterial infection caused by a foreign body introduced into the nose of a child (e.g. a small toy) is a well-recognized cause of halitosis, as are tonsillitis and sinusitis. The nasopharyngeal bacterial flora may include non-encapsulated or non-virulent strains of *Streptococcus pneumoniae*, *Neisseria meningitidis* and *Haemophilus influenzae*. These may cause meningitis. Pharyngitis can be caused by Group A streptococci (and can rarely lead to rheumatic fever and occasionally rheumatic carditis; Ch. 5) or pharyngitis can be caused by Epstein–Barr virus, in infectious mononucleosis.

VIRAL UPPER RESPIRATORY TRACT INFECTIONS

Viruses frequently evade the defences of the URT to produce infections; children have up to eight upper respiratory tract infections (UTRIs) per year, adolescents up to four. Most viral infections are contracted from other people via their sneezes, or by shaking their hands or touching things they have touched (and then touching the nose, mouth or conjunctivae; Table 14.1).

Viral URTI are highly infectious in the early stages. The incubation periods rarely exceed 14 days. The three main clinical patterns of URTI are the common cold syndrome (coryza),

Table 14.1 Main respiratory viruses

Viral respiratory pathogens	Presumed viral respiratory disease
Adenovirus	Coronaviruses
Para-influenza virus	Coxsackie viruses
Respiratory syncytial virus	Cytomegalovirus
Rhinovirus	ECHO viruses
	Epstein–Barr virus
	Herpes simplex viruses
	Influenza

pharyngitis and tonsillitis, and laryngotracheitis. Other URTI are discussed in Ch. 21.

THE COMMON COLD SYNDROME

General aspects

The common cold syndrome is usually caused by rhinoviruses, but can be caused by over 200 different viruses (Table 14.2), particularly by respiratory syncytial virus (RSV), coronaviruses, para-influenza and influenza.

Table 14.2 Upper respiratory tract infections and their main causes

Condition	Micro-organisms
Common cold	Corona virus Coxsackie viruses ECHO viruses Para-influenza virus Respiratory syncytial virus Rhinoviruses
Pharyngitis	Adenoviruses Coxsackie viruses ECHO viruses Epstein–Barr virus Beta-haemolytic streptococci Influenza viruses Candida
Tonsillitis	Adenoviruses Beta-haemolytic streptococci Enteroviruses Epstein–Barr virus Herpes simplex virus Influenza viruses Parainfluenza viruses
Influenza	Influenza viruses
Sinusitis	Streptococcus pneumoniae Streptococcus milleri Haemophilus influenzae Moraxella catarrhalis Aspergillus Mucormycosis

Clinical features

Sneezing, mucus overproduction with nasal obstruction, nasopharyngeal soreness and mild systemic upset are well-recognized features. Serious complications are rare in otherwise fit patients, but bacterial infection may supervene and cause sinusitis or infection of the middle ear (otitis media).

General management

Symptoms resembling the common cold can also precede other infections, such as measles or influenza. Only symptomatic treatment is available.

Dental aspects

Elective dental care is best deferred. General anaesthesia (GA) should be avoided since there is often some respiratory obstruction and infection can also be spread down to the lungs. If a GA is unavoidable, it is best to carry out intubation with a cuffed tube, so that nasal secretions do not enter the larynx. Antimicrobials may be indicated for prophylaxis. Xylitol chewing gum has been shown to reduce the risk of otitis media, presumably by inhibiting pneumococcal super-infection.

PHARYNGITIS AND TONSILLITIS

General aspects

Most pharyngitis and tonsillitis is caused by viruses (Table 14.1), some by streptococci.

Clinical features

The throat is sore with pain on swallowing (dysphagia) and sometimes fever and conjunctivitis. Prominent submucosal aggregates of lymphoid tissue may be evident in those with pharyngitis. Enlargement of the tonsils with an infected exudate from the crypts together with cervical lymphadenopathy is characteristic of tonsillitis.

Complications are rare, but may include peritonsillar abscess (quinsy), otitis media and rarely scarlet fever, acute glomerulonephritis or rheumatic fever.

General management

Infectious mononucleosis (glandular fever) or, rarely, diphtheria may need to be considered in the differential diagnosis.

Tonsillitis caused by bacterial infection is best treated with benzyl or phenoxymethyl penicillin or, if the patient is allergic, erythromycin or a cephalosporin. Ampicillin and amoxicillin should be avoided as they tend to cause rashes, especially if the sore throat is misdiagnosed as a streptococcal sore throat but due to glandular fever. As there is no evidence that antibiotics accelerate resolution or diminish septic complications, an increasing body of opinion advises simple analgesics for management of pharyngitis.

Dental aspects

Elective dental care is best deferred. GA should be avoided since there is often a degree of respiratory obstruction and infection may spread to the lungs.

SINUSITIS

General aspects

Infection of the paranasal air sinuses (maxillary most commonly, but also ethmoid, sphenoid and frontal) is usually bacterial but may be preceded by viral infection, or other factors (Box 14.1).

> **Box 14.1 Factors predisposing to sinusitis**
>
> - Diving – when water may be forced into the nose and sinuses or, conversely, barotrauma in air flight
> - Insertion of a foreign body in the nose
> - Periapical infection of upper posterior teeth or an oro-antral fistula
> - Prolonged endotracheal intubation and mechanical ventilation
> - Vasomotor or allergic rhinitis
> - Viral upper respiratory tract infection – commonly a cold

Sinusitis is classified as acute, chronic or recurrent. In acute sinusitis, the bacteria most commonly incriminated are *Streptococcus pneumoniae* and *Haemophilus influenzae*. Chronic sinusitis involves anaerobes, especially *Porphyromonas* (*Bacteroides*), and half are beta-lactamase producers. It may follow acute sinusitis, especially where there are local abnormalities, allergic rhinitis, or impaired defence mechanisms such as cystic fibrosis or HIV disease. Gram-positive cocci and bacilli as well as Gram-negative bacilli may also be found – especially in HIV/AIDS patients and those on prolonged endotracheal intubation. *Pseudomonas aeruginosa* (up to 5% of cases are caused by *Pseudomonas*, especially in cystic fibrosis), *Acinetobacter baumannii* and Enterobacteriaceae are also implicated. In immunocompromised persons, fungi may also be involved, including *Mucor*, *Aspergillus* or other species.

Clinical features

Headache on wakening is typical, with pain worse on tilting the head or lying down, and nasal obstruction with mucopurulent nasal discharge (Table 14.3).

Table 14.3	Paranasal sinusitis	
Location	**Location of pain**	**Other features**
Maxillary	Cheek and/or upper teeth, worsened by biting	Tenderness over antra
Frontal	Over frontal sinuses	Tenderness of sides of nose
Ethmoidal	Between eyes	Anosmia, eyelids swelling
Sphenoidal	Ear, neck, and at top or centre of head	–

General management

Diagnosis is from the history, plus tenderness over the sinus, dullness on transillumination, and radio-opacity or a fluid level on plain X-rays of the sinuses (sinus opacity may be due to mucosal thickening rather than infection, but a fluid level is highly suggestive of infection). Antral opacities in children can be difficult to evaluate since they are seen in up to 50% of healthy children under age 6 years. Computed tomography (CT) is now the standard of care, though magnetic resonance imaging (MRI) is indicated in some cases. Ultrasonography may be helpful. However, the gold standard for diagnosis remains sinus puncture and aspiration.

Acute sinusitis resolves spontaneously in about 50%, but analgesics are often indicated and antibiotics may be required if symptoms persist or there is a purulent discharge. Treatment is a > 7-day course of amoxicillin (or ampicillin or co-amoxiclav; erythromycin if penicillin-allergic), or a tetracycline, such as doxycycline, or clindamycin. Vasoconstrictor nasal drops, such as ephedrine or xylometazoline, can improve sinus drainage. Inhalations of warm, moist air, with benzoin, menthol or eucalyptus, may give symptomatic relief.

Chronic sinusitis responds better to drainage by functional endoscopic surgical techniques, plus antimicrobials – such as metronidazole with amoxicillin, erythromycin, clindamycin or a cephalosporin.

Recurrent sinusitis should be treated with drainage, plus antimicrobials, and investigation to determine whether there is any underlying cause.

Dental aspects

Dental treatment should be deferred until after recovery. GA should be avoided since there is often some respiratory obstruction and infection can spread to the lungs. Inhalational sedation may be impeded if the nasal airway is obstructed

Mycoses may infect the sinuses in immunocompromised persons (see Ch. 20).

OTITIS MEDIA

General aspects

Otitis media is a common middle-ear infection in children; three out of four experience it by age 3 years. The most important predisposing factor is Eustachian tube (ET) dysfunction but immune defects and palatal anomalies, such as cleft palate or submucous cleft, occasionally contribute. Interference with the ET mucosa by inflammatory oedema, adenoidal hypertrophy, negative intratympanic pressure or rarely a tumour, facilitates direct extension of infections from the nasopharynx to the middle ear. Oesophageal contents regurgitated into the nasopharynx can enter the middle ear through the ET if it is patulous. Otitis media usually follows a viral URTI, often followed by bacterial superinfection. The most common bacterial pathogen is *Streptococcus pneumoniae*, followed by non-typeable *Haemophilus influenzae* and *Moraxella catarrhalis*.

When the ears are infected, the ET become inflamed and swollen, the mucociliary pathways from the middle ear to the nasopharynx become paralysed or dysfunctional, and fluid gets trapped inside the middle-ear cleft. The adenoids can also become infected and can also block the openings of the ET, trapping air and fluid.

Clinical features

Acute otitis media is very painful, worse when the child is lying down, a feature recognized by parents when trying to get their pyrexial child to sleep. If the infection is not controlled, the eardrum ruptures and pus escapes through the perforation – otorrhoea – when there is an immediate decrease in pain. It may become evident that the child has lost hearing in that ear. If ET dysfunction merely prevents the normal drainage of the middle ear cleft, with or without previous acute infection, a condition referred to as otitis media with effusion or 'glue ear' becomes established. This also affects the hearing but is painless.

Temporary speech and language problems may become evident as a result of the hearing loss, but usually resolve spontaneously with time.

Complications that are rare but can be serious include mastoiditis, meningitis, brain abscess, lateral sinus thrombosis, otitic hydrocephalus, facial palsy, cholesteatoma and tympanosclerosis.

General management

Medical treatment includes antibiotics (usually penicillin) and decongestants and/or antihistamines together with analgesia. If fluids from otitis media stay in the ear for several months, drainage by surgery, usually myringotomy (incision of the ear drum) and grommets (small drainage tubes placed in the incision), may be recommended. Adenoidectomy may also be indicated.

LARYNGOTRACHEITIS

General aspects

Various microbes may be involved, such as respiratory syncytial virus (RSV) particularly in children.

Clinical features

Hoarseness, loss of voice and persistent cough are common. In children, partial laryngeal obstruction may cause noisy inspiration (stridor or croup) and is potentially dangerous.

General management

Symptomatic treatment only is available but, in RSV infection in infants who may otherwise subsequently develop bronchiolitis, ribavirin or palivizumab may be more appropriate.

Dental aspects

Dental treatment should be deferred until after recovery. GA must be avoided as it may exacerbate progression of infection to the lungs. Antimicrobials may be indicated for prophylaxis.

MALIGNANT NEOPLASMS

Most head and neck cancers are squamous cell carcinomas but other tumour types include lymphoepithelioma, spindle cell carcinoma, verrucous cancer, undifferentiated carcinoma and lymphoma.

MAXILLARY ANTRAL CARCINOMA

General aspects

Antral carcinoma is a rare neoplasm of unknown aetiology seen mainly in older people.

Clinical features

At the outset, antral carcinoma presents with severe maxillary pain. As the tumour increases in size, the effects of expansion and infiltration of adjacent tissues become apparent. There is intraoral alveolar swelling; ulceration of the palate or buccal sulcus; swelling of the cheek; unilateral nasal obstruction, often associated with a blood-stained discharge; obstruction of the nasolacrimal duct with consequent epiphora; hypoaesthesia or anaesthesia of the cheek in the infraorbital nerve distribution; proptosis and ophthalmoplegia consequent on invasion of the orbit; and trismus from infiltration of the muscles of mastication.

General management

Combinations of surgery and radio-chemotherapy are usually required. Further details can be found in standard textbooks of otorhinolaryngology or maxillofacial surgery.

NASOPHARYNGEAL CARCINOMA

General aspects

Nasopharyngeal carcinoma is a rare neoplasm that may be associated with Epstein–Barr virus and dietary nitrosamines, especially common amongst the Southern Chinese, some Inuit races and in parts of North Africa such as Tunisia. A similar tumour, undifferentiated carcinoma with lymphoid stroma, is one of the most common salivary gland cancers in Inuits and Southern Chinese.

Clinical features

Nasopharyngeal carcinoma is often asymptomatic for some time as it does not obstruct the nasopharynx. It presents in a variety of ways that include:

- isolated cervical lymph node enlargement
- unilateral conductive deafness (from obstruction of the Eustachian tube)
- abducens nerve palsy
- elevation and immobility of the soft palate
- ipsilateral pain, sometimes with anaesthesia, in the distribution of the major divisions of the trigeminal nerve, e.g. over the eye (ophthalmic division), the tongue, lower teeth and lower lip (mandibular division)
- a combination of the above - known as *Trotter's triad.*

General management

Treatment is usually by radiotherapy.

CANCER OF THE PHARYNX

Cancer can develop in the nasopharynx (see Ch. 22), oropharynx (consisting of the base of tongue, the tonsillar region, soft palate and back of the oral cavity) or the hypopharynx. Patients with pharyngeal cancer are at greater risk of cancer elsewhere in the upper aerodigestive tract.

Factors that increase the risk of pharyngeal cancers include smoking (both tobacco and marijuana) or chewing tobacco; alcohol use; leukoplakia; human papillomavirus (oropharyngeal carcinoma); Epstein–Barr virus (nasopharyngeal carcinoma); anaemia (Paterson–Brown-Kelly syndrome); radiation; and immune defects.

Pharyngeal cancer is treated by one, or a combination, of radiotherapy, chemotherapy or surgery.

CANCER OF THE LARYNX

Laryngeal cancer is found in the glottis, supraglottis or subglottis. It is most common in males, those over 55 and who smoke, drink alcohol, are infected with human papillomavirus or have immune defects. Risk factors may also include genetics (people of African descent are more likely than whites to be affected); a personal history of head and neck cancer; exposure to asbestos, sulfuric acid mist or nickel; or a diet low in vitamin A.

Clinical features

Symptoms and signs may include hoarseness, persistent sore throat, dysphagia, pain referred to the ear when swallowing, haemoptysis and cervical lymphadenopathy.

General management

Laryngoscopy, CT imaging and biopsy are required to confirm the diagnosis. Laryngeal cancer is treated by one, or a combination, of radiotherapy, chemotherapy or surgery. Laser surgery may be used for very early cancers of the larynx. A cordectomy removes the vocal cord. A supraglottic laryngectomy takes out only the supraglottis. A partial or hemi-laryngectomy removes only part of the larynx. A total laryngectomy removes the entire larynx and commits the patient to a permanent tracheostomy. Despite loss of part or all of the vocal apparatus, most patients are able to communicate by speech with or without further surgical procedures and electronic voice aids.

ORAL CANCER (CH. 22)
SALIVARY NEOPLASMS

General aspects

A wide range of different neoplasms can affect the salivary glands, but most are uncommon, are epithelial neoplasms, present as unilateral swelling of the parotid and are benign. The most common is pleomorphic salivary adenoma (PSA). The next most common is carcinoma. Other neoplasms of major salivary gland are usually monomorphic adenomas (such as adenolymphomas), mucoepidermoid tumours or acinic cell tumours. Neoplasms in the minor salivary glands are most commonly pleomorphic adenomas but carcinomas, particularly adenoid cystic carcinomas, account for about 50 per cent of all neoplasms. Most salivary gland neoplasms are seen in older people. There is a female predisposition. Salivary gland tumours are more common in certain geographical locations. Inuits, for example, have an increased prevalence. The aetiology of salivary gland tumours is unknown but there are various associations (Box 14.2).

Box 14.2 Risk factors for salivary neoplasms

Epstein–Barr virus infection
- At least in Asian patients and Inuits

Occupation
- Rubber manufacturing
- Plumbing industry
- Woodworking
- Hairdressing
- Asbestos exposure

Smoking
- At least for Warthin tumour

Other malignant disease
- Breast cancer
- Nasopharyngeal carcinoma
- Thyroid cancer

X-ray repair cross-complementing group 1 (XRCC1) single-nucleotide polymorphisms

Radiation exposure, as in
- Sun exposure
- Ionizing radiation exposure
  - survivors of atomic explosions in Japan (mucoepidermoid carcinomas and Warthin tumour)
  - survivors of childhood malignancies treated with radiation and chemotherapy
  - iodine-131 in the treatment of thyroid disease
  - radiotherapy to the head and neck
  - radiographs of the head and neck

A suggested association of parotid tumours with mobile phone use is controversial.

Apart from the above epithelial neoplasms, the next most common neoplasms found in salivary glands are lymphomas. Sjögren syndrome is recognized as predisposing to lymphomas, which have arisen in up to 6 per cent of patients over 10 years in some studies.

Clinical features

Salivary gland swelling is the main clinical feature of a neoplasm. A long history of gradual gland enlargement suggests a benign process while pain, facial palsy, rapid growth or change in growth pattern are ominous and suggest carcinoma.

General management

On clinical examination a mass is usually palpable. In the case of the parotid, this will often be in the retromandibular region but sometimes pre-tragal. Tumours confined to the deep lobe of the parotid present like other parapharyngeal tumours with medial displacement of the palate, tonsil and pharyngeal wall.

A few malignant neoplasms may be small, almost impalpable, and present with pain only. MRI is particularly helpful for diagnosing parotid and submandibular tumours. The use of sialography is nowadays largely reserved for the investigation of inflammatory disease. CT is often degraded in this region by amalgam artefacts. Ultrasonography has utility in determining whether a mass is in the tail of the parotid or posterior pole of the submandibular gland. Regardless of the image appearances, the precise diagnosis can only be firmly established by histological examination of either the operative specimen or, increasingly frequently, by fine-needle aspiration biopsy.

The treatment of choice for salivary gland neoplasms is surgical excision. Most salivary gland neoplasms are relatively radioresistant. Chemotherapy is used only on a very limited basis and as an adjunct in treatment of some malignant salivary gland neoplasms, such as adenocarcinoma or adenoid cystic carcinoma.

LYMPHOMAS (CH. 8)

PALATE

CLEFT LIP AND PALATE

General aspects

The primary palate or pre-maxilla forms during the fourth to seventh weeks of gestation and includes that portion of the alveolar ridge containing the four incisors. The secondary palate forms during the sixth to ninth weeks of gestation, and consists of the remaining hard palate and all the soft palate. The formation of the palate requires dynamic development in that the developing palatal shelves are vertical and lateral to the tongue. The shelves elevate over a relatively short period (24 h) to lie horizontally with eventual contact and fusion.

Orofacial clefts result from an embryopathy in which there is failure of the frontonasal process and/or fusion of the palatal shelves. In the submucous cleft palate, the palatal shelves may fail to join, but the overlying mucous membranes are intact and the muscle attachments of the soft palate are abnormal, causing velopharyngeal insufficiency.

The total incidence of clefting is between two and three per 1000 live births. A number of these do not develop as full-term fetuses. The common clefts are cleft lip with or without cleft palate (CL ± P) and cleft palate only (CP). Cleft palate is the fourth most common birth defect – affecting approximately 1 in 700–1000 live births – and is more prevalent in females, while cleft lip is more prevalent in males. There are also racial differences with a high incidence in South-East Asia and a low incidence in Afro-Caribbean races.

Facial clefts are associated with a syndrome in up to 15–60% of cases and are then termed syndromic clefts. More than 400 syndromes may include a facial cleft as one manifestation.

Cleft lip/palate (CLP) may be associated with many congenital syndromes. Van der Woude and Waardenberg syndromes are associated with CL, with or without CP. Common syndromes with CP include Apert, Stickler and Treacher Collins syndromes. CLP may also be seen in velocardiofacial, Pierre Robin and Klippel–Feil syndromes and in various chromosome anomalies (Down syndrome, Edwards syndrome; Appendix 14.1). A small subgroup of patients have cleft lip and palate with median facial dysplasia and cerebrofacial malformations, others with laryngotracheal oesophageal clefts (Opitz–Firas or G syndrome) or cranial asymmetry (Opitz or B syndrome).

The cause of non-syndromic cleft lip with or without cleft palate (NSCLP) is unclear but there is still a strong genetic component; there may be a family history of clefts and typically the same type of cleft is seen in affected members. In monozygotic twins, there is nearly 40% concordance. No single gene defect appears responsible, however. Several loci have been identified. Candidate genes in CLP include transforming growth factor alpha (*TGF*), poliovirus receptor-related 1 (*PVRL1*), retinoic acid receptor alpha (*RARA*), T-box transcription factor-22 (*TBX22*), specific isoforms of glutamic acid decarboxylase (*GAD*), interferon regulatory factor 6 (*IRF6*), *MSX1* (formerly homeobox 7 – encodes a member of the muscle segment homeobox gene family) and fibroblast growth factor (*FGF*) genes.

Cleft lip/palate is more prevalent in the lower socioeconomic classes. Maternal stress may increase the risk as may various lifestyle factors including teratogens. The teratogens incriminated include isotretinoin (Accutane), used to treat acne, which causes birth defects such as brain malformations, learning disability, heart problems, as well as facial abnormalities. Thalidomide given to pregnant mothers was, and anticonvulsants (phenytoin, valproic acid, lamotrigine, carbamazepine) and corticosteroids may be, associated with an increased incidence. Phenytoin may act via an effect causing fetal arrhythmias and hypoxia. Systemic corticosteroids increase the risk threefold (possibly acting via an effect on TGF) and there are also concerns about possible effects from topical steroids used in the first trimester. Other potential environmental factors include maternal upper respiratory infection in the first trimester, smoking [especially when the mother has glutathione-*S*-transferase theta 1 (GSTT1) – null variants], alcohol use, obesity and diabetes. Paternal smoking has also been implicated. There has been concern about aspirin and diazepam as possible causes but there is no real evidence. Folic acid given peri-conceptually may lower the risk, but the evidence is weak.

Clinical features

Clefts have a major impact from birth both from the aesthetic and functional viewpoints, since the neonate with a cleft palate is unable to suckle. Later, speech development is also impaired. A person may have a cleft lip, cleft palate, or both cleft lip and palate. A unilateral cleft lip occurs on one side of the upper lip. A bilateral cleft lip occurs on both sides of the upper lip. In its most severe form, the cleft may extend through the nose base.

Cleft palate may be incomplete involving only the uvula and the muscular soft palate (velum). A complete cleft palate extends the entire length of the palate. Cleft palates can be unilateral or bilateral. There may also be feeding difficulties and

associated congenital defects such as dental, hearing and speech defects. Dental abnormalities include malocclusion (almost 100%), hypodontia (50%), hypoplasia (30%) and supernumerary teeth (20%).

General management

Health care providers that frequently participate in a multidisciplinary cleft palate team include: audiologists; maxillofacial, ear, nose and throat, and plastic surgeons; geneticists; neurosurgeons; nurses; dentists (paediatric dentist/orthodontist/prosthodontist); paediatricians; social workers/psychologists, and speech and language pathologists.

A high percentage of patients with CP develop otitis media with effusion. Up to 20% have additional abnormalities that can affect management in various ways (Fig. 14.1). Systemic disorders are more frequent in patients with CP than in those with CL alone, and include especially skeletal, cardiac, renal and central nervous system defects.

Newborn to 12 months

Treatment of the airway takes priority and may be managed with positioning but, in severe cases, may need tracheostomy. There can be significant difficulties in management of the airway for anaesthesia in children under the age of 5 years, particularly in young infants and in those with feeding difficulties, bilateral clefts and/or retrognathia. Patients with mandibular dysostoses, or any requiring mid-face advancement (Le Fort II osteotomy) have the greatest problems. Difficulties are common in Pierre Robin, Treacher Collins and Goldenhar

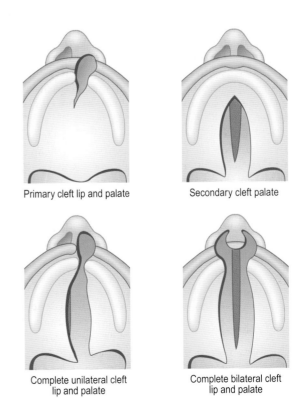

Primary cleft lip and palate

Secondary cleft palate

Complete unilateral cleft lip and palate

Complete bilateral cleft lip and palate

Fig. 14.1 Cleft palate

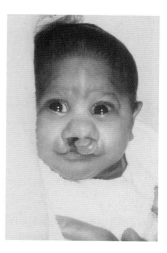

Fig. 14.2 Cleft lip

syndromes, and with the cervical spine in Klippel–Feil syndrome. The laryngeal mask has been recommended as a guide to fibreoptic endoscopic intubation. Aesthetics is a major issue for parents (Fig. 14.2). One of the problems for the child is feeding: a Rosti bottle with Gummi teat often helps. The timing of the initial cleft lip and palate repair is controversial. In general, when the lip alone is cleft, initial cosmetic repair is carried out at about 3–6 months of age, though earlier operations are becoming popular. Many repair cleft lip and palate within the first few days of life since, after repair, the appearance is dramatically improved, feeding difficulties are significantly minimized and speech develops better. If the palatal defect is too wide, it can be repaired 3 months later to allow for sufficient palatal growth. In any event, CP is now usually repaired before the child speaks, between 6 and 18 months, typically at 6–12 months of age.

Age 1–5 years is when it is important to have good hearing and normal appearance to avoid low self-esteem and help speech develop. These children need a hearing assessment, and if it is impaired, ear ventilation tubes (grommets) may be indicated.

Age 5–13 years is when the orthodontist can help correct malocclusion and alveolar bone grafting may be needed. Speech, if poor despite the best efforts by the child and the speech pathologist, may be corrected with pharyngoplasty.

Age 13–18 years is the time for final adjustments. Fine tuning such as scar revisions, rhinoplasty and orthognathic surgery is carried out to enable the child's appearance and speech to be restored to as near normal as possible.

Dental aspects

Palatal ulcers seen in neonates with cleft lip and palate appear to result from trauma from the tongue and resolve if a palatal plate is fitted. Children may have a higher prevalence of caries in both the primary and permanent dentitions, and significantly more gingivitis, especially in the maxillary anterior region. Adult cleft lip and palate patients may have poorer oral hygiene and more gingivitis. Prevention and continuity of care is essential and a high rate of success can be achieved.

Submucous cleft palate can be recognized by a notched posterior nasal spine, a translucent zone in the midline of the soft palate and a bifid uvula, but not all these features are necessarily present and a bifid uvula may be seen in isolation. About 1 in 1200 births are affected and feeding difficulties, speech defects and middle-ear infections may develop in 90% of affected children. Adenoidectomy is contraindicated as it may reveal latent velopharyngeal insufficiency.

VELOCARDIOFACIAL SYNDROME

General aspects

Velocardiofacial syndrome (VCFS; from the Latin *velum* – palate, *cardia* – heart, and *facies* – to do with the face) is a genetic disorder involving chromosome 22 (a deletion at 22q11 along with Cardiac defects, Abnormal facies, Thymic hypoplasia, Cleft palate and Hypocalcaemia – hence it is termed 'CATCH 22'). It affects approximately 5–8% of children born with CP and consists of characteristic facial appearance, minor learning problems and speech and feeding difficulties, and heart defects. It is inherited in only about 10–15% and, usually, neither parent has the syndrome or carries the defective gene.

Also known as Shprintzen syndrome, craniofacial syndrome, or conotruncal anomaly unusual face syndrome, at least 30 different defects have been associated with the 22q11 deletion of VCFS. DiGeorge syndrome is similar (Ch. 20).

Clinical features

There is great variation in the features (Box 14.3), although none of these problems occurs in all cases.

Box 14.3 Features of velocardiofacial syndrome (CATCH 22)

- Cleft palate, usually of the soft palate
- Heart disease
- Facies (elongated face, almond-shaped eyes, wide nose, small ears)
- Learning difficulties
- Eye defects
- Otitis media
- Hypoparathyroidism
- Immune defects
- Weak muscles
- Short height
- Curvature of the spine (scoliosis)
- Tapered fingers

Dental aspects

There may be problems associated with CLP, cardiac disease and immune defects.

ORO-ANTRAL FISTULA

Oro-antral fistula is discussed in surgical textbooks. Palatal perforations can be caused by trauma, malignant neoplasms or the use of cocaine.

OBSTRUCTIVE SLEEP APNOEA SYNDROME

General aspects

Obstructive sleep apnoea syndrome (OSAS) is characterized by periods of prolonged apnoea during sleep. Patients with OSAS snore extremely loudly, often termed 'heroic snoring'! The cause is airway obstruction, usually in the region of the oropharynx. Enlarged tonsils, nasal septum deformity, narrow dental arches and abnormalities in the larynx also contribute to this problem. As the patient relaxes in the early phase of sleep, their tongue falls back into the oropharynx and causes obstruction. Patients with significant obstructive sleep apnoea have daytime sleepiness that often culminates in road traffic accidents, an increased risk of acute cardiopulmonary complications and stroke. They are characteristically obese and most are middle-aged men.

Clinical features

Partial upper airways obstruction during sleep usually causes snoring. In some, apnoeic episodes are reported. During apnoea, arterial oxygen saturation falls and cardiac arrhythmias may develop. In more severe cases pulmonary hypertension and right ventricular failure result.

As stated above, there is an increased mortality rate in this group of patients, not least from road traffic accidents, since affected patients are constantly tired and drowsy.

A dangerous degree of dyspnoea and cyanosis has been noted in some weak senile patients, even when awake; oronasal obstruction resulting from blockage of the nose and lack of teeth or dentures causes the mouth to become over-closed. Hypoxia, thus caused, may contribute to the death of these vulnerable patients.

General management

Nasal continuous positive airways pressure (CPAP) has been shown to lower mortality and provides a rapid solution, but is less acceptable than some other measures.

Other measures may include appliances, orthognathic surgery (maxillary-mandibular and hyoid advancement; MMA), uvulopalatopharyngoplasty (UPPP), adenoidectomy, tonsillectomy or even tracheostomy. UPPP using scalpel surgery or lasers has been the standard treatment for OSAS, but is often overprescribed and its efficacy is under review.

Dental aspects

Recent work suggests that, where the obstruction is predominantly hypopharyngeal, surgical advancement of the facial skeleton and hyoid (MMA) may effectively expand the airway. When there is both oropharyngeal and hypopharyngeal obstruction, UPPP may need to be combined with MMA. Nasal obstruction may also have to be relieved, but maxillofacial surgery carried out in stages to assess the degree of improvement may relieve nocturnal hypoxia, snoring and daytime sleepiness.

Dental appliances that hold the mandible forward are claimed to be as effective as more drastic measures and should certainly be tried in the first instance.

USEFUL WEBSITES

http://www3.niaid.nih.gov/topics
http://www.entnet.org/
http://www.aaaai.org/professionals.stm
http://www.entuk.org/publications/
http://www.medicine.ox.ac.uk/bandolier/booth/booths/ent.html

FURTHER READING

Avila, J.R., Jezewski, P.A., Vieira, A.R., et al., 2006. PVRL1 variants contribute to non-syndromic cleft lip and palate in multiple populations. Am J Med Genet A 140, 2562–2570.

Azarbayjani, F., Danielsson, B.R., 2001. Phenytoin-induced cleft palate: evidence for embryonic cardiac bradyarrhythmia due to inhibition of delayed rectifier K+ channels resulting in hypoxia-reoxygenation damage. Teratology 63, 152–160.

Azarbayjani, F., Danielsson, B.R., 2002. Embryonic arrhythmia by inhibition of HERG channels: a common hypoxia-related teratogenic mechanism for antiepileptic drugs? Epilepsia 43, 457–468.

Bettega, G., Pepin, J.L., Veale, D., 2000. Obstructive sleep apnea syndrome. Am J Respir Crit Care Med 162, 641–649.

Bille, C., Olsen, J., Vach, W., et al., 2007. Oral clefts and life style factors – a case-cohort study based on prospective Danish data. Eur J Epidemiol 22, 173–181.

Bloch, K.E., Iseli, A., Zhang, J.N., 2000. A randomised, controlled crossover trial of two oral appliances for sleep apnea treatment. Am J Respir Crit Care Med 162, 246–251.

Boscolo-Rizzo, P., Maronato, F., Marchiori, C., Gava, A., Da Mosto, M.C., 2008. Long-term quality of life after total laryngectomy and postoperative radiotherapy versus concurrent chemoradiotherapy for laryngeal preservation. Laryngoscope 118, 300–306.

Boysen, T., Friborg, J., Andersen, A., Poulsen, G.N., Wohlfahrt, J., Melbye, M., 2008. The Inuit cancer pattern – the influence of migration. Int J Cancer 122, 2568–2572.

Carinci, F., Pezzetti, F., Scapoli, L., et al., 2003. Recent developments in orofacial cleft genetics. J Craniofac Surg 14, 130–143.

Carinci, F., Rullo, R., Farina, A., et al., 2005. Non-syndromic orofacial clefts in Southern Italy: pattern analysis according to gender, history of maternal smoking, folic acid intake and familial diabetes. J Craniomaxillofac Surg 33, 91–94.

Carmichael, S.L., Shaw, G.M., Yang, W., Abrams, B., Lammer, E.J., 2007. Maternal stressful life events and risks of birth defects. Epidemiology 18, 356–361.

Cedergren, M., Källén, B., 2005. Maternal obesity and the risk for orofacial clefts in the offspring. Cleft Palate Craniofac J 42, 367–371.

Chevrier, C., Bahuau, M., Perret, C., et al., 2008. Genetic susceptibilities in the association between maternal exposure to tobacco smoke and the risk of nonsyndromic oral cleft. Am J Med Genet A 146A, 2396–2406.

Clark, J.D., Mossey, P.A., Sharp, L., Little, J., 2003. Socioeconomic status and orofacial clefts in Scotland, 1989 to 1998. Cleft Palate Craniofac J 40, 481–485.

Cohen, M., Chhetri, D.K., Head, C., 2007. Isolated uvulitis. Ear Nose Throat J 86, 462, 464.

Cohen, M., Nabili, V., Chhetri, D.K., 2008. Palatal perforation from cocaine abuse. Ear Nose Throat J 87, 262.

de la Chaux R, Klemens C, Patscheider M, Dreher A., 2007. [Snoring: therapeutic options.] MMW Fortschr Med 149, 33–35.

Deacon, S., 2005. Maternal smoking during pregnancy is associated with a higher risk of non-syndromic orofacial clefts in infants. Evid Based Dent 6, 43–44.

Edwards, M.J., Agho, K., Attia, J., et al., 2003. Case-control study of cleft lip or palate after maternal use of topical corticosteroids during pregnancy. Am J Med Genet A 120A, 459–463.

Eng, C.Y., Evans, A.S., Quraishi, M.S., Harkness, P.A., 2007. A comparison of the incidence of facial palsy following parotidectomy performed by ENT and non-ENT surgeons. J Laryngol Otol 121, 40–43.

Eppley, B.L., van Aalst, J.A., Robey, A., Havlik, R.J., Sadove, A.M., 2005. The spectrum of orofacial clefting. Plast Reconstr Surg 115, 101e–114e.

Eros, E., Czeizel, A.E., Rockenbauer, M., Sorensen, H.T., Olsen, J., 2002. A population-based case-control teratologic study of nitrazepam, medazepam, tofisopam, alprazolum and clonazepam treatment during pregnancy. Eur J Obstet Gynecol Reprod Biol 101, 147–154.

Fallin, M.D., Hetmanski, J.B., Park, J., et al., 2003. Family-based analysis of MSX1 haplotypes for association with oral clefts. Genet Epidemiol 25, 168–175.

Gilgen-Anner, Y., Heim, M., Ledermann, H.P., Bircher, A.J., 2007. Iodide mumps after contrast media imaging: a rare adverse effect to iodine. Ann Allergy Asthma Immunol 99, 93–98.

Grewal, J., Carmichael, S.L., Ma, C., Lammer, E.J., Shaw, G.M., 2008. Maternal periconceptional smoking and alcohol consumption and risk for select congenital anomalies. Birth Defects Res A Clin Mol Teratol 82, 519–526.

Hardell, L., Hallquist, A., Hansson Mild, K., Carlberg, M., Gertzén, H., Schildt, E.B., Dahlqvist, A., 2004. No association between the use of cellular or cordless telephones and salivary gland tumours. Occup Environ Med 61, 675–679.

Hart, T.C., Marazita, M.L., Wright, J.T., 2000. The impact of molecular genetics on oral health paradigms. Crit Rev Oral Biol Med 11, 26–56.

Holmes, L.B., Baldwin, E.J., Smith, C.R., et al., 2008. Increased frequency of isolated cleft palate in infants exposed to lamotrigine during pregnancy. Neurology 70, 2152–2158.

Honein, M.A., Rasmussen, S.A., Reefhuis, J., et al., 2007. Maternal smoking and environmental tobacco smoke exposure and the risk of orofacial clefts. Epidemiology 18, 226–233.

Hughes, J.P., Tatla, T., Farrell, R., 2006. How we do it: changes in thyroid and salivary gland surgery since 1989: who's doing it and what are they doing? Clin Otolaryngol 31, 443–446.

Johnson, J.T., Vates, J., Wagner, R.L., 2008. Reduction of snoring with a plasma-mediated radiofrequency-based ablation (Coblation) device. Ear Nose Throat J 87, 40–43.

Källén, B., Otterblad Olausson, P., 2007. Use of anti-asthmatic drugs during pregnancy. 3. Congenital malformations in the infants. Eur J Clin Pharmacol 63, 383–388.

Kim, D.S., Cheang, P., Dover, S., Drake-Lee, A.B., 2007. Dental otalgia. J Laryngol Otol 121, 1129–1134.

Koch, M., Zenk, J., Iro, H., 2008. [Diagnostic and interventional sialoscopy in obstructive diseases of the salivary glands.] HNO 56, 139–144.

Kouwen, H.B., DeJonckere, P.H., 2007. Prevalence of OME is reduced in young children using chewing gum. Ear Hear 28, 451–455.

Kozer, E., Nikfar, S., Costei, A., Boskovic, R., Nulman, I., Koren, G., 2002. Aspirin consumption during the first trimester of pregnancy and congenital anomalies: a meta-analysis. Am J Obstet Gynecol 187, 1623–1630.

Krapels, I.P., Zielhuis, G.A., Vroom, F., et al.; Eurocran Gene-Environment Interaction Group, 2006. Periconceptional health and lifestyle factors of both parents affect the risk of live-born children with orofacial clefts. Birth Defects Res A Clin Mol Teratol 76, 613–620.

Lie, R.T., Wilcox, A.J., Taylor, J., et al., 2008. Maternal smoking and oral clefts: the role of detoxification pathway genes. Epidemiology 19, 606–615.

Little, J., Cardy, A., Munger, R.G., 2004. Tobacco smoking and oral clefts: a meta-analysis. Bull World Health Organ 82, 213–218.

Lönn, S., Ahlbom, A., Christensen, H.C., et al., 2006. Mobile phone use and risk of parotid gland tumor. Am J Epidemiol 164, 637–643.

Manrique, D., do Brasil Ode, O., Ramos, H., 2007. Drooling: analysis and evaluation of 31 children who underwent bilateral submandibular gland excision and parotid duct ligation. Braz J Otorhinolaryngol 73, 40–44.

Matalon, S., Schechtman, S., Goldzweig, G., Ornoy, A., 2002. The teratogenic effect of carbamazepine: a meta-analysis of 1255 exposures. Reprod Toxicol 16, 9–17.

Mueller, D.T., Callanan, V.P., 2007. Congenital malformations of the oral cavity. Otolaryngol Clin North Am 40, 141–160 , vii.

Nahlieli, O., Abramson, A., Shacham, R., Puterman, M.B., Baruchin, A.M., 2008. Endoscopic treatment of salivary gland injuries due to facial rejuvenation procedures. Laryngoscope 118, 763–767.

Nørgård, B., Puhó, E., Czeizel, A.E., Skriver, M.V., Sørensen, H.T., 2005. Aspirin use during early pregnancy and the risk of congenital abnormalities: a population-based case-control study. Am J Obstet Gynecol 192, 922–923.

Smith, S.D., 2007. Oral appliances in the treatment of obstructive sleep apnea. Atlas Oral Maxillofac Surg Clin North Am 15, 193–211.

Pavelec, V., Polenik, P., 2006. Use of Er,Cr:YSGG versus standard lasers in laser assisted uvulopalatoplasty for treatment of snoring. Laryngoscope 116, 1512–1516.

Perez-Aytes, A., Ledo, A., Boso, V., et al., 2008. In utero exposure to mycophenolate mofetil: a characteristic phenotype? Am J Med Genet A 146A, 1–7.

Puhó, E.H., Szunyogh, M., Métneki, J., Czeizel, A.E., 2007. Drug treatment during pregnancy and isolated orofacial clefts in hungary. Cleft Palate Craniofac J 44, 194–202.

Puraviappan, P., Dass, D.B., Narayanan, P., 2007. Efficacy of relocation of submandibular duct in cerebral palsy patients with drooling. Asian J Surg 30, 209–215.

Ramirez, D., Lammer, E.J., Iovannisci, D.M., Laurent, C., Finnell, R.H., Shaw, G.M., 2007. Maternal smoking during early pregnancy, GSTP1 and EPHX1 variants, and risk of isolated orofacial clefts. Cleft Palate Craniofac J 44, 366–373.

Ricciardiello, F., Martufi, S., Cardone, M., Cavaliere, M., D'Errico, P., Lengo, M., 2006. Otorhinolaryngology-related tuberculosis. Acta Otorhinolaryngol Ital 26, 38–42.

Rubino, C., de Vathaire, F., Dottorini, M.E., et al., 2003. Second primary malignancies in thyroid cancer patients. Br J Cancer 89, 1638–1644.

Sadetzki, S., Chetrit, A., Jarus-Hakak, A., et al., 2008. Cellular phone use and risk of benign and malignant parotid gland tumors – a nationwide case-control study. Am J Epidemiol 167, 457–467.

Sadetzki, S., Oberman, B., Mandelzweig, L., et al., 2008. Smoking and risk of parotid gland tumors: a nationwide case-control study. Cancer 112, 1974–1982. Erratum in Cancer 2008;113:662–663.

Sandow, P.L., Hejrat-Yazdi, M., Heft, M.W., 2006. Taste loss and recovery following radiation therapy. J Dent Res 85, 608–611.

Sandy, J.R., 2003. Molecular, clinical and political approaches to the problem of cleft lip and palate. J R Coll Surg Edinb Irel 1, 9–16.

Schüz, J., Jacobsen, R., Olsen, J.H., Boice Jr., J.D., McLaughlin, J.K., Johansen, C., 2006. Cellular telephone use and cancer risk: update of a nationwide Danish cohort. J Natl Cancer Inst 98, 1707–1713.

Shaw, G.M., Iovannisci, D.M., Yang, W., et al., 2005. Endothelial nitric oxide synthase (NOS3) genetic variants, maternal smoking, vitamin use, and risk of human orofacial clefts. Am J Epidemiol 162, 1207–1214.

Shi, M., Christensen, K., Weinberg, C.R., et al., 2007. Orofacial cleft risk is increased with maternal smoking and specific detoxification-gene variants. Am J Hum Genet 80, 76–90.

Shi, M., Wehby, G.L., Murray, J.C., 2008. Review on genetic variants and maternal smoking in the etiology of oral clefts and other birth defects. Birth Defects Res C Embryo Today 84, 16–29.

Sorrenti, G., Piccin, O., Mondini, S., Ceroni, A.R., 2006. One-phase management of severe obstructive sleep apnea: tongue base reduction with hyoepiglottoplasty plus uvulopalatopharyngoplasty. Otolaryngol Head Neck Surg 135, 906–910.

Vieira, A.R., 2008. Unraveling human cleft lip and palate research. J Dent Res 87, 119–125.

Webster, W.S., Howe, A.M., Abela, D., Oakes, D.J., 2006. The relationship between cleft lip, maxillary hypoplasia, hypoxia and phenytoin. Curr Pharm Des 12, 1431–1448.

Wikner, B.N., Stiller, C.O., Bergman, U., Asker, C., Källén, B., 2007. Use of benzodiazepines and benzodiazepine receptor agonists during pregnancy: neonatal outcome and congenital malformations. Pharmacoepidemiol Drug Saf 16, 1203–1210.

Wilcox, A.J., Lie, R.T., Solvoll, K., et al., 2007. Folic acid supplements and risk of facial clefts: national population based case-control study. BMJ 334, 464.

Wong, F.K., Hagg, U., 2004. An update on the aetiology of orofacial clefts. Hong Kong Med J 10, 331–336.

Yazdy, M.M., Honein, M.A., Xing, J., 2007. Reduction in orofacial clefts following folic acid fortification of the U.S. grain supply. Birth Defects Res A Clin Mol Teratol 79, 16–23.

Zeiger, J.S., Beaty, T.H., Liang, K.Y., 2005. Oral clefts, maternal smoking, and TGFA: a meta-analysis of gene-environment interaction. Cleft Palate Craniofac J 42, 58–63.

Appendix 14.1 Syndromes which may include cleft lip/palate

- Apert syndrome
- Basal cell carcinoma naevoid syndrome
- Carpenter syndrome
- Cleidocranial dysplasia
- Craniosynostosis Crouzon syndrome
- Freeman–Sheldon syndrome
- Goldenhar syndrome
- Hallerman–Streiff syndrome
- Hemifacial microsomia
- Hydrocephalus
- Microtia
- Miller syndrome
- Moebius syndrome
- Nager syndrome
- Nasal encephalocoeles
- Neurofibromatosis
- Orbital hypertelorism
- Parry–Romberg syndrome
- Pfeiffer syndrome
- Pierre Robin sequence
- Saethre–Chotzen syndrome
- Shprintzen syndrome
- Stickler syndrome
- Treacher Collins syndrome
- Van der Woude syndrome
- Waardenberg syndrome

RESPIRATORY MEDICINE

The respiratory tract consists of the upper respiratory tract (nose, paranasal sinuses, pharynx and larynx; discussed in Ch. 14) and the lower respiratory tract – the respiratory airways (trachea, bronchi and bronchioles) and lungs (respiratory bronchioles, alveolar ducts, alveolar sacs, and alveoli), discussed in this chapter.

Protective mechanisms in the respiratory tract include a mucociliary lining. Particles or pathogens are trapped in the mucus and driven by ciliary action (the ciliary elevator) to the pharynx. Mucociliary transport declines with age, but any effect on clinical infection has not been proved. Lymphoid tissues of Waldeyer ring (adenoids, palatine and lingual tonsils) are important in developing an immune response to pathogens. However, the best respiratory defence mechanism is the cough reflex, the components of which include cough receptors, afferent nerves, the cough centre and efferent nerves, and effector muscles. Impairment of any of these can weaken protection as may be seen in older patients or conditions associated with lowered consciousness (e.g. sedative use and neurological disease). Dysphagia or impaired oesophageal motility may exacerbate the tendency to aspirate foreign material. The alveolar defence mechanisms include macrophages, immunocytes, surfactant, phospholipids, immunoglobulin G (IgG), IgE, secretory IgA, complement components and Factor B.

Lung function is vital to gas exchange with the blood, absorbing oxygen and releasing carbon dioxide. Oxygen is transported combined with haemoglobin in erythrocytes and a small amount dissolved in plasma. The oxyhaemoglobin dissociation curve is sigmoidal: once the oxygen saturation falls below 95%, the amount of O_2 transported to the tissues and brain falls rapidly. High temperatures, acidosis, raised CO_2 and raised 2,3-diphosphoglycerate (2,3-DPG) levels encourage offloading of oxygen, whereas fetal haemoglobin and carboxyhaemoglobin have the opposite effect. Chronic hypoxaemia (e.g. at high altitudes) stimulates release of erythropoietin from the kidneys, with a rise in red cell production, and raised 2,3-DPG.

Normal gas exchange requires adequate alveolar ventilation, normal ventilation/blood flow relationships and adequate alveolar–capillary membrane surface area. Breathing (ventilation) depends on respiratory drive, which reacts to the respiratory load. This process requires work and results in gas exchange.

LOWER RESPIRATORY DISEASE

The most common lower respiratory disorders are asthma and chronic obstructive pulmonary disease.

GENERAL ASPECTS

Respiratory disorders are common, often caused or aggravated by tobacco smoking, and may significantly affect general anaesthesia (GA) and conscious sedation since they are often a contraindication to use of benzodiazepines, opioids and other respiratory depressants.

CLINICAL FEATURES

Impaired gas exchange leads to laboured breathing and can cause significant incapacity. Important features include cough, sputum production, wheeze, dyspnoea, chest pain, cyanosis, finger-clubbing (Fig. 15.1), use of accessory muscles of respiration with indrawing of the intercostal spaces (hyperinflation) and abnormalities in chest shape, movements, respiratory rate and breath sounds.

Cough may be a feature of any respiratory problem but, if chronic, may herald serious disease such as chronic obstructive airways disease, cancer or tuberculosis. Mucoid or mucopurulent sputum is often a feature of chronic bronchitis (Fig. 15.2); purulent sputum in acute bronchitis, bronchiectasis or lung abscess; and blood (haemoptysis) or blood-stained sputum, though common in acute infections (especially in pre-existing chronic obstructive pulmonary disease), bronchiectasis and pulmonary embolism, is usually a serious event possibly due to carcinoma or tuberculosis, for example. Wheezing is caused by airways obstruction and is a typical sign of asthma or bronchitis. Breathlessness (dyspnoea) is distressing, may be caused by respiratory or cardiovascular disease, or anaemia, and is particularly ominous if it persists at rest.

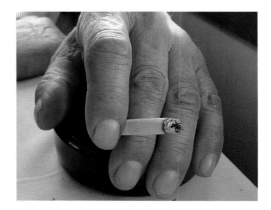

Fig. 15.1 Tobacco smoker with clubbing in lung cancer

Excessive resistive load, such as in asthma, chronic bronchitis and emphysema and cystic fibrosis, impairs airflow. Elastic load increases due, for example, to interstitial fibrosis, muscle paralysis and obesity.

GENERAL MANAGEMENT

Diagnosis of respiratory disorders is from the clinical features supported by imaging (especially chest radiography). Spiral computed tomography (CT) can now scan the lungs in a quick 20–30 s breath hold and therefore, instead of acquiring a stack of individual CT slices, which may be misaligned due to patient movement or breathing in between slices, provides high-resolution three-dimensional images.

Respiratory function tests can measure individual components of the respiratory process.

Spirometry is the basic screening test for assessing mechanical load problems, the quantification involving determining the vital capacity (VC) – slow vital capacity (SVC) and/or forced vital capacity (FVC) – and the speed of maximal expiratory flow (MEF; Fig. 15.3). Usually about 75% of a normal-sized VC is expelled in 1 second (FEV_1). The peak flow meter, which measures the peak expiratory flow rate (PEFR; the earliest portion of forced expiration), is a simple measure of airflow obstruction, when the FEV_1 is a much smaller fraction of the VC. In lung restriction, the diminished VC can be mostly expelled in about 1 s. Serial measurements (e.g. in asthma) provide valuable information about disease progress. The reversibility of airways obstruction is usually assessed by spirometry before and after use of a bronchodilator.

Arterial blood gas analysis yields considerable information about gas exchange efficiency. Arterial hypoxaemia in adults is defined as $PaO_2 < 10.7$ kPa breathing room air, although it is not usually treated as clinically important unless below 8 kPa, when oxygen saturation will be 90% or less (Table 15.1).

Arterial carbon dioxide tension (PaCO$_2$) is used as an inversely proportional index of 'effective' alveolar ventilation. Hence, a high $PaCO_2$ is taken to indicate poor alveolar ventilation. Alveolar hypoventilation (raised $PaCO_2$) with a normal pH probably represents a primary ventilatory change present long enough for renal mechanisms to compensate, as in chronic ventilatory failure. Ventilation/blood flow relationships are most simply assessed by considering the size of the difference between the amounts of oxygen and carbon dioxide in the blood and in the air: the differences are small if the lungs are working efficiently. Disparity between ventilation/blood flow ratios results in abnormally wide differences and then alveolar-arterial PO_2 and arterial-alveolar PCO_2 gradients will be abnormal.

Alveolar capillary surface area is assessed by measuring the uptake of carbon monoxide – usually abnormal in diffuse interstitial inflammatory and fibrotic processes and in emphysema.

Assessing bronchial reactivity and the exercise response can help evaluate breathlessness. Simple exercise testing provides information about overall fitness and the appropriateness of cardiorespiratory responses. Radionuclide lung scanning, blood gas analysis and sputum cytology or culture are sometimes needed in addition. Management can include oxygen by mask or nasal cannula (Figs 15.4 and 15.5).

DENTAL ASPECTS

Lower respiratory tract disorders can cause significant incapacity and are often a contraindication to GA, and even to conscious sedation.

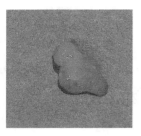

Fig. 15.2 Mucoid sputum from chronic obstructive pulmonary disease

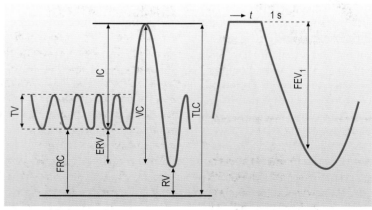

TV = Tidal volume
VC = Vital capacity (VC = IC + ERV)
FEV_1 = Forced expiratory volume in 1 s
FRC = Functional residual capacity
(FRC = ERV + RV)

TLC = Total lung capacity
RV = Residual volume (RV = TLC – VC)
IC = Inspiratory capacity
ERV = Expiratory reserve volume
(ERV = VC – IC)

Fig. 15.3 Spirometry

Table 15.1 Adult values for PaO₂ and oxygen saturation

	PaO₂ (kPa)	SaO₂ (%)
Normal (range)	13 (≥10.7)	97 (95–100)
Hypoxaemia	< 10.7	< 95
Mild hypoxaemia	8–10.5	90–94
Moderate hypoxaemia	5.3–7.9	75–89
Severe hypoxaemia	< 5.3	< 75

From Williams AJ. http://www.bmj.com/cgi/content/full/317/7167/1213

Table 15.2 Types of asthma

	Extrinsic asthma	Intrinsic asthma
Frequency	Most common	Least common
Aetiopathogenesis	Allergens causing IgE-mediated mast cell degranulation	Mast cell instability and airway hyper-responsivity
Association with atopy	+	–
Typical age of onset	Child	Adult

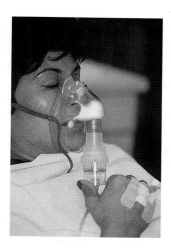

Fig. 15.4 Oxygen by mask in a patient with severe bronchospasm

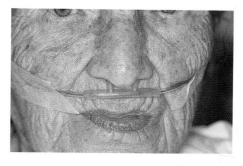

Fig. 15.5 Nasal catheter

ASTHMA

Asthma is a common condition, which affects 2–5% of the overall population and is increasing, particularly in childhood, with a frequency of up to 20% in some Western countries. Asthma usually begins in childhood or early adult life: about half the patients with asthma develop it before age 10.

Bronchial hyper-reactivity causes reversible airway obstruction from smooth muscle constriction (bronchospasm), mucosal oedema and hypersecretion of mucus. There are two main types, extrinsic (allergic) and intrinsic asthma (Table 15.2).

Extrinsic (allergic asthma), the main childhood type, may be precipitated by allergens in animal dander, feathers or hair, drugs [e.g. non-steroidal anti-inflammatory drugs (NSAIDs) and some antibiotics], food (e.g. eggs, fish, fruit, milk, nuts), house dust (allergens from mites) or moulds.

Patients are often asymptomatic between attacks, but frequently have or develop other allergic diseases, such as eczema, hay fever and drug sensitivities. This type of asthma is associated with IgE overproduction on exposure to allergens, and release of mast cell mediators (histamine, leukotrienes, prostaglandins, bradykinin and platelet activating factor), which cause bronchospasm and oedema. About 75% of asthmatic children lose their asthma or improve by adulthood.

Intrinsic asthma is usually of adult onset and is not allergic. Rather, it appears to be related to mast cell instability and airway hyper-responsivity, triggered by emotional stress, gastro-oesophageal reflux or vagally mediated responses.

Trigger factors for asthma of *either* type include: infections (especially viral, mycoplasmal or fungal); irritating fumes (e.g. traffic or cigarette smoke); exercise (possibly due to cold air); weather changes; emotional stress; foods (e.g. nuts, shellfish, strawberries or milk, or additives such as tartrazine); and drugs [e.g. aspirin and other NSAIDs, beta-blockers and angiotensin-converting enzyme (ACE) inhibitors].

CLINICAL FEATURES

In well-controlled patients with asthma, clinical features may be absent. During an asthmatic episode symptoms may include dyspnoea, cough and paroxysmal expiratory wheeziness with laboured expiration. Nasal polyps are common, especially in aspirin-sensitive asthmatics. Children with asthma initially suffer from repeated 'colds' with cough, malaise and fever, often at night. The frequency and severity of attacks vary widely between individuals (Table 15.3).

Patients may become distressed, anxious, tachycardic, have reduced chest expansion and be using accessory respiratory muscles to increase their ventilatory effort.

A prolonged asthmatic attack, which is refractory to treatment, may lead to life-threatening status asthmaticus (persists for more than 24 h). Failure of the patient to complete a sentence, indrawing of the intercostal muscles, a rapid pulse and a silent chest, and signs of exhaustion are suggestive of an impending respiratory arrest.

Table 15.3 Severity of asthma

Severity of asthma	Symptom duration	Attack frequency per week	Other comments	Typical therapy
Mild	< 1 h	< 2	Attacks follow exercise or exposure to trigger	Beta-agonist as required
Moderate	Days	> 2	Activity restricted	Beta-agonist plus steroid
Severe	Persistent	Persistent	Audible wheezing. Tachypnoea. Activity and sleep severely restricted	Beta agonist plus steroid plus theophylline

GENERAL MANAGEMENT

Diagnosis of asthma is based on clinical history and presentation. Investigations include chest radiography (to exclude other diagnoses, such as a pneumothorax, which may mimic an acute asthma attack), spirometry (serial PEFR), skin tests and blood examination (usually eosinophilia, raised total IgE and specific IgE antibody concentrations, which may help identify allergens). Occasionally a histamine or methacholine challenge is used if the diagnosis is unclear.

Management includes patient education, smoking cessation advice, the avoidance of identifiable irritants and allergens, and use of drugs. Treatment should be based on the amount by which peak flow is reduced (a PEFR diary should be kept). Home use of peak flow meters allows patients to monitor progress and detect any deterioration, that may require urgent modification of treatment.

Drugs used for management (Table 15.4) include oxygen β₂-agonists (such as salbutamol), corticosteroids, leukotriene receptor antagonists and omalizumab (a recombinant humanized monoclonal anti-IgE antibody that reduces the antigen-specific IgE).

Deaths from asthma are usually a result of failure to recognize deterioration or reluctance to use corticosteroids.

DENTAL ASPECTS

Elective dental care should be deferred in severe asthmatics until they are in a better phase; this can be advised by their own general practitioner.

Asthmatic patients should be asked to bring their usual medication with them when coming for dental treatment. Local anaesthesia (LA) is best used: occasional patients may react to the sulfites present as preservatives in vasoconstrictor-containing LA, so it may be better, where possible, to avoid solutions containing vasoconstrictor. Epinephrine may theoretically enhance the risk of arrhythmias with beta-agonists and is contraindicated in patients using theophylline as it may precipitate arrhythmias.

Relative analgesia with nitrous oxide and oxygen is preferable to intravenous sedation and gives more immediate control. Sedatives in general are better avoided as, in an acute asthmatic attack, even benzodiazepines can precipitate respiratory failure.

Table 15.4 Medical management of asthma[a]

Drug group	Examples	Comments
Beta-agonists	Selective β₂-agonists or stimulants (e.g. salbutamol). Others include:	Safest and most effective bronchodilators for routine control of asthma
	Terbutaline, fenoterol, rimiterol Pirbuterol, reproterol, tulobuterol Bambuterol, salmeterol, formoterol	Relax bronchial smooth muscle with little cardiac effect Act for 3–6 h Act for at least 12 h
Antimuscarinic bronchodilators	Ipratropium or oxitropium bromide	Useful particularly for those with asthma associated with bronchitis. Act for up to 8 h. Contraindicated in glaucoma and prostatic disease
Methylxanthines	Theophylline preparations (oral sustained release)	Prolonged action and useful for controlling nocturnal asthma
Corticosteroids	Corticosteroid (beclometasone, betametasone valerate, budesonide or fluticasone) aerosol inhalations	Effective inhaled along with a bronchodilator, but must be taken regularly. High-dose corticosteroid inhalants can cause some adrenal suppression
Mast cell stabilizers	Sodium cromoglicate (cromoglycate) or nedocromil	Occasionally used as inhalants for prophylaxis, mainly in children, but some fail to respond
Leukotriene receptor antagonists	Montelukast, zafirlukast	May impair liver function and increase INR. Given orally. Effective when used alone or with inhaled steroids but may precipitate, and should not be used in Churg–Strauss syndrome, where deterioration and cardiac complications may be seen
5-Lipoxygenase inhibitor (impairs leukotriene release)	Zileuton	
Recombinant humanized monoclonal anti-IgE antibody	Omalizumab	Safe, effective treatment for allergic asthma

[a]In addition to oxygen.
INR, international normalized ratio.

General anaesthesia is best avoided as it may be complicated by hypoxia and hypercapnia, which can cause pulmonary oedema even if cardiac function is normal, and cardiac failure if there is cardiac disease. The risk of post-operative lung collapse or pneumothorax is also increased. Halothane or, better, enflurane, isoflurane, desflurane or sevoflurane are the preferred anaesthetics, but ketamine may be useful in children.

Allergy to penicillin may be more frequent in asthmatics. Drugs to be avoided, since they may precipitate an asthmatic attack (see later), include those in Box 15.1.

Acute asthmatic attacks may also occasionally be precipitated by anxiety; it is important to attempt to lessen fear of dental treatment by gentle handling and reassurance. Even routine dental treatment can trigger a clinically significant decline in lung function in approximately 15% of asthmatics. Acute asthmatic attacks are usually self-limiting or respond to the patient's usual medication such as a beta-agonist inhaler but status asthmaticus is a potentially fatal emergency (see Ch. 1). There may be complications from the drugs (Table 15.5).

Gastro-oesophageal reflux is not uncommon, with occasional tooth erosion. Periodontal inflammation is greater in asthmatics than in those without respiratory disease.

Box 15.1 Agents that may precipitate asthmatic attack

- Acrylic monomer
- Aspirin (also increases serum zafirlukast levels) and other NSAIDs
- Barbiturates (e.g. methohexitone)
- Beta-blockers
- Colophony
- Cyanoacrylates
- Drugs causing histamine release directly
- Mefenamic acid
- Morphine and some other opioids
- Pancuronium
- Pentazocine
- Suxamethonium
- Tubocurarine

Table 15.5 Management complications from anti-asthmatic drugs

Anti-asthmatic drug	Possible complications
β_2-agonists	Dry mouth
Corticosteroids	Steroid complications and adrenal crisis. Corticosteroid inhalers occasionally causes oral or pharyngeal thrush and, rarely, angina bullosa haemorrhagica
Ipratropium bromide	Dry mouth
Leukotriene antagonists	Bleeding tendency (and prolonged INR) because of impaired liver metabolism
Theophylline	Levels increased by epinephrine, erythromycin, clindamycin, azithromycin, clarithromycin or ciprofloxacin

INR, international normalized ratio.

CHURG–STRAUSS SYNDROME (ALLERGIC GRANULOMATOSIS OR ANGIITIS)

GENERAL ASPECTS

Churg–Strauss syndrome (CSS) is a rare potentially fatal systemic vasculitis similar to polyarteritis nodosa (PAN) characterized by severe asthma-like attacks with peripheral eosinophilia, intravascular and extravascular granuloma formation with eosinophil infiltration and skin lesions in 70%. Cardiopulmonary involvement is the main cause of death.

Box 15.2 Features of Churg–Strauss syndrome

- Asthma
- Eosinophilia > 10%
- Neuropathy (mono- or poly-)
- Pulmonary infiltrates (non-fixed)
- Paranasal sinus abnormality
- Extravascular eosinophils

CLINICAL FEATURES

Churg–Strauss syndrome is diagnosed if at least four of the six criteria in Box 15.2 are positive.

GENERAL MANAGEMENT

The 5-year survival of untreated CSS is 25%. Combination treatment with cyclophosphamide and prednisolone provides a 5-year survival of 50%.

DENTAL ASPECTS

Management problems of patients with CSS may include respiratory impairment and corticosteroid treatment (Ch. 6).

CHRONIC OBSTRUCTIVE PULMONARY DISEASE

Chronic obstructive pulmonary disease (COPD; chronic obstructive airways disease; COAD) is a common, chronic, slowly progressive, irreversible disease (most frequently a combination of chronic bronchitis and emphysema) characterized by breathlessness and wheeze (airways obstruction), cough and sputum. The most important causes of COPD include cigarette smoking, and environmental pollution, dusts, or occupational exposures to chemicals. Exposure to smoke from home cooking or heating fuels may contribute. Deficiency of the anti-proteolytic enzyme alpha$_1$-antitrypsin is a rare cause of emphysema.

Chronic bronchitis is defined as the excessive production of mucus and persistent cough with sputum production, daily for more than 3 months in a year over more than 2 consecutive years. It leads to production of excessive, viscous mucus, which is ineffectively cleared from the airway, obstructs and stagnates, and becomes infected, usually with *Streptococcus pneumoniae*,

Moraxella catarrhalis and *Haemophilus influenzae*. Patchy areas of alveolar collapse can result.

Emphysema is dilatation of air spaces distal to the terminal bronchioles with destruction of alveoli, reducing the alveolar surface area available for respiratory exchange.

CLINICAL FEATURES

Chronic obstructive pulmonary disease is characterized by breathlessness and wheeze (airways obstruction), cough and an early morning mucoid sputum production. Progressive dyspnoea, low oxygen saturation, carbon dioxide accumulation (hypercapnia) and metabolic acidosis mean patients are ultimately dyspnoeic at rest ('respiratory cripples'), especially when recumbent (orthopnoea), and eventually develop respiratory failure, pulmonary hypertension, right ventricular hypertrophy and right-sided heart failure (cor pulmonale).

Two clinical patterns of COPD are recognized: *'pink puffers'* – patients with emphysema who manage to maintain normal blood gases by hyperventilation, and are always breathless but not cyanosed and rather they are pink from vasodilatation – and *'blue bloaters'*. The latter are patients with chronic bronchitis who lose the CO_2 drive, fail to maintain adequate ventilation and become both hypercapnic and hypoxic with central cyanosis, cor pulmonale and oedema. For these patients, the respiratory drive is from the low PO_2 and thus oxygen administration is contraindicated (Table 15.6).

Table 15.6 Comparison of chronic bronchitis and emphysema

	Chronic bronchitis	Emphysema
Cough	Chronic	Minimal
Sputum	Copious and mucoid	Minimal
Infections	Common	Uncommon
Dyspnoea	Mild	Severe
PO_2	Low	Low
PCO_2	Raised	Normal
Forced expiratory volume (FEV)	Low	Low
Clinical appearance	Blue bloater	Pink puffer

GENERAL MANAGEMENT

The diagnosis of COPD is based upon clinical history and presentation. Investigations include chest radiography (CXR; which may show hyperinflated lung fields with loss of vascular markings); arterial blood gases (which should be measured if pulse oximetry shows oxygen saturation less than 92%); and spirometry and lung function tests. Forced expiratory volume in one second (FEV_1) is reduced in all cases (FEV_1 of < 40% signifies severe COPD) and the flow–volume curve shows a typical pattern with reduced flow rates at mid and lower lung volumes. A ratio of FEV_1:forced vital capacity (FVC) of < 70% confirms airways obstruction.

Patients with COPD and their family should be educated about the disease, required lifestyle changes and medication.

Non-drug therapy includes: stopping smoking (nicotine replacement therapy or bupropion may help); exercise by pulmonary rehabilitation is of proven benefit; weight loss (improves exercise tolerance); and vaccination (pneumococcal and influenza vaccines).

Drug treatment includes bronchodilators [anticholinergic drugs (ipratropium bromide) and β_2-agonists (salbutamol) to treat the reversible component of airway disease]; corticosteroids (inhaled or systemic) and antibiotics (amoxicillin, trimethoprim or tetracycline). Mucolytics such as carbocisteine reduce acute exacerbations by almost one-third. Long-term oxygen therapy (LTOT) reduces mortality if given for 19 h/day every day at a flow rate of 1–3 L/min to maintain arterial oxygen saturation above 90%. Controlled oxygen administration in COPD patients is needed to avoid respiratory arrest. Advanced emphysema is occasionally treated with surgery – excision of large acquired bullae or, rarely, lung transplantation.

DENTAL ASPECTS

Patients with COPD who need dental care can be classified as follows.

- Patients at low risk – experience dyspnoea on effort but have normal blood gas levels; these patients can receive all dental treatment with minor modifications.
- Patients at moderate risk – experience dyspnoea on effort, are chronically treated with bronchodilators or recently with corticosteroids, and partial pressure of oxygen (PaO_2) lowered – then a medical consultation is advised to determine the level of control of the disease before any dental treatment.
- Patients at high risk – have symptomatic COPD that may be end-stage and poorly responsive to treatment. With these patients, a medical consultation is essential before any dental treatment is carried out.

Patients with COPD are best treated in an upright position at mid-morning or early afternoon, since they may become increasingly dyspnoeic if laid supine. It may be difficult to use a rubber dam, as some patients are mouth breathers and do not tolerate the additional obstruction. LA is preferred for dental treatment, but bilateral mandibular or palatal injections should be avoided. Patients with COPD should be given relative analgesia only if absolutely necessary, and only in hospital after full pre-operative assessment. Diazepam and midazolam should not be used as they are respiratory depressants. Patients should be given GA only if absolutely necessary, and intravenous barbiturates are contraindicated. Secretions reduce airway patency and, if lightly anaesthetized, the patient may cough and contaminate other areas of the lung. Post-operative respiratory complications are more prevalent in patients with pre-existing lung diseases, especially after prolonged operations and if there has been no pre-operative preparation. The most important single factor in pre-operative care is cessation of smoking for at least 1 week pre-operatively. Respiratory infections must also be eradicated, sputum should first be sent for culture and sensitivity, but antimicrobials such as amoxicillin should be started without awaiting results.

Patients taking corticosteroids should be treated with appropriate precautions (Ch. 6).

Interactions of theophylline with drugs, such as epinephrine, erythromycin, clindamycin, azithromycin, clarithromycin or ciprofloxacin, may result in dangerously high levels of theophylline. Ipratropium can cause dry mouth.

INFECTIONS

Respiratory viruses usually spread by airborne transmission and the very small particles (2–0.2 micrometres) can avoid the upper respiratory tract defences and the mucociliary elevator to reach the lung alveoli. A range of viruses can cause lower respiratory tract infections (LRTIs; Table 15.7).

Some viruses (e.g. influenza and respiratory syncytial) can spread from the upper to the lower respiratory tract via infection of the respiratory epithelium and can lead to bacterial superinfection and pneumonitis (pneumonia). Mycoplasmal (atypical) pneumonia and tuberculosis (TB) may be direct infections. More recently, a potentially fatal severe acute respiratory syndrome (SARS) due to a coronavirus has originated in south China and spread worldwide, H5N1 bird influenza arose as an epidemic and a similar epidemic, but of swine influenza (H1N1), has emanated from Mexico (see later).

Bacterial infections such as pneumonia or lung abscess can also result from material aspirated into the lungs, and are usually unilateral. Those who aspirate more than others have, as a result, more frequent LRTI and this is seen in alcohol and other drug abusers, and comatose patients. Exogenous penetration and contamination of the lung can result from trauma (e.g. a stab wound or road traffic accident) or surgery. *Entamoeba histolytica* can occasionally cause pneumonia – by direct extension from an amoebic liver abscess (Table 15.8). Patients with endocarditis, septic pelvic or jugular thrombophlebitis may experience LRTI acquired haematogenously and then often bilateral.

Immunocompromised persons [e.g. human immunodeficiency virus/acquired immune deficiency syndrome (HIV/AIDS) and transplant recipients] and people with bronchiectasis or cystic fibrosis are also susceptible to respiratory infections by a range of microbes, some of which are otherwise harmless. *Pneumocystis carinii* (*Pneumocystis jiroveci*), for example, is a common cause of fatal pneumonia in immunocompromised patients, especially those with HIV/AIDS (Ch. 21).

Table 15.7 Lower respiratory tract infections and their main causes (the most frequent are shown in bold)

Condition	Micro-organisms
Laryngo-tracheo-bronchitis (croup)	Influenza viruses Mycoplasma pneumoniae Parainfluenza viruses Respiratory syncytial virus
Acute bronchiolitis	Human metapneumovirus (HMPV) Influenza viruses Respiratory syncytial virus
Acute bronchitis	Adenovirus Bordetella pertussis Chlamydia pneumoniae [Taiwan acute respiratory (TWAR) agent] Coronaviruses Coxsackie virus Haemophilus influenzae (non-typeable) Herpes simplex virus Influenza viruses Moraxella catarrhalis Mycoplasma pneumoniae Parainfluenza virus Respiratory syncytial virus Rhinovirus
Acute pneumonitis (pneumonia)	Escherichia coli Haemophilus influenzae Klebsiella species Pseudomonas aeruginosa SARS-associated coronavirus (SARS-CoV) Streptococcus pneumoniae (pneumococcus)

SARS, severe acute respiratory syndrome.

Table 15.8 Causes of pneumonia

Infective route	Micro-organisms
Inhalation	Streptococcus pneumoniae, Streptococcus pyogenes Mycobacteria, Legionella, Coxiella burnetti (Q fever) Influenza, measles virus, adenovirus Coccidioides, Histoplasma, Cryptococcus
Aspiration	Anaerobes, Streptococcus pneumoniae, Staphylococcus aureus, Haemophilus influenzae, Gram-negative bacilli
Haematogenous	Staphylococcus aureus, Gram-negative bacilli (Pseudomonas aeruginosa) Candida Strongyloides, Ascaris
Contiguous spread	Anaerobes, Gram-negative bacilli Entamoeba histolytica
Reactivation	Mycobacteria Cytomegalovirus Coccidioides, Histoplasma, Blastomyces Toxoplasma, Strongyloides, Pneumocystis (carinii) jiroveci

CLINICAL FEATURES

Clinical features of LRTI vary according to the part of the respiratory tract mainly affected. Bronchitis causes cough, wheezing and sometimes dyspnoea. Bronchiolitis causes rapid respiration, wheezing, fever and dyspnoea but is restricted mainly to infants. Pneumonia causes cough, fever, rapid respiration, breathlessness, chest pain, dyspnoea and shivering.

GENERAL MANAGEMENT

Antimicrobial therapy is indicated, particularly for pneumonia. Antivirals have not been highly effective. Oxygen may be needed. Pneumococcal vaccine is indicated for older people.

DENTAL ASPECTS

The majority of LRTIs are severe illnesses, and contraindications to all but emergency dental treatment. GA is hazardous and absolutely contraindicated. Dental treatment should be deferred until recovery, or be limited to pain relief.

INFLUENZA ('FLU)

General aspects

Influenza is a contagious disease caused by the influenza virus types A, B or C. Type A has two main subtypes (H1N1 and H3N2), causes most of the widespread influenza epidemics and can occasionally be fatal; type B viruses generally cause regional outbreaks of moderate severity, and type C are of minor significance.

A person can spread influenza starting 1 day before they feel sick and for another 3–7 days after symptoms start. Influenza can be prevented or ameliorated by vaccination each autumn; this is especially indicated for older people, and those with cardiorespiratory disease.

Clinical features

Influenza attacks virtually the whole respiratory tract and symptoms appear suddenly after 1–4 days with fever, sore throat, nasal congestion, headache, tiredness, dry cough and muscle pains (myalgia).

Most people recover in 1–2 weeks but it can be life-threatening, mainly because primary influenzal viral pneumonia can lead to secondary bacterial pneumonia or exacerbate underlying conditions (e.g. pulmonary or cardiac disease). The old and very young, and those with chronic disorders, are more likely to suffer complications, such as pneumonia, bronchitis, sinusitis or otitis media.

Influenza has also been associated with depression, encephalopathy, myocarditis, myositis, pericarditis, Reye syndrome and transverse myelitis.

GENERAL MANAGEMENT

Zanamivir (antiviral against types A and B influenza) can shorten the symptoms by approximately 1 day, if treatment is started during the first 2 days of illness. Other antiviral drugs, which may help but are restricted mainly for immunocompromised persons since they can cause adverse effects, include amantadine, oseltamivir and rimantadine.

Rest, maintenance of fluid intake, analgesics, antipyretics, and avoidance of alcohol and tobacco help relieve symptoms. Aspirin must *never* be given to children under the age of 16 years who have 'flu-like symptoms, and particularly fever, as this can cause Reye syndrome.

Dental aspects

Influenza can be a severe illness and all but emergency dental treatment should be deferred until recovery. GA is hazardous and absolutely contraindicated.

Bird flu

Influenza type A subtype H5N1 can cause an illness known as 'avian influenza' or 'bird flu' in birds, humans and many other animal species. HPAI A(H5N1) – 'highly *pathogenic* avian influenza virus of type A of subtype H5N1' – is the causative agent and is *enzootic* in many bird populations, especially in South-East Asia. It spread globally and has resulted in the deaths of over 100 people and the slaughter of millions of chickens. A vaccine that could provide protection (Prepandrix) has been cleared for use in the European Union.

Swine flu

Swine influenza is common in pigs in the midwestern United States (and occasionally in other states), Mexico, Canada, South America, Europe (including the United Kingdom, Sweden and Italy), Kenya, Mainland China, Taiwan, Japan and other parts of eastern Asia. Transmission of swine influenza virus from pigs to humans is not common, but can produce symptoms similar to those of influenza. A 2009 outbreak in humans ('swine flu') was due to an apparently new strain of H1N1 arising from a reassortment produced from strains of human, avian and swine viruses. It can pass from human to human. Antiviral agents such as oseltamivir may help. Vaccines are now available.

SEVERE ACUTE RESPIRATORY SYNDROME

General aspects

An outbreak of a life-threatening febrile respiratory infection appeared in 2003 from Guangdong, China, and was named severe acute respiratory syndrome (SARS). Caused by a newly recognized coronavirus [SARS-associated coronavirus (SARS-CoV)], SARS spreads via close contact and has spread to many countries across the world. According to the World Health Organization, 8437 people worldwide became sick with SARS during the course of the first recognized outbreak and 813 died.

Clinical features

The incubation time of 2–7 days is followed by a high fever (> 38.0°C), malaise, headache and myalgia. Some people also experience mild upper respiratory symptoms and, after 2–7 days, lower respiratory signs – a dry cough and dyspnoea potentially progressing to hypoxaemia. SARS causes a pneumonia with a mortality approaching 10%, particularly in older or immunocompromised people.

General management

Artificial ventilation has been needed in 10–20% of cases. Antiviral agents such as oseltamivir or ribavirin may help.

Dental aspects

Severe acute respiratory syndrome is a severe illness, and all but emergency dental treatment should be deferred until recovery. GA is hazardous and absolutely contraindicated. For all contact with suspect SARS patients, careful hand hygiene is urged, including hand washing with soap and water; if hands are not visibly soiled, alcohol-based handrubs may be used as an alternative to hand washing. If a suspect SARS patient is admitted to hospital, infection control personnel should be notified immediately. Infection control measures (www.cdc. gov/ncidod/hip/isolat/isolat.htm) should include standard precautions (e.g. hand hygiene); health care personnel should wear eye protection for all patient contact; contact precautions (e.g. gown and gloves for contact with the patient or their environment) and airborne precautions (e.g. an isolation room with negative pressure relative to the surrounding area and use of an N-95 filtering disposable respirator for persons entering the room).

BACTERIAL PNEUMONIA

General aspects

Pneumonia is classed as 'primary' if it occurs in a previously healthy individual, and is usually lobar; or 'secondary' to some other disorder such as previous viral respiratory infections, aspiration of foreign material, lung disease (bronchiectasis or carcinoma), or depressed immunity (e.g. alcoholism or immunosuppression), or aspiration of oral bacteria (Table 15.9). It is usually bronchopneumonia.

Community-acquired pneumonia is often associated with *Strep. pneumoniae* or *Haemophilus influenzae* but Enterobacteriaceae, such as *Klebsiella* species, *Escherichia coli* and *Pseudomonas aeruginosa*, are especially likely in the very aged and infirm (Table 15.10). Poor oral hygiene and periodontal disease may promote oropharyngeal bacterial colonization. Early on, hospital-acquired pneumonia is often associated with *Strep. pneumoniae* or *Haemophilus influenzae*. In late hospital-acquired pneumonia, polymicrobial infections or meticillin-resistant *Staphylococcus aureus* (MRSA) are particular hazards.

Table 15.9 Factors predisposing to pneumonia

Exogenous	Endogenous
Viral respiratory infections, particularly influenza	Old age
Suppression of the cough reflex	Immobility
Aspiration of foreign material Mortality in patients in intensive care units (ventilator-associated pneumonia; VAP) can range from 20% to 50%	Respiratory depression or chest injury
Prolonged endotracheal intubation (increases risk by up to 20-fold)	Neurological disorders permitting aspiration of foreign material Underlying pulmonary disease such as carcinoma or emphysema Alcoholism Immunodeficiency (especially HIV/ AIDS) *Pneumocystis* (*carinii*) *jiroveci* pneumonia is discussed in Ch. 20

Table 15.10 Main causes of bacterial pneumonia

Pathogen	Comments
Chlamydia pneumoniae	Seen in persons in institutions
Chlamydia psittaci	Seen after contact with psittacine birds (parrots, etc.)
Coxiella burnetii	Seen after contact with farm animals
Gram-negative anaerobes	Seen after aspiration
Haemophilus influenzae	Seen at extremes of life
Klebsiella pneumoniae	Seen in the elderly, debilitated and in nursing homes
Legionella pneumoniae	Seen after exposure to water aerosols
Mycoplasma pneumoniae	Epidemics every 4 years
Staphylococcus aureus	Follows influenza
Streptococcus pneumoniae	Most common pathogen

Clinical features

Pneumonia causes cough, fever, rapid respiration, breathlessness, chest pain, dyspnoea and shivering. Complications can include lung abscess or empyema (pus in pleural cavity).

General management

It is important to avoid alcohol and tobacco, and use analgesics and antipyretics to relieve the symptoms. Broad-spectrum antimicrobials are given promptly and empirically usually a macrolide (azithromycin, clarithromycin or erythromycin) or quinolone (moxifloxacin, gatifloxacin or levofloxacin), or doxycycline for outpatients. For in-patients, cefuroxime or ceftriaxone plus a macrolide is used.

Prophylaxis includes smoking cessation, and immunization against influenza and pneumococci.

Dental aspects

Pneumonia is a severe illness and all but emergency dental treatment should be deferred until recovery. GA is hazardous and absolutely contraindicated.

LOEFFLER SYNDROME

This appears to be an allergic reaction, commonly to the parasitic worm *Ascaris lumbricoides*, or drugs such as sulfonamides. It manifests with pulmonary infiltrates (and an abnormal chest radiograph) and eosinophilia (eosinophilic pneumonia). The disease usually clears spontaneously.

LEGIONNAIRE'S DISEASE (LEGIONELLOSIS)

General aspects

The term Legionnaire's disease was coined as a result of an outbreak of the previously unrecognized respiratory disease in an American Legion meeting in Philadelphia in 1976, but it is now recognized worldwide, many infections being contracted during travel abroad, particularly to Spain, Turkey and some other Mediterranean areas.

Legionellosis is a respiratory infection with one of the family Legionellaceae, Gram-negative aerobic bacilli, ubiquitous in water and soil, but particularly preferring warm aquatic environments. Of over 30 Legionellaceae, most infections are by *Legionella pneumophila*. Infection spreads mainly (≈46%) through aerosolization of infected water in air-conditioning systems, hot-water systems, humidifiers, nebulizers, showers and spa pools. Many young people have been exposed to the infection and become seropositive but have remained healthy. Illness mainly affects males over 45, smokers, heavy drinkers, older people and the immunocompromised. Also vulnerable are travellers, especially middle-aged and older tourists, and conference or business groups, possibly because of tiredness or age. There is no evidence of person-to-person transmission of legionellosis.

Clinical features

Legionnaire's disease is typically a lobular type of pneumonia, which can be fatal, but is fortunately rare and can range from discrete patches of inflammation and consolidation to involvement of whole lobes.

Pontiac fever is milder, and usually rapidly subsides, often without treatment.

General management

The overall mortality may be as high as 10%, but over 25% in older people and up to 80% in the immunocompromised. Diagnosis can be by rapid urine molecular testing for *L. pneumophila*. Erythromycin is standard treatment.

Dental aspects

Legionella species are present in roughly two-thirds of potable water samples collected from domestic and institutional taps and drinking fountains, and from a similar percentage of dental units, but water from these dental units often has higher bacterial concentrations. Legionellae can be disseminated in the dental surgery during aerosolization of water from dental equipment such as air-turbine sprays or ultrasonic scalers. Serological studies of dental-school personnel have shown antibodies to *Legionella* species to rise with duration of work in the building, suggesting the bacteria could spread in this way, though it is not absolutely confirmed that the sources were dental equipment. Dental-unit systems should therefore be flushed through after treating patients and, when dental units have had to stand idle for long periods, such as over holidays or weekends. Dental water-line decontamination may be indicated.

TUBERCULOSIS

Tuberculosis (pulmonary TB), due to *Mycobacterium tuberculosis*, is usually transmitted by infected sputum, typically from close contacts such as family members. About 10% of those infected develop overt disease; of these, half will manifest within 5 years (primary TB), the remainder will develop post-primary disease. TB is unlikely to be transmitted between normal social contacts and is not spread by touch or by drinking glasses, dishes, sheets or clothing.

Tuberculosis can present an occupational risk to health care workers, including dental staff. One outbreak of drug-resistant TB in New York involved at least 357 patients, most of whom contracted the infection in one of 11 hospitals; nearly 90% of the patients were HIV-positive, and mostly young black or hispanic males.

Tuberculosis has also been transmitted between passengers during long-haul airline flights. The risk of transmitting TB though air circulation is now low because the high-efficiency particulate air (HEPA) filters on 'newer commercial aircraft' are the same type as that used in hospital respiratory isolation rooms, and the number of times air is cleaned each hour exceeds the recommendation for hospital isolation rooms.

Tuberculosis mainly affects medically neglected persons such as vagrants, alcoholics, intravenous drug abusers or older homeless people. Immunocompromised people, such as diabetics, severely immunodeficient patients, such as those with HIV/AIDS, and patients in prisons or institutions are also at risk. For example, about 30% of South Africans with HIV/AIDS also have TB.

Tuberculosis is a major global health problem affecting approximately one-third of the world's population (1.5 billion people) and some 2 million people die annually from it. TB is particularly widespread in developing countries and increasing: the highest rises in incidence are in South-East Asia, sub-Saharan Africa and Eastern Europe. In developed countries, the incidence is also rising, probably because of worsening social deprivation, homelessness, immigration, HIV infection and intravenous drug abuse. It is now as common in London as in the developing world, and is seen especially in immigrants, such as those from the Indian subcontinent, Africa and South Asia. This increase appears to be a result of TB disease developing in individuals who may have been infected for some time and new infections acquired in the UK, or as a result of travel to other countries where TB is common. Indian, Pakistani and Bangladeshi ethnic groups made up the highest proportion of UK cases reported in 2005 followed by black Africans and whites.

In some developing countries approximately 10% of cases are antibiotic resistant – multidrug-resistant (MDR) TB – but in the UK currently < 1% are in this category. MDR-TB is defined as resistance to rifampicin and isoniazide, may be atypical in presentation and the infection disseminates. More than 4% of people with TB worldwide have MDR-TB and Eastern Europe has the highest prevalence. MDR-TB and XDR-TB ('extensively drug-resistant' TB), defined as resistance to at least rifampicin and isoniazide plus any quinolone and an injectable second-line drug (capreomycin, amikacin, kanamycin), are seen mainly in people with HIV disease. XDR-TB is essentially untreatable, has been transmitted in health care facilities and by 2009 had been reported in 45 countries.

Tuberculosis from *Mycobacterium bovis* in milk has been virtually eliminated by the tuberculin testing of cattle, and pasteurization of milk.

Similar illnesses may also be caused by atypical (non-tuberculous) mycobacteria such as *M. avium* complex (MAC) (see below).

Clinical features

Initial infection is usually subclinical. Inhaled mycobacteria may cause subpleural lesions (primary lesion) and lesions in the regional lymph nodes (primary complex). Body defences usually localize the mycobacteria, though they remain viable and infected persons are not ill and are unlikely to know they are infected. However, in massive infections, acute active TB can result, typically causing a chronic productive cough, haemoptysis, weight loss, night sweats and fever. Extrapulmonary TB is less common, may appear as glandular involvement in the neck or elsewhere, and is less infectious than pulmonary TB. If body defences are impaired such as in ageing, drug or alcohol abuse, or HIV infection, active TB can develop shortly after mycobacteria enter the body. Otherwise, latent TB infection (LTBI) becomes active usually only after many years, when body defences become weakened (Box 15.3).

Box 15.3 Conditions in which tuberculosis may become activated

- Recent infection or young age
- HIV or immunosuppression
- Alcohol or drug abuse
- Cancer
- Chronic kidney disease
- Diabetes
- Gastric bypass/gastrectomy
- Leukaemia
- Silicosis

Post-primary TB follows reactivation of an old primary pulmonary lesion and results in lesions ranging from a chronic fibrotic lesion to fulminating tuberculous pneumonia. The pulmonary lesions may extend and result in a pleural effusion. Reactivation or progression of primary TB may also result in widespread haematogenous dissemination of mycobacteria – 'miliary TB'. Multiple lesions may involve the central nervous system, bones, joints, cardiovascular, gastrointestinal and genitourinary systems.

Clinical presentation is variable depending on the extent of spread and the organs involved. Active TB typically causes a chronic cough, haemoptysis, weight loss, night sweats and fever. Erythema nodosum may be associated. Lymph node TB may lead to lymphadenopathy, caseation of the nodes and pressure symptoms, for example on the bronchi. TB can thus have a very wide range of presentations and, because it frequently passes unrecognized for so long, the mortality is high.

General management

The diagnosis of TB is suggested by the history and confirmed by physical examination, a massively raised erythrocyte sedimentation rate (ESR), positive tuberculin skin tests [TSTs; Mantoux or Heaf test for a delayed hypersensitivity reaction to protein from *M. tuberculosis* (purified protein derivative; PPD)] and chest radiography.

Hypersensitivity develops with 2–8 weeks of infection and can be detected by conversion of the TST from negative to positive but TSTs are neither 100% sensitive nor specific. Positivity indicates infection, but not necessarily that the infection is active.

Chest radiography may show scarring and hilar lymphadenopathy. CT may show areas of calcification or highlight a tuberculous abscess. Smears and culture of sputum, blood, laryngeal swabs, bronchoalveolar lavage, gastric aspirates or pleural fluid may be tested for mycobacteria. Polymerase chain reaction (PCR) techniques have greatly accelerated the diagnosis and speciation, but Ziehl–Neelsen, auramine or rhodamine stains are still used. The mycobacteria growth indicator tube (MGIT) system gives results as early as 3–14 days. Blood assay for *M. tuberculosis* (BAMT) may be positive by interferon-gamma release assay (IGRA).

People who should be tested for TB include those who have symptoms, have had close day-to-day contact with active TB disease (family member, friend or co-worker), have HIV infection, or lowered immunity or who are required to for employment or school. The first priority of TB control programmes is to identify and completely treat all patients with active disease: TB is a notifiable disease and contact tracing is an important aspect of limiting the spread of disease.

Treatment with antibiotics is indicated for people who are sick with TB, those infected but not sick, and those who are close contacts to infectious TB cases. Treatment for 'symptomatic sputum-positive' patients, which should be instituted as soon as possible, is combination chemotherapy (isoniazid, rifampicin and either pyrazimamide and/or ethambutol for 2 months with continuation of daily isoniazid and rifampicin for a further 4 months). Treatment for 'asymptomatic' patients who are contacts believed to have been infected, but are not unwell, includes isoniazid for 6 months or isoniazid and rifampicin for 3 months. Rifapentine is a long-acting rifampicin used once weekly. Fluorquinolones (moxifloxacin) may also act against TB. Currently, given the potential risk of MDR-TB being present, four drugs are usually started, pending the results of cultures. Capreomycin has been used effectively to treat MDR-TB in HIV-positive individuals.

All antituberculous drugs (see Table 15.11) have potentially serious adverse effects and require careful monitoring. If patient compliance is considered to be poor, directly observed therapy, where drugs are dispensed by and taken in the presence of a health care professional, may be indicated.

Immunization using BCG (bacille Calmette–Guérin; live attenuated *M. bovis*) is advocated for schoolchildren, high-risk individuals and health care professionals – although its efficacy has been questioned. New vaccines are on the horizon.

Chemoprophylaxis with isoniazid and rifampicin is indicated in a number of situations (Box 15.4).

Dental aspects

Pulmonary TB is of high infectivity, as shown by cases of tuberculous infection of extraction sockets and cervical lymphadenitis in 15 patients treated by an infected member of staff at a dental clinic. Dental staff who themselves were HIV-positive, working in a dental clinic for HIV-infected persons

Table 15.11   Antitubercular therapy

Drug	Use	Main adverse effects
Ethambutol[a]	Initial therapy[b]	Ocular damage
Isoniazid	Initial therapy[b]	Peripheral neuropathy
		Hepatotoxicity
	Continuation therapy[c]	Hepatotoxicity
Pyrazinamide	Initial therapy[b]	
Rifampicin	Initial therapy[b]	Enhanced liver P450
	Continuation therapy[c]	drug-metabolizing enzymes
		Urine and saliva turn red
		Bullous lesions
		Hepatotoxicity
		Nephrotoxicity
Streptomycin[a]	Initial therapy[b]	Vestibular nerve damage
		Circumoral paraesthesiae

[a]Increasing resistance.

[b]Initial therapy, usually = isoniazid + rifampicin + pyrazimamide or ethambutol for 2 months.

[c]Continuation therapy = isoniazid + rifampicin for 4 months.

Box 15.4 Indications for tuberculosis (TB) chemoprophylaxis

- Previous inadequate treatment of TB
- Close contact with persons actively infected with TB
- Conversion of the tuberculin test within the past 2 years
- A positive tuberculin test in the following groups:
  - Immunocompromised persons (diabetes, renal failure, cancer, HIV infection)
  - Persons under 35 years, or intravenous drug users
  - A foreign-born person who has migrated from a region of high prevalence within the previous 2 years

Table 15.12   Dental management of patients with known or suspected tuberculosis (TB)

History of TB	Potential infectivity	Comment
Active sputum-positive TB	High	Urgent dental treatment only: use special infection control precautions. Defer elective dental care until TB treatment complete
Recent history of TB and sputum known positive for TB	High	
Past history of TB No history of TB but signs or symptoms suggestive No history of TB but positive tuberculin test	Refer to physician: needs confirmation	Use special infection control precautions for emergency dental care Defer elective dental care until medical advice received

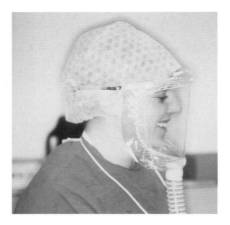

Fig. 15.6   Respirator

in New York, have died from TB contracted occupationally. Infection control is thus important, so staff with TB are usually precluded from their occupation until treated.

Management of a patient with TB depends upon the level of potential infectivity (Table 15.12). Patients with open pulmonary TB are contagious, and dental treatment is thus best deferred until the infection has been treated. Treatment with appropriate drugs for 2 weeks drastically reduces the infectivity of patients with pulmonary TB. If patients with open pulmonary TB must be treated, special precautions should be used to prevent the release of mycobacteria into the air, to remove any that are present and to stop the inhalation by other persons. Reduction of splatter and aerosols, by minimizing coughing and avoiding ultrasonic instruments, and use of a rubber dam, are important. Improved ventilation, ultraviolet germicidal light, new masks and personal respirators and other personal protective devices, such as HEPA filters, are indicated (Fig. 15.6). Mycobacteria are very resistant to disinfectants, so that heat sterilization should be used wherever possible.

Local anaesthesia is safe and satisfactory. Relative analgesia is contraindicated because of the risk of contamination of the apparatus. GA is also contraindicated for dental treatment because of the risk of contamination of the anaesthetic apparatus or because of impaired pulmonary function. Aminoglycosides such as streptomycin enhance the activity of

some neuromuscular blocking drugs and in large doses may alone cause a myasthenic syndrome.

Possible drug interactions are shown in Table 15.13.

Other factors, such as alcoholism or intravenous drug use (Ch. 34), hepatitis (Ch. 9) or HIV disease (Ch. 20), may also influence dental management.

Chronic ulcers, usually on the tongue dorsum, are the main oral manifestation of TB. They result from coughing of infected sputum from pulmonary TB, including HIV-infected persons with TB, but are rare and such cases (usually middle-aged males) may result from neglect of symptoms or default from treatment. Occasionally the diagnosis is made from the biopsy of an ulcer after granulomas are seen microscopically. Acid-fast bacilli are rarely seen in oral biopsies even with the help of special stains, so unfixed material should also be sent for culture if possible. Tuberculous cervical lymphadenopathy is the next most common form of the infection and is particularly common among those from South Asia. Most TB lymphadenitis is painless, with several enlarged, matted nodes, but systemic symptoms are present only in a minority and only about 15% have pulmonary manifestations on radiography (Fig. 15.7). Diagnosis relies on tuberculin testing, which can be positive in both tuberculous and NTM cervical lymphadenitis. Any person with lymphadenopathy and recent conversion from a negative to positive tuberculin test should be suspected

Table 15.13 Possible drug interactions in tuberculosis (TB)

Acetaminophen (paracetamol)	Isoniazid
Acetaminophen Azole antifungals Benzodiazepines Clarithromycin Diazepam	Rifampicin
Aspirin	Amikacin, capreomycin, kanamycin or streptomycin

Box 15.5 Mycobacteria other than tuberculosis

- *Mycobacterium avium*
- *M. intracellulare* (*M. avium–intracellulare* complex; MAC)
- *M. kansasii*
- *M. scrofulaceum*
- *M. fortuitum*
- *M. marinum*
- *M. ulcerans*
- *M. chelonae*
- *M. xenopi*

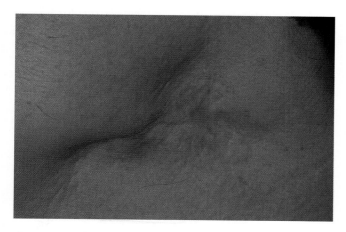

Fig. 15.7 Neck scarring from tuberculous lymphadenitis

to have mycobacterial infection and this should prompt biopsy (e.g. fine-needle aspiration biopsy), for culture or histological confirmation. PCR will improve diagnosis, as culture must wait 4–8 weeks for a result.

Non-tuberculous mycobacteria are a relatively common cause of cervical lymphadenitis in children under 12 years and in HIV disease.

Oral complications of antitubercular therapy are rare, but rifabutin and rifampicin can cause red saliva.

ATYPICAL MYCOBACTERIA (NON-TUBERCULOUS MYCOBACTERIA; NTM; MYCOBACTERIA OTHER THAN TUBERCULOSIS; MOTT)

General aspects

Atypical mycobacteria include *M. avium*, *M. intracellulare* (MAC) species and others (Box 15.5).

Mycobacteria other than tuberculosis (MOTT) are widely distributed in water, soil, animals and humans, and rarely cause disease. Severe MOTT infections, however, have been seen in individuals predisposed because of defects in the interleukin-12 (IL-12) and interferon-gamma (IFN-gamma) pathways.

Many people become infected with and harbour MOTT in their respiratory secretions without any symptoms or evidence of disease. Person-to-person transmission of atypical myco-bacteria is *not* important in acquisition of infection, except for skin infections. Individuals with respiratory disease from non-tuberculous mycobacteria do *not* readily infect others and, therefore, do not need to be isolated.

Clinical features

M. avium–intracellulare complex, *M. scrofulaceum* and *M. kansasii* are possible causes of tuberculous cervical lymphadenitis. MAC may infect the lungs (similar to TB), skin or lymph nodes. Lung disease is also occasionally caused by *M. kansasii*, mainly in middle-aged and older persons with underlying chronic lung conditions. *M. fortuitum* and *M. chelonae* may cause skin and wound infections and abscesses, frequently associated with trauma or surgery. *M. marinum* may cause 'swimming pool granuloma', a nodular lesion that may ulcerate, usually on an extremity. *M. ulcerans* may produce chronic ulcerative skin lesions, usually of an extremity.

An immune defect, underlying illness or tissue damage may result in disseminated MAC infection.

General management and dental aspects

Cervical lymphadenitis due to MAC, *M. scrofulaceum* and *M. kansasii* may affect otherwise healthy young children, most commonly pre-school females who have unilateral cervical lymphadenopathy, typically in the submandibular or jugulodigastric nodes, and they may form a 'cold abscess'. MOTT is the usual cause in children under 12 years, but TB is more common in older patients. Absence of fever or tuberculosis, a positive tuberculin test and failed response to conventional antimicrobials are highly suggestive of MOTT, but definitive diagnosis is by culture or PCR of biopsy material obtained by fine-needle aspiration or removal of nodes.

Treatment is based on results of laboratory testing, which should identify the appropriate antibiotic. Preventive treatment of close contacts of persons with disease caused by MOTT is *not* needed. Most MOTT are resistant to standard antitubercular medication and, though it is possible that clarithromycin or clofazimine may have some effect, excision of affected nodes is the usual recommended therapy.

Water from dental units may contain MOTT species; mycobacterial proliferation in biofilms may explain the extent of this contamination.

ASPIRATION SYNDROMES

Aspiration syndromes are conditions in which foreign substances are inhaled into the lungs and which can have consequences ranging from asphyxia to infection and lung abscess. Dental restorations or fragments of teeth, plaque, gastric contents and other materials may be aspirated, especially if material enters the pharynx, and particularly if the cough reflex is impaired for any reason.

Most commonly, aspiration syndromes involve oral or gastric contents associated with gastro-oesophageal reflux (GORD), swallowing dysfunction (Ch. 7), neurological disorders and structural abnormalities such as a pharyngeal pouch. Cricopharyngeal dysfunction involves cricopharyngeal muscle spasm or achalasia of the superior oesophageal sphincter, and can be seen in infants who have a normal sucking reflex but have incoordination during swallowing, possibly secondary to delayed development or cerebral palsy. Anatomic disorders, such as cleft palate, pharyngeal pouch, oesophageal atresia, tracheoesophageal fistula, duodenal obstruction or malrotation, and motility disorders, such as achalasia, may have an aspiration risk. Infirm older patients are also at risk of aspiration, especially if they are bedbound or have neurological disorders. Isolated superior laryngeal nerve damage, vocal cord paralysis, cerebral palsy, muscular dystrophy and Riley–Day syndrome (familial dysautonomia) are all associated with increased risk of aspiration.

LUNG ABSCESS

General aspects

Lung abscess is a localized infection leading to cavitation and necrosis. While some cases result from aspiration of foreign material, most result from pneumonia caused by infection with *Staph. aureus* or *Klebsiella pneumoniae*. Bronchial obstruction by carcinoma is another important cause.

Clinical features

Symptoms resemble those of suppurative pneumonia. There is a risk of infection spreading locally or leading, via septicaemia, to a brain abscess.

General management

Diagnosis rests mainly on the chest radiograph, which may sometimes show cavitation or a fluid level. Antimicrobial chemotherapy, postural drainage and relief by bronchoscopy of any obstruction are indicated.

Dental aspects

A well-recognized cause of lung abscess is inhalation of a tooth or fragment, a restoration, or rarely, an endodontic instrument. When undertaking endodontics or cementing restorations, such as inlays or crowns, a rubber dam or other protective device should always be used to avoid the danger of inhalation.

Lung abscesses may also result from aspiration of oral bacteria, particularly anaerobes, especially in infirm older patients or those who are intubated.

The other main dangers in dentistry are with GA, particularly if an inadequate throat pack has been used. Patients who inhale tooth fragments or dental instruments must have chest radiographs (lateral and postero-anterior) and, if necessary, bronchoscopy.

SARCOIDOSIS
GENERAL ASPECTS

Sarcoidosis, so named because skin lesions resembled a sarcoma, is a multisystem granulomatous disorder, seen most commonly in young adult females in northern Europe, especially in people of African heritage. The aetiology is unclear but *Propionobacterium acnes* and *P. granulosum* have been implicated and associations have been reported of exposure to inorganic particles, insecticides, moulds and occupations, such as firefighting and metal working. Serum samples contain antibodies directed against *Mycobacterium tuberculosis* antigens. Sarcoidosis is associated with HLA-DRB1 and DQB1, and a butyrophilin-like 2 (*BTNL2*) gene on chromosome 6. T helper 1 (Th1) cells release IL-2 and IFN-gamma, and augment macrophage tumour necrosis factor alpha (TNF-alpha) release. CD25 regulatory T cells cause a limited impairment of cell-mediated immune responses (partial anergy), but no obvious special susceptibility to infection.

CLINICAL FEATURES

Sarcoidosis affects the thorax in 90%, but has protean manifestations and can involve virtually any tissue (Table 15.14). Sarcoid most typically causes Löfgren syndrome (fever, bilateral hilar lymphadenopathy, arthralgia, erythema nodosum, especially around the ankles; Figs 15.8 and 15.9).

Other common presentations may include pulmonary infiltration and impaired respiratory efficiency, with cough and dyspnoea in severe cases, or acute uveitis, which can progress to blindness. Susceptibility to lymphomas has been suggested but not confirmed.

GENERAL MANAGEMENT

Because of its vague and protean manifestations, sarcoidosis is underdiagnosed. In the presence of suggestive clinical features, helpful investigations include: chest radiography (enlarged hilar lymph nodes); raised serum angiotensin-converting enzyme

Table 15.14 Sarcoidosis: possible clinical findings	
Dermatological	Erythema nodosum, infiltrates around eyes and nose (lupus pernio)
Hepatic	Asymptomatic hepatomegaly, sarcoid liver disease
Lymph nodes	Lymphadenopathy (rarely lymphoma)
Musculoskeletal	Arthralgia, effusions, cyst-like radiolucent areas
Neurological	Cranial or peripheral neuropathies
Oral/para-oral	Salivary gland or gingival swelling
Ocular	Acute uveitis, cataracts, glaucoma
Pulmonary	Hilar lymphadenopathy; widespread infiltration
Renal	Nephrocalcinosis, renal calculi
Spleen	Splenomegaly
Systemic symptoms	Fever, weight loss, fatigue

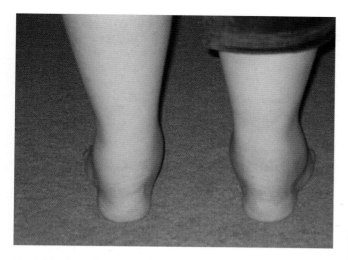

Fig. 15.8 Sarcoid causing ankle swelling in Lofgren syndrome

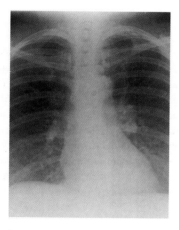

Fig. 15.9 Sarcoid lung image showing hilar adenopathy

Table 15.15 Sarcoidosis: laboratory findings	
Histological findings	Non-caseating tubercle-like granulomas
Immunological findings	Anergy (partial) Negative response to tuberculin and some other common antigens on skin testing Lymphopenia; low numbers of T cells Raised serum levels of immunoglobulins
Biochemical findings	Hypercalcaemia Raised serum levels of lysozyme, serum angiotensin-converting enzyme (SACE) and adenosine deaminase

(SACE; Table 15.15) in acute disease (this is insensitive, non-specific and a poor guide to therapy); positive gallium-67 citrate or gadolinium or positron emission tomography (PET) scans; labial salivary gland or transbronchial biopsy (for histological evidence of non-caseating epithelioid cell granulomas) – except in Löfgren syndrome, which is a classical clinical diagnosis. ^{18}F-deoxyglucose PET is helpful in identifying sites for biopsy.

Non-specific findings may include mild anaemia, leukopenia, eosinophilia, hypergammaglobulinaemia, raised ESR and low serum albumin. Hypercalcaemia is common because of extrarenal production of active vitamin D and can result in renal damage. Alkaline phosphatase, 5'-nucleotidase, lysozyme and adenosine deaminase levels are raised in hepatic sarcoidosis. Evidence of impaired delayed hypersensitivity reactions to some antigens may be useful. Kveim skin tests are not now used.

Half the patients with sarcoidosis remit within 3 years and about 66% remit by 10 years. Patients with only minor symptoms usually need no treatment but corticosteroids, sometimes with azathioprine, methotrexate, tetracyclines, hydroxychloroquine, infliximab or etanercept, are given if there is active organ disease (ocular disease, progressive lung disease, hypercalcaemia or cerebral involvement).

DENTAL ASPECTS

Management problems of patients with systemic sarcoidosis may include respiratory impairment, uveitis and visual impairment, renal disease, jaundice or corticosteroid treatment .

Local anaesthesia is safe and satisfactory. Conscious sedation is contraindicated if there is any respiratory impairment. GA should only be given in hospital.

Biopsy of the minor salivary glands frequently shows non-caseating granulomas and association with other features of sarcoidosis, particularly hilar lymphadenopathy. This is an important diagnostic finding that may obviate more invasive procedures. Sarcoidosis can involve any of the oral tissues but has a predilection for salivary glands. Asymptomatic swelling of the parotid glands or cervical nodes, and less frequently the lips, may accompany systemic disease. Superficial or deep-seated red submucosal nodules may develop intraorally and on the lips. Non-tender, well-circumscribed, brownish-red or violaceous nodules with superficial ulceration have also been reported. The oral and lip lesions may occasionally precede systemic involvement.

There is enlargement of the major salivary glands in about 6% of cases; some have xerostomia and the association of salivary and lacrimal gland enlargement with fever and uveitis is known as uveoparotid fever (Heerfordt syndrome). Salivary swelling may also be seen without other features of Heerfordt syndrome. The salivary gland swellings usually resolve on treatment of sarcoidosis but this may take up to 3 years.

Facial palsy and other cranial neuropathies may be seen. There is also an association with Sjögren syndrome, when SS-A and SS-B serum autoantibodies are found. Rarely there is an association of thyroiditis with Addison disease, Sjögren syndrome and sarcoidosis (TASS syndrome). There is a group of patients who have histological features of sarcoid in one or more sites in the mouth, such as the gingivae, but no systemic manifestations. A few of these patients may ultimately develop other more or less systematized disease but the majority probably have isolated lesions. Such cases, where no exogenous cause for the granulomatous reaction can be found, are regarded as having 'sarcoid-like' reactions (orofacial granulomatosis) and treatment is unnecessary. However, patients should be kept under observation for as long as possible.

LUNG CANCER

GENERAL ASPECTS

Lung cancer is the most common cancer in developed countries in males, and most frequently affects adult, urban, cigarette smokers. Bronchogenic carcinoma accounts for 95% of all primary lung cancer, and has also become increasingly common in women (because of increased tobacco use) to the extent that the mortality rate for the two sexes has become almost equal. Metastases from cancers elsewhere are also frequent in the lungs.

CLINICAL FEATURES

Recurrent cough, haemoptysis, dyspnoea, chest pain and recurrent chest infections are the predominant features. Local infiltration may cause pleural effusion, lesions of the cervical sympathetic chain (Horner syndrome), brachial neuritis, recurrent laryngeal nerve palsy or obstruction of the superior vena cava with facial cyanosis and oedema (superior vena cava syndrome).

There are many non-metastatic extrapulmonary effects of bronchogenic (or other) carcinomas, for example weight loss, anorexia, finger-clubbing, neuromyopathies, thromboses (thrombophlebitis migrans), muscle weakness, various skin manifestations and ectopic hormone production (of antidiuretic hormone, adrenocorticotropic hormone, parathyroid hormone, thyroid-stimulating hormone).

Metastases from bronchogenic cancer are common and typically form in the brain (which may manifest with headache, epilepsy, hemiplegia or visual disturbances), liver (hepatomegaly, jaundice or ascites) or bone (pain, swelling or pathological fracture).

GENERAL MANAGEMENT

The diagnosis is based on history and physical examination supported by radiography, CT and magnetic resonance imaging, sputum cytology, bronchoscopy and biopsy. Spiral CT appears to detect tumours at an early stage.

The overall 5-year survival rate is only 8%. Radiotherapy is the most common treatment. Only ≈25% of patients are suitable for surgery but, even then, the 5-year survival is only about 25%. Chemotherapy has been disappointing except in small cell carcinomas.

DENTAL ASPECTS

Dental treatment under LA should be uncomplicated. Conscious sedation should preferably be avoided. GA is a matter for specialist management in hospital: patients often have impaired respiratory function, especially after lobectomy or pneumonectomy. This, along with any muscle weakness (myasthenic syndrome, Eaton–Lambert syndrome) that can make the patient unduly sensitive to the action of muscle relaxants, makes GA hazardous.

Oral cancer may be associated with lung cancer, and vice versa, or develop at a later stage (Ch. 22). Such synchronous or metachronous primary tumours must always be ruled out.

Metastases can occasionally affect the orofacial region and cause enlargement of the lower cervical lymph nodes, epulis-like soft tissue swellings or labial hypoaesthesia or paraesthesia in the jaw. Soft palate pigmentation is a rare early oral manifestation.

Lung cancer is a fairly common cause of death in dental technicians, but it is unknown whether this is due to smoking alone or to dust inhalation.

OTHER RESPIRATORY DISORDERS

CYSTIC FIBROSIS (FIBROCYSTIC DISEASE; MUCOVISCIDOSIS)

General aspects

Cystic fibrosis (CF) is one of the most common fatal hereditary disorders. Inherited as an autosomal recessive trait, with an incidence of about 1 in 2000 births, it is the most common inherited error of metabolism and is seen mainly in people of European descent. The gene responsible is on chromosome 7q and encodes a membrane-associated protein called cystic fibrosis transmembrane regulator (CFTR), which appears to be part of a cyclic adenosine monophosphate (cAMP)-regulated chloride channel, regulating Cl^- and Na^+ transport across epithelial membranes. The basic defect in CF is abnormal chloride ion transport across the cell membrane of nearly all exocrine glands. Thus sweat and salivary sodium levels are raised and mucus, especially in the respiratory tract and pancreas, is viscid. Involved glands (the pancreas, intestinal glands, intrahepatic bile ducts, the gall bladder, submaxillary glands) may become obstructed by this viscid or solid eosinophilic material in their lumens. Heterozygotes may show subtle abnormalities of epithelial transport but are clinically unaffected.

Clinical features

Recurrent respiratory infections result in a persistent productive cough and bronchiectasis, with the lungs becoming infected with a variety of organisms including *Staph. aureus*, *Haemophilus influenzae*, *Pseudomonas aeruginosa*, *Strep. pneumoniae*, *Burkholderia cepacia*, and sometimes mycoses or mycobacteria. Viral infections, such as measles, can have severe sequelae.

Sinusitis is very common. Pancreatic duct obstruction leads to pancreatic insufficiency, with malabsorption and bulky, frequent, foul-smelling, fatty stools. Gallstones, diabetes, cirrhosis and pancreatitis may result.

Growth is frequently stunted. Fertility is impaired in most males with CF, secondary to maldevelopment of the vas deferens or to other forms of obstructive azoospermia. In women, fertility may be impaired by viscid cervical secretions, but many women have carried pregnancies to term.

General management

Most patients have a high concentration of sodium in their sweat (also reflected in the saliva) and a sweat test showing sodium and chloride values of > 60 mmol/l is considered positive, between 40 and 60 mmol/l equivocal, and < 40 mmol/l is negative.

Physiotherapy and postural drainage are crucially important. Clearance of sputum is helped by water aerosols and bronchodilators (terbutaline or salbutamol), but mucolytics such as carbocisteine, methyl cysteine and dornase alpha are of questionable effectiveness.

Amoxicillin and flucloxacillin are effective prophylactic antimicrobials, and may be given by aerosol. Vaccination against measles, whooping cough and influenza is important. A low fat intake, adequate vitamins and oral pancreatic enzyme replacement (pancreatin) are also necessary.

Double-lung or heart–lung transplantation may eventually become necessary.

Dental aspects

Lung disease, liver disease and diabetes may complicate treatment. LA is satisfactory but conscious sedation is usually contraindicated because of poor respiratory function. GA is contraindicated if respiratory function is poor.

Most patients have recurrent sinusitis and nasal polyps. The major salivary glands may become enlarged and xerostomia is sometimes a complaint. The low-fat, high-carbohydrate diet and dry mouth may predispose to caries but some studies have shown fewer caries in CF patients. Enamel hypoplasia and black stain may be seen, and both dental development and eruption are delayed. Tetracycline staining of the teeth was common, but should rarely be seen now. Pancreatin may cause oral ulceration if held in the mouth.

BRONCHIECTASIS

General aspects

Bronchiectasis is dilatation and distortion of the bronchi. In many cases, no cause is apparent, but in others it is often the consequence of childhood infections (such as measles, whooping cough, bronchiolitis or adenovirus), and some cases arise from cystic fibrosis, immunodeficiencies or bronchial obstruction.

The damaged and dilated bronchi lose their ciliated epithelium and therefore mucus tends to pool causing recurrent lower respiratory tract infections, typically with *Strep. pneumoniae, Haemophilus influenzae* or *Pseudomonas aeruginosa*.

Clinical features

Overproduction of sputum, which is purulent during exacerbations, a cough (especially during exercise or when lying down) and finger-clubbing are typical features, with recurrent episodes of bronchitis, pneumonia and pleurisy. Haemoptysis is not uncommon. In advanced bronchiectasis, chest pain, dyspnoea, cyanosis and respiratory failure may develop. Complications may include cerebral abscess and amyloid disease.

General management

Chest radiography and pulmonary function tests are required. High-resolution CT (HRCT) is useful. Postural drainage is important. Antimicrobials, such as amoxicillin, cephalosporins or ciprofloxacin, are given for acute exacerbations and for long-term maintenance treatment.

Dental aspects

General anaesthesia should be avoided where possible and is contraindicated in acute phases.

OCCUPATIONAL LUNG DISEASE (PNEUMOCONIOSES)

General aspects

Workers exposed to airborne particles may develop pulmonary disease (pneumoconiosis), which ranges from benign (e.g. siderosis) to malignant, as in mesothelioma from asbestosis (see Appendix 15.1), but any pneumoconiosis can cause significant incapacity.

Dental aspects

General anaesthesia may be contraindicated; the physician should be contacted before treatment.

Berylliosis may be a hazard in some dental technical laboratories, when lung cancer is more frequent.

POST-OPERATIVE RESPIRATORY COMPLICATIONS

Respiratory complications following surgical operations under GA include segmental or lobar pulmonary collapse and infection. They are more common after abdominal surgery or if there is pre-existent respiratory disease, or smoking (see also Ch. 3), and can be significantly reduced by stopping smoking, pre-operative physiotherapy and bronchodilators, such as salbutamol.

If post-operative pulmonary infection develops, sputum should be sent for culture, and physiotherapy and antibiotics should be given. The common microbial causes are *Strep. pneumoniae* and *Haemophilus influenzae*, when suitable antibiotics include amoxicillin or erythromycin. Hospital infections may include other micro-organisms, such as MRSA, *Klebsiella*, *Pseudomonas* and other Gram-negative bacteria.

Inhalation (aspiration) of gastric contents can cause pulmonary oedema and may be fatal (Mendelson syndrome); it is most likely if a GA is given to a patient who has a stomach that is not empty, has a hiatus hernia or is in the last trimester of pregnancy. Prevention is by ensuring the stomach is empty pre-operatively and by an anaesthetist passing an endotracheal tube if not. Antacids or an H_2-receptor blocker, such as cimetidine or ranitidine, may be given by mouth pre-operatively to lower gastric acidity.

If gastric contents are aspirated, the pharynx and larynx must be carefully sucked out. Systemic corticosteroids have been recommended, but probably do not reduce the mortality.

RESPIRATORY DISTRESS SYNDROMES

Respiratory distress in premature infants may be caused by immaturity of surfactant-producing cells, when the alveoli fail to expand fully, which necessitates endotracheal intubation for many weeks. This may, in turn, result in mid-face hypoplasia, palatal grooving or clefting, or defects in the primary dentition.

The same oral effects may be seen with prolonged use of oro-gastric feeding tubes. The degree to which subsequent growth corrects these deformations is currently unknown, though the palatal grooves typically regress by the age of 2 years. Using soft endotracheal tubes does not obviate this problem and, at present, the best means of avoiding palatal grooving appears to be the use of an intraoral acrylic plate to stabilize the tube and protect the palate.

Adult respiratory distress syndrome (ARDS) is a sequel to several types of pulmonary injury and some infections, including those with oral viridans streptococci.

LUNG TRANSPLANTATION

General aspects

Patients with end-stage pulmonary disease are considered for potential transplantation usually using a lung from a brain-dead organ donor. A combination of ciclosporin, aza-thioprine and glucocorticoids is usually given for lifelong immunosuppression to prevent a T-cell, alloimmune rejection response.

Inhaled nitric oxide modulates pulmonary vascular tone via smooth muscle relaxation and can improve ventilation/perfusion matching and oxygenation in diseased lungs. Early graft failure following lung transplantation has been described by various investigators as reimplantation oedema, reperfusion oedema, primary graft failure or allograft dysfunction. Pathologically, this entity is diffuse alveolar damage.

Dental aspects (in addition to those discussed in Ch. 35)

A meticulous pre-surgery oral assessment is required and dental treatment undertaken with particular attention to establish optimal oral hygiene and eradicate sources of potential infection. Dental treatment should be completed before surgery. For 6 months after surgery, elective dental care is best deferred. If surgical treatment is needed during that period, antibiotic prophylaxis is probably warranted.

HEART AND LUNG TRANSPLANTATION

General aspects

Cardiopulmonary transplantation (heart and lung transplantation) is the simultaneous surgical replacement of the heart and lungs in patients with end-stage cardiac and pulmonary disease, with organs from a cadaveric donor.

General management

All transplant recipients require lifelong immunosuppression to prevent a T-cell, alloimmune rejection response.

Dental aspects in addition to those discussed in Ch. 35

A meticulous pre-surgery oral assessment is required and dental treatment undertaken with particular attention to establishing optimal oral hygiene and eradicating sources of potential

infection. Dental treatment should be completed before surgery. For 6 months after surgery, elective dental care is best deferred. If surgical treatment is needed during that period, antibiotic prophylaxis is probably warranted.

OBSTRUCTIVE SLEEP APNOEA SYNDROME

General aspects

Obstructive sleep apnoea syndrome (OSAS) is the extreme end of a spectrum of sleep-disordered breathing (SDB), which may be related to weak activity of muscles in (or obstruction to) the tongue, palate and pharynx. Enlarged tonsils or tongue (macroglossia) are uncommon causes. Alcohol or other sedatives inducing muscle relaxation can aggravate the situation. SDB has as its minimal level simple snoring, then upper airways resistance syndrome (UARS) and, finally, OSAS, when there are periods of apnoea during sleep because of airways obstruction in the soft palate/tongue region. Each period of apnoea may last for up to a minute and episodes range from occasional to hundreds per night, awaking the patient and causing daytime tiredness, which is sometimes severe. This is not a trivial problem, since there is an association between OSAS, daytime sleepiness and cardiopulmonary complications.

Oronasal obstruction in weak senile patients may cause a dangerous degree of dyspnoea and cyanosis, even when awake. The oronasal obstruction results from blockage of the nose and lack of teeth or dentures, causing the mouth to become over-closed. Hypoxia, thus caused, may contribute to the death of these vulnerable patients.

Clinical features

Partial upper airways obstruction during sleep can cause snoring that is not OSAS. In OSAS, snoring is far more severe and, because there is apnoea, arterial oxygen saturation falls, and cardiac arrhythmias and stroke may develop, particularly in obese middle-aged men. In even more severe cases, pulmonary hypertension and right ventricular failure result. There is a raised mortality rate also from road traffic and other accidents since affected patients are constantly drowsy.

General management

Diagnosis is assisted by polysomnography and measurement of arterial blood oxygen. Severity is scored by an apnoea/hypopnea index calculated from the combined number of episodes per night (< 20 is mild, 20–40 is moderate and > 40 is classed as severe). Tiredness can be scored by the Epworth scale (Table 15.16): a score of 10 or more is considered 'sleepy'; 18 or more is 'very sleepy.'

Treatment includes reduction of obesity and nasal continuous positive airways pressure (CPAP). Other measures include various appliances (sometimes termed NADOs – non-sleep apnoea dental orthotics, e.g. *Silent nite, Klearway, Napa; Snore aid, Herbst, Silencer*), orthognathic surgery, uvulopalatopharyngoplasty (UPPP) or even tracheostomy. Although UPPP has been the standard treatment, its efficacy is currently under review.

Table 15.16 Score sheet for Epworth daytime sleepiness scale

Situation	Chance of dozing or sleeping[a]
Sitting and reading Watching TV Sitting inactive in a public place Being a passenger in a motor vehicle for an hour or more Lying down in the afternoon Sitting and talking to someone Sitting quietly after lunch (no alcohol) Stopped for a few minutes in traffic while driving	
	Total = Epworth score

[a]0, would *never* doze or sleep; 1, *slight* chance of dozing or sleeping; 2, *moderate* chance of dozing or sleeping; 3, *high* chance of dozing or sleeping.

Dental aspects

Recent work suggests that, where the obstruction is predominantly hypopharyngeal, surgical advancement of the facial skeleton and hyoid may effectively expand the airway. When there is both oropharyngeal and hypopharyngeal obstruction, UPPP may need to be combined with maxillary–mandibular and hyoid advancement (MMA). Nasal obstruction may also have to be relieved, but maxillofacial surgery carried out in stages to assess the degree of improvement may relieve nocturnal hypoxia, snoring and daytime sleepiness.

Dental appliances to hold the mandible forward are claimed to be as effective as more drastic measures. A nasal catheter provides a more rapid solution but is less likely to be acceptable.

USEFUL WEBSITES

http://www3.niaid.nih.gov/topics
http://www.aaaai.org/professionals.stm
http://www.library.nhs.uk/respiratory/
http://www.ers-education.org/pages/default.aspx
http://www.medic8.com/lung-disorders
http://www.lunguk.org/you-and-your-lungs/conditions-and-diseases/

FURTHER READING

Bettega, G., Pepin, J.L., Veale, D., 2000. Obstructive sleep apnea syndrome. Am J Respir Crit Care Med 162, 641–649.

Bloch, K.E., Iseli, A., Zhang, J.N., 2000. A randomised, controlled crossover trial of two oral appliances for sleep apnea treatment. Am J Respir Crit Care Med 162, 246–251.

Gandhi, N.R., Moll, A., Sturm, A.W., et al., 2006. Extensively drug-resistant tuberculosis as a cause of death in patients co-infected with tuberculosis and HIV in a rural area of South Africa. Lancet 368, 1575–1580.

Iannuzi, M.C., Rybicki, B.A., Teirstein, A.S., 2007. Sarcoidosis. N Engl J Med 357, 2153–2165.

Jensen, P.A., Lambert, L.A., Iademarco, M.F., Ridzon, R., 2005. Guidelines for preventing the transmission of Mycobacterium tuberculosis in health-care settings. MMWR 54, RR-17.

Maartens, G., Wilkinson, R.J., 2007. Tuberculosis. Lancet 370, 2030–2043.

Rinaggio, J., 2003. Tuberculosis. Dent Clin N Am 47, 449–465.

Sollecito, T.P., Tino, G., 2001. Asthma. Oral Surg 92, 485–490.

Scully C, Chaudhry S, 2009. Aspects of Human Disease 31. Tuberculosis Dental Update 36, 189.

Scully C, 2009. Aspects of Human Disease 32. Lung cancer Dental Update 36, 253 (2009)

Scully C, Chaudhry S, 2007. Aspects of Human Disease 8. Asthma Dental Update 34, 61.

Scully C, Chaudhry S, 2007. Aspects of Human Disease 9. Chronic obstructive pulmonary disease (COPD) Dental Update 34, 125.

Appendix 15.1 Occupational lung diseases

Disorder	Source of causal agent	Group at risk	Clinical significance of pneumoconiosis
Anthracosis	Soot, carbon smoke	Urban dwellers	Benign
Asbestosis	Asbestos, insulation, fertilizers, explosives	Asbestos workers	Pulmonary fibrosis (crocidolite) predispose to cor pulmonale) or amosite (bronchial carcinoma, mesothelioma)
Bagassosis	Mouldy sugar cane	Farmers	Acute pneumonia or fibre bronchiolitis
Barilosis	Barium	Barium miners	Benign
Berylliosis	Beryllium	Fluorescent lamps, various alloys	Chronic respiratory disease leading to cor pulmonale
Byssinosis	Cotton, flax or hemp	Cotton workers	Periodic bronchospasm leading to obstructive airways disease
Coal miner's lung	Coal dust	Coal miners	Largely asymptomatic but may cause fibrosis and emphysema
Kaolin	China clay	China clay workers	Resembles silicosis (q.v.)
Siderosis	Iron dust	Welders, grinders	Benign
Silicosis	Silica (quartz) dust	Miners, sandblasting, potters	Pulmonary fibrosis leading to cor pulmonale, tuberculosis
Stannosis	Tin dust	Tin refining	Benign

BONE

The organic matrix of bone consists largely of collagen produced by osteoblasts rich in alkaline phosphatase. When osteoblastic activity rises, the level of alkaline phosphatase rises in the serum. Osteoblasts secrete osteoid, which becomes mineralized by deposition of calcium phosphate, largely as hydroxyapatite, together with a smaller amount of amorphous calcium phosphate and smaller amounts of magnesium, sodium and other ions. Mineralization depends on the extracellular fluid calcium and phosphate levels. Bone stores buffer changes in their plasma levels. Bone is a dynamic tissue, constantly remodelling, with resorption mediated mainly by osteoclasts, but also by prostaglandins and some cytokines. When bone is resorbed, calcium and phosphate are removed and released into the extracellular fluid. Osteoclasts are rich in acid phosphatase (particularly tartrate-resistant acid phosphatase) which may also be released into the serum in significant amounts when there is widespread osteolysis. Bone formation, metabolism and blood calcium levels are affected mainly by parathyroid hormone, vitamin D and calcitonin. Bone morphogenetic proteins (BMPs) affect bone formation, and are available as recombinant proteins, sometimes used in repair of periodontal defects, other bone defects and in implantology.

Parathyroid hormone (PTH; parathormone) is regulated by blood calcium, vitamin D levels and phosphate levels. When PTH is secreted, intestinal transport of calcium and phosphate are promoted, and removal of calcium from bones accelerated.

Dietary vitamin D is fat-soluble and absorbed from the upper small intestine, promoting intestinal absorption of calcium and phosphate. Vitamin D is also synthesized in the skin from 7-dehydrocholesterol under the influence of sunlight, and converted by liver and then kidney to the most active metabolite 1,25-dihydroxycholecalciferol (DHCC: calcitriol – the hormonal form of vitamin D), a process enhanced by PTH and low phosphate levels. The active metabolite (active vitamin D or DHCC) controls bone metabolism and enhances calcium absorption (Fig. 16.1). It also, incidentally, affects the proliferation of various cells other than bone and enhances immunity.

Calcitonin opposes the action of PTH and lowers the blood calcium level, mainly by promoting deposition of calcium in the bones. Several other hormones affect bone formation and metabolism to varying degrees, especially during the first two decades of life, including growth hormone, oestrogens in females and testosterone in males.

Bone growth varies throughout life, it is rapid in the fetus and infant, but slows somewhat during childhood until an adolescent growth spurt. Adult levels of bone mass are achieved by age 18 or so. Lifestyle, especially physical activity and adequate nutrition, promote the formation of bone, whereas smoking may impair it. Osteoblasts are also less efficient at laying down bone than are osteoclasts at removing it and, although the difference is slight, there is a gradual loss of bone mineral density (BMD) as a person ages. Anything that accelerates the rate of bone remodelling ultimately leads to a more rapid loss of bone mass and thus, more fragile bones (osteoporosis).

BONE DISEASE

Many genetic disorders of the skeleton are rare; acquired disorders are more common. The more important examples are discussed here and the main features of others are summarized in Appendix 16.2.

GENETIC DISORDERS

Osteogenesis imperfecta (fragilitas ossium; brittle bone syndrome)

General aspects

Osteogenesis imperfecta is a rare, usually autosomal dominant, inherited condition characterized by brittle bones that are susceptible to fracture. The underlying defect appears to be in type I

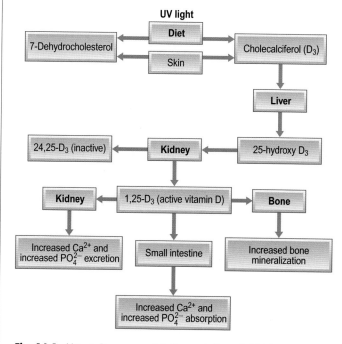

Fig. 16.1 Vitamin D sources metabolism and effects. 1,25-D3 acts as a hormone.

collagen formation, and, although osteoblasts are active, the total amount of bone formed is small and mostly woven in type. This disorder, with a frequency of 1 in 12 000 births, has several variants (Table 16.1).

The gene for dentinogenesis imperfecta, one of the more common heritable defects of the teeth, is closely related and some patients (types I and IV) have both conditions.

Clinical features

The long bones are typically normal in length, with epiphyses of normal width, but slender shafts, frequently giving a trumpet-shaped appearance. The bones are fragile and multiple fractures can follow minimal trauma; healing is rapid but usually causes distortion, so the ultimate effect in severe cases is gross deformity and dwarfism. The frequency of fractures usually tends to diminish after puberty.

The parietal regions of the skull may bulge outwards causing eversion of the upper part of the ear. Other defects are blue sclerae, deafness, easy bruising and weakness of tendons and ligaments causing loose-jointedness and often hernias. There may be cardiac complications such as mitral valve prolapse or aortic incompetence.

Dental aspects

It is important not to confuse children with brittle bone syndrome from those who have been subjected to physical abuse (Ch. 25). The management problems relate to bone fragility and careful handling of the patient. Despite the brittleness of most of the skeleton, the jaws rarely fracture and dental extractions can usually therefore be safely carried out, but care should obviously be taken to use minimal force, to support the jaws and to ensure haemostasis if there is any bleeding tendency (Ch. 8).

General anaesthesia is a risk if there are chest deformities or cardiac complications, such as mitral valve prolapse or aortic incompetence.

When dentinogenesis imperfecta is associated, the teeth may have the characteristic abnormal translucency, brown or purplish colour and subject to ready wear. The enamel may adhere poorly to the dentine and be progressively shed under the stress of mastication. By adolescence the teeth may be worn down to the gingival margins but obliteration of the pulp chamber by dentine usually prevents exposure of the pulp. The softness of the dentine makes the fitting of post crowns impractical so that steel crowns on primary molars and crowns in the permanent dentition, or even extraction and replacement by dentures, may be needed in severe cases.

Dentinogenesis imperfecta can also appear as an isolated abnormality without bone disease.

Achondroplasia

The achondrodysplasias are heritable disorders of skeletal growth, presenting typically with dwarfism, high forehead, cleft palate and various ocular anomalies.

Surgery is usually required for the cleft palate and other deformities.

General and clinical aspects

Achondroplasia is a defect in cartilaginous bone formation, often inherited as an autosomal dominant trait. The phenotypic appearance of dwarfism with a head of normal size but appearing large, and short limbs, has traditionally led to many achondroplastics becoming circus clowns. Nasal septal and base of skull growth are impaired so that the bridge is depressed and skull bossed. Lumbar lordosis can be severe and occasionally causes spinal cord compression.

Many patients with achondroplasia are otherwise completely healthy but diabetes is occasionally associated.

Dental aspects

The only significant dental aspects are orthodontic in nature as a result of malocclusion but short stature, diabetes and kyphosis may affect management.

Cleidocranial dysplasia (cleidocranial dysostosis)

General aspects

Cleidocranial dysplasia is a rare defect, mainly of membrane bone formation, mostly involving the skull and clavicle. It is an autosomal dominant trait related to chromosome 6, and a defect in the signal transduction SH3-binding protein. There are also sporadic cases.

Table 16.1	Osteogenesis imperfecta: subtypes				
Type	**Inheritance**	**Bone disease**	**Stature**	**Extraskeletal involvement**	
I[a]	AD	Mild: fractures in childhood	Almost normal	Common. Blue sclerae; otosclerosis; thin aortic valves; hypermobile joints; ± dentinogenesis imperfecta	
II	AR	Severe: skull virtually unossified; multiple fractures; lethal	Low	No dentinogenesis imperfecta	
III	AR, some sporadic	Progressive: few can walk unaided	Low	Blue sclerae; no dentinogenesis imperfecta	
IV	AD	Severe	Low	Sclerae not blue; dentinogenesis imperfecta common	
V	Variable	Mild	Almost normal	Loose-jointedness a prominent feature	

[a]Constitutes 80% of all cases.
AD, autosomal dominant; AR, autosomal recessive.

Clinical features

The clavicles are either absent or defective, thus conferring the unusual and pathognomonic ability to approximate the shoulders anteriorly (Fig. 16.2).

The head is large but brachycephalic, with persistent fontanelles, a persistent metopic (frontal) suture, numerous wormian bones and bulging frontal, parietal and occipital bones. The middle facial third is hypoplastic leading to a relative mandibular protrusion, and the nasal bridge is depressed. There is occasionally delayed closure of the mandibular symphysis. Abnormalities of the cranial base may be seen on lateral cephalograms, and clefts of the hard and soft palate have been recorded. Other skeletal defects may be associated, such as kyphoscoliosis or pelvic anomalies.

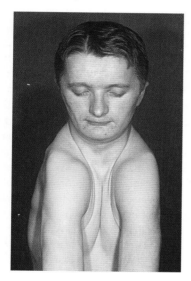

Fig. 16.2 Cleidocranial dystosis

Dental aspects

Apart from the facial anomalies there may be an excess number of teeth (hyperdontia, supernumeraries) with persistence of the deciduous dentition, multiple unerupted permanent teeth, twisted roots, malformed crowns and dentigerous cysts.

Osteopetrosis (Albers–Schönberg disease; marble-bone disease)

General aspects

Osteopetrosis is a rare genetic disorder of variable severity characterized by excessive bone density, probably as a result of a defect in osteoclastic activity and hence of bone remodelling. The bones, though abnormally dense, are weak and can fracture easily, but usually heal normally.

Clinical features

In mild osteopetrosis, there may be no symptoms and the diagnosis is made by chance by radiography. In severe osteopetrosis (malignant infantile osteopetrosis), patients may suffer bone pain, fractures or osteomyelitis and added complications can be cranial neuropathies leading, for example, to optic atrophy. Anaemia is common as the medullary cavities are filled with bone, despite extramedullary haemopoiesis in liver, spleen and lymph nodes and there is a susceptibility to infections, since macrophages and neutrophils are defective. Hydrocephalus, epilepsy and learning disability are less frequent.

General management

Serum levels of acid phosphatase are raised but calcium and phosphate levels are normal. Corticosteroid therapy may be of some help but bone marrow transplantation may be the only hope.

Dental aspects

Fracture of the jaw or osteomyelitis may complicate extractions. Once established, infection is difficult to eradicate, so that surgery should be minimally traumatic, mucoperiosteal flaps preferably not raised and antibiotic cover should be given. Eruption of posterior teeth may be complicated by osteomyelitis.

Management problems may include anaemia (Ch. 8) and corticosteroid therapy (Ch. 6).

The face may be broad, with hypertelorism, snub nose and frontal bossing. There may be retarded tooth eruption. Radiography shows excessive bone density and thickness, especially obvious in the skull. Trigeminal or facial neuropathies may complicate the disease.

ACQUIRED DISORDERS

Rickets and osteomalacia

General aspects

Rickets is a disease of childhood characterized by inadequate skeletal mineralization. Osteomalacia has the same pathogenesis but affects adults in whom there is failure of mineralization of replacement bone (osteoid) in the normal process of bone turnover.

Both rickets and osteomalacia are largely related to a lack of vitamin D or calcium, due to the causes shown in Box 16.1.

Rickets and osteomalacia are commonly now results of a dietary deficiency in poorly nourished communities: South Asian immigrants living in northern Europe are particularly at risk. Contributory factors may be lack of sunshine exposure and eating chapattis of wholemeal flour, containing phytates, which impair calcium absorption.

Clinical features

In rickets, the bones are weak, readily deformed and fracture easily but incompletely (greenstick or pseudofractures). Affected infants and young children are often listless and irritable, the muscles are weak and hypotonic, and they suffer bone pains. Excess formation of osteoid matrix causes a 'rachitic rosary' (swellings at the costochondral junctions).

385

General management

The plasma alkaline phosphatase levels are usually raised, calcium levels tend to be low in about 50%, and phosphate levels may be normal or low.

The underlying cause should be rectified where possible. Vitamin D and calcium should be given.

Dental aspects

The teeth usually escape surprisingly well from the effects of rickets. Dental defects are seen only in unusually severe cases, but eruption may be retarded. Vitamin D deficiency is not a contributory cause of dental caries. The jaws may show abnormal radiolucency.

In malabsorption syndromes there may be secondary hyperparathyroidism or vitamin K deficiency, with endocrine or bleeding disorders, respectively, and oral manifestations of malabsorption.

In vitamin D-resistant rickets (familial hypophosphataemia), the skull sutures are wide and there may be frontal bossing, but dental complaints frequently bring attention to the disease. The teeth have large pulp chambers, abnormal dentine calcification, and are liable to pulpitis and multiple, apparently spontaneous, dental abscesses. Since even minimal caries or attrition can lead to pulpitis, preventive care and fissure sealing or prophylactic occlusal coverage are needed.

Osteoporosis

General aspects

Osteoporosis (brittle bone disease) is a very common condition of diminished bone mass and low bone density, which leads to fragile bones, usually in the elderly. Factors that lead to limited formation of bone early in life or loss of bone structure later in life lead to osteoporosis. The same factors that encourage bone formation in youth affect the maintenance of bone mass during the adult years, particularly calcium intake, reproductive hormone status, normal parathyroid gland function and physical activity (Fig. 16.3). The difference between how much healthy bone is formed during the first 28 or so years of life and the rate at which it is remodelled and removed later determines how much osteoporosis or osteopenia (see later) results. From age 30 years, about 1% bone is lost per year, rising to about 5% after the menopause. During the first 20 years of life, formation of bone is the most important factor preventing osteoporosis, but after that point it is prevention of bone loss that becomes most important.

Risk factors for osteoporosis are shown in Box 16.2.

Clinical features

Mildly traumatic or non-traumatic injuries in osteoporosis can cause fractures. The chief complications are fractures of the neck of the femur, distal radius or humerus, or of the vertebral bodies causing gradual collapse of the spine (hence the shrinking size of some older women). Low back pain is common.

General management

Diagnosis of osteoporosis is mainly from bone densitometry – a radiographic technique that gives accurate and precise measurements of the amount of bone (not the *quality*), termed 'bone mineral density'. Poor bone mineral density and raised serum alkaline phosphatase are risk markers. Dual X-ray energy absorptiometry (DXA) or sometimes dual photon absorptiometry (DPA) are used. BMD values that fall well below the average for the 25-year-old female (stated statistically as 2.5 standard deviations below the average) are diagnosed as 'osteoporotic'. BMD values less than those in the normal

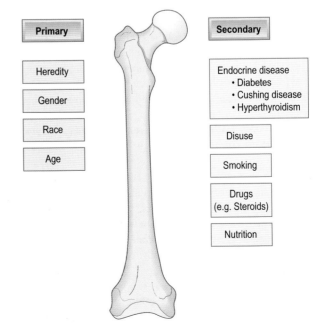

Fig. 16.3 Osteoporosis

Box 16.2 Risk factors for osteoporosis

- Advanced age: over the age of 60 years, nearly one-third of the population has osteoporosis – at least one in three women and one in 12 men
- Female gender and early menopause. The most common form of osteoporosis is post-menopausal and affects 50% of women over 70 years of age. It is due to loss of oestrogen production by the ovaries, which accelerates bone loss. In terms of bone remodelling, the lack of oestrogen promotes the ability of osteoclasts to absorb bone
- Positive family history
- Lifestyle factors
  - Lack of exercise. When the normal stresses placed upon bones by normal physical activity are removed, bones lose density, best illustrated in a significant loss of bone density in patients with spinal injuries. Athletes have stronger bones than normal sedentary adults
  - Diet low in calcium or vitamin D
  - Excess alcohol intake
  - Smoking
- Drugs and disease
  - Drugs such as corticosteroids, heparin, ciclosporin and anticonvulsants
  - Malignant disease
  - Chronic inflammatory states, such as rheumatoid arthritis or ulcerative colitis
  - Endocrine disorders (Cushing syndrome, hyperthyroidism, hypogonadism)

Table 16.2   Recommended calcium intake

Age	Amount of daily calcium
Infants	
Birth to 6 months	400 mg
6 months to 1 year	600 mg
Children/young adults	
1–10 years	800–1200 mg
11–24 years	1200–1500 mg
Adult women	
Pregnant or lactating	1200–1500 mg
25–49 years (pre-menopausal)	1000 mg
50–64 years (post-menopausal taking oestrogen or similar hormone)	1000 mg
50–64 years (post-menopausal not taking oestrogen or similar hormone)	1500 mg
Over 65 years old	1500 mg
Adult men	
25–64 years old	1000 mg
Over 65 years old	1500 mg

25-year-old female, but not 2.5 standard deviations below the average, are diagnosed as 'osteopenic'.

There are often no biochemical abnormalities, but there may be raised alkaline phosphatase levels, and urinary loss of calcium and hydroxyproline. In women who lose bone particularly fast, urinary tests can be informative. Bone biopsy is neither practical nor necessary.

The best management of osteoporosis is to avoid falls and injuries, and to consider use of hip protectors. Exercise has a positive effect on bone density (and therefore the risk of osteoporosis) particularly in adults who have been sedentary and begin to exercise. Weight-bearing exercises, such as walking, running, jogging and dancing, are recommended.

Additional calcium and 1-alpha-hydroxyvitamin D may also be helpful. The main sources of calcium are dairy products and green vegetables. The main sources of vitamin D are sun exposure (15 min exposure daily from April to October in the northern hemisphere is sufficient), margarine, breakfast cereals, oily fish, eggs and meat. Several forms of oral calcium are readily available and can help. Table 16.2 shows the recommended calcium intake according to age, gender and hormone status.

Hormone replacement therapy (HRT) may be effective in post-menopausal women and may also help to relieve other symptoms, such as flushing (see Ch. 25), but oestrogens can cause vaginal bleeding and there is a slightly greater risk of breast cancer. Oestrogen replacement during menopause protects bone mass and lessens the risk of osteoporotic fractures. The role of androgens (testosterone) in males is less clear, but the loss of testosterone promotes osteoporosis.

Raloxifene, given post-menopausally, may help to maintain bone density and the kidneys to produce vitamin D. Raloxifene also behaves like natural oestrogen in the liver where it raises production of 'good' cholesterol (high-density lipoprotein; HDL) and lowers 'bad' cholesterol (low-density lipoprotein; LDL). This drug appears to have no effect on the uterine endometrial lining growth, so there is no need for progestogen and there is no periodic bleeding. Raloxifene may also lower the risk of breast cancer.

Anti-resorption drugs' that lower the rate at which osteoclasts reabsorb bone include calcitonin and bisphosphonates. Calcitonin is a hormone produced in the thyroid and a powerful inhibitor of osteoclastic activity that produces modest improvements in bone mass. A disadvantage has been that calcitonin had to be injected but recently a nasal spray has been developed.

Bisphosphonates are adsorbed on to hydroxyapatite and can prevent or significantly slow the normal osteoclastic activity responsible for the resorption of bone; they can lead to a 50% reduction in fractures (including hip and spine) compared with women taking calcium only. Strontium ranelate may inhibit osteoporosis but can cause serious drug rashes with eosinophilia and systemic symptoms (DRESS). There is considerable controversy as to any benefits of fluorides on osteoporosis and consequent fractures.

Dental aspects

Patients with osteoporosis may have any of the problems of older people (Ch. 25). They may be at risk during general anaesthesia (GA) if there has been vertebral collapse and chest deformities.

There seems to be a correlation between osteoporosis and excessive alveolar bone loss in the elderly. Jaw osteoporosis is particularly a problem in women. Systemic treatment of osteoporosis may improve jaw bone density.

Alendronate may induce oral ulceration or osteonecrosis. Bisphosphonates, especially if used intravenously, may induce osteonecrosis of the jaws.

Bisphosphonates are used not only to treat osteopenia/osteoporosis but also hypercalcaemia of malignancy, metabolic bone disease (hyperparathyroidism, Paget disease) and osteogenesis imperfecta, Gaucher disease and Langerhans histiocytosis. Bisphosphonates are pyrophosphate analogues that block the 3-hydroxy-3-methylglutaryl-coenzyme A (HMG-CoA) reductase pathway (mevalonate path) and inhibit osteoclasts, thereby decreasing bone resorption. However, bisphosphonates remain in bone for years and have an extremely long-lasting effect. Bisphosphonate potency varies enormously, from the lowest potency (etidronate, clodronate and tiludronate) to the highest nitrogenous bisphosphonates (risedronate, ibandronate and zoledronate).

Intravenous bisphosphonates such as pamidronate and zoledronate used in cancer patients are a particularly high risk for producing bisphosphonate-induced osteonecrosis of the jaws (BIONJ; ranging from one in ten to one in 100 patients). However, in osteoporosis, in which the doses used are an order of magnitude lower, the prevalence appears to be very much lower. Oral bisphosphonates such as alendronate used for > 3 years have a risk between one in 10 000 to one in 100 000, the lowest risk being with the lower potency agents etidronate and tiludronate.

A working party from US National Institutes of Health and Canadian Institutes of Health Research have published recommendations (Khosla et al., 2007; see 'Further reading') and defined a *confirmed case of BIONJ* as

> an area of exposed bone in the maxillofacial region
> that did not heal within 8 weeks after identification by
> a health care worker, in a patient who was receiving or
> had been exposed to a bisphosphonate and had not had
> radiation therapy to the craniofacial region

and a *suspected case* as

> an area of exposed bone in the maxillofacial region that
> had been identified by a health care provider and had
> been present for < 8 weeks in a patient who was receiv-
> ing or had been exposed to a bisphosphonate and had
> not had radiation therapy to the craniofacial region.

Eighty per cent of cases of BIONJ present after surgery, as exposed necrotic bone, primarily mandibular alveolar bone (Box 16.3). Lamina dura sclerosis or loss, and widening of the periodontal ligament space may well be early manifestations.

Prevention of BIONJ is by avoiding elective oral surgery, or treatment should be carried out well before commencing

---

Box 16.3 Osteonecrosis of the jaws

- Exposed bone
- Loose teeth
- Foul discharge
- Pain ±
- Fistula

---

bisphosphonates or after a drug holiday for 6 months. The patient must be counselled about risks and a risk assessment carried out. Risk factors include bisphosphonate type and dose (intravenous is worst), and dental co-morbidities (increase risk). Bone turnover tests – low turnover as shown by low CTX (C-terminal cross-linking type 1 collagen telopeptides) increases risk. Recommendations for managing bisphosphonate patients are shown in Table 16.3.

If dental extractions become unavoidable in a patient taking bisphosphonates, the use of prophylactic antibiotics may be considered, but there are no controlled studies to support their use. The decision depends on the clinician's level of concern relative to the individual patient and his or her specific situation, including concomitant risk factors (e.g. prolonged use of oral bisphosphonates, intravenous bisphosphonates, older age, concomitant use of oestrogen or glucocorticoids).

Therefore, whenever possible, dentists should avoid performing extractions and elective oral surgery in patients taking bisphosphonates. If surgery is essential, the dentist must counsel the patient about the risks of use of intravenous or oral bisphosphonates taken for more than 3 years.

Osteoradionecrosis (see Ch. 22)

Osteomyelitis

General aspects

Osteomyelitis literally means 'inflammation of the bone marrow', although sometimes the subperiosteal bone is mainly affected.

Haematogenous osteomyelitis is an infection caused by bacterial seeding from the blood, involves a single species of micro-organism (typically a bacterium), occurs primarily in children and the most common site is in the rapidly growing and highly vascular metaphysis of growing bones.

Table 16.3 Recommendations for bisphosphonate patients (Khosla et al., 2007)

	Patients with non-malignant disease on bisphosphonates > 3 years	Patients with malignancy, starting or already on bisphosphonates
Surgery	Conventional orthograde endodontics recommended rather than extraction where possible	Conventional orthograde endodontics recommended rather than extraction where possible
Periodontics	Periodontal surgery is appropriate if it reduces or eliminates disease	No periodontal surgery
Endodontics	No apical surgery	No apical surgery
Implants	Currently not contraindicated if taking bisphosphonates but prudent to gain informed consent which should be documented (risk assessment)	Not recommended

Direct or contiguous inoculation osteomyelitis is usually caused by trauma or surgery, and tends to involve multiple micro-organisms.

Acute osteomyelitis of the jaws primarily affects the mandible, usually in adults and is essentially an osteolytic, destructive process, but an osteoblastic response is typical of sclerosing osteomyelitis. In children, proliferative periostitis may occur. Predisposing factors are sources from which bacteria can spread to bone:

- from local odontogenic infections (the commonest cause)
- from other adjacent structures (e.g. otitis media, tonsillitis, suppurative sialadenitis)
- haematogenous spread of organisms (this is rare in relation to the jaws).

When osteomyelitis of the mandible does occur, it may be a sign of an underlying debilitating disease, such as diabetes mellitus, an immune defect, an autoinflammatory condition, or the effects of alcoholism. Alternatively, it may be related to reduced vascularity such as after irradiation, or in rare conditions such as Paget disease or osteopetrosis.

Staphylococcus aureus is the commonest organism causing jaw osteomyelitis, but streptococci (both α- and β-haemolytic) and anaerobic organisms (e.g. *Bacteroides* and *Peptostreptococcus* species) are occasionally implicated.

In acute osteomyelitis, the organisms excite acute inflammation in the medullary bone and the consequent oedema and exudation causes pus to be forced under pressure through the medullary bone. The pressure causes thrombosis of intrabony blood vessels (i.e. the inferior dental artery), reducing the vascular supply to the bone, which then necroses. Eventually pus bursts through the cortical plate to drain via sinuses in the skin or mucosa. Where pus penetrates the cortex it may spread subperiosteally, stripping the periosteum and thus further reducing the blood supply. Necrotic bone becomes sequestrae surrounded by pus, which either spontaneously discharge or remain and perpetuate infection. The periosteum lays down new bone to form an involucrum encasing the infected and sequestrated bone. The involucrum may prevent sequestra from being shed. Finally, if little new bone is formed, a pathological fracture may occur.

Clinical features

Osteomyelitis in the jaw presents with a deep-seated, boring pain and swelling. Teeth in the affected segment are mobile and tender to percussion, and pus oozes from the gingival crevices. Once pus penetrates the cortical plate the pain improves and discharges intraorally or extraorally, often through several sinuses. Labial anaesthesia is a characteristic feature because of pressure on the inferior alveolar nerve. The patient is often febrile and toxic with enlarged regional lymph nodes.

General management

Diagnosis is clinical, supported by radiographs which, in established cases, show marked bony destruction and sequestration. However, since radiographic changes are seen only after there has been significant decalcification of bone, early cases may not be detected; in these, isotope bone scanning using technetium diphosphonate may show increased uptake. Blood tests show a leukocytosis with neutrophilia and a raised erythrocyte sedimentation rate.

Treatment is with antibiotics and usually drainage. Penicillin is the drug of choice, but many staphylococci are now penicillin-resistant, and for these flucloxacillin or fusidic acid may be used. Lincomycin and clindamycin also give high bone levels but, because of a high incidence of pseudomembranous colitis, are now regarded as second-line drugs. Metronidazole gives good bone levels and is indicated for anaerobic infections. Drainage of established pus follows the same guidelines used for other infections. When dead bone is exposed in the mouth, it can often be left to sequestrate without surgical interference, but sequestrectomy should be undertaken if the separated dead bone fails to discharge and decortication of the mandible may be needed in order to allow this and drainage. Hyperbaric oxygen is an effective adjunct for recalcitrant osteomyelitis, especially where anaerobic organisms are involved.

Acute maxillary osteomyelitis is rare, and usually seen in infants, presumably because the lack of development of the antrum at this age makes the maxilla a dense bone.

Chronic osteomyelitis presents with intermittent pain and swelling, relieved by the discharge of pus through long-standing sinuses. Bone destruction is localized and often a single sequestrum may be the source of chronic infection. Removal of the sequestrum and curettage of the associated granulation tissue usually produces complete resolution.

Focal sclerosing osteomyelitis is usually asymptomatic and is revealed as an incidental radiographic finding. Most common in young adults, it is usually associated with apical infection of a mandibular molar. Radiographically there is a dense, radio-opaque area of sclerotic bone related to the apical area, caused by formation of endosteal bone. This appears to be a response to low-grade infection in a highly immune host. Following tooth extraction the infection usually resolves (but the area of sclerotic bone often remains).

Diffuse sclerosing osteomyelitis is a sclerotic endosteal reaction, which, like focal sclerosing osteomyelitis, appears to be a response to low-grade infection. However, the area of bone involved is widespread and sometimes involves most of the mandible or occasionally the maxilla. Sometimes the infection arises in an abnormally osteosclerotic mandible, such as in Paget disease, osteopetrosis or fibrous dysplasia. Intermittent swelling, pain and discharge of pus may go on for years. Management is difficult because of the extensive nature of the disease process. Long-term antibiotics, curettage and limited sequestrectomy all have their place.

Proliferative periostitis (Garré osteomyelitis) is more common in children than adults. The cellular osteogenic periosteum of the child responds to low-grade infection, such as apical infection of a lower first molar tooth, by proliferation and deposition of subperiosteal new bone. The subperiosteal bone may be deposited in layers, producing an onion-skin appearance radiologically, which can simulate Ewing sarcoma. The endosteal bone, however, may appear to be completely normal, but in severe cases also appears moth-eaten radiologically. Removal of the infective source is usually followed by complete resolution, although subsequent bone remodelling can take a considerable time.

Tumoral calcinosis

This rare disease is characterized by ectopic, soft tissue calcifications but normocalcaemia. Early-onset periodontitis may be a feature.

Fibrous dysplasia

General aspects

Fibrous dysplasia consists of replacement of an area of bone by fibrous tissue and production of a localized swelling. Fibrous dysplasia may affect a single bone (monostotic) or is less commonly multiple (polyostotic).

The aetiology of fibrous dysplasia is unknown. The process typically starts in childhood and, as the skeleton matures, the lesions ossify progressively and ultimately, when skeletal growth ceases, usually become stabilized.

The natural history of cherubism also has some features in common with fibrous dysplasia but may cause bilateral lesions of the maxilla causing the eyes to 'up-turn towards heaven'.

Clinical features

Monostotic fibrous dysplasia is more common in females, and frequently involves the jaws, particularly the maxilla.

Polyostotic fibrous dysplasia may affect either sex and may involve over 50% of the skeleton, but is uncommon. The lesions may be unilateral and 50% have abnormal skin hyperpigmentation of a café-au-lait colour, especially over the dorsum of the trunk and limbs, usually on the same side as the bone lesions (Jaffe syndrome). Albright syndrome is polyostotic fibrous dysplasia with skin hyperpigmentation and precocious puberty in females. There are episodic rises in serum oestrogen and falls in gonadotropin levels.

General management

Radiography typically shows a ground-glass appearance with no defined margins. Serum calcium and phosphate levels are normal with, in many, raised serum alkaline phosphatase level and raised urinary hydroxyproline.

Fibrous dysplasia is typically self-limiting and usually ceases to progress after adolescence. Patients are sometimes managed with calcitonin. Testolactone is effective for the precocious puberty of Albright syndrome.

Surgery can be used to correct any residual cosmetic defect but the bone tends to bleed a great deal. Radiotherapy should be avoided because of the risk of inducing osteosarcomas.

Dental aspects

The facial bones are frequently involved in monostotic fibrous dysplasia and, in 25% of cases of polyostotic disease, facial deformity is the presenting feature. Monostotic fibrous dysplasia is not a medical problem but it is possible for the polyostotic type of the disease to be unrecognized when the facial lesions are the most obvious feature.

Hyperthyroidism or diabetes mellitus may occasionally be associated with polyostotic fibrous dysplasia and therefore may, rarely, complicate treatment.

Mucosal pigmentation is rare in Albright syndrome. In the differential diagnosis, it may be confused with that of Addison disease while the skin pigmentation may simulate that of neurofibromatosis.

Paget disease of bone (osteitis deformans)

General aspects

Paget disease is a common disorder in northern Europeans, characterized by progressive deformity and enlargement of bones related to overactivity of osteoclasts and osteoblasts. There appears to be considerable geographic variation in the prevalence, but there is always a male predominance.

In the earlier stages, resorption predominates (osteolytic phase) but later bone apposition takes over and, as disease activity declines, the affected bones become enlarged and dense (sclerotic stage). The essential features are total disorganization of the normal orderly replacement of bone, and an anarchic alternation of bone resorption and apposition.

The aetiology of Paget disease is unknown but a slow virus and, in some, a genetic factor may be involved.

Clinical features

Symptoms are absent in the early stages, which can only be detected radiologically. Bone pain is the most common feature in the elderly, is usually felt around the hips or knees, but is non-specific. One or many bones may be affected and, in the polyostotic type, the axial skeleton is mainly involved. The hands and feet are usually spared (Fig. 16. 4).

Other possible complications of Paget disease are deformities or pathological fractures, and sometimes compression of cranial nerves with such effects as deafness or impairment of vision. Rarely there is brainstem or spinal compression.

If Paget disease is widespread, hypervascularity of the bones can produce, in effect, an arteriovenous fistula and high-output cardiac failure.

Development of osteosarcoma is a recognized, but uncommon, complication.

General management

Radiographs of affected bones show predominantly radiolucencies due to osteolysis early on but mixed areas of lysis with sclerosis later. Affected bones become thicker. Radionuclide bone scanning shows increased uptake of technetium diphosphonate.

The serum total alkaline phosphatase level is grossly raised when many bones are affected, but usually there is little or no change in calcium or phosphate levels. More specific is a rise in bone-specific alkaline phosphatase and osteocalcin. There is then also raised urinary hydroxyproline and pyridinoline excretion.

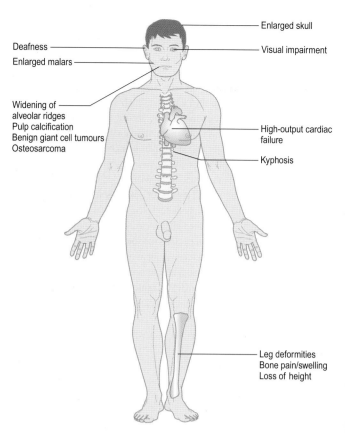

Fig. 16.4 Paget disease of bone

Labels on figure:
- Deafness
- Enlarged malars
- Enlarged skull
- Visual impairment
- Widening of alveolar ridges
- Pulp calcification
- Benign giant cell tumours
- Osteosarcoma
- High-output cardiac failure
- Kyphosis
- Leg deformities
- Bone pain/swelling
- Loss of height

Currently the most effective treatment of Paget disease is with bisphosphonates. Calcitonin is given by injection or intranasally to relieve bone pain and deafness but may be immunogenic.

Dental aspects

If the patient is in heart failure, the usual precautions have to be taken but, since general anaesthesia may be needed for extractions, this aspect of the disease needs to be kept in mind. Chest deformity may also complicate general anaesthesia.

When the skull is affected a typical early feature is a large irregular area of relative radiolucency (osteoporosis circumscripta; Fig. 16.5). Later, there is radio-opacity, with loss of the normal landmarks and an irregular cotton-wool appearance. Basilar invagination may be seen. The maxilla is involved occasionally and the mandible rarely. Typically, enlargement of the maxilla causes symmetrical bulging in the malar region (leontiasis ossea; Fig. 16.6). The intraoral features are gross symmetrical widening of the alveolar ridges and sometimes loss of lamina dura. Hypercementosis often forms enormous craggy masses which may become fused to the surrounding bone. Pulpal calcification may be seen.

Serious complications follow efforts to extract severely hypercementosed teeth. Attempts using forceps may fail to move the tooth, or cause fracture of the alveolar bone. Alternatively, the tooth may be mobilized but retained as if in a ball-and-socket

joint. In the early stages of the disease, the highly vascular bone may bleed freely; later, the poor blood supply to the bone makes it susceptible to chronic suppurative osteomyelitis. If hypercementosis is severe, a surgical approach with adequate exposure should be used for extractions. Prophylactic administration of an antibiotic such as penicillin (immediately before and for 3 or 4 days after the operation) may help prevent postoperative infection. Dentures have to be replaced as the alveolar ridge enlarges. Benign giant cell tumours may be seen.

Patients with Paget disease involving facial or maxillomandibular parts of the skeleton have a higher prevalence of heart disease and of deteriorating hearing, sight and smell.

Osteosarcoma is rare in the jaws but a few fully authenticated cases have been reported.

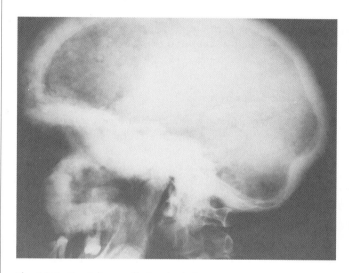

Fig. 16.5 Paget disease affecting the skull

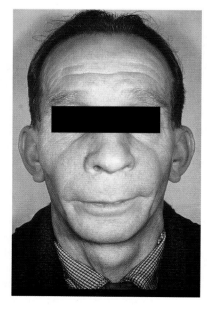

Fig. 16.6 Leontiasis ossea in Paget disease

Hyperparathyroidism (Ch. 6)

Guided bone regeneration

Guided bone regeneration (GBR) is a surgical procedure that uses barrier membranes to direct growth of new bone at sites having insufficient volumes or dimensions for function or prosthesis placement. Barrier membranes have been derived from a variety of sources, both natural and synthetic, and are marketed under various trade names. Membranes used in GBR and grafting may be of two principal varieties, non-resorbable (expanded polytetrafluoroethylene) and resorbable [collagen from various sources, ox caecum *cargile membrane*, polylactic acid, polyacetic acid, polyglycolic acid, polyglactin 910 (Vicryl), synthetic skin (Biobrane) and freeze-dried dura mater]. A range of materials – from demineralized bone matrix formulations and bone morphogenic proteins to synthetic ceramic materials – are now being used. Animal studies have even enabled a hybrid tooth–bone construct to be developed.

Distraction osteogenesis

Distraction osteogenesis is a surgical process involving the gradual, controlled displacement of surgically created fractures, which results in simultaneous expansion of bone and soft tissue, used to reconstruct combined deficiencies in bone and soft tissue. Developed in orthopaedics, it is also effective in orofacial skeletal reconstruction including in cleft palate reconstruction and alveolar ridge augmentation for placement of osseointegrated implants. The most frequent complications are infection, loosening and breaking of the introduced pins, osteomyelitis and fracture of the newly generated bone. Disadvantages are its expense and technical difficulty, and the long training required.

JOINT DISORDERS

Joints are considerably more frequently affected by disease than the bones or muscles. The jaws and temporomandibular joints are rarely involved in systemic disease. Patients with arthritis may experience restricted manual dexterity, which may compromise their ability to maintain adequate oral hygiene. These patients may need toothbrushes with specially adapted handles (such as a handle with a ball added to help the patient grip) or may benefit from using electric toothbrushes. Since joint stiffness tends to improve during the day, short appointments in the late morning or in the early afternoon are recommended for patients with arthritis. Supine positioning may be uncomfortable for them, and they may need neck and leg supports. Dentists should consider a patient's tendency to bleed and any need for corticosteroid supplementation or antibiotic coverage before performing any invasive procedures. There is no reliable evidence of a need for antibiotic prophylaxis before dental treatment in most patients with prosthetic joints, and the risks from adverse reactions to antibiotics probably exceed any benefit.

GENETIC CONDITIONS

The Marfan syndrome

The Marfan syndrome is an autosomal dominant disorder of connective tissue, a defect in fibrillin, with skeletal, cardiovascular and ocular manifestations. Rare, with a prevalence of about one in 10 000 and of such variable expression, the diagnosis may be difficult (Table 16.4). A Marfanoid body build may also be a feature of the benign joint hypermobility syndrome or multiple endocrine adenoma syndrome (MEA III; Ch. 6). The Marfan syndrome shares the features of loose-jointedness, cardiac valvular defects and ocular lesions with various of the subtypes of Ehlers–Danlos syndrome; there can also be confusion with other rare disorders, particularly homocystinuria and congenital contractural arachnodactyly. However, the most obvious distinguishing feature of the Marfan syndrome is the long, thin body habitus and long slender fingers. It has been suggested that Abraham Lincoln may have had the Marfan syndrome. His facial appearance and build suggest a mild case. However, casts of his hands, which were broad and strong, disprove this idea.

Table 16.4 Marfan syndrome

Skeletal defects	Cardiovascular defects	Neuro-ocular defects
Disproportionately long limbs	Dilatation of ascending aorta	Ectopia lentis
Arachnodactyly (spider fingers)	Dissecting aneurysm	Blue sclerae in some
Loose joints	Aortic regurgitation	Learning impairment (sometimes)
Pectus excavatum	Mitral valve prolapse	
Temporomandibular joint subluxation		

Clinical features

Skeletal manifestations are excessive length of tubular bones so that patients are tall with wide arm span and long spider-like fingers (arachnodactyly). The arm span often exceeds the patient's height by a ratio of > 1.03.

Cardiovascular abnormalities affect 90% of patients, and aortic dissection can be life-threatening. There is often severe aortic and mild mitral incompetence. Death in the fifth decade is common. Mitral valve prolapse can lead to arrhythmias, embolism or sudden death and, if it causes a systolic murmur, can predispose to infective endocarditis, particularly in older persons.

Ligaments are lax, predisposing to joint hyperextensibility, subluxation or dislocation, and hernias are common. Visual impairment is common due to lens subluxation or dislocation in 80%. Survival has been greatly improved with aortic graft surgery and the use of beta-blockers.

Lung function can be impaired by cysts which lead to spontaneous pneumothorax and kyphoscoliosis.

Dental aspects

Management may be complicated by chest deformities and cardiovascular abnormalities, which may be contraindications to general anaesthesia, and a risk of infective endocarditis (Ch. 5).

The palatal vault is high and temporomandibular joint dysfunction or recurrent subluxation may be troublesome. Bite problems may occur from malocclusion.

Ehlers–Danlos syndrome

General aspects

Ehlers–Danlos syndrome (EDS) is a group of rare disorders of collagen formation characterized by hyperextensible skin, propensity to bruising and loose-jointedness. The most common forms are inherited as autosomal dominant traits, while the remainder are recessive and there is wide variation in the clinical features of the different types (Table 16.5).

Clinical features

Hypermobility of the joints is the best known manifestation of EDS and may be extreme (India-rubber man) but the severity varies in the different subtypes. Recurrent, semi-spontaneous dislocation may result. It may be possible to hyperextend the fingers until they are at right angles to the back of the hand and the diagnosis is often made by the unusual ability of the patient to pull their thumb back to their forearm (Fig. 16.7).

The skin is typically soft, abnormally extensible, feels fine and thin and may appear lax; wounds tend to gape or to split after slight trauma. Healing is slow and may leave fragile scars with a tissue-paper texture. Even when it appears normal, it may be possible to pull the skin out for one or two inches (Fig. 16.8). Other, incidental oddities that may be seen in EDS may include the ability to touch the nose with the tip of the tongue (Gorlan's sign).

Weakness of the connective tissue component may cause lesions in the gastrointestinal tract, urinary tract and respiratory system. In the vascular type (type IV), spontaneous rupture of major arteries can cause fatal haemorrhage and internal bleeding.

Easy ('spontaneous') bruising, though of vascular origin, may mimic purpura caused by haematological diseases but, unlike any of the latter, there is a combination of subcutaneous, submucosal and deep bleeding. Although platelet defects have occasionally been reported, haemostatic function is often normal, except in type IV. Mitral valve prolapse (floppy valve syndrome) is seen in many types of EDS, particularly type III, and may confer susceptibility to infective endocarditis or lead to rapid development of mitral insufficiency and heart failure. Cardiac conduction defects may be present.

Dental aspects

Patients with mitral valve prolapse may develop heart failure with attendant risks during anaesthesia (Ch. 5).

Post-extraction bleeding is likely to be most severe in type IV (vascular type), in which there are also the most severe vascular

Table 16.5 Ehlers–Danlos syndrome: subtypes

Types	Inheritance	Hyper-extensibility	Skin fragility and bruising	Joint hypermobility	Special features
I (gravis) Classical type	AD	++	++	++	Parrot face. Frequent musculoskeletal disorders. Mitral valve prolapse
II (mitis) Classical type	AD	+	+	+ Hands and feet only	Mitral valve prolapse. Bruising common
III (benign hypermobility) Hypermobility type	AD	±	+	++	Dislocations, haemarthrosis, early-onset arthritis. Mitral valve prolapse
IV Vascular type	AR	±	+++	± Digits only	Bleeding from major arteries
V (sex-linked)	X-linked	++	+	±	Frequent musculoskeletal disorders. Males only
VI (ocular or hydroxylysine deficient)	AR	++	±	++	Fragile cornea and sclera. Multiple ocular defects, deafness, often early loss of sight
VII (multiple congenital dislocation or arthrochalasis multiplex congenita)	AR	+	±	++	Early onset of multiple dislocations. Some laxity of ligaments, short stature
VIII (periodontal)	AD	±	±	±	Severe early-onset periodontitis and loss of teeth. Blue sclerae
IX (skeletal and urinary tract dysplasia)*	AR	–	±	±	Occipital exosfoses, low copper levels
X (fibronectin deficiency)	AR	±	±	±	Bleeding tendency

AD, autosomal dominant; AR, autosomal recessive.
*No longer classified as Ehlers-Danlos syndrome

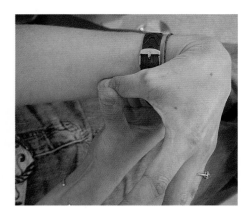

Fig. 16.7 Ehlers–Danlos syndrome: a typical party trick

abnormalities. There is then severe semi-spontaneous purpura with extensive ecchymoses and also weakness of arterial walls. Severe bleeding from the gingivae, especially after toothbrushing, or from extraction sockets, may sometimes be the main complaint.

Hypermobility of joints is severe in types I, VI and VII and, in all of these, subluxation and dislocation of the temporomandibular joint is a possibility. In type VIII EDS, and possibly type IV, there is early onset of periodontal disease, with early loss of teeth.

In type III EDS, local anaesthetics may have less effect, though there is no satisfactory explanation.

The teeth in EDS may be small with short or abnormally shaped roots, and many pulp stones. Orofacial features in type VII include micrognathia, an anterior open bite and gingival hyperplasia with varying degrees of hyperkeratosis. The deciduous dentition shows abnormal morphology of the molars, obliteration of the tooth pulp and severe enamel attrition. The permanent dentition shows agenesis and microdontia of several teeth. Tooth discoloration, dysplastic roots, and tooth pulp obliteration are present in a restricted number of permanent teeth.

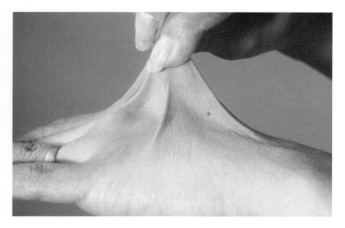

Fig. 16.8 Extensible skin in Ehlers–Danlos syndrome

Recurrent temporomandibular joint dislocation

Chronic recurrent temporomandibular joint (TMJ) dislocation is defined as the complete loss of articular relationships, during mouth wide opening, between the articular fossa of the

temporal bone and the condyle–disc complex. This may be seen in EDS, those with internal derangement and other conditions. The classic treatment was the Dautrey operation (eminectomy), which modifies the bony obstacle, preventing condylar locking, but does not have a therapeutic effect on TMJ ligament and capsular laxity or masticatory muscle incoordination, which seem to be the real cause of TMJ dislocation in most cases. Plication of the joint capsule may help.

ARTHRITIS

Osteoarthritis (osteoarthrosis)

General aspects

Osteoarthritis (OA) is the most common form of arthritis and is most common in adults over age 45 years. Osteoarthritis is especially painful in frequently used, weight-bearing or traumatized joints. OA is characterized by degeneration of articular cartilage with compensatory thickening of the exposed underlying bone and development of peri-articular cysts. Collapse of these peri-articular cysts, together with continued peripheral bone proliferation, causes progressive joint deformity.

Risk factors for OA are shown in Box 16.4.

Box 16.4 Risk factors for osteoarthritis

- Age: most in people > 45 years
- Gender: females more commonly affected
- Genetic predisposition
- Obesity
- Malformed joints (hereditary or acquired)
- Occupation (athletes)
- Haemochromatosis
- Paget disease
- Gout

Osteoarthritis may affect any joint, but especially affects frequently used, weight-bearing or traumatized joints such as those in the fingers, hips, knees, lower back and feet. Initially it tends to strike only one joint, but if the fingers are affected multiple hand joints may become arthritic, but sometimes painlessly.

The essential change in osteoarthritis is degeneration of articular cartilage with compensatory thickening of the underlying bone, which becomes exposed and is at first smooth and shiny but later becomes roughened. Cystic spaces form beneath and bone proliferates at the joint margins. Exposure and collapse of the cystic cavities, together with continued peripheral proliferation, cause progressive deformity.

Clinical features

In contrast to rheumatoid arthritis, in osteoarthritis there are no systemic symptoms, no obvious inflammation of affected joints or serological changes (Table 16.6). Features may include: pain with stiffness, progressively diminished function and deformity particularly of the larger joints, such as the hips or knees; pain swelling and stiffness in a joint during or

Table 16.6 Comparison of osteoarthritis and rheumatoid arthritis

	Osteoarthritis	Rheumatoid arthritis
Age of onset	Late middle age or elderly	Middle age
Pain and disability	+	++
Main joints affected	Weight-bearing or frequently used joints (hip, spine, knee, fingers)	Bilateral, interphalangeal
Clinical inflammation over joints	–	+
Joint deformities	Heberden or Bouchard nodes	Swelling and deviations
Morning stiffness	Some	Pronounced
Systemic problems, malaise, fatigue	–	+
Erythrocyte sedimentation rate	Normal	Raised
Rheumatoid factor	–	+ Usually

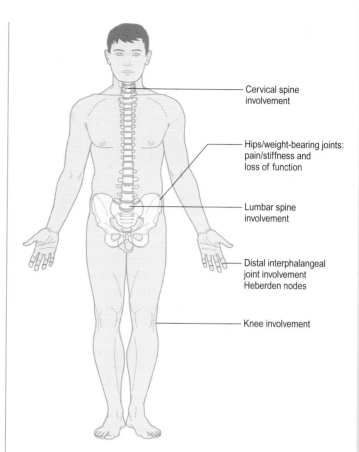

Fig. 16.10 Osteoarthritis

- Cervical spine involvement
- Hips/weight-bearing joints: pain/stiffness and loss of function
- Lumbar spine involvement
- Distal interphalangeal joint involvement Heberden nodes
- Knee involvement

after use, or pain before or during a change in weather; loss of joint flexibility; bony lumps on the fingers, on the middle (Bouchard nodes) or end joints (Heberden node; Fig. 16.9), or the first metacarpo-phalangeal joint at the thumb base (Fig. 16.10).

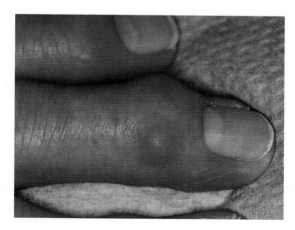

Fig. 16.9 Heberden nodes

General management

The diagnosis is usually on clinical grounds, supported by imaging. The characteristic radiographic features include narrowing of the joint space, marginal osteophyte formation (lipping), subchondral bone sclerosis, bone 'cysts' (rounded areas of radiolucency just beneath the joint surface) and deformity.

Physical methods of treatment include a number of factors shown in Box 16.5.

Medical methods of treatment include: topical pain relievers (counterirritant medications such as trolamine salicylate, methyl salicylate, menthol and camphor, or capsaicin), which may relieve pain in joints close to the skin surface, such as fingers, knees and elbows; anti-inflammatory drugs (non-steroidal anti-inflammatory drugs; NSAIDs) or licofelone, or cyclo-oxygenase 2 (COX-2) inhibitors, such as celecoxib; glucosamine as a food supplement – said to provide moderate pain relief comparable to that from NSAIDs; antidepressants, independent of their antidepressant properties, can help lessen chronic pain; and intra-articular injections with a corticosteroid or hyaluronate, which can give pain relief for a time.

Surgical methods of treatment include joint replacement surgery – the most important surgical treatment for arthritis. The damaged joint is removed and replaced with a plastic or metal prosthesis. The hip joint is most commonly replaced, but implants are available for knee, shoulder, elbow, finger or ankle joints. Completely normal function is usually restored. Arthroscopy can be used to remove loose fragments of bone or cartilage that may cause pain or cause mechanical symptoms such as 'locking'. However, there is no significant improvement in pain relief or function 2 years afterwards. Surgery can reposition bones to help correct deformities and can permanently fuse bones in a joint to improve stability and reduce pain.

Box 16.5 Physical aids to osteoarthitis

- Regular exercise – to help maintain joint mobility
- Weight control – to minimize stress on joints
- Appropriate footwear if there is arthritis in weight-bearing joints or back
- A walking stick to ease the load on a damaged joint
- Heat application to ease pain, relax tense, painful muscles and increase the regional flow of blood
- Cold application for occasional flare-ups

Table 16.7 Prophylactic antibiotics in patients with prosthetic joints: based on AAOS/ADA guidelines[a]

	Comments
Dental at-risk procedure	Tooth removal Oral or periodontal surgery or raising mucogingival flaps for any other purpose (including implants) Subgingival procedures including probing, scaling, root planing, subgingival fibre placement or any form of periodontal surgery Intraligamentary injections Reimplantation of avulsed teeth Endodontic manipulation beyond the root apex Orthodontic banding
Joint at risk	Joint placed within previous 2 years Joint with history of previous infection Joint in patient with haemophilia Joint in patient with type 1 diabetes Joint in patient with rheumatoid arthritis Joint in patient on immunosuppressive therapy
Antibiotic prophylaxis regimens	Cefalexin 2 g or Clindamycin 600 mg or Azithromycin 500 mg or Clarithromycin 500 mg or Amoxicillin 2 g

[a]Modified from American Association of Orthopedic Surgeons and American Dental Association.

Dental aspects

Age and immobility may influence access to dental care. Infections of prosthetic joints are usually due to non-oral organisms such as staphylococci and only exceptionally rarely to oral bacteria. Even where viridans streptococci have been found in infected joints, they could have come from non-oral sources, or simply have come from a bacteraemia associated with chewing. The same arguments as to the risk:benefit of antimicrobial prophylaxis for endocarditis (Ch. 5) apply. Antibiotic prophylaxis is therefore not indicated for dental surgery on most patients with bone pins, plates and screws or with total joint replacements.

However, antibiotic prophylaxis 1–1.5 h before dental treatment likely to initiate a bacteraemia (Table 16.7) may be considered where dental at-risk procedures are to be carried out in patients who have recent new joints (within 2 years), or in haemophiliacs, or where the joint has previously been infected, or where the patient is immunocompromised, such as those with diabetes or rheumatoid disease.

Antibiotic regimens are shown in Table 16.7; cephradine 1 g orally or intravenously is a further choice. Although the evidence may be questionable, medicolegal and other considerations suggest that one should act on the side of caution and fully inform and discuss with the patient; take medical advice in any case of doubt; and give antibiotic prophylaxis for at-risk procedures in patients at high risk for infection.

Dental management may be complicated by a bleeding tendency if the patient is anticoagulated or takes high doses of aspirin (Ch. 8).

Osteoarthritis affects the TMJ in some older patients but typically painlessly. Those with osteoarthritis of other joints also do not appear to have significantly more involvement of the TMJ than controls. The radiographic severity of TMJ osteoarthritis does not correlate with symptoms and it is frequently only a post-mortem finding. Since TMJ osteoarthritis is rarely clinically significant, patients should not be made unnecessarily anxious.

A syndrome of dry mouth and osteoarthritis has been described (sialoadenitis, osteoarthritis, xerostomia – SOX) but needs confirmation.

Rheumatoid arthritis

Rheumatoid arthritis (RA) affects about 2% of the population in the West, women approximately three times as frequently as men, typically between the ages of 30 and 40 years. It is a multisystem, immunologically mediated disease and occurs in genetically predisposed individuals (HLA-DR4 genotype). RA is characterized by the presence of rheumatoid factor (RF) – an IgM antibody directed against abnormal IgG that forms immune complexes and leads to activation of complement, synovial inflammation and destructive joint disease.

Clinical features

The onset of RA is often insidious, with increasing stiffness of the hands or feet, worse in the morning. In the acute stage, there is aching, swelling, redness, tenderness and limitation of movement of small joints of the wrists, hands and feet, which are typically affected first. The metacarpophalangeal and interphalangeal joints typically become spindle-shaped as a result of joint swelling with muscle wasting on either side (Fig. 16.11). Ulnar deviation of the fingers may develop later. Eventually the wrists, elbows, ankles and knees also may be involved and the patient becomes disabled (Fig. 16.12). Other common manifestations are tenosynovitis or subcutaneous nodules. The cervical spine is involved in 30% and there may be atlanto-axial subluxation (Fig. 16.13).

Clinically apparent effects on other systems are less common (Table 16.8).

General management

Rheumatoid arthritis is diagnosed if at least four of the features shown in Box 16.6 are present.

The diagnosis is confirmed by raised erythrocyte sedimentation rate (ESR) and other inflammatory markers, and positive rheumatoid factor, present in about 70%, is usually immunoglobulin M (IgM) and a sensitive marker of RA but is not

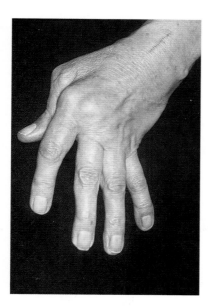

Fig. 16.11 Rheumatoid arthritis

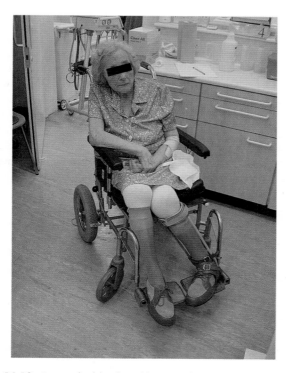

Fig. 16.12 Patient wheelchair-bound by severe rheumatoid disease

specific. In so-called seronegative cases, the RF may be IgG, and therefore not detected by the routine agglutination tests (latex and sheep-cell agglutination test; SCAT), which detect only IgM RF. Radioimmunoassay (RIA) and enzyme-linked immunosorbent assay (ELISA) detect any class of RF. Antinuclear antibodies are also often found but usually in low titre (Table 16.9).

Radiographic features include widening of the joint space (early) followed by narrowing later; joint erosion, destruction and deformity; and peri-articular osteoporosis. Later there is narrowing of the joint spaces, cyst-like spaces in the bone, and subluxation. Ultimately there may be severe bone destruction and deformity, but ankylosis does not follow.

Factors associated with a poor prognosis in RA include positive RF, extra-articular disease, HLA DR4, early erosions and severe disability at presentation. The main aspects of treatment are rest in acute phases, but between these episodes maintenance of mobility of affected joints.

Drugs used include symptom-modifying drugs such as simple analgesics or NSAIDs, and corticosteroids (given via intra-articular injections in acute phases). Disease-modifying anti-rheumatic drugs (DMARDs), which may relieve painful, swollen joints and slow joint damage, include sulfasalazine, gold, penicillamine, minocycline, antimalarials, methotrexate, corticosteroids, azathioprine, ciclosporin, cyclophosphamide and leflunomide. Biological response modifiers such as anakinra – a direct and selective blocker of interleukin-1 (IL-1) receptor –etanercept, tocilizumab (anti–IL-6), adalimumb and infliximab, which act against tumour necrosis factor alpha (TNF-alpha), and rituximab – a monoclonal antibody against CD20 antigen on B lymphocytes – may be given for severe active disease, but are costly and can cause severe toxic effects. A Prosorba column, a blood-filtering technique used weekly to remove autoantibodies, is sometimes available.

Management of RA also includes general supportive measures such as splints and appliances to facilitate mobility, reduce pain and preserve function. Surgery may be indicated for replacement of severely damaged joints.

Dental aspects

In some patients dislocation of the atlant-oaxial joint or fracture of the odontoid peg can readily follow sudden jerking extension of the neck, as a result of weakness of the ligaments. Disastrous accidents of this sort have been known to follow adjustment of the headrest of older types of dental chair, or sudden extension of the neck during the induction of GA.

Sjögren syndrome is the main oral complication. There is a predilection of RA for small joints, including the TMJ, but though there may be limitation of opening or stiffness, these are often painless. Radiographic changes are common in the TMJ and consist of erosions, flattening of the joint surfaces and marginal proliferation. Even when the disease is severe, pain from the TMJ appears to trouble only a minority. Occasionally an anterior open bite or even sleep apnoea may result. Intubation for GA can be difficult.

Patients with joint prostheses because of RA may possibly require antibiotic cover before surgical procedures since they are regarded as mildly immunocompromised. A few patients are treated with corticosteroids.

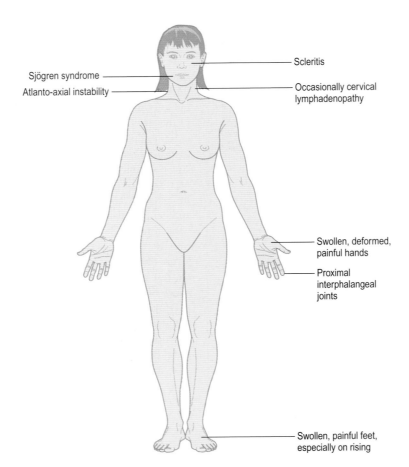

Fig. 16.13 Rheumatoid arthritis

Some treatments induce neutropenia, thrombocytopenia or a bleeding tendency.

Patients may also have severely restricted manual dexterity and consequent difficulty maintaining adequate oral hygiene. Toothbrushes may need specially adapted handles (e.g. by adding a plastic or rubber ball to help the patient grip the brush) or an electric brush may solve this problem.

The drugs used in rheumatoid arthritis can be a cause of oral side-effects such as ulcers and lichenoid reactions (Table 16.10). NSAIDs, gold and low-dose methotrexate may cause ulceration.

Felty syndrome

Felty syndrome comprises RA, splenomegaly and lymphadenopathy, and is managed as RA. These patients are at risk from infections because of leukopenia. Management can also be complicated by anaemia and mild thrombocytopenia. Orofacial manifestations may include severe ulceration or oropharyngeal infections, including chronic sinusitis.

Juvenile arthritis

General aspects

There are many types of juvenile arthritis, one of which resembles adult rheumatoid arthritis, another has features in common with ankylosing spondylitis. Juvenile rheumatoid arthritis

(JRA) is uncommon compared with adult RA but can be considerably more severe.

Clinical features

One important form of JRA predominantly affects girls in late childhood, affects virtually any joint and is associated with rheumatoid nodules, mild fever, anaemia and malaise. Over 50% develop severe arthritis and deformity.

General management

Rheumatoid factor is positive in most cases and antinuclear antibodies are present in 75%. Management is as for RA.

Dental aspects

Damage to the TMJ of various types has occasionally been described. Complete bony ankylosis has been reported and micrognathia may develop in 4–25%. Chronic use of aspirin may occasionally cause tooth erosion.

Psoriatic arthritis

Psoriatic arthritis can affect particularly the lower spine and sacro-iliac joints. Joint disease can closely resemble RA but is usually milder. There are no characteristic serological abnormalities.

Table 16.8 Rheumatoid arthritis: features and complications

Cardiovascular	Cardiac conduction defects Myocarditis Pericarditis Valvulitis Vasculitis
Dermal, oral and para-oral	Oral drug lesions Palmar erythema Sjögren syndrome Subcutaneous rheumatoid nodules Temporomandibular arthritis Vasculitis and various rashes
Haematological	Anaemia Leukopenia Thrombocytopenia
Hepatic	Abnormal liver function
Joints	Arthritis Laxity of ligaments Spinal nerve root compression Subluxation Tenosynovitis
Muscular	Wasting Weakness
Neurological	Benign trigeminal neuropathy Carpal tunnel syndrome Glove-and-stocking anaesthesia Various neuropathies
Non-specific features	Fatigue Fever Malaise Weight loss
Ocular	Episcleritis, scleritis or scleromalacia Sjögren syndrome
Osseous	Osteoporosis
Renal	Amyloidosis Various nephropathies
Respiratory	Bronchiolitis Fibrosis Lung nodules (rheumatoid lung disease) Pleurisy and pleural effusion

Table 16.9 Laboratory findings in rheumatoid arthritis

Test	Typical findings
Full blood count	Normocytic anaemia Mild leukocytosis (or leukopenia) Mild thrombocytopenia
Erythrocyte sedimentation rate	Raised
Protein electrophoresis	Hypergammaglobulinaemia
Rheumatoid factor – latex agglutination	Positive usually
Antinuclear antibodies	Positive in 20–60%

Table 16.10 Drugs in rheumatoid arthritis: oral adverse effects

Drugs	Adverse effects
Antimalarials	Lichenoid reactions
Corticosteroids	Candidosis
Gold	Lichenoid reactions
	Ulceration
Leflunomide	Candidosis
	Salivary swelling
	Taste disturbance
Methotrexate	Ulceration
NSAIDs	Lichenoid reactions
	Ulceration
Pencillamine	Lichenoid reactions
	Loss of taste
	Severe ulceration

NSAIDs, non-steroidal anti-inflammatory drugs.

General management is with NSAIDs.

Psoriatic arthritis of the TMJ is rare. oral mucosal lesions, histologically verified as oral psoriasis, are occasionally seen. Methotrexate may cause oral ulcers. Anti-TNF agents are now available and approved for use in psoriatic arthritis.

Temporomandibular pain-dysfunction syndrome (Ch. 13)

Gout

In gout, deposits of sodium urate monohydrate crystals in the joints result in the release of lysosomal enzymes from polymorphonuclear leukocytes, causing acute inflammation.

Primary gout is an inborn error of metabolism causing raised plasma urate levels (hyperuricaemia). It mainly affects adult men in whom food or drink rich in purines (e.g. fish roe) can precipitate an attack in those with the underlying metabolic disorder. Ethanol favours conversion of pyruvate to lactate, which impairs renal excretion of urate, so an alcoholic 'binge' (especially with beer) can precipitate an attack. Some forms of primary gout are inherited in an autosomal dominant manner, while in others there is evidence of polygenic inheritance.

Secondary gout is usually caused by cell breakdown from drug treatment or radiotherapy for myeloproliferative diseases releasing large amounts of purines into the blood. Hyperuricaemia is common but usually symptomless.

Gout of either type is aggravated or can be caused by diuretics (thiazides and loop diuretics), which impair renal excretion of uric acid. Women are not significantly at risk from gout until after the menopause.

Lesch–Nyhan syndrome, deficiency of hypoxanthine–guanine phosphoribosyltransferase (HGPRT), is a rare cause of gout, associated with learning impairment, choreoathetosis and compulsive self-mutilation. The lips are chewed and self-inflicted injuries, especially to the face and head, despite the pain it obviously causes, are typical.

Clinical features

An acute attack of gout causes sudden and intensely severe joint pain, usually in the big toe, associated with fever, leukocytosis and raised serum uric acid levels. Many gouty patients are obese, and there is a high incidence of hyperlipidaemia, hypertension, diabetes and atherosclerosis.

Chronic tophaceous gout is often associated with renal disease (gouty nephropathy), which, unless treated, leads to fatal renal failure in up to 25%.

Gouty tophi are masses of urate crystals, which, in joints, interfere mechanically with function and also destroy bone and cartilage to cause a severe deforming arthritis. Extra-articular tophi typically form in the helix of the ear as conspicuous, almost white, hard, subcutaneous nodules.

Renal disease (gouty nephropathy), unless treated, can lead to fatal renal failure.

General management

Blood chemistry shows raised uric acid levels. Secondary gout should be investigated for the underlying disorder.

Colchicine, etoricoxib, naproxen and indometacin relieve an acute attack but can cause severe adverse effects. Anti-inflammatory analgesics are therefore used but aspirin, which interferes with uricosuric agents, should not be given. Allopurinol reduces the frequency of acute gouty attacks by inhibiting xanthine oxidase, conversion of xanthine to uric acid and purine synthesis. In severe cases, uricosuric agents, such as probenecid or sulfinpyrazone, can be used in addition to increase urate excretion. In very few patients (< 1%) with diminished HGPRT activity, allopurinol does not work and the drug can, rarely, cause xanthine renal stones to form. Activation of 6-mercaptopurine and azathioprine, both purine antimetabolites, depends on HGPRT; consequently, these drugs are not effective in Lesch–Nyhan syndrome.

Dental aspects

Hypertension, ischaemic heart disease, cerebrovascular disease, diabetes and renal disease may affect dental management. Gout affects the TMJ only rarely.

Aspirin is contraindicated as it interferes with uricosuric drugs. The incidence of rashes with ampicillin, but not other penicillin allergies, is greater in patients on allopurinol. Drugs used for the treatment of gout, particularly allopurinol, can occasionally cause oral ulceration.

Calcium pyrophosphate deposition disease involves deposition of calcium pyrophosphate in and around joints in conditions of high plasma calcium, low phosphate or low magnesium. It manifests similarly to gout and is treated with NSAIDs, and by correction of the metabolic disturbance.

Ankylosing spondylitis

General aspects

Ankylosing spondylitis is a seronegative spondyloarthropathy (predominantly affecting the spine) seen mainly in young males. The inflammation involves the insertions of ligaments and tendons and is followed by ossification, forming bony bridges that fuse adjacent vertebral bodies or other joints.

Ankylosing spondylitis is partly genetically determined: the family history may be positive and in Caucasians over 90% are HLA-B27.

Clinical features

The onset is usually insidious, with low back pain (spondylitis) and stiffness followed by worsening pain and tenderness in the sacroiliac region due to sacroiliitis. Hip joints may also be involved. Over the course of years the back becomes fixed (Fig. 16.14), usually in extreme flexion, and chest expansion becomes limited and respiration impaired. About 25% develop eye lesions (acute uveitis or iridocyclitis). About 10% develop cardiac disease (aortic incompetence or conduction defects; Fig. 16.15).

General management

Erythrocyte sedimentation rate is raised, HLA-B27 is often positive and there is a mild anaemia, but no other significant laboratory findings – and no autoantibodies. Radiography shows progressive squaring-off of vertebrae (which become rectangular), intervertebral ossification ('bamboo spine'), calcification of tendon/ligament insertions and obliteration of the sacroiliac joints.

Treatment consists of: physiotherapy and exercises; anti-inflammatory analgesics to control pain and allow the back to be kept as mobile as possible (indometacin may be used); anti-TNF agents; radiotherapy to the spine is occasionally given, but carries the risk of leukaemia.

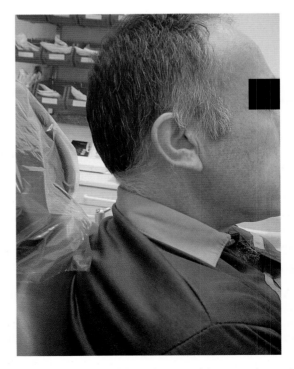

Fig. 16.14 Ankylosing spondylitis in this patient did not permit him to place his neck on the headrest

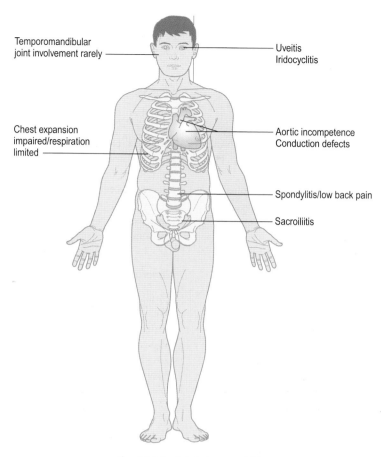

Temporomandibular
joint involvement rarely

Uveitis
Iridocyclitis

Chest expansion
impaired/respiration
limited

Aortic incompetence
Conduction defects

Spondylitis/low back pain

Sacroiliitis

Fig. 16.15 Ankylosing spondylitis

Dental aspects

General anaesthesia can be hazardous because of severely restricted opening of the mouth, impaired respiratory exchange associated with severe spinal deformity or cardiac disease (aortic insufficiency). Ankylosing spondylitis can affect the TMJ in about 10%, especially those over 40 with widespread disease, but symptoms are usually mild.

Reactive arthritis or seronegative spondyloarthropathy (Reiter disease)

This comprises arthritis, urethritis and conjunctivitis, but there are numerous other effects and it is more appropriate to speak of reactive arthritis or seronegative spondyloarthropathy. It may follow a range on infections (Box 16.7).

Reactive arthritis typically begins about 1–3 weeks after infection, is itself not contagious, but the causative bacteria can be passed from person to person or affect many persons who acquire it from the same source. It most often affects males

> **Box 16.7 Aetiology of reactive arthritis**
>
> - Sexually transmitted infections with *Chlamydia trachomatis* (urogenital reactive arthritis)
> - Gut infections, such as by *Shigella flexneri*, *Salmonella typhimurium*, *Yersinia* or *Campylobacter* (enteric or gastrointestinal reactive arthritis)
> - Respiratory infections with *Chlamydia pneumoniae*

between 20 and 40 years of age, about 80% of whom are HLA-B27 positive.

Clinical features

Seronegative spondyloarthropathy often affects and causes symptoms from the urogenital tract, particularly the prostate or urethra in men and the urethra, or rarely, the uterus or vagina in women. Joint symptoms typically include pain and swelling in the knees, ankles and feet. Approximately 50% have low-back and buttock pain. Eye involvement is usually conjunctivitis and uveitis, with eye redness, pain and irritation, and blurred vision. Characteristic skin lesions are small, hard nodules of hyperkeratotic thickening, which can be gross, and affect the palms and soles (keratoderma blenorrhagica). The penis may show painless circinate lesions (circinate balanitis) and similar lesions may be seen in the mouth. The symptoms usually last 3–12 months, although they can return or develop into long-term disease in a few.

General management

There is no specific diagnostic test for seronegative spondyloarthropathy, which is usually diagnosed by the exclusion of other arthritides, the finding of a raised ESR and leukocytosis, and the demonstration of causal micro-organisms or antibodies to them.

Treatment may include antibiotics for up to 3 months to eliminate the triggering of bacterial infection. Anti-inflammatory analgesics help control the acute phase. Corticosteroid injections are used if NSAIDs are unsuccessful. Other immunosuppressives, TNF inhibitors, sulfasalazine, methotrexate, etanercept or infliximab, may be effective if other treatments fail.

Dental aspects

The most characteristic lesion is a pattern of painless scalloped white lines surrounding reddish areas and closely resembling one variant of migratory glossitis (geographic tongue), but affecting any part of the mouth.

Oral ulcers or other lesions may be frequent but are transient and often unnoticed.

Infective arthritides

Infective (pyogenic) arthritides are rare but may follow penetrating wounds, extension from adjacent septic areas or by bloodstream spread. Possible causal agents include *Neisseria gonorrhoeae*, *Haemophilus influenzae*, *Staphylococcus aureus*, *Mycobacterium tuberculosis*, *Salmonella* or *Borrelia* (Lyme disease). Oral micro-organisms are only rarely implicated.

Pain, limitation of movement, swelling and erythema may be evident (Fig. 16.16). Ankylosis can be a complication.

Infective arthritides are an emergency; joint fluid should be sent for microbiological examination and culture, and antibiotics given. Empirical treatment, given until the causal agent is known, is flucloxacillin intravenously plus fusidic acid or, in penicillin-allergic patients, clindamycin. Gentamicin is added if the patient is immunocompromised.

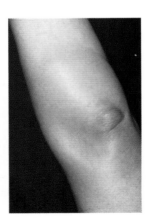

Fig. 16.16 Infective arthritis

Lyme disease

General aspects

Lyme disease is caused by the spirochaete *Borrelia burgdorferi* transmitted mainly by insects (*Ixodes* ticks from deer mainly). It is considerably more common in the USA (first described in Lyme, Connecticut) than in other countries, but cases are seen in most parts of the world and it is spreading in most areas, possibly as global warming increases the range of habitats of the vectors.

The risk of Lyme disease is mainly to those who live or work in or close to areas surrounded by tick-infested woods or overgrown brush. Lyme disease is not transmitted between humans.

Clinical features

The first sign is usually a red 'bull's-eye' rash (erythema migrans) that spreads outwards from the site of the insect bite. Tiredness, fever, headache, stiff neck and muscle aches are common. Arthritis may develop in the acute phase and be transient, or later persistent, most typically severely affecting the knees. Chronic arthritis can be a late complication. Neurological involvement may result in facial palsy. Cardiac disease, such as atrioventricular block, myopericarditis or cardiomegaly, is uncommon.

General management

Antibiotic treatment for 3–4 weeks with doxycycline or amoxicillin is generally effective in early disease. Cefuroxime axetil or erythromycin can be used for persons allergic to penicillin or who cannot take tetracyclines.

Early treatment does not necessarily prevent development of chronic arthritis.

Dental aspects

Facial palsy and lymphadenitis may be seen. TMJ involvement is rare even in endemic areas.

MUSCLE

Muscle cells are embedded in a basal lamina of collagen and large glycoproteins. In between are satellite cells important in the growth and repair of the fibre. Muscle fibres contain specialized structures for excitation–contraction coupling to ensure that a contractile stimulus (received at the synapse) is quickly and evenly communicated to the whole fibre. Force production occurs in the *myofibrils*, which are chains of sarcomeres running from one end of the fibre to the other. Contractile forces are closely linked to the myosin heavy chain isoform expressed by the fibre responsible for force generation. Myosin is a protein composed of a globular head with adenosine triphosphate (ATP) and actin binding sites, and a long tail involved in its polymerization into myosin filaments. Actin is the other major protein in force production. Troponin is the major regulator of force production. Titin maintains the neatly ordered striation pattern of skeletal (striped) muscles by anchoring myosin to actin. Nebulin acts as a molecular ruler – regulating the length of actin filaments.

Adenosine triphosphate is the immediate source of energy for muscle contraction. Energy for contraction comes from the metabolism of fatty acids and sugars. Fatty acids are the major source of energy during normal activities and derived from fats broken down to acetyl coenzyme A, which is then oxidized by the same citric acid cycle involved in the metabolism of glucose. Blood glucose diffuses into the muscle cytoplasm and is locked there by phosphorylation. A glucose molecule is then rearranged slightly to fructose and phosphorylated again to fructose diphosphate. Glucose is metabolized anaerobically in the cytoplasm but this is only moderately efficient. Aerobic metabolism is more efficient, but requires oxygen and takes place in the mitochondria. Creatine phosphate is one of the other important energy stores, a source for high-energy phosphate groups with which to replenish *ATP*, particularly in fast-twitch glycolytic fibres.

Anabolic steroids work by increasing synthesis of muscle proteins.

MUSCLE DISEASES

Weakness that affects muscles of the upper arms and legs more than the hands and feet may indicate a disorder that affects all muscles (myopathy). Myopathies tend to affect the largest muscles first: the person may have difficulty combing hair or climbing stairs.

When the hand and feet are weaker than the upper arms and legs, the problem is often a polyneuropathy, which tends to affect the longest nerves first (those in the hands and feet). The affected person may thus have the most trouble with fine finger movements. Strength that decreases with repetitive activity suggests myasthenia gravis.

When weakness is limited to one side of the body, a stroke may be responsible (Ch. 13). Weakness that affects the body below a certain level may be caused by a spinal cord disorder (Ch. 13).

Muscle diseases (myopathies) are uncommon and rarely cause oral manifestations or affect dental management. The genetic myopathies, which comprise the muscular dystrophies and the myotonic disorders, have the most significance. Acquired myopathies are rare but significant; metabolic myopathies are tabulated in Appendix 16.1.

GENETIC MYOPATHIES

Muscular dystrophies

General and clinical aspects

Muscular dystrophies, the main crippling diseases of childhood, are a group of uncommon genetically determined diseases characterized by degeneration of muscle leading to progressive weakness (Table 16.11).

Duchenne muscular dystrophy – a recessive sex-linked disorder that results from lack of a specific muscle protein, dystrophin – is the most common. Complications include loss of ability to walk, deterioration of lung and cardiac function and, often, early death. The pelvic girdle is affected first and the disease appears as the infant begins to walk with a waddling gait and severe lumbar lordosis. The child has difficulty in standing and, after lying down, typically has to climb up his legs in order to stand (Gower's sign). The shoulder girdle is also weak, and winging of the scapulae is characteristic. Weakness spreads to all other muscles but tends to spare those of the head, neck and hands.

The affected muscles enlarge (pseudohypertrophy) but the child is crippled and, before puberty, becomes confined to a wheelchair. Cardiac disease (cardiomyopathy), respiratory impairment and intellectual deterioration appear at an early stage, and patients usually die in their twenties.

Dental aspects

Cardiomyopathies and respiratory disease are contraindications to general anaesthesia. Muscular dystrophy may also predispose to malignant hyperthermia.

In those muscular dystrophies where there is facial myopathy (classically in the facioscapulohumeral type), there is lack of facial expression and, often, inability to whistle. Malocclusions,

Type	Inheritance	Muscles affected	Pseudo-hypertrophy	Onset	Progress	Other features
Duchenne	X	All	Usual	Early childhood	Rapid	Cardiomyopathy Death in early adulthood
Becker	X	All	Usual	Late childhood	Variable	More benign than Duchenne type
Childhood	AR	All	Usual	Late childhood	Variable	More benign than Duchenne type
Limb girdle	AR	Pelvic and shoulder girdles	Occasional	Adolescence	Variable	Severely disabling May be cardiomyopathy
Facioscapulohumeral	AD	Starts in face and shoulder	Rare	Adolescence	Slow	Most benign type Normal life expectancy Pouting of lips with facial weakness
Scapuloperoneal	AD or X	Scapular Peroneal All	Occasional	Adolescence	Slow	Cardiac conduction defects Relatively benign
Congenital muscular	AR	All	Rare	Birth	Variable	Possible joint deformities
Distal myopathy	AD	Distal	Rare	Any age	Slow	–
Oculopharyngeal	AD	Facial and sternomastoid	Rare	Adult	Slow	Dysphagia may be prominent Weakness of masticatory muscles and tongue

Table 16.11 Muscular dystrophies

AD, autosomal dominant; AR, autosomal recessive; X, X-linked.

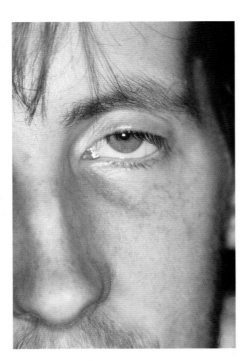

Fig. 16.17 Ptosis in dystrophia myotonica

especially expansion of the arches, may be seen, but there is no abnormal susceptibility to dental disease.

Myotonic disorders

Myotonic disorders are characterized by abnormally slow relaxation after muscle contraction. *Dystrophia myotonica* – the most disabling form – can lead to ptosis (Fig. 16.17), progressive facial weakness, cataracts, testicular atrophy and frontal baldness. The onset is typically in the third decade. Other complications include cardiac conduction defects, respiratory impairment, mild endocrinopathies, intellectual deterioration and personality changes.

Myotonia congenita (Becker type) appears late in childhood and is characterized by muscle hypertrophy. Myotonia congenita (Thomsen disease), a generalized myotonia without weakness, starts in infancy.

Paramyotonia congenita causes myotonia and weakness after exposure to cold.

Dental aspects

General anaesthesia may be a risk because of cardiac conduction defects, suxamethonium sensitivity, respiratory impairment, behavioural problems or malignant hyperthermia (Ch. 23).

Patients may have dental management problems resulting from treatment with corticosteroids or phenytoin. In dystrophia myotonica, there is atrophy of the temporalis, masseter and sternomastoid muscles (producing a swan-neck appearance), and sometimes distal limb weakness and wasting. Myotonia in the tongue causes difficulty in speaking (dysarthria) and there may also be difficulty in masticating food.

Atrophy of the masticatory muscles leads to an open mouth posture. There may also be dysphagia, dysarthria and dental caries.

ACQUIRED MYOPATHIES

Polymyalgia rheumatica

General aspects

Polymyalgia rheumatica is an uncommon disorder characterized by muscle pain and stiffness, which is sometimes accompanied by cranial arteritis (see later). Women are predominantly affected, usually after the age of 55.

Clinical features

There is pain, stiffness and weakness across the shoulders, in the upper arms and in the pelvic region radiating into the thighs.

General management

There is no non-invasive diagnostic test but the ESR is typically raised and electromyography (EMG) normal. Biopsy may be helpful. Small doses of corticosteroids usually give rapid relief.

In most cases the disease is ultimately self-limiting though it frequently persists for 1–2 years or longer.

Dental aspects

Local anaesthesia is safe. Conscious sedation can be given if required. Corticosteroid treatment may be associated with its usual problems (Ch. 6).

Orofacial manifestations are present if cranial arteritis is associated.

Myasthenia gravis

General aspects

Myasthenia gravis (MG) is a chronic autoimmune disorder that causes weakness and rapid fatigue of voluntary muscles, and usually affects women between 20 and 30. Circulating autoantibodies to the nicotinic acetylcholine (ACh) receptor proteins on the post-synaptic membrane of the neuromuscular junction can be detected in at least 85% and these damage the receptor so that the response of the muscle to ACh is weak. These autoantibodies are associated in 75% of cases with thymic hyperplasia and, in the remainder, a thymoma.

Occasional cases of MG are associated with carcinoma (Eaton–Lambert syndrome), drugs (penicillamine can also result in anti-ACh receptor antibodies) or other diseases.

Clinical features

Typically the extraocular muscles and the muscles of face, tongue, neck and extremities are severely affected. Ptosis and diplopia are common early features. Disability is worsened by fatigue of the muscles, particularly towards the end of the day,

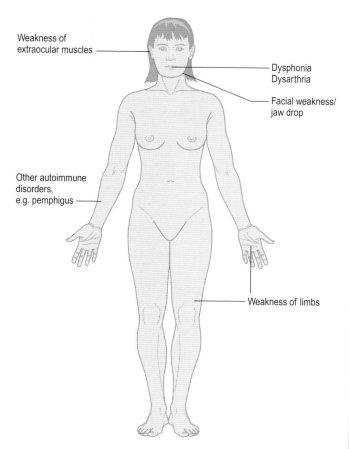

but improves with rest. Other factors that can make MG worse include illnesses such as a cold, stress and overexertion.

Myasthenia gravis can cause difficulties with speech, chewing and swallowing, as well as weakness of limbs. Speech may have a nasal quality. Difficulties in swallowing with nasal regurgitation of food and drink may also develop (Fig. 16.18).

A potentially fatal complication of MG is involvement of the respiratory muscles, particularly in the elderly, and respiratory insufficiency may result from either the disease itself (myasthenic crisis) or treatment (cholinergic crisis).

Thymic disease is common and can also depress immunological responses. There is an uncommon syndrome of thymoma, myasthenia gravis, depressed cell-mediated immunity, chronic mucocutaneous candidosis and haematological disease (Good syndrome; Ch. **20**).

General management

The diagnosis is made from the clinical features and an edrophonium (anticholinesterase) test, sometimes supported by electrodiagnostic tests and detection of serum antibodies to ACh receptors.

Thymic disease should be excluded by mediastinal computed tomography (CT) or magnetic resonance imaging (MRI), and autoimmune disorders should be sought.

Myasthenia gravis very occasionally remits spontaneously but in those with thymoma the prognosis is poor. Treatment may include cholinesterase inhibitors (neostigmine, pyridostigmine),

which improve muscle contraction and muscle strength. Corticosteroids, preferably in combination with azathioprine or ciclosporin, are also effective. Thymectomy brings great relief to more than 50% of patients with severe MG. However, the effect is often delayed for many years and the response is more dramatic in younger people. Plasmapheresis can remedy life-threatening stages of the disease.

Dental aspects

Dental treatment is best carried out during a remission, best early in the day, within 1–2 h of routine medication with anticholinesterases, and with short appointments, since weakness increases during the day and fatigue or emotional stress may precipitate a myasthenic crisis.

Local anaesthesia is preferred but minimal doses should be given. Lidocaine, prilocaine or mepivacaine can safely be used. A small oral dose of a benzodiazepine may be given if the patient is anxious, but intravenous sedation must not be given in the dental surgery since bulbar or respiratory involvement impairs respiration.

Many drugs used in GA, such as opioids, barbiturates, suxamethonium, curare or anaesthetic agents, are potentiated by or aggravate the myasthenic state. Post-operative respiratory infection can result and may also cause myasthenia to worsen. Lithium can impair synaptic transmission, and drugs such as aminoglycosides, beta-blockers, phenytoin and others can also worsen myasthenia. Other drugs that may increase weakness and should be avoided include tetracyclines, clindamycin, lincomycin, quinolones, sulfonamides and aminoglycosides. Penicillin or erythromycin can safely be used. Occasionally, aspirin has caused a cholinergic crisis in those on anticholinesterases; acetaminophen and codeine do not have this potential disadvantage.

Corticosteroids, other immunosuppressants or emotional lability may also complicate dental treatment.

Facial weakness causes a snarling appearance as the patient attempts to smile. Weakness of the masticatory muscles causing the mouth to hang open (hanging or lantern jaw sign) is characteristic and patients typically tend to support the jaw with their hand. Occasionally there is also furrowing, atrophy or paresis of the tongue or uvula palsy. Occasionally, Sjögren syndrome or other autoimmune disorders, particularly pemphigus, may be associated. If there is a thymoma there may be chronic candidosis.

Salivation is increased if an anticholinesterase is being taken.

Myositis ossificans

Myositis ossificans is a rare condition in which there is ossification in muscles (muscles turn to bone). Two types are recognized.

Myositis ossificans is an autosomal dominant genetic disorder with overexpression of bone morphogenetic protein 4 (BMP4) mapped to chromosome 14. The most common sites affected are the sternomastoid, paraspinal, masticatory, and shoulder and pelvic girdle muscles. The abdominal muscles, extraocular muscles and gastrintestinal tract and tongue muscles are spared. Electrocardiogram (ECG) findings may be abnormal, while spirometry may demonstrate a restrictive pattern.

Myositis ossificans circumscripta develops in response to soft tissue injury (blunt trauma, stab wound, fracture/dislocation or surgical incision) or without known injury. Non-documented trauma, repeated small mechanical injuries and non-mechanical injuries caused by ischaemia or inflammation may also be implicated.

Most ossifications (80%) arise in the thigh or arm but intercostals, erector spinae, pectoralis and gluteal muscles may be affected.

General management

In both types, the diagnosis is made by serial radiography. There is no definitive treatment: immediate immobilization of the patient with a regime of gradually increased exercise should be arranged. Analgesics, cortisone and adrenocorticotropin may be indicated. Genetic counselling is indicated.

USEFUL WEBSITES

http://www.nlm.nih.gov/medlineplus/encyclopedia.html
http://www.arthritis.org/conditions/DiseaseCenter/ra.asp
http://www.niams.nih.gov/Health_Info/Bone/

FURTHER READING

Abel, M.D., Carrasco, L.R., 2006. Ehlers–Danlos syndrome: classifications, oral manifestations, and dental considerations. Oral Surg Oral Med Oral Pathol Oral Radiol Endod 102, 582–590.

Bagan, J.V., Murillo, J., Jimenez, Y., et al., 2005. Avascular jaw osteonecrosis in association with cancer chemotherapy: series of 10 cases. J Oral Med Pathol 34, 120–123.

Bagan, J.V., Jimenez, Y., Murillo, J., et al., 2006. Jaw osteonecrosis associated with bisphosphonates: multiple exposed areas and its relationship to teeth extractions. Study of 20 cases. Oral Oncol 42, 327–329.

Bagan, J., Jiménez, Y., Gómez, D., Sirera, R., Poveda, R., Scully, C., 2008. Collagen telopeptide (serum CTX) and its relationship with the size and number of lesions in osteonecrosis of the jaws in cancer patients on intravenous bisphosphonates. Oral Oncol 44, 1088–1089.

Baltali, E., Zhao, K.D., Koff, M.F., Durmus, E., An, K.N., Keller, E.E., 2008. A method for quantifying condylar motion in patients with osteoarthritis using an electromagnetic tracking device and computed tomography imaging. J Oral Maxillofac Surg 66, 848–857.

Baltali, E., Zhao, K.D., Koff, M.F., Durmus, E., An, K.N., Keller, E.E., 2008. Kinematic assessment of the temporomandibular joint before and after partial metal fossa eminence replacement surgery: a prospective study. J Oral Maxillofac Surg 66, 1383–1389.

Cagla Ozbakis Akkurt, B., Guler, H., Inanoglu, K., Dicle Turhanoglu, A., Turhanoglu, S., Asfuroglu, Z., 2008. Disease activity in rheumatoid arthritis as a predictor of difficult intubation?. Eur J Anaesthesiol 19, 1–5.

Cascone, P., Ungari, C., Paparo, F., Marianetti, T.M., Ramieri, V., Fatone, M., 2008. A new surgical approach for the treatment of chronic recurrent temporomandibular joint dislocation. J Craniofac Surg 19, 510–512.

De Paepe, A., Malfait, F., 2004. Bleeding and bruising in patients with Ehlers–Danlos syndrome and other collagen vascular disorders. Br J Haematol 127, 491–500.

Eppley, B.L., Pietrzak, W.S., Blanton, M.W., 2005. Allograft and alloplastic bone substitutes: a review of science and technology for the craniomaxillofacial surgeon. J Craniofac Surg 16, 981–989.

Expert panel recommendations, 2006. Dental management of patients receiving oral bisphosphonate therapy. Am Dent Assoc 137, 1144–1150.

Kao, S.T., Scott, D.D., 2007. A review of bone substitutes. Oral Maxillofac Surg Clin North Am 19, 513–521 vi.

Karrer, S., Landthaler, M., Schmalz, G., 2000. Ehlers–Danlos type VIII. Review of the literature. Clin Oral Investig 4, 66–69.

Kent, J.N., Carlton, D.M., Zide, M.F., 1986. Rheumatoid disease and related arthropathies. II. Surgical rehabilitation of the temporomandibular joint. Oral Surg Oral Med Oral Pathol 61, 423–439.

Khosla, S., Burr, D., Cauley, J., et al., 2007. Bisphosphonate-associated osteonecrosis of the jaw: report of a task force of the American Society for Bone and Mineral Research. J Bone Miner Res 22, 1479–1491.

Malfait, F., De Coster, P., Hausser, I., et al., 2004. The natural history, including orofacial features of three patients with Ehlers–Danlos syndrome, dermatosparaxis type (EDS type VIIC). Am J Med Genet A 131, 18–28.

Marx, R.E., 2006. Oral and intravenous bisphosphonate-induced osteonecrosis of the jaws; history, etiology, prevention and treatment. Quintessence Publishing, Illinois.

Meyle, J., Gonzáles, J.R., 2000. Influences of systemic diseases on periodontitis in children and adolescents. Periodontol 2001 (26), 92–112.

National Institute for Health and Clinical Excellence (NICE), 2005. Bisphosphonates (alendronate, etidronate, risedronate), selective oestrogen receptor modulators (raloxifene) and parathyroid hormone (teriparatide) for the secondary prevention of osteoporotic fractures in postmenopausal women. Technology appraisal guidance 87. NICE, London.

Ozcan, I., Ozcan, K.M., Keskin, D., Bahar, S., Boyacigil, S., Dere, H., 2008. Temporomandibular joint involvement in rheumatoid arthritis: correlation of clinical, laboratory and magnetic resonance imaging findings. B-ENT 4, 19–24.

Scully C, Chaudhry S, 2008 Aspects of Human Disease 28. Osteoarthritis Dental Update 35, 709.

Scully C, Chaudhry S, 2009 Aspects of Human Disease 29. Rheumatoid arthritis Dental Update 36, 61.

Scully, C., Diz Dios, P., Kumar, N., 2007. Special care in dentistry: handbook of oral healthcare. Churchill Livingstone Elsevier, Edinburgh.

Scully, C., Madrid, C., Bagan, J., 2006. Dental endosseous implants in patients on bisphosphonate therapy. Implant Dent 15, 212–218.

Shirota, Y., Illei, G.G., Nikolov, N.P., 2008. Biologic treatments for systemic rheumatic diseases. Oral Dis 14, 206–216.

Straub, A.M., Grahame, R., Scully, C., Tonetti, M.S., 2002. Severe periodontitis in Marfan's syndrome: a case report. J Periodontol 73 (7), 823–826.

Thyne, G.M., Ferguson, J.W., 1991. Antibiotic prophylaxis during dental treatment in patients with prosthetic joints. J Bone Joint Surg 73B, 191–194.

Van Sickels, J.E., 2007. Distraction osteogenesis: advancements in the last 10 years. Oral Maxillofac Surg Clin North Am 19, 565–574 vii.

Von Wowern, N., 2001. General and oral aspects of osteoporosis; a review. Clin Oral Invest 5, 71–82.

Appendix 16.1 Metabolic myopathies

Endocrine
- Acromegaly
- Hyperthyroidism
- Hypothyroidism
- Cushing syndrome and steroid therapy
- Hyperaldosteronism
- Diabetes mellitus

Bone disease
- Hyperparathyroidism
- Osteomalacia
- Chronic renal failure

Drugs
- Alcohol
- Diuretics
- Carbenoxolone
- Vincristine
- Cimetidine
- Tryptophan

Malignant hyperthermia

Neuromuscular disorders
- Peroneal muscular atrophy (Charcot–Marie–Tooth disease)
- Hypertrophic polyneuritis (Dejerine–Sottas disease)
- Glycogen storage diseases

Mitochondrial myopathies

Appendix 16.2 Some genetically determined skeletal disorders

Achondroplasia	See Ch. 37
Albers–Schönberg syndrome	See Ch. 37
Albright syndrome	See Ch. 37
Apert syndrome	Craniostenosis; syndactyly
Cheney syndrome	Osteoporosis; early loss of teeth
Cherubism	Familial symmetrical self-limiting soft-tissue jaw lesions
Cleidocranial dysplasia	See Ch. 16
Congenital hyperphosphatasia	Thickened calvarium; early loss of teeth; visual or hearing defects; blue sclerae
Crouzon syndrome	Hypoplastic mid-face; proptosis; craniostenosis; hearing defects
Ellis–van Creveld syndrome	Atrial septal defect; dwarfism; polydactyly
Gardner syndrome	See Ch. 37
Gaucher disease	See Ch. 37
Goldenhar syndrome	Same as Treacher Collins syndrome plus epibulbar dermoids
Gorlin syndrome	See Ch. 37
Hallermann–Streiff syndrome	Cataracts; mandibular retrognathism; scanty hair
Holt–Oram syndrome	Abnormalities of thumb, wrist and clavicle; atrial septal defect
Hypophosphataemia	Vitamin D-resistant rickets; dentinal anomalies leading to early pulp involvement in caries
Klippel–Feil deformity	See Ch. 37
Maffuci syndrome	See Ch. 37
Mucopolysaccharidoses	See Ch. 23
Noonan syndrome	See Ch. 37
Odontomatosis	Multiple odontomas; cirrhosis; oesophageal stenosis
Ollier disease	Multiple enchondromas
Orofacial digital syndromes	Facial anomalies; fraenal hyperplasia; tongue hamartomas; digital anomalies
Osteogenesis imperfecta	See Ch. 16
Pierre Robin syndrome	Micrognathia; cleft palate; glossoptosis
Rubinstein–Taybi syndrome	Broad thumbs and toes; maxillary hypoplasia; patent ductus arteriosus
TAR syndrome	Thrombocytopenia, absent radius; atrial septal defect or tetralogy of Fallot
Treacher–Collins syndrome	Hypoplastic malars and mandible; palpebral fissures slope down and out; colobomas; hearing defects
van Buchem syndrome	Generalized cortical hyperostosis; facial palsy; optic atrophy; hearing defects

SECTION C

OTHER SYSTEMS MEDICINE

Autoimmune disease 425
Immunity, inflammatory disorders, immunosuppressive and
anti-inflammatory agents 439
Immunodeficiencies 451
Infections and infestations 475
Malignant disease 517
Metabolic disorders 539
Trauma and burns 552

GENERAL ASPECTS OF ALLERGIES

Allergy is an abnormal immune response (usually a type I or type IV hypersensitivity response) to an antigen – a protein or allergen. Many allergies have a hereditary component but the prevalence of allergies appears to be increasing. People who suffer allergies to one type of substance are more likely to suffer allergies to others.

Hypersensitivity responses are summarized in Table 17.1 and common allergens are shown in Table 17.2.

Table 17.1   Hypersensitivity reactions

Type	Alternative nomenclature	Mechanisms	Examples
I	Immediate (anaphylactic)	IgE-mediated via mast cell degranulation	Atopic disorders Anaphylaxis
II	Cytotoxic	Antibody against membrane-bound surface antigens	Pemphigus Idiopathic thrombo-cytopenic purpura Blood transfusion reactions
III	Immune complex	Immune complexes deposited in tissues	Systemic lupus erythematosus Rheumatoid arthritis
IV	Cell mediated	T-lymphocyte mediated	Contact allergies Graft rejection

IgE, immunoglobulin E.

Common allergens are pollen, dust mites, mould, pet dander, milk and egg proteins but, in many cases, the allergen cannot be reliably identified. The most common types of allergic type I hypersensitivity reactions include allergic rhinitis (hay fever), some asthma, eczema and urticaria – so-called 'atopic reactions' which affect about 10% of the population, have a strong genetic basis (and family history) and are related to antibody of immunoglobulin E class. The first time an allergy-prone person is exposed to the allergen, T helper (Th2) lymphocytes produce interleukin-4 (IL-4) and interact with B cells, stimulating them to produce large amounts of immunoglobulin E (IgE) antibody. This attaches to receptors on basophils (in the circulation) and mast cells (in the lungs, skin, tongue and linings

Table 17.2   Common allergens

Source of allergen	Hypersensitivity	Examples
Food products	I	Milk, nuts, egg, shellfish
Drugs	I, III	Aspirin, penicillins, sulfonamides
Environmental	I, IV	Animal hair, dust mite, pollen
Latex	IV, I (rare)	Condoms, dressings, elastic bands, gloves
Dental materials	IV	Amalgam alloy, gold, mercury, resin-based materials

of the nose and intestinal tract; Fig. 17.1). When the specific allergen is again encountered, the IgE antibody–antigen reaction on basophils and/or mast cells signals them to synthesize chemical mediators (prostaglandins and leukotrienes) and to release others (histamine and heparin, as well as substances that activate platelets and later on attract eosinophils and neutrophils). This produces a rapid type I hypersensitivity response within minutes, which may be anaphylactic and cause bronchospasm and hypotension (Fig. 17.2).

Type IV (delayed) hypersensitivity, seen mainly in contact allergies, arises more slowly and less dramatically, often more than 24 h after exposure to the allergen and is mediated by sensitized T lymphocytes, which release cytokines that attract macrophages to the site of exposure. Table 17.3 shows common contact allergens.

Type IV reactions also appear to be involved in the pathogenesis of some chronic diseases that result in granulomas (e.g. tuberculosis, leprosy, sarcoidosis, orofacial granulomatosis and Crohn disease) characterized by foci of chronic inflammatory cells, especially macrophages, that may fuse to produce giant cells, which arise in response to certain antigens (sometimes of an unidentified nature; Box 17.1).

Why allergies appear to be increasing is unclear, but alterations in exposure to micro-organisms may be an explanation. Children who live in crowded households, or who attend day care, have fewer allergies, a fact that has been attributed to microbial exposure somehow protecting against allergies. Exposure to bacterial endotoxins reduces release of inflammatory cytokines such as tumour necrosis factor alpha (TNF-alpha), interferon gamma (IFN-gamma), IL-10 and IL-12. Toll-like receptors, which respond to micro-organisms, may also be involved.

CLINICAL FEATURES OF ALLERGIES

Clinical manifestations of an allergic reaction are dependent upon the nature of the response, the antigenic challenge and the individual's allergic predisposition. Early symptoms

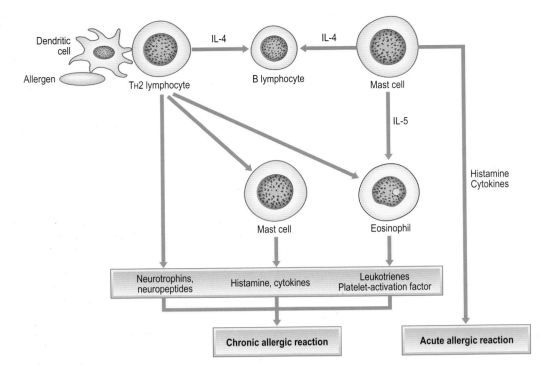

Fig. 17.1 Immunopathogenesis of allergic reactions

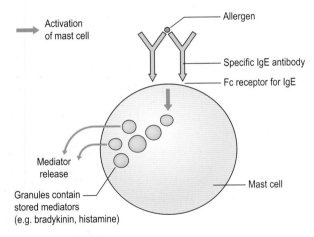

Fig. 17.2 Mast cell involvement in allergies

Box 17.1 Granulomatous disorders

Infections

- Tuberculosis and non-tuberculous mycobacteria
- Leprosy
- Syphilis
- Deep mycoses
- Cat-scratch disease
- Toxoplasmosis

Foreign body reactions

- To zirconium, beryllium, silicone or others

Disorders of uncertain aetiology

- Crohn disease
- Orofacial granulomatosis, cheilitis granulomatosa and Melkersson–Rosenthal syndrome
- Sarcoidosis
- Wegener granulomatosis

Some malignant diseases

and signs of a type I (immediate) hypersensitivity reaction include wheezing, breathlessness, sneezing, runny eyes, itching and urticaria, which typically occur within a few minutes to an hour. As the reaction progresses, bronchospasm, acute hypotension and angioedema of the face and laryngopharynx may result in life-threatening anaphylactic shock (Table 17.4).

Contact allergy (type IV delayed hypersensitivity), being a T cell-mediated process, is characterized by local inflammation at the allergen contact site (skin or mucous membrane), is usually slower and less profound. Metals, disinfectants, rubber, detergents and bonding agents can cause allergic contact (and irritant contact) dermatitis. Rashes are seen in many allergies (Fig 17.3)

GENERAL MANAGEMENT OF ALLERGIES

Physical factors (thermal stimuli, sunlight, water, pressure) and drugs may also release histamine in susceptible individuals and cause features similar to allergies. For example, morphine can directly trigger mast cell histamine release and occasionally causes anaphylactoid reactions.

Diagnosis of an allergy is based on clinical history and presentation, including a family history of allergy; skinprick or patch testing to identify contact allergens using a battery of test allergens (*European Standard Contact Dermatitis Testing Series*; Table 17.5); or an elimination diet to identify food allergens. Patch testing is usually carried out with Finn chambers

Table 17.3 Common contact allergens

Allergens	Sources
Balsam of Peru	Cosmetics, perfumes
Chromate	Bleaches, cement, dental alloys, leather, matches, tattoos
Cobalt	Dental alloys, dental and other prostheses, jewellery, polish stripper
Colophony	Polish, solder flux, sticking plaster, varnishes
Epoxy resins	Glues, resins, PVC products, surface coatings
Ethylenediamine	Antifreeze, creams, paints, rubber
Formaldehyde	Clothing, cosmetics, deodorant, newsprint, shampoo
Mercaptobenzothiazole	Catheters, glues, rubber boots and gloves
Nickel	Clothing clasps, coins, dental alloys, ear rings, jewellery, spectacles
Parabens	Cosmetics, skin creams
Paraphenylenediamine	Clothing colour, hair dyes, henna, rubber
Plant allergens	Blister bush (*Diplolophium buchananii*), dahlia, garlic, onion, poison ivy, primula, sesquiterpene lactones (artichoke, boneset, burdock, chamomile, chrysanthemum, cockle-bur, gailladrin, lettuce, marsh elder, mugwort, parthenium, poverty weed, pyrethrum, ragweed, sagebrush, sneezeweed, spinach, sunflower, wormwood), tulip bulbs
Plant phototoxins	Celery, fennel, orange, parsley, parsnip
Thiurams	Clothing dyes, fungicides, hair dye, rubber, stockings
Topical medications	Antihistamines (antazoline), benzocaine, chloramphenicol, neomycin, quinoline
Wool alcohols	Cosmetics, skin creams, emollients, lanolin

Table 17.4 Common features of allergy

Affected organ	Features
Nose	Sneezing, congested or runny nose and rhinorrhoea (allergic rhinitis)
Sinuses	Post-nasal drip and pain (allergic sinusitis)
Airways	Coughing, wheezing and dyspnoea, sometimes asthma or angioedema
Eyes	Red, itchy, runny eyes (allergic conjunctivitis)
Ears	Discomfort and impaired hearing, due to blocked Eustachian tube
Skin	Eczema and hives (urticaria)
Gastrointestinal	Abdominal pain, bloating, vomiting, diarrhoea

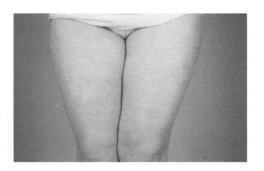

Fig. 17.3 Rash from penicillin allergy

Table 17.5 The European Standard Contact Dermatitis Testing Series: some allergens and their sources

Allergen	Source
Benzocaine	Benzocaine (local anaesthetic)
Cl + Me-isothiazolinone (Kathon CG, 100 ppm)	Isothiazolinone (preservative)
Clioquinol (Chinoform and Vioform)	Clioquinol (antibacterial)
Colophonium	Rosin and colophony (adhesive)
Cobalt chloride	Cobalt (metal)
Epoxy resin	Epoxy resin (adhesive)
Formaldehyde	Formaldehyde and formalin (in clothing, cosmetics, household products)
Fragrance mix	Fragrance and perfume
Lanolin alcohol	Wool fat
Mercaptobenzothiazole	Rubber
Mercapto mix	Rubber
Methyldibromo-glutaronitrile	Preservative
Myroxylon pereirae resin	Balsam of Peru (fragrance)
Neomycin sulfate	Neomycin (topical antibiotic)
Nickel sulfate	Nickel (metal, coins, jewellery)
N-isopropyl-N-phenyl-4-phenylenediamine	Rubber
Parabens mix	Parabens (preservative)
4-Phenylenediamine base	Hair dye
Potassium dichromate	Chrome (cement, shoes, metal)
Primin	*Primula obconica* (plant)
Quaternium-15 (Dowicil 200)	Quaternium-15 (preservative)
Sesquiterpene lactone mix	Plant dermatitis (daisies)
4-tert-butylphenol formaldehyde resin	Para-tertiary butylphenol formaldehyde resin (adhesive)
Thiuram mix	Rubber
Budesonide	Topical corticosteroid
Tixocortol pivalate	Topical corticosteroid

on Scanpor, a non-woven adhesive skin-friendly tape that contains no colophony. Assays of serum IgE levels (PRIST: **p**aper **r**adio-**i**mmuno**s**orbent **t**est) and serum specific IgE antibodies (RAST: **r**adio**a**llergo**s**orbent **t**est) can help. In the RAST, purified extracts of a range of allergens are coupled to cellulose or paper discs to which the patient's serum is applied. Its ability to react with one or more of these allergens is tested by adding rabbit anti-IgE labelled with radioactive iodine. The level of radioactivity then indicates the levels of specific IgE antibodies.

The *British standard series* of 12 allergens, used in addition to those already in the European standard series, includes methyl dibromoglutaronitrile, carba mix, ethylenediamine, cetearyl alcohol, 2-bromo-2-nitropane-1,3-diol, diazolidinyl urea, chlorocresol, fusidic acid, imidazolidinyl urea and chloroxylenol.

The *Dental series* typically includes amalgam, amalgam alloying metals, ammoniated mercury, ammonium tetrachloroplatinate, benzoyl peroxide, bisphenol A (Bis-GMA), diurethane dimethacrylate, ethylene glycol dimethacrylate, eugenol, 2-hydroxyethyl methacrylate (2-HEMA), hydroquinone, menthol, methyl methacrylate, palladium chloride peppermint oil, potassium dicyanoaurate, *N,N*-dimethyl-*p*-toluidine, sodium thiosulfatoaurate, and triethylene glycol dimethacrylate.

No tests, however, can *reliably* predict the possibility of allergic or anaphylactic reactions. Many cases of 'local anaesthesia (LA) allergy' represent untoward events such as the unintended intravenous injection of the drug, while many cases of 'food allergy' are of food intolerance or occasionally food poisoning only. Supposed phenomena such as systemic 'allergy' to amalgam restorations, 'candida syndrome' and 'total allergy syndrome' are myths.

Medications such as antihistamines or antidepressants that interfere with allergy tests must be stopped from 2 days to 6 weeks or more before testing. Resuscitation facilities must be available during allergy testing, since anaphylactic reactions can occasionally follow intradermal skin test doses, particularly of penicillin. The test procedure includes a positive control (usually histamine), a negative control – a solution without allergens, and then the test – the various suspect allergens. If the test substance provokes an allergic reaction, a raised, red, itchy wheal may develop within about 20 min and, in general, the larger the reaction, the more sensitive is the patient. A negative skin test means that the patient is not allergic to that particular allergen. A complication of skin testing is that it can induce sensitivity to the test compound.

To avoid future allergic reactions, known allergens should be avoided, which is easier said than done, since sensitive individuals may react to minute traces and allergens can be present in the most unexpected places (more likely in commercially prepared foods and drinks than in natural products).

Individuals with a complex history of allergy should be referred to a specialist allergy clinic for careful assessment and management. Treatments include drugs to block allergic mediators, or the activation of cells and degranulation (Table 17.6). These include antihistamines, corticosteroids and cromoglicate. Anti-leukotrienes (leukotriene receptor antagonists; e.g. montelukast or zafirlukast) are also effective. Intravenous injection of monoclonal anti-IgE antibodies (omalizumab), which bind to free and B cell-associated IgE, causes their destruction. Immunotherapy by desensitization or hyposensitization is a treatment in which the patient is gradually vaccinated with progressively larger doses of the responsible allergen for at least a year – but it is potentially hazardous as it can induce anaphylaxis.

Patients who have had serious allergic reactions are also usually advised *always* to carry adrenaline (epinephrine) with them,

Table 17.6 Management of allergies

Allergen	Avoidance	Other measures
Any	Medic-Alert bracelets detailing an individual's allergies	Epinephrine (adrenaline) Patients at risk of anaphylaxis should carry an EpiPen, Anapen or Twinject for immediate self-administration
Drugs	Accurate documentation of drug allergies in medical notes	Anti-leukotrienes (leukotriene receptor antagonists), such as montelukast or zafirlukast
Food products	Systematic elimination diets	Corticosteroids
House dust mite	Mite-proof bed linen and wooden floors	Cromoglicate to prevent mediator release
Pets	Avoid or exclude	Antihistamines to relieve itching and oedema
Pollens	Windows should be kept shut and grassy spaces avoided	Bronchodilators for the management of bronchospasm

for subcutaneous self-administration in the event of a reaction (e.g. EpiPen).

There is no reliable evidence that supports the use of alternative medicine in the control of allergies.

ANAPHYLAXIS
GENERAL ASPECTS

Anaphylaxis is a severe life-threatening type I hypersensitivity reaction, which may affect up to 15% of the population. It is predisposed to by hyper-IgE syndromes and caused mainly by food, drugs, latex and insect stings (Table 17.7).

Table 17.7 Main precipitants of anaphylaxis (see table 17.8)

Foods	Drugs	Latex	Hymenoptera stings
Eggs	Radiocontrast media		Ants
Fish	Chemotherapeutic agents		Bumble bees
Milk	Penicillins		Honey bees
Peanuts	Cephalosporins, tetracyclines,		Hornets
Shellfish	sulfonamides, ciprofloxacin		Wasps
Soy	Vancomycin		
Tree nuts	Asparaginase		
Wheat	Vinca		
	Ciclosporin		
	Methotrexate		
	Fluorouracil		
	NSAIDs, local anaesthetics, intravenous anaesthetics, heparin, vaccines, immune globulins, insulin, opiates		

*a*Mainly iodide containing reactions exacerbated by use of beta-blockers. NSAIDs, non-steroidal anti-inflammatory drugs.

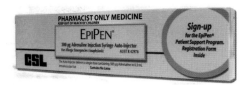

Fig. 17.4 EpiPen

CLINICAL FEATURES

Bronchospasm, acute hypotension and angioedema of the face and laryngopharynx are the critical features, but there may also be flushing, dizziness and urticaria. The condition may progress to arrhythmias or cardiac arrest. The time to onset is usually indicative of the severity of the reaction (i.e. the more rapid the onset, the more severe the reaction). Most reactions occur within seconds to 30 min of exposure to the responsible precipitant.

GENERAL MANAGEMENT

People at risk *must* avoid the allergens responsible, and carry adrenaline for immediate use (Fig. 17.4).

HAY FEVER (ALLERGIC RHINITIS)

GENERAL ASPECTS

There is often a positive family history and the common specific allergens are inhaled and include pollen, mould, dust mites and pet dander. Pollen from trees such as birch, alder, cedar, hazel, hornbeam, horse chestnut, willow, poplar, plane, linden/lime and olive can be responsible: in northern latitudes, birch is the most important. Grasses, especially ryegrass and timothy, may be responsible, as may various weeds.

CLINICAL FEATURES

Features typically include: itchy eyes, nose, roof of mouth or throat; frequent sneezing, nasal congestion and discharge; lacrimation and cough. Nasal polyps often develop. In the northern hemisphere, symptoms are particularly prevalent from late May to the end of June.

GENERAL MANAGEMENT

The best management is to avoid the allergens, if possible, but this can be difficult. Medications include: topical cromoglicate (which inhibits mast cell release of chemicals) as prophylaxis to nose and eyes or lungs; corticosteroids such as beclometasone (which suppress the response but take 3–10 days to provide maximum relief); leukotriene receptor antagonists; or antihistamines (which suppress the symptoms but many cause sedation). Non-sedating preparations include fexofenadine, loratadine and terfenadine.

DENTAL ASPECTS

Patients with allergic rhinitis may be mouth-breathers and develop mild gingival hyperplasia. No oral diseases are known to have any significant direct association with atopic disease, although aphthae and geographic tongue may possibly be more frequent. Antihistamines can cause a dry mouth. Cromoglicate was once used in an attempt to control aphthae. Corticosteroids occasionally induce candidosis.

Azole antifungals, macrolide antibiotics such as erythromycin, human immunodeficiency virus (HIV) protease inhibitors and grapefruit juice can impair metabolism of the antihistamine terfenadine and can lead to arrhythmias (torsade de pointes).

ASTHMA (SEE CH. 15)

ECZEMA (SEE CH. 11)

URTICARIA AND ACUTE ALLERGIC ANGIOEDEMA

GENERAL ASPECTS

Acute urticaria ('nettle rash') and angioedema are potentially dangerous reactions, which can be triggered when mast cells release histamine and other chemicals into the bloodstream, causing increased blood vessel dilatation and permeability. About one in five people will experience one of these at one time or another. The risk of urticaria and angioedema is greater if there is a history of urticaria and angioedema, other allergies or a positive family history of allergies.

Angioedema can be life-threatening if swelling blocks the airway.

Allergens that precipitate acute angioedema and urticaria can be: latex; foods (shellfish, peanuts, eggs and milk); drugs [e.g. penicillin, aspirin, ibuprofen, angiotensin-converting enzyme (ACE) inhibitors, and opioids]; and animal allergens (mainly pollen, animal dander and insect stings). Physical factors that can release histamine in susceptible individuals (heat, cold, sunlight, water, pressure on the skin, emotional stress and exercise) and immune factors (e.g. blood transfusions, immune disorders, such as lupus or cancer, thyroid disorders and infections, such as hepatitis A or B) are occasionally responsible.

CLINICAL FEATURES

Features of urticaria include raised, red, often itchy, skin wheals that appear and disappear most commonly where clothes rub the skin. Features of angioedema include large wheals or swellings, especially near the eyes and lips, but also on hands and feet and inside the throat (Fig. 17.5). Complications can include dyspnoea and anaphylaxis – bronchospasm, and hypotension, sometimes causing loss of consciousness or death.

GENERAL MANAGEMENT

Allergy tests should be made to determine the cause. The standard treatment is with antihistamines such as loratidine. H_2-receptor antagonists such as cimetidine and ranitidine may

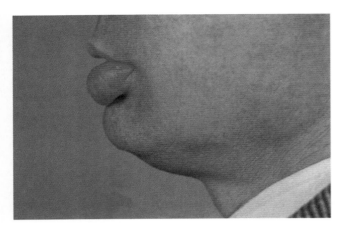

Fig. 17.5 Angioedema

help control symptoms. Occasionally, for severe urticaria, systemic corticosteroids may be indicated.

DENTAL ASPECTS

Angioedema is characterized by rapid development of oedematous swelling, particularly of the head and neck region. It is the only type of allergy that can involve the oral tissues by causing swelling, particularly the lips or the floor of the mouth. When oedema involves the neck and extends to the larynx, it can cause rapidly fatal respiratory obstruction.

There is possibly a greater risk of sensitization or of acute allergic reactions to drugs used in dentistry. Dental materials (such as mercury), which accidentally come into contact with the patient's skin, can very occasionally provoke contact dermatitis, but do *not* affect the oral mucosa.

There are anaesthetic hazards in asthma, and severe asthma or anaphylaxis can occur in the dental surgery (Ch. 15). Problems may be caused by drugs, particularly corticosteroids. Beclometasone dipropionate and betamethasone valerate inhalers can cause oropharyngeal thrush in a minority. Corticosteroids absorbed from ointments used for eczema can cause adrenal suppression. Dry mouth and drowsiness affect patients taking antihistamines.

Although there may be a slightly greater prevalence of allergic diseases associated with aphthous stomatitis, there is little evidence for an allergic mechanism (Ch. 11), though in a very few patients ulceration appears to be precipitated by foods – especially walnuts, chocolate or citrus fruits.

FOOD ALLERGY AND INTOLERANCE

True food allergy, primarily mediated by IgE antibodies to food proteins, is present in 3–4% of adults and the incidence appears to be increasing. There may be a positive family history but the cause is otherwise unclear. There is evidence that breast-feeding for at least 4 months prevents or delays the occurrence of cows' milk allergy as well as childhood atopic dermatitis and wheezing. Symptoms range from mild mouth-itching ('oral allergy syndrome') to anaphylaxis. Peanut and shellfish allergies, in particular, can be dangerous or even fatal. However, many

Table 17.8 Important allergens in food

Food	Main types implicated
Eggs	Hens'
Fish	Cod
Fruit	Apple, cherry, peach and nectarine
Gluten	Wheat, barley, rye
Milk	Cows'
Moulds	
Mustard	
Nuts	Peanuts and tree nuts (e.g. walnuts, brazil nuts, almonds, hazelnut)
Sesame	
Shellfish	Crab, crayfish, lobster, mussels, prawns, shrimp, squid
Soya	
Sulfites	
Vegetables	Carrot, celery, potato

cases of suspected 'food allergy' are actually due to food intolerance or occasionally food poisoning.

GENERAL ASPECTS

Food allergy is an abnormal immune response to a food but is comparatively rare. There may be a positive family history of atopic disease. The most common food allergens are eggs, milk and peanuts in children; shellfish, fish, nuts and eggs in adults (Table 17.8). Gluten intolerance is discussed in Ch. 7.

Food allergens are proteins that usually are not broken down by the heat of cooking or by gastric acid or digestive enzymes and, as a result, they enter the bloodstream, to reach target organs.

Other reactions include allergic eosinophilic reactions present with oesophagitis, gastritis or gastroenteritis; reactions such as food protein-induced enteropathy (e.g. coeliac disease; Ch. 7), proctocolitis or enterocolitis syndrome (FPIES); milk soy protein intolerance (MSPI); and Heiner syndrome – a lung disease resulting from formation of milk protein/IgG antibody immune complexes.

CLINICAL FEATURES OF FOOD ALLERGY

The symptoms may begin as itching in the mouth as the person starts to eat the food responsible, followed by abdominal symptoms (vomiting, diarrhoea or pain). Then, as the food allergens enter the bloodstream, hypotension, urticaria or eczema and bronchospasm can appear.

GENERAL MANAGEMENT

A detailed patient history, diet diary or an elimination diet together with skin tests, PRIST and RAST are needed, but confirmation is by double-blind food challenge. Food allergy is treated by dietary avoidance, which is possible if labels are read carefully and care is taken in choosing restaurant-prepared foods. However, many allergy-inducing foods, such as peanuts, eggs and milk, can appear unsuspected in prepared dishes.

Symptoms can be relieved by antihistamines and bronchodilators, but patients with severe food allergies can react to minute traces of the allergen. Such patients must always avoid the allergen and should wear medical alert bracelets or necklaces stating that they have a food allergy. If subject to severe reactions, they should always carry a syringe of epinephrine to self-administer and be prepared to treat an inadvertent exposure instantly.

ORAL ALLERGY SYNDROME

GENERAL ASPECTS

Oral allergy syndrome is an uncommon variant of the reactions described above, usually preceded by hay fever typically associated with birch-pollen allergies, but it can also affect people with allergies to the pollens of grass, mugwort (more common in Europe) and ragweed (more common in North America; Table 17.9).

Table 17.9 Foods most commonly associated with oral allergy	
Pollen allergy	**Foods which may also trigger an allergic reaction**
Birch	*Fruits:* apple, apricot, cherry, kiwi, nectarine, peach, pear, plum, prune *Nuts:* almond, hazelnut, walnut *Seeds:* sunflower *Vegetables:* anise, beans, caraway, carrot, celery, coriander, cumin, dill, fennel, green pepper, lentils, parsnips, parsley, peas, peanuts, potato, tomato
Grass	*Fruits:* kiwi, melon, orange, tomato, watermelon
Mugwort	*Fruits:* apple, melon, watermelon *Vegetables:* celery, carrot
Ragweed	*Fruits:* banana, cantaloupe, honeydew, watermelon *Vegetables:* cucumber, zucchini

It can also arise as a cross-reaction to proteins in a variety of fresh fruits or their juices (mainly apple, orange, grape and strawberries), vegetables (particularly tomatoes) and nuts. Cooking often destroys the allergens (except with celery and nuts, which may cause reactions even after being cooked).

Oral allergy syndrome occasionally causes urticaria or anaphylaxis; beans, celery, cumin, hazelnut, kiwi fruit, parsley and white potato are then implicated.

CLINICAL FEATURES

Symptoms usually develop within minutes but occasionally more than an hour later. Irritation, pruritus and swelling of the lips, tongue, palate and throat are sometimes associated with other allergic features such as rhinoconjunctivitis, asthma, urticaria–angioedema and anaphylactic shock.

Some individuals, after peeling or touching the offending foods, may develop a rash, itching or swelling where the juice touches the skin.

GENERAL MANAGEMENT

Individuals hypersensitive to the foods in Table 17.9 usually find that they can eat them provided that they are well cooked, canned or microwaved. People who develop symptoms when touching or peeling these foods may prevent them by wearing gloves. Consultation with an allergologist is recommended.

FOOD INTOLERANCE

Food intolerance symptoms can resemble food allergy but enzyme defects, chemicals, additives, toxins or infections are implicated rather than the immune system.

Lactase (a gut enzyme that degrades milk lactose) deficiency is the most common, almost universal in people of Chinese origin, common in people of southern European or African descent and affecting at least one out of ten other people. In lactase deficiency, lactose cannot be digested and remains in the gut to be used by bacteria, which produce gas, causing bloating, pain, and sometimes diarrhoea.

Histamine (often along with tyramine) is a chemical present in foods such as some cheese, wines and fish (particularly tuna and mackerel); it can provoke a reaction mimicking food allergy.

Additives that may cause reactions that can be confused with food allergy include mainly caffeine, yellow dye number E5, benzoates, salicylates, tartrazine, monosodium glutamate (MSG) and sulfites.

Toxins found in some foods, such as mushrooms and potatoes, and from bacteria in putrefying meat and fish, can cause similar symptoms.

Infections are discussed in Ch. 21.

HYPERSENSITIVITY TO DRUGS AND MATERIALS USED IN DENTISTRY

Latex allergy has become a significant clinical problem, along with **i**odine, **E**lastoplast and **d**rug allergies (hence the acronym LIED). The drugs causing the most severe and potentially fatal reactions are penicillins and intravenous anaesthetic agents. Allergies to other drugs and materials are uncommon.

Patients may be more likely to develop hypersensitivities if they are from an affected family, have atopic disease, have HIV disease, or have Sjögren syndrome.

ANAESTHETIC AND RELATED AGENTS

Intravenous anaesthetic agents and muscle relaxants can cause anaphylactic-type reactions, either because of hypersensitivity or by directly inducing histamine release (when the term 'anaphylactoid' rather than anaphylaxis may be more appropriate). Such reactions have been reported particularly for thiopental, and have sometimes been fatal, probably because of failure to recognize their nature since the loss of consciousness that results must be distinguished from the onset of anaesthesia. Many intravenous agents have been discontinued because of this risk. Suxamethonium is the muscle relaxant most commonly responsible, but alcuronium, tubocurarine and other relaxants are sometimes implicated and, as there does not need to be previous exposure to the agent, cross-reacting antigens are presumably implicated.

Tachycardia, vascular collapse and skin reactions (flushing, oedema or urticaria) are the most frequent signs, but reactions can range from minor symptoms to bronchospasm and a sharp fall in blood pressure. Treatment is as for anaphylaxis.

Halothane hypersensitivity may be a cause of 'halothane hepatitis' (Ch. 9). Local anaesthetic allergies are rare (Ch. 3).

ANTIBIOTICS

Anaphylaxis to antibiotics has been estimated to have caused approximately 300 deaths annually in the USA. Hypersensitivity reactions to beta-lactams (in penicillin and cephalosporins) are the most common type of reaction and are more likely to follow parenteral rather than oral administration. Patients allergic to penicillin usually react to any other penicillin except aztreonam and sometimes also react to cephalosporins. However, some allergic reactions can be selective for certain semi-synthetic penicillins, and some patients tolerant of benzylpenicillin can show delayed reactions to aminopenicillins.

The major antigenic determinant appears to be the penicilloyl group: this forms from metabolic cleavage of the beta-lactam ring and acts as a hapten binding to body proteins to become antigenic. Specific IgE antibodies to penicillin are the cause of the anaphylactic reactions by binding to mast cells and triggering release of mediators. There appears to be *no* association between penicillin anaphylaxis and atopic disease, even though the latter is mediated by the same mechanisms.

The most common reactions are urticarial and irritating rashes; sometimes a serum sickness type of reaction with joint pains and fever can follow days or weeks after administration; or anaphylaxis can occur. A history of previous reactions to penicillin suggests a greater risk of acute anaphylaxis – but there is no completely reliable method of prediction. Unfortunately, the first manifestation of sensitivity can occasionally be anaphylaxis and, rarely, a patient who has had penicillins on several occasions without ill-effect can suddenly develop anaphylaxis. A negative history therefore reduces the chances but does not exclude the possibility of anaphylaxis when the patient claims to be allergic to penicillin and, from the practical and medicolegal viewpoints therefore, reliance has to be placed on the history and an alternative antimicrobial used – but not one of the many penicillin derivatives (except aztreonam).

On the very rare occasions when no other antibiotic than a penicillin is indicated for a life-threatening infection, it may be possible to predict the possibility of an IgE-mediated response and anaphylactic reaction, by skin testing with benzylpenicilloyl polylysine, which, if there is allergy, gives a wheal and flare reaction within 10 min. Fewer than 5% of those who claim to be allergic to penicillin react positively in this way and anaphylaxis is virtually unknown in those who give negative reactions to this test.

Since a negative history of reactions to penicillin does not totally exclude the possibility of anaphylaxis, it is arguable that penicillin should not be given immediately before a general anaesthetic (GA). Admittedly the chances are small, but acute anaphylactic reactions during anaesthesia have been reported and, clearly, their recognition under such circumstances can be difficult. If penicillin has to be given, 30 min should be allowed to elapse before induction of GA – after such a period a severe reaction is unlikely.

Depot penicillins, which are slowly excreted, can maintain the antigenic challenge so that treatment of an allergic reaction may have to be continued until all the antigen is used up. Procaine penicillin can also occasionally cause vertigo, hallucinations and acute anxiety reactions if given intravenously (or if it accidentally enters a vein), reactions which may be mistaken for anaphylaxis.

A patient should of course be lying down when any injections are given, as fainting after injections is common and may be confused with anaphylaxis.

About 10% of those sensitized to penicillin are said to be also sensitive to the cephalosporins. However, much of the literature describing this cross-reactivity was established based on non-allergic adverse reactions or *in vitro* studies. Oral rechallenge and skin-testing data support the relationship of the beta-lactam side-chain structures of these drugs as a predictor of cross-reactivity. Nevertheless, it is best not to give cephalosporins to a patient severely allergic to penicillin unless there is a specific bacteriological indication.

Cefaclor may cause a serum sickness-like reaction.

NON-STEROIDAL ANTI-INFLAMMATORY DRUGS

Aspirin can provoke allergic reactions but, in relation to the scale of its use, the incidence is almost negligible. Aspirin-induced asthma is a rare possibility, mainly in patients with nasal polyps ('triad asthma' – asthma, nasal polyps and aspirin sensitivity). Other NSAIDs may, even more rarely, induce allergic reactions.

If there is a history of allergy to a drug it should not be given.

DENTAL MATERIALS AND ORAL HEALTH CARE PRODUCTS

Of dental materials that can induce allergic reactions (Box 17.2), latex is particularly important. Iodine and iodides present in some radiological contrast media and antiseptics such as povidone–iodine can also provoke dangerous reactions.

Box 17.2 Dental materials and health care products that may cause allergic reactions

- Denture fixatives
- Essential oils
- Iodides
- Latex
- Metals (amalgam, gold and other alloys, wires)
- Methylmethacrylate
- Oral health care products – mouthwashes, toothpastes
- Periodontal dressings
- Resins (colophony, composite and epoxy)
- Rubber base materials

LATEX (SEE ALSO APPENDIX 17.1)

Latex allergy affects ≈1% of the general population, is usually due to a contact allergy (type IV delayed hypersensitivity) and only rarely to a type I immediate hypersensitivity reaction. Natural rubber latex (NRL) is manufactured from the sap (latex) of *Havea brasiliensis*, which is allergenic, as are some of the chemicals added during production. NRL products that are dipped or stretchy (e.g. balloons, condoms, gloves, rubber bands) more frequently cause allergic reactions than do dry rubber products (e.g. tubing, tyres) but by far the most common sensitizer is the rubber in the soles of shoes.

Latex products are common in the home and workplace including clinics, wards and operating theatres, where allergy is an important occupational problem, especially with abrasive hand washing, which increases the risk of sensitization. Allergic reactions have become increasingly common since the widespread use of protective medical/dental gloves following the advent of HIV/AIDS. Latex allergies are also now common in patients who have been frequently exposed to rubber gloves or long-term indwelling urinary catheters (Box 17.3).

Box 17.3 People at high risk of latex allergy

- People with regular occupational exposure: health care workers, car mechanics, caterers and electronics tradespeople
- People with atopy or dermatitis/eczema (can facilitate the transfer of antigens across the skin)
- Patients frequently exposed to latex: pre-term infants; after multiple surgical procedures; spina bifida (up to 60% may be allergic), urogenital anomalies, imperforate anus, tracheo-oesophageal fistula, ventriculo-peritoneal shunts, paraplegia, learning impairment and cerebral palsy
- People allergic to foods with known latex cross-reactivity (Box 17.4)

Latex exposure may occur via the skin, mucous membranes or bronchial tree with inhalation of latex glove powder (NRL allergens may attach to lubricating powder, and become aerosolized, causing sensitization or, in those allergic, respiratory, ocular or nasal symptoms). 'Low-allergen' latex gloves are available but there is little certainty that these offer any real benefit.

Patients with latex allergy may react to foods with allergen cross-reactivity such as avocado, banana, chestnut and kiwi (Box 17.4).

Clinical features

Latex causes immediate type I allergic reactions ranging from pruritus to urticaria and, rarely, anaphylaxis or, more commonly, slower contact dermatitis reactions (type IV), which appear after 24–48 h and are eczematous.

Management

Persons with symptoms of type I latex hypersensitivity should be regarded as truly allergic, since testing for latex allergy is problematic: intradermal injection carries the risk of inducing anaphylactic shock and false positives are not uncommon in patients with RAST. Persons with type IV reactions can have

---

Box 17.4 Foods sometimes cross-reacting with latex

- Apricots
- Avocados
- Bananas
- Celery
- Cherries
- Chestnuts
- Figs
- Grapes
- Kiwi fruit
- Melons
- Nectarines
- Papaya
- Passion fruit
- Peaches
- Pineapples
- Pistachios
- Plums
- Potatoes
- Strawberries
- Tomatoes

---

patch testing, but this is difficult to standardize because of variations in latex preparations. Skinprick tests or RAST assays can also be used.

Anything containing, or contaminated by, latex should be avoided: a latex-free clinic is ideal. Latex is found in many items used in hospital clinics, wards and operating theatres (Box 17.5) and even equipment and laboratory work previously handled with latex gloves may elicit an allergic response.

Many items used in dental practice can contain latex (Box 17.6).

Box 17.5 Latex in medical items

- Equipment previously handled with latex gloves
- Anaesthetic masks, props, intubation tubes, airways and other equipment
- Catheters and cannulae
- Tourniquets
- Rubber gloves
- Rubber surgical drains
- Sphygmomanometer cuffs
- Stethoscopes

Patients with latex type I hypersensitivity

Latex antigens must particularly be avoided for type I hypersensitivity patients, who should therefore only be treated with latex avoidance and where staff are confident in their ability to manage such problems, particularly anaphylaxis. NRL-free gloves and equipment *must* be used, which may mean specialist management in a hospital latex-free environment, and the individual should be advised to wear a Medic-Alert or similar device. Affected persons should contact only latex-free vinyl (polyvinyl chloride), nitrile (acrylonitrile butadiene), vitrile (a blend of vinyl and nitrile), polychloroprene (neolon), polystyrene–poly(ethylene–butylene)–polystyrene (tactylon), styrene butadiene, polyurethane or other polymer gloves, medical or dental products.

Box 17.6 Latex in dental items

- Equipment and laboratory work previously handled with latex gloves
- Adhesive dressings and their packaging
- Amalgam carrier tips
- Bandages and tapes
- Chip syringes
- Dappens pot
- Endodontic stops
- Gloves
- Gutta percha and gutta balata
- Headgear and head positioners
- Induction masks
- Latex ties on face masks
- Local anaesthetic cartridges^a
- Mixing bowls
- Needle guards
- Orthodontic elastics
- Prophylaxis cups and polishing wheels and points
- Protective eyewear
- Rubber dam
- Rubber gloves
- Rubber sleeves on props and bite blocks
- Spatula
- Suction tips
- Surgical face masks and other protective items of clothing (e.g. gowns, overshoes)
- Tourniquets and blood pressure cuffs
- Wedges

^aLatex is present in some rubber dental LA cartridges, stoppers or plungers – where either the harpoon penetrates or where the flat piston end of a self-aspirating syringe rests. At the other end of the cartridge is the diaphragm, which the needle penetrates. Any of these components may contain latex. Although there are no documented reports of allergy due to the latex component of cartridges of dental LA, the UK preparation of prilocaine (Citanest) contains no latex.

If there is any possibility of contact with traces of latex, pre-medication prophylaxis with corticosteroids and/or antihistamines may be indicated (Table 17.10).

Patients with unproven latex hypersensitivity

If the history of latex allergy is dubious, treatment is best carried out as above but without pre-medication. In the absence of a latex-free clinic, care is best offered at the beginning of the day, before environmental levels of latex allergens rise, as activity in the surgery continues.

ORAL HEALTH CARE PRODUCTS

Contact dermatitis can occasionally be precipitated on the lip vermilion or, more frequently, perioral skin by components of toothpastes, impression materials, lipsticks and some foods (notably mangoes and oranges). Toothpastes or chewing gum components, especially cinnamon, can also cause plasma cell gingivitis or inflammation of other parts of the oral mucosa. Gingivitis, cheilitis, perioral dermatitis and other lesions have been described in patients using tartar-control toothpastes that contain cinnamonaldehyde or pyrophosphates.

Some substances (e.g. zirconium) occasionally cause granulomatous oral reactions and allergic reactions may underlie orofacial granulomatosis.

Table 17.10 Treatment of latex-sensitive patients

History of latex allergy	Drug prophylaxis	Drug regimen
Previous anaphylaxis	Methylprednisolone	1 mg/kg 6-hourly i.v. Max. dose 50 mg
	Chlorphenamine	1 month–1 year 250 µg/kg 1–5 years 2.5–5 mg 6–12 years 5-10 mg
Previous allergy with no anaphylaxis (e.g. urticaria, central dermatitis, eye swelling, bronchospasm)	Methylprednisolone	1 mg/kg 6-hourly i.v. Max. dose 50 mg
	Chlorphenamine	1 month–1 year 250 µg /kg 1–5 years 2.5–5 mg 6–12 years 5-10 mg

DENTAL MATERIALS

Dental alloys, bonding, cements, plastics, primers, resins and other materials can cause allergies leading to dermatitis, rashes, blistering, itching or burning, though these features are usually seen only in people highly sensitive to epoxy resins. Illustrative of the difference in response between skin and mucosa to sensitizing agents is that a substance, to which the patient is sensitized when put in the mouth, can occasionally induce the typical rash on the skin. This has been reported in the case of nickel sensitivity when a nickel-containing denture caused a rash but no oral reaction.

Alloys

With few exceptions, metals used in dentistry are alloys – solid mixtures of two or more metals. Nickel-containing alloys, such as nickel–titanium and stainless steel, are widely used in orthodontic appliances. Nickel–titanium alloys may contain more than 50% nickel and can cause allergic reactions. Stainless steel has a much lower nickel content, bound in a crystal lattice not available to react, and is therefore unlikely to cause allergic reactions.

Dental amalgam is a combination of mercury with a specially prepared silver alloy. The American Dental Association (ADA) specification states that the alloy must include a minimum of 65% silver, a maximum of 29% tin, a maximum of 6–13% copper, and a maximum of 2% zinc by weight. Alloys with high copper content usually have lower creep values than the conventional silver–tin alloys. Some alloys are completely zinc free and can therefore be used more successfully in a moisture-contaminated environment.

Dental amalgam has been reported to cause mucosal reactions such as lichenoid lesions, but the evidence is controversial and mercury absorbed from amalgams into the mucosa frequently causes no histological reaction. In people sensitized to mercury, amalgam restorations can safely be inserted provided that stray amalgam is not allowed to touch the patient's skin.

Gold alloys may be used for dental restorations or occasionally prostheses. Pure gold, because of its softness, is not indicated for use in the mouth except as gold foil. The basic alloys used are casting gold, gold solder, wrought gold and gold plate, and may contain silver, copper, platinum, palladium or zinc. Lichenoid reactions have been described.

Cements

Dental cements include zinc phosphate, zinc oxide and eugenol, polycarboxylate (zinc oxide powder mixed with polyacrylic acid), and glass ionomer cements (GICs). Allergic reactions to dental cements are rare but GICs contain a polyalkeonic acid such as polyacrylic acid plus a fluoride-containing silicate glass (fluoro-aluminosilicate) powder and occasionally cause reactions. Resin-modified glass-ionomer cements (RMGICs) usually contain HEMA (hydrophilic monomer) plus a fluoride-containing glass and polyacrylic acid. Tri-cure GICs also incorporate a chemical curing tertiary amine-peroxide reaction to polymerize the methacrylate along with the photo-initiation and acid–base ionic reaction.

Plastics and Resins

Some chemicals in plastics may cause reactions and some may leach from set material at least for a few days, as may degradation products (e.g. formaldehyde). A few individuals may react to potential allergens shown in Box 17.7.

Box 17.7 Potential allergens in dental resins

- 1,4-Butanediol dimethacrylate (BUDMA)
- 1,7,7-Trimethylbicyclo-2,2,1-heptane
- 2-Hydroxyethyl methacrylate (2-HEMA)
- 2-Hydroxypropyl methacrylate (2-HPMA)
- 2,2-Dimethoxy-1,2-diphenyletanone (DMBZ)
- 4-Dimethylaminobenzoic acid ethyl ester (DMABEE)
- Acrylated epoxy oligomer
- DL-Camphorquinone
- Ethylene glycol dimethacrylate (EGDMA)
- Methyl methacrylate (MMA)
- Triethylene glycol dimethacrylate (TEGDMA)
- Urethane dimethacrylate (UDMA)

Plastics include polymethyl methacrylate (PMMA), polystyrene, polyvinylchloride (PVC), etc., which contain potential allergens such as long hydrocarbon-based chains produced from small monomer units (e.g. methyl methacrylate, styrene, vinyl chloride, etc.).

Methyl methacrylate

Polymethyl methacrylate used for acrylic clothing, plastic items or denture base is probably inert. Dental methyl methacrylate contains a wide range of components, however, which are potentially sensitizing (Table 17.11); there are rare cases, particularly in dental staff, of allergic contact reactions to methyl methacrylate monomer and associated chemicals. Affected persons should avoid exposure. Surgical rubber, latex or vinyl gloves offer little if any protection, as they are quickly penetrated by the chemicals, but commercial laminated disposable protective gloves are available.

Resins

Resins are used in dentistry as bonding agents, composite resins, pit and fissure sealants and resin-based cements. Often referred to as direct-filling resins, they are of several types: the older

Table 17.11 Typical components of dental methyl methacrylate

Liquid	Powder
Dimethacrylate (cross-linker)	Organic peroxides (initiators)
Hydroquinone (inhibitor)	Pigments
Methyl methacrylate (monomer)	Polymethyl methacrylate
Organic amines (accelerator)	Titanium dioxide
Ultraviolet absorber	

type was an unfilled polymethacrylate (acrylic resin, Perspex or PMMA); the newer type is the composite resin based mainly on dimethacrylates. Composites consist of hydrophobic methacrylate monomers plus silanated glass. Acid-modified composites (compomers) consist of acidic hydrophobic methacrylate monomers, such as urethane dimethacrylate (UDMA) and fluoride-containing glass. The monomers most commonly used are 2,2,-bis[4(2-hydroxyl-3-methacryloxyloxypropoxy)-phenyl] propane – more commonly termed BisGMA (bisphenol A glycidal methacrylate)–and UDMA, which are combined with lower molecular weight monomers such as triethylene glycol dimethacrylate (TEGDMA). Photo-initiators such as camphoroquinone facilitate polymerization via light curing.

The major sensitizers appear to be EGDMA, 2-HEMA, 2-HPMA, MMA and acrylated epoxy oligomer. BUDMA and UDMA seem to be only weak sensitizers. Allergic reactions in the mouth are typically lichenoid but occasionally urticarial or anaphylactoid, and dermatological reactions in health care workers are usually contact dermatitis or eczema – so direct skin contact is best avoided.

Allergic reactions may be produced by the catalyst methyldichlorobenzene sulfonate in dibenzyltoluol present in *Impregum* and by the catalyst methyl *p*-toluene sulfonate in dibenzyltoluol present in *Scutan*.

Some patients are sensitive to colophony resins: in wound sticking plasters, periodontal dressings, impression materials, cements, fix adhesives and some fluoride varnishes (e.g. Duraphat). Eugenol and resin in periodontal dressings can be contact allergens.

USEFUL WEBSITES

http://www.3niaid.nih.gov/topics
http://www.allergyuk.org/
http://www.bbc.co.uk/health/conditions/allergies/allergicconditions_food.shtml
http://www.bad.org.uk/public/leaflets/bad_patient_information_gateway_leaflets/latex/
http://www.hse.gov.uk/latex
http://www.anaphylaxis.org.uk/information/basic_facts.html
http://www.nda.ox.ac.uk

FURTHER READING

Auzerie, V., Mahé, E., Marck, Y., Auffret, N., Descamps, V., Crickx, B., 2002. Oral lichenoid eruption due to methacrylate allergy. Contact Dermatitis 45, 241.

Aziz, S.R., Tin, P., 2002. Spontaneous angioedema of oral cavity after dental impressions. N Y State Dent J 68, 42–45.

Bismil, Q., Bowles, C., Edwards, M., Arastu, M., Ricketts, D.M., Solan, M.C., 2007. Detecting patient allergy: beware the LIE. Ann R Coll Surg Engl 89, 603–604.

Bush, R.K., 2008. Approach to patients with symptoms of food allergy. Am J Med 121, 376–378.

Chin, S.M., Ferguson, J.W., Bajurnows, T., 2004. Latex allergy in dentistry. Review and report of case presenting as a serious reaction to latex dental dam. Aust Dent J 49, 146–148.

Clarke, A., 2004. The provision of dental care for patients with natural rubber latex allergy: are patients able to obtain safe care?. Br Dent J 197, 749–752.

DePestel, D.D., Benninger, M.S., Danziger, L., et al., 2003. Cephalosporin use in treatment of patients with penicillin allergies. J Am Pharm Assoc 2008 (48), 530–540.

Desai, S.V., 2007. Natural rubber latex allergy and dental practice. N Z Dent J 103, 101–107.

Fan, P.L., Meyer, D.M., 2007. FDI report on adverse reactions to resin-based materials. Int Dent J 57, 9–12.

García, J.A., 2007. Type I latex allergy: a follow-up study. J Invest Allergol Clin Immunol 17, 164–167.

Garn, H., Renz, H., 2007. Epidemiological and immunological evidence for the hygiene hypothesis. Immunobiology 212, 441–452.

Greer, F.R., Sicherer, S.H., Wesley Burks, A and the Committee on Nutrition and Section on Allergy and Immunology, 2008. Effects of early nutritional interventions on the development of atopic disease in infants and children: the role of maternal dietary restriction, breastfeeding, timing of introduction of complementary foods, and hydrolyzed formulas. Pediatrics 121, 183–191.

Hain, M.A., Longman, L.P., Field, E.A., Harrison, J.E., 2007. Natural rubber latex allergy: implications for the orthodontist. J Orthod 34, 6–11.

Hamann, C.P., DePaola, L.G., Rodgers, P.A., 2005. Occupation-related allergies in dentistry. J Am Dent Assoc 136, 500–510.

Huber, M.A., Terezhalmy, G.T., 2006. Adverse reactions to latex products: preventive and therapeutic strategies. J Contemp Dent Pract 7, 97–106.

Issa, Y., Duxbury, A.J., Macfarlane, T.V., Brunton, P.A., 2005. Oral lichenoid lesions related to dental restorative materials. Br Dent J 198, 361–366.

Karabucak, B., Stoopler, E.T., 2007. Root canal treatment on a patient with zinc oxide allergy: a case report. Int Endod J 40, 800–807.

Kelso, J.M., 2007. Allergic contact stomatitis from orthodontic rubber bands. Ann Allergy Asthma Immunol 98, 99–100.

Kerosuo, H.M., Dahl, J.E., 2007. Adverse patient reactions during orthodontic treatment with fixed appliances. Am J Orthod Dentofacial Orthop 132, 789–795.

Kitaura, H., Fujimura, Y., Nakao, N., Eguchi, T., Yoshida, N., 2007. Treatment of a patient with metal hypersensitivity after orthognathic surgery. Angle Orthod 77, 923–930.

Leggat, P.A., Kedjarune, U., 2003. Toxicity of methyl methacrylate in dentistry. Int Dent J 53, 126–131.

Möller, H., 2002. Dental gold alloys and contact allergy. Contact Dermatitis 47, 63–66.

Morris, D.A., 2004. Contact dermatiotis. Curr Allergy Clin Immunol 17, 190–191.

Nainar, S.M.H., 2001. Dental management of children with latex allergy. Int J Paediatr Dent 11, 322–326.

Neugut, A.I., Ghatak, A.T., Miller, R.I., 2001. Anaphylaxis in the United States. Arch Intern Med 161, 15–21.

Noble, J., Ahing, S.I., Karaiskos, N.E., Wiltshire, W.A., 2008. Nickel allergy and orthodontics. a review and report of two cases. Br Dent J 204, 297–300.

Örtengren, U., 2000. On composite resin materials – degradation, erosion and possible adverse effects in dentists. Swed Dent J (Suppl 141), 1–61.

Pandis, N., Pandis, B.D., Pandis, V., Eliades, T., 2007. Occupational hazards in orthodontics: a review of risks and associated pathology. Am J Orthod Dentofacial Orthop 132, 280–292.

Schweikl, H., Spagnuolo, G., Schmaltz, G., 2006. Genetic and cellular toxicology of dental resin monomers. J Dent Res 85, 870–877.

Scully C, Chaudhry S, 2006. Aspects of Human Disease 7. Allergy Dental Update 33, 637.

Sharma, P.R., 2006. Allergic contact stomatitis from colophony. Dent Update 33, 440–442.

Todd, G., 2000. Contact dermatitis. ALLSA Information Sheet.

Torgerson, R.R., Davis, M.D., Bruce, A.J., Farmer, S.A., Rogers 3rd, R.S., 2007. Contact allergy in oral disease. J Am Acad Dermatol 57, 315–321.

Trattner, A., David, M., Lazarov, A., 2008. Occupational contact dermatitis due to essential oils. Contact Dermatitis 58, 282–284.

Vamnes, J.S., Lygre, G.B., Grönningsæter, A.G., Gjerdet, N.R., 2004. Four years of clinical experience with adverse reaction unit for dental biomaterials. Community Dent Oral Epidemiol 32, 150–157.

Vozza, I., Ranghi, G., Quaranta, A., 2005. Allergy and desensibilization to latex. Clinical study on 50 dentistry subjects. Minerva Stomatol 54, 237–245.

Wallenhammar, L.-M., Örtengren, U., Andreasson, H., et al., 2000. Contact allergy and hand eczema in Swedish dentists. Contact Dermatitis 43, 192–199.

Appendix 17.1 Latex Allergy

(From http://www.hse.gov.uk/latex/dental.htm)

Natural rubber latex products may impact on dental health care workers (i.e. dentists, nurses, hygienists) because:

1 they are at greater risk of developing NRL allergy through the frequent use of NRL gloves
2 they may need to manage NRL-sensitive patients, which may be either known in advance or previously undiagnosed
3 they have a statutory responsibility to reduce risk of sensitization in themselves, their colleagues and their patients.

Ensure you have and are familiar with:

- a written *policy* – on action to protect staff from developing NRL allergy; on safe accommodation of NRL-sensitive members of staff; for the safe dental management of patients with known or suspected NRL allergy
- an *education programme* to inform new and existing staff
- posters for patient and staff information, clearly displayed and on file
- an *occupational health* surveillance programme, which includes pre-employment screening
- a named responsible person for managing health and safety.

PREVENTION OF NRL ALLERGIES

It is important that you protect yourself against breaches of the skin barrier that can result from frequent use of skin cleansers and occlusive glove-wear, especially if you have an atopic background (asthma, hay fever or flexural eczema) where damage to the skin from irritants is more common. A compromised skin barrier will increase your chances of developing type IV rubber chemical or type I NRL allergy. Hand-disinfectant agents and protective gloves need to be selected with great care and it is also important to use a suitable aqueous-based emollient at the end of the session and also at other times if your skin has any tendency to dry out.

The British Dental Association offers the following tips on hand care:

- don't wear jewellery (e.g. rings)
- wash and disinfect hands at the beginning and end of each session, as well as between each glove change

- use cool/tepid water when washing, to keep hand temperature down
- use hand-wash agents sparingly
- rinse thoroughly to remove all traces of hand wash
- pat skin dry rather than rubbing it
- use soft towels (disposable)
- ensure hands are dry before putting on gloves
- use non-powdered gloves with low levels of NRL proteins and residual chemicals
- choose the right size of gloves
- minimize contact with other potential irritants/allergens in the surgery (e.g. acrylic powders/antimicrobial solutions)
- outside work, don't forget to protect hands when gardening/doing household chores, etc.

The Faculty of General Dental Practice UK is presently developing NRL guidelines.

If you or your patient are not NRL-sensitive and you choose to wear NRL gloves to protect yourself from blood-borne pathogens, choose powder-free and low-protein (< 50 µg/g) gloves only.

Ensure that gloves comply with national and international standards of performance (British and European Standard BSEN 455, 1993). These should carry the 'CE' mark.

(See Hand dermatitis and latex allergy, British Dental Association (BDA) Fact File, Nov 2000.)

MANAGEMENT OF SENSITIZED WORKERS

If you suspect that you may be allergic to NRL, it is best to seek a referral to a dermatologist or immunologist via your GP or occupational health physician so that this can be appropriately investigated as soon as signs and symptoms develop.

If you are found to be NRL-sensitive, then it is essential that your work environment is adapted as soon as possible to avoid unnecessary exposure to NRL, which would increase your sensitivity and put you at risk of more severe reactions.

TYPE I NRL ALLERGY

If you are diagnosed with type I allergy, it may be possible for you to continue to work in the clinical environment, although this depends on the severity of reactions you experience (see earlier).

It is important that you learn to avoid NRL proteins in consumer and medical products both at home and at work. As gloves are the main cause of allergic reactions to NRL, it is essential that you replace NRL gloves with suitable *NRL-free gloves* for yourself and ensure that you are not working in powdered NRL environments (i.e. from the use of powdered NRL gloves worn by colleagues).

A minority of allergic workers can only work symptom free in a strict NRL-free glove environment so it may become necessary for colleagues to switch to using NRL-free gloves also or that other modifications to the work environment are required.

It is recommended that you wear a Medic-Alert® bracelet.

If you have been advised to carry adrenaline for self-administration (e.g. EpiPen® or Anapen®), colleagues should be instructed on how to use it.

TYPE IV ALLERGY

If you are diagnosed with type IV allergy to a rubber chemical, then you need to find a glove that does not contain the chemical to which you are allergic. The dermatologist who has diagnosed this should be able to help you with appropriate glove selection.

MANAGEMENT OF A PATIENT WITH TYPE 1 NRL ALLERGY

(See Field EA, Longman LP, Al-Sharkawi M, Perrin L, Davies M. The dental management of patients with natural rubber latex allergy. Br Dent J 1998;185:65–9.)

Establish a *patient history* to identify whether your patient needs to be treated in an NRL-safe environment. Questions include:

- has the patient ever experienced an adverse reaction (itch or swelling) to balloons, condoms, household gloves, or associated with surgery, internal examination or dental treatment?
- does the patient have an allergy to foods cross-reacting with NRL (e.g. banana, kiwi, avocado, chestnut)?
- has the patient experienced hives, asthma or hay-fever symptoms as a result of their work, where latex gloves are used?

Contact with natural rubber latex in dental equipment and products (including medicines) must be avoided in patients with diagnosed or suspected Type 1 NRL allergy and NRL-free alternatives used instead.

Treatment at the beginning of the working day is preferred, before environmental levels of NRL allergens rise with increased activity in the surgery.

Patients with NRL allergy have often been treated in a general dental practice without significant problems when adjustments have been made by the dental team to manage the patient's allergy. However, if the dentist is in doubt or lacks confidence (e.g. managing a highly reactive patient), the patient may need to be referred for appropriate management, possibly in a community CDS or PDS (Community and Primary Dental Services) or in a hospital setting.

All forward planning and documentation should inform future carers of the patient's sensitization by effective recording in notes and the use of *Labels for patient notes*.

Possible sources of NRL in dental practice include the following.

General:
- Gloves
- Rubber dam and some wedges
- Local anaesthetic cartridges
- Prophylaxis polishing cups
- Orthodontic elastics

- GA/sedation equipment, including tubing, face masks, props
- Endodontic stops
- Amalgam carrier tips
- Adhesives and dressings and their packaging
- Equipment and laboratory work previously handled with latex gloves

Emergency equipment:
- Oral and nasal airways
- Oxygen masks and nasal cannulae
- Self-inflating bag
- Blood pressure monitor
- Emergency medication

For the more reactive patient or member of staff, other items should be checked for their latex content (e.g. mixing bowls, spatula, chip syringes, needle guards, dappens pot).

MANAGEMENT OF ALLERGIC REACTIONS DURING DENTAL TREATMENT

Ensure that NRL-free emergency equipment and medicines are readily available to treat any allergic reaction from mild (e.g. urticaria and asthma) to severe (i.e. laryngeal oedema/bronchospasm/cardiovascular collapse from anaphylaxis) and that staff are fully trained in resuscitation techniques.

AUTOIMMUNE DISEASE

The normal immune response and tests are summarized in Ch. 19. Many diseases are immunologically mediated and this is especially notable in allergies and autoimmunity.

A genetically determined susceptibility to immunologically mediated diseases is often suggested by a positive family history, and also by significant associations with certain major histocompatibility complex (MHC) histocompatibility (human lymphocyte antigen or HLA) antigens. The genes for histocompatibility antigens are identified by a letter (A–D) and a number (e.g. HLA-D2). The causes of autoimmune disease are unclear. Heredity appears to play a role: autoimmune reactions are influenced by MHC genes, and a proportion of human patients with autoimmune disease have particular HLA types. Several polymorphic genes [i.e. HLA-DRB1, tumour necrosis factor (TNF) and PTPN22] influence the susceptibility to different autoimmune diseases. Many organ-specific autoimmune diseases are associated with HLA-B8 and DR3, but the association is not sufficiently strong to help in the diagnosis. Rheumatoid arthritis, by contrast, is associated with HLA-DR4, but any genetic predisposition is controversial. HLA specificities are therefore still of limited value in diagnosis.

This chapter discusses autoimmune disorders – mainly those that affect multiple tissues; organ-specific disorders are discussed in the appropriate chapters (Table 18.1).

AUTOIMMUNE DISEASES

GENERAL ASPECTS

Autoimmune diseases are due to antibodies and T cells directed against self, produced when immune system recognition fails or malfunctions. Autoimmune diseases may be initiated by virsuses, drugs, chemicals or other factors and affect the immune system at several levels. In patients with systemic lupus erythematosus, for instance – B cells are hyperactive while suppressor cells are underactive; it is not clear which defect comes first. Moreover, production of interleukin-2 (IL-2) is low, while levels of interferon-gamma are high. Patients with rheumatoid arthritis, who have defective suppressor T cells, continue to make antibodies to common viruses, a response that would normally cease after about 14 days. Some autoantibodies are directed against specific antigens and cause localized disease (e.g. autoantibodies to desmoglein in epithelial intercellular cement, which cause

Table 18.1 Types of autoimmune disease

Non-organ-specific autoantibodies: the connective tissue diseases[a]	Organ or cell-specific autoantibodies[b]
Raynaud disease	Autoimmune haemolytic anaemia
Lupus erythematosus	Chronic atrophic gastritis (pernicious anaemia)[c]
Rheumatoid arthritis	Hashimoto thyroiditis
Sjögren syndrome	Idiopathic Addison disease
Scleroderma	Idiopathic hypoparathyroidism
Dermatomyositis	Idiopathic thrombocytopenic purpura
Mixed connective tissue disease	Myasthenia gravis
Antiphospholipid syndrome	Pemphigoid
	Pemphigus vulgaris

[a]Probably mediated by immune complex reactions: discussed in this chapter.
[b]Discussed elsewhere in this book (section B).
[c]Not all chronic atrophic gastritis.
Note: only the more important and typical examples are given.

pemphigus; autoantibodies to red blood cells, which cause anaemia; autoantibodies to pancreatic islet cells, which contribute to juvenile diabetes; and autoantibodies to acetylcholine receptors, which are present in myasthenia gravis). Polyglandular autoimmune diseases are examples of autoimmune attack on many organs.

Where autoantibodies are directed against several types of cell and cellular components, including nuclear components such as deoxyribonucleic acid (DNA), ribonucleic acid (RNA) or proteins, then generalized disease, such as systemic lupus erythematosus, may result (Table 18.1).

CLINICAL FEATURES

Autoimmune diseases sharse common features (Table 18.2).

GENERAL MANAGEMENT

The blood picture may show results of autoantibodies against haematological factors (e.g. haemolytic anaemia, thrombocytopenia or leukopenia). Alternatively, there may be leukocytosis associated with inflammatory processes. The erythrocyte sedimentation rate (ESR) is often raised. Serum protein levels are also typically raised because of immunoglobulin overproduction. Specific tests for autoimmune disease include assays for serum autoantibodies (see Ch. 2 and Table 18.3). Specific autoantibodies can be identified by special tests but often an autoantibody profile is carried out (includes the most common abnormalities, namely rheumatoid and antinuclear factors and thyroid microsomal, gastric parietal cell, mitochondrial,

Table 18.2 Typical features of autoimmune diseases

Clinical features	Laboratory features
Female predisposition	Hypergammaglobulinaemia
Family history positive often	Autoantibodies specific to tissue under attack sometimes present in the circulation. Circulating autoantibodies often detectable in apparently unaffected relatives. Multiple autoantibodies often detectable but frequently without clinical effect
Response to immuno-suppressive treatment in many	Immunoglobulin and complement deposits sometimes detectable by immunofluorescence microscopy at sites of tissue damage (e.g. damaged blood vessels)
Patients especially liable to develop further autoimmune diseases	Associations with HLA-B8 and DR3 in some

smooth muscle and reticulin antibodies). Serum complement levels may show the complement consumed when the cascade is activated by antigen/antibody reactions or other triggering factors, with complement levels (CH50) often depressed. Biopsy and tissue immunostaining may show immunoglobulin or complement deposits. Vasculitis with deposits of immunoglobulins and complement in the damaged vessel walls strongly suggests immune complex injury.

Treatments for autoimmune diseases include mainly anti-inflammatory and immunosuppressive drugs or plasmapheresis (removal of the antibodies).

THE CONNECTIVE TISSUE DISEASES

The connective tissue diseases (collagen diseases) are autoimmune diseases that share, to a variable degree, common features, such as: multiple autoantibodies, often against nuclear components (Table 18.3); immune complex reactions; associations with Raynaud phenomenon and Sjögren syndrome; responsiveness to immunosuppressives; and cancer as a possible late complication.

RAYNAUD DISEASE AND RAYNAUD PHENOMENON

Raynaud disease and phenomenon are characterized by skin arteries that over-respond to cold, contracting briefly, limiting blood flow (vasospasm) so that the skin first turns white then blue and, as the arteries relax and blood flows again, it turns red. Women mainly are affected. Raynaud disease (primary or idiopathic Raynaud disease) has no predisposing factor, is mild, and causes few complications – but approximately 30% eventually progress to secondary Raynaud disease. Raynaud phenomenon (secondary Raynaud disease) has the same clinical features but occurs in individuals with a predisposing factor, is often more complicated and severe, and is more likely to deteriorate. Predisposing factors include: connective tissue disorders mainly; smoking; injuries such as frostbite, surgery, regular use of vibrating machinery such as chain saws and drills, or other activities such as regular typing or piano playing; drugs (e.g. some cardiovascular drugs and ergotamine); arteriosclerosis or pulmonary hypertension.

Clinical features

Symptoms include changes in skin colour (white to blue to red) and coldness. Both hands and feet are usually affected. Raynaud can sometimes also attack other areas such as the nose and ears. It is common for the affected area to feel numb or prickly. Raynaud disease usually affects both hands and both feet, while Raynaud phenomenon usually affects either both hands or both feet only.

Raynaud tends to be slowly progressive with more frequent and prolonged episodes of spasm. Ischaemia can cause atrophy of the fat pads or ulceration at the tips of the fingers or toes, sometimes with the loss of more tissue (Fig. 18.1).

Table 18.3 Significance of the more common autoantibodies related to connective tissue diseases (see Appendix 2.5)

Autoantibodies			Main associations
Anti-Jo 1 antibody (GAD65)			Polymyositis, dermatomyositis
Anti-Ku antibody			Polymyositis/scleroderma (PM/Scl) overlap syndrome
Antinuclear antibody (ANA)	Anti-ds (double-stranded) DNA antibody		Antibody with the highest specificity for systemic lupus erythematosus (SLE) and found in most patients
	Anti-extractable nuclear antigen antibodies (anti-ENA antibodies)	Anti-Ro (Robair) antibody	Sjögren syndrome
		Anti-La (Lattimer) antibody	Sjögren syndrome
Anti-PM/Scl (anti-exosome) antibody			PM/Scl overlap syndrome
Anti-Scl 70 antibody	Anti-topoisomerase antibodies		Scleroderma
	Anti-centromere antibodies		CREST syndrome
Rheumatoid factor (RF)			Rheumatoid arthritis (high rate of false-positives in SLE and other conditions)
Lupus anticoagulant	Anti-thrombin antibodies		SLE

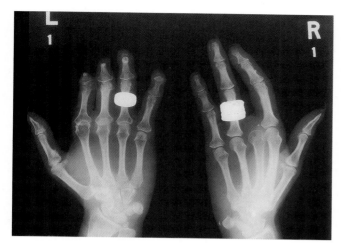

Fig. 18.1 Loss of digit and atrophy of distal phalanges in severe Raynaud syndrome

General management

People suffering from Raynaud should stop smoking and protect themselves from cold and keep all parts of their body warm – not just their extremities – and guard against cuts, bruises, and other injuries to the affected areas.

Medications such as calcium-channel blockers (e.g. nifedipine), reserpine or nitroglycerin may relax artery walls and improve blood flow. Naftidrofuryl or inositol nicotinate may also help symptomatically.

Dental aspects

The dental facility should be kept at a temperature and humidity that the patient finds comfortable. Nifedipine may cause gingival swelling.

LUPUS ERYTHEMATOSUS

Lupus can be categorized as systemic lupus erythematosus, drug-induced systemic lupus erythematosus or discoid lupus erythematosus.

Systemic lupus erythematosus

General aspects

Systemic lupus erythematosus (SLE) is a potentially fatal disease – the archetypal autoimmune disease – characterized by autoantibodies to DNA, which may initiate immune complex reactions, in particular vasculitis, resulting in multisystem disease. Lupus susceptibility relates to several genes including HLA-DR3 and B8, HLA-DR2, complement C4 genes and a polymorphism of the T-cell receptor, which has been associated with Ro antibodies.

Clinical features

Depending on the organs predominantly affected, SLE can cause a variety of clinical manifestations which range greatly in severity, from mild to those with significant and potentially fatal lesions. The onset may be acute, resembling an infection, or vague symptoms which may progress over many years (Table 18.4).

Table 18.4 Manifestations of systemic lupus erythematosus

System	Main lesions
Skin	Rash
Joints	Arthritis Polyarthralgia
Serous membranes	Pericarditis Pleurisy
Cardiovascular	Endocarditis (Libman–Sacks) Myocarditis Raynaud syndrome
Lungs	Pneumonitis
Kidney	Nephritis
Neurological	Cranial nerve palsies Neuroses Psychoses Strokes
Eye	Conjunctivitis Retinal damage
Gastrointestinal	Hepatomegaly Pancreatitis Sjögren syndrome
Blood	Anaemia Purpura

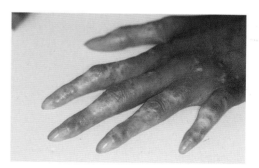

Fig. 18.2 Raynaud syndrome in lupus

The classic picture of SLE is that of a young woman with fever, malaise, anaemia, joint pains, Raynaud syndrome and a rash variable in character but erythematous, often with raised margins and scaling (Fig. 18.2). The well-known rash with a butterfly pattern extending over both cheeks and bridge of the nose is relatively uncommon, and actually not specific to lupus erythematosus. Photosensitivity rashes are common. Renal involvement (proteinuria and haematuria) is common and often associated with hypertension. Relatively minor disturbances of mood, and depressive or hysterical behaviour are common, while central nervous system (CNS) involvement is potentially fatal. Ocular lesions may affect 20–25% and serositis can cause pleurisy or occasionally pericarditis and peritonitis (polyserositis) (Fig 18.3).

Cardiac lesions typically cause myocarditis, which leads to cardiac failure; there is a higher risk of infarction and a characteristic (Libman–Sacks) endocarditis can also develop. Murmurs are more often caused by anaemia.

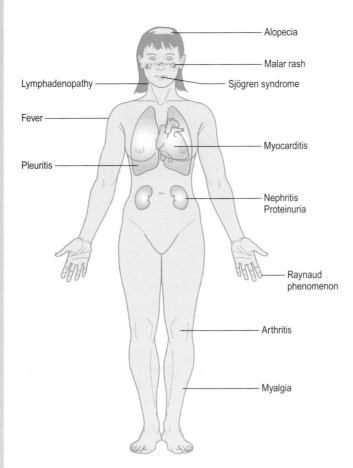

Fig. 18.3 Lupus erythematosus

Women who have SLE can pass antibodies across the placenta, which can cause fetal heart block (see Sjögren syndrome).

General management

The American College of Rheumatology diagnostic criteria for diagnosis of SLE are based on the presence of at least four of the following: malar rash; discoid rash; photosensitivity; oral ulcers; arthritis; serositis (pleuritis or pericarditis); renal disorder (persistent proteinuria or cellular casts); neurological disorder (seizures or psychosis); haematological disorder (anaemia, leukopenia or lymphopenia on two or more occasions, thrombocytopenia); or immunological disorder [positive LE (lupus erythematosus) cell preparation, anti-DNA or anti-Sm, false-positive VDRL (Venereal Disease Reference Laboratory)].

Initial screening includes ESR, tests for specific autoantibodies (e.g. antinuclear antibodies; ANA; Box 18.1), a full blood count, liver and kidney function tests, a syphilis test (VDRL), LE cell test, urinalysis and blood chemistries.

No single laboratory test can definitely prove or exclude SLE, but high-titre anti-native DNA antibody or anti-Sm antibody are important indications (Table 18.3). Anti-double-stranded DNA (anti-dsDNA) is peculiar to SLE, and about 70% of patients form antibodies against double-stranded RNA (anti-dsRNA), or against hybrid RNA/DNA molecules. Other autoantibodies (e.g. anti-SS-A and anti-SS-B) may be

---

Box 18.1 Investigation findings in systemic lupus erythematosus

- Antinuclear antibodies
    Anti-DNA antibodies, especially anti-double strandard DNA (Crithidial)
    Anti-RNA antibodies
- Circulating antibodies to platelets and other blood cells
- ESR raised
- Hypergammaglobulinaemia
- Hypocomplementaemia
- LE cell phenomenon
- Rheumatoid factor (30%)
- VDRL false-positive

helpful. About 40% of patients also have antibodies directed against phospholipid – about 15% of patients have antiphospholipid syndrome (APS, see later). Biopsies of skin or kidney using immunofluorescent staining techniques can support the diagnosis.

Systemic lupus erythematosus is characterized by 'flares' of activity interspersed with periods of improvement or remission, and it tends to remit over time. The titre of anti-DNA antibodies correlates well with disease activity.

Most patients appear to do well in the long term either with non-steroidal anti-inflammatory drugs (NSAIDs) or, if these are ineffective, on low doses of corticosteroids taken on alternate days. Antimalarials such as chloroquine appear to be effective for skin and joint lesions. Corticosteroids are useful to control acute manifestations and, together with immunosuppressive drugs (e.g. azathioprine), are used for potentially fatal complications such as renal involvement. Ciclosporin, 2-chlorodeoxyadenosine and rituximab may also be used. SLE has a 5-year survival rate of more than 90%.

Dental aspects

Surgery may exacerbate the symptoms and, if elective, should therefore be postponed until lupus activity subsides. Hospitalization may be required for otherwise minor procedures and post-operative discharge may be delayed.

Tetracyclines may cause photosensitivity rashes while sulfonamides or penicillins may cause deterioration in SLE. Bleeding tendencies are caused by thrombocytopenia: circulating anticoagulants rarely cause a bleeding tendency – rather they predispose to thrombosis. Other aspects to consider are corticosteroid or other immunosuppressive therapy (Ch. 35) renal disease (Ch. 12) and anaemia (Ch. 8).

Oral lesions, which typically consist of erythematous areas, erosions or white patches fairly symmetrically distributed, and resembling lichen planus, may be seen in 10–20% of patients with SLE and are rarely an early feature. Slit-like ulcers may also be seen near the gingival margins. The best management of erosive lesions of SLE in the oral mucosa is uncertain but corticosteroids, often in high doses, may be the only effective treatment. Biopsies of oral lesions show irregular epithelial thinning and acanthosis, basement membrane thickening, liquefaction degeneration of the basal cell layer and an irregularly distributed chronic inflammatory infiltrate. Vasculitis is inconstant. Immunofluorescent staining shows lumpy deposits of immunoglobulins and complement perivascularly and along the basement membrane of lesions, and under normal skin or mucosa in up to 90% of patients with SLE. Sjögren syndrome is associated in up to 30%. Antimalarials sometimes used to control SLE can cause lichenoid oral lesions or occasionally oral hyperpigmentation.

Drug-induced systemic lupus erythematosus

Drug-induced lupus (Table 18.5) has some features similar to those of SLE, particularly pleuropericardial inflammation, fever, rash, and arthritis and serological changes. The clinical and serological signs of LE usually subside gradually after the offending drug is discontinued.

Discoid lupus erythematosus

General aspects

Discoid lupus erythematosus (DLE) is essentially a mucocutaneous disease in which the rashes may be indistinguishable from those of SLE, but serological abnormalities are typically absent or minor, there are no serious systemic effects and it only rarely progresses to SLE.

Clinical features

Discoid lupus erythematosus is characterized by a rash, usually on the face or other sun-exposed areas, or mucosal lesions. The skin lesions are patchy, crusty, sharply defined skin plaques that may scar. DLE may cause patchy, bald areas on the scalp, and hypopigmentation or hyperpigmentation in older lesions. Arthralgia is a frequent complaint.

General management

Lesional biopsy will usually confirm the diagnosis. Topical and intralesional corticosteroids are usually effective for localized lesions; antimalarial drugs may be needed for more generalized lesions.

Table 18.5 Drugs associated with lupoid reactions	
Drugs with proven association with LE	**Drugs with possible association with LE**
Chlorpromazine	Beta-blockers
Hydralazine	Captopril
Isoniazid	Carbamazepine
Methyldopa	Cimetidine
Procainamide	Diphenylhydantoin (phenytoin)
	Ethosuximide
	Etanercept
	Methimazole
	Phenazine
	Quinidine

LE, lupus erythematosus.

Dental aspects

Oral mucosal lesions can be a feature of DLE and may also simulate lichen planus, but the lesions are less often symmetrically distributed and the pattern of striae is typically less well defined or conspicuous. Nevertheless, differentiation can be difficult and biopsy is essential. Even this may not be diagnostic and, occasionally, histological appearances intermediate between those of lichen planus and lupus erythematosus are seen. Management is as for the oral lesions of SLE but DLE may have some malignant potential.

RHEUMATOID ARTHRITIS (SEE CH. 16)

SJÖGREN SYNDROME

General aspects

Sjögren syndrome (SS) is the association of dry mouth (xerostomia) with dry eyes. It mainly affects middle-aged or older women. SS affects up to 5% of women and 0.5% of men.

Primary SS ('sicca syndrome') is the association of dry mouth with dry eyes (keratoconjunctivitis sicca) in the absence of any connective tissue disease. Secondary SS refers to the association of dry mouth and dry eyes, with another connective tissue disease – usually rheumatoid arthritis; less frequently, thyroiditis, primary biliary cirrhosis, systemic lupus erythematosus, progressive systemic sclerosis or polymyositis form part of this syndrome.

Sjögren syndrome is an autoimmune exocrinopathy. Lacrimal, salivary and other exocrine glands are infiltrated by lymphocytes and plasma cells, causing progressive acinar destruction and often multisystem disease. The aetiology may involve genetic factors: a range of loci have been implicated (Box 18.2).

> **Box 18.2 Some gene loci implicated in Sjögren syndrome**
>
> - HLA DQ DQ1, DQ2 and DQB1*02/DQB1*0602
> - Interleukin-10
> - Immunoglobulin kappa-chain allotype KM1
> - SS-A1
> - STAT4
> - Tumour necrosis factor

Anti-Ro and anti-La autoantibodies activate caspase-3 and apoptosis, which could be responsible for impaired salivary secretory function. In SS, several neuroendocrine system functions are also impaired. Raised T helper 1 (Th1) cytokines (IL-10 and IL-6) are seen in SS and correlate with the clinical manifestations of disease. High levels of cytokines from Th1 (IL-2, IL-2) and Th2 (IL-6, IL-10), and chemokines (CKs) CXCL13, CCL21 and CXCL12, which play roles in lymphoid tissue organization and the development of lymphoid malignancies, are expressed in salivary glands of patients with SS and mucosa-associated lymphoid tissue (MALT) lymphoma. CXCL13 is a B cell-attracting chemokine expressed in Sjögren syndrome.

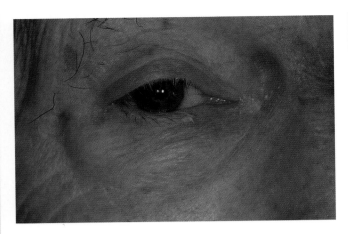

Fig. 18.4 Sjögren syndrome: dry eyes

Table 18.6 Sjögren syndrome				
Ocular	**Oral**	**Vaginal**	**Autoimmune disorders**	**Extraglandular disease**
Kerato-conjunc-tivitis sicca	Xerostomia Lobulated tongue Infections (candidosis, caries, sialadenitis)	Vaginal dryness	Mainly rheumatoid arthritis	Cutaneous Gastrointestinal Haematological Joints Neurological Pancreatic Psychiatric Pulmonary Renal Respiratory Reticuloendo-thelial Vascular

Clinical features

Sjögren syndrome is characterized by dryness of all mucosae but the most important effects are on the eyes, where drying causes keratoconjunctivitis sicca. This can lead ultimately to impairment or loss of sight. Patients with dry eyes may have no symptoms or may complain of grittiness, burning, soreness, itching or inability to cry. They may wake in the morning with a pustular exudate in the eyes, crusting at the canthus, or have infections of the lids (Fig. 18.4). Lacrimal and salivary glands may swell. Dry mouth can be a real complaint. Raynaud phenomenon or other autoimmune manifestations are common.

Multisystem disease can manifest with extraglandular complications, as shown in Table 18.6 and Fig. 18.5.

Extraglandular disease may precede exocrine problems by years and is found in 50% of SS-1. Fatiguability, fever and Raynaud disease are common early on; late complications include glomerulonephritis, lymphoma and skin problems (itching or cracking). Vaginal dryness causing painful intercourse is a frequent complaint. Lung disease can result from aspiration, or bronchial dryness. Bronchitis, tracheobronchitis and laryngotracheobronchitis are common. Renal disease (interstitial nephritis) is an important complication. Peripheral nervous system involvement may present with carpal tunnel syndrome, peripheral neuropathy and cranial neuropathy.

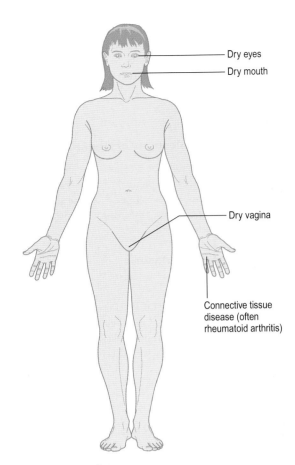

Fig. 18.5 Sjögren syndrome

Gastrointestinal complaints may include dysphagia, heartburn, abdominal pain and swelling, anorexia, diarrhoea and weight loss.

Autoimmune thyroid disorders can appear as either an overactive thyroid (Graves disease) or an underactive thyroid (Hashimoto thyroiditis). Nearly half of the people with autoimmune thyroid disorder also have SS, and many people with SS show evidence of thyroid disease.

Women who have SS can pass autoantibodies across the placenta into the fetal circulation, which can lead to heart block. Though it can be fatal, the long-term outlook for the child with heart block is generally good, but most require pacemakers, usually for life.

About 5% of people with SS develop lymphomas, mainly people with SS-1. Most (45–75%) are MALT lymphomas, usually affecting the parotid salivary glands. Risk factors for lymphoma are shown in Box 18.3.

Allergic drug reactions are frequent to penicillins and cephalosporins. Systemic reactions to trimethoprim present with CNS symptoms or aseptic meningitis. There are also rare associations of SS with a number of conditions (Box 18.4).

General management

Screening questions to assess oral and ocular symptoms (Box 18.5) may help identify patients with sicca syndrome. Dehydration, drugs, irradiation and infections can also cause dry mouth and dry eyes, and should be ruled out (Box 18.6).

Box 18.3 Risk factors for lymphoma in Sjögren syndrome

- Cryoglobulinaemia
- Hypocomplementaemia C4
- Monoclonal gammopathy
- Palpable purpura
- Peripheral neuropathy
- Persistent bilateral parotid swelling
- Reduced CD4 lymphocytes
- Vasculitis

Box 18.4 Rare associations with Sjögren syndrome

- Hereditary angioedema
- Primary amyloidosis
- Phenytoin
- Sarcoidosis
- Sweet syndrome
- Ulcerative colitis and selective IgA deficiency

Box 18.5 Screening questions for dry mouth and dry eyes

- Have you had a daily feeling of dry mouth for > 3 months?
- Have you had recurrently or persistently swollen salivary glands as an adult?
- Do you frequently drink liquids to aid in swallowing dry foods?
- Have you had a daily feeling of persistent troublesome dry eyes for > 3 months?
- Do you have a recurrent sensation of sand or gravel in the eyes?
- Do you use a tear substitute > 3 times a day?

Box 18.6 Conditions to be differentiated from Sjögren syndrome

- Drugs
- Irradiation
- Infections (hepatitis C, HIV and HTLV-1)
- Infiltrative diseases:
  - Amyloidosis
  - Haemochromatosis
  - Hyperlipoproteinaemias (types II, IV, V)
  - Sarcoidosis
  - Graft versus host disease

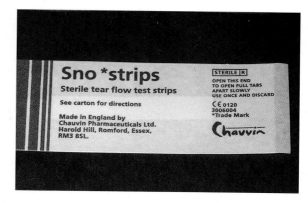

Fig. 18.6 Schirmer strip to test lacrimal flow

Labial gland biopsy is one of the most specific investigations. The parotid glands are chiefly affected but the changes are also usually present in the other glands, including the minor labial glands (such as in the lower lip). Labial gland biopsy is easier, safer and usually reflects the parotid changes.

Other investigations that may be helpful include sialography, magnetic resonance imaging (MRI) and ultrasound. Sialography, though non-specific and time-consuming, is helpful but is of course contraindicated if there is acute parotitis. Hydrostatic instillation of contrast medium typically shows a snowstorm appearance (punctate sialectasis) in well-established cases. Scintigraphy measures radioactive pertechnetate uptake and concentration in the major glands, but involves the use of radioisotopes, depends on the availability of specialized equipment and appears to have little place. Sialochemistry is theoretically helpful; SS alters the protein profile and brings about a change in the composition of saliva with an increase in the levels of lactoferrin, beta$_2$-microglobulin, sodium, lysozyme C and cystatin C, and a decrease in salivary amylase and carbonic anhydrase.

Diagnosis is based on criteria developed and revised by the American–European Consensus (Table 18.7).

Primary SS (SS-1) tends to be a more aggressive disorder than secondary SS (SS-2; Table 18.8). Management is largely symptomatic though there have been attempts at immunosuppression to control the disease process. This may increase the risk of lymphomatous change. Cyclophosphamide may help control renal and vascular disease, and polyneuropathy. Mizoribine, a nucleoside produced by *Eupenicillium brefedianum* with antibiotic, cytotoxic and immunosuppressive activity, may be effective. Mycophenolate, epratuzumab (anti-CD22 monoclonal antibody) and rituximab may be helpful. Of no real value are anti-TNF (infliximab), etanercept, ciclosporin, azathioprine, hydroxychloroquine, methotrexate and NSAIDs.

Lymphomas may best be diagnosed with high-resolution CT, MRI, MRI contrast sialography (gadolinium MRI with fat subtraction) or ultrasonography. They may respond to chemotherapy. Rituximab may also be used.

Dental aspects

Oral involvement in Sjögren syndrome results in discomfort caused by the poor salivary flow, obvious dryness of the mucosa in severe cases, and erythema and lobulation of the tongue.

No single investigation will reliably establish the diagnosis of Sjögren syndrome. An ophthalmological examination is important; a Schirmer test shows impaired lacrimation (Fig. 18.6). Salivary flow rates will confirm the presence and degree of xerostomia. Whole saliva collected without stimulation by allowing the patient to dribble into a sterile container over a measured period is now regarded as the best form of sialometry. A value below 1.5 ml/15 min is regarded as abnormal. Parotid output after stimulation with 10% citric acid can also be objectively determined using a suction (Lashley or Carlsson-Crittenden) cup over the parotid duct orifice or by cannulation of the duct but has no advantage. A value below 1.0 ml/min is regarded as abnormal.

Serum autoantibodies, especially antinuclear antibodies SS-A (Ro: Robair) or SS-B (La: Lattimer), are common and helpful diagnostically. Hypergammaglobulinaemia is seen mainly as a result of rheumatoid factor.

Table 18.7   Diagnostic criteria (American–European) for Sjögren syndrome

		Criteria
I Ocular symptoms	A positive response to at least one of the following questions:	1 Have you had daily ocular symptoms or persistent, troublesome dry eyes for > 3 months? 2 Do you have a recurrent sensation of sand or gravel in the eyes? 3 Do you use tear substitutes > 3 times a day?
II Oral symptoms	A positive response to at least one of the following questions:	1 Have you had a daily feeling of dry mouth for > 3 months? 2 Have you had recurrently or persistently swollen salivary glands as an adult? 3 Do you frequently drink liquids to aid in swallowing dry food?
III Ocular signs	That is, objective evidence of ocular involvement defined as a positive result for at least one of:	1 Schirmer's 1 test, performed without anaesthesia (< 5 mm in 5 min) 2 Rose Bengal score or other ocular dye score (> 4 according to van Bijsterveld's scoring system)
IV Histopathology	In minor salivary glands (obtained through normal-appearing mucosa)	Focal lymphocytic sialadenitis evaluated by an expert histopathologist, with a focus score > 1, defined as a number of lymphocytic foci (which are adjacent to normal-appearing mucous acini and contain more than 50 lymphocytes) per 4 mm² of glandular tissue
V Salivary gland involvement	Objective evidence of salivary gland involvement, defined by a positive result for one of the following:	1 Unstimulated whole salivary flow, 1.5 ml in 15 min 2 Parotid sialography showing the presence of ductal sialectasis (punctate, cavitary or destructive pattern) without evidence of obstruction in the major ducts 3 Salivary scintigraphy showing delayed uptake, reduced concentration and/or delayed excretion of tracer
VI Autoantibodies	Presence in the serum of the following autoantibodies:	Antibodies to Ro (SS-A) or La (SS-B) antigens, or both

For primary Sjögren syndrome (SS)
In patients without any potentially associated disease, primary SS may be defined as follows:
a The presence of any four of the six items is indicative of primary SS as long as item IV (histopathology) is positive, or
b The presence of any three of the four objective criteria items (i.e. items III, IV, V, VI)
c The classification tree method represents a valid alternative method for classification, although it should be used in a clinico-epidemiologic survey
For secondary Sjögren syndrome
In patients with a potentially associated disease (for instance, another well-defined connective tissue disease), the presence of item I or item II plus any two from among items III, IV and V may be considered as indicative of secondary SS.
Exclusion criteria
- Past head and neck radiation treatment
- Hepatitis C infection
- AIDS
- Pre-existing lymphoma
- Sarcoidosis
- Graft-versus-host disease
- Use of anticholinergic drugs (since a time shorter than fourfold the half-life of the drug)

Apart from its dryness, the oral mucosa may appear normal but the supervention of candidal infection causes redness and soreness.

The other main effects of persistent xerostomia can include difficulty in speaking, swallowing, or managing dentures, disturbed taste sensation and accelerated caries, and susceptibility to oral candidosis and to ascending (bacterial) sialadenitis.

Swelling of the parotid salivary glands is seen in a minority. Rarely, these glands can also be persistently painful. Late onset of salivary gland swelling, especially in sicca syndrome, may indicate development of a lymphoma (Box 18.3).

Dry mouth may be helped symptomatically by simple methods. Frequently sipping water or sugar-free drinks, sucking ice or using frequent, liberal rinses of a salivary substitute containing carboxymethyl cellulose or mucin may help.

Salivation may be stimulated by sialogogues. Pilocarpine 5 mg three times daily with meals, or pyridostigmine, may improve salivation if any functional tissue remains, but systemic effects such as diarrhoea and blurred vision may be troublesome and there may be dysrhythmias. Cevimeline is a newer alternative.

Simply chewing sugar-free gum or sucking citrus or malic acid lozenges may help salivation.

Preventive dental care is important. Patients have a tendency to consume a cariogenic diet because of the impaired sense of taste. This must be avoided and caries should also be controlled by fluoride applications. Use of a 0.2% chlorhexidine mouthwash will help to control periodontal disease and other infections. Denture hygiene is important because of susceptibility to candidosis; antifungal treatment is often also needed.

Infections should be treated. Generalized soreness and redness of a dry oral mucosa is typically caused by *Candida albicans* and often associated with angular stomatitis. Antifungal treatment is given as rinses of nystatin, or amphotericin mixture. Acute complications such as ascending parotitis should be treated with antibiotics. Pus should be sent for culture and antibiotic sensitivities but, in the interim, a penicillinase-resistant penicillin, such as flucloxacillin in combination with metronidazole, should be started because of the possible presence of anaerobes.

No crowns should be constructed until caries is controlled and there are no new lesions for more than 1 year.

Table 18.8 Sjögren syndrome – comparison of subtypes

Feature	Primary	Secondary
Other connective tissue disease	–	+
Ocular involvement	More severe	Less severe
Extraglandular manifestations	More common	Less common
Oral involvement	More severe	Less severe
Recurrent sialadenitis	More common	Less common
Risk of lymphoma	More common	Less common
HLA associations	HLA-DR3	HLA-DR4, HLA-B8
Rheumatoid factor	50%	90%
Anti-SS-A (Ro)	5–10%	50–80%
Anti-SS-B (La)	50–75%	1–5%
Rheumatoid arthritis precipitin (RAP)[a]	5%	75%

[a]Also known as SS-C.

Patients with SS who need dental treatment may not be good candidates for general anaesthesia because of the tendency to respiratory infections. It is important to lubricate the eyes and throat, to humidify the gases, to avoid drying agents (atropine, phenergan), to be conscious of the possibility of cervical spine involvement in rheumatoid arthritis, to maintain body heat (because of Raynaud disease) and to consider renal function.

There may also be problems in management related to the associated connective tissue disease and complicating factors such as anaemia (Ch. 8).

There is a higher incidence of drug allergies. Trimethoprim may induce a systemic reaction of fever, headache, backache and meningeal irritation (trimethoprim-induced aseptic meningitis).

MIKULICZ DISEASE

Mikulicz disease (MD) has been included in the differential diagnosis of SS-1, but it represents a unique condition with persistent lacrimal and salivary gland enlargement, few autoimmune reactions and good responsiveness to glucocorticoids, leading to the recovery of gland function. The diagnostic features are shown in Box 18.7.

> **Box 18.7 Diagnostic features of Mikulicz disease**
> - Visual confirmation of symmetrical and persistent swelling in more than two lacrimal and major salivary glands
> - Prominent mononuclear cell infiltration of lacrimal and salivary glands
> - Exclusion of other diseases that present with glandular swelling, such as SS, sarcoidosis and lymphoproliferative disease

Complications of Mikulicz disease include autoimmune pancreatitis, retroperitoneal fibrosis, tubulo-interstitial nephritis, autoimmune hypophysitis, and Riedel thyroiditis, in all of which immunoglobulin G_4 (IgG_4) is involved. Mikulicz disease thus differs from SS, and is associated with raised serum IgG_4 concentrations and a prominent infiltration of IgG_4-expressing plasmacytes in the lacrimal and salivary glands. Mikulicz disease is therefore now termed systemic IgG_4-related plasmacytic disease.

SCLERODERMA

General aspects

Scleroderma, from the Greek, means hard skin (*skleros* – hard; *derma* – skin), and is an uncommon disorder affecting about two in 10 000 people. It results from antinuclear antibodies against topoisomerase or centromeres causing fibroblasts to produce excess collagen. A gene that codes for fibrillin-1 may put some people at risk for scleroderma. Perivascular macrophage infiltration and endothelial cell damage with increased collagen and extracellular matrix are the main features.

Suspected triggers for scleroderma include viral infections (especially cytomegalovirus), drugs (e.g. taxanes or bleomycin), and adhesive and coating materials or organic solvents (e.g. vinyl chloride or trichloroethylene).

Women develop scleroderma at a rate up to ten times higher than men, possibly because of oestrogen: silicone breast implants have been blamed, but evidence has not been found for this.

Clinical features

Scleroderma can be localized, which can be incapacitating, or systemic, which affects a number of organs and can be life-threatening. *Localized scleroderma* is limited to the skin and related tissues and, in some cases, the underlying muscle, but never progresses to a systemic form.

Localized types of scleroderma are recognized. *Morphoea* (from the Greek for 'form' or 'structure') is characterized by local patches of scleroderma. The first signs of the disease are reddish patches of skin most often on the chest, stomach and back that thicken into firm oval-shaped areas. The centre of each patch becomes whitish with violet borders. These patches sweat very little and have little hair growth. Morphoea generally fades out in 3–5 years, but patients are often left with darkened skin patches and, in rare cases, muscle weakness.

Linear scleroderma (*coup de sabre* or 'sword cut') has a single line or band of thickened and/or abnormally coloured skin that usually runs down an arm or leg, but in some runs down the side of the face (Fig. 18.7).

Scleroderma (systemic sclerosis; SSc) involves deeper tissues (blood vessels and major organs) and often the skin. It appears in one of three forms.

Limited scleroderma typically comes on gradually and affects the skin only in certain areas: the fingers, hands, face, lower arms and legs, and many people with limited disease have CREST: calcinosis – calcium deposits typically on the fingers, hands, face and trunk, and on the skin above the elbows and knees; Raynaud phenomenon; (o)esophageal dysfunction; sclerodactyly – thick and tight skin on the fingers making it difficult to bend or straighten the fingers; and telangiectasias (Fig. 18.8).

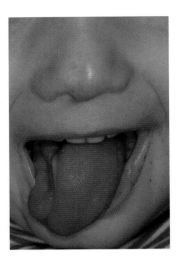

Fig. 18.7 Coup de sabre

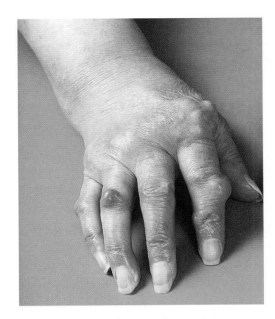

Fig. 18.8 CREST syndrome: calcinosis and Raynaud phenomenon are shown here

Diffuse scleroderma typically develops suddenly, affecting the hands, face, upper arms, upper legs, chest and stomach in a symmetrical fashion (e.g. if one arm or one side of the trunk is affected, the other is also affected). About one-third develop severe renal, pulmonary, gastrointestinal or cardiac disease.

Sine scleroderma resembles either limited or diffuse systemic sclerosis, causing changes in the lungs, kidneys and blood vessels, but not the skin. However, it is heterogeneous with two main subsets. One is a diffuse cutaneous form with early onset of pulmonary, cardiac and renal complications and associated in 30% with antitopoisomerase antibodies. The other is a limited cutaneous form of disease with somewhat similar features but with sclerosis limited to the skin, such as CRST, with late visceral complications, and often (70%) associated with anticentromere antibodies.

Systemic scleroderma classically presents with Raynaud phenomenon, often associated with joint pains (polyarthralgia), skin becoming thinned, stiff, tethered, pigmented and marked by prominent fine blood vessels (telangiectases or spider naevi) and eventually limiting movement. There is also dysphagia and reflux oesophagitis, and pulmonary involvement, which leads to impaired respiratory exchange and, eventually, dyspnoea and pulmonary hypertension, and renal damage secondary to vascular disease – typically a late feature leading to hypertension, and an important cause of death (Fig. 18.9). There appears also to be an increased incidence of cancer of the oesophagus and of oral cancer.

General management

Scleroderma should be differentiated from undifferentiated connective tissue disease, overlap syndromes, and eosinophilic fasciitis (EF; which involves the fascia causing muscles to become encased in collagen, with contractures, sometimes causing disfigurement and problems with joint motion and function).

Diagnostically useful autoantibodies include anticentromere antibodies (in up to 90% of people with limited systemic sclerosis) and antitopoisomerase-1 antibodies (in 40% of people with diffuse systemic sclerosis). PM-Scl antibodies suggest muscle involvement. Other laboratory findings are a raised ESR, normochromic anaemia and abnormal nailfold capillaroscopy.

There is no specific treatment, though hydroxychloroquine, methotrexate, ciclosporin, interferon-alpha and mycophenolate have been used; newer therapies include anti-transforming growth factor-beta (anti-TGF-beta), stem cell transplantation and antagonists to endothelin. Medications for specific problems include iloprost to treat pulmonary hypertension, cyclophosphamide for lung fibrosis, ACE inhibitors for scleroderma-related kidney disease and nifedipine for Raynaud phenomenon.

The 5-year survival rate in severe forms is about 50%.

Dental aspects

Some 80% of patients have manifestations in the head and neck region; in 30% the symptoms start there. Involvement of the face causes characteristic changes in appearance, notably narrowing of the eyes and mask-like restriction of facial movement (Mona Lisa face). Constriction of the oral orifice can cause progressively limited opening of the mouth (fish-mouth; Fig. 18.10). The submucosal connective tissue may also be affected and the tongue may become stiff and less mobile (chicken tongue).

The mandibular angle, condyle or coronoid process may be resorbed or rarely there is gross extensive resorption of the jaw. Occasionally, involvement of the peri-articular tissues of the temporomandibular joint together with the microstomia so limit access to the mouth as to make dental care and/or treatment more or less impracticable.

Sjögren syndrome develops in a significant minority, but very frequently when systemic sclerosis is associated with primary biliary cirrhosis. Since self-care can be challenging, and there may be xerostomia, it is not surprising that there are often more decayed, missing or filled teeth. Toothbrush handle

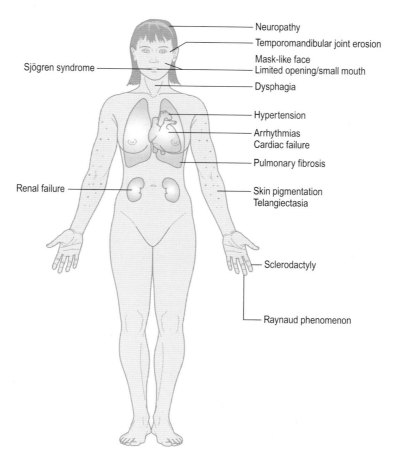

- Neuropathy
- Temporomandibular joint erosion
- Mask-like face
- Limited opening/small mouth
- Dysphagia
- Hypertension
- Arrhythmias
- Cardiac failure
- Pulmonary fibrosis
- Skin pigmentation
- Telangiectasia
- Sclerodactyly
- Raynaud phenomenon

Sjögren syndrome

Renal failure

Fig. 18.9 Scleroderma

modifications or powered brushes and flosses, fluorides, dietary control and management of dry mouth may help. The dental facility should be kept at a temperature and humidity that the patient finds comfortable. Otherwise, the main problems of systemic sclerosis are caused by dysphagia and pulmonary, cardiac or renal disease as potential contraindications for general anaesthesia.

A recognized but uncommon feature seen in fewer than 10% of cases is widening of the periodontal membrane space without tooth mobility. Trigeminal neuropathy may occur. There may be a predilection to carcinoma of the tongue.

Penicillamine therapy may cause loss of taste, oral ulceration, lichenoid reactions and other complications. Nifedipine for Raynaud phenomenon may cause gingival swelling.

A typical manifestation of morphoea is involvement of the side of the face causing an area of scar-like contraction aptly described as *coup de sabre*. Morphoea in childhood is believed to be one cause of facial hemiatrophy.

POLYMYOSITIS AND DERMATOMYOSITIS

General aspects

Polymyositis and dermatomyositis are rare immunologically mediated inflammatory myopathies. Polymyositis, if associated with skin lesions, is known as dermatomyositis. The conditions usually develop between the fifth and sixth decades, women being affected twice as often as men.

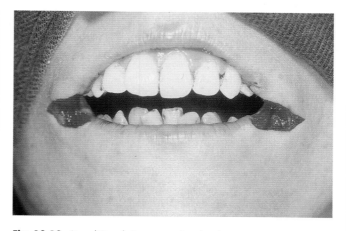

Fig. 18.10 Lip splitting during surgery in scleroderma

Clinical features

Polymyositis onset is characteristically insidious with pain and weakness, usually of the pelvic girdle and proximal limb muscles, especially the legs. Eventually, in severe cases, speaking and swallowing may become difficult and weakness may make patients bedridden. Ultimately, atrophy, contracture and calcinosis of muscles can develop. Other complications may include myocarditis and fibrosing alveolitis.

Dermatomyositis is characterized by a dusky and violaceous (Gottron, or heliotrope) rash with a butterfly distribution across the bridge of the nose and adjacent cheeks. This may spread to the upper part of the body or hands. Small ulcerated skin lesions may develop over bony prominences. In a minority, Raynaud phenomenon is associated and there can be features of other connective tissue diseases, particularly scleroderma, myasthenia gravis or Hashimoto thyroiditis, especially in those with dermatomyositis.

Malignant disease may arise, particularly in dermatomyositis, typically ovarian, lung, pancreatic, stomach and colorectal cancers, Waldenstrom macroglobulinaemia or non-Hodgkin lymphoma.

General management

Serum enzymes [aldolase, creatinine phosphokinase (CPK) and aspartate transaminase (AST)] may be raised, but the diagnosis is confirmed by electromyography (EMG) and muscle biopsy (shows muscle necrosis and regeneration and inflammation).

Treatment is with immunosuppressants (corticosteroids or others) but these are less effective when there is malignant disease.

Dental aspects

Dental management may be complicated by corticosteroid therapy or associated disorders such as other connective tissue diseases, including Sjögren syndrome. A minority have pharyngeal weakness.

Oral lesions in polymyositis/dermatomyositis may present in 10–20%, are variable in character and mainly comprise dark or purplish mucosal erythema and oedema. Small whitish patches occasionally with shallow ulceration may also develop and bear some resemblance to lichen planus or lupus erythematosus.

MIXED CONNECTIVE TISSUE DISEASE

Mixed connective tissue disease (MCTD) is an undifferentiated connective tissue disease presenting as a multisystem disorder with Raynaud phenomenon and features of two or more of the following connective tissue diseases: SLE, scleroderma and polymyositis. MCTD may evolve into one of several major connective tissue diseases or to an overlap syndrome.

Patients have anti-ribonucleoprotein antibody (anti-U1-68 kD antibody) but no anti-Smith autoantibody (anti-Sm Ab). Sjögren syndrome is the main complication of dental interest, but mouth ulcers or sensory changes may be seen.

ANTIPHOSPHOLIPID SYNDROME (HUGHES SYNDROME)

Antiphospholipid syndrome (APS) is characterized by persistently raised antibodies against membrane anionic phospholipids [i.e. the antiphospholipid antibodies (aPL), anticardiolipin antibody (aCL) and antiphosphatidylserine) or their associated plasma proteins, predominantly beta-2 glycoprotein I (apolipoprotein H). The antibodies are deposited in small vessels, leading to intimal hyperplasia and hypercoagulability due to lupus 'anticoagulant', causing venous or arterial thromboses in cerebral, renal, pulmonary, cutaneous and cardiac arteries.

Transient ischaemic attacks, migrainous headaches, Raynaud syndrome and livedo reticularis are thus common.

Primary APS is seen in isolation; secondary APS is associated with SLE or another connective tissue disease such as Sjögren syndrome.

Warfarin is the most effective treatment known. Thromboses or a bleeding tendency, pulmonary and systemic hypertension are the main factors possibly complicating dental care.

VASCULITIS

Immune complexes are complexes of interlocking antigens and antibodies that, under normal conditions, are rapidly removed from the bloodstream by splenic macrophages and liver Kupffer cells. When they continue to circulate, they become trapped in the kidneys, lung, skin, joints or blood vessels, activating complement and thus initiating vasculitis and tissue damage. Immune complexes may form in autoimmune diseases; in persistent low-grade infections (e.g malaria and viral hepatitis); or in response to environmental antigens, such as mouldy hay (e.g. farmer's lung) or drugs (e.g. serum sickness).

POLYARTERITIS NODOSA (PERIARTERITIS NODOSA)

General aspects

Polyarteritis nodosa (PAN) is a multisystem immune-complex disease characterized by necrotizing vasculitis affecting mainly small and medium-sized arteries, most frequent in middle-aged men. Antineutrophil cytoplasmic antibodies (ANCAs) appear to play a significant role in causing endothelial damage; perinuclear antineutrophil cytoplasmic antibodies (p-ANCAs; antimyeloperoxidase) are often are found in microscopic polyarteritis (MPA). Cytoplasmic ANCAs (c-ANCAs; antiproteinase 3) have also been described but are more often seen in Wegener granulomatosis. Increased serum interferon-alpha and IL-2, and a moderate rise in TNF-alpha and IL-1beta, may enhance endothelial damage by activating endothelial cells and polymorphonuclear neutrophil leukocytes (PMNLs).

The precipitating factor is often unidentified, but may be microbial or a drug. Hepatitis B virus has been implicated in up to 40% of patients, and other infective agents occasionally implicated include hepatitis C virus, human immunodeficiency virus (HIV), cytomegalovirus, parvovirus B19, human T-lymphotropic virus 1 (HTLV-1) or *Streptococcus* spp. Drugs (e.g. thiouracil, iodides and sulfonamides) may occasionally be responsible.

Clinical features

Polyarteritis nodosa has protean manifestations as a result of the capricious distribution of the lesions anywhere in the body. Fever, anorexia, weight loss, myalgia, arthralgia and peripheral neuropathies are common but non-specific. Abdominal involvement, with pain, nausea, vomiting or diarrhoea, is seen in over 60%. Renal disease affects 50%. Tender skin nodules may be palpable over inflamed vessels. Hypertension and angina are common.

General management

Leukocytosis, eosinophilia, raised ESR, pANCA hypergammaglobulinaemia and sometimes a false-positive test for rheumatoid factor may be found. Albuminuria or haematuria is common. Angiography may demonstrate arterial aneurysms (early PAN) or vascular occlusions (late PAN). Histological examination of clinically involved tissue is needed to confirm the diagnosis.

The prognosis is poor in untreated disease: up to 60% die within 1 year. Systemic corticosteroids give a 5-year survival of over 40%. Cyclophosphamide may also be of value.

Allergic granulomatosis is a closely related disease characterized by fever, asthma and eosinophilia.

Dental aspects

Dental management may be complicated by corticosteroid therapy and immunosuppression; hepatitis B antigen carriage; hypertension and cardiac disease; or renal disease. Submucosal nodules, haemorrhage or oral ulcers are rare manifestations. Facial palsy or other cranial neuropathies may be occasional complications.

WEGENER GRANULOMATOSIS

General aspects

Wegener granulomatosis (WG) is an uncommon, potentially fatal disease characterized by vasculitis associated with giant cells, necrotizing granulomatous lesions in the respiratory tract and glomerulonephritis. A limited form of the disease is confined primarily to the lung or oral cavity.

Wegener granulomatosis is an autoimmune inflammatory disease, involving antineutrophil cytoplasmic antibodies (c-ANCAs) directed at neutrophil proteinase 3 (PR-3). Neutrophils and endothelial cells are involved in early lesions as both targets and promoters of inflammation.

Many patients are nasal carriers of *Staphylococcus aureus*.

Clinical features

Wegener granulomatosis comprises the triad of nasopharyngeal inflammation, pulmonary cavitation and renal disease. Upper respiratory involvement typically presents as chronic sinusitis that fails to respond to treatment. The lungs are involved in more than 90% and the kidneys in 75%. It typically terminates in a focal necrotizing glomerulonephritis.

General management

In WG the cytoplasmic type of c-ANCA is found in more than 88% of patients and is virtually diagnostic. p-ANCA (directed at myeloperoxidase) is not found. Chest radiography and examination of urine for blood or sediment can indicate pulmonary or renal involvement. Biopsy shows inflammatory changes with giant cells. A necrotizing vasculitis is the main pathological feature but is not seen in gingival biopsies, where small arteries are lacking. This arteritis may, however, be seen in palatal lesions caused by downward spread of the disease from the nasopharynx. Granuloma formation is characteristic but the granulomas may be difficult to see.

Corticosteroids and cyclophosphamide are effective if given early enough. Trimethoprim–sulfamethoxazole may be effective used alone in disease restricted to the upper aerodigestive tract. In others it may mitigate some of the adverse effects of cytotoxic agents, and may prevent relapse. Etanercept and infliximab are under trial as therapies.

Dental aspects

Wegener granulomatosis can occasionally produce a characteristic and apparently pathognomonic form of gingivitis, where the gingivae are swollen, red and have a strawberry-like texture, as its initial manifestation,. Mucosal ulceration or delayed healing of extraction sockets are complications of the later stages of disease, particularly if renal failure develops.

Dental management may be complicated by renal failure, respiratory disease, or corticosteroid, other immunosuppressive or cytotoxic therapy.

FURTHER READING

Amital, H., Govoni, M., Maya, R., et al., 2008. Role of infectious agents in systemic rheumatic diseases. Clin Exp Rheumatol 26 (1 Suppl 48), S27–S32.

Barone, F., Bombardieri, M., Rosado, M.M., et al., 2008. CXCL13, CCL21, and CXCL12 expression in salivary glands of patients with Sjögren's syndrome and MALT lymphoma: association with reactive and malignant areas of lymphoid organization. J Immunol 180, 5130–5140.

Barry, R.J., Sutcliffe, N., Isenberg, D.A., et al., 2008. The Sjögren's Syndrome Damage Index – a damage index for use in clinical trials and observational studies in primary Sjögren's syndrome. Rheumatology (Oxford) 47, 1193–1198.

Bischoff, L., Derk, C.T., 2008. Eosinophilic fasciitis: demographics, disease pattern and response to treatment: report of 12 cases and review of the literature. Int J Dermatol 47, 29–35.

Boström, E.A., d'Elia, H.F., Dahlgren, U., et al., 2008. Salivary resistin reflects local inflammation in Sjögren's syndrome. J Rheumatol 35, 2005–2011.

Ceribelli, A., Cavazzana, I., Cattaneo, R., Franceschini, F., 2008. Hepatitis C virus infection and primary Sjögren's syndrome: a clinical and serologic description of 9 patients. Autoimmun Rev 8, 92–94.

Coaccioli, S., Giuliani, M., Puxeddu, A., 2007. The therapy of Sjögren's syndrome: a review. Clin Ter 158 (5), 453–456.

Derk, C.T., Rasheed, M., Artlett, C.M., Jimenez, S.A., 2006. A cohort study of cancer incidence in systemic sclerosis. J Rheumatol 33, 1113–1116.

Derk, C.T., Rasheed, M., Spiegel, J.R., Jimenez, S.A., 2005. Increased incidence of carcinoma of the tongue in patients with systemic sclerosis. J Rheumatol 32, 637–641.

Fedele, S., Wolff, A., Strietzel, F., López, R.M., Porter, S.R., Konttinen, Y.T., 2008. Neuroelectrostimulation in treatment of hyposalivation and xerostomia in Sjögren's syndrome: a salivary pacemaker. J Rheumatol 35, 1489–1494.

Hansen, A., Lipsky, P.E., Dörner, T., 2003. New concepts in the pathogenesis of Sjögren syndrome: many questions, fewer answers. Curr Opin Rheumatol 15, 563–570.

Ittah, M., Miceli-Richard, C., Gottenberg, J.E., et al., 2008. Viruses induce high expression of BAFF by salivary gland epithelial cells through TLR- and type-I IFN-dependent and -independent pathways. Eur J Immunol 38, 1058–1064.

Jorkjend, L., Bergenholtz, A., Johansson, A.K., Johansson, A., 2008. Effect of pilocarpine on impaired salivary secretion in patients with Sjögren's syndrome. Swed Dent J 32, 49–56.

Mathews, S.A., Kurien, B.T., Scofield, R.H., 2008. Oral manifestations of Sjögren's syndrome. J Dent Res 87 (4), 308–318.

Mignogna, M.D., Fedele, S., Lo Russo, L., Lo Muzio, L., Wolff, A., 2005. Sjögren's syndrome: the diagnostic potential of early oral manifestations preceding hyposalivation/xerostomia. J Oral Pathol Med 34, 1–6.

Moutsopoulos, H.M., Fragoulis, G.E., 2008. Is mizoribine a new therapeutic agent for Sjögren's syndrome? Nat Clin Pract Rheumatol 4, 350–351.

Porter, S., Scully, C., 2008. Connective tissue disorders and the mouth. Dent Update 35, 294–296, 298–300, 302.

Sakai, A., Sugawara, Y., Kuroishi, T., Sasano, T., Sugawara, S., 2008. Identification of IL-18 and Th17 cells in salivary glands of patients with Sjögren's syndrome, and amplification of IL-17-mediated secretion of inflammatory cytokines from salivary gland cells by IL-18. J Immunol 181, 2898–2906.

Salaffi, F., Carotti, M., Iagnocco, A., et al., 2008. Ultrasonography of salivary glands in primary Sjögren's syndrome: a comparison with contrast sialography and scintigraphy. Rheumatology (Oxford) 47, 1244–1249.

Shenin, M., Naik, M., Derk, C.T., 2008. The use of mycophenolate mofetil for the treatment of systemic sclerosis. Endocr Metab Immune Disord Drug Targets 8, 11–14.

Stewart, C.M., Bhattacharyya, I., Berg, K., et al., 2008. Labial salivary gland biopsies in Sjögren's syndrome: still the gold standard? Oral Surg Oral Med Oral Pathol Oral Radiol Endod 106, 392–402.

Thieblemont, C., de la Fouchardière, A., Coiffier, B., 2003. Nongastric mucosa-associated lymphoid tissue lymphomas. Clin Lymphoma 3, 212–224.

Triantafyllopoulou, A., Moutsopoulos, H., 2007. Persistent viral infection in primary Sjogren's syndrome: review and perspectives. Clin Rev Allergy Immunol 32, 210–214.

Triantafyllopoulou, A., Moutsopoulos, H.M., 2005. Autoimmunity and coxsackievirus infection in primary Sjogren's syndrome. Ann N Y Acad Sci 1050, 389–396.

Tzioufas, A.G., Tsonis, J., Moutsopoulos, H.M., 2008. Neuroendocrine dysfunction in Sjogren's syndrome. Neuroimmunomodulation 15, 37–45.

Tzioufas, A.G., Voulgarelis, M., 2007. Update on Sjögren's syndrome autoimmune epithelitis: from classification to increased neoplasias. Best Pract Res Clin Rheumatol 21, 989–1010.

Yamamoto, M., Takahashi, H., Ohara, M., et al., 2006. A new conceptualization for Mikulicz's disease as an IgG4-related plasmacytic disease. Mod Rheumatol 16, 335–340.

IMMUNITY, INFLAMMATORY DISORDERS, IMMUNOSUPPRESSIVE AND ANTI-INFLAMMATORY AGENTS

This chapter discusses innate and acquired immunity and inflammation, autoinflamatory disorders and immunosuppressive therapy.

INNATE IMMUNITY AND INFLAMMATION

Innate immunity includes basic mechanisms of resistance to infection such as epithelial anatomical barriers of skin and mucous membranes, cilia, secretions such as saliva and tears, and the innate inflammatory response. The latter is characterized by increased localized blood flow and capillary permeability (inflammation), releasing soluble factors which recruit phagocytes (neutrophils and macrophages) that restrict and engulf invasive micro-organisms.

Inflammation is initiated and maintained by mediators, especially complement and cytokines – small proteins that specifically also affect the behaviour of immune cells (immunocytes). Cytokines, including interleukins, lymphokines and cell signal molecules such as tumour necrosis factors and interferons, regulate the intensity or duration of immune responses by stimulating or inhibiting proliferation of various immunocytes, or by modulating their secretion of other cytokines or antibodies.

COMPLEMENT

The complement system is a plasma protein sequence (cascade) involving at least nine plasma proteins. When activated, this sequence releases important mediators of inflammation and chemotaxis (C3a and C5a), compounds capable of opsonizing micro-organisms for phagocytosis (C3b) and an attack complex (C5–9) capable of damaging cell membranes (Fig. 19.1). There are three complement pathways – classical, lectin and alternative – that differ in the manner in which they are activated [triggering agents include bacterial lipopolysaccharides (LPS), and immune (antigen/antibody) complexes], though all produce C3 convertase – the key enzyme. The system is controlled by inhibitors such as C1 esterase inhibitor, decay accelerating factor (DAF), membrane inhibitor of reactive lysis (MIRL) and homologous restriction factor (HRF).

CYTOKINES

Cytokines are a family of proteins – interferons, tumour necrosis factors, transforming growth factors (TGFs), interleukins (ILs), chemokines and colony-stimulating factors – which act in concert with inhibitors and soluble receptors to regulate immune responses.

Interferons (IFNs) are one of the most important natural defences against viral infection. IFN-alpha and IFN-beta are antiproliferative for virally infected and other cell types. IFN-gamma is involved in cell-mediated immune responses, via Th1 lymphocytes; is antagonistic to IL-4; activates macrophages; and induces expression of class II major histocompatibility complex (MHC) antigens.

Tumour necrosis factors (TNFs) are important in inflammation and antitumour immunity. *TNF-alpha* is secreted by a variety of cells, including T and B lymphocytes, macrophages, natural killer (NK) cells, endothelial cells and keratinocytes. TNF-alpha primes both endothelial cells and neutrophils for adhesion, is chemotactic for inflammatory cells and can signal cells to begin apoptosis (programmed cell death). It is a death activator, triggering the proteolytic caspase cascade that culminates in apoptosis. It can also activate NF-kB (nuclear

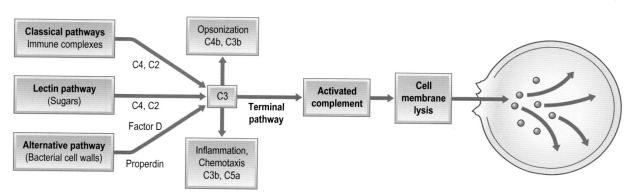

Fig. 19.1 Complement pathways

factor kappa B) and activator protein 1 (AP-1) leading to the induction of several genes and inflammation. It can also initiate and perpetuate an inflammatory response through up-regulating adhesion molecules on microvascular endothelial cells and enhance expression of MHC class I and II antigens, and co-stimulatory molecules on dendritic cells (DCs) and macrophages. Matrix metalloproteinase (MMP) production by stromal cells is induced, which may lead to tissue remodelling and the enhanced TNF-mediated secretion of keratinocyte growth factor (KGF). TNF can also induce fever, either directly via stimulation of prostaglandin E_2 (PGE_2) synthesis by the hypothalamic vascular endothelium, or indirectly by inducing release of the pyrogen interleukin 1 (IL-1) and can stimulate collagenase and PGE_2 production. TNF also induces hepatic acute-phase reactant protein production.

TNF-beta – from T and B cells, NK cells and astrocytes – mediates fibroblast and endothelial cell proliferation, important in wound healing.

Transforming growth factor beta (TGF-beta) is part of a protein superfamily that includes inhibins, activins and bone morphogenetic protein (BMP), which can affect development, haemopoiesis, wound healing and tissue repair. TGF-beta has a crucial role in cell-cycle regulation and apoptosis (regulated cell death), via the SMAD or the DAXX (death domain-associated protein) pathways.

Interleukins and their functions are diverse. Over 33 interleukins have been identified, most originating from T cells, some macrophages, mast cells, or from B cells or other cells (Appendix 19.1).

Cytokines that promote inflammation are termed pro-inflammatory cytokines; others are anti-inflammatory (Table 19.1).

Table 19.1 Main cytokines

Pro-inflammatory cytokines	Anti-inflammatory cytokines

Tumour necrosis factor (TNF-alpha)
Interferons (IFNs)
  – Alpha
  – Beta
Interleukins (ILs)
  – 1
  – 6, 15, 17 and 18
	IL-4, IL-10 and IL-11

CHEMOKINES (CHEMOATTRACTANT CYTOKINES)

Historically known under names such as the SIS family of cytokines, SIG family of cytokines, SCY family of cytokines, platelet factor-4 superfamily or intercrines, chemokines are classified into four groups (Box 19.1).

Box 19.1 Chemokines

- C chemokines – attract T-cell precursors to the thymus
- CC chemokines – induce migration of monocytes, dendritic and NK cells
- CXC chemokines – specifically induce the migration of neutrophils
- CX3C chemokines – chemoattractant and as an adhesion molecule

Colony-stimulating factors (CSFs) are glycoproteins that bind to haematopoietic cell receptors to drive differentiation. Those most relevant to the immune response are shown in Box 19.2.

Box 19.2 Colony-stimulating factors (CSFs)

- CSF1: macrophage CSF (M-CSF)
- CSF2: granulocyte–macrophage CSF (GM-CSF; sargramostin)
- CSF3: granulocyte CSF (G-CSF; filgrastim)

ACUTE-PHASE RESPONSE

In response to injury, infection, physical trauma or malignancy, neutrophils and macrophages secrete several cytokines (most notably IL-1, IL-6, IL-8 and TNF-alpha), which cause the liver to produce *acute-phase reactants* – proteins whose plasma concentrations increase in response to, and suppress, inflammation (Table 19.2).

C-reactive protein (CRP) and serum amyloid A protein (SAA) are critical in the innate immune response. CRP can bind to some bacteria and fungi, activating complement and inflammation, as can SAA, which can also stimulate macrophages to phagocytose debris. Most organisms that tend to be invasive are ingested by phagocytes, including blood neutrophils (polymorphonuclear neutrophilic leukocytes) and tissue macrophages ('phage' = eating up), which kill most organisms. However, some (i.e. all viruses, and bacteria such as those causing tuberculosis or brucellosis) survive inside cells, including phagocytes, and then the immune system is the main defence. Clinically, this positive acute-phase response appears within 12 h and can be measured by determining CRP levels or the erythrocyte sedimentation rate (ESR). The acute-phase

Table 19.2 Acute-phase reactants

Protein	Main functions
Alpha$_1$-antichymotrypsin	A serpin, which down-regulates inflammation
Alpha$_1$-antitrypsin	A serpin, which down-regulates inflammation
Alpha$_2$-macroglobulin	Inhibits coagulation and fibrinolysis
Caeruloplasmin	Inhibits microbial iron uptake
Complement	See text
C-reactive protein (CRP)	Binds to phosphorylcholine in bacterial membranes and phosphatidyl ethenolamine in fungal membranes activating the classical complement pathway
D-dimer protein	Fibrin degradation product
Factor VIII	Coagulation factor
Ferritin	Inhibits microbial iron uptake
Fibrinogen	Coagulation factor
Haptoglobin	Inhibits microbial iron uptake
Mannan-binding protein (MBP) or lectin (MBL)	Binds to microbial mannose-rich glycans to act as an opsonin, and also activates the lectin pathway
Plasminogen	Coagulation factor
Prothrombin	Coagulation factor
Serum amyloid A	Recruits immunocytes to inflammatory sites
von Willebrand factor	Coagulation factor

response is also characterized by leukocytosis, fever, and alterations in the metabolism of many organs. In contrast, there is a negative acute-phase response with decreases in albumin, transferrin, transthyretin and insulin growth factor I.

ACQUIRED IMMUNE RESPONSE

The main activity of the immune system is protection against infections. Immunocytes (leukocytes) are mainly lymphocytes and they produce humoral (antibody; mainly B-cell) or cell-mediated (mainly T-cell) responses that are central to the immune defences. B lymphocytes evolve into plasma cells, which produce antibodies to protect against extracellular organisms (Fig. 19.2). Antigens are processed by antigen-presenting cells (APC) and presented to T lymphocytes, which fulfil most other immune functions (i.e. cell-mediated immunity). Macrophages and polymorphs are the main professional phagocytes; macrophages and macrophage-like cells are widely distributed in the lymphoreticular (reticuloendothelial) system (Fig. 19.3).

More than 70 types of leukocyte are recognized and defined by their cluster of differentiation (CD) antigens, which in turn are recognized by monoclonal antibodies.

Immunocytes are, in large part, regulated by cytokines produced by a variety of cells. Cytokines produced by lymphocytes are termed lymphokines, and those that act between leukocytes are called interleukins (see Appendix 19.1). Cytokines may also induce systemic effects such as the acute-phase response (see above).

The movement of leukocytes between the blood and tissues depends on leukocyte–endothelial cell adhesion molecules known as selectins, integrins and the immunoglobulin gene superfamily [IgSF; intercellular adhesion molecules (ICAMs) and lymphocyte functional antigen 3], and over 20 other proteins.

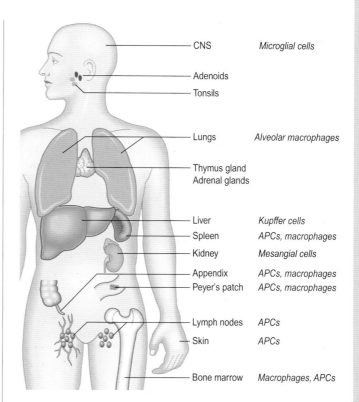

Fig. 19.3 Reticuloendothelial system. APCs, antigen processing cells

HUMORAL IMMUNITY

Antibodies are immunoglobulins. B cells carry surface immunoglobulins and also receptors for immunoglobulin G (IgG; CD32) and complement-activated components C3d (CD21) and C3b (CD35). Antibody production is modulated by T lymphocytes, which either assist (T-helper cells) or moderate (T-suppressor cells). The many cytokines involved include IL-1 to IL-7 and B-cell growth factor (BCGF). Immunoglobulins (antibodies) are of different classes (Table 19.3).

Complement and polymorphonuclear leukocytes (PMNLs) are essential to phagocytosis and inflammation. Cell-mediated responses are usually protective, and macrophages are also phagocytic.

PHAGOCYTES AND OTHER CELLS

Macrophages and dendritic cells intimately involved in antigen processing and the transference of information to lymphocytes are called antigen-processing cells (APCs). Phagocytes (PMNLs and macrophages) are attracted towards antigens, via activated

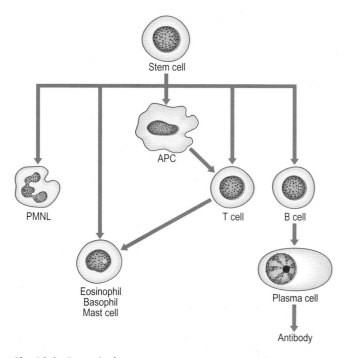

Fig. 19.2 Essentials of immunity

Table 19.3 Immunoglobulins

	Comments
IgA	Secreted by exocrine glands and helps to protect mucosal surfaces
IgD	Of unclear function
IgE	Important in the mediation of atopic allergy but has a role in the defence against parasites
IgG	Essential for protection against bacterial infections, by such functions as neutralizing toxins, activating complement, or promoting phagocytosis (opsonization)
IgM	

Table 19.4   Important prostaglandins (PGs)

Prostaglandin	Site of origin	Effects
PGD_2	Mast cells	Bronchoconstriction, vasodilatation and inhibition of platelet aggregation
PGI_2 (prostacyclin)	Endothelium	Vasodilatation and inhibits platelet aggregation
PGE_2	Epithelium, Dendritic cells	Inhibits lymphocyte proliferation, cytokine production and neutrophil function

Table 19.5   Leukotrienes (LTs)

Leukotriene	Causes
LTB_4	Neutrophil chemotaxis, mucus secretion, cell growth
LTC_4 (formerly termed slow-reacting substance A)	Vascular permeability, smooth muscle contraction, mucus production
LTD_4	
LTE_4	

complement after an antigen–antibody reaction, and can ingest and often kill microbes that are opsonized (i.e. coated by specific antibody and activated complement components). During phagocytosis or attempted phagocytosis of, for example, immune complexes, these phagocytes may discharge degradative enzymes (lysosomal enzymes), which can cause local tissue damage.

Large granular lymphocytes (LGLs; or null cells) are non-phagocytic cells that mediate natural killer (NK) cell activity and antibody-dependent cellular cytotoxicity (ADCC) – the binding and lysis of antibody-coated target cells. NK cells recognize malignant or foreign cells by a non-immune mechanism.

Basophils and mast cells have surface receptors for IgE, and contain histamine, prostaglandins, leukotrienes and proteases. They are involved in immune responses to parasites and in the immediate type of hypersensitivity responses (Ch. 17).

Prostaglandins (Table 19.4) and leukotrienes (Table 19.5) are produced from eicosanoids – lipids produced by the oxygenation of arachidonic acid from omega-3 fatty acids in fish oils, or released from cells by phospholipase A_2. The enzyme cyclooxygenase (COX) produces prostaglandins and thromboxane, while the enzyme 5-lipoxygenase produces leukotrienes.

CELL-MEDIATED IMMUNITY

Antigens are processed by antigen-presenting cells such as macrophages and Langerhans cells in epithelia and presented to T cells in association with class I or II MHC molecules. T lymphocytes originate in bone marrow but differentiate within and are under the control of the thymus (hence T), acquiring immunological competence there, a process which requires the normal functioning of purine metabolism. T cells all have T-cell receptors, highlighted by the CD3 surface marker. When

activated by antigens, T lymphocytes produce lymphokines, which, among other activities, can modulate nearby cells, particularly macrophages, resulting in cell-mediated immunity (type IV immune responses). These are particularly important in the defence against some intracellular bacteria, such as mycobacteria, and against viruses and fungi, graft rejection, graft-versus-host reaction, delayed hypersensitivity and defences against cancer cells.

Circulating T lymphocytes differentiate into CD4 cells – mainly helper T cells that are antigen-processing and can recognize MHC class II antigens, and can induce B-cell differentiation, induce CD8 cytotoxic T-cell proliferation, produce various soluble mediators (lymphokines) and regulate erythropoiesis. Healthy adults usually have CD4+ T-cell counts of 1000 or more per mm^3 of blood. CD4 helper T cells are either Th1 or Th2. Th1 cells secrete IL-2 and IFN-gamma, and provide help for the generation of cytotoxic T cells involved in type IV immune responses (Ch. 17) and are suppressed by IL-10. Th2 secrete IL-4, 5, 6 and 10, which both help B cells to produce IgG, IgA and IgE, and regulate the production of other cytokines – and thereby the immune response. Th2 cells are involved in type II and type III immune reactions and are suppressed by interferon.

Circulating T lymphocytes can also differentiate into CD8 cells, which recognize MHC class I antigens and are one type of cytotoxic or suppressor T cell, and are important in eliminating virus-infected cells.

To summarize, T-cell proliferation and differentiation is regulated by many cytokines, including interleukins, interferons, tumour necrosis factors and transforming growth factors. Cytokines generally function as local signals for cell growth, differentiation, activation, inhibition, apoptosis or chemotaxis, but may also induce systemic effects such as acute-phase responses (fever, CRP, osteoclast activation, platelet release) induced by IL-1, IL-6 and TNF.

EVALUATION OF B-LYMPHOCYTE FUNCTION

The initial screening for B-lymphocyte function is an assay of serum IgG, IgA and IgM. There are four subclasses of IgG, and selective deficiencies of these can develop. Thus, when there is a strong suspicion of a humoral immunodeficiency based on clinical grounds but the total IgG is normal, quantitative measurement of individual subclasses is indicated.

Assessment of antibody function is necessary. Antibody titres after immunization with protein antigens (e.g. tetanus or diphtheria toxoids) and polysaccharide (e.g. pneumococcal capsular polysaccharides) are most convenient (immunization with live viral vaccines must be avoided as the person may be immunocompromised). If immunoglobulin levels and/or antibody titres are low, more advanced tests of B-lymphocyte numbers and function are needed.

EVALUATION OF T-LYMPHOCYTE FUNCTION

Indirect information about T-lymphocyte function may be obtained by counting peripheral blood T lymphocytes. The total number of T lymphocytes (CD2 or CD3), T-helper lymphocytes (CD4) and T-suppressor/cytotoxic lymphocytes

(CD8) in peripheral blood can be quantified with appropriate monoclonal antibodies.

Delayed-type hypersensitivity (DTH) skin tests use a panel of ubiquitous antigens to screen for T-cell function. A positive test generally indicates intact T-cell function and cell-mediated immunity, but requires prior exposure and sensitization to the antigen, which may not have happened. Also, a positive DTH skin test to some antigens does not guarantee that the patient will have normal cell-mediated immunity (CMI) to all. Furthermore, some normal individuals may have transiently depressed DTH reactions during viral infections. Skin testing for DTH measures not only T-lymphocyte responses but also the afferent (receptor) arc of the cell-mediated immune response. Thus, most adults show DTH to tuberculin in the tuberculin (Mantoux) test, since they have had previous contact with *Mycobacterium tuberculosis* or BCG. A positive response in apparently well people is generally an index of 'waiting immunity' to the disease and usually does not mean that mycobacteria are actively causing cell-mediated tissue damage. A recent change from negative to positive in the absence of vaccination implies recent exposure, and prophylactic treatment may be indicated. By contrast, a negative tuberculin reaction indicates susceptibility to infection or occasionally that overwhelming infection is established – all CMI has been used up in an attempt to combat the infection. In such cases, successful treatment may allow CMI to return and a negative Mantoux test can then become positive.

It is possible also, in specialized laboratories, to measure several different cytokines involved in T- and B-lymphocyte regulation (e.g. IL-2, IFN-gamma).

EVALUATION OF PHAGOCYTIC FUNCTION

A white blood cell count and differential are the first essentials. Assessment of phagocyte function requires *in vitro* assays of directed cell movement (chemotaxis), ingestion (phagocytosis) and intracellular killing (bactericidal activity).

EVALUATION OF THE COMPLEMENT SYSTEM

Most complement components can be detected using antibody-sensitized sheep erythrocytes in a total haemolytic complement assay (CH50 assay), since this assay requires the functional integrity of C1 to C9. Deficiencies of alternative pathway components factors D, H and I and properdin can be detected by a haemolytic assay using activators of the alternative pathway, such as unsensitized rabbit erythrocytes. Individual components are detected by specialized functional and immunochemical tests.

AUTOINFLAMMATORY DISEASES (PERIODIC SYNDROMES)
GENERAL ASPECTS

The autoinflammatory diseases (periodic syndromes) are rare disorders of innate immunity, often hereditary, which involve an ongoing imbalance between factors promoting and those inhibiting inflammation. The abnormalities seen include aberrant responses to pathogen-associated molecular patterns (PAMPs), including lipopolysaccharide (LPS) and peptidoglycan; neutrophilia; and dysregulation of the pro-inflammatory cytokines IL-1beta, and/or TNF-alpha, or the receptors for these cytokines.

CLINICAL FEATURES

Periodic syndromes usually begin from childhood and are characterized by fluctuating or recurrent episodes of fever and generalized inflammation, affecting the surfaces, joints, eyes and/or skin.

Patients with the autoinflammatory syndromes generally are well between abrupt episodes of fever and systemic inflammation, but some develop amyloidosis.

GENERAL MANAGEMENT

Diagnosis is supported by evidence of elevated acute-phase response during attacks, and often a positive family history and ethnic background. Genetic testing is indicated. Many of the syndromes have a specific treatment (Table 19.6).

DENTAL ASPECTS

Aphthous-like oral ulceration has been reported as one manifestation in PFAPA (periodic fever, aphthous stomatitis, pharyngitis, adenitis), familial Mediterranean fever (FMF), hyperimmunoglobulinaemia D and periodic fever syndrome, TRAPS (tumour necrosis factor receptor-associated periodic syndrome) and PAPA (pyogenic sterile arthritis, pyoderma gangrenosum, acne).

Chronic recurrent osteomyelitis has been recorded in the jaws in chronic recurrent multifocal osteomyelitis. There is a suggested association of FMF with Behçet disease.

PERIODIC FEVER, APHTHOUS STOMATITIS, PHARYNGITIS, ADENITIS (MARSHALL SYNDROME)

PFAPA is not a familial disease. Attacks usually appear in pre-school children as recurrent fever with aphthous-like stomatitis, pharyngitis and cervical lymphadenitis. Long-term sequelae have not been reported and most children eventually grow out of it. Diagnostically, raised ESR, leukocyte count, fibrinogen and serum IgD have been found. PFAPA often responds well to corticosteroids, cimetidine or tonsillectomy.

IMMUNOSUPPRESSIVE THERAPY (SEE ALSO CHAPTER 35)

Where inflammation can become harmful, attempts can be made to suppress the immune response or block cytokine action. Most immunosuppressive drugs predominantly depress cell-mediated responses and autoantibody production more strongly than normal antibody production.

Immunosuppressive therapy is widely used especially to suppress rejection in transplant recipients (bone marrow, kidney,

Table 19.6 Main autoinflammatory syndromes

Disease	Inheritance	Acronym	Gene and protein defect	Main features apart from fever and rashes	Management
Familial Mediterranean fever	AR	FMF	MEFV	Serositis and synovitis, amyloidosis	Colchicine
Tumour necrosis factor receptor-associated periodic syndrome	AD	TRAPS	TNFRS1A	Abdominal pain, migratory myalgia, rash, and periorbital oedema, mouth ulcers, amyloidosis	Corticosteroids Etanercept (TNF inhibitor) Colchicine
Hyperimmunoglobulin D syndrome	AR	HIDS	MVK	Abdominal pain, diarrhoea, arthralgia, mouth ulcers	Simvastatin, anakinra (IL-1 receptor antagonist)
Mevalonate aciduria	AD	MA		Learning disability, failure to thrive, progressive visual impairment and cerebellar ataxia, dysmorphic features	Corticosteroids
Neonatal-onset multisystem inflammatory disease	AD	NOMID	CIAS1	Chronic meningitis, hearing and vision loss	Anakinra
Muckle–Wells syndrome	AD	MWS		Urticaria, arthralgia, deafness, amyloidosis	
Familial cold autoinflammatory syndrome	AD	FCAS		Urticaria, amyloidosis	
Pyogenic sterile arthritis, pyoderma gangrenosum, acne	AD	PAPA	PSTPIP1/CD2BP1	Arthritis, headache, abdominal pain, mouth ulcers	Anakinra Etanercept
Blau syndrome	AD	–	CARD15 or NOD2	Arthritis, uveitis	Anakinra
Periodic fever, aphthous stomatitis, pharyngitis, adenitis	Not known	PFAPA	Not known	Pharyngitis, adenitis, mouth ulcers	Corticosteroids Cimetidine
Chronic recurrent multifocal osteomyelitis	AD	CRMO	LPIN2 and Lipin2	Chronic recurrent multifocal osteomyelitis	Antimicrobials

AD, autosomal dominant; AR, autosomal recessive; IL, interleukin; TNF, tumour necrosis factor.
MIM, Mendelian inheritance in man classification; from OMIM (http://www.ncbi.nlm.nih.gov/sites/entrez?db=OMIM) and Scully et al. (2008).

liver, pancreas, heart and heart–lung; Ch. 35), to treat autoimmune and connective tissue diseases, and to control tumours – especially lymphoproliferative neoplasms (Ch. 8).

Immunosuppressive therapy inevitably predisposes patients significantly to infections, particularly viral, fungal, mycobacterial and protozoal infections, since T-cell immunity is largely depressed, and to malignant disease (Kaposi sarcoma, lymphomas and squamous cell carcinomas of the skin, cervix and lip), most of which are virally related. Infections may be opportunistic (i.e. involve micro-organisms that are normally commensal), spread rapidly and often may be clinically silent or atypical.

Now immunosuppressive strategies attempt to be more selective in their effects on the immune response using biologic agents designed to inhibit the harmful effects of up-regulated pro-inflammatory cytokines (e.g. TNF-alpha, IL-1 and receptor, IFN-beta, IFN-alpha, IL-6, IL-15, IL-17 and IL-18). Biologic agents are also termed targeted immune modulators (TIMs), and biological response modifiers (BRMs). Successful cytokine antagonists inhibit the effects of TNF. Examples of other successful agents are interferons and haematopoietic growth factors (colony-stimulating factors). Potential therapeutic strategies augment the activity of anti-inflammatory cytokines (e.g. IL-4, IL-10 and IL-11). However, biological response modifiers can have a high cost and significant adverse effects (infusion reactions, and liability to infection, including reactivation of latent tuberculosis and hepatitis B). The efficacy of murine human monoclonal antibodies can also be limited by the development of human antichimeric antibodies.

IMMUNOSUPPRESSIVE AND ANTI-INFLAMMATORY DRUGS

The main immunosuppressive agents include antimitotic drugs, anti-inflammatory drugs and biological response modifiers.

Antimitotic agents

Drugs such as azathioprine, cyclophosphamide and chlorambucil are cytotoxic to cells, including some immunocytes, act thus as fairly crude immunosuppressive agents and adverse effects are common (Table 19.7). Thiopurine methyltransferase (TPMT) should be measured before azathioprine therapy because, if this enzyme is depressed, bone marrow toxicity may result at low drug doses.

Anti-inflammatory drugs

Corticosteroids are anti-inflammatory by influencing glucocorticoid response elements to up-regulate anti-inflammatory genes/molecules such as lipocortin-1, IL-10 and IL-1ra. Lipocortin (macrocortin), a member of the annexin superfamily of proteins, acts to inhibit phospholipase A2 and so prevent

Table 19.7 Commonly used immunosuppressive agents

Drug	Mode of action	Main adverse effects	Main interactions with
Azathioprine	6-Mercaptopurine pro-drug. Metabolized by TPMT to the active mercaptopurine, which acts as a purine analogue that blocks nucleotides and DNA – reducing DNA synthesis and inhibiting lymphocyte division	Myelosuppression hepatotoxicity, leukopenia thrombocytopenia. Low TPMT increases myelosuppression risk. Infections, lymphoproliferative disorders, malignancies, teratogenicity	Allopurinol, cytostatic drugs, muscle relaxants, warfarin
Basiliximab	Antibody against CD25 T cells Anti-IL2R	Hypersensitivity reactions	–
Ciclosporin	Calcineurin inhibitor. Highly lipid-soluble drug, metabolized in the liver by cytochrome P450 enzymes (CYP3A4). Ciclosporin prevents dephosphorylation of NFAT (nuclear translocation of nuclear factor of activated T cells) and thus blocks cytokine IL-2	Neurotoxicity, hypertension, tremulousness, hypertrichosis, gingival swelling, hepatotoxicity, and nephrotoxicity with hyperkalaemia and/or renal tubular acidosis. No bone marrow effect, infections, lymphoproliferative disorders, malignancies, teratogenicity	Carbamazepine, phenytoin, isoniazid, rifampin, phenobarbital and other drugs that induce CYP3A4 may lower ciclosporin concentrations. Drugs may inhibit CYP3A4 may raise ciclosporin levels and risks of toxicity. Acute renal failure, rhabdomyolysis, myositis, and myalgias when taken concurrently with statin
Corticosteroids	May reduce inflammation by reversing increased capillary permeability suppressing PMNLs, and decreasing inflammatory cytokines	Hypertension, diabetes, osteoporosis and fractures, hip necrosis, cataracts, acne and obesity. Psychiatric effects, infections, lymphoproliferative disorders, malignancies, teratogenicity	–
Daclizumab	Antibody against IL-2 receptors	Hypersensitivity reactions	–
Dapsone	Blocks PMNL adherence, chemotaxis, prostaglandin E2 release, lysosomal enzyme release, and myeloperoxidase–hydrogen peroxide–halide-mediated cytotoxicity	Mainly haematological	Acetohydroxamic acid, Aminobenzoate potassium, Aminobenzoic acid, Clofazimine, Didanosine, Furazolidone, Methyldopa, Nitrofurantoin, Oral antidiabetics, Primaquine, Probenecid, Procainamide, Pyrimethamine, Quinidine, Quinine, Rifampin, Sulfonamides, Trimethoprim, Vitamin K
Mycophenolate mofetil	Inhibits inosine monophosphate dehydrogenase. Impairs cytotoxic T cells	Nausea, vomiting. No liver or kidney damage. More gastrointestinal, haematological effects and infections than azathioprine	Aciclovir, antacids, ganciclovir, cholestyramine
Sirolimus	A non-calcineurin inhibitor. Inhibits lymphocyte proliferation and impairs cytotoxic T cells	Hyperlipidaemia	Ch. 29
Tacrolimus	Calcineurin inhibitor similar to ciclosporin. Inhibits IL-2, IFN-gamma and IL-3 production; transferrin and IL-2 receptor expression; and cytotoxic T-cell generation through an immunophilin protein – the FK-binding protein (FKBP), which inhibits nuclear translocation of NFAT. Metabolized by same P450 system as ciclosporin	Hyperglycaemia, neurotoxicity and nephrotoxicity. Cardiomyopathy, if given with ciclosporin to children	Aciclovir, antacids, azathioprine, cholestyramine, probenecid Ch. 29

IFN, interferon; IL, interleukin; PMNL polymorphonuclear leukocyte; TPMT, thiopurine methyltransferase.

conversion of arachidonic acid to inflammatory substances, leukotrienes, prostaglandins and thromboxanes. COX-1 and COX-2 expression is also suppressed. Corticosteroids also induce the inhibitor of NF-kB subtype a (IkBa), reducing NF-KkB translocation to the nucleus and thus decreasing pro-inflammatory cytokines. Glucocorticoids also reduce microvascular permeability, mast cells and eosinophils. Adverse effects of steroids are shown in Box 19.3.

Box 19.3 Corticosteroid adverse effects

- Immunity: immunosuppression
- Adrenal: insufficiency
- Glucose: hyperglycaemia (increased gluconeogenesis, insulin resistance and impaired glucose tolerance – 'steroid diabetes')
- Obesity: appetite stimulation and weight gain – visceral and truncal fat deposition (central obesity), expansion of malar fat pads, increased plasma amino acids, increased urea formation, negative nitrogen balance
- Blood pressure: raised
- Skin: increased fragility, dilatation of small blood vessels and easy bruising
- Bone: reduced density (osteoporosis, osteonecrosis, higher fracture risk)
- Muscle: breakdown (proteolysis), weakness
- Reproductive: anovulation, menstrual period irregularity, pubertal delay
- Growth: failure
- Central nervous system excitation (euphoria, psychosis)
- Eyes: glaucoma, cataracts

Other drugs

Calcineurin inhibitors bind to immunophilins (cyclophilin and macrophilin) and block APC receptor expression, T-cell activation and cytokine release.

Ciclosporin has poor penetration when used topically and has a number of adverse effects if used systemically (nephrotoxicity, hypertension, gingival swelling) and may be co-carcinogenic.

Tacrolimus blocks APC receptor expression, T-cell activation, cytokines (IL-2, 3, 4, 5, 8; TNF, IFN, GM-CSF, ICAM-1, E selectin), IL-8 and IL-8R, PMNLs, mast cell/eosinophil recruitment and histamine release. Metabolized by liver CYP1A and CYP111A, it does not accumulate in blood or skin, and there are no drug interactions.

Pimecrolimus is a more potent immunosuppressant than ciclosporin, less potent than tacrolimus. It targets mast cells, and reduces serotonin and beta-hexosaminidase release.

Dapsone is anti-inflammatory by interfering with neutrophil adherence, chemotaxis, prostaglandin E2 release, lysosomal enzyme release or myeloperoxidase–hydrogen peroxide–halide-mediated cytotoxicity. Adverse effects are mainly haematological and can be pharmacological, dose-dependent, allergic or idiosyncratic (Table 19.8).

Mycophenolate mofetil, derived from *Penicillium stoloniferum*, is metabolized in the liver to the active mycophenolic acid, which inhibits inosine monophosphate dehydrogenase, in the *de novo* pathway of purine synthesis necessary for B and T cell proliferation. Common adverse reactions include diarrhoea, nausea, vomiting, infections, leukopenia, anaemia,

---

Table 19.8 Dapsone adverse effects and contraindications

Adverse effects	Haemolysis; more likely in glucose-6-phosphate dehydrogenase or methaemoglobin reductase deficiencies Long-term dapsone at standard doses (up to 100 mg/day) in normal patients causes methaemoglobinaemia of 15% (not clinically significant) via liver production of hydroxylamine Agranulocytosis; unpredictable and idiosyncratic: risk 25-fold greater in dermatitis herpetiformis, liver dysfunction, renal dysfunction, drug hypersensitivity syndrome; idiosyncratic, presents with fever Lymphadenopathy, rash, internal organ involvement (most commonly liver and haematological) Headaches, photosensitivity
Contraindications	Glucose-6-phosphate dehydrogenase deficiency, methaemoglobin reductase deficiency, anaemia, porphyria, liver disease, pregnancy and breast-feeding, allergies (to dapsone, naphthalene, niridazole, nitrofurantoin, phenylhydrazine, sulfa drugs, primaquine)

---

fatigue, headache and/or cough. Intravenous administration is commonly associated with thrombophlebitis and thrombosis. Infrequent adverse effects include oesophagitis, gastritis, gastrointestinal tract haemorrhage and/or invasive cytomegalovirus infection. Mycophenolate is usually used as part of a three-compound regimen of immunosuppressants, also including prednisolone and a calcineurin inhibitor.

Tetracyclines are anti-inflammatory by down-regulating pro-inflammatory cytokines; inhibiting matrix metalloproteinases (including collagenases MMP-1, MMP-8 and MMP-13); inhibiting prostaglandin synthesis; and inhibiting nitric oxide release (and minocycline inhibits caspase activation).

Zinc, iron and antacids can inhibit absorption. Tetracyclines can cause gastrointestinal discomfort, nausea, anorexia, photosensitivity, hypersensitivity, lupoid reactions or a serum sickness-type reaction. Tetracyclines are contraindicated in children, liver disease, lupus erythematosus, myasthenia gravis and porphyria.

Biological response modifiers (see also Chapter 35)

Biological response modifiers (BRMs) block the inflammatory and immune responses, acting on immunocytes directly or via cytokines. They inhibit cytokine behaviour, cellular activation and inflammatory gene transcription by various means. Some are antibodies, soluble receptors or natural antagonists; others are small molecules that specifically inhibit intracellular, cell–cell and cell–matrix interactions intrinsic to inflammatory and immune processes. Examples are shown in Table 19.9.

Labelled indications for use of BRMs include rheumatoid arthritis, ankylosing spondylitis, psoriasis, Crohn disease, ulcerative colitis and malignancies such as non-Hodgkin lymphoma. Off-label applications include pemphigus, recurrent aphthous stomatitis and Behçet disease ulceration, mucous membrane pemphigoid, lichen planus, orofacial granulomatosis and Sjögren syndrome. Epratuzumab may be a promising treatment for Sjögren syndrome. One of the advantages of BRMs is that they act specifically to neutralize targeted immune components so there *should be* relatively few adverse effects. They are administered by injection or infusion, and the most common adverse effect is a mild skin reaction at the injection site. Some patients have headaches during infusion, and there may be an increased susceptibility to infection – a serious risk to patients already prone to infection (e.g. diabetics) or who have an active infection (Table 19.10). Other long-term effects are not yet clear (see also Chs 29 and 35).

Table 19.9 Some biological response modifiers

Actions	Examples	Names
Antibodies against immunocytes	Anti-B-lymphocyte CD20, proliferation and activation	Rituximab
	Anti-T-lymphocyte migration and cytotoxicity	Alefacept Efalizumab
	Anti-CD3	Vizilumab
	Anti-T-cell activation	Abatacept
	Anti-CD22	Epratuzumab
Cytokine inhibitors	Anti-TNF	Adalimumab CDO571 Certolizumab Etanercept Infliximab Onercept
	Anti-IFN-gamma	Apilimod Fontolizumab
	IL-1 inhibitors	Anakinra
Others	Anti-IL-2 receptors	Basiliximab Daclizumab
	Anti-alpha$_4$-integrin	Natalizumab
	Selectin inhibitors	Efomycine

IFN, interferon; IL, interleukin; TNF, tumour necrosis factor.

Table 19.10 Biological response modifiers in current clinical use

Agent	Actions	Administration	Adverse effects	Monitoring
Adalimumab	TNF-alpha inhibitor (initiates complement-mediated cell lysis)	Subcutaneous	Respiratory tract infections, dizziness, headache, neurological sensation disorders, cough, nasopharyngeal pain, diarrhoea, abdominal pain, mouth ulcers, hepatic enzymes increased, rash, pruritus, musculoskeletal pain, injection site reaction, pyrexia, fatigue	Pre-treatment PPD screening, other recommended screening LFTs, FBC ANA, anti-ds DNA HBV, HCV, HIV
Alefacept	CD2 antagonist fusion protein impairs memory T cells	Intramuscular	Lymphopenia, malignancies, infections, hypersensitivity reactions	CD4+ T lymphocyte counts every 2 weeks
Anakinra	IL-1 inhibitor	Subcutaneous	Neutropenia, 'flu-like symptoms, infections	Pre-treatment PPD screening Blood platelets WBC Haemoglobin and haematocrit LFTs CRP Other

Table 19.10 Biological response modifiers in current clinical use—cont'd

Agent	Actions	Administration	Adverse effects	Monitoring
Efalizumab	CD11a inhibitor blocks interaction of LFA-1 and ICAM-1	Subcutaneous	Leukocytosis and lymphocytosis, 'flu-like symptoms, infections, hypersensitivity, psoriasis, arthralgia, arthritis, back pain, raised alkaline phosphatase, thrombocytopenia injection site reactions	Pre-treatment PPD screening Blood platelets WBC Haemoglobin and haematocrit LFTs CRP Other
Etanercept	TNF-alpha inhibitor; blocks TNF receptor	Subcutaneous	Infections, reactions at injection site, infections, allergic reactions, cardiac failure, lupus-like syndrome	Pre-treatment PPD screening/possible screening for FBC, LFTs, ANA and anti-ds DNA
Infliximab	TNF-alpha inhibitor (initiates complement-mediated cell lysis)	Intravenous	Infusion reaction and hypersensitivity, infections, respiratory infection, hepatitis B reactivation, serum sickness-like reaction, headache, vertigo, dizziness, nausea, abdominal pain, raised hepatic transaminases, urticaria, rash, hyperhidrosis, lymphoma and other malignancies	Pre-treatment PPD screening Possible monitoring and screening for: LFTs ANA and anti-DNA, HBV, HCV, HIV, FBC
Rituximab	Anti-CD 20 (depletes B cells)	Intravenous	Infections, HACAs (human anti-chimaeric antibodies), leukopenia, neutropenia, infusion-related reactions, angioedema, nausea Cardiac reactions, dyspnoea, bronchospasm, gastrointestinal effects, progressive multifocal leukoencephalopathy (PML) due to JC virus	FBC with differential and platelets, peripheral CD20+ cells HBV screening Signs or symptoms of PML (focal neurological deficits: hemiparesis, visual field deficits, cognitive impairment, aphasia, ataxia and/or cranial nerve deficits) Cardiac monitoring

ANA, antinuclear antibody; CRP, C-reactive protein; FBC, full blood count; HBV, hepatitis B virus; HCV, hepatitis C virus; ICAM, intercellular adhesion molecule; IL, interleukin; LFA, leukocyte functional antigen; LFT, liver function test; PPD, purified protein derivative, TNF, tumour necrosis factor; WBC, white blood cells.

USEFUL WEBSITES

http://en.wikipedia.org/wiki/Inflammation
http://users.rcn.com/jkimball.ma.ultranet/BiologyPages/I/Inflammation.html
http://www.textbookofbacteriology.net/innate.html
http://aids.about.com/od/otherconditions/a/immunerecon.htm
http://www.emedicine.com/emerg/TOPIC341.HTM
http://en.wikipedia.org/wiki/Immunosuppressive_drug

FURTHER READING

Ahmed, A.R., Spigelman, Z., Cavacini, L.A., Posner, M.R., 2006. Treatment of pemphigus vulgaris with rituximab and intravenous immunoglobulin. N Engl J Med 26 (355), 1772–1779.

Almoznino, G., Ben-Chetrit, E., 2007. Infliximab for the treatment of resistant oral ulcers in Behçet's disease: a case report and review of the literature. Clin Exp Rheumatol 25 (4 Suppl 45) S99–S102.

Antonucci, A., Negosanti, M., Tabanelli, M., Varotti, C., 2007. Treatment of refractory pemphigus vulgaris with antiCD20 monoclonal antibody (rituximab): five cases. J Dermatol Treat 18, 178–183.

Arin, M.J., Engert, A., Krieg, T., Hunzelmann, N., 2005. AntiCD20 monoclonal antibody (rituximab) in the treatment of pemphigus. Br J Dermatol 153, 620–625.

Arin, M.J., Hunzelmann, N., 2005. AntiB-cell-directed immunotherapy (rituximab) in the treatment of refractory pemphigus – an update. Eur J Dermatol 15, 224–230.

Atzeni, F., Sarzi-Puttini, P., Capsoni, F., Mecchia, M., Marrazza, M.G., Carrabba, M., 2005. Successful treatment of resistant Behçet's disease with etanercept. Clin Exp Rheumatol 23, 729.

Barnadas, M., Roe, E., Brunet, S., et al., 2006. Therapy of paraneoplastic pemphigus with rituximab: a case report and review of literature. J Eur Acad Dermatol Venereol 20, 69–74.

Berookhim, B., Fischer, H.D., Weinberg, J.M., 2004. Treatment of recalcitrant pemphigus vulgaris with the tumor necrosis factor alpha antagonist etanercep Cutis 74, 245–247.

Böhm, M., Luger, T.A., 2007. Lichen planus responding to efalizumab. J Am Acad Dermatol 56 (Suppl 5), S92–S93.

Bonilla, F.A., Bernstein, I.L., Khan, D.A., et al., 2005. Practice parameter for the diagnosis and management of primary immunodeficiency. Ann Allergy Asthma Immunol 94 (5 Suppl 1), S1–S63.

Canizares, M.J., Smith, D.I., Conners, M.S., Maverick, K.J., Heffernan, M.P., 2006. Successful treatment of mucous membrane pemphigoid with etanercept in 3 patients. Arch Dermatol 142, 1457–1461.

Chang, A.L., Badger, J., Rehmus, W., Kimball, A.B., 2008. Alefacept for erosive lichen planus: a case series. J Drugs Dermatol 7, 379–383.

Cheng, A., Mann, C., 2006. Oral erosive lichen planus treated with efalizumab. Arch Dermatol 142, 680–682.

Cianchini, G., Corona, R., Frezzolini, A., Ruffelli, M., Didona, B., Puddu, P., 2007. Treatment of severe pemphigus with rituximab: report of 12 cases and a review of the literature. Arch Dermatol 143, 1033–1038.

Devauchelle-Pensec, V., Pennec, Y., Morvan, J., et al., 2007. Improvement of Sjögren's syndrome after two infusions of rituximab (antiCD20). Arthritis Rheum 57, 310–317.

Diaz, L.A., 2007. Rituximab and pemphigus – a therapeutic advance. N Engl J Med 357, 605–607.

Dupuy, A., Viguier, M., Bédane, C., et al., 2004. Treatment of refractory pemphigus vulgaris with rituximab (antiCD20 monoclonal antibody). Arch Dermatol 140, 91–96.

España, A., Fernández-Galar, M., Lloret, P., Sánchez-Ibarrola, A., Panizo, C., 2004. Long-term complete remission of severe pemphigus vulgaris with monoclonal antiCD20 antibody therapy and immunophenotype correlations. J Am Acad Dermatol 50, 974–976.

Esposito, M., Capriotti, E., Giunta, A., Bianchi, L., Chimenti, S., 2006. Long-lasting remission of pemphigus vulgaris treated with rituximab. Acta Derm Venereol 86, 87–89.

Faurschou, A., Gniadecki, R., 2008. Two courses of rituximab (antiCD20 monoclonal antibody) for recalcitrant pemphigus vulgaris. Int J Dermatol 47, 292–294.

Fivenson, D.P., Mathes, B., 2006. Treatment of generalized lichen planus with alefacept. Arch Dermatol 142, 151–152.

Foulon, G., and others., 2004. Sarcoidosis in HIV-infected patients in the era of highly active antiretroviral therapy. Clin Infect Dis 38, 418–415.

Gartehner, G., Hansen, R.A., Thieda, P., Jonas, B., Lohr, K.N., Carey, T., 2005. Drug class review on targeted immune modulators. http://www.ohsu.edu/drugeffectiveness.

Gaya, D.R., Aitken, S., Fennell, J., Satsangi, J., Shand, A.G., 2006. AntiTNF-alpha therapy for orofacial granulomatosis: proceed with caution. Gut 55, 1524–1525.

Goh, M.S., McCormack, C., Dinh, H.V., Welsh, B., Foley, P., Prince, H.M., 2007. Rituximab in the adjuvant treatment of pemphigus vulgaris: a prospective open-label pilot study in five patients. Br J Dermatol 156, 990–996.

Gottenberg, J.E., Guillevin, L., Lambotte, O., et al., 2005. Club Rheumatismes et Inflammation (CRI). Tolerance and short term efficacy of rituximab in 43 patients with systemic autoimmune diseases. Ann Rheum Dis. 64, 913–920.

Graves, J.E., Nunley, K., Heffernan, M.P., 2007. Off-label uses of biologics in dermatology: rituximab, omalizumab, infliximab, etanercept, adalimumab, efalizumab, and alefacept (part 2 of 2). J Am Acad Dermatol 56, e55–e79.

Heffernan, M.P., Bentley, D.D., 2006. Successful treatment of mucous membrane pemphigoid with infliximab. Arch Dermatol 142, 1268–1270.

Heffernan, M.P., Smith, D.I., Bentley, D., Tabacchi, M., Graves, J.E., 2007. A single-center, open-label, prospective pilot study of subcutaneous efalizumab for oral erosive lichen planus. J Drugs Dermatol 6, 310–314.

Huang, W., Cordoro, K.M., Taylor, S.L., Feldman, S.R., 2008. To test or not to test? An evidence-based assessment of the value of screening and monitoring tests when using systemic biologic agents to treat psoriasis. J Am Acad Dermatol 58, 970–977.

Jackson, J.M., 2007. TNF-alpha inhibitors. Dermatol Ther 20, 251–264.

Jacobi, A., Shuler, G., Hertl, M., 2005. Rapid control of therapy-refractory pemphigus vulgaris by treatment with the tumour necrosis factor-alpha inhibitor infliximab. Br J Dermatol 153, 448–449.

Joly, P., Mouquet, H., Roujeau, J.C., et al., 2007. A single cycle of rituximab for the treatment of severe pemphigus. N Engl J Med 9 (357), 545–552.

Mariette, X., Ravaud, P., Steinfeld, S., et al., 2004. Inefficacy of infliximab in primary Sjögren's syndrome: results of the randomized, controlled Trial of Remicade in Primary Sjögren's Syndrome (TRIPSS). Arthritis Rheum 50, 1270–1276.

McAdam, A.J., Greenward, R.J., Levin, M.A., et al., 2001. ICOS is critical for CD40-mediated antibody class switching. Nature 409, 102.

Meijer, J.M., Pijpe, J., Bootsma, H., Vissink, A., Kallenberg, C.G., 2007. The future of biologic agents in the treatment of Sjögren's syndrome. Clin Rev Allergy Immunol 32, 292–297.

Mestas, J., Hughes, C.W., 2004. Of mice and men: differences between mouse and human immunology. J Immunol 172, 2731–2738.

Morrison, L.H., 2004. Therapy of refractory pemphigus vulgaris with monoclonal antiCD20 antibody (rituximab). J Am Acad Dermatol 51, 817–819.

Moutsopoulos, N.M., Katsifis, G.E., Angelov, N., et al., 2008. Lack of efficacy of etanercept in Sjögren syndrome correlates with failed suppression of tumour necrosis factor alpha and systemic immune activation. Ann Rheum Dis 67, 1437–1443.

Niedermeier, A., Wörl, P., Barth, S., Schuler, G., Hertl, M., 2006. Delayed response of oral pemphigus vulgaris to rituximab treatment. Eur J Dermatol 16, 266–270.

Pardo, J., Mercader, P., Mahiques, L., Sanchez-Carazo, J.L., Oliver, V., Fortea, J.M., 2005. Infliximab in the management of severe pemphigus vulgaris. Br J Dermatol 153, 222–223.

Peitsch, W.K., Kemmler, N., Goerdt, S., Goebeler, M., 2007. Infliximab: a novel treatment option for refractory orofacial granulomatosis. Acta Derm Venereol 87, 265–266.

Pijpe, J., van Imhoff, G.W., Spijkervet, F.K., et al., 2005. Rituximab treatment in patients with primary Sjögren's syndrome: an open-label phase II study. Arthritis Rheum 52, 2740–2750.

Robinson, N.D., Guitart, J., 2003. Recalcitrant, recurrent aphthous stomatitis treated with etanercept. Arch Dermatol 139, 1259–1262.

Sacher, C., Rubbert, A., König, C., Scharffetter-Kochanek, K., Krieg, T., Hunzelmann, N., 2002. Treatment of recalcitrant cicatricial pemphigoid with the tumor necrosis factor alpha antagonist etanercept. J Am Acad Dermatol 46, 113–115.

Sankar, V., Brennan, M.T., Kok, M.R., et al., 2004. Etanercept in Sjögren's syndrome: a twelve-week randomized, double-blind, placebo-controlled pilot clinical trial. Arthritis Rheum 50, 2240–2245.

Scheinberg, M.A., 2002. Treatment of recurrent oral aphthous ulcers with etanercept. Clin Exp Rheumatol 20, 733–734.

Schmidt, E., Herzog, S., Bröcker, E.B., Zillikens, D., Goebeler, M., 2005. Long-standing remission of recalcitrant juvenile pemphigus vulgaris after adjuvant therapy with rituximab. Br J Dermatol 153, 449–451.

Schmidt, E., Seitz, C.S., Benoit, S., Bröcker, E.B., Goebeler, M., 2007. Rituximab in autoimmune bullous diseases: mixed responses and adverse effects. Br J Dermatol 156, 352–356.

Scully, C., Diz Dios, P., Kumar, N., 2007. Special care in dentistry: handbook of oral healthcare. Churchill Livingstone Elsevier, Edinburgh.

Scully, C., Hodgson, T., Lachmann, H., 2008. Auto-inflammatory syndromes and oral health. Oral Diseases 14, 690–699.

Seror, R., Sordet, C., Guillevin, L., et al., 2007. Tolerance and efficacy of rituximab and changes in serum B cell biomarkers in patients with systemic complications of primary Sjögren's syndrome. Ann Rheum Dis 66, 351–357.

Sfikakis, P.P., Markomichelakis, N., Alpsoy, E., et al., 2007. AntiTNF therapy in the management of Behcet's disease – review and basis for recommendations. Rheumatology (Oxford) 46, 736–741.

Shetty, K., Achong, R., 2005. Dental implants in the HIV-positive patient – case report and review of the literature. Gen Dent 53, 434–437, quiz 438, 446.

Sommer, A., Altmeyer, P., Kreuter, A., 2005. A case of mucocutaneous Behçet's disease responding to etanercept. J Am Acad Dermatol 52, 717–719.

Steinfeld, S.D., Demols, P., Appelboom, T., 2002. Infliximab in primary Sjögren's syndrome: one-year follow up. Arthritis Rheum 46, 3301–3303.

Steinfeld, S.D., Demols, P., Salmon, I., Kiss, R., Appelboom, T., 2001. Infliximab in patients with primary Sjögren's syndrome: a pilot study. Arthritis Rheum 44, 2371–2375.

Steinfeld, S.D., Tant, L., Burmester, G.R., et al., 2006. Epratuzumab (humanised antiCD22 antibody) in primary Sjögren's syndrome: an open-label phase I/II study. Arthritis Res Ther 8, R129.

Stevenson, G.C., Riano, P.C., Moretti, A.J., Nichols, C.M., Engelmeier, R.L., Flaitz, C.M., 2007. Short-term success of osseointegrated dental implants in HIV-positive individuals: a prospective study. J Contemp Dent Pract 8, 1–10.

Strietzel, F.P., Rothe, S., Reichart, P.A., Schmidt-Westhausen, A.M., 2006. Implant-prosthetic treatment in HIV-infected patients receiving highly active antiretroviral therapy: report of cases. Int J Oral Maxillofac Implants 21, 951–956.

Tayal, V., Kalra, B.S., 2008. Cytokines and anticytokines as therapeutics – an update. Eur J Pharmacol 579, 1–12.

Vinuesa, C.G., Goodnow, C.C., 2004. Illuminating autoimmune regulators through controlled variation of the mouse genome sequence. Immunity 20, 669–679.

Vujevich, J., Zirwas, M., 2005. Treatment of severe, recalcitrant, major aphthous stomatitis with adalimumab. Cutis 76, 129–132.2

Appendix 19.1 Interleukins (ILs; modified from Wikipedia)

Name	Main sources	Functions
IL-1	Macrophages	Activates T cells. Induces IL-6. Generates prostaglandins. Induces acute-phase reaction, and fever
IL-2	Th1 cells	T-cell growth and apoptosis
IL-3	T cells	Haematopoietic cell growth
IL-4	Th2 cells, just activated naive CD4+ cell, memory CD4+ cells Mast cells	Proliferation of B cells, and development of T cells and mast cells. Important role in allergic response (IgE)
IL-5	Th2 cells	B-cell and eosinophil differentiation and IgA production
IL-6	Macrophages, Th2 cells	Activates many cells inducing acute-phase reaction and inflammation
IL-7	Stromal cells of the red marrow and thymus	B-, T- and NK-cell survival, development and homeostasis
IL-8	Macrophages, epithelial cells, endothelial cells	Neutrophil chemotaxis
IL-9	T cells, specifically by CD4+ helper cells	T-cell and mast cell growth
IL-10	Monocytes, Th2 cells, mast cells	T-cell and mast cell growth
IL-11	Bone marrow stroma	Plasma cell growth
IL-12	Macrophages	Induces interferon-gamma
IL-13	Th2 cells	Induces IgE
IL-14	T cells and certain malignant B cells	B-cell growth
IL-15	Mononuclear phagocytes (and some other cells) following infection by virus(es)	Induces production of T and B cells and NK-cell growth
IL-16	A variety of cells (including lymphocytes and some epithelial cells)	CD4 cell chemoattractant.
IL-17	T cells	Induces IL-6, IL-8 and granulocyte colony-stimulating factor inflammatory cytokines
IL-18	Macrophages, liver	Induces production of interferon-gamma
IL-19	T cells	–
IL-20	Monocytes	Regulates keratinocyte proliferation and differentiation
IL-21	T cells	Induces proliferation in NK cells and cytotoxic T cells
IL-22	T cells	Activates signal transducers and activators of transcription (STAT)1 and STAT3 and increases production of acute-phase proteins such as serum amyloid A, alpha$_1$-antichymotrypsin and haptoglobin in hepatoma cell lines
IL-23	Macrophages	Increases angiogenesis but reduces CD8 T-cell infiltration
IL-24	T cells, macrophages	Tumour suppression, wound healing and psoriasis
IL-25	Mast cells	Induces IL-4, IL-5 and IL-13 production, which stimulates eosinophil expansion
IL-26	T cells	Enhances IL-10 and IL-8 secretion and epithelial cell expression of CD54
IL-27	Dendritic cells	Regulates B- and T-lymphocyte activity
IL-28	Dendritic cells	Defence against viruses
IL-29	Dendritic cells	Defences against microbes
IL-30		Is one chain of IL-27
IL-31	T cells	Possible role in skin inflammation
IL-32	T cells	Induces monocytes and macrophages to secrete tumour necrosis factor-alpha, IL-8 and CXCL2
IL-33	Stroma cells, fibroblasts	Induces helper T cells to produce cytokines

-, Unknown; Ig, immunoglobulin; NK, natural killer.

IMMUNODEFICIENCIES

INTRODUCTION

Immunodeficiencies are states that result from a defect in the immune response. They are usually acquired (secondary immune defects) and rarely genetic (primary immune defects). They predispose to recurrent infections, especially of the skin, mucosae and respiratory tract (Fig. 20.1).

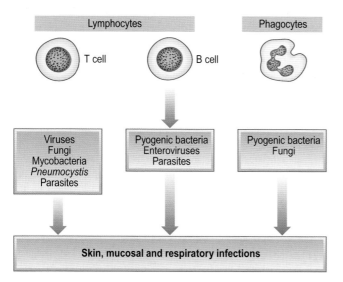

Fig. 20.1 Immune defects and infections

Human immunodeficiency virus (HIV) disease and the resultant acquired immune deficiency syndrome (AIDS) is a major immunodeficiency and public health issue worldwide. Other important causes of secondary immune defects are malnutrition and immunosuppressive therapy (Table 20.1).

Table 20.1 Causes of immunodeficiency

PRIMARY	SECONDARY	
Genetic	**Disease causes**	**Iatrogenic causes**
	Diabetes mellitus	Chemotherapy
	HIV disease	Immunosuppressive drugs
	Leukaemias	Radiotherapy
	Lymphomas	Splenectomy
	Neutrophil defects	

An immunodeficient patient is often somewhat ponderously referred to as an 'immunocompromised host'. The most important consequence of immunodeficiency is an abnormal susceptibility to infections, frequently caused by organisms of such low pathogenicity as rarely to affect the normal individual (opportunistic infections). Common infections are candidosis, herpetic infections and *Pneumocystis carinii* (*Pneumocystis jiroveci*) pneumonia (PCP; Table 20.2). Immunocompromised people are also prone to various neoplasms.

Infections vary in character as a consequence of the nature of the immune defect; the kinds of micro-organisms to which the patient is exposed; and attempts at treatment; for example, broad-spectrum antibiotics used to control bacterial infections increase the hazard of fungal infections.

Immunodeficiency diseases can affect any component of the immune system but often do not produce clinical pictures precisely predictable from the immune defect. Thus, in T-cell disorders (such as HIV disease), cell-mediated immunity is principally affected but antibody production may also be impaired.

HIV INFECTION AND AIDS

GENERAL ASPECTS

HIV (a lentivirus or retrovirus) infects CD4+ helper T lymphocytes causing AIDS after an average of 10 years in the untreated and has spread worldwide to create a global pandemic. AIDS was first recognized in 1981 in young male homosexuals in the USA. Sporadic cases have been identified as long ago as 1959 in central Africa (where the virus appears to have crossed the species barrier from chimpanzee monkeys). HIV is found worldwide and disease patterns are changing as a result of growing travel, and the emergence of new pathogens such as multidrug-resistant tuberculosis and exotic infections now appearing in temperate zones. Untreated, AIDS mortality rate is virtually 100%, although antiviral drugs can significantly impede its progress.

TRANSMISSION

HIV is transmitted mainly by body fluids, mostly by:

- sexual intercourse – saliva, semen and blood may contain HIV
- contaminated blood, blood products and donated organs
- contaminated needles – intravenous drug users and needlestick injuries in health care workers
- vertical transmission (mother to child) – *in utero*, during childbirth and via breast milk.

The virus is transmitted mainly by intimate sexual contact and can infect anyone who practises risky behaviours such as having sexual contact with an infected person or someone whose HIV status is unknown without using a condom. Sexual transmission of HIV is more likely during HIV seroconversion or in advanced AIDS, by receptive anal intercourse, or where

Table 20.2 Complications in immunodeficient or immunosuppressed patients

INFECTIONS				NEOPLASMS	OTHERS
Mucocutaneous	**Gastrointestinal**	**Respiratory**	**Meningitis; encephalitis**		
Herpes simplex	Cryptosporidiosis	*Pneumocystis carinii* (*Pneumocystis jiroveci*)	Creutzfeldt–Jakob agent	Kaposi sarcoma (KSHV)	Thrombocytopenia
Herpes zoster	Microsporidiosis	Aspergillosis	Papovaviruses	Lymphomas (EBV)	Lupus erythematosus
Cytomegalovirus	Isosporiasis	Candidosis	*Cryptococcus neoformans*	Squamous cell carcinoma (cervix, anus) (HPV)	Encephalopathy
Epstein–Barr virus (EBV)	Giardiasis	Cryptococcosis	*Toxoplasma gondii*		Drug allergies
Human herpesvirus 8		Histoplasmosis			
Human papillomaviruses		Zygomycosis (mucormycosis)			
Molluscum contagiosum		Strongyloidosis			
Non-tuberculous mycobacteria		Tuberculosis			
Candida species		Non-tuberculous mycobacterioses			
Staphylococcus aureus		Legionellosis			
Histoplasmosis		*Pseudomonas aeruginosa*			
		Staphylococcus aureus			
		Streptococcus pneumoniae			
		Haemophilus influenzae			
		Toxoplasmosis			
		Cytomegalovirus (CMV)			

there is genital ulceration. Saliva and breast milk may contain HIV, but transmission via the orogenital route is uncommon. Reports that HIV virions are present in a cell-free state in saliva have not been confirmed and saliva contains inhibitory factors. However, saliva transmission may result from human bites.

Heterosexual intercourse is the main transmission route worldwide, is an important route in developing countries in Africa and Asia, and is an increasingly important mode of transmission in the developed world, where it is responsible for 25–50% of cases. A major risk group in developed countries is still men who have sex with men (MSM). In the UK, the number of young men diagnosed with HIV has more than doubled in the last decade and, in 2008, almost half of new cases were infected through sex between men. With antiretroviral therapy, more people with HIV now survive and this, along with increasing use of the Internet to make contact with new partners; increasing substance abuse and use of medications to treat erectile dysfunction, and an increase in unsafe sexual practices, has resulted in a rise in the number of new cases of HIV infection – especially in MSM. Unfortunately, multidrug-resistant HIV (MDR-HIV) has now been recognized, with a rapid progression to AIDS.

HIV spread by contaminated needles and syringes is an important route in injecting drug users. Persons infected with HIV, especially those who abuse drugs intravenously or/and who are sexually promiscuous, may also be co-infected with other agents, including viruses, such as human T-lymphotropic viruses 1 and 2 (HTLV-1 and HTLV-2), hepatitis viruses and

other sexually transmitted infections (Ch. 32). Transmission by needlestick injury is an occasional risk for health care workers (see later).

Transmission of HIV can also occur via infected blood or blood products, including plasma, or tissues, such as in transplantation, but, in developed countries, screening of blood and plasma for HIV antibody, and heat-treatment of clotting factor concentrates has substantially reduced the risk. All HIV antibody-positive individuals are potentially infective and must not be allowed to donate blood, organs for transplantation or semen for artificial insemination. Some seronegative but infected blood (collected during the incubation period before antibodies are detectable) can still rarely transmit HIV. Haemophiliacs, initially a risk group for HIV, now form only a small proportion of HIV patients.

Children can contract HIV intrapartum or via breast milk; approximately one-quarter of all untreated pregnant women infected with HIV pass the infection to their babies, and the figure rises to one-third if the infant is breast-fed. Antiretroviral drugs reduce this transmission.

There is no reliable evidence for transmission of HIV by non-sexual social contact or by insect vectors such as mosquitoes or bedbugs. Studies of families of HIV-infected people have shown clearly that HIV is not spread through casual contact, such as the sharing of food utensils, towels and bedding, swimming pools, spas, telephones or lavatory seats.

Prevention of HIV/AIDS can thus be achieved by measures such as the use of condoms, the cessation of needle-sharing, screening blood and tissue before transfer to a recipient, and the use of antiretroviral drugs for children born to HIV-infected mothers.

EPIDEMIOLOGY

HIV-1, the most common virus, has spread to all continents to create a global pandemic with the most devastating consequences ever known to humankind. A further virus, HIV-2, which originated in Sooty Mangabee monkeys, predominates in West Africa, and has also now spread to many countries including Central Africa, Europe, the USA and South America, though at present there are few HIV-2 infections in developed countries.

An estimated 20 million people have died from AIDS since the epidemic was recognized. Estimates are that over 40 million HIV cases had developed worldwide by 2008 – more than one in every 100 sexually active adults. The difference between numbers estimated and reported is due to underdiagnosis (especially in the developing world), under-reporting and delayed reporting, and false extrapolation of basic information derived from Africa and men who have sex with men (MSMs).

Probably 75% of the cases worldwide are located in Africa, about 10% are in Latin America, about 7% in the USA, about 5% in Asia and slightly less in Europe. However, epidemics are progressing in Asia, especially India and China, and in Eastern Europe. In the USA, the Centers for Disease Control and Prevention (CDC) estimated that, by 2008, gay and bisexual men of all races were the group most heavily affected by HIV, accounting for 53% of all new infections, and the impact of HIV was greater among blacks than any other racial or ethnic group, with an HIV incidence rate seven times higher than that of whites and almost three times higher than that of Latinos. Currently, HIV infection is the commonest cause of death in US men aged 25–44 years, and the third commonest cause of death in women of this age. In the UK, by 2008 there were estimated to be 102,333 people infected with HIV and HIV infection is the fourth most common cause of death in men aged 25–44 years. Africa bears the greatest burden of disease.

PATHOGENESIS

The HIV viruses are ribonucleic acid (RNA) viruses. HIV-1 and HIV-2 differ in antigens and nucleic acids, but are transmitted similarly, have similar biological properties, and both are capable of causing disease. HIV-2 may progress more slowly and cause less profound immunosuppression. HIV-1/HIV-2 co-infection can occasionally be acquired. However, the remaining discussion relates to HIV-1.

HIV-1 can be classified into two major groups: M, which contains ten genetically distinct subtypes (A to J), and O, which contains several very heterogeneous viruses. The B virus is found in USA, Europe, and Central Africa.

HIV contains several so-called 'core' proteins and is surrounded by an envelope containing 'coat' proteins, one of which, env, recognizes the host cell CD4 receptor. HIV then binds to, and later damages, host cells bearing the T4 or CD4 receptor via the gp120 protein. CD4 cells are mainly helper-inducer T lymphocytes, monocytes and macrophages, Langerhans cells, brain glial cells and some colonic cells. Brain tissue, in particular the cells of monocyte–macrophage lineage, can become infected with HIV. Neurological damage may also be mediated by the production by HIV-infected macrophages of factors that affect neuronal cell function or neural transmitters. Most HIV is tropic for various chemokines such as CC CKR-5 (CCR5-tropic virus or R5), involved in HIV–cell attachment; a few patients appear able to resist infection, because of altered expression of this chemokine or the emergence of CXCR4-tropic virus strains (X4). Some HIV strains show dual-tropism. HIV-1 subtype B, CXCR4 co-receptor use ranges from approximately 20% in early infection to approximately 50% in advanced disease. HIV-1 subtype D does not use CXCR4. HIV-1 variants that use the co-receptor CCR5 for entry (R5; macrophage tropic) predominate in early infection, while variants that use CXCR4 emerge during disease progression. Some late-stage variants use CXCR4 alone (X4; T-cell tropic), while others use both CXCR4 and CCR5 (R5X4; dual tropic).

One coat protein, p24, is particularly antigenic. Antibodies to p24 form the basis for most serological testing (the HIV test). The coat proteins are subject to considerable variability, making vaccine development difficult. HIV also contains enzymes involved in its pathogenicity – reverse transcriptase (which can transcribe DNA from RNA, i.e. in the reverse direction, hence 'retrovirus') and proteases. These can be targets for therapy.

After primary infection with HIV, acute viraemia results in widespread dissemination of HIV and, in one third, in a clinical seroconversion illness resembling glandular fever (Table 20.3 and Fig. 20.2). The virus is trapped in follicular dendritic cells in lymphoid tissue germinal centres and there is expansion of a subset of CD8 cells that are precursors of HIV-specific cytotoxic T cells. Pro-inflammatory cytokines including interleukin-6 (IL-6), tumour necrosis factor, gamma-interferon and IL-10 are also overexpressed and may represent an unsuccessful attempt at protective response. Dendritic cells are involved in the initiation and propagation of HIV infection in CD4 cells.

Antibodies to HIV develop and appear in the serum within 6 weeks to 6 months from infection (seroconversion) but, within this window, the patient may be seronegative (though HIV may be detected by the polymerase chain reaction; PCR). The seroconversion clinical illness is a battle between the virus and the host. Usually the virus has been proliferating unchecked prior to this and therefore infectivity is maximal and thereafter wanes (although never dropping to zero).

After infection of CD4+ cells, there is usually a long asymptomatic period, but as HIV damages CD4 cells in the immune and nervous systems the risk of development of severe immunodeficiency, and symptoms of disease, rises with time. HIV damage to CD4+ lymphocytes leads to a lymphopenia over about 6 months to 10 years, a fall in the ratio of helper (CD4+) to suppressor (CD8+) lymphocytes, a profound defect in cell-mediated immune reactivity, and HIV disease, which manifests with infections (Fig. 20.2).

CLINICAL FEATURES

Infection with HIV may be staged according to its clinical features (Table 20.3). After primary infection with HIV an acute viraemia results in widespread dissemination of the virus. Antibodies to HIV develop and appear in the serum within

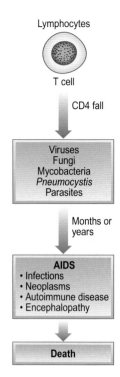

Fig. 20.2 HIV progression

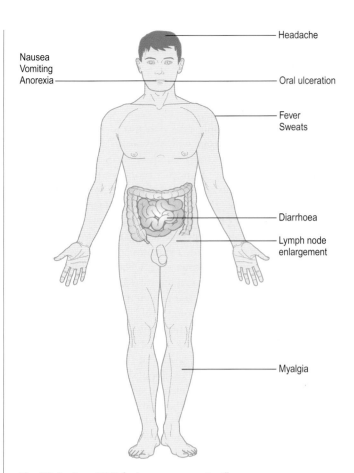

Fig. 20.3 Acute HIV infection – seroconversion illness

Table 20.3	CDC classification of HIV infection
CDC stage	**Presentation**
1	Primary seroconversion illness
2	Asymptomatic disease
3	Persistent generalized lymphadenopathy (PGL)
4a	AIDS-related complex (ARC) but no AIDS-defining conditions
4b–d	AIDS (AIDS-defining illness)

CDC, Centers for Disease Control and Prevention, Atlanta, Georgia, USA.

6 weeks to 6 months of infection (seroconversion). One-third of individuals develop a clinical seroconversion illness 3–6 weeks after infection, resembling glandular fever, sometimes with neurological involvement or with a rash or mouth ulcers. HIV infection may then remain asymptomatic for a median time of about 10 years. However, despite having circulating (and thus diagnostic) antibodies, people are also able to transmit the disease in the interim. Persistent generalized lymphadenopathy may become evident (Fig. 20.3).

As HIV infection of CD4+ cells leads to lymphopenia and the CD4 count falls to about 500/mm³, a variety of clinical syndromes appears (HIV disease). The CD4+ to CD8+ T-lymphocyte ratio falls. The common manifestations are mainly infections (Fig. 20.4), neoplasms, neurological and autoimmune disorders (Table 20.4).

The CDC definition of AIDS comprises a CD4 count of < 200/mm³ of blood in a patient infected with HIV and 26 clinical conditions that affect people with advanced HIV disease such as pulmonary tuberculosis (TB), *Pneumocystis*

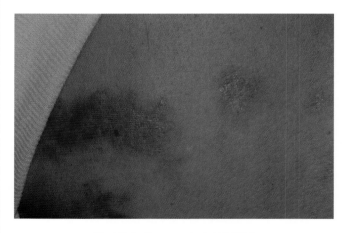

Fig. 20.4 Herpes zoster in HIV/AIDS

Table 20.4	Main manifestations of HIV/AIDS
Main manifestations	**Comments**
Opportunistic infections	Mainly fungal and viral
Neoplasms	Mainly Kaposi sarcoma and lymphoma
Neurological disorders	Mainly dementia
Autoimmune disorders	Mainly purpura

pneumonia, recurrent episodes of pneumonia or invasive cervical carcinoma.

Patients can develop a range of infections (viral, mycobacterial, fungal and parasitic), malignancies (malignant neoplasms, including melanoma, basal cell carcinoma, Kaposi sarcoma, lymphomas and squamous cell carcinomas of the skin and lip, and carcinoma of the cervix, external genitalia and perineum) and encephalopathy. Loss of weight and wasting is common in AIDS, and in Africa is called 'slim disease' (Figs 20.5 and 20.6).

The onset of AIDS may be influenced by the titre of HIV virus, patient age, gender, drug habits, immunogenetics and other factors. Clinical disease is most likely to appear when the CD4 counts fall to low levels, where the infected person has depressed defences for other reasons, such as malnutrition, and where there is exposure to potential pathogens.

In the developed world, about 20% develop AIDS within 5 years but a very few (about 2%) appear not to develop AIDS over periods as long as 15 years, mostly because they retain active cytotoxic T cells. Untreated, 50% of those infected have developed AIDS at 10 years. Nearly all the untreated will have developed AIDS at 20 years.

Some HIV-infected individuals have, or are vulnerable to, a host of co-morbid conditions, including other infections (e.g. fungal/viral infections, hepatitis, sexually transmitted infections, TB), substance abuse, mental illness and homelessness.

OPPORTUNISTIC INFECTIONS

Opportunistic infections are common and resistant to treatment.

Pneumocystis carinii (*Pneumocystis jiroveci*) pneumonia (PCP) is a lung infection seen in up to 80% of patients and is the immediate cause of death in up to 20% of patients dying with AIDS. Features include cough, dyspnoea, fever and malaise. Treatment of this fungus (previously thought to be a protozoon) is often with co-trimoxazole or pentamidine. Clindamycin/primaquine, atovaquone or dapsone/trimethoprim are alternatives. PCP is the most common opportunistic infection in people with HIV disease. People with CD4 cell counts under 200/mm³ have the highest risk of developing PCP.

Tuberculosis is particularly common in Africa and is spreading in the West where some 5% of patients now have lung infection with *M. tuberculosis*, which is increasingly multidrug resistant. TB can affect other sites, including the central nervous system (CNS). Since TB can spread by droplets, it is becoming a major public health problem.

Atypical mycobacteria are found in about 40% of AIDS patients in the West, though double that number are actually infected. Over 95% of these are *Mycobacterium avium* complex (MAC) infections – *M. avium* and *M. intracellulare*.

Toxoplasmosis, due to the protozoon *Toxoplasma gondii*, affects about 15% of AIDS patients, and particularly involves the CNS. It is treated with pyrimethamine and sulfadiazine.

Gastrointestinal protozoal infections (cryptosporidia, microsporidia, *Isospora belli*) often cause intractable diarrhoea.

Candidosis is extremely common in the mouth (Fig. 20.7) and vagina, and virtually all patients experience it. HIV infection should be suspected in a young or youngish person who develops thrush without any apparent precipitating factor.

Cryptococcus neoformans is a mycosis that is the main cause of meningitis in AIDS and is especially common in Africa. It is treated with amphotericin or/and an azole.

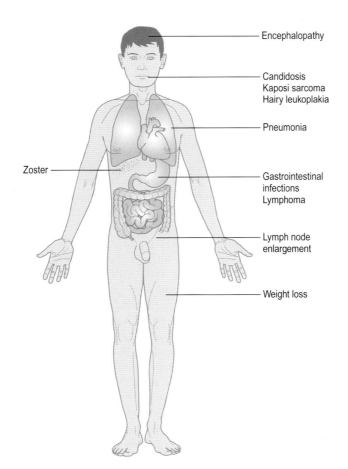

Fig. 20.5 AIDS

Encephalopathy

Candidosis
Kaposi sarcoma
Hairy leukoplakia

Pneumonia

Zoster

Gastrointestinal
infections
Lymphoma

Lymph node
enlargement

Weight loss

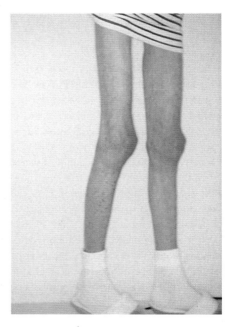

Fig. 20.6 Slim disease

455

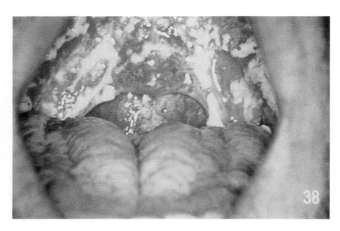

Fig. 20.7 Thrush

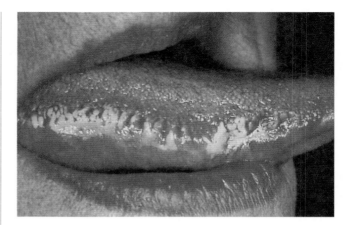

Fig. 20.8 Hairy leukoplakia

Histoplasmosis, usually as disseminated disease, affects mainly persons from endemic areas in the Americas. The same applies to coccidioidomycosis. They are treated with amphotericin or/ and an azole.

Penicillosis (infection with *Penicillium marneffei*) is seen in some areas of Thailand.

Herpes simplex can produce severe erosive lesions around the mouth, genitals, anus or other orifices and may be seen intra-orally and in the oesophagus. It can involve the skin and eyes. It is treated with aciclovir or foscarnet.

Herpes zoster can be severe, painful and incapacitating. It is treated with aciclovir or foscarnet.

Cytomegalovirus (CMV) is the most dangerous viral infection, capable of widespread lesions, especially ulceration throughout the gastrointestinal tract, and retinitis. It is treated with ganciclovir, foscarnet or cidofovir.

Epstein–Barr virus (EBV) is associated with oral hairy leuko-plakia (Fig. 20.8) and with lymphomas.

The pattern of infections associated with HIV infection varies geographically and with time. For example, histoplasmosis affects mainly AIDS patients from endemic areas of the USA and tuberculosis is seen mainly in AIDS in Africa.

NEOPLASMS

Various virally related neoplasms are seen in HIV/AIDS. *Kaposi sarcoma* (an otherwise exceedingly rare tumour of endothelial cells among elderly persons) is seen almost exclusively in sexually transmitted HIV infection in male homosexuals with AIDS and is associated with human herpesvirus-8 (HHV-8 or Kaposi sarcoma Herpes virus, KSHV). It accounts for about 80% of neoplasms in AIDS and often affects the gastrointestinal tract and skin, respiratory tract, mouth or lymph nodes. It is atypical in its early age of onset, distribution (particularly in the head and neck area) and greater malignancy (Fig. 20.9).

Lymphomas are also seen in AIDS, frequently affect the brain and are often related to EBV. Because the B cells are polyclonally stimulated by HIV, most lymphomas are non-Hodgkin B cell in type. A diffuse infiltrative lymphocytosis syndrome (DILS) can cause asymptomatic bilateral parotid swelling. Since patients with DILS can develop lymphomas, periodic observation is mandatory.

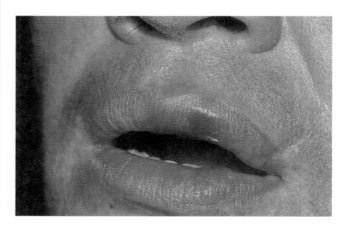

Fig. 20.9 Kaposi sarcoma

Carcinomas of the cervix and of the anus are increased in HIV disease, and due to human papillomaviruses (HPVs).

NEUROLOGICAL DISORDERS

HIV can cause a wide variety of neurological symptoms culminating in encephalopathy (AIDS-related dementia) and death. In addition, intracranial infections of many kinds (mainly parasitic, viral or fungal) are common. Up to two-thirds of AIDS patients develop a dementia complex, with personality changes, ataxia and convulsions; about 15% of AIDS patients develop CNS toxoplasmosis, while 10% develop cryptococcal meningitis. Spinal cord disease is seen in about 20% and may progress to bladder and bowel dysfunction.

Neurological manifestations can be acute, with fever, malaise, depression, fits, facial palsy and neuropathies affecting the extremities. Myelopathy or neuropathy can cause weakness of the legs, sometimes paraesthesiae and, in severe cases, ataxia and incontinence. Subacute encephalopathy affects about 30% of AIDS patients, who gradually develop a confusional state associated with fever and depression; the patient eventually may become bedridden and incontinent. Chronic meningitis may precede more typical features of AIDS and is characterized by fever, headache, meningeal signs and cranial nerve palsies (typically affecting nerves V, VII and VIII). Brain tumours, particularly lymphomas, are also common complications of

HIV/AIDS. Peripheral and cranial neuropathies, and myopathy, are relatively common.

AUTOIMMUNE DISORDERS

Autoimmune disorders, particularly thrombocytopenic purpura, are relatively common in HIV disease. Drug reactions are common, probably attributable to B-cell overstimulation and overproduction of antibodies, some of which form immune complexes to give rise to rashes and other manifestations of allergy. Most reactions are to co-trimoxazole and may cause erythema multiforme.

HIV INFECTION IN CHILDREN

Infection with HIV in children causes them to appear ill and stunted, and promotes staphylococcal and streptococcal infections, such as otitis media, rashes and diarrhoea as well as fungal and viral infections.

Normal CD4/CD8 ratios may persist late in the disease and lymphopenia is uncommon. Humoral immunity is more severely affected than in adult HIV disease and may long precede changes in T-lymphocyte subsets. Bacterial infections are relatively more common because of depressed humoral immunity. Generalized lymphadenopathy and hepatosplenomegaly are often the first signs and chronic parotitis is a common presenting feature. Neurological disease develops in the great majority. Interstitial lymphoid pneumonitis is particularly characteristic. Hypergammaglobulinaemia is also severe and 13% have thrombocytopenic purpura.

B-cell lymphomas are the most common tumours but Kaposi sarcoma is rare and particularly rarely affects the skin.

Other systemic effects of HIV infection in children include renal disease and cardiomyopathy.

GENERAL MANAGEMENT

The diagnosis of HIV infection is based upon a history of potential exposure to HIV (which may not be apparent) and the pattern of clinical presentation.

Preliminary screening comprises straightforward, routine investigations, which can identify gross abnormalities, such as full blood picture, including a differential leukocyte count, low CD4 count and reduced CD4:CD8 ratio and total serum protein levels. More specific investigation is by serology: serum antibodies to HIV may be detected by ELISA (enzyme-linked immunosorbent assay) or agglutination screening tests and a supplemental confirmatory test such as western immunoblotting.

Many infections are totally asymptomatic and the risk history may be unsuspected, being that of a partner. Diagnosis of HIV infection is from suspicion, especially if there is a supportive history, clinical criteria if present and, after appropriate professional counselling, by laboratory investigations. Lymphopenia, low CD4 counts in the blood and a low CD4:CD8 ratio from a normal value of about 2, to about 0.5 in AIDS, are typical but not specific findings. HIV infection must be confirmed by testing for HIV (with appropriate counselling of patients) and all results must be kept confidential. Relatives *cannot* give consent for an HIV test.

The 'AIDS test' is for serum HIV antibodies and usually involves ELISA and western blot assays. The ELISA or agglutination screening tests for serum antibodies to HIV are the first step. Antibodies are usually detectable from about 6–8 weeks after infection, and most persist for life. The ELISA test has a sensitivity of about 98% and a specificity of about 99% under optimal conditions. It is rapid and easy to use, but there may be false-positive or false-negative results, and therefore a positive ELISA result must be retested in duplicate samples and, if two or more of these three ELISA results are positive, a supplemental (confirmatory) test such as western immunoblotting must be used. A positive ELISA result with an indeterminate western blot result is not uncommon, and should be explored using nucleic acid assays. False-positives in both ELISA and western blotting are found in only about 1 in 100 000 tests.

Indirect immunofluorescence assay (IFA) can allow detection of HIV-specific immunoglobulin M (IgM) antibodies as soon as 5 days after the onset of acute HIV illness. IFA is as sensitive and specific as western blot, but does not permit precise delineation of specific patterns of antibody reactivity. Absence of HIV antibody usually, but not invariably, excludes HIV infection: there is a 'window' period when virus is present but the antibodies are not yet detectable. Some patients are infected with HIV but do not appear to produce detectable antibody to it, or lose it as AIDS develops. Therefore, antibody to HIV means that the patient has been infected with the virus; it implies a carrier state but does not indicate immunity to HIV. Conversely, the absence of antibody to HIV clearly does not always mean that infection is absent. In cases of doubt, HIV antigens or nucleic acid can be detected in the blood and earlier than antibodies. Techniques available to detect HIV nucleic acid can be used to clarify indeterminate western blot results. For example, PCR is very sensitive and able to detect HIV in seronegative persons. HIV can also be detected by viral culture or testing for the HIV reverse transcriptase enzyme (RT) but these are more difficult and lack the sensitivity and reproducibility needed for clinical work. However, they can reveal HIV-1/HIV-2 dual infection. It is important for diagnosis of HIV to apply at least two methodologically different assays for HIV infection; and repeat the test 2–3 months later. No patient with signs of HIV infection should be discharged as uninfected solely on the basis of one negative HIV test result and no patient should be told that they are HIV infected without the knowledge that the laboratory has confirmed the result of the test using the above criteria. Treat the results of any of HIV tests and a diagnosis of HIV infection or AIDS with confidentiality. Considerable care is needed regarding the social and psychological consequences of HIV infection.

ANTIRETROVIRAL MEDICATION

The mortality rate from AIDS was virtually 100% but, although there is still no effective treatment for the underlying immune defect, antiretroviral drugs which can significantly impede the progress of HIV infection include nucleoside analogues, non-nucleoside reverse transcriptase inhibitors, protease inhibitors, entry/fusion inhibitors and integrase inhibitors. Treatment with a combination of these drugs is termed active antiretroviral therapy (ART) or highly active antiretroviral therapy (HAART).

Early intervention with these drugs (Table 20.5) is usually beneficial.

Table 20.5 Antiretroviral agents most commonly used for HIV infection

Class	Examples
Combined formulations	Atripla, Combivir, Epzicom, Kaletra, Trizivir, Truvada
Entry/fusion inhibitors	Enfuvirtide, maraviroc
Integrase inhibitors	Raltegravir
Nucleoside and nucleotide reverse transcriptase inhibitors (NRTI)	Abacavir (ABC), didanosine, emtricitabine, lamivudine (3TC), stavudine, tenofovir, zalcitabine, zidovudine (AZT)
Non-nucleoside reverse transcriptase inhibitors (NNRTI)	Delavirdine, efavirenz, etravirine, loviride, nevirapine
Protease inhibitors (PI)	Amprenavir, atazanavir, darunavir, fosamprenavir, indinavir, lopinavir, ritonavir, saquinavir, tipranavir

See also http://aidsinfo.nih.gov/DrugsNew/Default.aspx and http://www.fda.gov/oashi/aids/virals.html

Patients on antiretroviral therapy are monitored by regular CD4 counts and plasma viral load levels, which correlate well with clinical response. Adverse effects are common and adherence to therapy is important to avoid the development of drug-resistant variants.

Patients with low CD4 counts are given antimicrobials as prophylaxis against opportunistic infections. Individuals should also be offered psychological support to help them come to terms with their illness and should be educated on measures necessary to prevent further spread of infection. At CD4 counts below 200/microlitre, patients are at high risk of *Pneumocystis carinii* infection, and at counts below 100/microlitre, CMV and *Mycobacterium avium–intracellulare* are risks.

ANTIMICROBIAL PROPHYLAXIS

Antimicrobial prophylaxis, therapeutic and supportive treatment may help prolong and improve the quality of life in HIV disease. Drugs available to help treat opportunistic infections are shown in Table 20.6.

Table 20.6 Antimicrobial agents for infections in HIV disease

Antimicrobial	Used for
Aciclovir	Herpes simplex and zoster infections
Foscarnet and ganciclovir	Cytomegalovirus infections
Fluconazole	Yeast and other fungal infections
Trimethoprim/sulfamethoxazole (TMP/SMX), atovaquone or pentamidine	*Pneumocystis carinii* pneumonia
Rifabutin	Prophylaxis against MAC infection
Isoniazid	Tuberculosis

MAC, *Mycobacterium avium* complex.

VACCINES

Attempts to produce a safe and effective vaccine against HIV encounter development problems not least because the proteins of HIV can undergo changes. Some candidate vaccines are currently in the initial phases of testing in humans. Post-exposure vaccination (e.g. with killed virus, envelope subunits or recombinant vaccinia vectors in combination with viral subunits) may have provided some clinical benefit, but long-term detailed trials are still required before it is known if such vaccines can provide reliable control of HIV.

IMMUNE RECONSTITUTION SYNDROME

General aspects

HIV damages the immune system, and so the inflammatory process is inhibited. However, this will return as the immune system is reconstituted by antiretroviral therapy sometimes with the appearance of symptoms that often resemble an AIDS-defining illness or other condition seen in people with HIV/AIDS. This is known as the immune reconstitution syndrome (IRS) or immune reconstitution inflammatory syndrome (IRIS). IRS development appears linked not only to increases in CD4 cells, but also to higher CD8 cell counts induced by HAART. Raised CD8 cells may be a prime factor contributing to worsening of both herpes zoster and hepatitis B or C symptoms after the initiation of HAART. Increased activity of IL-2 and IL-12 may contribute. Though most individuals starting HAART are not likely to experience IRIS, AIDS patients are more at risk if they are put on HAART for the first time, or if they have recently been treated for an opportunistic infection.

Clinical features

While IRS by definition heralds a return to a healthier immune system, a range of common conditions can occur or be exacerbated (Table 20.7) that can be serious, even fatal.

Table 20.7 Manifestations of immune reconstitution syndrome

Known infections	Other conditions
Cytomegalovirus	Aphthous-like ulcers
Cryptococcus	Castleman disease
Hepatitis viruses	Eosinophilic folliculitis
Herpes simplex	Graves disease
Herpes zoster	Myopathy
Histoplasmosis	Non-Hodgkin lymphoma (NHL)
Human herpesvirus 8	Progressive multifocal leukoencephalopathy
Leprosy	Sarcoidosis
Mycobacterium avium	Systemic lupus erythematosus
Papillomavirus	
Pneumocystis	
Tuberculosis	

The two common IRIS scenarios are the 'unmasking' of occult opportunistic infectious pathogens, which needs appropriate antimicrobial therapy, and the 'paradoxical' symptomatic relapse of a prior infection despite microbiological treatment success, which usually resolves spontaneously. Many cases of IRIS have atypical presentations. For example, the hallmarks of IRIS in a person previously responding to treatment for TB might be a new or worsening fever, new effusions, new or worsening lymphadenopathy, and other uncharacteristic reactions, rather than progression of lung disease itself. Mild shingles or a local *M. avium* infection without bacteraemia, both seen in IRIS, would be unusual in an HIV-positive person not taking HAART.

General management

Treatment of IRIS is continuation of the current HIV medication regimen; antimicrobial medications to treat infection and corticosteroids to temporarily suppress the inflammatory process.

POST-EXPOSURE PROPHYLAXIS (PEP)

Regular supervision in health care settings can help to diminish risk of occupational hazards in the workplace. The proper use of supplies, staff education and supervision needs should be firmly established in institutional policies and guidelines.

The risk of transmission of HIV from an infected patient through a needlestick (inoculation) injury is less than 1%, around one in 300 – far lower than the nearly 26% of persons who develop hepatitis B virus (HBV) or the 10% who contract hepatitis C virus (HCV) infection after needlestick injuries involving those agents. The risk for transmission from exposure to infected fluids or tissues is believed to be lower than from exposure to infected blood. If injury or contamination results in exposure to HIV-infected material, first aid, post-exposure counselling, treatment, follow-up and care should be provided (Fig. 20.10).

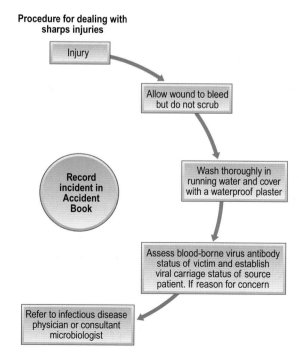

Procedure for dealing with sharps injuries

Injury

↓

Allow wound to bleed but do not scrub

↓

Wash thoroughly in running water and cover with a waterproof plaster

↓

Assess blood-borne virus antibody status of victim and establish viral carriage status of source patient. If reason for concern

↓

Refer to infectious disease physician or consultant microbiologist

Record incident in Accident Book

Fig. 20.10 Needlestick injury protocol

First aid should be given immediately after the injury. Wounds and skin sites exposed to blood or body fluids should be washed and mucous membranes flushed with water.

The exposure should be evaluated for potential to transmit HIV infection. The exposure source should be evaluated for HIV infection only after obtaining informed consent, and should include appropriate counselling and case referral. Clinical evaluation and baseline testing of the exposed health care worker should proceed only after informed consent.

PEP is by short-term antiretroviral treatment to lessen the likelihood of HIV infection after potential exposure and should be provided when a person has been exposed to HIV (or it is likely that the source person is infected with HIV). There may also need to be consideration of exposure to other blood-borne infections such as HBV.

PEP should be started as soon as possible after exposure to HIV. The medications used in HIV PEP depend on the level of exposure to HIV, and the selection of a drug regimen must balance the risk for infection against the potential toxicities of the agent(s) used. Because of the complexity of selection of HIV PEP regimens, consultation with persons having expertise in antiretroviral therapy and HIV transmission is strongly recommended. The following situations are considered dangerous exposure – for which PEP with antiretroviral drugs for 4 weeks is recommended:

- exposure to a large amount of blood
- blood contact with cuts or open sores on the skin
- blood visible on a needle that has been used on a patient
- exposure to blood from someone with a high viral load (a large amount of HIV in the blood).

The current UK Health Department recommended regimen for PEP provides updated guidance.

- PEP should be initiated as soon as possible after the exposure, ideally within an hour, following a careful risk assessment. In a change to previous guidelines, PEP is now generally not recommended after 72 h post-exposure.
- The recommended follow-up period after occupational exposure to HIV has been shortened and is now a minimum of 12 weeks after the HIV exposure or, if PEP has been taken, a minimum of 12 weeks from when PEP was stopped.
- The PEP regimen for starter packs is: Truvada (245 mg tenofovir and 200 mg emtricitabine (FTC)) once a day plus Kaletra (200 mg lopinavir and 50 mg ritonavir) twice a day is now recommended.
- A recommendation for good practice is that hospitals should have the capacity to obtain a source patient HIV test result within 8 h (ideally) and no longer than 24 h after blood is obtained. This is to minimize health care workers' exposure to PEP drugs where the source is found to be uninfected.

(See http://www.dh.gov.uk/en/Publicationsandstatistics/ Publications/PublicationsPolicyAndGuidance/DH_088185)

Current CDC guidance is similar and nelfinavir, which was once used, is no longer recommended, since some preparations are known to contain ethyl methane mesylate (EMS), a known animal carcinogen, mutagen and teratogen. This might be relevant to the choice of drugs included in an HIV PEP regimen because many health care personnel are female and many are of child-bearing age.

Confidentiality must be maintained. An exposure report should be made.

Exposure risk reduction education should be provided with counsellors reviewing the sequence of events that preceded the exposure in a sensitive and non-judgemental way.

DENTAL ASPECTS

It is unethical to withhold treatment from any patient on the basis of a moral judgement that the patient's activities or lifestyle might have contributed to the condition for which treatment was being sought.

The chief occupational risk of acquiring infection is as a result of injury by a sharp instrument, particularly a LA needle, which can contain a significant amount of contaminated fluid. Though needlestick injuries can transmit the virus, infection among dental health personnel caring for HIV-infected patients is rare despite reports of many such injuries. In most health care workers who have acquired HIV, the infection has been sexually transmitted. There have been, as yet (2008), only two reports of dental staff contracting HIV as a consequence of occupation, even in endemic areas.

The virus does appear to have been transmitted within health care facilities on rare occasions. One dentist with HIV infection in Florida, USA, appears to have transmitted it to at least six patients as a consequence of invasive dental procedures. That the dentist was the source of the infection was suggested by the fact that the strain of the virus was the same; the circumstances surrounding transmission remains uncertain as the dentist has since died. An outbreak of 14 cases of HIV infection was discovered in May 1993 among haemodialysis patients at a university hospital in Bucaramanga, Colombia, and seems most likely to have been transmitted by contaminated dental instruments. Many other studies, however, have shown no evidence of any transmission of HIV from HIV-infected dentists to patients.

Regarding orofacial manifestations, most patients with HIV disease have head and neck and oral manifestations at some time (Table 20.8). Oral lesions in HIV/AIDS are most likely to appear when the CD4 cell count is low and are often controlled, at least temporarily, by antiretroviral treatment. Oral features are classified as strongly, less commonly or possibly associated with HIV infection (Table 20.9). Cervical lymphadenopathy is an almost invariable feature at some stage of HIV disease and AIDS. Persistent generalized lymphadenopathy (PGL) is common.

Oral candidosis (usually thrush or erythematous candidosis) is common, often the initial manifestation and seen in 50% of patients. Oral candidosis is frequently associated with oesophageal candidosis and is also a predictor of liability to systemic opportunistic infections; the latter, but not the former, is an AIDS-defining illness. Conventional antifungal treatment is indicated initially, although fluconazole may be required, especially if there is oesophageal infection. Azole resistance is a growing problem.

Infections with herpes simplex virus, varicella zoster virus, cytomegalovirus, EBV, human herpesvirus 6 (HHV-6) and a herpesvirus associated with Kaposi sarcoma (KSHV or herpesvirus 8) are common. Herpes simplex infections are usually intraoral, sometimes severe and persistent, but rarely disseminate; they usually respond well to aciclovir. Severe herpes zoster may be seen. CMV may cause mouth ulcers. EBV has been implicated in hairy leukoplakia and some lymphomas (see later).

Hairy leukoplakia, though characteristic of HIV, can be seen very rarely in other patients, mainly those who are immunocompromised. It derives its name from the raised white areas of thickening, usually on the lateral borders of the tongue. The

Table 20.9 World Health Organization classification of oral lesions in HIV/AIDS

Group I lesions strongly associated with HIV infection	Group II lesions less commonly associated with HIV infection	Group III lesions possibly associated with HIV infection
Candidosis • Erythematous • Hyperplastic • Thrush (pseudo-membranous) Hairy leukoplakia (EBV) HIV gingivitis Necrotizing ulcerative gingivitis HIV periodontitis Kaposi sarcoma (HHV-8) Non-Hodgkin lymphoma (EBV)	Atypical ulceration (oropharyngeal) Idiopathic thrombocytopenic purpura Dry mouth • Salivary gland diseases • Unilateral or bilateral swelling of major salivary glands Viral infections (other than EBV) • Cytomegalovirus (CMV) • Herpes simplex virus (HSV) • Human papillomavirus (warty-like lesions; HPV): condyloma acuminatum, focal epithelial hyperplasia and verruca vulgaris • Varicella-zoster virus: herpes zoster and varicella	A miscellany of rare diseases

EBV, Epstein–Barr virus; HHV-8, human herpesvirus-8.

Table 20.8 Orofacial manifestations in HIV disease

Common	Less common	Rare
Cervical lymph-adenopathy	Herpes simplex	Mycobacterial ulcers
Candidosis	Herpes zoster	Cryptococcal ulcers
Hairy leukoplakia	Cytomegalovirus	Histoplasmal ulcers
Kaposi sarcoma	Human papillomavirus	Addisonian pigmentation
	Periodontitis and gingivitis	Osteomyelitis
	Aphthous-like ulcers	Cranial neuropathies
	Lymphomas	Other infections
	Parotitis	
	Xerostomia	

EBV capsid antigen can be identified in the prickle cell layer. It appears not to be pre-malignant. Less common oral and peri-oral infections include venereal warts. Mycobacterial oral ulcers and oral histoplasmosis or cryptococcosis, as well as sinusitis, gingivitis or periodontitis, may be seen. Major aphthae increase in frequency and severity with the severity of the immunodeficiency. Giant persistent aphthous-like ulcers respond to thalidomide (which needs to be given with caution and never to potentially pregnant women). Post-extraction infections, osteomyelitis after jaw fractures and cancrum oris (noma) have very occasionally been seen.

Kaposi sarcoma in 50% of patients is oral or perioral, and often an early oral manifestation, presenting as a red or purple macule or a nodule, usually on the palate. Oral and salivary gland lymphomas also develop more frequently in patients with AIDS than in a normal population; EBV is implicated.

In childhood HIV disease, chronic parotitis is common and virtually pathognomonic (Table 20.10). Chronic oral candidosis is present in 75% and is the single most common mucocutaneous manifestation. Most types of oral candidosis may be seen but most frequently in the form of persistent thrush. Difficulties in swallowing usually indicate candidosis of the oesophagus.

Unlike normal children, those with AIDS are frequently subject to recurrent intraoral as well as labial herpetic infection. Initially the infection responds to intravenous aciclovir but becomes more resistant as AIDS progresses. Shingles is rare in normal children, but can be an early sign of AIDS in a child, and tends to be more severe and painful.

HAART may affect the prevalence of some orofacial manifestations (Table 20.11) but may also cause adverse reactions (Table 20.12).

There is a move towards normalization and mainstreaming of oral health care provision, but many HIV-infected individuals have concerns about privacy; the additional stigma and social implications of their infection may prevent them from accessing general dental services – at least in their locality. It is therefore critical to ensure that there is a strict adherence to data protection and patient confidentiality – the patient should be reassured that any of their details will not be discussed, even with their physicians, unless permission is sought from the patient.

Caution is advised to minimize the risk of needlestick injury with LA. There is a theoretical interaction of LA with protease inhibitors, and protease inhibitors such as indinavir and nelfinavir can enhance benzodiazepine activity. Bleeding can be aggravated by non-steroidal anti-inflammatory drugs (NSAIDs) such as aspirin or indometacin; codeine and acetaminophen are safer analgesics (the interaction between acetaminophen and zidovudine, inducing granulocytopenia, appears rarely to be clinically significant).

Table 20.11 Effect of HAART on orofacial manifestations of HIV/AIDS

Declined	Increased
Candidosis	Salivary gland disease
Hairy leukoplakia	Warts and zoster
Kaposi sarcoma	Drug adverse effects

HAART, highly active antiretroviral therapy.

Table 20.10 Features, diagnosis and management of the more common orofacial lesions of HIV infection

Condition	Clinical features	Diagnosis	Management
Candidosis[a]	White removable lesions or red lesions, typically in the palate	Clinical plus investigations; smear, culture, rinse or biopsy	Antifungals (fluconazole most effective)
Hairy leukoplakia[a]	White non-removable lesions almost invariably bilaterally on the tongue	Clinical plus cytology; deoxyribonucleic acid (DNA) studies or biopsy	None usually but podophyllin or aciclovir effective
Periodontal disease	Linear gingival erythema, necrotizing gingivitis or periodontitis	Clinical	Oral hygiene, plaque removal, chlorhexidine, metronidazole
Herpesvirus ulcers	Chronic ulcers often on tongue, hard palate or gingivae. Zoster increased by HAART	Clinical plus investigations; cytology, electron microscopy, DNA studies or biopsy	Antivirals
Aphthous-like ulcers	Recurrent ulcers anywhere but especially on mobile mucosae	Clinical plus investigations; possibly biopsy	Corticosteroids or thalidomide or granulocyte colony-stimulating factor
Papillomavirus infections	Warty lesions, increased by HAART	Clinical plus investigations; DNA studies, possibly biopsy	Excise or remove with heat, laser or cryoprobe, imiquimod, interferon-alpha or podophyllin
Salivary gland disease	Xerostomia and sometimes salivary gland enlargement	Clinical plus investigations; sialometry, possibly biopsy	Salivary substitutes and/or pilocarpine or cevimeline
Kaposi sarcoma[a]	Purple macules leading to nodules, seen mainly in the palate	Clinical plus investigations; biopsy	Liposomal anthracyclines or paclitaxel chemotherapy. Vinblastine intralesionally. Alitretinoin gel, interferon-alpha intralesionally; cryotherapy and photodynamic therapy reportedly effective
Lymphomas	Lump or ulcer in fauces or gingivae	Clinical plus investigations; biopsy	Chemotherapy or radiation or both. Ifosfamide, mesna and rituximab on trial

[a]HAART (highly active antiretroviral therapy) or ART (active antiretroviral therapy) reduces manifestations.

Table 20.12 Most common orofacial adverse effects of antiretroviral treatment

	Erythema multiforme	Ulcers	Xerostomia	Taste alteration	Perioral paraesthesia	Facial lipodystrophy	Others
Zidovudine	+						Hp
Didanosine	+	+	+			+	
Zalcitabine	+	+	+			+	
Estavudine	+						
Lamivudine							
Abacavir							
Nevirapine	+	+					
Delavirdine	+		+	+			
Efavirenz	+						
Saquinavir	+	+	+		+	+	Ch
Ritonavir			+	+	+	+	
Indinavir			+	+	+	+	
Nelfinavir			+	+	+	+	
Amprenavir			+			+	
Lopinavir						+	

Hp, hyperpigmentation; Ch, cheilitis.

Of note, HIV disease has become a major risk factor for adverse drug reactions; the incidence of reactions to ampicillin is inversely proportional to CD4+ cell counts.

Medical consultation is mandatory for symptomatic HIV-infected patients before any dental surgical procedure, although no serious post-operative complications have been found in most instances. There have been no systematic studies involving dental implants, orthognathic surgery, periodontal therapy, prophylaxis, or scaling and root planing, and only one study on endodontics, which reported few immediate complications. Prospective studies on implants showed a 100% success rate at 6 months for both HIV and controls, with no difference in clinical outcomes. The prevalence of complications following tooth extractions in HIV-infected persons overall is estimated at about 5%, similar to that achieved in HIV-negative patients, and most complications are mild (alveolitis and delayed healing) and easily treated. Post-operative bleeding is unusual, even in thrombocytopenic patients. Factors increasing the potential for post-operative complications are shown in Box 20.1.

Immunologically stable (undetectable viral load and T-cell (CD4) count > 200/ml) HIV-positive patients on HAART may be considered low risk. However, patients with profound immunodeficiency (those with neutropenia and/or CD4 T-lymphocyte count < 200×10^6/L), may require antibiotic cover with metronidazole, amoxicillin plus clavulanic acid, or clindamycin before surgery or after maxillofacial injuries. Dental treatment should be carried out with the standard precautions and additional attention given to the possibility, though small, of post-operative infection and prolonged haemorrhage.

Patients with profound immunodeficiency may require antibiotic cover before surgery or after maxillofacial injuries.

Possible drug interactions with drugs used in oral health care are shown in Table 20.13.

Box 20.1 Factors increasing potential for post-operative complications

- Low CD4 count
- High viral load
- Low lymphocyte count
- Neutropenia
- Bleeding tendency (i.e. thrombocytopenia, liver damage, etc.)
- Another concomitant infection

Table 20.13 Possible drug interactions in HIV-infected patients

Drug used in oral health care	May interact with	Possible consequence
Miconazole Fluconazole Itraconazole Ketoconazole	Terfenadine (Astemizole and cisapride withdrawn because of interaction)	Arrhythmias and cardiotoxicity
Miconazole Fluconazole Itraconazole Ketoconazole	Anticoagulants	Anticoagulants potentiated
Miconazole Fluconazole Itraconazole Ketoconazole	Antacids Didanosine (DDI) H$_2$ antagonists Omeprazole	All impair absorption of the azoles
Benzodiazepines	Azoles Indinavir Ritonavir	All enhance benzodiazepines
Fluconazole	Rifabutin	Uveitis from rifabutin toxicity
Metronidazole	Ritonavir	Disulfiram-like reaction

IDIOPATHIC CD4 T-LYMPHOCYTOPENIA (ICL)

Idiopathic CD4 T-lymphocytopenia (ICL) is a rare syndrome that appears to represent a variety of disorders not related to HIV or any known transmissible agent but causes a generalized immunodeficiency state similar to that seen with HIV infection, with CD4 counts around 300/microlitre, but differs from HIV infection in that all lymphocyte cell lines tend to fall (low CD8 and B cells), and the lymphopenia is usually transient. In addition, immunoglobulin levels are normal or low.

There is no evidence for transmissibility, but ICL has been associated with many infectious entities not related to AIDS and with non-infectious diseases, such as autoimmune disorders, malnutrition, drugs and skin disorders. A total of 40% of patients with ICL have developed AIDS-defining illnesses, including cryptococcal meningitis, histoplasmosis and *M. avium* complex. Some persons are healthy but have had idiopathic CD4+ lymphocytopenia diagnosed by the more frequent screening for lymphocyte subsets. Finally, ICL does not progress and may even improve spontaneously.

OTHER SECONDARY IMMUNODEFICIENCIES

Worldwide, most immune defects are secondary and one of the most common causes is malnutrition. Immunosuppressive and other drugs, other iatrogenic causes and various chronic diseases are increasingly important (Table 20.14). Immunodeficiency can also be caused by hypercatabolism of immunoglobulin or excessive loss of immunoglobulins (nephrosis, severe burns, lymphangiectasia, severe diarrhoea).

AGRANULOCYTOSIS, LEUKOPENIA AND NEUTROPENIA

General aspects

Agranulocytosis – the name given to the clinical syndrome resulting from leukopenia or neutropenia – is characterized by abnormal susceptibility to infection and oropharyngeal ulceration.

Leukopenia – low levels of circulating functional leukocytes, either in absolute numbers or as functionally effective cells – is a feature of cytotoxic drug therapy and many diseases.

Neutropenia – low levels of circulating functional polymorphonuclear leukocytes, either in absolute numbers or as functionally effective cells – is also a feature of cytotoxic drug therapy and many diseases. Some cases are genetically determined.

These states can develop in isolation or they can be associated with other effects of depressed marrow function, notably anaemia and bleeding tendencies, as in acute leukaemia and aplastic anaemia (Table 20.15).

Clinical features

There is often sudden in onset and characterized by fever, weakness or prostration and sore throat. Gingival, oral and pharyngeal ulceration with pseudomembrane formation are typical features but ulceration can affect any mucous membrane. Lymphadenopathy and sometimes rashes are also features. Later, haemorrhagic necrosis of mucous membranes and respiratory infection may go on to septicaemia as the terminal event. Purpura and bleeding as a result of thrombocytopenia is also a common first manifestation.

General management

The diagnosis is confirmed by blood examination and bone marrow biopsy.

Treatment depends on the underlying cause. In the case of drugs, the triggering agent must be stopped and this may sometimes allow bone marrow function to recover. The main measure is to control infections. Septicaemia is a hazard, particularly in neonates and patients treated with cytotoxic chemotherapy.

Gram-negative infections should be treated with antibiotics such as ticarcillin, mecillinam or one of the third-generation cephalosporins such as ceftazidime or cefotaxime. Complications of septicaemia include adult respiratory distress syndrome, pneumonia, or shock, but endocarditis is rare. Mortality rates may be as high as 30%. Patients should therefore be nursed in laminar-airflow rooms and surgical procedures should be carried out under antibiotic cover.

Gram-positive oral micro-organisms such as viridans streptococci, mainly *Streptococcus mitis* and *S. sanguis,* are increasingly frequently implicated and may lead to serious morbidity and mortality. Predisposing factors appear to be mucositis, the use of high doses of cytosine arabinoside and the failure to use intravenous antibiotics at the time of bacteraemia. Viridans

Table 20.14 Some causes of white cell defects					
CONGENITAL DEFECTS	ACQUIRED DEFECTS				
	Bone marrow disease	Drugs	Autoimmune disorders	Viral infections	Others
See Appendix 20.1	Leukaemia, other marrow infiltrations and myelofibrosis Aplastic anaemia (Ch. 08)	Antithyroid drugs Cephalothin Chloramphenicol Cytotoxic agents Phenothiazines Phenylbutazone Phenytoin Sulfonamides	Systemic lupus erythematosus Felty syndrome Others	HIV infection Others	Diabetes Crohn disease

Table 20.15 Main immune defects[a]

Main defect	Includes	Manifestations
Severe combined immune deficiencies	Includes mutations in relation to DNA ligase IV and CD3δ deficiencies	Recurrent serious infections
Predominantly T-cell deficiencies	Chronic mucocutaneous candidiasis DiGeorge anomaly	Usually present as recurrent or persistent fungal infections
Predominantly B-cell deficiencies	Autosomal recessive agammaglobulinaemia X-linked agammaglobulinaemia Common variable immunodeficiency Inducible co-stimulator (ICOS) deficiency Selective antibody deficiency (such as IgA deficiency) Hyper-IgM syndrome – includes activation-induced cytidine deaminase (AID) and uracil-DNA glycosylase (UNG) deficiencies	Usually present as recurrent bacterial infections
Other well-defined immuno-deficiency syndromes in which there are non-immunological features	Includes syndromes with defects in DNA repair mechanisms. This group has included Bloom syndrome	The immune defects associated with non-immunological features, such as Wiskott–Aldrich syndrome, DNA repair defects and thymic defects, have traditionally been classified together
Diseases of immune dysregulation	Includes defects of apoptosis resulting in lymphoproliferative or auto-immune syndromes. Autoimmune lymphoproliferative syndrome (ALPS). Immune dysregulation, polyendocrinopathy, enteropathy, X-linked syndrome (IPEX) – a recessive disorder	ALPS presents with lymphadenopathy, autoimmunity and expansion of a normally infrequent population of CD4⁻ CD8⁻ T cells. IPEX presents with protracted diarrhoea, ichthyosiform dermatitis, insulin-dependent diabetes mellitus, thyroiditis and haemolytic anaemia
Defects of phagocytic cell number, function or both	Chédiak–Higashi syndrome Chronic granulomatous disease Hyperimmunoglobulinaemia E (Job) syndrome Leukocyte glucose-6-phosphate dehydrogenase deficiency Myeloperoxidase deficiency Leukocyte adhesion defects include LAD types 1–3, Rac2 deficiency, β-actin deficiency and localized juvenile periodontitis Papillon–Lefevre syndrome	Ranges from defects of wound healing or localized infections or periodontitis, to severe clinical pheno-types requiring bone marrow transplantation
Defects of innate immunity relating to monocyte and dendritic cell functions	Defects in NF-kB or other signals	Various
Autoinflammatory disorders	Periodic fever, aphthous stomatitis, pharyngitis, adenitis (PFAPA) syn-drome) – not inherited Hereditary conditions, including: 1 Familial Mediterranean fever (FMF) 2 Mevalonate kinase deficiencies (including hyperimmunoglobulinae-mia D and periodic fever syndrome (HIDS) and mevalonate aciduria) 3 Tumour necrosis factor receptor-associated periodic syndrome (TRAPS) 4 Pyogenic sterile arthritis, pyoderma gangrenosum, acne (PAPA) 5 Chronic recurrent multifocal osteomyelitis (CRMO) 6 Blau syndrome 7 Cryopyrin-associated periodic syndromes (CAPS)	The periodic fevers
Complement deficiencies	Complement component 1 (C1) inhibitor deficiency (hereditary angio-edema) C3 deficiency C6 deficiency C7 deficiency C8 deficiency New complement-related deficiencies – mannose-binding protein (MBP) deficiency and MBP-associated serine protease 2 (MASP2) deficiency	Various

[a]For fine detail see Notarangelo L, Casanova JL, Fischer A, Puck J, Rosen F, Seger R, Geha R. International Union of Immunological Societies Primary Immunodefi-ciency Diseases Classification Committee. Primary immunodeficiency diseases: an update. J Allergy Clin Immunol 2004;114:677–87.

streptococci are sensitive to many antibiotics but there is increas-ing resistance to penicillin after prolonged exposure. Penicillin, vancomycin and roxithromycin are usually effective in lower-ing the incidence of viridans streptococcus bacteraemia but co-trimoxazole is not.

If patients develop a fever, samples of blood, urine, sputum and faeces should be taken for culture lest there be septicaemia, and the patient started on systemic antibiotics, usually initially piperacillin/tazobactam plus gentamicin or, if penicillin-allergic, ceftazidime.

Granulocyte colony-stimulating factors (filgrastim, lenograstim, molgramostim) are now available and may be of benefit.

Dental aspects

Infections and ulcers are the main oral manifestations; periodontal disease may be accelerated and minor oral infections may result in gangrenous stomatitis in severe cases. Oral infections can be painful and a potential source of metastatic infections or septicaemia, sometimes fatal. Oral infections can usually be controlled with topical or systemic antibiotic therapy or sometimes with antiseptics such as chlorhexidine. Mixed infections can often be controlled by a broad-spectrum antibiotic such as topical tetracycline, but this should be given together with an antifungal drug because of the risk of candidal superinfection. Failure to respond to such treatment indicates that the causative bacteria are not sensitive and bacteriological investigation is required. Clindamycin may be a more suitable choice for anaerobic infections.

Dental surgical procedures should be covered with an antibiotic and particular attention should be paid to the possibility of thrombocytopenia with haemorrhagic tendencies and to the risks associated with corticosteroid treatment.

CHRONIC DISEASES WITH IMMUNE DEFECTS

Diabetes mellitus is the most common chronic disease associated with immune defects, mainly defective phagocytosis. Cancers of lymphoid or haemopoietic tissues are also associated with immune defects, as shown in Table 20.16, especially as a consequence of their treatment. Many infections, particularly viral, produce some degree of immune defect.

For dental surgical procedures, particular attention should be paid to the possibility of thrombocytopenia with haemorrhagic tendencies and to the risks associated with corticosteroid treatment.

ASPLENIC PATIENTS

General aspects

The spleen is essential for controlling the quality of erythrocytes in the circulation by sequestrating effete erythrocytes. It is also essential for the production of opsonins, thereby having an important function in antibody production and phagocytosis of micro-organisms. The opsonins properdin and tuftsin protect against bacteria such as pneumococci.

Asplenia may be caused by splenectomy (e.g. after serious splenic injuries in abdominal trauma, for some haemolytic anaemias, in idiopathic thrombocytopenic purpura and in some lymphomas). The spleen becomes hypofunctional in sickle cell disease and other disorders.

Clinical features

Asplenia predisposes to infections, which usually appear within the first 2 years after splenectomy, though up to one-third may manifest at least 5 years later, and some have developed more than 20 years later. Children are ten times more likely than adults to develop sepsis. Patients may become predisposed to infection

Fig. 20.11 Asplenia

with encapsulated bacteria and other microbes. *Streptococcus pneumoniae* (pneumococcus) is the most common pathogen and, together with *H. influenzae* and *N. meningitidis* (meningococcus), accounts for 70–90% of cases. Other infections can include *Capnocytophaga canimorsus* (from dog bites), babesiosis (from tick bites), hepatitis C, tuberculosis and malaria. Infection after splenectomy only rarely emanates from the oral flora.

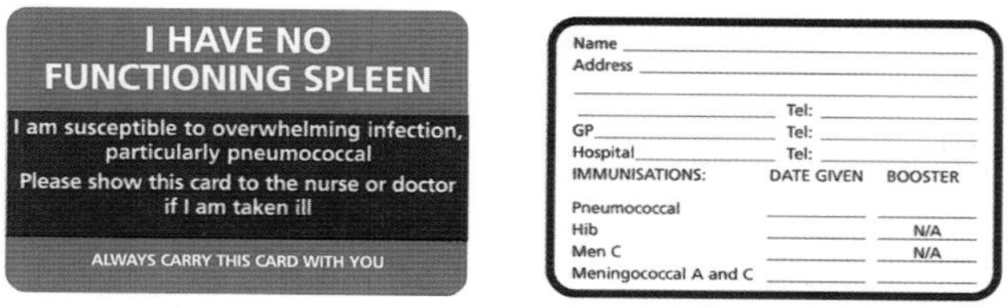

After splenectomy, patients may also be predisposed to develop malignant neoplasms.

General management

Patients having splenectomy, therefore, should be immunized 2 weeks beforehand, against pneumococci, *Haemophilus influenzae* type b and meningococcus. Post-splenectomy, for at least the first 2 years, especially for other immunocompromised patients and for children under 16, daily penicillin or erythromycin prophylaxis is advised. Patients are usually advised to carry a warning card (Fig. 20.11).

Patients having had splenectomy in the past, if becoming acutely unwell, should promptly be given benzylpenicillin.

Dental aspects

There is no indication for antimicrobial prophylaxis before dental procedures unless there are other reasons and, in any event, such prophylaxis might fail.

It is important, however, to exclude thrombocytopenia and corticosteroid therapy.

PRIMARY (CONGENITAL) IMMUNODEFICIENCY DISEASES

GENERAL ASPECTS

Primary immunodeficiency diseases are due to abnormalities of one or more genes important in immunity. There are over 100 different immune defects, mostly rare, and most can be categorized according to the main type of immune cell that is defective (Table 20.15 and Fig. 20.12).

Some primary immune defects are inherited as autosomal recessive traits, some as X-linked recessive traits, and at least one as an autosomal dominant trait. Others are not inherited as single gene defects. Two of the most common primary immunodeficiency diseases, selective IgA deficiency, and common variable immunodeficiency, considered later, are frequently sporadic.

Immune defects are also common in some chromosomal anomalies, including Down syndrome (Ch. 28), Fanconi anaemia and Bloom syndrome, and in various rare hereditary metabolic defects.

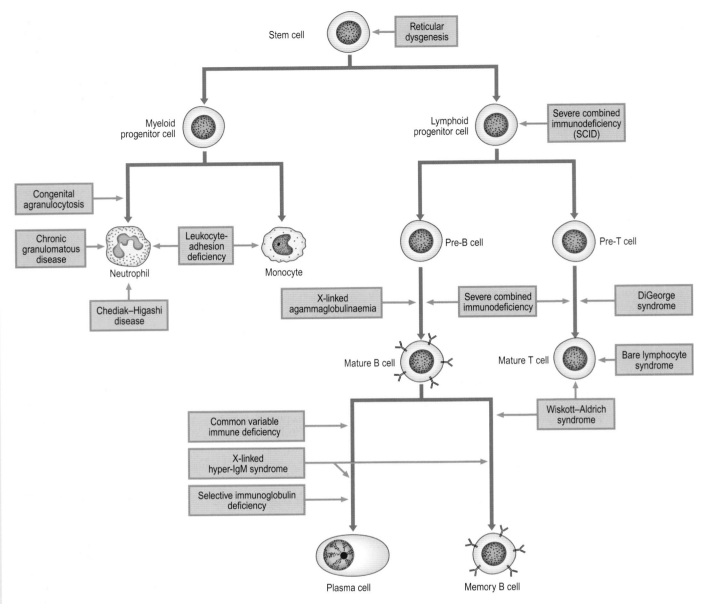

Fig. 20.12 Primary immune defects

CLINICAL FEATURES

Primary immune defects should be suspected if there are recurrent or persistent infections or other features (Box 20.2).

Box 20.2 Features suggestive of a primary immune defect

- A family history of primary immune deficiency
- Eight or more new ear infections within 1 year
- Failure of an infant to gain weight or grow normally
- Need for intravenous antibiotics to clear infection
- Persistent thrush in the mouth or elsewhere on the skin, after age 1
- Recurrent, deep skin or organ abscesses
- Two or more deep-seated infections, such as sepsis, meningitis or cellulitis
- Two or more months on antibiotics with little effect
- Two or more pneumonias within 1 year
- Two or more serious sinus infections within 1 year

http://www.pia.org.uk/publications/10_signs_of_pia/10_signs_01.htm

The main features of primary immune defects are summarized in Appendix 20.1.

GENERAL MANAGEMENT

Antibody deficiency is most frequently encountered and commonly presents with sinopulmonary bacterial infections. If these are the only types of infection under consideration, screening for antibody deficiency is appropriate. Other forms of primary immunodeficiency may present with distinct infectious complications with or without sinopulmonary bacterial disease. Some of these forms of infection are more or less characteristic of specific categories of immunodeficiency.

Some primary immune defects are treated by replacement of defective immunocytes or their products with immunoglobulin or bone marrow transplantation, and gene transfer is being developed to correct several defects. Immune system molecules, such as interferon-gamma, can be injected to improve immune function and control infection.

Infections must be treated by accepted means.

DENTAL ASPECTS

The more severe congenital immune defects often cause early death, so that they are not relevant to dental care, except in so far as some are treated by bone marrow transplantation.

T-LYMPHOCYTE DEFECTS

Chronic mucocutaneous candidosis

General and clinical aspects

Chronic mucocutaneous candidosis (CMC or CMCC) is a group of disorders in which candidosis is the main or a prominent feature. Defects of cell-mediated immunity can sometimes be detected, particularly in the more severe cases (Table 20.16).

Table 20.16 Chronic mucocutaneous candidosis syndromes	
Type	**Clinical features**
1. Familial	Persistent oral candidosis Often iron deficiency
2. Diffuse (candida granuloma)	Severe chronic candidosis Susceptibility to bacterial infections
3. Candidosis–endocrinopathy syndrome (polyendocrinopathy syndrome)	Mild chronic oral candidosis Hypoparathyroidism Hypoadrenocorticism
4. Candidosis–thymoma syndrome	Chronic oral candidosis Myasthenia gravis Haematological disorders
5. CMC in HIV disease or hyperimmunoglobulin E syndrome	Recurrent candidosis

Early-onset chronic mucocutaneous candidosis (CMC types 1–3) typically has an onset in infancy, often as persistent thrush; the candidosis is mainly or entirely oral and immunological defects are sometimes associated.

Familial candidosis in an adult with chronic oral candidosis can escape diagnosis until middle age. Enquiry should be made as to whether siblings are affected and whether there was any parental consanguinity, as the disease appears to be autosomal recessive. In familial candidosis, investigation for iron deficiency should be carried out, and treatment with iron may improve the response to antifungal drugs.

Diffuse type of CMC presents with particularly severe candidosis that can give rise to gross proliferative and disfiguring lesions of the skin (so-called granulomas) as well as widespread oral lesions. Immunological defects are frequently found and there is also susceptibility to bacterial infections of the respiratory tract or elsewhere. Even in this unusually severe form of the disease, candidosis remains superficial and does not progress to candidal septicaemia or other types of disseminated infection.

Candidosis–endocrinopathy syndrome (Autoimmune Polyendocrinopathy Candidosis-Ectodermal Dystrophy [APECED]) has usually mild but persistent candidosis as the initial feature, and endocrine disorders appear but often not until 10 or 15 years later. Occasionally this sequence is reversed. There is no evidence that candidosis causes the endocrine disorders or vice versa. Hypoparathyroidism or Addison disease, or both, are the most commonly associated endocrinopathies. The endocrine disorders in candidosis–endocrinopathy syndrome are associated with multiple organ-specific autoantibodies both in patients and in unaffected relatives. Patients may for long appear to be quite well apart from chronic oral candidosis. If, therefore, a patient, particularly a child or adolescent with chronic oral candidosis, has a family history of any of the associated disorders, and autoantibodies (particularly to glandular tissues) are found, endocrine disease will probably develop in the future.

Candidosis–thymoma syndrome presents with late-onset chronic mucocutaneous candidosis, when evidence of impaired cell-mediated immunity, particularly to *C. albicans*, may be found. In such a case investigation for a thymoma should be carried out, as early excision may improve the prognosis.

General management

Candidosis is persistent and responds poorly to topical treatment with nystatin or amphotericin but may respond to topical antifungal agents, such as miconazole, or to systemic ketoconazole, fluconazole, itraconazole or voriconazole.

DiGeorge anomaly

The coincidental association between chronic candidosis and hypoparathyroidism (type I polyendocrinopathy syndrome), also seen in the DiGeorge syndrome (CATCH 22), has given rise to the myth that hypoparathyroidism predisposes to candidosis. However, treatment of hypoparathyroidism has no effect on candidosis and hypoparathyroidism from any other cause is not associated with candidosis. Branchial arch defects in DiGeorge syndrome affect both thymus (and thymocytes) and parathyroids.

ANTIBODY DEFICIENCY SYNDROMES

Hypoimmunoglobulinaemia can have several causes and can also be caused by hypercatabolism, or excessive loss of, immunoglobulins (Table 20.17).

Common variable immunodeficiency (adult-onset agammaglobulinaemia, late-onset hypogammaglobulinaemia or acquired agammaglobulinaemia)

General aspects

Common variable immunodeficiency (CVID) is relatively common. Serum IgG is low with a marked decrease in IgM or IgA. The serum IgM concentration is normal in about half of the patients. Most patients have normal B-cell numbers, though some do have low or absent B cells. Abnormalities in T-cell numbers or function are common.

Table 20.17 Differential diagnosis of hypogammoglobulinaemia

Genetic disorders	Drug-induced	Infections	Malignancy	Immunoglobulin loss or degradation
Ataxia telangiectasia	Antimalarials	Congenital rubella	Chronic lymphocytic leukaemia	Lymphangiectasia
Autosomal SCID	Captopril	or cytomegalovirus	Immunodeficiency with	Nephrosis
Hyper IgM immunodeficiency	Carbamazepine	or *Toxoplasma gondii*	thymoma	Severe burns
Transcobalamin II deficiency and	Glucocorticoids	HIV	Non-Hodgkin lymphoma	Severe diarrhoea
hypogammaglobulinaemia	Fenclofenac	Epstein–Barr virus	B-cell malignancy	
X-linked agammaglobulinaemia	Gold salts			
X-linked lymphoproliferative	Penicillamine			
disorder	Phenytoin			
X-linked SCID	Sulfasalazine			
Chromosome 18q- syndrome				
Monosomy 22				
Trisomy 8				
Trisomy 21				

Clinical features

Symptoms are mainly frequent bacterial infections of ears, sinuses, bronchi and lungs. Viral, fungal and parasitic infections as well as bacterial infections may be problematic. Pneumonias are common and approximately 50% of patients have autoimmune disease. Gastrointestinal disease, including chronic diarrhoea, affects as many as 30% and there is a high incidence of inflammatory bowel disease, gluten-sensitive enteropathy and nodular lymphoid hyperplasia. *Giardia lamblia* and bacterial overgrowth of the small bowel are the most frequently identified pathogens. Haematological abnormalities may include autoimmune haemolytic anaemia, immune thrombocytopenia, leukopenia and pernicious anaemia. Arthralgia in the knee, ankle, elbow or wrist is common, and rheumatoid arthritis and other collagen vascular diseases are also more common than expected. Splenomegaly and lymphadenopathy may be seen. Patients are usually recognized to be immunodeficient by the second, third or fourth decade of life.

General management

Diagnosis is confirmed by finding low serum IgG, IgA and possibly IgM. B cells still produce antibodies after a common vaccination such as tetanus. Antibody levels can be normalized by intravenous immunoglobulin every 3–4 weeks. Bacterial infections are treated with antibiotics. Physical therapy and daily postural drainage may help clear respiratory infections.

Selective IgA deficiency

General aspects

Selective IgA deficiency is the most common congenital immunodeficiency, affecting one in 600 in the normal population. IgA is deficient in both serum and secretions.

Clinical features

Many individuals with IgA deficiency are asymptomatic if the levels of other classes of immunoglobulin are normal or raised. Others have persistent or recurrent infections and some develop CVID over time. Some have an increased incidence of upper respiratory tract infections, allergies and autoimmune disease but a normal IgG antibody response to vaccination.

Where IgA deficiency is associated with deficiency of IgG$_2$, there is a definite predisposition to recurrent bacterial or viral respiratory infections, and small intestine infections – usually *Giardia lamblia* (a protozoon causing diarrhoea and malabsorption, although the disease is often unrecognized because the symptoms are chronic and indolent). Atopic disease, coeliac disease, lupus erythematosus, rheumatoid arthritis and Sjögren syndrome are abnormally frequent.

General management

IgA replacement is difficult since autoantibodies frequently form against IgA when blood transfusions or immunoglobulins are given, and can sometimes cause anaphylactic reactions.

Bacterial infections should be treated with antibiotics. Giardiasis needs treatment with metronidazole or quinacrine hydrochloride.

Dental aspects

Despite the fact that IgA is the main salivary antibody, reported effects of IgA deficiency on dental caries and other oral disease are conflicting. Part of the reason for this apparently anomalous situation is that other immunoglobulins may be secreted in saliva. IgA deficiency may be associated occasionally with oral ulcers and herpes labialis.

X-linked agammaglobulinaemia (Bruton syndrome)

Patients with X-linked agammaglobulinaemia (XLA) are male with low CD19+ B cells and low serum IgG, IgM and IgA, no isohaemagglutinins and/or a poor response to vaccines. They develop recurrent bacterial infections in the first 5 years of life, particularly otitis, sinusitis and pneumonia. The most common organisms are *Streptococcus pneumoniae* and *Haemophilus influenzae*. Approximately 20% of patients present with a dramatic, overwhelming infection, often also with neutropenia. Another 10–15% have higher concentrations of serum immunoglobulin than expected or are not recognized to have immunodeficiency until after 5 years of age.

B- AND T-LYMPHOCYTE DEFECTS

Ataxia telangiectasia

Ataxia telangiectasia (AT) is progressive cerebellar ataxia with walking difficulty presenting at the end of the first year of life and, by the teenage years, most patients are wheelchair bound. Ocular or facial telangiectasia are usually seen at 4–8 years of life. Serum IgA is low and alpha-fetoprotein high. Many patients have recurrent respiratory infections. Radiation-induced chromosomal breakages may culminate in leukaemia or lymphomas.

Severe combined immunodeficiency (SCID)

Patients with SCID have low CD3+ T cells. They usually fail to thrive, and develop persistent diarrhoea, respiratory infections and/or thrush in the first 7 months of life. *Pneumocystis* pneumonia, significant bacterial infections and disseminated bacille Calmette-Guérin (BCG) infection are common. SCID is fatal in the first 2 years of life unless the patient is treated with extremely restrictive isolation, haematopoietic stem cell transplant or therapy that replaces the abnormal gene or gene product.

Wiskott–Aldrich syndrome

Wiskott–Aldrich syndrome (WAS) presents in males with congenital thrombocytopenia, small platelets and abnormal antibody response to polysaccharide antigens. Many patients have increased IgE and IgA, with low IgM, and T-cell numbers and function decline with age. The main features include eczema, recurrent bacterial or viral infections, autoimmune diseases (vasculitis, haemolytic anaemia and glomerulonephritis) and lymphoma, leukaemia or brain tumour. Otitis and sinusitis, and infections due to herpes simplex virus and EBV are particularly troublesome.

X-linked lymphoproliferative syndrome

Males with X-linked lymphoproliferative syndrome (XLP) are usually asymptomatic until they develop EBV infection, which may cause fulminant hepatitis (60% of patients), particularly in young children. Lymphoma/Hodgkin disease, immunodeficiency, aplastic anaemia or lymphohistiocytic disorders may be fatal in childhood. Less common manifestations include EBV-associated haemophagocytic syndrome and vasculitis.

PHAGOCYTE DEFECTS

Chediak–Higashi syndrome

Chediak–Higashi syndrome (CHS) is caused by impaired polymorphonuclear leukocyte function related to abnormal microtubular assembly. It is a rare autosomal recessive disorder that manifests with: hypopigmentation of skin, eyes and hair; bleeding tendency and easy bruisability; recurrent infections; abnormal natural killer (NK) cell function; and peripheral

neuropathy. Most patients who do not undergo bone marrow transplantation die from a lymphoproliferative syndrome.

Chronic granulomatous disease

Patients with the X-linked form of chronic granulomatous disease (CGD; 60–70%) usually present earlier and with more severe disease than patients with autosomal recessive forms. Abnormal respiratory burst in activated neutrophils characterizes CGD. Clinically, deep-seated infections (liver, perirectal or lung abscess; lymphadenitis; or osteomyelitis) due to catalase-positive organisms such as staphylococci, *Serratia marcescens*, *Candida* or *Aspergillus*; diffuse granulomas in the respiratory, gastrointestinal or urogenital tracts; failure to thrive; and hepatosplenomegaly or lymphadenopathy are seen.

Hyperimmunoglobulinaemia E syndrome (Job syndrome; Buckley syndrome)

Patients with hyperimmunoglobulinaemia E syndrome (HIES) appear to have T-cell abnormalities, including a decrease in interferon-gamma and an increase in IL-4, and an inadequate inflammatory response that may delay recognition of infections. HIES is characterized by eczema, recurrent skin abscesses, cystic lung infections [primarily *Staphylococcus aureus* and *Candida* species (chronic mucocutaneous candidosis)], eosinophilia and raised IgE. Non-immunological features include multiple bone fractures, joint hyperextensibility and other skeletal abnormalities, coarse facial features, retained primary teeth, palatal keratosis or ridging, and tongue-fissuring.

Leukocyte adhesion deficiency (LAD)

Decreased expression of CD18 on neutrophils with mutation in the beta$_2$-integrin gene leads to recurrent or persistent bacterial or fungal infections, leukocytosis, and delayed separation of the umbilical cord and/or defective wound healing. Infections with *Staphylococcus*, Gram-negative enteric bacteria and fungi are particularly troublesome. Periodontitis is a common finding. In the severe form of LAD, with no CD18 expression on neutrophils, the patient usually succumbs without bone marrow transplantation (BMT). In the moderate form, patients can survive to adulthood.

Leukocyte glucose-6-phosphate dehydrogenase deficiency

Glucose-6-phosphate dehydrogenase (G6PD) is one of the pentose phosphate pathway enzymes, involved in maintaining adequate coenzyme nicotinamide–adenine dinucleotide phosphate (NADPH) in cells. G6PD deficiency can lead to meningitis, septicaemia or osteomyelitis.

Myeloperoxidase deficiency

Myeloperoxidase (MPO) is an enzyme in the neutrophil azurophilic granules and in lysosomes of monocytes, which has a major role in killing some bacteria (*Staphylococcus aureus*,

Serratia species and *Escherichia coli*), fungi, parasites, protozoa, viruses and tumour cells. Most individuals with partial or total MPO deficiency have no increased frequency of infections but recurrent infections may be seen, especially where there is coexistent diabetes.

COMPLEMENT DEFECTS

Defects in complement components tend to be associated with autoimmune disease, especially lupus erythematosus, and increased susceptibility to meningococcal and gonococcal infections.

Hereditary angioedema (C1 esterase inhibitor deficiency)

General aspects

Hereditary angioedema (HANE) is caused by continued complement activation resulting from a genetically determined deficiency of an inhibitor of the enzyme C1 esterase (Fig. 20.13); thus C4 is consumed and its plasma level falls. The level of C3 is usually normal. Complement activation is associated with release of kinin-like substances, which are the probable cause of the sudden increase in capillary permeability.

Despite its hereditary nature, usually as an autosomal dominant trait, the disease may not present until later childhood or adolescence, and nearly 20% of cases are caused by spontaneous mutation. Rare cases are acquired.

Clinical features

Blunt injury is the most consistent precipitating event and the trauma of dental treatment is a potent trigger of attacks. Some attacks follow emotional stress.

Hereditary angioedema mimics allergic angioedema, though it causes a more severe reaction. Abdominal pain, nausea or vomiting, diarrhoea, rashes and peripheral oedema sometimes herald an attack. Oedema typically affects the mouth, face and neck region, can persist for up to 4 days and may involve the airway. The extremities and gastrointestinal tract may be involved.

The mortality may be as high as 30% in some families but the disease is compatible with prolonged survival if emergencies are effectively treated.

General management

In 85% of cases the C1 esterase levels are low (type 1 HANE) but in 15% this inhibitor is present but dysfunctional (type 2 HANE); in both types the C4 level falls. C1 esterase inhibitor concentrates are available for replacement of the missing factor. The androgenic steroids, danazol and stanazolol, raise plasma C1 esterase inhibitor levels to normal. Stanazolol needs to be given for 5 days to be effective and it should not be given during pregnancy. Oligomenorrhoea may be induced in women and there may be acne, hirsutism, hypercalcaemia or headache. Plasma or plasminogen inhibitors, such as tranexamic acid, can also mitigate attacks and may be life-saving.

MUCOCILIARY SYNDROMES

Cilia in the respiratory tract normally clear mucus and act as a defence mechanism. If they are impaired, as in some genetic and acquired disorders, this may lead to chronic sinusitis or other respiratory infections. Examples are Kartagener syndrome (mucociliary disease and dextrocardia) and intolerance of NSAIDs in the Fernand–Widal syndrome.

USEFUL WEBSITES

http://www.eupidconference.com
http://www.guideline.gov
http://www.allergy.org.au
http://www.doh.gov.uk/ab/index
http://www.info.dh.gov.uk
http://www.dh.gov.uk/en
http://www.aidsportal.org
http://www.pia.org.uk
http://www.esid.org
http://www.hivdent.org
http://www.hivatis.org
http://www.cdc.gov/hiv

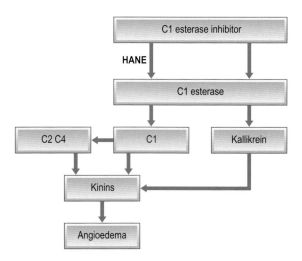

Fig. 20.13 Hereditary angioedema (HANE)

FURTHER READING

Achong, R.M., Shetty, K., Arribas, A., Block, M.S., 2006. Implants in HIV-positive patients: 3 case reports. J Oral Maxillofac Surg 64 (8), 1199–1203.

Bohjanen, P.R., Boulware, D.R., 2007. Chapter 18: Immune reconstitution inflammatory syndrome. In: Volberding, P., Sande, M.A., Lange, J., Greene, W. (eds), Global HIV/AIDS medicine, Elsevier, Philadelphia, pp. 193–205.

Bonilla, F.A., Bernstein, I.L., Khan, D.A., et al., 2005. Practice parameter for the diagnosis and management of primary immunodeficiency. Ann Allergy Asthma Immunol 94 (5 Suppl 1), S1–63.

Campo-Trapero, J., Cano-Sanchez, J., del Romero-Guerrero, J., Moreno-Lopez, L.A., Cerero-Lapiedra, R., Bascones-Martinez, A., 2003. Dental management of patients with human immunodeficiency virus. Quintessence Int 34, 515–525.

CDC, 2007. Notice to readers: updated information regarding antiretroviral agents used as HIV postexposure prophylaxis for occupational HIV exposures. MMWR 56 (49), 1291–1292.

Chaisson RE. Immune reconstitution syndrome. Johns Hopkins AIDS Service: Clinician Forum. http://qa.hopkins-aids.org/forum/view_question.html?section_id=62 &id=42969&category_id=113. October 14, 2001.

Chapel, H.M., 2005. Primary immune deficiencies – improving our understanding of their role in immunological disease. Clin Exp Immunol 139, 11–12.

Chapel, H.M., 2003. IUIS report on immunodeficiency disease: an update. Clin Exp Immunol 132, 9–15.

DeSimone, J.A., 2000. Inflammatory reactions in HIV-1-infected persons after initiation of highly active antiretroviral therapy. Ann Intern Med 133, 447–454.

Dios, P.D., Scully, C., 2002. Adverse effects of antiretroviral therapies: focus on orofacial effects. Expert Opin Drug Safety 1, 304–317.

Dios, D., Ocampo Hermida, A., Miralles Alvarez, C., Limeres Posse, J., Tomás Carmona, I., 2000. Changing prevalence of human immunodeficiency virus-associated oral lesions. Oral Surg Oral Med Oral Pathol Oral Radiol Endod 90, 403–404.

Freeman, A.F., Domingo, D.L., Holland, S.M., 2009. Hyper IgE (Job's) syndrome: a primary immune deficiency with oral manifestations. Oral Dis 15, 2–7.

Fukui, N., Amano, A., Akiyama, S., Daikoku, H., Wakisaka, S., Morisaki, I., 2000. Oral findings in DiGeorge syndrome: clinical features and histologic study of primary teeth. Oral Surg Oral Med Oral Pathol Oral Radiol Endod 89, 208–215.

Grimbacher, B., Hutloff, A., Schlesier, M., et al., 2003. Homozygous loss of ICOS is associated with adult-onset common variable immunodeficiency. Nat Immunol 4, 261.

HPA Centre for Infection, November 2007. Testing times – HIV and other sexually transmitted infection in the United Kingdom 2007. The UK Collaborative Group for HIV and STI Surveillance, London.

Markowitz, M., Mohri, H., Mehandru, S., 2005. Infection with multi-drug resistant dual-tropic HIV-1 and rapid progression to AIDS: a case report. Lancet 365, 1031–1038.

Mazer, B., Nelson Jr., R.P., Orange, J.S., Routes, J.M., Shearer, W.T., Sorensen, R.U., 2005. Practice parameter for the diagnosis and management of primary immunodeficiency. Ann Allergy Asthma Immunol 94 (5 Suppl 1), S1–63.

McAdam, A.J., Greenward, R.J., Levin, M.A., et al., 2001. ICOS is critical for CD40-mediated antibody class switching. Nature 409, 102.

Minegishi, Y., Rohrer, J., Coustan-Smith, E., et al., 1999. An essential role for BLNK in human B cell development. Science 286, 1954.

Nguyen, Q.D., 2000. Immune recovery uveitis in patients with AIDS and cytomegalovirus retinitis after highly active antiretroviral therapy. Am J Ophthalmol 129, 634–639.

Notarangelo, L., Casanova, J.L., Fischer, A., et al., 2004. Primary immunodeficiency diseases: an update. J Allergy Clin Immunol 114, 677–687.

Pappu, R., Cheng, A.M., Li, B., et al., 1999. Requirements for B cell linker protein (BLNK) in B cell development. Science 286, 1949.

Parisi, E., Glick, M., 2003. Immune suppression and considerations for dental care. Dental Clin N Am 47, 709–731.

Patel, A.S., Glick, M., 2003. Oral manifestations associated with HIV infection: evaluation, assessment, and significance. Gen Dent 51, 153–156.

Patton, L.L., Shugars, D.A., Bonito, A.J., 2002. A systematic review of complication risks for HIV-positive patients undergoing invasive dental procedures. J Am Dent Assoc 133, 195–203.

Peschon, J.J., Morrissey, P.J., Grabstein, K.H., et al., 1994. Early lymphocyte expansion is severely impaired in interleukin 7 receptor-deficient mice. J Exp Med 180, 1955.

Price, P., Morahan, G., Huang, D., et al., 2002. Polymorphisms in cytokine genes define subpopulations of HIV-1 patients who experienced immune restoration diseases. AIDS 16, 2043–2047.

Satterthwaite, A.B., White, O.N., 2000. The role of Bruton's tyrosine kinase in B-cell development and function: a genetic perspective. Immunol Rev 175, 120.

Saurborn, D., Boiselle, P.M., 2003. Recognizing the radiologic signs of mycobacterial infections: pleural effusion may be the only sign in some patients. J Resp Dis 24 454–451.

Scully C. Chaudhry S., 2009. Aspects of Human Disease 30. HIV infection and AIDS Dental Update 36, 125.

Scully, C., Dios, P.D., 2001. HIV topic update; orofacial effects of antiretroviral therapies. Oral Dis 7, 205–210.

Scully, C., Diz Dios, P., Kumar, N., 2007. Special care in dentistry: handbook of oral healthcare. Churchill Livingstone Elsevier, Edinburgh.

Scully C., Hodgson, T., Lachmann, H., 2008. Autoinflammatory syndromes and oral health. Oral Diseases 14, 690–699.

Scully, C., Watt-Smith, P., Dios, P., Giangrande, P.L.F., 2002. Complications in HIV-infected and non-HIV-infected hemophiliacs and other patients after oral surgery. Int J Oral Maxillofac Surg, 31634–31640.

Shelburne, S.A., Visnegarwala, F., Darcourt, J., et al., 2005. Incidence and risk factors for immune reconstitution inflammatory syndrome during highly active antiretroviral therapy. AIDS 19, 399–406.

Shetty, K., Achong, R., 2005. Dental implants in the HIV-positive patient – case report and review of the literature. Gen Dent 53, 434–437, quiz 438, 446.

Stevenson, G.C., Riano, P.C., Moretti, A.J., Nichols, C.M., Engelmeier, R.L., Flaitz, C.M., 2007. Short-term success of osseointegrated dental implants in HIV-positive individuals: a prospective study. J Contemp Dent Pract 8, 1–10.

Strietzel, F.P., Rothe, S., Reichart, P.A., Schmidt-Westhausen, A.M., 2006. Implant-prosthetic treatment in HIV-infected patients receiving highly active antiretroviral therapy: report of cases. Int J Oral Maxillofac Implants 21, 951–956.

The, UK Collaborative Group for HIV and STI Surveillance, 2006. A complex picture. HIV and other sexually transmitted infections in the United Kingdom. Health Protection Agency, Centre for Infections, London.

Vinuesa, C.G., Goodnow, C.C., 2004. Illuminating autoimmune regulators through controlled variation of the mouse genome sequence. Immunity 20, 669–679.

Walker BD. Immune reconstitution and immunotherapy in HIV infection. Medscape Clinical Update. www.medscape.com/viewprogram/2435_pnt. June 12, 2003.

Yin, M.T., Dobkin, J.F., Grbic, J.T., 2007. Epidemiology, pathogenesis, and management of human immunodeficiency virus infection in patients with periodontal disease. Periodontology 2007 44, 55–81.

Appendix 20.1 Main features of major primary (genetically determined) immunodeficiency disorders

Type or name of syndrome	Immunological phenomena	Clinical effects	Possible orofacial features
Predominantly B-cell defects			
Transient hypog-ammaglobulinaemia of infancy	Hypogammaglobulinaemia in early childhood only	Eczema, food allergies	NR
X-linked infantile hypogamma-globulinaemia (XLA; Bruton syndrome)	Immunoglobulins of all classes deficient or absent	Recurrent pyogenic infections Infants develop pus-producing infections of the inner ear and lungs Hepatitis, CNS viral infections	Sinusitis, absent tonsils, cervical lymph node enlargement, ulcers
X-linked hyper IgM syndrome	IgA, IgG and IgE low	Recurring upper and lower respiratory infections within first year of life. Enlarged liver and spleen, chronic diarrhoea, and increased risk of unusual or opportunistic infections and non-Hodgkin lymphoma. • Recurrent bacterial infections in the first 5 years of life • *Pneumocystis carinii* infection in the first year of life • Neutropenia • *Cryptosporidium*-related diarrhoea. *Cryptosporidium* infection may lead to severe bile duct disease and hepatic cancer • Sclerosing cholangitis • Parvovirus-induced aplastic anaemia	Enlarged tonsils Over 50% of patients have chronic or intermit-tent neutropenia, often associated with oral ulcers
Non-X-linked hyper-IgM syndrome	IgA and IgE low	Neutropenia, thrombocytopenia, liver disease	Mouth ulcers
Nijmegen breakage syndrome	Serum IgG and IgA more than 2 SD below normal for age	Increased radiation-induced chromosomal breakage on chromo-some 8q21 Additional features are café-au-lait spots, vitiligo and clinodactyly and syndactyly More than 50% develop B- or T-origin lymphomas before 18 years of age. Many patients have recurrent bacterial and viral respiratory infections (56%) associated with antibody deficiencies	Microcephaly Typical facial appearance (receding forehead, promi-nent midface with long nose and long philtrum and a receding mandible)
WHIM (warts, hypogammaglobu-linaemia, infections, myelokathexis) syndrome	Chronic neutropenia (absolute neutrophil count <500/L) Myelokathexis (retention of senescent neutrophils in the bone marrow) Chronic lymphopenia (absolute lymphocyte count <1500/L) Serum IgG at or below the normal range for age Hypogammaglobulinaemia may be present, but the serum immunoglobulin concentrations do not correlate with the number of B cells	Male or female patient Autosomal dominant disorder Most patients present with recurrent infections at less than 3 years of age Warts generally begin to appear after 5 years of age and some patients have hundreds of warts Increased susceptibility to infection from members of the herpesvirus family can be seen Most patients develop a normal neutrophil count during infection	Facial warts
Common variable immunodeficiency	Variable deficiency of different immunoglobulins	Respiratory infections starting in childhood	Sinusitis, hyperplastic tonsils, cervical lymph node enlargement, oral ulceration
Wiskott–Aldrich syndrome	Deficiency mainly of IgM and IgA IgE may be increased	Recurrent infections especially by pneumococci, meningococci and *H. influenzae*, thrombocytopenia, eczema Severe infections with herpesviruses and *Pneumocystis carinii* High incidence of malignancies, particularly lymphomas and autoimmune diseases	Purpura, candidosis, herpetic infections
Hypogamma-globulinaemia after intrauterine viral infections (e.g. rubella)	Deficiency usually of only one Ig class (e.g. IgA)	Occasionally increased susceptibility to infection	Enamel hypoplasia

Appendix 20.1—cont'd

Type or name of syndrome	Immunological phenomena	Clinical effects	Possible orofacial features
IgA deficiency	Variable. Deficient IgA and sometimes IgE or IgG$_2$	Recurrent respiratory infections or atopic allergy or autoimmune disease or normal health	Tonsillar hyperplasia, possibly oral ulceration, herpetic infections
IgG2 subclass deficiency	Defective humoral immunity	Recurrent respiratory infections	Sinusitis
T- and B-cell defects			
Congenital thymic aplasia (DiGeorge syndrome)	Deletion of chromosome 22q11.2 Defective cell-mediated immunity; reduced numbers of CD3+ T cells (less than 500/mm^3). Ig production also impaired	Viral and fungal infections starting in infancy Cardiovascular defects. Conotruncal cardiac defect (truncus arteriosus, tetralogy of Fallot, interrupted aortic arch or aberrant right subclavian) Hypoparathyroidism with hypocalcaemia of > 3 weeks' duration The severity of the T-cell defect varies greatly: in many patients the immunodeficiency resolves in the first few years of life Autoimmune disorders may be seen in older patients	Dysmorphic facies or palatal abnormalities, bifid uvula Candidosis, herpetic infection
MHC class II deficiency (Base lymphocyte syndrome)	Subtype of SCID	Seen most often in patients from around the Mediterranean Sea, results in a clinical phenotype similar to SCID with severe infections and protracted diarrhoea in the first 6 months of life Pseudomonas, CMV and Cryptosporidium infections are common Hepatic abnormalities, particularly sclerosing cholangitis, are frequent	Candidosis
Severe combined immunodeficiency (SCID)	Defective cell-mediated immunity and hypogammaglobulinaemia. There are two types: • Patients lack adenosine deaminase (ADA) or • Patients lack the ability to produce interleukin-2 receptor gamma chain, a molecule that T cells need to communicate with B cells	Lack of resistance to all types of infection Within the first 3 months of life, babies get serious or life-threatening infections, especially pneumonia, meningitis and sepsis Common infections like chickenpox, measles or herpes can overwhelm them Chronic skin infections, candidosis, chronic hepatitis, diarrhoea and blood disorders	Candidosis, herpetic infections Oral ulceration
X-linked SCID	Defective cell-mediated immunity and hypogammaglobulinaemia	Onset of failure to thrive before 1 year of age, serum IgG and IgA more than 2 SD below normal for age Persistent or recurrent diarrhoea, UTI or thrush Many patients have normal serum IgM Some show signs of GVHD	Thrush
Deficiencies of MHC class II CD3, ZAP-70 or TAP-2	Decreased CD4 cells, CD8 cells	Recurrent infections	NR
Immunodeficiency with ataxia telangiectasia	Defective cell-mediated immunity Ig production impaired	Respiratory infections starting in infancy Ataxia telangiectasia, learning impairment	Sinusitis, oral ulceration
Late-onset immunodeficiency	Defective cell-mediated or hypogammaglobulinaemia	Susceptibility to various infections starting late in life	Chronic candidosis
Complement deficiencies			
C1, C2 or C4 deficiencies	Defects in complement pathways	Autoimmune disease, especially lupus erythematosus	Possibly oral lesions of lupus erythematosus
C1, C3 or C5 deficiencies	Defects in complement pathways	Increased susceptibility to meningococcal and gonococcal infections	NR
C1 esterase inhibitor deficiency	Abnormal complement activation	Swelling of face and neck Airway obstruction	Swellings

Continued

Appendix 20.1—cont'd

Type or name of syndrome	Immunological phenomena	Clinical effects	Possible orofacial features
Granulocyte defects			
Interferon-gamma receptor (IFNGR) deficiency	Granulocytes have protein that rejects interferon	Infections with mycobacteria and *Salmonella*	NR
Cyclical neutropenia	Depression of neutrophil count at 21-day intervals	Periodic infections – especially bacterial	Recurrent oral ulceration Periodontitis
Chronic granuloma-tous disease	Leukocyte killing defect	Catalase-positive bacterial infections. *E. coli, Staphylococcus aureus, Pseudomonas, Serratia* and *Aspergillus* Lymph node abscesses	Cervical lymphadenopathy and suppuration. Enamel hypoplasia
Myeloperoxidase deficiency	Leukocyte killing defect	Candidosis	Candidosis
Chediak–Higashi syndrome	Leukocyte defect of chemotaxis and phagocytosis	Albinism, recurrent infections, hepatosplenomegaly, thrombocyto-penia	Cervical lymph node enlargement, oral ulcer-ation, periodontitis
Leukocyte adhesion defect (LAD) 1	Adhesion defect (deficiency of beta$_2$-integrin; also called CD18, Mac1, or p150, 95)	Umbilical cord does not detach Severe infections of soft tissue Eroding skin sores without pus Infections of the gastrointestinal tract Wounds that heal slowly and may leave scars Poor prognosis	Periodontitis
LAD 2	Adhesion defect (failure to con-vert mannose to fucose)	Recurrent infection	Periodontitis
Papillon–Lefevre syndrome	Chemotactic defect	Recurrent infection	Periodontitis
Job syndrome Hyperimmunoglobu-linaemia E (HIE)	Hyperimmunoglobulinaemia E with neutrophil defects In about half of the cases, linked to chromosome 4. In most cases, it is autosomal dominant	Recurrent infection by *Staphylococcus aureus* HIE patients may also have scoliosis (curvature of the spine), weak bones and recurrent bone fractures, strokes or other brain prob-lems, severe itching and inflamed skin	Asymmetry or uneven facial features Prominent forehead Deep-set eyes Broad nasal bridge Wide, fleshy nasal tip Protruding lower jaw Periodontitis Ulcers
Glycogen storage disease b	Leukopenia and defect of chemotaxis	Recurrent infection	Periodontitis Ulcers
Schwachman syndrome (lazy leukocyte syndrome)	Leukocyte defect of chemotaxis	Recurrent infection	Periodontitis Ulcers

CMV, cytomegalovirus; CNS, central nervous system; GVHD, graft-versus-host disease; NR, not recorded; SD, standard deviation.

Bacteria, viruses and fungi are in the external and internal environment, and cause problems only if they secrete noxious substances, become invasive or elicit inappropriate host defence responses. Protection against most bacteria involves largely B cells, and plasma cell production of antibodies, together with phagocytes (neutrophils and macrophages). Protection against mycobacteria, and viruses and fungi is largely via T lymphocytes.

An enormous range of infections is recognized; many are prevalent in the tropics and developing countries and some are fatal. Global travel and global warming increasingly bring contact with these infections to the rest of the world. Concern has recently been expressed about a dozen fatal infections that appear to be increasing in their geographical range (Box 21.1).

Infection control guidelines to prevent transmission of infections are found at http://www.udp.org.uk/resources/bda-cross-infection.pdf. Diseases that are notifiable to the local authorities in UK are shown in Box 21.2.

Box 21.1 Possible imminent fatal diseases increasing with global warming

- Avian flu
- Babesiosis
- Cholera
- Ebola fever
- Lyme disease
- Parasites
- Plague
- Red tides
- Rift valley fever
- Sleeping sickness
- Tuberculosis
- Yellow fever

BACTERIAL INFECTIONS

Bacterial infections are discussed here and in other chapters (see Table 21.1) and in Appendices 21.4 and 21.5.

Bacterial infections are common. Most are transient with few untoward sequelae but some can cause serious, recurrent, disseminated or persistent lesions – especially in immunocompromised persons [particularly in neutropenic patients, those with organ transplants, and in human immunodeficiency virus/acquired immune deficiency syndrome (HIV/AIDS)],

or can be life-threatening immediately (e.g. meningococcal meningitis), less immediately (e.g. diphtheria) or in the longer term (e.g. tuberculosis, syphilis).

Bacterial infections are often diagnosed on clinical grounds, supported by smears, culture, testing for immune responses (serology) and, increasingly, by examining for nucleic acids.

Antibacterial drugs can often be effective therapy (Appendices 21.3 and 21.4) but drainage of pus is often more important. Antibiotic resistance is increasingly a serious problem (e.g. *Staphylococcus aureus; Clostridium difficile, Mycobacterium tuberculosis*) and is encouraged by unwarranted use of antibiotics. Immunization against various bacteria is available, and should be taken up (Appendix 21.6).

There is a wide range of bacterial infections recognized (Table 21.1) – this chapter discusses odontogenic and orofacial bacterial infections; most cause lesions of limited duration, but some are life-threatening. Nosocomial infections (health care associated infections; HCAI), tetanus, puncture wounds and bites and other infections not discussed elsewhere are then summarized.

Box 21.2 Notifiable diseases

- Anthrax
- Cholera
- Diphtheria
- Dysentery
- Encephalitis
- Food poisoning
- Haemorrhagic fever
- Hepatitis
- Leprosy
- Leptospirosis
- Malaria
- Measles
- Meningitis
- Meningococcal septicaemia
- Mumps
- Ophthalmia neonatorum
- Paratyphoid
- Plague
- Poliomyelitis
- Rabies
- Relapsing fever
- Rubella
- Scarlet fever
- Smallpox
- Tetanus
- Tuberculosis
- Typhoid
- Typhus
- Whooping cough
- Yellow fever

Table 21.1 Bacterial infections

Bacterial infection	Chapter location
Bartonella infections (*Rochalimaea*)	This chapter
Brucellosis	This chapter
Chlamydia	Ch. 32
Cholera	This chapter
Diphtheria	This chapter
Gonorrhoea	Ch. 32
Granuloma inguinale	Ch. 32
Haemophilus	This chapter
Legionella	Ch. 15
Leprosy	This chapter
Leptospirosis	This chapter
Lyme disease	This chapter
Listeria	This chapter
Meningococci	Ch. 13
Paratyphoid	This chapter
Pertussis	This chapter
Plague	This chapter
Pneumococci	This chapter
Q fever	This chapter
Rickettsia	This chapter
Salmonella	This chapter
Staphylococci	This chapter
Streptococci	This chapter
Syphilis	Ch. 32
Tetanus	This chapter
Trichomoniasis	Ch. 32
Tuberculosis	Ch. 15
Tularaemia	This chapter
Typhoid	This chapter
Yersinia	This chapter

OROFACIAL AND ODONTOGENIC BACTERIAL INFECTIONS

Periodontal infections

Abscesses

A gingival abscess may arise from infection or a foreign body. A lateral periodontal abscess (parodontal abscess) is seen almost exclusively in patients with chronic periodontitis, but may follow impaction of a foreign body or, rarely, can be related to a lateral root canal on a non-vital tooth.

Clinical features

Erythema and swelling are the main features. Lateral periodontal abscesses may be painful, and eventually may discharge – either through the pocket or buccally, but more coronally than a periapical abscess.

General management

Drainage, and sometimes antibiotics (Table 21.2; after British National Formulary 2009).

Acute necrotizing ulcerative gingivitis

Acute necrotizing ulcerative gingivitis (ANUG) is a non-contagious anaerobic infection associated with proliferation of *Borrelia vincentii* and fusiform bacteria. Typically an infection of young adults, especially in institutions, armed forces, etc., predisposing factors include poor oral hygiene, smoking, viral respiratory infections and immune defects such as in HIV/AIDS.

Clinical features

Characteristic features of ANUG include profuse gingival bleeding, severe soreness from gingival ulceration, halitosis and a bad taste. Malaise, fever and cervical lymph node enlargement are rare.

General management

Diagnosis is usually clinical. Smears show fusospirochaetal bacteria and leukocytes. Occasionally there may be confusion with acute leukaemia or herpetic stomatitis and a full blood picture may be needed. HIV infection may need to be considered.

Management is by oral debridement, metronidazole (penicillin, if pregnant) and improved oral hygiene.

Noma (cancrum oris; gangrenous stomatitis)

Noma can result from ANUG in malnourished, debilitated or immunocompromised patients, especially in children in developing areas. Anaerobes, particularly *Bacteroides* (*Porphyromonas*) species, *Fusobacterium necrophorum* (an animal pathogen), *Prevotella intermedia*, *Actinomyces* and alpha-haemolytic streptococci, have been implicated. In cases following ANUG, *Streptococcus anginosus* and *Abiotrophia* spp. are predominant species. In early noma, predominant species include *Ochrobactrum anthropi*, *Stenotrophomonas maltophilia*, an uncharacterized species of *Dialister*, and an uncultivated phylotype of *Leptotrichia*. A range of species or phylotypes is found in advanced noma, including *Propionibacterium acnes*, *Staphylococcus* spp., *Stenotrophomonas maltophilia*, *Ochrobactrum anthropi*, *Achromobacter* spp., *Afipia* spp., *Brevundimonas diminuta*, *Capnocytophaga* spp., *Cardiobacterium* spp., *Eikenella corrodens*, *Fusobacterium* spp., *Gemella haemoylsans* and *Neisseria* spp. Phylotypes unique to noma infections include those in the genera *Eubacterium*, *Flavobacterium*, *Kocuria*, *Microbacterium* and *Porphyromonas*, and the related *Streptococcus salivarius* and genera *Sphingomonas* and *Treponema*. Spreading necrosis penetrates the buccal mucosa, leading to gangrene and an orocutaneous fistula and scarring.

Table 21.2 Antimicrobials for odontogenic and antral infections

Condition	In non-allergic individuals, antimicrobial for > 3 days or until symptoms resolve	Comments
Acute necrotizing gingivitis	Metronidazole or amoxicillin	Only if systemic involvement
Bites	Co-amoxiclav	Ch. 24
Cellulitis	Benzylpenicillin plus flucloxacillin	
Periapical abscess	Amoxicillin or metronidazole for 5 days	Only if systemic involvement or cellulitis
Pericoronitis	Metronidazole or amoxicillin	Only if systemic involvement or trismus
Periodontal abscess	Amoxicillin or metronidazole for 5 days	Only if systemic involvement or cellulitis
Periodontitis	Metronidazole or doxycycline	Only for severe disease
Sinusitis	Amoxicillin, or doxycycline or erythromycin for 7 days	Only for symptoms > 7 days

Diagnosis is clinical; an immune defect should always be excluded. Management includes improving nutrition, systemic antibiotics (clindamycin, penicillin, tetracyclines or metronidazole) and plastic surgery.

Pericoronitis

Acute pericoronitis is inflammation of the operculum over an erupting or impacted tooth, usually a mandibular third molar. It appears in relation to the accumulation of plaque and trauma from the opposing tooth. A mixed flora with *Fusobacterium* and *Bacteroides* is recognized to be important. Immune defects may predispose.

Clinical features

Acute pericoronitis manifests with pain, trismus, swelling and halitosis. The operculum is swollen, red and often ulcerated, and there may be fever and regional lymphadenitis. Pus usually drains from beneath the operculum but, in a migratory abscess of the buccal sulcus, may track anteriorly.

General management

Diagnosis is from clinical features. Radiology is usually indicated to confirm the position and root formation of the underlying partially erupted tooth.

Initial management comprises local debridement and application of antiseptics such as chlorhexidine. Reduction of the occlusal surface (or extraction) of an opposing tooth may be helpful if there is local trauma. Pyrexia, trismus or cervical lymphadenopathy may be indications for use of systemic antibiotics, typically metronidazole. Long-term treatment may include extraction of the associated impacted tooth, particularly when this is a lower third molar.

Dental abscess (periapical abscess, odontogenic abscess)

General aspects

A dental abscess is often a sequel of pulpitis caused by dental caries, but may arise in relation to any non-vital tooth. A mixed bacterial flora, especially anaerobes such as *Fusobacterium* and *Bacteroides* (*Porphyromonas*), is implicated.

Clinical features

The causal tooth is non-vital but tender to palpation. Most dental abscesses produce an intraoral swelling, typically on the labial or buccal gingival; those on maxillary lateral incisors and those from palatal roots of the first molar tend to present palatally. Occasionally, abscesses track or discharge elsewhere; for example, lower incisors or molars may discharge extraorally, maxillary premolars and molars may discharge into the maxillary sinus (Fig. 21.1). Pain and facial swelling are characteristic but, once the abscess discharges, the acute inflammation, pain and swelling resolve and a chronic abscess develops discharging from a sinus – usually buccally and intraorally.

General management

Diagnosis is from clinical features plus imaging. Extraction or endodontic therapy of the affected tooth removes the source of infection. Analgesics may be indicated. Antimicrobials are indicated only in the circumstances outlined below.

Odontogenic infections

Odontogenic infections are mainly a consequence of pulpitis leading initially to periapical infection and a dental abscess. Most odontogenic (and many orofacial) infections arise from the commensal oral mixed flora, with a substantial proportion of anaerobes. Most odontogenic and orofacial infections respond to drainage, by either endodontic treatment, incision or tooth extraction. Analgesics also may be required. Antimicrobials may be indicated in a number of circumstances (Table 21.3).

Most odontogenic infections respond well to penicillin or metronidazole, but increasing rates of resistance due to production of beta-lactamase (an enzyme that degrades penicillins) have lowered the usefulness of penicillins. Co-amoxiclav and clindamycin, because of their broad-spectrum of activity and resistance to beta-lactamase, are increasingly used as first-line antimicrobials.

Anaerobic infections

Most head and neck infections are endogenous and mixed, with anaerobes, two-thirds containing more than one anaerobic species. Predominant anaerobes include *Prevotella*, *Fusobacterium*

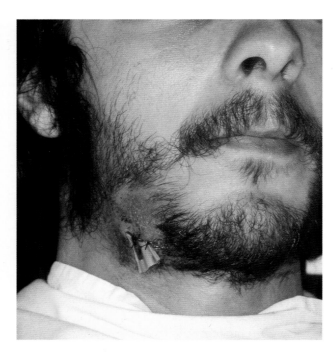

Fig. 21.1 Odontogenic infection

Table 21.3 Indications for antimicrobial therapy

Patient status	Infections
Any patient with:	Fascial space infections in the neck Necrotizing fasciitis Osteomyelitis; removal of affected tissue is mandatory Serious or life-threatening infections
Ill or immunocompromised persons with:	Acute sinusitis Acute ulcerative gingivitis Dental abscess Dry socket Oral surgery Pericoronitis

species, *Actinomyces* spp. (about 50% are *Actinomyces odontolyticus*), anaerobic cocci and *Eubacterium* spp. *Prevotella intermedia*, *Fusobacterium nucleatum*, *Prevotella melaninogenica* and the *Bacteroides fragilis* group are the most common Gram-negative anaerobic species. Microaerophilic streptococci are often associated with anaerobes. Gram-positive anaerobic cocci (GPAC) are detected in about 15% specimens – *Finegoldia magna* accounting for about one-third. Among aerobic/facultative isolates are Gram-positive cocci, Gram-negative bacteria and *Candida* species.

Treatment involves surgical procedures and antibacterial agents, which should cover both aerobes and anaerobes. Resistance rates to some agents (such as ampicillin/sulbactam and clindamycin) have increased.

Streptococcal infections

Streptococcal oral or head and neck infections are shown in Table 21.4. Most streptococci are highly susceptible to penicillin. Some pneumococci (mostly imported) are increasingly resistant.

Table 21.4 Streptococcal infections in the head and neck

Bacteria	Found in/on	May cause
Streptococcus viridans	Normal oral flora	Caries and, rarely, infective endocarditis
Strep. pyogenes	Skin and pharynx	Cellulitis, impetigo, necrotizing fasciitis, pharyngitis, scarlet fever or erysipelas, rheumatic fever and carditis
Strep. pneumoniae (pneumococci)	Upper respiratory tract	Acute glomerulonephritis, meningitis, sinusitis, otitis media, bronchitis and pneumonia

Staphylococcal infections

Staphylococcal oral or head and neck infections may be caused by *Staphylococcus aureus*, most are minor (such as furuncles and boils) and most can be treated without antibiotics, but *S. aureus* can also cause serious infections such as surgical wound infections, sinusitis, tonsillitis, otitis externa or media, tracheitis, cellulitis, necrotizing fasciitis and toxic shock syndrome (caused by a staphylococcal-produced toxin that has resulted from nasal packing, and tampon use) is characterized by fever, hypotension, flushing of the skin followed by desquamation, shock and sometimes death.

Up to 80% of the *S. aureus* isolates in the West are resistant to penicillin, primarily due to production of beta-lactamase, but these will usually respond to lactamase-stable antibiotics such as flucloxacillin and meticillin, though meticillin-resistant *S. aureus* (MRSA) is resistant to these, and often to other antibiotics. Culture is essential to guide treatment of MRSA infections.

Serious sequelae of odontogenic or orofacial infections

Cellulitis

Cellulitis is usually an acute streptococcal or staphylococcal skin infection. It usually resolves with treatment with benzylpenicillin plus flucloxacillin or, if penicillin allergic, clarithromycin, or erythromycin, clindamycin or vancomycin/teicoplanin. Cellulitis can spread locally or systemically.

Buccal cellulitis is usually caused by *Haemophilus influenzae* type B, spread by bacteraemia, by lymphatics from, for example, otitis media, or more probably from direct invasion through the oral mucosa. It is an uncommon but distinctive infection characterized by swelling, tenderness, induration and warmth of the cheek soft tissues in the absence of an adjacent oral or skin lesion, which almost invariably affects children under the age of 5 years. A minority develop meningitis. Blood and cerebrospinal fluid cultures should be taken and treatment with intravenous cefuroxime started.

Lymphangitis

Lymphangitis (inflammation of the lymphatics with pain and systemic symptoms) is commonly secondary to an acute streptococcal or staphylococcal cellulitis, or abscess in the skin or soft tissues. Lymphangitis may be confused with thrombophlebitis and suggests an infection is progressing, and may lead to bacteriaemia, septicaemia and life-threatening infection.

Fascial space infections

Fascial space infections of the neck are dangerous, since they can embarrass the airway, erode the carotid vessels, cause toxicity, or spread to the mediastinum or intracranially. They usually arise from the oral flora and are polymicrobial, involving predominantly anaerobes, including Gram-positive cocci and bacilli as well as Gram-negative bacilli.

Patients with fascial space infections must be admitted for hospital care, which may involve drainage and usually high-dose antibiotics.

Necrotizing fasciitis (Fournier gangrene, Meleney ulcer, post-operative progressive bacterial synergistic gangrene, flesh-eating bacteria, Cullen ulcer)

General aspects

This is a dangerous, progressive, rapidly spreading infection in the deep fascia, with secondary necrosis of subcutaneous tissues. The speed of spread along the deep fascial plane is directly proportional to the thickness of the subcutaneous layer. Most patients are middle-aged or older but, though the condition has become more frequent because of an increase in immuno-compromised patients with diabetes, cancer, alcoholism, vascular insufficiencies, transplants, neutropenia or HIV, few have such detectable underlying predisposing factors.

Group A haemolytic streptococci and *Staph. aureus*, alone or in synergism, are often the initiating infecting bacteria, but other aerobic and anaerobic pathogens, such as *Bacteroides (Porphyromonas)*, *Clostridium*, *Peptostreptococcus*, Enterobacteriaceae, coliforms, *Proteus*, *Prevotella*, *Pseudomonas*, *Klebsiella*, *Bacteroides fragilis*, *Fusobacterium necrophormans* and *Escherichia coli* may be present. Some men who have sex with men (MSM) have suffered outbreaks of necrotizing fasciitis caused by community-associated MRSA – distinct from health care-associated strains. Anaerobic streptococci, occasionally seen in drug addicts, cause many forms of non-clostridial myonecrosis. Necrotizing fasciitis can also be caused by *Vibrio vulnificus*, often following the consumption of raw seafood – especially in patients with chronic liver disease. There may be a relationship between the use of non-steroidal anti-inflammatory drugs and the development of necrotizing fasciitis during varicella infections.

Clinical features

There is often a history of trauma or recent surgery to the area. The lesion begins with an area of thrombosis and skin necrosis, which is initially red, painful and oedematous. Erythema quickly spreads over hours to days, and rapidly turns purplish, dusky and then black, with gas and exudate, and pain disproportionate to the clinical appearance. The margins of the infection move into surrounding skin without being raised or sharply demarcated. Over the next several hours to days, despite severe pain there may be cutaneous anaesthesia – an unusual combination as (the cutaneous nerves are damaged by the infection

(hence anaesthesia), but the proximal stump is irritated (hence the pain). Multiple patches develop to produce a large area of gangrenous skin.

Early on the patient may look deceptively well but, within 24–48 h, fever appears with rapidly spreading tissue necrosis, so that the patient usually appears moderately to severely toxic.

General management

Necrotizing fasciitis is uncommon but potentially fatal and, if from a dental source, can also spread and may threaten the airway. The mortality can sometimes reach 30%.

The gas-forming organisms may release subcutaneous gas that may be seen on radiography. Absence of gadolinium contrast enhancement in magnetic resonance imaging (MRI) T1 images reliably detects fascial necrosis. Thoracic computed tomography (CT) may be required to detect mediastinal spread.

Necrotizing fasciitis requires early aggressive treatment: the patient should be admitted to hospital and intubated, the affected area opened to drain, necrotic tissue excised and the patient given high doses of penicillin or clindamycin, plus metronidazole or a cephalosporin, or gentamicin, combined with clindamycin or chloramphenicol. Hyperbaric oxygen, if available, should be given.

Lemierre syndrome (post-anginal septicaemia)

Lemierre syndrome is a rare, potentially fatal, acute anaerobic oropharyngeal infection, typically seen in apparently healthy young adults, leading to septic thrombophlebitis of the internal jugular vein infection, and often complicated by septic pulmonary emboli and distant metastatic infections. Surgical drainage and intravenous antibiotics are indicated.

Septicaemia

Septicaemia can arise from odontogenic or orofacial infections, but more commonly from infections of the urinary tract, gall bladder or chest. Immunosuppressed patients are particularly susceptible and oral bacteria are sometimes responsible.

Blood, urine and sputum should be cultured and the patient started on ceftriaxone (a once-daily dose) or cefuroxime plus metronidazole if anaerobic sepsis is suspected.

Actinomycosis (lumpy jaw)

Actinomycosis is a rare chronic infection, usually of the face and neck, caused by *Actinomyces israelii*, a Gram-positive non-contagious anaerobic bacillus with filamentous growth and mycelia-like colonies bearing a striking resemblance to fungi, which is primarily a commensal found in normal oral cavities, in tonsillar crypts, in dental plaque and in carious teeth. There are three main presentations.

Cervicofacial actinomycosis is the most common and typically causes a red or purplish, somewhat indurated, subcutaneous mass of abscesses and open draining sinuses, usually in the submandibular area near the angle of the mandible, arising a few weeks after an antecedent local lesion (dental or periodontal infection or tooth extraction). Tenderness is slight or absent. Microscopic examination of drained fluid shows 'sulfur granules' and *Actinomyces*, and culture of the fluid or tissue shows *Actinomyces* species.

Pulmonary actinomycosis causes fever and general malaise, cough and purulent sputum. Cutaneous sinuses may form.

Abdominal actinomycosis may cause pain and a palpable mass in the abdomen.

Treatment of actinomycosis is at least 1–2 months of penicillin or tetracycline. Surgical drainage may be indicated.

Osteomyelitis (Ch. 16)
ANTIBIOTIC COVER

Antibiotic cover is sometimes suggested for various procedures or in various conditions, but this is rarely indicated (Box 21.3).

> **Box 21.3 Patients for whom antibiotic cover is *not* usually considered essential**
>
> - Immunosuppressed (including transplant patients) or immunodeficient
> - Indwelling intraperitoneal catheters
> - Intraocular lenses
> - Local tissue augmentation materials
> - Pacemakers
> - Penile prostheses
> - Prosthetic joint implants
> - Ventriculo-peritoneal shunts

HEALTH CARE ASSOCIATED (HCAI; NOSOCOMIAL) INFECTIONS

HCAI are an increasing problem across the world. Box 21.4 summarizes steps that can be taken to prevent infection transmission.

A number of micro-organisms can be involved, often bacteria, and many are becoming antimicrobial-resistant ('super bugs'; see Table 21.6).

WOUND INFECTIONS

General aspects

Infections (surgical wound infections; surgical site infections; SSIs) can be a problem in terms of morbidity and mortality. Post-operative bacterial infection rates vary from 3% to 21%, with SSIs accounting for up to 34% of the total (probably underestimated since most wound infections start after the patient is discharged). SSIs have significant morbidity and mortality accounting for ≈77% of deaths of general surgical patients.

Surgical wounds have been classified as clean, clean-contaminated, contaminated and dirty-infected (Table 21.5). Most head and neck surgery involves Class I or II wounds.

Most SSIs arise from the patient's own flora or from health care workers and articles brought into the operative field, and the operating room air. The usual pathogens on skin surfaces are Gram-positive aerobic cocci (mainly staphy-

> **Box 21.4 Prevention of health care-associated infection transmission**
>
> - Follow good hygiene and standard infection control procedures
> - Avoid contact with wounds or material contaminated from wounds
> - Use alcohol-based waterless antiseptic agents for routinely decontaminating hands, when hands are not visibly soiled
> - Wash hands thoroughly with a non-antimicrobial soap and water, or an antimicrobial soap and water, when hands are visibly dirty or contaminated with proteinaceous material such as blood
> - Keep cuts and abrasions clean and covered with a proper dressing until healed, when hands are cut or abraded
> - Use a moisturizer to prevent skin cracking

lococci), but anaerobes and Gram-negative aerobes may be involved. The normal oral flora is 90% anaerobes and 10% Gram-positive aerobic cocci. Gram-negative aerobes may be a problem in patients who have been hospitalized or treated with radiotherapy. Factors promoting wound infection include pre-operative removal of hair, especially when there is skin abrasion, inadequate skin preparation with bactericidal solution, poor surgical technique, lengthy operation (> 2 h), intraoperative contamination, prolonged stay in hospital, hypothermia, trauma, non-viable tissue in the wound, haematoma, foreign material (including drains and sutures), dead space, pre-existing sepsis (local or distant), immunocompromised or malnourished host, hypovolaemia, poor tissue perfusion, or obesity, and delayed prophylaxis with, or incorrect choice of, antibiotics.

PROPHYLAXIS

Prophylactic antibiotics are indicated for clean-contaminated and contaminated trauma, for clean procedures in which prosthetic devices are inserted and, more controversially, for clean procedures such as orthognathic surgery.

The concentration of prophylactic antibiotic should be at therapeutic levels by the time of incision, during the surgical procedure, and for a few hours post-operatively, and this is achieved by intravenous administration of the antibiotic, 30 min before incision (not more than 2 h before surgery). For head and neck surgery, *Staph. aureus*, streptococci, anaerobes and streptococci can be present in an oropharyngeal approach; examples of antibiotics shown to be effective in Class II head and neck wound prophylaxis include cefazolin 1–2 g alone or in combination with metronidazole, or clindamycin alone or with gentamicin or amikacin, amoxicillin/clavulanate, ampicillin/sulbactam, and ticarcillin/clavulanate.

Clinical features

Surgical site infection is suggested by features such as pus draining from the wound, the wound becoming excessively tender, progressive swelling starting about 48 h after surgery, increasing redness around the wound (cellulitis), a red streak from the wound toward the heart (lymphangitis), lymphadenitis or fever. The wound may fail to heal within 10 days after the injury, the scab increases in size and a pimple or yellow crust may form on the wound (impetigo).

Table 21.5 Surgical wound classification and subsequent risk of infection – (no antibiotics used (Cruse PJ. Surgical wound sepsis. Can Med Assoc J 1970;102:251–8. Cruse PJ, Foord R. The epidemiology of wound infection. A 10-year prospective study of 62,939 wounds. Surg Clin North Am 1980;60:27–40.)

Classification	Oral or perioral example	Description	Infective risk (%)
Clean (Class I)	Excision of a facial skin lesion	Uninfected operative wound No acute inflammation Closed primarily Respiratory, gastrointestinal, biliary and urinary tracts not entered No break in aseptic technique Closed drainage used if necessary	< 2
Clean-contaminated (Class II)	Parotid surgery	Elective entry into respiratory, biliary, gastro-intestinal, urinary tracts and with minimal spillage No evidence of infection or major break in aseptic technique	< 10
Contaminated (Class III)	Third molar surgical removal	Non-purulent inflammation present Spillage from gastrointestinal tract Penetrating traumatic wounds < 4 h Major break in aseptic technique	About 20
Dirty-infected (Class IV)	Incision and drainage of a submandibular abscess	Purulent inflammation present Pre-operative perforation of viscera Penetrating traumatic wounds > 4 h	About 40

General management

Treatment of SSI often involves antibiotics after opening the wound, evacuating pus and cleansing the wound – inspecting deeper tissues for integrity and for deep space infection or source. Dressing changes allow the tissues to granulate, and the wound heals by secondary intention over several weeks.

The antibiotic choice depends on the known or probable infecting micro-organism, and factors such as severity of SSI, patient's age, hepatic and renal function, allergies and other medication(s). First choices are flucloxacillin in the absence of allergy if staphylococci or streptococci are implicated; metronidazole or clindamycin for anaerobic infections; cefuroxime for Gram-negative organisms; amoxicillin or co-amoxiclav for enterococcal infection. For pain relief, acetaminophen/paracetamol, ibuprofen or an opioid is indicated.

ANTIBIOTIC-RESISTANT INFECTIONS

The main antibiotic-resistant infections are meticillin-resistant *Staph. aureus* (MRSA) and *Clostridium difficile*, but there are several others (Table 21.6). Six bacteria of this type have been dubbed ESKAPE (*Enterococcus faccium, Staph. aureus; Klebsiella* specias, Acinetobacter *baumannii, Pseudomonas aeruginosa* and *Enterobacter* species.

MRSA

MRSA (sometimes referred to as 'the superbug') stands for meticillin-resistant *Staphylococcus aureus* (also resistant to flucloxacillin). The most common clones are E(pidemic)-MRSA 15 and E-MRSA16. Strains of *Staph. aureus* producing Panton–Valentine leukocidin (PVL) are especially virulent.

About one in three people carry *Staph. aureus* on the skin surface or in the nose; if this enters the body through a break in the skin, it can cause infections such as abscesses, or impetigo. MRSA is no more infectious than other types of *Staph. aureus*, but infections are more difficult to treat owing to their antibiotic resistance, and mortality is increased.

The infection may simply require a much higher dose over a much longer period, or the use of an agent to which the MRSA is not resistant.

MRSA is usually spread through person-to-person contact with someone who has an MRSA infection, or who is colonized. It can also spread through contact with towels, sheets, clothes, dressings or other objects that have been used by someone with MRSA. *Staph. aureus* can also survive on objects or surfaces such as door handles, sinks, floors and cleaning equipment. MRSA infections are far more common in people who are in hospital; risk factors are shown in Box 21.5.

Community-associated MRSA infections are typically skin infections, usually transmitted from people with active MRSA skin infections. The strains causing these infections, designated community-associated MRSA (CA-MRSA), are distinct from health care-associated strains (HA-MRSA). Infection with multidrug-resistant USA300 MRSA has emerged among men who have sex with men. Infection is most often of buttocks, genitals or perineum. The risk is independent of HIV infection but the infection might be sexually transmitted in this population.

Community-associated MRSA spreads especially to:

- intravenous drug users
- children in day care
- athletes
- military personnel
- prison inmates.

Table 21.6 Main antibiotic-resistant nosocomial infections

Infection	Found	Transmission by	Consequences	UK epidemiology
MRSA	On skin or in nose of 25–30% of healthy people	Close contact with infected people, usually direct physical contact, not through air. Also by indirect contact with contaminated objects (towels, sheets, wound dressings, clothes, work-out areas, sports equipment)	Wound and other infections	Increasing since 1993 1652 deaths in 2006
VRE	In mouths of 66%	Direct contact, health care staff or contaminated environment	Diarrhoea, wound infection, urinary tract infection, endocarditis and bacteraemia	Increasing
ESBL	Respiratory or urinary tract	Direct contact, health care staff or contaminated environment	Diarrhoea, urinary tract infection	Increasing since 2003 Affects 30 000 annually in UK
Clostridium difficile	In gut of 5% of healthy adult people	Direct contact, health care staff or contaminated environment	Diarrhoea and colitis	Increasing since 2005 6480 deaths in 2006
Stenotrophomonas maltophilia	Frequently colonizes fluids	Invasive medical devices	Various	≈1000 cases annually

ESBL, extended spectrum beta-lactamase; MRSA, meticillin-resistant *Staphylococcus aureus*; VRE, vancomycin-resistant enterococci.

Box 21.5 Risk factors for MRSA

- Immune incompetence (e.g. elderly, newborn babies, diabetes, cancer or HIV/AIDS)
- An open wound, catheter or intravenous tube
- A severe skin condition (e.g. burn or cut, ulcer or psoriasis)
- Recently had surgery
- Have to take frequent courses of antibiotics.
- Prolonged hospital stay
- Asymptomatic nasal carriage of MRSA

Clinical features

Symptoms depend on the type of infection. Most *Staph. aureus* infections are skin infections, including boils, abscesses, styes, carbuncles, cellulitis and impetigo, but infections are able to enter the bloodstream (bacteraemia), can cause septicaemia, septic shock, septic arthritis, osteomyelitis, abscesses, meningitis, pneumonia and endocarditis, and can be fatal. *Staph. aureus* can also cause scalded skin syndrome and, very occasionally, toxic shock syndrome.

General management

Many hospitals now test all people being admitted to see if they are colonized; swabs from the skin and nose, urine and blood samples may be tested. It can take 3–5 days for the results. People colonized with MRSA may still be admitted to hospital, but treated to reduce or remove it by using antibiotic cream applied to skin or the inside of the nose, and washing skin and hair with antiseptic shampoo and lotion. Health care workers should use fast-acting, special alcohol rubs or gels, and wear disposable gloves when there will be physical contact with open wounds, for example when

changing dressings, handling needles or inserting intravenous lines.

MRSA infections are diagnosed by testing blood, urine or a tissue sample for the presence of MRSA. Patients who are only *colonized* with MRSA usually do not need treatment. Infections often require hospital treatment in isolation for several weeks. Frank MRSA infections can sometimes be treated without antibiotics by draining and, in reality, most are resistant to multiple antibiotics as well as to meticillin.

A number of agents may be used to treat MRSA infections, normally given by injection or intravenously. Vancomycin, quinupristin combined with dalfopristin or linezolid may be effective, but resistance has been reported. Linezolid can also cause cytopenias, including pancytopenia, and optic neuropathy and acts as a monoamine oxidase inhibitor. Teicoplanin, rifampicin and streptogramin may also be effective.

People more at risk of MRSA are best advised not to visit an infected person and all visitors must wash hands thoroughly before and after visiting.

MRSA has rarely been transmitted to dental patients but oral infections have now been reported.

Vancomycin-resistant *Staphylococcus aureus* and vancomycin-intermediate *Staphylococcus aureus*

Vancomycin-resistant (VRSA) and reduced susceptibility (vancomycin-intermediate) *S. aureus* (VISA) infections are starting to appear.

Clostridium difficile

Clostridium difficile is the major cause of antibiotic-associated diarrhoea and colitis, a health care-associated intestinal infection that mostly affects elderly patients with other underlying diseases. In most cases, the disease develops after cross-infection from a patient, either through direct contact, or via health care staff, or via a contaminated environment. It is thus a problem in hospital environments in particular.

Diagnosis is from the presence of *C. difficile* toxins in a faecal sample. Type 027 produces much more of the toxins than most other types.

Prevention and control of *C. difficile* is by reduction of the use of broad-spectrum antibiotics, isolation of patients with *C. difficile* diarrhoea, good infection control nursing (alcohol gel does not destroy the spores), and enhanced environmental cleaning using a chlorine-containing disinfectant.

Vancomycin-resistant enterococci (VRE)

Enterococci are commensals in the gastrointestinal and urinary tracts, acquired from other people or from contaminated food or water. Up to 66% carry enterococci in the mouth, especially in patients undergoing endodontic treatment. VRE may be associated with endodontic failures. Enterococci can cause diarrhoea, wound infection, bacteraemia or urinary tract infections, mainly in immunocompromised and medically ill patients. Most infections are seen in hospital. They may also give rise to endocarditis.

Extended-spectrum beta-lactamase (ESBL) producers

Gram-negative enteric bacilli (Enterobacteriaceae), which destroy beta-lactam antibiotics, are producers of ESBL enzymes that mediate resistance to extended-spectrum (third-generation) cephalosporins (e.g. ceftazidime, cefotaxime and ceftriaxone) and oxyimino-monobactams (e.g. aztreonam) but do not affect cephamycins (e.g. cefoxitin and cefotetan) or carbapenems (e.g. meropenem or imipenem). ESBL enzymes are most commonly produced by *Escherichia coli* and *Klebsiella pneumoniae*, but other bacteria that may produce them include *E. cloacae*, *C. freundii*, *S. marcescens*, *P. aeruginosa*, *Salmonella* spp. and *P. mirabilis*.

Infection with ESBL may originate in infected chicken meat. Persistent oral carriage may be seen in immunocompromised persons, in advanced age and in xerostomia. Outbreaks have occurred in hospitals and nursing homes, and increasingly in the community, typically with urinary tract infections and bacteraemia. Carbapenems, such as meropenem, are usually effective treatment.

Stenotrophomonas maltophilia ('steno')

Stenotrophomonas (Pseudomonas) maltophilia is an aerobic, non-fermentative, Gram-negative bacterium of low virulence found in aquatic environments. It frequently colonizes fluids used in hospitals (e.g. irrigation solutions, intravenous fluids) and is found in patient secretions (e.g. secretions, urine, exudates).

Stenotrophomonas maltophilia rarely causes disease in healthy hosts unless invasive medical devices are present. Antimicrobial treatment is usually unnecessary and may be potentially harmful. Infections are in any event difficult to treat, but *Stenotrophomonas maltophilia* is susceptible to trimethoprim–sulfamethoxazole, meropenem, minocycline, quinolones and colistin/polymyxin B.

TETANUS, PUNCTURE WOUNDS AND BITES

Tetanus

General aspects

Tetanus is a non-communicable infection caused by wound contamination with *Clostridium tetani* spores with mortality up to 60%. The spores are ubiquitous in soil or dust, particularly where there is faecal contamination, as on agricultural land. Tetanus is most likely to follow contaminated deep wounds, such as puncture wounds, especially if there is tissue necrosis, but it may also follow trivial wounds, or even bites or burns. The elderly, particularly women, are at greatest risk. Neonates may develop tetanus from contamination of the umbilical stump, a condition only found in the developing world.

Clinical features

The incubation period is between 4 and 21 days, commonly about 10 days.

Clostridium tetani produces a neurotoxin (tetanospasmin) responsible for violent muscular spasms: trismus (lockjaw) due to masseteric spasm is the single most common early sign. Facial spasm produces a so-called sardonic smile (risus sardonicus) where the eyebrows are raised with eyes closed and the lips are drawn back over clenched teeth. Spinal muscle spasm produces arching of the back (opisthotonos), while laryngeal spasm can lead to asphyxiation. Autonomic dysfunction can cause cardiac arrhythmias and fluctuations in blood pressure. Death may follow within 10 days of the onset of tetanus, usually from asphyxia, autonomic dysfunction or bronchopneumonia.

General management

Patients who have contaminated wounds, such as those associated with maxillofacial injuries caused by road traffic or riding accidents, are at greatest risk from tetanus. Wounds that are considered tetanus-prone include any wound or burn sustained more than 6 h before surgical treatment of the injury, or that shows a significant degree of devitalized tissue; a puncture wound; contact with manure or soil; or clinical sepsis.

Management of wounds where tetanus is likely includes active immunization with tetanus toxoid, but it is *not* good practice to give toxoid after every *minor* injury, as severe allergic reactions can occasionally follow (see Table 21.7).

The diagnosis of tetanus is clinical. There are no immediate tests that will help the diagnosis. Patients with tetanus should be admitted to an intensive care unit for protection of the airway (tracheostomy should be carried out if the airway is endangered) and to facilitate artificial respiration should it become necessary; for anti-tetanus immunoglobulin (give early as it is ineffective after the toxin has become bound to nervous tissue) – human anti-tetanus immunoglobulin (ATG; Humotet, 500 units or more) or, if this is not available, animal anti-tetanus serum (ATS; after testing for hypersensitivity and with epinephrine and corticosteroids available in case a severe reaction develops); for control of muscle spasms by

Table 21.7 Management of wounded patients at risk from tetanus

Wound type	Immune status	Course of action[a]
Superficial wound or abrasion	Immune[b]	–
	Not known to be immune	Active immunization with toxoid. Full three-dose course or, if partially immune, a reinforcing dose
Deep wounds, puncture wounds, or bites or burns	Immune	Give toxoid booster[c]
	Not known to be immune	Give antibiotics (metronidazole or penicillin) and start immunization with toxoid and: (1) if seen after 4 h give 250–500 units HTIG i.m.; (2) if seen after 24 h give 500 units HTIG i.m.

[a]Wound debridement in all.
[b]Last of three-dose course or reinforcing dose within past 10 years.
[c]Human tetanus immunoglobulin (250–500 units HTIG i.m.) should also be given if wound is highly contaminated or there is any doubt about immune status.
HTIG, human tetanus immunoglobulin.

heavy sedation or, in severe cases, using general anaesthesia, muscle relaxants and mechanical ventilation; and for wound debridement, the purpose of which is to remove the source of toxin, as antibiotics alone are ineffective. Metronidazole is usually given.

Survivors suffer no after-effects but should have active immunization with toxoid.

Prophylaxis

Prophylaxis is active immunization in childhood, given as a triple vaccine (diphtheria, pertussis and tetanus antigens) starting at the age of 12 weeks, followed by further injections 6–8 weeks later and then after a further 4–6 months. Booster immunization (diphtheria plus tetanus) is given on starting primary school and at 15–19 years. The duration of immunity after such an immunization schedule is not known but current practice is to boost it every 10 years. Groups at highest risk (e.g. farm workers) should be given boosters every 5 years. Most cases of tetanus in the developed world are now seen in those who were never immunized, or in those whose immunity has declined – hence the risk in the elderly.

Dental aspects

Trismus is usually caused by local irritation such as pericoronitis or temporomandibular pain-dysfunction syndrome but, in the absence of a local cause, tetanus must always be considered. Such patients should therefore be asked whether they have had any recent wounds, particularly if farm workers or gardeners.

Dyskinesias due to phenothiazines include facial grimacing but rarely trismus – the mouth is usually forcefully opened.

Puncture wounds

A puncture wound is caused by an object *piercing* the skin and creating a small hole. Some punctures can be very deep and do not often result in obvious excessive bleeding, and tend to close fairly quickly spontaneously. A puncture wound from a cause such as stepping on a nail can become infected. Treatment may be necessary to prevent tetanus or other infections. Most healthy people without signs of infection do not require antibiotics, but these may be given to people with diabetes, peripheral vascular disease, contaminated wounds or deep wounds to the foot.

Bites

Dogs and cats cause most animal bites. Dog bites may cause severe tissue injury to tissues as well as infections. Cat bites are more frequently (approximately 50%) infected. Animal bite infections are usually bacterial – typically polymicrobial (staphylococci and anaerobes). Tetanus is rarely transmitted.

Bites from non-immunized domestic animals and wild animals may carry the risk of rabies, which is more common in raccoons, skunks, bats and foxes than in cats and dogs. Rabbits, squirrels and other rodents rarely carry rabies.

Treatment includes consideration of the possibilities of tetanus and rabies, debridement, and antibiotic coverage for staphylococci (co-amoxiclav) and anaerobes.

Human bites are discussed in Ch. 24.

OTHER BACTERIAL INFECTIONS

Many other infections are seen, especially in the developing world (Appendix 24.1).

VIRAL INFECTIONS

Viral infections are often readily transmitted in saliva and other body fluids, and where general hygiene is low and there is close contact with other persons or their secretions, infections are common. They thus mainly affect young children, who often thereby acquire immunity. In developed countries, children may not contract these infections and thus are non-immune, and may have a primary infection as adolescents and adults.

Rashes (exanthemata) are common in some viral infections (Table 21.8).

Most viral infections are transient with few untoward sequelae, though many cause malaise, fever and depression of the immune system. Some viral infections can be immediately life-threatening (e.g. severe acute respiratory syndrome; SARS), others can result in tumours (e.g. hepatitis C and B and liver cancer), and others can seriously damage the immune system (e.g. HIV/AIDS; Ch. 20). Many viral infections can cause severe, recurrent, disseminated or persistent lesions in immunocompromised persons, such as those with organ transplants, or HIV/AIDS.

Table 21.8 Common childhood infections with rashes		
	Name	**Alternative term**
First disease	Measles	Rubeola
Second disease	Scarlet fever	Streptococci
Third disease	German measles	Rubella
Fourth disease	Filatov–Dukes disease	Doubt exists over the existence of this
Fifth disease	Erythema infectiosum ('slapped cheek syndrome')	Parvovirus
Sixth disease	Herpesvirus 6 infection ('exanthem subitum')	Roseola infantum

Viral infections are often diagnosed on clinical grounds, supported by testing for immune responses (serology) and, increasingly, by examining for viral nucleic acids.

Anti-herpetic and anti-retroviral drugs can be effective (Appendices Ch. 21) but relatively few other effective antiviral agents are available. Immunization against various viruses is available, and should be taken up.

There is a wide range of infections recognized (Table 21.9).

This chapter discusses the important common viral infections, alphabetically; see Appendix 21.7 for serious life-threatening but fortunately uncommon viral infections.

Table 21.9 Viral infections	
Viral infection	**Chapter location**
Arborviruses	This chapter
Arenaviruses	This chapter
Enteroviruses	This chapter
Hantaviruses	This chapter
Hepatitis	Ch. 9
Herpesviruses	This chapter
Human immunodeficiency viruses	Ch. 20
Influenza	Ch. 15
Measles	This chapter
Molluscum contagiosum	This chapter
Mumps	This chapter
Papillomaviruses	This chapter
Parvovirus	This chapter
Poliomyelitis	Ch. 13
Rabies	This chapter
Rhabdoviruses	This chapter
Rubella	This chapter
Severe acute respiratory syndrome (SARS)	Ch. 15

ENTEROVIRUSES

Enteroviruses multiply in the gut mucosa and are transmitted from person to person by the faecal–oral route. Most infections are in childhood, often as small epidemics. Enterovirus infections are usually transient but produce lifelong immunity to the strain. Clinical syndromes are generally mild, but occasional infections may cause serious disease such as paralytic poliomyelitis, meningitis or myocarditis.

Enterovirus diseases relevant to dentistry include hepatitis A (Ch. 9), poliomyelitis (Ch. 13), herpangina, and hand, foot and mouth disease.

Herpangina

Coxsackie viruses, usually A7 or B1, or echoviruses 9 or 17 cause infections, often subclinically. After an incubation of 2–9 days, clinical features may include mouth ulcers affecting the posterior mouth alone (soft palate and uvula) and causing sore throat, cervical lymphadenitis, fever, malaise, irritability, anorexia and sometimes vomiting. Diagnosis is from the clinical features. Management is symptomatic (see Herpes simplex).

Hand, foot and mouth disease

Picornaviruses [Coxsackie A and Enterovirus (EV) 71] are responsible for most hand, foot and mouth disease (HFMD). Coxsackie (usually A16; rarely A5 or 10) virus infections are often subclinical. However, the World Health Organization reported one outbreak in 2008 in China involving a total of 1884 cases including 20 deaths due to enterovirus EV-71.

Clinical features, after an incubation of 2–6 days, include mouth ulcers, resembling herpetic stomatitis, mild fever, malaise and anorexia, and a rash. Red papules that evolve to superficial vesicles in a few days form mainly on the palms and soles. Diagnosis is from the clinical features. Management is symptomatic (see Herpes simplex).

HERPESVIRUSES

The herpesviruses are DNA viruses, transmitted mainly in saliva and other body fluids (Table 21.10). They typically cause a short-lived primary clinical, or more often subclinical, infection, and remain latent thereafter. Reactivation is often because of immunosuppression and recrudescence can lead to protracted illness. Some herpesviruses can be oncogenic.

Herpes simplex virus (HSV; human herpesvirus types 1 and 2) infections

General aspects

Type 1 HSV typically causes primary oral infection with acute gingivostomatitis but may cause primary anogenital infection. Type 2 HSV typically causes anogenital infections but may cause oral or oropharyngeal infections. HSV thereafter remains latent in the sensory ganglia but if reactivated may cause lesions. Recurrent infections typically affect the mucocutaneous junctions and are often precipitated by factors such as exposure to

Table 21.10	The herpesviruses	
Herpesvirus type	Standard nomenclature	Abbreviation
1	Herpes simplex type 1	HSV-1
2	Herpes simplex type 2	HSV-2
3	Herpes varicella-zoster	VZV
4	Epstein–Barr virus	EBV
5	Cytomegalovirus	CMV
6	Human herpesvirus type 6	HHV-6
7	Human herpesvirus type 7	HHV-7
8	Human herpesvirus type 8 (kaposi sarcoma herpesvirus)	HHV-8 (KSHV)

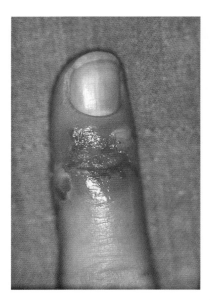

Fig. 21.3 Herpetic whitlow

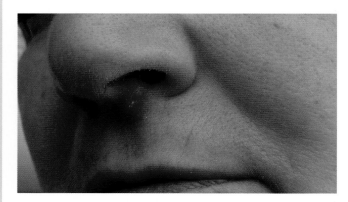

Fig. 21.2 Herpes simplex recurrent infection

systemic infections, sunlight, trauma, stress, menstruation or immune incompetence (Figs 21.2).

Clinical features

Primary oral infection with HSV, usually type 1, typically causes acute gingivostomatitis, ulcers, fever, cervical lymph node enlargement and irritability. It is common in young children and sometimes misdiagnosed as 'teething', or may be subclinical. Primary herpetic gingivostomatitis is limited to the mouth and resolves within about 10 days but, in immunosuppressed patients or in those with eczema, disseminated infection may result.

Thereafter HSV remains latent, often in the trigeminal ganglia, but reactivates from time to time, appears in the saliva and may cause lesions. The virus can be spread by saliva and occasionally causes painful whitlows in dental staff not previously exposed to it (Fig. 21.3). A growing number of oral or oropharyngeal infections appear to be caused by HSV-2, which otherwise causes genital infections. Diagnosis is typically clinical.

Aciclovir is effective against HSV but many patients present with disease too far advanced to really benefit. Aciclovir, famciclovir or other antivirals are essential to control infection in immunocompromised patients (Table 21.11). Treatment is supplemented with supportive care such as adequate fluid intake, antipyretics and analgesics (usually acetaminophen)

and good oral hygiene by mouth cleansing and use of aqueous chlorhexidine mouthwashes.

Recurrent infections appear in up to 30% of patients, typically at the mucocutaneous junction of the lip (herpes labialis; cold sores) or nose, and are often precipitated by exposure to systemic infections, sunlight, trauma, stress or menstruation. These factors stimulate HSV to reactivate by more than one mechanism. One way is by direct induction of viral genes such as *ICP4* and *VP16*. Heat can induce these viral genes either directly or via the by-products of heat. The activated viral gene products then overcome the effects of latent (LAT) RNAs. Another mechanism is an indirect one involving immunosuppression. Ultraviolet light is immunosuppressive and also induces cytokines that can trigger inflammation. These cytokines may affect dendrites that communicate the signal back to the neuron where the viral DNA is residing; *ICP4* and *VP16* are viral genes critical for reactivation.

Diagnosis is clinical. Recurrent labial infections respond well to penciclovir or aciclovir cream applied early.

Intraoral recurrences appear as ulcers, and seem to be more likely after trauma, such as in the palate, or in immunocompromised patients (e.g. leukaemia or HIV/AIDS). Aciclovir may be indicated but HSV is now showing starting to show resistance. Famciclovir, valaciclovir or even forscarnet may then be required.

Genital herpes

A person almost always contracts HSV-2 infection by sexual contact. HSV-1 infection of the genitals is almost always caused by oral–genital contact with a person who has oral HSV-1 infection. One out of five of the total adolescent and adult population in the USA are infected with HSV-2; the prevalence is rising but few have signs or symptoms. When signs of genital herpes do appear, they are typically as blisters on or around the genitals or rectum. The blisters break, leaving tender ulcers that may take 2–4 weeks to heal. It is important that women avoid contracting HSV-2 during pregnancy because a first episode during pregnancy causes a greater risk of transmission

Table 21.11   Antiviral therapy considerations in common herpesvirus infections

Virus	Disease	Otherwise healthy patient	Immunocompromised patient
Herpes simplex	Primary	Consider oral aciclovir[a] 100–200 mg, five times daily as suspension (200 mg/5 ml) or tablets	Aciclovir 250 mg/m^2 i.v. every 8 h
	Recurrent herpetic ulcers	Consider oral aciclovir[a] 100–200 mg, five times daily as suspension (200 mg/5 ml) or tablets	Consider aciclovir 250 mg/m^2 i.v. every 8 h
	Recurrent herpes labialis	Penciclovir 1% cream or aciclovir 5% cream every 2 h	Consider aciclovir 250 mg/m^2 i.v. every 8 h
Herpes varicella	Chickenpox	–	Aciclovir 500 mg/m^2 (5 mg/kg) i.v. every 8 h
	Zoster (shingles)	3% aciclovir ophthalmic ointment for shingles of ophthalmic division of trigeminal	Aciclovir 500 mg/m^2 (5 mg/kg) i.v. every 8 h or famciclovir 250 mg three times daily, or 750 mg daily

[a]In neonate, treat as if immunocompromised.

Aciclovir: systemic preparations, caution in renal disease and pregnancy, occasional rise in liver enzymes and urea, rashes, central nervous system effects.

Famciclovir: caution in renal disease and pregnancy. Occasional nausea and headache.

to the newborn. HSV-2 can cause potentially fatal infections in infants if the mother is shedding virus at the time of delivery. If a woman has active genital herpes at delivery, a Caesarean delivery is therefore usually performed.

Antiviral medications, such as aciclovir or famciclovir, can shorten and prevent outbreaks during the period the medication is being taken.

Varicella and zoster (human herpesvirus 3)

Chickenpox

General aspects

Varicella (chickenpox) is a highly contagious disease caused by the varicella-zoster virus (VZV), spread readily by droplets. Patients are infectious from 1 to 2 days before the rash, until the rash scabs and dries.

Varicella-zoster virus then remains latent within dorsal root ganglia and, if reactivated, as can happen in the elderly or the immunocompromised, can lead to shingles (zoster) – a painful unilateral rash.

Clinical features

Varicella is most common in children below the age of 10 years. There is fever, malaise and a centripetal rash (mainly on trunk and face), which passes through macular, papular, vesicular and pustular stages before scabbing. There are about 3–5 crops of lesions. There may be mouth ulcers.

Infants, adolescents, adults and immunocompromised persons are at higher risk for complications, such as disseminated or haemorrhagic varicella. Adults, especially those who are pregnant or who smoke, are at risk from fulminating varicella pneumonia. There is also a risk to the fetus and neonate if the mother contracts chickenpox. In the first 20 weeks of pregnancy, a congenital varicella syndrome with microcephaly, cataracts, growth retardation and limb hypoplasia may result, and the mortality rate is high. Later in pregnancy, chickenpox may result in zoster in an otherwise healthy infant. Chickenpox

around the time of delivery may cause severe and even fatal infection of the neonate.

General management

Diagnosis is clinical. Varicella-zoster immunoglobulin, or aciclovir, valaciclovir or famciclovir, may be indicated for non-immune persons who are pregnant or immunocompromised. Varicella vaccine is effective in preventing illness or modifying varicella severity if used within 3 days, and possibly up to 5 days of exposure.

Zoster

General aspects

Varicella-zoster virus remains latent within dorsal root ganglia and may be reactivated, especially in the elderly or immunocompromised, leading to shingles (zoster). In about 8–10%, zoster may reflect an underlying immunodeficiency state, sometimes as a result of HIV/AIDS or a neoplasm, particularly a lymphoma.

Clinical features

Zoster involves one or more contiguous sensory dermatomes, usually of the face or the chest, and causes severe pain and a rash similar to chickenpox, but localized to the dermatome (Fig. 21.4). Trigeminal ophthalmic zoster may cause facial rash and pain and ulcerate the cornea (Fig. 21.5). Zoster of the maxillary or mandibular divisions of the trigeminal nerve may cause facial rash and pain (sometimes simulating toothache) and oral ulceration – unilateral and in the nerve distribution.

General management

Diagnosis is clinical. Patients with ophthalmic zoster should have an urgent ophthalmological opinion. Treatment of zoster is with aciclovir, valaciclovir or famciclovir by mouth, given within 3 days of the appearance of the rash. Intravenous administration is needed in immunodeficient patients, particularly in those with HIV/AIDS for whom it can be a life-threatening disease.

The pain of herpetic neuralgia may not respond well to analgesics, but may respond to tricyclic antidepressants, carbamazepine

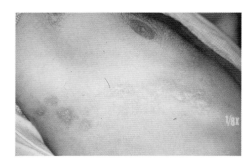

Fig. 21.4 Thoracic zoster

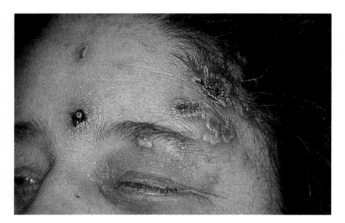

Fig. 21.5 Ophthalmic zoster

or capsaicin. Other treatments for post-herpetic pain include skin stimulation of the painful area by prolonged rubbing with a soft cloth; firm pressure with the flat of the hand or the ball of the thumb; massage; acupuncture; local heat; a cold spray; or transcutaneous electric nerve stimulation (TENS).

Immunization of children against VZV reduces the risk of zoster at a later age. However, if immunity wanes with age, there may be epidemics of chickenpox in the middle-aged and, if the middle-aged who have had chickenpox do not get occasional boosts of their immunity by exposure to chickenpox (which has been prevented in children by vaccination), the incidence of shingles may rise. In immunocompromised patients who are exposed to VZV, it may be desirable to give zoster immunoglobulin or vaccine.

Epstein–Barr virus (human herpesvirus 4)

General aspects

Epstein–Barr virus (EBV) causes infectious mononucleosis (IM; classic glandular fever). EBV also has epidemiological associations with Burkitt and some other lymphomas, and nasopharyngeal carcinoma. EBV may also cause sialadenitis (see later) and, in immunocompromised patients, EBV may be associated with hairy leukoplakia (Ch. 20) or lymphomas.

Clinical features

Epstein–Barr virus is found in saliva during infectious mononucleosis and for several months thereafter. EBV is also often in the saliva of immunocompromised persons. Though infectivity

is low, EBV appears to be spread by close oral contact, such as kissing.

Infection is common among young adults and is often subclinical or unrecognized, especially in children. Infectious mononucleosis causes mainly lymphadenopathy, sore throat and fever but is protean in its manifestations (glandular fever). Glandular fever is a syndrome in which fever, malaise and lymph node enlargement are the main features and, though typically caused by EBV, other infectious agents are occasionally responsible (Box 21.6).

Box 21.6 Causes of glandular fever syndrome

- Cytomegalovirus infection
- HIV infection
- Human herpesvirus 6 infection
- Infectious lymphocytosis
- Infectious mononucleosis (Epstein–Barr virus)
- Toxoplasmosis
- Rarely: acute leukaemia; brucellosis; drug-induced hypersensitivity syndrome [DIHS; drug reaction with eosinophilia and systemic symptoms (DRESS) syndrome]

Infectious mononucleosis can appear in many forms.

- *Febrile type IM* – high fever with rubelliform rashes and occasionally jaundice.
- *Anginose type IM* – sore throat with soft palate petechiae and a whitish exudate confined to the tonsils, and pharyngeal oedema that may threaten the airway (to be distinguished from diphtheria) and petechiae on the palate. The latter are occasionally seen in other viral infections such as rubella and HIV. Occasionally there is mouth ulceration.
- *Glandular type IM* – generalized, especially cervical, lymph node enlargement and splenomegaly. IM is an important cause of enlarged cervical lymph nodes. Unfortunately, the lymph node histopathological changes closely resemble those in lymphomas and an expert opinion is needed.

Complications of IM include persistent fatigue, mild liver dysfunction, ECG changes, depression, neurological syndromes and, rarely, nephritis, pancreatitis or lung infiltration. Ampicillin and amoxicillin frequently cause a maculopapular rash (which is not an allergy), affecting the extensor surfaces of limbs (Fig. 21.6).

General management

Serological changes diagnostic of IM include heterophile antibodies (Paul–Bunnell test) and EBV antibodies. Heterophile antibodies are immunoglobulin M (IgM) antibodies that agglutinate sheep and horse red blood cells. The Paul–Bunnell test uses sheep erythrocytes but more rapid methods are available to detect heterophile antibodies to horse red blood cells by detecting agglutination on a glass slide (Monospot test).

Heterophil antibodies usually develop during the first or second week of the illness (60% of patients), and by 4 weeks up to 90% of patients have a titre before absorption of 224 (or 28 after absorption). The titre then declines and disappears over 3–6 months. EBV antibodies include those to viral capsid antigen (VCA), which are produced early, peak at about

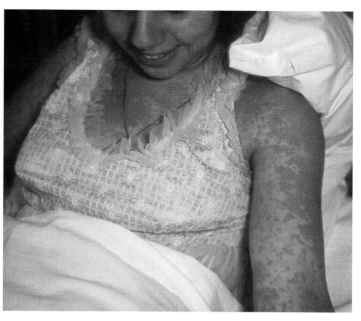

Fig. 21.6 Infectious mononucleosis

4 weeks and persist for many years. EBV IgM testing is used if there is any diagnostic doubt.

There may be a false-positive Wassermann reaction. Characteristic blood changes of IM are an excess of atypical lymphocytes (mononucleosis) that may cause confusion with leukaemia but for the absence of anaemia. Occasionally there is also mild neutropenia or thrombocytopenia.

Infection with EBV is usually acute and self-limiting, and no reliably effective specific treatment is available. However, as there frequently is malaise and fatigue, the patient may benefit from bed rest. Systemic corticosteroids are required if there is severe pharyngeal oedema that hazards the airway. Nearly 20% of patients have concurrent beta-haemolytic streptococcal pharyngeal infection, for which penicillin may be given. Tinidazole may improve the sore throat.

Burkitt lymphoma

Burkitt lymphoma, found predominantly in Africa, in children before the age of 12 years, presents with massive swellings affecting particularly the mandible, with pain, paraesthesia and bone destruction causing tooth mobility, jaw radiolucencies and destruction of the lamina dura. It appears to be related to EBV in association with malaria. Burkitt lymphoma may also be seen outside of Africa and can be a complication of HIV/AIDS. Chemotherapy is remarkably effective but relapse is common.

Hairy leukoplakia in HIV/AIDS (see Ch. 20)

Lymphomas (see Ch. 80)

Nasopharyngeal carcinoma (see Chs. 14 and 22)

Cytomegalovirus (human herpesvirus 5)

Cytomegalovirus (CMV) is a ubiquitous herpesvirus found in large quantities in the saliva and urine of infected persons.

Primary infections are mostly asymptomatic but some cause a glandular fever-like illness. Thereafter CMV remains latent in oropharyngeal and other epithelial cells and may be reactivated by immunosuppression and other factors. Under these circumstances, disseminated infection can cause CMV retinitis in particular, often leading to blindness. CMV infection is a particular problem in HIV/AIDS (Ch. 20).

The other main problem identified in relation to CMV is its potential to cause fetal damage. A range of infections of the pregnant mother, especially in the first trimester, can cause fetal damage, sometimes fatal. These include *t*oxoplasmosis, *r*ubella, *c*ytomegalovirus and *h*erpes simplex virus (TORCH syndrome). When less severe these may cause mild hearing loss, or result in learning disability, pneumonitis, cardiac malformations, micro-ophthalmia, microcephaly, jaundice and low birthweight. CMV is thereafter excreted by the neonate in urine and saliva for many months.

Antiviral therapy for CMV includes ganciclovir or foscarnet.

Human herpesvirus 6

Human herpesvirus 6 (HHV-6) is a T-cell lymphotropic herpesvirus that is almost invariably contracted via oropharyngeal secretions and within the first 2 years of life.

Human herpesvirus 6 causes a febrile illness, sometimes with a macular or papular rash on the face and/or trunk (exanthema subitum; roseola infantum; sixth disease), mild diarrhoea, cough, oedematous eyelids and occasionally hepatitis, meningitis or meningo-encephalitis or blood dyscrasias (particularly granulocytopenia). Erythematous papules (Nagayama's spots) may appear on the soft palate and uvula and pharynx. Cervical lymphadenopathy is detectable in about one-third of patients. HHV-6 infection in later life may produce a glandular fever syndrome, persistent lymphadenopathy, chronic fatigue syndrome, or hepatitis.

Thereafter HHV-6 remains latent. Immunocompromised patients may suffer reactivation of HHV-6 with pneumonitis, retinitis, encephalitis or bone marrow failure, and it may have a cofactorial role in HIV infection. There are suggested but certainly unproven associations with multiple sclerosis and various neoplasms.

Human herpesvirus 6 is inhibited by ganciclovir, phosphono-formate (foscarnet, PFA) and phosphonoacetic acid (PAA), but it is relatively resistant to aciclovir.

Human herpesvirus 7

Human herpesvirus 7 (HHV-7) is T lymphotropic, not known to be related to any human disease, but might be a cofactor in HHV-6-related syndromes and may cause rashes.

Human herpesvirus 8

Human herpesvirus 8 (HHV-8: kaposi sarcoma herpes virus, KSHV) is a B-lymphotropic DNA virus, transmitted mainly by sexual contact. HHV-8 is strongly associated with Kaposi sarcoma and body cavity-based lymphomas. It is present in saliva, but there are as yet no documented cases of nosocomial transmission to health care workers. There is no specific effective treatment, but HAART (Ch. 20) may play an indirect role in clearing HHV-8 from HIV-infected patients.

MEASLES

Measles is an acute infection with the measles virus, transmitted by droplet infection, with an incubation period of about 10–14 days. Whitish spots in the buccal mucosa (Koplik spots) herald the onset. The illness consists of fever, coryza, conjunctivitis and a maculopapular rash. Complications include bronchitis, pneumonia, otitis media, convulsions and encephalitis (which has a mortality of 15% – highest in infants – and leaves a neurological deficit in up to 40%). Subacute sclerosing panencephalitis (SSPE) is a late complication.

Immunization is indicated in early childhood (Appendix 21.6) and had almost abolished measles, until the decline recently over concerns about immunization.

MOLLUSCUM CONTAGIOSUM

Molluscum contagiosum is a viral infection that spreads easily among children, and in adults may be sexually transmitted. Molluscum contagiosum is common in HIV/AIDS. Characteristic umbilicated papules may be seen on the face and elsewhere. Local application of trichloracetic acid effectively burns the lesions off.

MUMPS

Mumps was a common infection, usually caused by the mumps virus spread by droplet infection, and now mostly eliminated by vaccination. Mumps-like illnesses are occasionally caused by adenoviruses or echoviruses.

The incubation period is 14–21 days and mumps is transmissible from 2 or 3 days before parotitis appears until several days afterwards. Mumps causes swellings involving particularly the major salivary glands, usually the parotids (Fig. 21.7). One or both parotids become enlarged and tender (parotitis) with

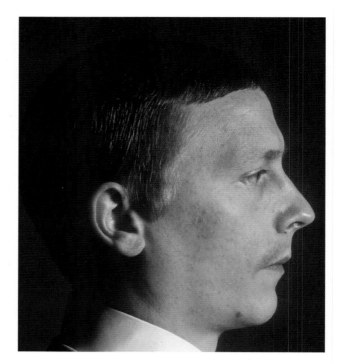

Fig. 21.7 Mumps

trismus, and oedema and erythema of the orifice of the parotid duct (papillitis). The other major salivary glands may also be affected, but rarely in the absence of parotitis. Mumps should always be considered in the differential diagnosis of acute swellings of salivary glands, particularly in the young. Complications of mumps are uncommon but include particularly deafness, pancreatitis, meningo-encephalitis, orchitis and oophoritis. The latter conditions rarely cause sterility, even if bilateral.

There is no antiviral agent available for use against mumps. Mumps immunization is carried out in childhood.

PAPILLOMAVIRUSES

Human papillomaviruses (HPVs) are ubiquitous DNA viruses. Over 100 HPV types are now recognized, are transmissible and mostly cause benign warts and other epithelial lesions, affecting skin and mucosae, including mouth and genitals. Skin warts (verruca vulgaris) are common (Fig. 21.8), especially in children, and spread mainly from close contact or in wet environments such as changing rooms. Genital warts (condylomata acuminata) are caused by HPV and may be found on the penis,

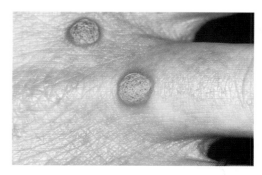

Fig. 21.8 Human papillomavirus infection: common warts

vulva or vagina or perianally, or may be unseen in the urethral meatus or cervix. Around one-third of young American women have genital HPV infection. About 65% of sexual contacts of patients with genital warts develop warts after an incubation period that may exceed 2 years.

Some HPVs cause oral warts (verruca vulgaris) and papillomas. Heck disease (focal epithelial hyperplasia) is an unusual oral condition, caused by specific HPV (types 13 and 32), mainly in ethnic groups such as Inuits and American Indians.

Some HPVs are closely associated with malignant disease; for example, HPV-16, 18 and 33 appear to be associated with cervical carcinoma. HPVs may also be associated with some oropharyngeal carcinomas.

Local surgery or podophyllum resin has been the usual treatments for non-malignant HPV-related lesions. Immune stimulators such as interferon-alpha and imiquimod are now available.

A vaccine against HPV-16 and HPV-18 is now offered free of charge in the UK to girls aged 12–13 years.

PARVOVIRUS

Parvoviruses are among the smallest, simplest DNA viruses and cause infections in a variety of birds and mammals. The only known human parvovirus is B19, which is transmitted by droplets, touch and occasionally in blood and has an incubation period usually of 4–14 days. Parvoviruses tend to infect rapidly dividing tissues, most commonly the fetus, the intestinal epithelium or the haematopoietic system. A total of 70–90% of most adult populations are seropositive for B19.

Parvovirus commonly causes fifth disease (erythema infectiosum; slapped cheek syndrome), a mild illness with a lace-like rash on the face, trunk and extremities, usually in children. In ≈80% of patients, there is also arthropathy – temporary arthritis-like joint involvement (particularly in adults). Since the vaccination-induced disappearance of rubella, parvovirus is the commonest cause of infection-related transitory arthritis, particularly if it affects the hands.

B19 also causes acute depression of red blood cell production, a transient event of little clinical significance, except in patients with other haematological diseases, particularly sickle cell disease, when haemolytic crises may be precipitated. B19 infection in pregnancy is associated with early fetal loss, although the probability of this appears to be low (< 10%). There is no specific therapy for parvoviruses.

RUBELLA (GERMAN MEASLES)

Acquired rubella

Rubella, caused by rubella virus, is a highly infectious, usually mild, disease spread by droplet infection, with an incubation period of about 14–21 days.

In children, rubella causes a minor macular rash starting on the face and behind the ears, mild fever, sore throat and enlarged lymph nodes (including the posterior auricular and suboccipital posterior cervical nodes). In adults, rubella may cause arthritis or arthralgia.

No antiviral treatment is available for rubella. Immunization against rubella is available and indicated for health care workers. After rubella immunization, immunity is long-lasting.

Congenital rubella

Rubella infection during the first trimester of pregnancy can damage the fetus causing problems ranging from deafness to death. If the fetus survives, learning disability, retinopathy and cataracts, cardiac malformations and deafness may result (major rubella syndrome). The infant may also have liver damage, bone defects and thrombocytopenic purpura. The virus is excreted, particularly in the urine, for months after birth (see TORCH syndrome). Pregnant females should thus consider whether or not they are immune to rubella. Rashes resembling rubella (rubelliform rashes) are also common in enterovirus and other infections, and thus a *clinical* diagnosis of rubella may not always be accurate unless confirmed serologically. Females who believe they have had rubella (and thus think they are immune) may in fact be non-immune and they and any fetus may be at risk. Antibody titres should be assayed to determine their actual immune status.

Rubella immunization of non-immune pre-pubertal females is the most effective prophylaxis and should be given to female health care staff who are not known to be immune, who are seronegative, and who are not pregnant and are unlikely to become pregnant within the following 2 months. Rubella immunization should also be given to males who, as health care workers, may come into contact with pregnant women.

Because of the danger to the fetus, pregnant patients exposed to, or developing, rubella or a similar rash should have serological investigation. The haemagglutination inhibition (HAI) test for rubella antibodies is rapid, reliable, rises within 48 h of illness or immunization and persists for years, and is useful to differentiate past infection from acute illness. Serum should be obtained within 2 days of the onset of the illness or within 2 weeks of exposure to the virus. If this acute serum is not available, complement fixation tests or assay of rubella-specific IgM antibody is required (Table 21.12).

Table 21.12 Confirmation of diagnosis of rubella

Suspected rubella infection of patient	Suspected rubella contact
1 Test acute serum for HAI antibody to rubella	1 Test acute serum for HAI antibody to rubella
2 If HAI-positive in acute serum, reassure. If HAI continues negative, reassure	2 Test serum of the contact for rubella. If HAI-negative, reassure
3 If HAI-negative but then rises, offer termination or rubella immunoglobulin	3 If pregnant woman has rubella antibodies already, reassure
	4 If pregnant woman has no immunity and contact is rubella or suspected, retest patient's sera for HAI. If HAI continues negative, reassure. If HAI becomes positive, offer termination or rubella immunoglobulin

HAI, haemagglutination inhibition.
http://www.hpa.org.uk/cdph/issues/CDPHVol5/No1/rash_illness_guidelines.pdf

MYCOSES

Fungi are widespread and sometimes commensals, but infections may occur where general hygiene is low, where suitable local conditions (humid sites) are present and where people are immunocompromised, such as those with organ transplants or HIV/AIDS.

Most fungal infections have few untoward sequelae in otherwise healthy people but some can cause severe, recurrent, disseminated or persistent lesions in immunocompromised person. Fungal infections (Table 21.13) are often diagnosed on clinical grounds, supported by culture. Antifungal drugs can be effective therapy but resistance may arise, especially in long-term use or HIV/AIDS.

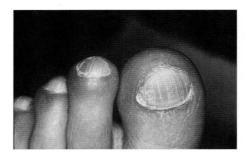

Fig. 21.9 Candidosis

Table 21.13 Fungal infections	
Fungal infection	**Chapter location**
Aspergillosis	This chapter
Blastomycosis (North American blastomycosis)	This chapter
Candidosis	This chapter
Coccidioidomycosis	This chapter
Cryptococcosis	This chapter
Histoplasmosis	This chapter
Mucormycosis	This chapter
Paracoccidioidomycosis (South American blastomycosis)	This chapter
Pneumocystosis	This chapter
Rhinosporidiosis	This chapter
Sporotrichosis	This chapter
Tinea	This chapter

Table 21.14 *Candida* species	
Most common	**Less common**
Candida albicans	Candida zeylanoides
Candida tropicalis	Candida viswanathii
Candida glabrata	Candida rugosa
Candida parapsilosis	Candida lambica
Candida krusei	Candida norvegensis
Candida lusitaniae	Candida lipolytica
Candida kefyr	Candida famata
Candida guilliermondii	Candida ciferrii
Candida dubliniensis	

SUPERFICIAL MYCOSES

The common superficial mycoses (fungal infections) are candidosis and tinea.

Candidosis

Candidosis (candidiasis) is infection with *Candida* species, usually *Candida albicans*. Candidosis can produce a variety of clinical pictures but thrush is the best-known type. Thrush was aptly described in the nineteenth century as a 'disease of the diseased', and candidosis can undoubtedly be a reflection of impaired immune responses. This has become particularly evident since HIV/AIDS was first recognized. *Candida* is one of many other fungi that can cause severe, recurrent, disseminated or persistent lesions in immunocompromised persons, such as those with AIDS (Fig. 21.9).

Candida species other than *C. albicans* can cause candidosis (Table 21.14), particularly in immunocompromised individuals, and some, particularly *C. krusei*, are resistant to conventional antifungal agents. Correction of any underlying local cause, and use of antifungals, is the usual treatment for candidosis.

Thrush

General and clinical aspects

Thrush produces a highly characteristic picture of soft, creamy-coloured, slightly raised patches that *can be wiped off the mucosa* leaving red areas. These lesions may form isolated flecks or large confluent areas. Typical sites are the vagina or mouth.

Thrush is common in the newborn, in whom it does not usually indicate any immunodeficiency and may resolve spontaneously or in response to topical antifungal treatment. In adults, unless known to be having immunosuppressive treatment, thrush is rare and should prompt investigation for an underlying cause. Thrush in a young or middle-aged adult must be regarded as a possible sign of HIV infection until proved otherwise. The other main predisposing factors are antibiotic treatment, anaemia, diabetes mellitus or an immunological defect, as shown in Table 21.15.

General management

The diagnosis is usually clinical but can be readily confirmed by taking a Gram-stained smear, which shows long tangled masses of candidal hyphae.

Superficial fungal infections often respond readily to topical treatment but deep-seated infections often require protracted systemic therapy. In addition to treatment of any underlying disorder, localized thrush should be manageable with topical antifungal drugs such as nystatin, or amphotericin. Alternatively, a nystatin suspension or systemic fluconazole or suspension may be indicated.

Table 21.15 Factors predisposing to mycoses

Predisposing factor	Aetiological agent(s)
Cell-mediated immune defects	*Candida* spp., *Cryptococcus neoformans*, *Histoplasma capsulatum*, *Coccidioides immitis* *Paracoccidioides brasiliensis*, *Blastomyces dermatitidis*
Chronic granulomatous disease	*Aspergillus* spp., *Candida albicans*, *Torulopsis glabrata*
Desferrioxamine therapy	Agents of zygomycosis
Intravenous drug abuse	*Candida* spp., agents of zygomycosis
Ketoacidosis	Agents of zygomycosis
Malnutrition	*Candida* spp., agents of zygomycosis
Moisture	*Trichophyton* spp.
Neutropenia	*Candida* spp., *Aspergillus* spp., agents of zygomycosis, *Pseudallescheria boydii*, *Trichosporon* spp., *Fusarium* spp.
Traumatized skin	*Candida* spp., *Torulopsis glabrata*, *Malassezia furfur*

Erythematous candidosis

General and clinical aspects

Erythematous candidosis appears as mucosal erythema, in the mouth due to coverage of the mucosa with a denture (denture-related stomatitis; denture sore mouth), antibiotic treatment, xerostomia or immunodeficiency. Denture-related stomatitis (denture-associated stomatitis) is a common infection secondary to long-standing occlusion of part of the oral mucosa by a denture. Denture-related stomatitis typically develops beneath a well-fitting upper denture which effectively cuts off the mucous membrane from the normal oral defence mechanisms. Denture-related stomatitis is not seen under a lower denture, in spite of the fact that the latter is a common cause of trauma. The characteristic feature is uniform bright erythema of the whole of the upper denture-bearing area and limited by the denture margin. Occasionally the erythema is patchy or there may be flecks of thrush. Symptoms are typically absent but occasionally there is soreness. Angular stomatitis is frequently associated. The vast majority of patients are healthy, as local factors alone determine the pathogenesis. Occasionally, patients may be anaemic but less frequently than might be expected from the fact that angular stomatitis is often regarded as a typical sign of iron deficiency. Other occasional contributory factors are dry mouth, diabetes mellitus or immune defects. It is, however, unjustifiable to screen all patients with denture-related stomatitis but investigation should be considered if the patient has any other complaints suggestive of such disorders or if the infection is particularly severe or intractable. Treatment includes leaving dentures out of the mouth at night and storing them in hypochlorite to clear the fungus from the denture surface. Topical antifungals should also be used, as suggested above, or the fitting surface of the denture can be coated with miconazole.

Antibiotic stomatitis occasionally follows the use of broad-spectrum antibiotics, particularly tetracycline used topically in the mouth. The whole of the oral mucosa is then typically red, oedematous and sore. One or two flecks of thrush may be found in protected situations, such as the posterior upper buccal sulcus. A similar picture of generalized redness and soreness of the oral mucosa is the typical manifestation of candidosis associated with xerostomia. As with any other type of candidosis, angular stomatitis may be associated.

Xerostomia may also underlie erythematous candidosis. In HIV infection a patch of erythematous candidosis is sometimes seen on the palate or tongue.

General management

The treatment of erythematous candidosis is to treat the underlying problem, if feasible, and to give antifungal drugs as described earlier.

Angular stomatitis

General and clinical aspects

Angular stomatitis (angular cheilitis; cheilosis) is most frequently seen as a complication of denture-related stomatitis, but can be associated with any type of intraoral candidosis and, in addition, is a 'classic' sign of a deficiency anaemia.

General management

It is important to consider the possibility of underlying systemic disease, and treat it where possible.

Clearance of intraoral candidosis with adequate antifungal treatment typically leads to healing of the lesions at the angles of the mouth without any local treatment but miconazole cream applied to the lesion may be useful. Occasionally, bacteriological examination may be necessary, as the cause may be staphylococcal, but imidazoles such as miconazole or clotrimazole also have antibacterial activity and may be effective.

Candidal leukoplakia

General and clinical aspects

Candidal leukoplakia (chronic hyperplastic candidosis) appears as white plaques clinically indistinguishable from other types of keratotic lesion though they may be speckled and tough and firmly adherent, and are seen mainly in men of middle age or over, many of whom are heavy smokers. Typical sites are the buccal mucosa just within the commissures, or the dorsum or edges of the tongue. Long-standing angular stomatitis and occasionally also denture-related stomatitis may be associated. Patients are usually otherwise well.

Candidal leukoplakia may account for up to 10% of leukoplakias and several reports of malignant transformation have appeared. However, the prevalence of candidal leukoplakia and its potentialities remain uncertain.

General management

Diagnosis depends on biopsy, showing *Candida albicans* hyphae and a characteristic inflammatory reaction in the superficial epithelial plaque. Investigations should include a family history and haematological examination. Investigations for cell-mediated responses to *C. albicans* may be needed to exclude one of the rare mucocutaneous candidosis syndromes that show similar oral lesions as described below, but in most cases no abnormality is detectable.

Treatment is difficult since the response to topical antifungal drugs such as nystatin or amphotericin is poor, and excision is also followed by recurrence. Antifungals such as miconazole topically or ketoconazole or fluconazole systemically appear to be more effective.

Persistent candidosis

General and clinical aspects

Persistent candidosis is a well-recognized complication of defective cell-mediated immunity (Box 21.7).

> **Box 21.7 Causes of persistent candidosis**
>
> - HIV infection
> - Primary immunodeficiencies, especially severe combined (Swiss) type or DiGeorge syndrome
> - Chronic mucocutaneous candidosis (CMCC)
> - Intense immunosuppression, particularly for organ grafts

Both thrush and herpetic infection may be present together and produce confluent lesions.

General management

Candidal infection usually responds eventually to antifungal drugs but sometimes immunosuppressive treatment has to be moderated for a time. Patients on long-term corticosteroid treatment for any of the immunologically mediated diseases are also susceptible to oral candidosis, but not often as a serious complication.

Chronic mucocutaneous candidosis (CMC or CMCC; Ch. 20)

'Chronic candidiasis syndrome'

Many normal persons, around half the population, harbour *Candida albicans* as part of their normal microflora. This finding has been exploited as a supposed explanation of such symptoms as headaches, fatigue and lassitude, rashes and gastrointestinal symptoms, but this so-called syndrome has absolutely no scientific basis, and there is no evidence that antifungal treatment is warranted. A controlled trial has shown that it has no effect on the symptoms.

Tinea

General and clinical aspects

Tinea is a term for a range of common skin infections seen worldwide, caused by dermatophytes, usually *Trichophyton* (Table 21.16). Dermatophytes, specifically *Trichophyton*, *Epidermophyton* and *Microsporum* species, are responsible for most superficial fungal infections. Fungal transmission occurs through direct contact with infected persons, animals, soil or fomites.

Table 21.16 Forms of tinea

Tinea	Features	Organisms
Barbae	Beard area	*Trichophyton verrucosum*
Capitis ('ringworm')	Head itchy, red areas, leaving bald patches	*Trichophyton tonsurans* *Microsporum andouinii* *Microsporum canis*
Corporis	Red spots growing into large rings on arms, legs or chest.	*Trichophyton rubrum* *M. canis* *T. tonsurans* *T. verrucosum*
Cruris	Itchy erythema in moist, warm areas, e.g. the groin ('jock itch') or beneath the breasts (Fig. 21.10). Second most common tinea	*T. rubrum* *Epidermophyton floccosum*
Pedis (athlete's foot)	Most common tinea. Itchy and red moist skin between toes (Fig. 21.11), with a white, wet surface. Infection may spread to the toenails (tinea unguium – 'unguium', from Latin for nail). Toenails become thick and crumbly	*T. rubrum* *Trichophyton mentagrophytes* var *interdigitale* *E. floccosum*
Versicolor	Patchy skin discoloration. Areas of infected face, for example, may appear lighter in colour (hypopig-mented). Seen primarily in young adults	*Malassezia furfur*

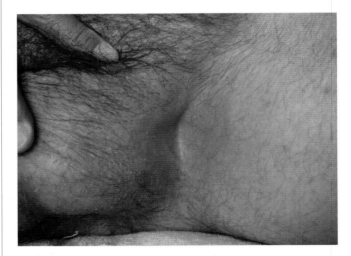

Fig. 21.10 Tinea cruris

General management

Treatment of tinea is with topical clotrimazole, miconazole or terbinafine, or oral fluconazole or itraconazole or terbinafine.

Dental aspects

Terbinafine may disturb taste. Azoles may enhance the effects of warfarin (Ch. 8).

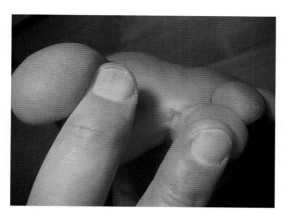

Fig. 21.11 Tinea pedis

SYSTEMIC MYCOSES (DEEP MYCOSES)

Healthy individuals in endemic areas (often in the developing world) are often infected with fungi, typically involving the lungs, but often asymptomatic. Even acute pulmonary and primary mucocutaneous symptomatic mycotic lesions, in otherwise healthy persons, may resolve spontaneously. Chronic pulmonary infections tend to progress and disseminated infections can be fatal. Immunocompromised persons are at particular risk from clinical disease. Equally, clinical infection with mycoses may be an indication of an underlying immune defect. Severe, recurrent, disseminated or persistent lesions appear in immunocompromised persons, particularly those with HIV/AIDS, organ transplants, leukaemia, leukopenia, solid tumours, burns and in premature infants.

The proliferation of mycoses in immunocompromised persons includes 'new' opportunists such as new *Candida* species, *Torulopsis glabrata*, *Fusarium* and *Trichosporon beigelii*.

Orofacial lesions caused by the main systemic mycoses may occasionally be seen in isolation but they are typically associated with lesions elsewhere, often in the respiratory tract. The diagnosis may be suggested by a tumour-like nodule or mass, chronic oral ulceration, chronic sinus infection, or bizarre mouth lesions, especially in immunocompromised patients, or in those who have been in endemic areas, or where there is granuloma formation found on biopsy. Investigations include smear, biopsy, culture, sometimes serology, physical examination and chest radiography. Tissue forms of the fungus may be visible but special stains are often required.

Patients should be managed in consultation with a physician with appropriate expertise, usually with systemic anti-mycotics. Most systemic mycoses can be treated with systemic amphotericin given orally, liposomally, or slowly intravenously, or azoles. Adverse effects from intravenous amphotericin include thrombophlebitis, nephrotoxicity, chills, nausea, anaemia and hypokalaemia. The azoles are less toxic, but the cost is prohibitive where they are most needed – in the developing world. Given orally, the adverse effects of ketoconazole include nausea, gynaecomastia and liver damage. The main adverse effects of miconazole include thrombophlebitis and ventricular tachycardia. Fluconazole and itraconazole are therefore now being used but fluconazole resistance can be a significant problem.

Systemic candidosis

Candidosis is typically a superficial mycosis but, nevertheless, increasingly frequently causes invasion of deep organs, particularly in immunocompromised persons. Many *Candida* species are now responsible; some are resistant to fluconazole but voriconazole or caspofungin may be effective.

Pneumocystis (carinii) jiroveci

General and clinical aspects

Pneumocystis (carinii) jiroveci is now recognized to be a fungus rather than a protozoan. Some of the first patients recognized in the HIV epidemic were revealed because of *Pneumocystis* pneumonia (PCP); it is a common infection in AIDS and other severely immunocompromised patients.

General management

Treatment is with co-trimoxazole, inhaled pentamidine isetionate or atovaquone.

Aspergillosis

General and clinical aspects

Aspergillus species are the most common environmental fungi and are prolific saprophytes in soil and decaying vegetation.

Aspergillosis is found worldwide, increasing in frequency, and is the most prevalent mycosis, second only to candidosis. Inhalation of *Aspergillus* spores and colonization of the respiratory tract is common but disease is rare. Types of aspergillosis include the following.

- *Allergic bronchopulmonary aspergillosis* – the most common disease.
- *Invasive aspergillosis* – a rare lung infection which may spread to brain, bone or endocardium. Invasive sinus aspergillosis affects mainly immunocompromised hosts, though it is also seen in some apparently healthy individuals in subtropical countries, such as Sudan, Saudi Arabia or India.
- *Aspergillus fumigatus* is the usual cause of invasive sinus aspergillosis, but *A. flavus* appears to predominate in immunocompromised patients. There is destruction of the antral wall and often antral pain, swelling or sequelae from orbital invasion (impaired ocular motility, exophthalmos, or impaired vision) or intracranial extension (headaches, meningism).
- *Aspergillomas* – fungus balls that grow in pre-existing cavities such as tuberculous lung cavities. Aspergilloma of the maxillary antrum is uncommon, typically appearing in a healthy host as a hyphal ball in a chronically obstructed sinus.
- *Chronic sinus aspergillosis* – an uncommon cause of a diffusely radio-opaque antrum, sometimes with dense punctate radio-opacities. It is unresponsive to treatment used for bacterial sinusitis. Occasional cases of sinus aspergillosis are a result of metastasis from pulmonary aspergillosis or are iatrogenic, following dental procedures such as extractions.
- *Allergic fungal sinusitis* – an uncommon problem, usually due to fungi other than *Aspergillus*.

General management

Diagnosis of antral aspergillosis is supported by MRI and CT (which are more sensitive than conventional radiography in detecting bone erosion) and confirmed by smear and lesional microscopy, staining with periodic acid–Schiff (PAS) or Gomori methenamine silver. Immunostains may help definitive diagnosis.

Prolonged conservative therapy may worsen the prognosis. Topical ketoconazole or clotrimazole may clear superficial infections. If there is no resolution in 72 h, a course of systemic amphotericin should be tried. Miconazole is not active, and ketoconazole is not particularly active against *Aspergillus*, but itraconazole may have a place in treatment. Fluconazole is under trial.

Non-invasive antral forms usually need treatment by antral debridement and drainage. Corticosteroids may also be indicated in allergic sinusitis.

Invasive aspergillosis should be treated by surgical debridement supplemented with amphotericin and, possibly, hyperbaric oxygen.

Blastomycoses

General and clinical aspects

Blastomyces dermatitidis causes North American blastomycosis, seen predominantly in the USA and Canada. *Paracoccidioides brasiliensis* causes the South American form, seen especially in Brazil. Inhalation of spores, found in soil, leads to subclinical infection in up to 90% of the population in endemic areas. Outdoor workers are particularly affected.

Clinical illness is typically pulmonary. HIV infection and other immunocompromising states predispose to pulmonary and disseminated disease.

General management

Diagnosis is based on biopsy, smear or culture. Amphotericin, ketoconazole, miconazole, itraconazole and voriconazole can be effective.

Coccidioidomycosis

General and clinical aspects

Coccidioidomycosis is seen mainly in hot dry areas of South West USA, Mexico, Central America and parts of South America. Inhalation of spores of *Coccidioides immitis*, found in soil, produces subclinical infection in up to 90% of the population. Clinical illness is typically acute pulmonary disease and fever (San Joaquin valley fever). Chronic pulmonary disease is less common but pregnant women, blacks, Filipinos and Mexicans and immunocompromised persons are susceptible.

General management

Diagnosis is mainly by history and examination supported by histology and the spherulin or coccidioidin skin tests. Management is with systemic amphotericin, sometimes supplemented with ketoconazole, itraconazole, fluconazole or voriconazole.

Cryptococcosis

General and clinical aspects

Cryptococcosis is seen worldwide. Aspiration of spores of *Cryptococcus neoformans*, a yeast found especially in pigeon faeces and soil, may lead to infection. In healthy persons, infection is typically pulmonary and subclinical. Immunocompromised persons are liable to dissemination of infection to meninges, heart, spleen, pancreas, adrenals, ovaries, muscles, bones, liver and gastrointestinal tract. Most patients with disseminated cryptococcosis have meningoencephalitis and, untreated, this is fatal in over 70%.

Cryptococcosis is the most common systemic mycosis in AIDS.

General management

Diagnosis is confirmed by microscopy, culture and assay of serum or cerebrospinal fluid for capsular antigen and antibody. Systemic amphotericin is effective, best supplemented with flucytosine. Ketoconazole and itraconazole may be effective.

Histoplasmosis

General and clinical aspects

Histoplasmosis is found worldwide and is the most frequent systemic mycosis in the USA. *Histoplasma capsulatum* is present especially in bird and bat faeces and is a soil saprophyte found particularly in the Ohio and Mississippi valleys, in Latin America, India, the Far East and in Australia. In endemic areas, over 70% of adults are infected, typically subclinically, by inhaling spores. Clinical histoplasmosis includes acute and chronic pulmonary and cutaneous forms. Disseminated and potentially fatal histoplasmosis, which can affect the reticuloendothelial system, lungs, kidneys and gastrointestinal tract, is rare and seen typically in immunocompromised patients, especially in HIV/AIDS.

General management

Diagnosis is confirmed by microscopy, culture and serotests. Amphotericin is the first line for treatment, followed by ketoconazole, fluconazole, itraconazole or voriconazole.

Mucormycosis (zygomycosis; phycomycosis)

General and clinical aspects

Mucorales are responsible for most mucormycosis. *Mucor, Rhizopus* and many other species of the class Zygomycetes can be responsible, and the condition is probably, therefore, better termed zygomycosis. These fungi are ubiquitous worldwide in soil, manure and decaying organic matter, and can commonly be cultured from the nose, throat, mouth and faeces of healthy individuals.

Immunocompromising conditions underlie most zygomycosis; diabetes mellitus and leukaemia are the most important underlying causes, but cases are now appearing in HIV/AIDS and malnutrition. Rhinocerebral and pulmonary zygomycosis are the most common forms.

Rhinocerebral zygomycosis is usually caused by *Rhizopus oryzae*, typically starts in the nasal cavity or paranasal sinuses with pain and nasal discharge, and fever, and may then invade the palate, orbit or skull. Orbital invasion may cause orbital cellulitis, impaired ocular movements, proptosis and ptosis. Intracranial invasion follows penetration of ophthalmic vessels or the cribriform plate.

General management

Zygomycosis used to be almost uniformly fatal and still has a mortality approaching 20%. Radiography or MRI typically show thickening of the antral mucosa with patchy destruction of the walls, and may define the extent of the lesion.

Diagnosis is confirmed by smears and histological demonstration of tissue invasion by hyphae. Control of underlying disease is essential, if possible, together with systemic amphotericin and surgical debridement.

Rhinosporidiosis

Rhinosporidium seeberi can infect the nasal and other mucosae. Particularly common in India and Sri Lanka, but also found in Latin America, Africa and South-East Asia, mouth lesions are usually proliferative lumps on the palate. Diagnosis is by biopsy. Surgery is required for treatment.

Sporotrichosis

Sporothrix schenckii is found throughout the world mainly as a saprophyte on plants and shrubs. Disease is seen almost exclusively in visitors to tropical and subtropical countries. Infection follows an injury to the epithelium resulting in a primary lesion – a sporotrichotic chancre. Lesions may then spread by the lymphatics. Pulmonary and disseminated sporotrichosis are rare and of uncertain origin.

Diagnosis is confirmed by histology and culture. Potassium iodide is effective treatment for superficial sporotrichosis, itraconazole or amphotericin for other forms.

INFESTATIONS

Parasitic infestations are endemic in the tropics and developing world and increasingly frequently seen in the developed world, in travellers or immigrants, having usually been acquired from animals (zoonotic parasites), water or improperly prepared food. Common parasitic infestations include fleas, lice, mites and ticks, all transmitted between humans, particularly in conditions of poor hygiene, close-living and in war areas, and sometimes transmitting disease that can be fatal. Serious parasitic infections are shown in Box 21.8 and Appendix 21.19.

Since the appearance of the HIV/AIDS pandemic, parasitic infestations, especially toxoplasmosis and leishmaniasis, are now being recognized in HIV-infected patients.

Many parasitic infestations can be prevented by avoidance of insect bites (avoiding areas of high prevalence, good hand and food hygiene, and using protective clothing and insect repellants), and avoiding high-risk times (dusk is the worst time for many mosquitoes, though dengue is transmitted by

---

> **Box 21.8 Main parasitic infestations**
>
> - Amoebiasis – common in the developing world; causes gastrointestinal disease
> - Giardiasis – common worldwide; causes gastrointestinal disease
> - Leishmaniasis – common in the tropics and around the Mediterranean
> - Malaria – one of the more serious worldwide; common in the tropics where anopheline mosquitoes survive, and causes haemolysis. Hundreds of cases are imported into the West in travellers; not all of those infected survive
> - Toxoplasmosis – one of the more serious; endemic in the developing world, and relatively common in the developed world
> - Worms, mites and maggots

mosquitoes that bite during the day). Many parasitic infestations are difficult to diagnose unless there is a high index of suspicion. Clinicians and pathologists should be vigilant therefore, especially when examining lesions in travellers or immigrants. Treatments include a range of medications, and patients should be managed in consultation with a specialist physician.

AMOEBIASIS

General and clinical aspects

Entamoeba histolytica can cause amoebic dysentery or amoebic liver abscesses.

General management

Metronidazole is used. Diloxanide furoate clears cysts from symptomless patients.

GIARDIASIS

General and clinical aspects

Giardia lamblia is a protozoon, cysts of which may be found in unfiltered drinking and recreational waters contaminated by faeces of humans or animals in many parts of the world. Features include anorexia, chronic diarrhoea, abdominal cramps, bloating, frequent loose greasy stools, fatigue and weight loss.

General management

Treatment is with metronidazole, tinidazole or mepacrine.

LEISHMANIASIS

General and clinical aspects

A bloodsucking sandfly is the intermediate host; humans or other vertebrates, including dogs and cats, are the definitive hosts. The developmental stage is the amastigote in the vertebrate host and promastigote in the arthropod host. After inoculation into the skin, leishmanias multiply within histiocytes. Leishmaniasis is one of the most common HIV/AIDS-associated opportunistic infections in Spain. Human *Leishmania* species, although similar in morphology and life cycle to one another, produce different types of infection.

Mucocutaneous leishmaniasis has an incubation period usually of 2–8 weeks but can be as long as 3 years. An itching papule at the site of the sandfly bite (usually on the face) becomes surrounded by gradually spreading erythema and induration. In a few days, the surface crusts, then breaks down to form a slowly extending ulcer that discharges fluid. Healing usually begins in 3–12 months, leaving a scar. Secondary lesions develop at the mucocutaneous junctions many years after the primary infection, and are destructive. The nose is the site of predilection.

Visceral leishmaniasis causes fever, splenomegaly, anaemia, wasting, cough and diarrhoea and is potentially fatal.

General management

Clinical and serological tests are useful diagnostically but the demonstration of the parasite in biopsies or smears is definitive. A leishmanin skin test is also available. Mucocutaneous leishmaniasis may heal spontaneously but, since there can be extensive destruction of tissue, chemotherapy is indicated.

Pentavalent antimony as sodium stibogluconate or meglumine antimonate is usually effective. Alternatives are amphotericin or pentamidine isethionate.

MALARIA

General and clinical aspects

Malaria is the most serious and common parasitic infection worldwide; it still infects over 100 million persons in the world, mainly in tropical areas of Africa, Latin America and Asia, is transmitted by mosquito bites and is potentially fatal.

There are four main species of the protozoon, usually *Plasmodium falciparum* or *P. vivax*, sometimes *P. ovale*, or *P. malariae*. In highly endemic areas, the patient may become infected with one, two or even more species of the malarial parasite. In India, 4–8% is due to mixed infection. The plasmodium infects erythrocytes and damages them, causing haemolysis, as well as fever, myalgia, headaches and in some cases cerebral involvement. Infection with *P. falciparum* is the most dangerous (Table 21.17) and often fatal (malignant malaria) due to haemolysis and sludging in intracerebral vessels. Infection with *P. vivax*, *P. ovale* or *P. malariae* is usually benign.

Typical features of malaria are incapacitating episodes of hyperexia, rigors and chills, sometimes recurring for years.

General management

Diagnosis is made from the history of travel to a malarial area and clinical features, confirmed by demonstrating the parasite in a blood smear. Repeated smears may be required.

Treatment of *P. malariae* malaria, is usually chloroquine; of *P. ovale and P. vivax* is usually chloroquine followed by primaquine; and of *P. falciparum* (infections are often drug resistant, particularly in Asia and Latin America) is currently with quinine, mefloquine or artesunate or artemether or artemether with lumefantrine.

Prophylaxis

Specialist advice should always be sought before travel to the tropics. Transmitted by the bite of an infected mosquito, clothing, insect repellants and nets reduce the risk. Prophylactic chemotherapy does not guarantee total protection but may be life-saving. It may be with chloroquine and/or proguanil, but mefloquine or doxycycline or proguanil plus atovaquone are recommended where the malaria risk is high and chloroquine resistance likely and should commence well before entering and continued for 6 weeks after leaving the malarial area.

TOXOPLASMOSIS

General and clinical aspects

Toxoplasma gondii is a common intestinal parasite of many animals, particularly cats. Infection is contracted mainly from the ingestion of cysts, either from animal faeces or in inadequately cooked food (up to 10% of lamb and pork contains cysts). *Toxoplasma* may also occasionally be transmitted in infected blood or blood products.

T. gondii may cause a glandular fever type of illness with fever, and cervical lymphadenopathy, sometimes with fever, rash, hepatosplenomegaly, myalgia and other minor features. Some patients may develop chorioretinitis, which threatens sight, severe pneumonia, necrotizing encephalitis or myocarditis, but such untoward sequelae are seen mainly if the patient is immunocompromised. Central nervous system (CNS) involvement is common, and can cause changes in mental status,

Table 21.17	Malaria	
Plasmodium	**Comments**	**Chloroquine resistance**
falciparum	Widespread. Results in the most severe infections and responsible for nearly all malaria-related deaths. 'Severe' and 'complicated' are the terms used more frequently than 'malignant' to describe this type of malaria	Chloroquine-resistant strains found in South America, Central America east of the Panama Canal, the Western Pacific, East Asia and sub-Saharan Africa. Resistance to combination of pyrimethamine and sulfadoxine in South-East Asia, Amazon Basin and sub-Saharan Africa. Variable degrees of resistance to quinine and quinidine in South-East Asia and Oceania and in sub-Saharan Africa
malariae	Restricted distribution in India and responsible for less than 1% of infections	No chloroquine resistance
ovale	A rare parasite of humans; mostly confined to tropical Africa	No chloroquine resistance
vivax	The widest geographical distribution throughout the world. Causes much debilitating but relatively mild disease, which is seldom fatal. Also called benign or uncomplicated malaria	High levels of chloroquine resistance in Indonesia and Papua New Guinea, also Solomon Islands, Myanmar, Brazil, Colombia. Resistance to pyrimethamine and sulfadoxine particularly in South-East Asia

headache, neurological defects and epilepsy. CT or MRI scans may demonstrate the lesions.

Toxoplasmosis in pregnancy may lead to chorioretinitis, or transplacental spread and fetal infection, with resultant congenital defects and blindness (TORCH syndrome; Fig. 21.12).

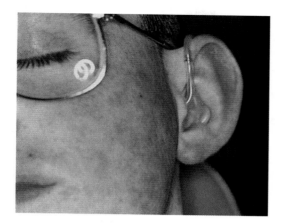

Fig. 21.12 Congenital toxoplasmosis causing learning impairment with visual and hearing defects

General management

Toxoplasmosis is confirmed serologically by the Sabin–Feldman dye test, enzyme-linked immunosorbent assay (ELISA), indirect fluorescent antibody test or indirect haemagglutination test. The organism may be demonstrable in tissue sections or smears. Treatment is *not* usually required for asymptomatic healthy infected persons who are not pregnant. For immunocompromised patients with toxoplasmosis, treatment is a combination of pyrimethamine and sulfadiazine, together with folic acid (pyrimethamine is a folate antagonist), continued for at least 1 month after clinical resolution. Weekly full blood counts are essential.

For pregnant patients with toxoplasmosis, since pyrimethamine may be teratogenic, sulfadiazine alone is used. Clindamycin, clarithromycin and azithromycin are alternatives.

WORMS

A range of helminths can occasionally infect humans (Table 21.18).

CYSTICERCOSIS

Cysticercus cellulosae (encysted larva of *Taenia solium*) can cause cysticercosis, which prevails in regions of poverty and where hygiene is insufficient, particularly Africa, Far East, India, Latin America, Eastern Europe and the Iberian peninsula. It is rare in Jews and Muslims since they avoid pork.

General and clinical aspects

The adult *Taenia solium* lives in the intestine of humans, the only definitive host. The stools release eggs, which, if they contaminate the ground, can be swallowed by pigs. The eggs hatch in the pig's intestine releasing oncospheres that enter the bloodstream, and become encysted as cysticerci in muscle. Pork is then the intermediate host. The life cycle is completed

Table 21.18 Worms (helminths)

Usual helminth	Geographical distribution	Therapy
Cestodes		
Cysticercus cellulosae (*Taenia solium* larvae)	Worldwide	Niclosamide Praziquantel
Echinococcus granulosus	Middle East, North and East Africa, Asia, Latin America, Australasia	Albendazole
Nematodes		
Ancylostoma duodenale	Mediterranean littoral, Middle East, China, India, South America	Mebendazole
Ascaris lumbricoides	Worldwide	Mebendazole Levamisole
Filariae	South-East Asia, India, East Africa, South America	Diethylcarbamazine Ivermectin
Gnathostoma spinigerum	South-East Asia	Albendazole Ivermectin
Gongylonema pulchrum	Former USSR, China, Sri Lanka	Albendazole
Onchocerca volvulus	Africa, Central America	Ivermectin Diethylcarbamazine
Schistosoma mansonii, *S. haematobium* or *S. japonicum*	Middle and Far East, Latin America, sub-Saharan Africa	Praziquantel
Trichinella spiralis	Worldwide	Mebendazole
Trichuris trichiuria	South-East Asia	Mebendazole

when humans ingest inadequately cooked pork containing cysticerci (measly pork), which, upon reaching the human intestine, release the oncospheres. Oncospheres also penetrate the gut mucosa and are distributed to various tissues and organs, particularly muscles, where they develop into cysticerci, most commonly in the brain and eye, striated muscles in the tongue, neck and trunk, and skin and subcutaneous tissues.

General management

Prevention relies on thorough cooking of pork meat and good hygiene.

Diagnosis usually relies upon identification of the parasite. The appearance of the translucent membrane, with its central milky spot, is characteristic.

Praziquantel plus prednisolone, or albendazole, or niclosamide can be curative. Single or even multiple parasites may be excised from tissues and organs.

ECHINOCOCCOSIS (ECHINOCOCCIASIS)

Echinococcosis (hydatid disease) is caused most often by larvae (cestodes) of the tapeworm *Echinococcus granulosus*. Echinococcosis has been a serious problem in many sheep-raising regions, most prevalently in Australia, New Zealand, South,

East and North Africa, Mediterranean countries and in parts of the Russian Federation, Middle East and Americas.

General and clinical aspects

The adult tapeworm *E. granulosus* lives in the small intestine mainly of sheep, though many mammals can serve as intermediate hosts. The eggs hatch in the sheep's intestine, releasing oncospheres that penetrate the intestinal mucosa, enter the bloodstream and develop into hydatid cysts in various organs, particularly the liver and the lungs. Daughter cysts pass in the faeces. Dogs and wolves are infected by eating the discarded offal of sheep, and deposit eggs in their faeces. Humans are an accidental intermediate host, usually infected by ingestion of eggs from the faeces of dogs, usually from improper hand washing and, less often, by ingestion of contaminated water or food such as lamb or mutton containing cysts or eggs. The incubation is from 10 to 30 years. Only the larval stage, the hydatid cyst, develops in humans and there are no specific clinical signs until a cyst becomes large enough to act as a space-occupying lesion causing compression of adjacent structures. Typically the liver and sometimes the lungs, bone or brain are affected.

General management

A skin test (Casoni test) is available but not specific. Serology may be helpful. Eosinophilia is merely suggestive of a parasitic disease and not specific. The hydatid cyst can sometimes be demonstrated radiographically or by MRI or ultrasound, but a definitive diagnosis is often made only by identifying it at operation.

Prevention relies on the protection of definitive hosts (dogs) as well as intermediate hosts (sheep) from becoming contaminated. Thorough hand washing, and washing of vegetables and wild berries located close to the ground, and the elimination of contact with potentially contaminated dogs, are the best protection. High doses of albendazole, mebendazole or flubendazole interfere with larval growth but are not curative. Only surgery is curative.

FILARIASIS

General and clinical aspects

Filariae are helminths transmitted by the bite of blood-sucking insects, usually mosquitoes or black flies, whose adult and larval forms are found in humans. The main filariasis is onchocerciasis, seen mainly in tropical Africa, but also in Saudi Arabia, the Yemen and Latin America. It may involve the face, and eye lesions remain a major problem in Africa (river blindness). The diagnosis is made by identifying the worm in biopsies. Treatment is with ivermectin.

Lymphatic filariasis is infestation particularly by *Wuchereria bancrofti* or *Brugia malayi*, transmitted by blood-sucking mosquitoes and most common in India, South-East Asia, the South Pacific, Latin America, East Africa and Egypt. The lymphatics are affected causing obstructive oedema or elephantiasis. Diagnosis is from blood examination for filariae. Diethylcarbamazine is the treatment of choice.

GNATHOSTOMIASIS

Gnathostomiasis is a rare benign infestation, seen mainly in southern and South-East Asia, caused by larvae of the nematode *Gnathostoma spinigerum*, harboured in chicken, snails or fish. The worm may cause swellings in the skin or mouth, or occasionally bleeding. Skin tests and serology help the diagnosis. Metronidazole may be of some benefit or the worm can be excised.

LARVA MIGRANS

General and clinical aspects

Adult hookworms live mainly in animal intestines and they release ova into the faeces, which are then found in sand or soil contaminated by the animals. The ova hatch into infective larvae, which can infect human skin, where they fail to develop fully but may wander in the tissues, causing 'larva migrans'. Larva migrans is thus common in tropical climates, along the US coast from southern New Jersey to Florida, around the Caribbean and around the Mediterranean. It is seen especially in those working or playing in warm, moist, shaded sandy places.

There are two types of larva migrans as detailed below.

- *Visceral larva migrans* is synonymous with toxocariasis – infection by larvae from roundworms of dogs, cats or wild carnivores.
- *Cutaneous larva migrans* (creeping eruption) is caused by hookworms of dogs, cats and other mammals and characterized by itching serpiginous tracks, mainly on the feet, hands or buttocks. Larva migrans is self-limiting but nearly 50% of patients can develop transient migratory pulmonary infiltrates with eosinophilia (Loeffler syndrome).

General management

Larva migrans can be prevented by stopping dogs, cats and other animals contaminating play areas. Treatments include thiabendazole, albendazole, ivermectin or mebendazole. Local application of 10% thiabendazole, ethyl chloride, chloroform, electrocoagulation and cryotherapy have been tried for cutaneous lesions.

THREADWORMS

General and clinical aspects

Threadworms (*Enterobius vermicularis*, pinworms) are common infestations worldwide. The ova are swallowed and worms develop when exposed to digestive juices of the upper gastrointestinal tract. Female worms lay ova on the anal skin, which cause intense peri-anal itching.

General management

Treatment must involve the whole family and includes mebendazole (or piperazine) and improved hygiene.

TRICHINOSIS

General and clinical aspects

Trichinosis is the most frequent roundworm infestation to affect muscles.

Trichinella spiralis is a nematode acquired through the ingestion of contaminated meat, usually pork products. Trichinosis is more prevalent in central Europe and North America, where pork is widely consumed, than in Islamic or Jewish cultures or tropical countries. Both larval and adult forms of *T. spiralis* can parasitize humans as the definitive host but later they become the intermediate host when the larvae are established in the muscles. The same host sustains the adult worm temporarily, but the larvae for a long period of time. After ingestion of infected meat, the larvae mature to adult forms in the intestine in approximately 1 week. Adult female nematodes then deposit larvae in the gastrointestinal mucosa. The larvae penetrate and subsequently enter the bloodstream and pass to muscles such as the tongue, masseter, gastrocnemius, deltoid and diaphragm where they grow and develop, and become encapsulated. Many infestations are subclinical but they can calcify and appear as radio-opaque nodules.

Clinical features

In mild infections, symptoms are often vague and transient. Acute trichinosis is characterized by myalgia, facial and palpebral oedema and fever with eosinophilia. Myocarditis is present in up to 20% and there may be involvement of lungs, kidneys, pancreas and CNS.

General management

The diagnosis is clinical, supported by a history of ingestion of poorly cooked meat, and by investigations. There is eosinophilic leukocytosis, serodiagnosis is feasible after the third week and. serum levels of muscle enzymes (such as creatine phosphokinase) are also raised. However, definitive diagnosis relies on biopsies from affected muscle or blind biopsies from the deltoid or gastrocnemius muscles.

Treatment is mebendazole or thiabendazole. Prevention requires meat to be cooked throughout at a temperature above 65°C.

TRICHURIASIS

General and clinical aspects

Trichuriasis, infestation of the large intestine by the whipworm *Trichuris trichiura*, is common in the Caribbean and South-East Asia, especially in children, who contract the condition by ingesting eggs from contaminated soil.

General management

Trichuriasis is diagnosed by faecal examination for the worms. Treatment is mebendazole or albendazole.

MITES

General and clinical aspects

Scabies is a common infestation with the mite *Sarcoptes scabiei*, which is transmitted by close contact, particularly in bed. The mite burrows into the superficial skin and lays eggs which excite an inflammatory response and an itchy rash, typically interdigitally and on the wrists.

General management

Patient and family/partners need improved hygiene and treatment with malathion or permethrin.

MAGGOTS

General and clinical aspects

Myiasis is the condition when fly maggots invade living tissue, most commonly the nose, or when they are harboured in the intestine or any part of the body and feed on the host's organs. Human myiasis is most common in the tropics.

Various flies can cause human myiasis; most troublesome in the New World is *Cochliomyia hominovorax* (screwworm). *Chrysomyia bezziana* is seen in Africa, Asia, the Pacific Islands and the Old World.

Larvae burrow through tissue and may produce a type of larva migrans creeping eruption (see earlier), and when they mature they migrate out of the host in an effort to reach soil to pupate, and may then be visible.

General management

A few drops of turpentine or 15% chloroform in light vegetable oil should be instilled in the lesion and larvae should be removed with blunt tweezers.

PRIONS (see Ch 13)

USEFUL WEBSITES

http://www.cdc.gov/Diseasesconditions
http://medlineplus.gov/
http://www.fitfortravel.nhs.uk/
http://www.mic.ki.se/Diseases/C01.html
http://www.mercksharpdohme.com/pro/fungal_disease/info/facts/opportunistic/home.html
http://www.merck.com/mmhe/index.html

FURTHER READING

Almeida, O.D.P., Jacks, J., Scully, C., 2003. Paracoccidioidomycosis of the mouth; an emerging deep mycosis. Crit Rev Oral Biol Med 14, 377–383.
Bedi, R., Scully, C., 2009. Tropical oral health. In: Cook, G.C., Zumla, A. (eds), Manson's tropical diseases, 22nd edn. WB Saunders, Elsevier, Edinburgh, pp. 499–514.
Berman, J., 2003. Current treatment approaches to leishmaniasis. Curr Opin Infect Dis 16, 397–401.

Beyari, M.M., Hodgson, T.A., Cook, R.D., et al., 2003. Multiple human herpesvirus-8 infection. J Infect Dis 188, 678–689.

Bez, C., Lodi, G., Scully, C., Porter, S.R., 2000. Genoprevalence of TT virus among clinical and auxiliary UK dental health care workers: a pilot study. Br Dent J 189, 554–555.

Boyanova, L., Kolarov, R., Gergova, G., et al., 2006. Anaerobic bacteria in 118 patients with deep-space head and neck infections from the University Hospital of Maxillofacial Surgery, Sotia, Bulgaria. J Med Microbiol 55, 1759–1760.

Centers for Disease Control and Prevention, 2003. Guidelines for infection control in dental health care settings. MMWR 52, 10–11.

Cleveland, J.L., Cardo, D.M., 2003. Occupational exposures to human immunodeficiency virus, hepatitis B virus, and hepatitis C virus: risk, prevention and management. Dent Clin N Am 47, 681–696.

Cousin, G.C., 2002. Potentially fatal oro-facial infections: five cautionary tales. J R Coll Surg Edinb 47, 585–586.

Dawson, M.P., Smith, A.J., 2006. Superbugs and the dentist; an update. Dent Update 33, 198–208.

Department of Health's consultation draft of HTM 01-05 on Decontamination in primary care dental facilities. Health Estates and Facilities Management Association (http://www.hefma.org.uk/consultations.php).

Epstein, J.B., Hancock, P.J., Nantel, S., 2003. Oral candidiasis in hematopoietic cell transplantation patients: an outcome-based analysis. Oral Surg Oral Med Oral Pathol Oral Radiol Endod 96, 154–163.

Garcia-Pola, M.J., Gonzalez-Garcia, M., Garcia-Martin, J.M., Villalain, L., De los Heros, C., 2002. Submaxillary adenopathy as sole manifestation of toxoplasmosis: case report and literature review. J Otolaryngol 31, 122–125.

Groll, A.H., 2002. Itraconazole – perspectives for the management of invasive aspergillosis. Mycoses 45 (Suppl 3), 48–55.

Gupta, A.K., Tomas, E., 2003. New antifungal agents. Dermatol Clin 21, 565–576.

Hay, R.J., 2003. Antifungal drugs used for systemic mycoses. Dermatol Clin 21, 577–587.

Hegarty, A.M., Chaudhry, S.I., Hodgson, T.A., 2008. Oral health care for HIV-infected patients: an international perspective. Expert Opin Pharmacother 9, 387–404.

Hodgson, T.A., Rachanis, C.C., 2002. Oral fungal and bacterial infections in HIV-infected individuals: an overview in Africa. Oral Dis 8 (Suppl 2), 80–87.

Holmstrup, P., Poulsen, A.H., Andersen, L., Skuldbol, T., Fiehn, N.E., 2003. Oral infections and systemic diseases. Dent Clin North Am 47, 575–598.

Knouse, M.C., Madeira, R.G., Celani, V.J., 2002. Pseudomonas aeruginosa causing a right carotid artery mycotic aneurysm after a dental extraction procedure. Mayo Clin Proc 77, 1125–1130.

Martin, S., 2001. Congenital toxoplasmosis. Neonatal Netw 20, 23–30.

Martins, M.D., Russo, M.P., Lemos, J.B., et al., 2007. Orofacial lesions in treated southeast Brazilian leprosy patients: a cross-sectional study. Oral Dis 13, 270–273.

Milian, M.A., Bagan, J.V., Jimenez, Y., Perez, A., Scully, C., 2002. Oral leishmaniasis in an HIV-positive patient. Report of a case involving the palate. Oral Dis 8, 59–61.

Moraru, R.A., Grossman, M.E., 2000. Palatal necrosis in an AIDS patient: a case of mucormycosis. Cutis 66, 15–18.

Motta, A.C.F., Lopes, M.A., Ito, F.A., Carlos-Bregni, R., de Almeida, O.P., Roselino, A.M., 2007. Oral leishmaniasis: a clinicopathological study of 11 cases. Oral Dis 13, 335–340.

Nakamura, S., Inui, M., Nakase, M., et al., 2002. Clostridial deep neck infection developed after extraction of a tooth: a case report and review of the literature in Japan. Oral Dis 8, 224–226.

Nunez-Marti, J.M., Bagan, J.V., Scully, C, Peñarrocha, M., 2004. Leprosy: dental and periodontal status of the anterior maxilla in 76 patients. Oral Dis 10, 19–21.

Ochandiano S., 2000. Leprosy. Med Oral 5, 316–323.

Phelan, J.A., 2003. Viruses and neoplastic growth. Dent Clin North Am 47, 533–543.

Reichart, P.A., Samaranayake, L.P., Bendick, C., Schmidt-Westhausen, A.M., Jayatilake, J.A., 2007. Prevalence of oral Candida species in leprosy patients from Cambodia and Thailand. J Oral Pathol Med 36, 342–346.

Reichart, P.A., Samaranayake, L.P., Samaranayake, Y.H., Grote, M., Pow, E., Cheung, B., 2002. High oral prevalence of Candida krusei in leprosy patients in northern Thailand. J Clin Microbiol 40, 4479–4485.

Scott, L.A., Stone, M.S., 2003. Viral exanthems. Dermatol Online J 9, 4.

Silverman, S., Scully, C., 2000. Infectious diseases. In: Millard, D., Mason, D.K. (eds), 3rd World Workshop in Oral Medicine, University of Michigan Press, Ann Arbor, MI.

Sitheeque, M.A., Samaranayake, L.P., 2003. Chronic hyperplastic candidosis/candidiasis (candidal leukoplakia). Crit Rev Oral Biol Med 14, 253–267.

Vargas, P.A., Mauad, T., Bohm, G.M., Saldiva, P.H., Almeida, O.P., 2003. Parotid gland involvement in advanced AIDS. Oral Dis 9, 55–61.

Welsby, P.D., 2006. Chickenpox, chickenpox vaccination, and shingles. Postgrad Med J 82, 351–352.

Appendix 21.1 Infectious diseases: incubation times and period of infectivity

Incubation period	Disease	Incubation period	Period of infectivity
< 1 week	Diphtheria	2–5 days	Until treated[a]
	Gonorrhoea	2–5 days	Until treated[a]
	Influenza	1–2 days	Until fever gone
	Scarlet fever	1–3 days	3 weeks after onset of rash
	Hand, foot and mouth	3–6 days	Until rash gone
1–2 weeks	Herpes	2–12 days	Until lesions gone[a]
	Measles	7–14 days	4 days after onset of rash
	Pertussis	7–10 days	21 days after onset of symptoms
2–3 weeks	Chickenpox	14–21 days	Until all lesions scab[a]
	Mumps	12–21 days	7 days after onset of sialadenitis
	Rubella	14–21 days	7 days after onset of rash
> 3 weeks	Hepatitis A	2–6 weeks	Usually non-infective at diagnosis
	Hepatitis B	2–6 months	3 months after jaundice resolves[a]
	Hepatitis C	2–26 weeks	3 months after jaundice resolves[a]
	HIV	Up to 5 years	Persists[a]. Average time from infection to AIDS is 10 years in the untreated
	HPV	30–180 days	While lesions present
	Infectious mononucleosis (EBV)	30–50 days	Until fever resolved[a]. Once infected we intermittently excrete the virus asymptomatically for the rest of our lives. Thus most people who develop IM have not had contact with someone who has had a recent illness
	Syphilis	10–90 days	Until treated[a]
	Tuberculosis	14–70 days	Until treated[a]

[a]Carrier states exist.

AIDS, acquired immune deficiency syndrome; EBV, Epstein–Barr virus; HIV, human immunodeficiency virus; HPV, human papillomavirus; IM, infectious mononucleosis.

Appendix 21.2 Some antibacterials

Penicillins	Benzyl and phenoxymethyl penicillin	
	Penicillinase-resistant penicillins	Flucloxacillin, temocillin
	Broad-spectrum penicillins	Ampicillin, amoxicillin, co-amoxiclav, co-fluampicil
	Anti-pseudomonal penicillins	Piperacillin, ticarcillin
	Mecillinams	Pivmecillinam
Cephalosporins and other beta-lactams	Cephalosporins	Second generation (cefuroxime, cefamandole) Third generation (cefotaxime, ceftazidime, ceftriaxone)
	Carbapenems	Imipenem–cilastatin, ertapenem, meropenem
	Monobactams	Aztreonam
Nitroimidazoles	Metronidazole	
Glycopeptides	Teicoplanin Vancomycin	

Sulfonamides and trimethoprim		
Macrolides	Azithromycin Clarithromycin Erythromycin Spiramycin Telithromycin	
Lincosamides	Clindamycin	
Oxazolidinones	Linezolid	
Aminoglycosides	Amikacin Gentamicin Neomycin Streptomycin Tobramycin	
Quinolones (Fluoroquinolones; 4-quinolones)	Ciprofloxacin Norfloxacin Ofloxacin	
Tetracyclines	Doxycycline Minocycline Tetracycline	Tigecycline is related

Appendix 21.3   Summary of antibacterial agents used in dentistry

		Comments	Cautions and contraindications
Penicillins	Amoxicillin	Given by mouth (absorption better than ampicillin) Broad-spectrum (effective against many Gram-negative bacilli) *Staphylococcus aureus* often resistant Not resistant to penicillinase	Contraindicated in penicillin allergy Rashes, particularly in infectious mononucleosis, lymphoid leukaemia, or during allopurinol treatment May cause diarrhoea
	Ampicillin	Less well absorbed than amoxicillin, otherwise similar. (Many analogues, such as bacampicillin and pivampicillin – but few advantages) Available with cloxacillin (Ampiclox) or flucloxacillin (co-fluampicil)	Contraindicated in penicillin allergy. Causes transient rashes if given to patients with glandular fever or leukaemia or CMV infection
	Benzylpenicillin	Given i.m. or i.v. Most effective penicillin when organism is sensitive. Not resistant to penicillinase	Contraindicated in penicillin allergy Large doses may cause K^+ to fall, Na^+ to rise
	Co-amoxiclav	Mixture of amoxicillin and potassium clavulanate: inhibits some penicillinases (beta-lactamases) and therefore active against most *Staphylococcus aureus*; also active against some Gram-negative bacilli	Contraindicated in penicillin allergy. May cause cholestatic jaundice
	Flucloxacillin	Given by mouth Effective against most penicillin-resistant staphylococci	Contraindicated in penicillin allergy. Treatment in elderly, or for more than 2 weeks, may result in cholestatic jaundice
	Phenoxymethyl penicillin (penicillin V)	Given by mouth. Not resistant to penicillinase. Used for prophylaxis of rheumatic fever, in sickle cell disease, and after splenectomy	Contraindicated in penicillin allergy
	Procaine penicillin	Depot penicillin Not resistant to penicillinase	Contraindicated in penicillin allergy. Rarely, psychotic reaction due to procaine
	Temocillin	Given by intramuscular or intravenous injection Active against penicillinase-producing Gram-negative bacteria	Contraindicated in penicillin allergy
	Triplopen	Depot penicillin (benzylpenicillin 300 mg, procaine penicillin 250 mg, and benethamine penicillin 475 mg) Not resistant to penicillinase	Contraindicated in penicillin allergy
Tetracyclines	Tetracyclines	Very broad antibacterial spectrum. Little to choose between the many preparations, but doxycycline and minocycline (see later) are safer for patients with renal failure. Given by mouth. Many bacteria now resistant, but still useful for infections with *Chlamydia*, *Rickettsia*, *Brucella*, Lyme disease, acne, leptospirosis, *Haemophilus influenzae*, MRSA	Absorption impaired by iron, antacids, milk, etc. Use of tetracyclines may predispose to candidosis. In children, tetracyclines cause dental discoloration. Contraindicated in pregnancy and children up to at least 7 years (tooth discoloration) Reduce dose in renal failure, liver disease and elderly Frequent mild gastrointestinal upsets May rarely cause intracranial hypertension
	Doxycycline	Given by mouth in a single daily dose	Contraindicated in pregnancy and children up to at least 7 years (tooth discoloration) Safer than other tetracyclines in renal failure; may rarely cause intracranial hypertension Reduce dose in liver disease and elderly. Mild gastrointestinal effects
	Minocycline	Given by mouth Active against some meningococci Absorption not reduced by milk	Safer than tetracycline in renal disease May cause dizziness and vertigo Contraindicated in pregnancy and children up to at least 7 years (tooth discoloration) May also cause bone pigmentation
Macrolides	Azithromycin	Slightly less active than erythromycin against Gram-positive bacteria. Long half-life (single daily dose) Fewer gastrointestinal effects than erythromycin	Reduced dose indicated in liver disease With terfenadine and pimozide may cause arrhythmias Interacts with theophyline and lithium Caution in pregnancy

			Comments	Cautions and contraindications
		Erythromycin	Given by mouth, but absorption erratic and unpredictable Similar antibacterial spectrum to penicillin. Often used for penicillin-allergic patients. Avoid erythromycin estolate, which may cause liver disturbance Useful in those hypersensitive to penicillin Effective against some staphylococci and most streptococci May cause nausea or hearing loss in large doses Rapid development of resistance	Reduced dose indicated in liver disease With terfenadine and pimozide may cause arrhythmias Interacts with theophylline and lithium Caution in pregnancy
		Clarithromycin	Fewer gastrointestinal effects than with erythromycin	Reduced dose indicated in liver disease With terfenadine and pimozide may cause arrhythmias Interacts with theophylline and lithium Caution in pregnancy
Others		Cephalosporins cephamycins and other beta-lactams	These agents are rarely needed in dentistry; they are expensive	May cross-react with penicillins, causing hypersensitivity reactions in those allergic to penicillins Caution in pregnancy
		Clindamycin	Given by mouth, very reliably absorbed	Cross-resistance with erythromycin Mild diarrhoea common Repeated doses may cause pseudomembranous colitis (antibiotic-associated colitis), especially in the elderly and in combination with other drugs Caution in pregnancy
		Gentamicin	Reserved for serious infections and prophylaxis of endocarditis	Can cause vestibular and renal damage Contraindicated in pregnancy and myasthenia gravis
		Metronidazole	Given by mouth Effective only against anaerobes Available as i.v. preparation but expensive	Use only for 7 days (or peripheral neuropathy may develop, particularly in patients with liver disease) Avoid alcohol (disulfiram-type reaction) May increase warfarin effect Avoid in pregnancy
		Rifampicin	Reserved mainly for treatment of tuberculosis May be used in prophylaxis of meningitis after head injury since *Neisseria meningitidis* and *Staphylococcus aureus* frequently resistant to sulfonamides	May interfere with oral contraception Occasional rashes, jaundice or blood dyscrasias Safe and effective but resistance rapidly develops Body secretions turn red
		Sulfonamides	Main indication is for prophylaxis of post-traumatic meningitis but meningococci increasingly resistant Adequate hydration essential to prevent (rare) crystalluria Other adverse reactions include rashes, erythema multiforme and blood dyscrasias	Contraindicated in pregnancy and in renal disease
		Teicoplanin	Reserved mainly for endocarditis and serious *Staphylococcus aureus* infections including some MRSA Occasional rashes, nausea, fever, anaphylaxis May cause hearing loss or tinnitus	Reduce dose in renal failure and elderly
		Vancomycin	Reserved for serious infections (including MRSA) or prophylaxis of endocarditis; given by slow (100 min) i.v. infusion. Extravenous extravasation causes necrosis and phlebitis Effective by mouth for pseudomembranous colitis	Contraindicated in renal disease or deafness May cause nausea, rashes, 'red man syndrome', tinnitus, deafness when given i.v.
		Quinolones	Can induce fits Can cause tendon damage	Contraindicated in patients with tendonitis, the elderly or on steroids; epilepsy; diabetes; pregnancy; myasthenia gravis

Warn patients taking an oral contraceptive to use additional precautions if on antimicrobials for more than a single dose.
CMV, cytomegalovirus; MRSA, meticillin-resistant *Staphylococcus aureus*.

Appendix 21.4 Bacterial infections seen mainly in the developing world

Disease	Micro-organism or parasite (areas of greatest risk)	Infection via	Possible outcomes	Prevention	Diagnostic aids	Management
Anthrax	*Bacillus anthracis* (Central Asia and worldwide)	Contact with contaminated products from or soil infected by animals (mainly cattle, goats, sheep). Spores survive for decades	Untreated infections may spread to regional lymph nodes and bloodstream, and may be fatal	Avoid direct contact with soil and products of animal origin (e.g. souvenirs made from animal skins). Vaccine available for people at high risk	Isolation from blood, skin or respiratory secretions	Ciprofloxacin, doxycycline or erythromycin
Bartonella	*Bartonella (Rochali-maea)henselae*, Gram-negative bacilli which appear to be transmitted by ectoparasites (worldwide)	Contact with cats	Cat scratch disease lymphadenitis Most common in children, in the cervical region, the typical case presents with a tender papule about 3–10 days after contact with the animal, and this is followed by cervical lymphadenopathy after up to 6 weeks Systemic features vary from none to a mild 'flu-like illness and only very rarely are there more serious sequelae such as encephalitis. *Bartonella henselae* or sometimes *B. quintana* in immunodeficient patients may cause epithelioid (bacillary) angiomatosis; clinical resemblance of the lesions to Kaposi sarcoma, but they are benign	Avoid cats	Warthin–Starry silver stain may show the causal organisms, or they may be identified by *in vitro* DNA amplification or serological testing	Treatment, if required, involves use of tetra-cyclines, doxycycline, or chloramphenicol, or erythromycin or other macrolides
	B. bacilliformis (in some valleys of Colombia, Ecuador and Peru)	Transmitted by sandflies The bacterial reservoir is in humans only	Carrion disease is either acute with severe infectious haemolytic anaemia (or Oroya fever), or appears as benign cutaneous tumours (verruga peruana). Healthy blood carriers of the bacterium exist	Avoid sand flies		
	B. quintana (worldwide)	Transmitted by body louse Humans seem to be the reservoir of that bacterium	Trench fever, first described during the First World War, is a non-fatal disease of recurrent attacks of fever and bone pains. Can also cause endocarditis, bacillary angiomatosis and chronic or recurrent bacteraemia	Avoid lice		
Brucellosis	*Brucella* species (worldwide, mainly in developing countries and around the Mediterranean)	From cattle (*Brucella abortus*), dogs (*B. canis*), pigs (*B. suis*), or sheep and goats (*B. melitensis*), by direct contact with animals, skin or unpasteurized milk or cheese	Continuous or intermittent fever and malaise In the *acute form*, symptoms are non-specific and 'flu-like, particularly fever, sweats, malaise, anorexia, headache, myalgia, and back pain In the *undulant form* (< 1 year from illness onset), symptoms include undulant fevers, arthritis and epididymoorchitis in males. Neurological symptoms may develop rapidly in up to 5% In the *chronic form* (> 1 year from onset), symptoms may include chronic fatigue syndrome-like depressive episodes, and arthritis Brucellosis may be associated with chronic or intermittent lymphadenopathy	Avoid unpasteurized milk and milk products and direct contact with animals, particularly cattle, goats and sheep	Blood or bone marrow culture and serology are required for diagnosis	Doxycycline and rifampicin are used in combination for 6 weeks to prevent recurring infection

APPENDICES

Cholera	*Vibrio cholerae*, serogroups O1 and O139 from contaminated water, occasionally from food	Ingestion of food or water contaminated directly or indirectly by faeces or vomitus of infected persons. Endemic in Bangladesh and common throughout the tropics, currently in South America, the Middle East, Africa and Asia	An acute enteric disease varying in severity Cholera can cause massive diarrhoea with depletion of water and electrolytes and can be fatal	Oral cholera vaccines gave little protection and have been abandoned. All care should be taken to avoid consumption of potentially contaminated food, drink and drinking water	Stool culture	Treatment is with electrolyte-containing solutions and if necessary ciprofloxacin
Diphtheria	*Corynebacterium diphtheriae*. Human to human transmission by droplet infection and fomites. Patients infectious for up to 4 weeks but carriers may shed for longer. Three biotypes – gravis, intermedius and mitis, the most severe disease being caused by the gravis biotype, but any strain may produce neurotoxin	Where immunization has been neglected, diphtheria continues to re-emerge, as in Eastern Europe (e.g. Ukraine 2008)	*C. diphtheriae* multiplies mainly on the nasal, pharyngeal or laryngeal mucous membranes to cause inflammation, surface necrosis and exudate (pseudomembrane). There is a mild sore throat but disproportionate cervical lymph node enlargement, which in severe cases produces a bull neck. Nasal, laryngeal or tracheal diphtheria are variants. Exotoxin causes potentially fatal myocardial, adrenal and neurological damage. Palatal paralysis is a possible manifestation	Diphtheria immunization carried out in early childhood	Swabs should be taken for bacterial culture and for Gram and Kenyon staining	Antibiotics (usually penicillin or erythromycin) immediately. Diphtheria antitoxin if the patient has not been actively immunized. Household contacts may need immunization
Haemophilus meningitis	*Haemophilus influenzae* type b (Hib) (worldwide where vaccination against Hib is not practised)	Direct contact with infected person	Meningitis in infants and young children; may also cause epiglottitis, osteomyelitis, pneumonia, sepsis and septic arthritis	Vaccination against Hib	White cell count Hib culture from blood	
Leprosy	*Mycobacterium leprae* (India alone accounts for 78% of new cases detected, worldwide. Endemic in tropical and subtropical areas of Asia, Africa, and Latin America, it is also seen occasionally all around the Mediterranean and Black Sea and in southern Europe)	*M. leprae* transmitted by direct contact and via the respiratory tract	Outcome of infection highly dependent upon cell-mediated immune reactions, which, if intact, result in localized form (tuberculoid leprosy) but, if deficient, generalized (lepromatous) leprosy. Tuberculoid leprosy is a benign form and causes thickening of cutaneous nerves, flat and hypopigmented or raised and erythematous skin lesions, and enlarged lymph nodes. Lepromatous leprosy affects nerves (with hypoaesthesia); skin with macules progressing to papules and nodules or infiltration; lymph nodes; and other tissues including bones, eyes, testes, kidneys and bone marrow	Hygiene	Based on one or more of three cardinal signs: hypopigmented or reddish hypo- or anaesthetic skin lesion(s); peripheral nerve involvement; and a positive smear from an open lesion, or biopsy, for acid-fast bacilli. The lepromim test is of dubious value. Serological diagnostic tests capable of identifying and allowing treatment of early-stage leprosy are appearing	Multidrug therapy (MDT), with clofazimine, rifampicin and prothionamide over 2 or more years; second-line drugs include ofloxacin, minocycline and clarithromycin

(Continued)

INFECTIONS AND INFESTATIONS

Appendix 21.4 Bacterial infections seen mainly in the developing world—cont'd

Disease	Micro-organism or parasite(areas of greatest risk)	Infection via	Possible outcomes	Prevention	Diagnostic aids	Mangement
Leptospirosis	Spirochaetes of the genus *Leptospira* (worldwide; most common in tropics)	Contact between the skin or mucosae and water, wet soil or vegetation contaminated by animal urine, notably rats and foxes	Sudden fever, headache, myalgia, chills, conjunctival suffusion and rash. May progress to meningitis, haemolytic anaemia, jaundice, haemorrhages and hepatorenal failure	Avoid contact with rodents and contaminated waters including canals, ponds, rivers, streams and swamps	ELISA serology	Doxycycline, penicillin
Listeriosis	*Listeria monocytogenes* (worldwide)	*Listeria* multiplies readily in refrigerated foods that have been contaminated (e.g. unpasteurized milk, soft cheeses, vegetables and prepared meat products)	Newborn infants, pregnant women, the elderly and immunocompromised individuals are particularly susceptible. In pregnancy, causes fever and abortion. Meningoencephalitis and/or septicaemia in adults and newborn infants. In others, disease may be limited to a mild acute febrile episode	Avoid unpasteurized milk and milk products	Culture blood, urine, CSF or amniotic fluid	Ampicillin plus gentamicin
Lyme disease	*Borrelia burgdorferi*. (first recognized in 1977 when arthritis was noted in children in and around Lyme, Connecticut, USA. British Lyme disease differs from the USA version, in having fewer complications)	Bite of infected deer ticks, which have become infected by feeding on small rodents, such as white-footed mice	Spirochaetes disseminate from the tick bite via lymphatics and blood to nervous or musculoskeletal systems, or heart. Some individuals have subclinical infection but most often presents with a 'bull's-eye' rash (erythema migrans), and non-specific features such as fever, malaise, fatigue, headache, muscle aches (myalgia) and joint aches (arthralgia). The rash usually appears 7–14 days following tick exposure Early neurological manifestations may include lymphocytic meningitis, cranial neuropathy (especially facial nerve palsy) and radiculoneuritis Musculoskeletal manifestations may include migratory joint and muscle pains Cardiac manifestations rare but may include myocarditis and transient atrioventricular blocks	Avoid areas where there could be deer	Serological testing initially with a sensitive enzyme-linked immunosorbent assay (ELISA) or indirect fluorescent antibody (IFA) test, followed by testing with the more specific western immunoblot (WB), which is confirmatory	Doxycycline or amoxicillin for 3–4 weeks. Cefuroxime or erythromycin for persons allergic to penicillin
Paratyphoid	*Salmonella paratyphi* *Salmonella cholerasuis* or *Salmonella enteritidis*	Poultry, eggs, dairy products, other foods	Similar to typhoid but usually less severe	Hygiene	Culture stool	Supportive therapy
Pertussis	*Bartonella pertussis*	Nasopharyngeal secreations	Catassh, recurrent cough	Hygiene	Culture nasopharyngeal swab	Erythromycin, azithromycin
Plague	*Yersinia pestis* (Asia, Africa, South America; epidemics in Asia, Africa and South America)	*Xenopsylla cheopis* (oriental rat flea) is primary vector. Other routes of spread include direct contact with infected tissues or fluids from handling sick or dead animals or by droplets from cats Direct person-to-person transmission only in pneumonic plague	Bubonic plague: lymphadenitis, with swelling, and suppuration – buboes. Untreated, often fatal. Septicaemic plague may develop from bubonic plague or occur in the absence of lymphadenitis. Dissemination of infection in bloodstream causes meningitis, endotoxic shock and disseminated intravascular coagulation. Pneumonic plague results from secondary infection of lungs following dissemination from other sites. Direct infection of others may result. Untreated septicaemic and pneumonic plague are invariably fatal	Avoid contact with rodents. Antibiotics for prophylaxis with tetracyclines or sulfonamides	Immunostain smear from affected tissues serology	Aminoglycosides such as streptomycin and gentamicin

Disease	Organism	Source	Symptoms	Prevention	Diagnosis	Treatment
Q fever	Coxiella burnetii (worldwide)	Excreta or milk of cattle, sheep and goats. Ticks	Fever headache, malaise, myalgia, sore throat, chills, sweats, cough, nausea, vomiting, diarrhoea, abdominal and chest pain	Avoid contact with excreta or unpasteurized milk	Serology	Tetracycline, doxycycline
Salmonellosis	Salmonella serotype Typhimurium and Salmonella serotype Enteritidis	Contaminated foods are often of animal origin, such as beef, poultry, milk, or eggs, but any food, including vegetables, may become contaminated. Thorough cooking kills Salmonella Outbreaks in developing world mainly (e.g. Kenya 2008) but also in developed world (e.g. USA 2008)	Diarrhoea, fever or abdominal cramps	Avoid contact with uncooked food and do not eat raw or undercooked eggs, poultry or meat. Reptiles (turtles, iguanas, lizards, snakes) may harbour Salmonella. Chicks and birds may carry Salmonella in their faeces. Always wash hands immediately after handling reptiles or birds	Laboratory tests that identify Salmonella in the stool of an infected person	Usually resolve in 5–7 days and often do not require treatment other than oral fluids. Persons with severe diarrhoea may require rehydration with intravenous fluids. Antibiotics, such as ampicillin, trimethoprim–sulfamethoxazole or ciprofloxacin, are not usually necessary
Sodoku	Spirillum minus (Asia mainly)	From rat bites or scratches	High fever, headache and regionally swollen lymph nodes	Avoid rats, mice or squirrels	Darkfield microscopy	Penicillin
Tularaemia	Francisella tularensis (USA and other countries)	From ticks, water contaminated by rats, undercooked meat from an infected animal such as rabbit, and also from contaminated soil	High fever, generalized aching and swollen lymph nodes	Avoid rats	Serology	Aminoglycosides (e.g. gentamicin and streptomycin), chloramphenicol, fluoroquinolones and tetracyclines
Typhoid fever	Salmonella typhi (worldwide, especially north and west Africa, south Asia and Peru)	Contaminated water or food. A strict human pathogen, typhoid is always acquired from a human. Contact tracing is important	Fever, rash, splenomegaly and leukopenia, and intestinal bleeding or perforation	Vaccination. Hygiene. Avoid contaminated water or food	Culture blood, vomit and stool	Chloramphenicol effective but toxic. S. typhi may be resistant in India, the Middle East and South–East Asia, when ciprofloxacin is indicated
Typhus fever (epidemic louse-borne typhus)	Rickettsia prowazekii (colder, i.e. mountainous, regions of central and East Africa, Central and South America and Asia. In recent years, most outbreaks have taken place in Burundi, Ethiopia and Rwanda)	Human body louse, rat or cat flea	Sudden fever, headache, chills, prostration, coughing and muscular pains. After 5–6 days, a macular skin eruption (dark spots) on the upper trunk and then rest of the body except face, palms or soles. Case fatality rate up to 40%	Avoid infestation by body lice	Serology after the first week. PCR.	Doxycycline, azithromycin, rifamificin
Yersiniosis	Y. enterocolitica (worldwide)	Eating contaminated food, especially raw or undercooked pork products	Features typically develop 4–7 days after exposure and may last 1–3 weeks or longer. Fever, abdominal pain, bloody diarrhoea, and sometimes cervical lymphadenopathy	Hygine	Culture stool or body fluids	Uncomplicated cases usually resolve spontaneously In severe or complicated infections, use aminoglycosides, doxycycline, trimethoprim–sulfamethoxazole, or fluoroquinolones

Appendix 21.5   Bacterial infections and antiviral agents that rarely may have implications in dentistry

Bacterial infections			
Infecting organism	**Main features**	**Orofacial lesions**	**Treatment**
Bacillus anthracis	Anthrax	Painful or ulcerated swellings mainly on palate	Penicillin
Brucella melitensis, suis and *abortus*	Brucellosis	Rare infections or cranial nerve palsies	Tetracycline with streptomycin
Clostridium botulinum	Botulism	Xerostomia, parotitis Muscle weakness	Antitoxin
Clostridium perfringens (C. welchii), C. sporogenes, C. oedematiens, C. septicum	Gas gangrene	Gas gangrene	Antitoxin Penicillin Surgery
Escherichia coli	Enteric infections mainly Also urinary tract, wound, and other infection	Found in some oral infections, especially in denture wearers and immunocompromised	Ampicillin Cefalexin Cephalothin Co-trimoxazole
Francisella tularensis	Tularaemia	Pharyngitis Stomatitis (often ulcerative) Faucial membrane Cervical lymphadenopathy	Streptomycin
Mycoplasma hominis and *pneumoniae*	Pneumonia	Rare infections or cranial nerve palsies? Reiter syndrome	Tetracyclines Erythromycins
Neisseria meningitidis	Meningitis Septicaemia	Petechiae Occasionally: herpes labialis Facial palsy	Penicillin
Nocardia asteroides, brasiliensis and *caviae*	Nocardiosis	Ulceration Cheek or gingivae	Co-trimoxazole
Proteus vulgaris	urinary tract and wonds	Occasional infections	Ciprofloxacin
Pseudomonas aeruginosa	Skin and lungs	Opportunistic infections	Sulfadiazine Aminoglycosides
Pseudomonas mallei	Glanders (acute pneumonia)	Ulceration from nasal glanders Ulcers	Penicillin Cephalosporins
Pseudomonas pseudomallei	Melioidosis (lung or other or other localized infections or septicaemia)	Oral abscesses, or other infections Parotitis	Tetracyclines
Rickettsia ricketssiae	Rocky mountain spotted fever	Faucial gangrene	Tetracyclines
Rickettsia akari	Rickettsialpox	Vesicles	Tetracyclines
Salmonellae typhi, paratyphi, choleraesuis and *enteritidis*	Typhoid and paratyphoid fever	Occasional infections	Co-trimoxazole Ampicillin

Appendix 21.6   Bacterial infections and antiviral agents that rarely may have implications in dentistry

Antiviral agents		
Virus	**Type of infection treated**	**Antivirals that may have a role**
Cytomegalovirus	Immunocompromised persons	Ganciclovir Foscarnet Valganciclovir
Epstein–Barr virus	Immunocompromised persons	Aciclovir Ganciclovir
Hepatitis B	Chronic infection or immunocompromised persons	Interferon-alpha 2b
Hepatitis C	Chronic infection or immunocompromised persons	Interferon-alpha 2b

Virus	Type of infection treated	Antivirals that may have a role
Herpes simplex	Primary infections	Aciclovir
	Recurrent oral	Aciclovir
	Recurrent peri-oral	Penciclovir Aciclovir
	Recurrent ano-genital	Aciclovir
	Encephalitis	Aciclovir
HIV	Any	Ch. 20
Influenza	Elderly or immunocompromised persons	Amantadine Oseltamivir Rimantadine Zanamivir
Papillomaviruses	Any	Interferon-alpha 2b Imiquimod
Respiratory syncytial virus	Young or immunocompromised persons	Ribavirin
Severe acute respiratory syndrome corona virus	Elderly or immunocompromised persons	Ribavirin
Vanicella-Zoster virus	Chickenpox	Aciclovir
	Zoster	Famciclovir Valacyclovir
	Zoster in immunocompromised	Aciclovir

Appendix 21.7   Immunization schedules (UK)

Age for immunization	Vaccines and routine
2 months	Diphtheria, tetanus, pertussis (DTP), poliomyelitis (polio) and *Haemophilus influenzae* B (Hib) Pneumococcal conjugate vaccine
3 months	2nd dose DTP, polio and Hib Group C meningococcus
4 months	DTP, polio, HIB and Group C meningococcus Pneumococcal conjugate vaccine
12 months	Hib, measles, mumps and rubella (MMR), Group C meningococcus and pneumococcal conjugate vaccine
4–5 years	'Pre-school' boosters of DTP and MMR
14–18 years	Booster DTP
Certain groups	
10–14 years	BCG (bacille Calmette–Guérin; against tuberculosis) for at-risk groups
Adults	Tetanus, diphtheria and polio, if not fully immunized as a child
Special risk groups	

Further immunization in the UK is recommended for the following:
1 *Influenza* – recommended yearly to those who suffer from bad chests (e.g. asthma, chronic bronchitis, etc.), heart disease, kidney disease, diabetes and those who are elderly.
2 *Pneumococcus* – considered important for people over the age of 2 who are more likely to acquire this infection (those who have had their spleen removed or have a non-functioning spleen, sickle cell disease, severe kidney disease, heart disease, lung disease, liver disease, diabetes and HIV infection).
3 *Hepatitis B* – considered important for people at increased risk because of occupation or lifestyle and at birth for babies whose mothers are hepatitis B positive.
4 *Others* – workers who handle animals may be offered rabies immunization. Those in very close contact with people who have certain forms of meningitis may be offered specific immunizations.
5 *Adults* – adults who are not fully immunized against polio and tetanus.
6 *Varicella* – for health care workers caring for vulnerable patients.
7 *Tuberculosis* (TB) – at birth for babies who are more likely to come into contact with TB than the general population.

Immunization is not recommended in:
1 Pregnancy *if live organisms* are involved.
2 Immune defects, for example in people with HIV infection (though some vaccines are indicated, such as pneumococcal – not a live vaccine), people with primary immune deficiency, people undergoing chemotherapy or those who have had transplants or are receiving high doses of corticosteroids.
3 Where there is a confirmed anaphylactic reaction to a previous vaccine, to neomycin, streptomycin or polymixin B.
There is no reliable evidence linking MMR vaccine with autism or inflammatory bowel disease.

http://www.fitfortravel.nhs.uk/advice/travellers/britishnationalvaccinationschedule.htm

Appendix 21.8 Life-threatening virus infections[a]

Disease	Micro-organism or parasite	Infection via	Possible outcomes	Areas of greatest risk	Prevention
Arboviruses	Many different arboviruses	Transmitted to humans by arthropods, mostly mosquitoes, sandflies or ticks	Fever, with rashes, arthralgias, lymphadenopathy, CNS involvement or haemorrhagic features	Worldwide, especially Latin America, the southern USA, South-East Asia and Africa Chikungunya virus, endemic in Africa, South-East Asia and the Indian subcontinent, has been found in Italy, around Ravenna (2007)	Avoid insect bites (wear protective clothing and use insect repellants), and use prophylactic measures such as vaccination
Dengue	Dengue virus – a flavivirus	*Aedes aegypti* mosquito, which bites during day. There is no direct person-to-person transmission. Monkeys act as a reservoir host in South-East Asia and West Africa	Dengue fever – an acute febrile illness, macular skin rash and muscle pains, 'breakbone fever' Dengue haemorrhagic fever Dengue shock syndrome	Endemic in tropical and subtropical regions of Latin America (e.g. Brazil 2008) and South and South-East Asia and Africa below 600 m	Avoid mosquito bites
Ebola fever	See Haemorrhagic fevers				
Encephalitis (viral)	Togaviridae or flaviviruses *Eastern equine encephalitis* (EEE) is caused by a Togaviridae, genus *Alphavirus* *Western equine encephalitis*	Mosquito bites	Infections range from mild 'flu-like illness to frank encephalitis, coma and death, leaving mild to severe neurological deficits in survivors	Worldwide *tick-borne encephalitis* is seen in forested areas of Austria, northern Europe and Scandinavia. *Japanese encephalitis* (JE) virus is a flavivirus *St Louis encephalitis* virus is a flavivirus seen in southern USA and the Caribbean	Avoid bites of mosquitoes. A vaccine against tick-borne encephalitis is available for those walking or camping in forests in areas at risk. Travellers to monsoon areas of South-East Asia may require immunization against JE
Haemorrhagic fevers Crimean–Congo haemorrhagic fever (CCHF), dengue, Ebola and Marburg haemorrhagic fevers, Lassa fever, Rift Valley fever (RVF) and yellow fever	Most haemorrhagic fevers, including dengue and yellow fever, caused by flaviviruses; Ebola and Marburg caused by filoviruses, CCHF by bunyavirus, Lassa fever by arenavirus, RVF by phlebovirus	Most viruses transmitted by mosquitoes. Ebola or Marburg viruses acquired from bats or monkeys or direct contact with body fluids of infected patients. CCHF is transmitted by a tick bite. Lassa fever virus carried by rodents and transmitted by excreta, either as aerosol or direct contact. RVF acquired by either mosquito bite or direct contact with blood or tissues of infected animals	Sudden fever, malaise, headache, myalgia, rash and multiple haemorrhages including from the mouth	Tropics and subtropical regions. Ebola and Marburg haemorrhagic fevers and Lassa fever in sub-Saharan Africa. Lassa fever, the most infamous arenavirus, is named from Nigerian town where infection was first recorded in 1969. Cases since then reported from Liberia, Sierra Leone, Uganda RVF in Africa and Saudi Arabia. CCHF in central Asia and central Europe (including Greece and Turkey 2008), tropical and southern Africa Other viral haemorrhagic fevers in central and south America. Marburg virus has been of concern since first reports in 1967 in persons working with monkeys in Germany and Yugoslavia. Other Arenavirus infections include Korean, Argentinian and Bolivian fevers	Avoid mosquitoes and ticks and rodents. Filoviruses have very high transmissibility, morbidity and mortality

Disease	Cause	Transmission	Clinical features	Distribution	Prevention
Hantavirus diseases [Haemorrhagic fever with renal syndrome (HFRS) and hantavirus pulmonary syndrome (HPS)]	Hantaviruses – family bunyaviruses. HPS caused by Sin Nombre virus (SNV)	Direct contact with the faeces, saliva or urine of infected rodents such as deer mice or by inhalation of the virus. In North America there is no evidence of person-to-person transmission. In South America person-to-person transmission may be a factor in disease spread	1–5 weeks after exposure there is fever and muscle aches, followed by dyspnoea and coughing. Then the disease progresses rapidly, necessitating hospitalization and often ventilation within 24h. Vascular endothelium is damaged, leading to vascular permeability, hypotension, haemorrhages and shock. Impaired renal function with oliguria characterizes HFRS. Fatal in up to 15%. Respiratory distress due to pulmonary oedema in HPS. Fatal in up to 50%	A pan-American zoonosis, with an expanding clinical spectrum, caused by many novel New World hantaviruses with distinct rodent hosts	Avoid exposure to rodents and their excreta
Hepatitis viruses	Ch. 9				
HIV	Ch. 20				
Influenza	Ch. 15				
Japanese encephalitis	Japanese encephalitis (JE) virus – a flavivirus	Various mosquitoes of the genus Culex. Infects pigs and wild birds as well as humans	Fever, headache or aseptic meningitis. Severe cases: rapid onset with headache, high fever and meningeal signs. May be neurological sequelae. Approximately 50% of severe cases are fatal	Asia, especially monsoon areas of South-East Asia	Vaccination. Avoid mosquito bites
Lassa fever	See Haemorrhagic fevers				
Marburg disease	See Haemorrhagic fevers				
Poliomyelitis	Ch. 13				
Rabies	Rhabdovirus of genus Lyssavirus	Bite of an infected animal such as dogs, cats, foxes, racoons, wolves or bats transmitted in saliva mainly by bites	Acute encephalomyelitis, which is almost invariably fatal. Initial signs include sense of apprehension, headache, fever, malaise and sensory changes around bite site. Excitability, hallucinations and aerophobia common, followed in some cases by fear of water (hydrophobia) due to spasms of swallowing muscles, progressing to delirium, convulsions and death	Worldwide, especially in developing countries but also in Europe (e.g. France 2008) and North America	Avoid contact with both wild and domestic animals, including dogs and cats. Vaccination
Severe acute respiratory syndrome (SARS)	Ch. 15				

(Continued)

Appendix 21.8 Life-threatening virus infections[a]—cont'd

Disease	Micro-organism or parasite	Infection via	Possible outcomes	Areas of greatest risk	Prevention
Tick-borne encephalitis (spring–summer encephalitis)	Tick-borne encephalitis (TBE) virus – a flavivirus	Bite of infected ticks	Influenza-like illness, with a second phase of fever in 10% of cases. Encephalitis develops during second phase and may result in paralysis, or death	Below 1000 m in Eastern Europe, particularly Austria, Baltic States, Czech Republic, Hungary and Russian Federation	Avoid bites by ticks by wearing long trousers and closed footwear when hiking or camping in endemic areas
West Nile fever	West Nile virus	Bite of an infected mosquito, and can infect people, horses, many types of birds, and some other animals	After a 3–15-day incubation, no symptoms or only mild 'flu-like illness with pharyngitis, lymph-adenopathy and rash usually. Sometimes severe and sometimes fatal encephalitis: in USA in 2002, of 4161 people infected, 277 died	Africa, North America, Europe (France and Spain)	Avoid mosquito bites
Yellow fever	Yellow fever virus – an arbovirus of the *Flavivirus* genus	Bite of *Aedes aegypti* mosquitoes Yellow fever virus infects humans and monkeys	Acute illness characterized initially by fever, chills, headache, muscular pain, anorexia, nausea and/or vomiting, with bradycardia. About 15% progress to second phase, with fever resurgence, jaundice, abdominal pain, vomiting and haemorrhages. 50% die after 10–14 days	Tropical areas of Africa and Latin America below 2500 m (e.g. Paraguay and Argentina 2008)	Vaccination Avoid mosquito bites during the day as well as at night

[a]Now that the African tiger mosquito has arrived in Europe, there is a risk of these infections being spread.

Appendix 21.9 Main antifungal drugs

Group	Examples	Comments	Oral dose
Polyenes	Amphotericin[a]	Active topically. Negligible absorption from gastrointestinal tract. Given i.v. for deep mycoses	10–100 mg, 6-hourly
	Nystatin[a]	Active topically. Negligible absorption from gastrointestinal tract. Pastilles taste better than lozenges	500 000 unit lozenge, 100 000 unit pastille or 100 000 unit per ml of suspension 6-hourly
Imidazoles	Ketoconazole	Absorbed from gastrointestinal tract. Useful in intractable candidosis. Contraindicated in pregnancy and liver disease. May cause nausea, rashes, pruritus and liver damage. Interacts with anticoagulants, terfenadine, cisapride and astemizole	200–400 mg once daily with meal, for 14 days
	Miconazole[a]	Active topically. Also has antibacterial activity. Absorption from gastrointestinal tract. Theoretically the best antifungal to treat angular stomatitis. Interacts with anticoagulants, terfenadine, cisapride and astemizole. Avoid in pregnancy and porphyria	250 mg tablet 6-hourly or 25 mg/ml gel used as 5 ml 6-hourly, for 14 days
Triazoles	Fluconazole	Absorbed from gastrointestinal tract. Useful in intractable candidosis. Contraindicated in pregnancy and lactation, liver and renal disease. Interacts with anticoagulants, terfenadine, cisapride and astemizole	50–100 mg daily for 14 days
	Itraconazole	Absorbed from gastrointestinal tract. Useful in intractable candidosis. May cause nausea, neuropathy, diarrhoea, rash. Implicated in cardiac failure in high dose, or in older people or cardiac disease, or those on calcium channel blockers. Contraindicated in heart disease, pregnancy, liver disease. Interacts with terfenadine, cisapride and astemizole	100 mg daily for 14 days
	Posaconazole	Caution with cardiac patients. Contraindicated in porphyria	400 mg bd
	Voriconazole	Caution with cardiac patients, liver or renal disease. Contraindicated in porphyria and breast-feeding	200 mg bd

[a]Dissolve in mouth slowly.

Appendix 21.10 Important systemic (deep) mycoses

Disease	Organism	Source	Main endemic areas	Clinical forms	Prognosis
Aspergillosis	*Aspergillus fumigatus, A. flavus, A. niger* and other *Aspergillus* spp.	Ubiquitous	Worldwide	Allergic bronchopulmonary, pulmonary, disseminated, aspergilloma	Variable
Blastomycosis	*Blastomyces dermatiditis*	Soil	Mississippi and Ohio valleys in USA, Canada, North Africa and Venezuela	Cavitary, pulmonary, disseminated, others	Often good, except in disseminated form
Coccidioidomycosis	*Coccidiodes immitis*	Soil	Southwestern USA, Mexico, Latin America	Acute pulmonary, disseminated, chronic pulmonary, meningitis	Often good, except in disseminated or meningeal form
Cryptococcosis	*Cryptococcus neoformans*	Soil, pigeon droppings	Worldwide	Pneumonia, meningitis, disseminated, cryptococcoma	Poor in disseminated form
Histoplasmosis	*Histoplasma capsulatum*	Soil, bird and bat droppings	Mississippi and Ohio valleys in USA, Latin America, Africa, India, Far East, Australia	Benign pulmonary, disseminated, chronic pulmonary, cutaneous	Often good, except in disseminated form
Mucormycosis	*Mucor, Rhizopus* and *Absidia*	Ubiquitous	Worldwide	Rhinocerebral, pulmonary, gastrointestinal	Variable
Paracoccidioidomycosis (South American blastomycosis)	*Paracoccidioides brasiliensis*	Soil	South America, esp. Brazil	Pulmonary, disseminated	Good in young patients
Pneumocystosis	*Pneumocystis carinii (jerovici)*	Ubiquitous	Worldwide	Pulmonary, disseminated	Variable
Sporotrichosis	*Sporothrix schenkii*	Associated with thorny plants, wood, sphagnum moss	Worldwide	Lymphocutaneous, localized cutaneous, pulmonary, disseminated	Good

Appendix 21.11 Parasitic infestations

Disease	Micro-organism or parasite	Infection via	Consequence	Areas of greatest risk	Prevention	Treatment
Filariasis	Nematodes (roundworms) of family Filarioidea	Lymphatic filariasis transmitted through bite of mosquitoes. Onchocerciasis transmitted through bite of blackflies	Lymphatic filariasis and onchocerciasis (river blindness)	Lymphatic filariasis throughout sub-Saharan Africa and South-East Asia. Onchocerciasis in western and Central Africa, Central and South America	Avoid bites of mosquitoes and/or blackflies	Diethylcarbamazine, ivermectin
Giardiasis	Protozoan parasite *Giardia lamblia*	Ingestion of *Giardia* cysts in water (unfiltered drinking and recreational waters) contaminated by faeces of humans or animals	Anorexia, chronic diarrhoea, abdominal cramps, bloating, frequent loose greasy stools, fatigue and weight loss	Worldwide	Avoid ingesting any potentially contaminated (i.e. unfiltered) drinking water or recreational water	Metronidazole
Leishmaniasis	See text *					
Malaria	See text *					
Schistosomiasis (bilharziasis)	Parasitic blood flukes (trematodes), of which the most important are *Schistosoma mansoni*, *S. japonicum* and *S. haematobium*	Infection occurs in fresh water containing larval forms (cercariae) of schistosomes, which develop in snails infected as a result of excretion of eggs in human urine or faeces. The free-swimming larvae enter the skin of individuals swimming or wading in water	*S. mansoni* and *S. japonicum* cause hepatic and intestinal signs. *S. haematobium* causes urinary dysfunction	*S. mansoni* in sub-Saharan Africa, the Arabian peninsula, Brazil, Surinam and Venezuela. *S. japonicum* in China, Indonesia and Philippines (not Japan). *S. haematobium* in sub-Saharan Africa and eastern Mediterranean areas	Avoid swimming or wading in fresh water in endemic areas	Praziquantel
Strongyloidiasis	*Strongyloides stercoralis*, *Strongyloides fulleborni*	Infection acquired by walking barefoot in contaminated soil. Larvae enter the body by burrowing into the skin. Humans are principal host. Dogs, cats, and other mammals also	At the entry site, larvae petechial haemorrhages and intense pruritus. Larvae migrate into pulmonary circulation via the lymphatic system and venules, produce haemorrhages and an alveolar inflammatory response with eosinophilic infiltration (pneumonitis). Larvae migrate up pulmonary tree, are swallowed, and reach gastrointestinal system, where they embed and can produce an inflammatory reaction and malabsorption syndrome	*Strongyloides* species distributed worldwide but endemic in tropical and subtropical regions. Most prevalent in South-East Asia, Sahara desert, Colombia and tropical Brazil. Infection rates in these areas can be 60%	Avoid walking barefoot. Persons in household contact not at risk for infection. Proper disposal of human excreta reduces prevalence	Albendazole Tiabendazole
Trypanosomiasis African trypanosomiasis (sleeping sickness)	Protozoan parasites *Trypanosoma brucei* (T. b.) *gambiense* and *T. b. rhodesiense*	Bite of infected tsetse flies	*T. b. gambiense* causes chronic illness after a prolonged incubation period of weeks or months. *T. b. rhodesiense* causes a more acute illness, with onset a few days or weeks after the infected bite; often, a striking inoculation chancre. Initial signs include headache, insomnia, enlarged lymph nodes, anaemia and rash. In late stages, there is loss of weight and involvement of CNS. Without treatment, it is invariably fatal	*T. b. gambiense* present in foci in tropical countries of western and central Africa. *T. b. rhodesiense* in East Africa, extending south as far as Botswana	Avoid contact with tsetse flies since bites are difficult to avoid because tsetse flies bite during the day; can penetrate clothing and are not repelled by insect repellents	Consult experts
Trypanosomiasis American trypanosomiasis (Chagas disease)	Protozoan parasite *Trypanosoma cruzi*	Blood-sucking triatomine bugs ('kissing bugs'). Also by transfusion if blood is from infected donor	Chronic illness, progressive myocardial damage leading to cardiac arrhythmias and dilatation, and mega-oesophagus and megacolon	Mexico, Central and South America (to central Argentina and Chile)	Avoid exposure to blood-sucking bugs. Use bednets in houses and camps	Consult experts

* see text

MALIGNANT DISEASE

GENERAL ASPECTS

Malignant disease (neoplasms or 'cancers') develop as a consequence of deoxyribonucleic acid (DNA) mutations (mutagenesis). Some mutations are spontaneous (possibly due to oxygen radicals) but mutagens such as chemical carcinogens (e.g. from tobacco, alcohol or betel), ionizing and ultraviolet radiation or oncogenic micro-organisms (e.g. hepatitis, herpes and human papilloma viruses; HPVs; Fig. 22.1) can also induce mutations.

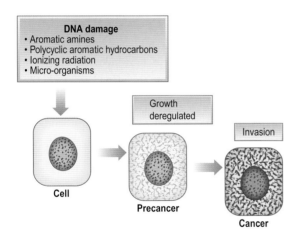

Fig. 22.1 Diagrammatic simplification of the process of carcinogenesis

Important carcinogens are aromatic amines (including arylamines and heterocyclic amines) found in tobacco smoke and cooked foods But the list of carcinogens is long, and the most important relevant carcinogens and pro-carcinogens in tobacco and alcoholic beverages are shown in Box 22.1.

Box 22.1 Some known common carcinogens

- Acetal dehyde
- Alkyl halides
- Arylamines
- Nitrosamines
- Polycyclic aromatic hydrocarbon
- Urethane

Various enzymes, found especially in the liver, are involved in the activation or degradation of carcinogens or pro-carcinogens. These are termed xenobiotic-metabolizing enzymes (XME; Table 22.1); several are polymorphic.

DNA repair enzymes can reverse or repair some of the damage from mutations but, when mutations involve genes such as tumour suppressor genes, the cell may become autonomous, despite attempts at DNA and cell repair, and the cell then proliferates and invades – the hallmark of cancer. Eventually the tumour spreads elsewhere (metastasizes) to lymph nodes and through the blood to the brain, liver, bones and elsewhere.

Carcinomas arise from epithelia and are a leading cause of morbidity and mortality, mainly in persons middle-aged or older, and are most common in the lung, breast, colon, cervix, stomach, pancreas, ovary, prostate and skin. They metastasize mainly to the brain liver, and bones. Younger people may be affected, but more particularly by haematological malignancies (Ch. 8) and occasionally by rare tumours.

Lung tumours are discussed in Ch. 15, breast in Ch. 25, gastrointestinal and pancreatic in Ch. 7, ovary and prostate in Ch. 25, brain in Ch. 13, liver in Ch. 7 and skin in Ch. 11.

Oral cancer is discussed below.

Table 22.1 Main xenometabolizing enzymes

Enzyme	Abbreviation	Main activities of some genotypes
Alcohol dehydrogenases	ADH	Activate ethanol
Aldehyde dehydrogenases	ALDH	Inactivate ethanol
Cytochrome P450	CYP	Activate ethanol, benzpyrene and nitrosamines
Glutathione S-transferases	GST	Metabolize benzpyrene, alkyl halides, epoxides, lipid peroxides
N-acetyl transferases	NAT	Acetylate arylamines

CANCER PREVENTION

The prognosis of much malignant disease is poor and treatment can also unfortunately have significant adverse effects, so prevention and early detection of cancer are important. The European Code Against Cancer, summarizes the preventive aspects (Box 22.2; Boyle et al 2003).

Tobacco and alcohol use, and other lifestyle habits are vitally important in carcinogenesis. The World Cancer Research Fund advocates measures in addition to not using tobacco, as in Table 22.2.

AVOIDING TOBACCO

Tobacco smoke is a complex mixture of at least 50 compounds including polycyclic aromatic hydrocarbons, nitrosamines, aldehydes and aromatic amines.

Tobacco use is best avoided.

Between 25% and 30% of all cancers in developed countries are tobacco-related. Tobacco, acting either singly or jointly with the consumption of alcohol, is responsible for 87% of lung cancer, and between 43% and 60% of cancers in the oesophagus, larynx and oral cavity. Tobacco consumption is also linked to cancers of bladder and pancreas, and a minority of cancers of kidney, stomach, cervix and nose, and myeloid leukaemia. On stopping smoking, the risk of cancer rapidly declines: benefit is evident within 5 years and is progressively greater with the passage of time. Tobacco smoke released to the environment by smokers, commonly referred to as environmental tobacco smoke (ETS) and which is responsible for 'passive smoking', has several deleterious effects on people who inhale it. It causes a small rise in the risk of lung cancer, and also some increase in the risk of heart disease and respiratory disease. It is particularly harmful to small children.

Although the greatest cancer hazard is caused by cigarette smoking, cigars can cause similar hazards, and both cigar and pipe smoking cause comparable hazards of cancers of the oral cavity, pharynx, larynx and oesophagus. Bidi, a type of cigarette made of tobacco rolled in a dried temburni leaf, is smoked in India and is associated with a high incidence of oral leukoplakia and oral cancer.

Tobacco-chewing in peoples from parts of Asia, along with a variety of ingredients in a 'betel quid' (betel vine leaf, areca nut, catechu, and slaked lime together with tobacco)

appears to predispose to oral squamous cell carcinoma (OSCC; Ch. 11). Smokeless tobacco, for example snuff-dipping in women in south-eastern USA who place snuff in the buccal sulcus, has been shown to predispose to gingival and alveolar carcinoma close to where the snuff is placed, but the risk is low.

AVOIDING ALCOHOL

Alcoholic beverages may contain carcinogens or pro-carcinogens, including ethanol, nitrosamines and urethane contaminants. Acetaldehyde is the main carcinogenic metabolite of ethanol. There does not seem to be a different effect of beer, wine or spirits on cancer risk; rather the total amount of ethanol ingested appears to be the key factor.

Alcoholic beverages increase the risk of squamous cell cancers of oral cavity, pharynx, larynx and oesophagus. The risks tend to increase with the amount of ethanol drunk. Alcohol drinking raises the risk of neoplasms, even in the absence of smoking, but alcohol drinking and tobacco smoking together greatly increase the risk. Compared to never-smokers and non-alcohol drinkers, the relative risk of these neoplasms is raised between 10- and 100-fold in people who drink and smoke heavily. A probable carcinogenic mechanism of alcohol is by facilitating the carcinogenic effect of tobacco and possibly of other carcinogens to which the upper digestive and respiratory tract are exposed, particularly those of dietary origin. However, a direct carcinogenic effect of acetaldehyde, the main metabolite of ethanol, and of other agents present in alcoholic beverages is likely. A diet poor in fruits and vegetables, typical of heavy drinkers, may also play an important role.

Alcohol drinking is also strongly associated with risk of primary liver cancer; particularly among smokers and among people chronically infected with hepatitis C virus. A higher risk of colorectal cancer has been observed in many cohort and case–control studies, and seems to be linearly correlated with the amount of alcohol consumed, and independent of the type of alcohol.

A greater risk of breast cancer has been consistently reported. More cases of breast cancer than of any other cancer are attributable to alcohol drinking among European women. It has been suggested that alcohol acts on hormonal factors involved in breast carcinogenesis.

Few studies have analysed the relation between stopping alcohol drinking and the risk of cancers of the upper respiratory and digestive tract, but there is clear evidence that the risk of oesophageal cancer falls by 60%, 10 years or more after drinking cessation. The pattern of risk reduction is less clear for oral and laryngeal cancers.

OTHER FACTORS

Weight reduction

Obesity is associated with a greater risk of cancer of the colon, breast (post-menopausal), endometrium, kidney and oesophagus (adenocarcinoma). In Western Europe, it has been estimated that being overweight or obese accounts for approximately 11% of all colon cancers, 9–11% of breast cancers, 39%

Table 22.2 10 rules for reducing cancer risk

1 Be as lean as possible without becoming underweight	Convincing evidence shows that weight gain and obesity increases the risk of a number of cancers, including bowel and breast cancer. Maintain a healthy weight through a balanced diet and regular physical activity to help keep your risk lower
2 Be physically active for at least 30 min every day	There is strong evidence that physical activity protects against cancers, including bowel and breast cancer. Being physically active is also key to maintaining a healthy weight. Any type of activity counts – the more you do the better! Try to build some into your everyday life
3 Avoid sugary drinks. Limit consumption of energy-dense foods (particularly processed foods high in added sugar, or low in fibre or high in fat)	Energy-dense foods are high in fats, sugars and can be low in nutrients. These foods, especially when consumed frequently or in large portions, increase the risk of obesity, which increases the risk of cancer. Fast foods like burgers, chips, fried chicken and most pizzas, and snack foods like chocolate, crisps and biscuits, tend to be energy dense Some energy-dense foods, such as nuts, seeds and some vegetable oils are important sources of nutrients, and have not been linked with weight gain as part of a typical diet
4 Eat more of a variety of vegetables, fruits, wholegrains and pulses such as beans	Evidence shows that vegetables, fruits and other foods containing dietary fibre (such as wholegrains and pulses) may protect against a range of cancers including mouth, stomach and bowel cancer. They also help to protect against weight gain and obesity. As well as eating your five a day, try to include wholegrains (e.g. brown rice, wholemeal bread and pasta) and/or pulses with every meal. Sugary drinks, such as colas and fruit squashes, can also contribute to weight gain. Fruit juices, even without added sugar, are likely to have a similar effect, so try not to drink them in large quantities. Try to eat lower energy-dense foods such as vegetables, fruits and wholegrains instead. Opt for water or unsweetened tea or coffee in place of sugary drinks
5 Limit consumption of red meats (such as beef, pork and lamb) and avoid processed meats	There is strong evidence that red and processed meats are causes of bowel cancer, and that there is no amount of processed meat that can be confidently shown not to increase risk. Aim to limit intake of red meat to less than 500 g cooked weight (about 700–750 g raw weight) a week. Try to avoid processed meats such as bacon, ham, salami, corned beef and some sausages
6 If consumed at all, limit alcoholic drinks to two for men and one for women a day	Since the 1997 report, the evidence that alcoholic drinks can increase the risk of a number of cancers, including breast and colon cancer, is much stronger. Any alcohol consumption can increase your risk of cancer, though there is some evidence to suggest that small amounts of alcohol can help protect against heart disease. Therefore, if you choose to drink, do so in moderation
7 Limit consumption of salty foods and food processed with salt (sodium)	Evidence shows that salt and salt-preserved foods probably cause stomach cancer. Try to use herbs and spices to flavour your food and remember that processed foods, including bread and breakfast cereals, can contain large amounts of salt
8 Don't use supplements to protect against cancer	Research shows that high-dose nutrient supplements can affect our risk of cancer, so it's best to opt for a balanced diet without supplements. However, supplements are advisable for some groups of people
9 It's best for mothers to breast-feed exclusively for up to 6 months and then add other liquids and foods	Strong evidence shows that breast-feeding protects mothers against breast cancer and babies from excess weight gain
10 After treatment, cancer survivors should follow the recommendations for cancer prevention	Maintaining a healthy weight through diet and physical activity may help to reduce the risk of cancer recurrence

See http://www.wcrf-uk.org/research_science/recommendations.lasso

of endometrial cancers, 27% of oesophageal adenocarcinomas and 25% of renal cell cancers.

A body mass index of below 25 kg/m^2 should, if possible, be maintained.

Greater physical activity

There is consistent evidence that regular physical activity is associated with a 40% reduction in the risk of colorectal cancer, and a 20–40% reduction in the risk of breast and oesophageal cancer and may possibly also lower the risk of prostate cancer. The protective effect of physical activity improves with increasing levels of activity. One hour per day of moderate physical activity such as walking may also be needed to maintain a healthy body weight, particularly for people with sedentary lifestyles. More vigorous activity, such as fast walking, several times per week may give some additional benefits.

Greater intake of fruit and vegetables

A low-fat diet with at least 11 servings of fruits, vegetables, whole grains and beans daily may reduce the chances of colon cancer by 75%, breast cancer by 50% and lung cancer by 30%. There may also be a protective effect on the risk of a wide variety of other cancers, in particular oral, oesophagus, stomach, rectum and pancreas. So far the best evidence for the benefits of a low-fat diet is in protecting against breast cancer. Vegetables and fruits contain many potentially anti-carcinogenic agents. Antioxidant activity seems important in cancer protection but the exact molecule(s) in vegetables and fruits that confers protection is unknown and their mechanism of action unclear.

'Five-a-day' (minimum 400 g/day, i.e. two pieces of fruit and 200 g of vegetables) is advocated to lead to a lower cancer risk.

Avoiding sun exposure

Ninety per cent of skin cancers are seen in white-skinned peoples and are caused by the sun's ultraviolet rays (Ch. 11). Squamous cell carcinoma of the skin or lip shows the clearest relationship between cumulative sun exposure and the risk is greatest in outdoor workers. The recipients of transplanted organs are particularly at risk as a result of the combined effects of the unchecked growth of HPV due to immunosuppression, and exposure to the sun (Ch. 35).

Basal cell carcinoma is the commonest type of skin cancer but, in this, intermittency of sun exposure seems to be important.

Malignant melanoma is more common in people of high socioeconomic status who work inside but who have the opportunity to spend leisure time in the sun, and this includes dentists. The incidence of melanoma has doubled in Europe between the 1960s and the 1990s, and this is attributed to longer intense sun exposure. The fair-skinned are more susceptible, particularly those with red hair, freckles and a tendency to burn in the sun. These characteristics are genetically determined at least partially by the *MCIR* gene, which codes for the melanocyte-stimulating hormone receptor. Variants in the *MCIR* gene control the ratio of black melanin (eumelanin) to red (phaeomelanin) in the skin. The strongest phenotypic risk factor for melanoma, however, is the presence of large numbers of moles or melanocytic naevi, which may be normal in appearance but are also usually accompanied by so-called atypical moles. The latter are larger than 5 mm in diameter with variable colour and an irregular shape. The phenotype, described as the atypical mole syndrome phenotype (AMS), is present in approximately 2% of the Caucasian population and is associated with an approximately tenfold higher risk of melanoma. Advice about sun protection is particularly of importance to this population.

The best protection from the summer sun is to stay out of it. If outdoors, keep out of the sun between 11am and 3pm, wear close-weave heavy cotton and use sunscreens with high sun protection factor (SPF). Do not rely upon sunscreens for protection, however useful they may be to protect skin sites such as the ears.

Avoiding occupational exposures

The cancers that have most frequently been associated with occupational exposures are those of the lung, urinary bladder, mesothelioma, larynx, leukaemia, liver, nose and nasal cavity and skin (non-melanoma). For several other neoplasms also associated with occupational exposures, the evidence is less strong. They include cancers of the oral cavity, nasopharynx, oesophagus, stomach, colon and rectum, pancreas, breast, testis, kidney, prostate, brain, bones, soft-tissue sarcoma, lymphomas and multiple myeloma.

The more common occupational exposures are solar radiation, passive smoking, crystalline silica, diesel exhaust, radon, wood dust, benzene, asbestos, formaldehyde, polycyclic aromatic hydrocarbons (PAHs), chromium, cadmium and nickel compounds. There is no reliable evidence of a risk from power plants, or power lines or mobile telephones.

Many chemicals are known or suspect carcinogens. Many of the agents in this group are still widely used, for example 1,3-butadiene and formaldehyde. Twenty-nine chemical or physical agents, groups of agents or mixtures that appear predominantly in the workplace have been classified as human carcinogens. More than 200 agents, groups of agents or exposure circumstances are classified as 'possibly carcinogenic' to humans largely on the basis of data from animal experiments. Thirty-five agents or industrial processes are classified as probably carcinogenic. The rubber industry, and painting and decorating are examples. The effect of specific occupational carcinogens such as aromatic amines or PAHs is also mediated by genetic factors such as genetic polymorphisms of the *NAT2* or the *GSTMI* genes.

Prevention of workplace exposures can be effective. Occupational bladder cancer fell after the ban on the use of beta-naphthylamine in the rubber and chemical industries.

Avoiding environmental exposures

Environmental exposures usually refer to exposures of the general population that cannot be directly controlled by the individual and include air pollution, drinking water contaminants, passive smoking, radon gas in buildings, exposure to solar radiation, food contaminants such as pesticide residues, dioxins or environmental oestrogens, chemicals from industrial emissions, ionizing radiation and waste from nuclear processes, and others. These exposures have been associated with a variety of neoplasms including cancers of the lung, urinary bladder, leukaemia and skin. The impact of several exposures that are widespread, such as disinfection by-products in drinking water, is still inconclusive.

Agents in the general environment to which many are exposed for long periods (such as passive smoking or air pollution) may increase only modestly the relative risk for certain cancers, but may overall be responsible for a significant number of cases.

Avoiding hormones that may play a role

Hormone replacement therapy (HRT) for menopausal symptoms appears to raise the risk of breast cancer.

CANCER SCREENING

Table 22.3 shows cancer screening methods.

CLINICAL FEATURES

There is a range of different cancers (Box 22.3), each with specific manifestations (see relevant chapters). Features that may raise suspicion of cancer are shown in Box 22.4.

Table 22.3 Cancer screening (from Boyle et al., 2003)

Cancer site	Methods
Breast	Self-examination/mammography/*BRCA1* and *BRAC2* mutation in Jewish women
Cervix	Cervical cytology/human papilloma virus testing
Colon/rectum	Faecal occult blood/flexible sigmoidoscopy
Lung	Spiral computed tomography (CT) or chest radiography
Neuroblastoma	Urinary homovanillic acid (HVA) and vanillylmandelic acid (VMA)
Oral	Examination of the mouth
Ovary	CA125 and/or ultrasonography
Prostate	Prostate-specific antigen (PSA)
Skin (melanoma)	Examination for moles
Stomach	*Helicobacter pylori* testing; breath test/endoscopy
Testis	Self-examination

Box 22.3 Common cancer types

- Bladder cancer
- Breast cancer
- Colon and rectal cancer
- Endometrial (cervical) cancer
- Kidney (renal cell) cancer
- Leukaemia
- Lung cancer
- Melanoma
- Non-Hodgkin lymphoma
- Oral cancer
- Pancreatic cancer
- Prostate cancer
- Skin cancer (non-melanoma)
- Thyroid cancer

MANAGEMENT

Clinical examination supplemented with imaging and biopsy is invariably indicated to diagnose malignant disease. There is also considerable interest in tumour markers in blood or other body fluids, or tissues; unfortunately, none of these tumour markers, including CEA (carcinoembryonic antigen), meets the goal of *reliably* finding cancer at an early stage. The reasons for this are that: most people have small amounts of these markers in their blood; the levels of these markers tend to be higher than normal only when there is a large tumour present; some people with cancer never have higher levels of markers; and even when marker levels are high, they are often not adequately specific. For example, CA125 can be high in women with ovarian cancer but also in other gynaecological conditions. Because of this, "tumour markers" are used mainly in patients who have already been diagnosed with cancer in order to monitor treatment response or detect recurrences.

The most widely accepted tumour marker is the prostate-specific antigen (PSA) blood test, which is used (along with the digital rectal examination) to screen for prostate cancer but it

Box 22.4 Features that may suggest cancer

- Abdominal pain
- Abnormal vaginal bleeding
- Anorexia
- Blood in faeces
- Blood in sputum
- Blood in urine
- Change in bowel habits
- Change in size or colour of a skin lump
- Change in urination
- Chronic backache
- Chronic headaches
- Dysphagia
- Fever
- Finger clubbing
- Hoarseness
- Lump in breast
- Lump in testicle
- Lymph node enlargement
- Night sweats
- Persistent cough
- Unexplained anaemia
- Weight loss

also suffers from the drawbacks outlined above (Ch. 25). Others are shown in Table 22.4.

Surgery, radiotherapy and chemotherapy are the main types of treatment for cancer.

ORAL CANCER
GENERAL ASPECTS

Oral cancer is usually squamous cell carcinoma (OSCC) and is mainly a disease of older males. It is the predominant cancer in the head and neck region. High rates of OSCC are seen particularly in India, Sri Lanka and Brazil, but high rates also occur in Hungary and France and there is a wide geographical variation in incidence. Risk factors are shown in Box 22.5.

The results of many studies of lifestyle risk factors have been summarized by the International Agency for Research on Cancer (IARC) showing the importance of specific risk factors (i.e. tobacco, betel and alcohol use).

Tobacco contains a number of addictive components, especially nicotine, and releases acetaldehyde and also many other carcinogens (see above). Tobacco use in all forms appears to carry a risk of OSCC. Oral cancer risks show a clear decline after stopping tobacco use.

Betel quid (BQ) is probably used by 20% of the world's population. Snuff is finely powdered plant material, principally tobacco, used orally or nasally, and is a risk factor for OSCC. Increased consumption of any alcohol-containing beverages is associated with a risk of OSCC. The risk decreases after stopping alcohol use but the effects appear to persist for several years. The type of alcoholic beverage appears to influence the risk – hard liquors confer higher risks. The combined effect of alcohol and tobacco is far greater than the sum of the two effects and is multiplicative. There have been reports of oral cancer in marijuana smokers and in users of alcohol containing mouthwashes but any relationships have yet to be containing by full epidemiological studies.

Table 22.4 Tumour markers

Marker	Abbreviation	Comments
Alpha-fetoprotein	AFP	Useful to follow treatment response and follow-up in liver cancer (hepatocellular carcinoma), testicular cancers (embryonal cell and endodermal sinus types). Raised AFP levels are also seen in rare ovarian and testicular cancers (yolk sac tumour or mixed germ cell cancer)
Beta$_2$-microglobulin	B2M	Raised in multiple myeloma, chronic lymphocytic leukaemia (CLL), and some lymphomas
Bladder tumour antigen	BTA	Found in urine in bladder cancer
Calcitonin	–	Raised blood levels in cancer of parafollicular C cells (medullary thyroid carcinoma; MTC)
Cancer antigens	CA15-3 CA19-9 CA27.29 CA72-4 CA125	Breast cancer Developed to detect colorectal cancer, but more sensitive for pancreatic cancer Breast cancer Ovarian and pancreatic cancer and digestive tract cancers, especially stomach Ovarian cancer
Carcinoembryonic antigen	CEA	Used to monitor treatment and recurrence of colorectal carcinoma and breast, lung, pancreatic and gastric malignancies
Chromogranin A	CgA	Neuroendocrine tumours (carcinoid tumours, neuroblastoma and small cell lung cancer)
Immunoglobulins	Igs	Bone marrow cancers (e.g. multiple myeloma and Waldenstrom macroglobulinaemia)
Neuron-specific enolase	NSE	Neuroendocrine tumours (small cell lung cancer, neuroblastoma and carcinoid tumours)
Soluble 100% in ammonium sulfate	S-100	Found in most melanoma cells
Tissue polypeptide antigen	TPA	Follow-up of patients treated for cancers in lung, bladder
Thyroglobulin	–	Thyroid diseases, including some cancer

Breast cancer markers are discussed in Ch. 25.
See http://www.cancer.org/docroot/PED/content/PED_2_3X_Tumor_Markers.asp

---

Box 22.5 Risk factors for oral cancer

- Old age
- Male gender
- Tobacco, smoked and/or chewed
- Alcohol
- Betel (areca) use, as in betel chewing
- Sun exposure
- Ionizing radiation
- Immunosuppression and graft-versus-host disease
- Infections with human papillomavirus, *Candida* or syphilis
- Low socioeconomic status
- Diet law in fruit and vegetables

Charcoal-grilled red meat and fried foods have been implicated as risk factors. An increased consumption of fruits and vegetables, however, is associated with lower risk of OSCC. Raised risks of oral cancer have also been found in a number of occupations (Table 22.5).

Micro-organisms implicated in the aetiology of OSCC include syphilis, *Candida albicans* and viruses such as herpesviruses and human papillomaviruses. Syphilis is discussed in Ch. 32. Candidal leukoplakias are potentially malignant and autoimmune polyendocrinopathy–candidiasis–ectodermal dystrophy (APECED), an autosomal recessive disease associated with a limited T-lymphocyte defect, seems to favour the growth of *Candida albicans* and predisposes to OSCC.

Viral infections, particularly with oncogenic HPV subtypes and possibly Epstein–Barr virus (EBV), can have a tumorigenic

Table 22.5 Occupations associated with risk of oral cancer

Occupations	Main Countries
Exposure to wood-stove fumes	Brazil
Building industry Electricity production Machinery operations Plumbers Textile industry	Italy
Carpet installation Exposure to fossil fuels Furniture industry Machining Metal working Painting Petroleum industry Woodworkers	USA
Blacksmithing Butchering Driving Electricity working Masonary Railway working	Uruguay
Metal working	Brazil
Exposure to horses on farms, employment on construction work, pesticide use, grain production	Norway
Exposure to benzene	UK

effect. Oropharyngeal cancer is significantly associated with oral HPV type 16 and also associated with a high lifetime number of vaginal-sex partners and oral-sex partners; HPV-16 DNA is detected in most.

Lip cancer is seen mainly in males with chronic sun exposure and in smokers. Ionizing radiation exposure is a possible risk factor for second primary cancers.

Persons with poor oral hygiene appear to have increased risk of OSCC, independent of any effect of tobacco, alcohol, or other well-proven risk factors; not all workers agree, so further studies are required. Polymicrobial supragingival plaque is a possible independent factor, as it possesses a relevant mutagenic interaction with saliva, and individual oral health is a cofactor in the development of OSCC. Viridans group streptococci of normal oral flora can produce acetaldehyde *in vitro* during ethanol incubation via alcohol dehydrogenase. In particular, clinical strain of *Streptococcus salivarius*, both clinical and culture collection strains of *Streptococcus intermedius* and culture collection strain of *Streptococcus mitis* produced high amounts of acetaldehyde.

SYSTEMIC HEALTH AND ORAL SQUAMOUS CELL CARCINOMA

There is a highly significant increase in the incidence of OSCC in dyskeratosis congenita and systemic sclerosis, and an increase of potentially malignant lesions and OSCC in transplant recipients and in people with similar lesions elsewhere in the upper oeso digestive tract. There is a putative association of diabetes mellitus with oral cancer.

POTENTIALLY MALIGNANT DISORDERS

Some potentially malignant (pre-cancerous) oral clinical lesions which can progress to OSCC include the following in particular.

- Erythroplasia (erythroplakia) – the most likely lesion to progress to severe dysplasia or carcinoma.
- Leukoplakia, particularly where admixed with red lesions as in speckled leukoplakia, and proliferative verrucous leukoplakia, sublingual leukoplakia, candidal leukoplakia and syphilitic leukoplakia (exceptionally rare now).
- Lichen planus.
- Oral submucous fibrosis.

Apart from these lesions, most other potentially malignant lesions or conditions have only a very low incidence of dysplasia or malignant change (Table 22.6).

CLINICAL FEATURES

Common sites for OSCC are the lips, the lateral border of the tongue and the floor of the mouth. There may be widespread dysplastic mucosa ('field change') or even a second neoplasm anywhere in the oral cavity, oropharynx or upper aerodigestive tract. *Second primary neoplasms* in the aerodigestive tract may be seen in those with OSCC over 3 years in up to 25%, and in up to 40% of those who continue to smoke.

Many OSCCs can be detected visually but early OSCC can be asymptomatic, may appear innocuous, and can be overlooked

Table 22.6 Potentially malignant oral disorders

Approximate malignant potential	Lesion	Known aetiological factors
Very high (85%+)	Erythroplasia	Tobacco/alcohol
High in some instances (30%+)	Actinic cheilitis	Sunlight
	Chronic candidosis (candidal leukoplakia)	Candida albicans
	Dyskeratosis congenita	Genetic
	Leukoplakia (non-homogeneous)	Tobacco/alcohol
	Proliferative verrucous leukoplakia	Tobacco/alcohol/human papillomavirus (HPV)
	Sublingual keratosis	Tobacco/alcohol
	Submucous fibrosis	Areca nut
	Syphilitic leukoplakia	Syphilis
Low (< 5%)	Atypia in immunocompromised patients	? HPV
	Leukoplakia (homogeneous)	Friction/tobacco/alcohol
	Discoid lupus erythematosus	Autoimmune
	Lichen planus	Idiopathic
	Paterson–Brown-Kelly syndrome (Plummer–Vinson syndrome)	Iron deficiency

especially if the examination is not thorough. The whole oral mucosa should be examined, often along with examination of the rest of the upper aerodigestive tract – and the cervical lymph nodes must always be carefully examined by palpation (Fig. 22.2). Cancer must be suspected, especially when there is a single oral lesion persisting for more than 3 weeks, and particularly when having features as shown in Box 22.6.

CLASSIFICATION/GRADING

Oral cancer is a term which usually includes cancer of the lip, tongue, salivary glands and other sites in the mouth (gum, floor of the mouth and other unspecified parts of the mouth). Pharyngeal cancer is a term that includes cancers of the nasopharynx, oropharynx and hypopharynx.

Staging of OSCC should be made according to the TNM classification of the International Union Against Cancer (UICC) – tumour size (T), nodal metastases (N) and distant metastases (M; Table 22.7) – since this classification relates well to overall survival rate (i.e. the earlier the tumour, the better the prognosis and the less complicated the treatment). It is generally accepted that prognosis is best in early carcinomas, especially those that are well differentiated and not metastasized (Table 22.8).

GENERAL MANAGEMENT

Any lesion of a potentially malignant or dubious nature persisting for more than 3 weeks should be biopsied and second primary tumours should be excluded by chest radiography and endoscopy. Tumours are staged using the TNM system (tumour, nodes, metastases).

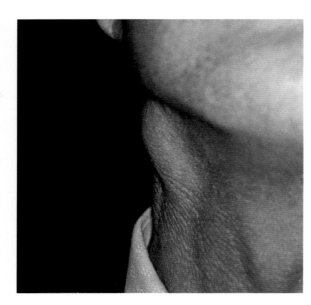

Fig. 22.2 Cervical lymph node enlargement in oral carcinoma

Box 22.6 Warning features of oral carcinoma

- Red lesion (erythroplasia)
- Mixed red/white lesion, irregular white lesion
- Lump
- Ulcer with fissuring or raised exophytic margins
- Pain or numbness
- Abnormal blood vessels supplying a lump
- Loose tooth
- Extraction socket not healing
- Induration beneath a lesion (i.e. a firm infiltration beneath the mucosa)
- Fixation of lesion to deeper tissues or to overlying skin or mucosa
- Lymph node enlargement
- Dysphagia
- Weight loss

Oral squamous cell carcinomas are routinely discovered late and have one of the lowest 5-year survival rates of any major cancer site, at ~50%, and this has not changed in the past 30 years. Localized cancers have the highest 5-year relative survival rates (80%), those with regional disease intermediate (40%) and cancers with distant metastasis the lowest (20%). OSCC is also particularly dangerous because it maybe associated with second, primary tumours.

The reliable differentiation of malignant lesions from benign lesions by clinical inspection alone is not possible. Also, malignant transformation of potentially malignant lesions cannot be accurately excluded based solely upon clinical characteristics. The only method currently available to determine the diagnosis and give an indication of prognosis reliably is the laboratory histopathological examination of a biopsy tissue sample since it is accepted that dysplasia may precede malignant change. The golden rule is therefore to biopsy any persistent mucosal lesion where there is not absolute confidence that the diagnosis is of a benign lesion. There should be a high index of suspicion, especially of a solitary lesion present for over 3 weeks, when biopsy is invariably indicated. In practice, therefore, all ulcerated, red, white or mixed persistent solitary lesions require biopsy evaluation. Early diagnosis and treatment are the goals.

Table 22.7 TNM classification of malignant neoplasms[a]

Primary tumour size (T)	
Tx	No available information
T0	No evidence of primary tumour
Tis	Only carcinoma *in situ*
T1, T2, T3, T4[b]	Increasing size of tumour
Regional lymph node involvement (N)	
Nx	Nodes could not or were not assessed
N0	No clinically positive nodes
N1	Single ipsilateral node less than 3 cm in diameter
N2a	Single ipsilateral node 3–6 cm
N2b	Multiple ipsilateral nodes less than 6 cm
N2c	Bilateral or contralateral nodes less than 6 cm
N3	Any node greater than 6 cm
Involvement by distant metastases (M)	
Mx	Distant metastasis was not assessed
M0	No evidence of distant metastasis
M1	Distant metastasis is present

[a]Several other classifications are available, e.g. STNM (S = site).
[b]T1, maximum diameter 2 cm; T2, maximum diameter 4 cm; T3, maximum diameter over 4 cm; T4, massive tumour greater than 4 cm in diameter, with involvement of adjacent anatomical structures.

Table 22.8 Prognosis for intraoral carcinoma (adapted from Woolgar et al., 1995, and Sciubba, 2001)

Stage	TNM	Approximate % survival at 5 years
I	T1 N0 M0	85
II	T2 N0 M0	65
III	T3 N0 M0, or T1, T2 or T3 N1 M0	40
IV	Any T4, N2, N3 or M1	10

Since red rather than white areas are most likely to show any dysplasia present in the lesion, a biopsy should include the former.

Patients with oral cancer are best managed by a team of specialists. They include dental and maxillofacial surgeons, as well as oncologists, nurses, speech therapists and hygienists.

Cancer treatment can be with surgery, radiotherapy, chemotherapy (cytotoxic drugs singly or in combination), targetted therapy stem cell transplantation, immunotherapy (monoclonal antibodies and, on the horizon, vaccines) and now gene therapy. Surgery can lead to complications, which are discussed in standard textbooks of surgery, not least some defects of aesthetics and function (Fig. 22.3).

Radiotherapy and chemotherapy are used mainly to damage or destroy proliferating malignant cells, (particularly in malignant disease affecting blood cells (Ch. 8) and lymphomas (Ch. 8)),

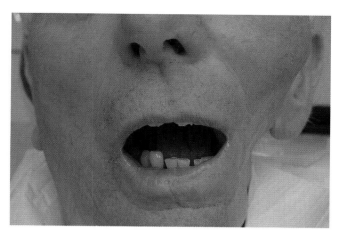

Fig. 22.3 Deformity after tumour resection

but also for some more solid tumours such as OSCC. They can affect many tissues, and can have severe adverse effects on health, health care and quality of life. These treatments can also damage the developing fetus.

Radiotherapy and cytotoxic chemotherapy can also have profound adverse effects on oral health and quality of life, and can give rise to the major complaints of the patient undergoing cancer treatment – especially when the radiotherapy field affects the head and neck and involves the oral cavity and salivary glands. Opinion varies as to the relative value of radiotherapy or surgery.

Treatment of patients with oral and oropharyngeal tongue cancers has not shown a significant improvement in 5-year disease-specific survival over decades. Poorer survival is significantly associated with age 45 years or older, oropharyngeal tongue cancers and advanced stage disease. A multimodal approach of surgery for the primary tumour and the neck, followed by post-operative radio(chemo)therapy seems superior to non-surgical treatment protocols, since it results in better disease-free and overall survival.

Many early carcinomas can be treated by either surgery or radiotherapy, but in later stages surgery is the first option. Cancer of the floor of the mouth presents considerable problems in surgery and may necessitate partial mandibulectomy. Lingual and labial cancers are often managed with radiotherapy, which may also provide the best palliation in patients with advanced disease. Cytotoxic chemotherapy has offered any better prognosis and, indeed, may cause a greater morbidity and mortality but newer drugs may help, as discussed below.

SURGERY

Surgery is the oldest form of treatment for oral cancer (see http://www.oralcancerfoundation.org/facts/surgery.htm) and is often done to achieve more than one of the following goals.

• *Curative surgery* – the removal of a tumour when it appears to be confined to one area. It may be used along with radiation therapy or chemotherapy, which can be given before or after the operation. In some cases, radiation therapy is actually used during an operation (intraoperative radiation therapy).

• *Debulking (or cytoreductive) surgery* is done in some cases when removing a tumour entirely would cause too much damage to an organ or surrounding areas. In these cases, radiation therapy or chemotherapy are also typically used.

• *Palliative surgery* is used to treat complications of advanced disease. It is not intended to cure the cancer.

• *Supportive surgery* is used to help with other types of treatment. For example, a vascular access device, such as a catheter port, can be placed into a vein to facilitate chemotherapy.

• *Restorative (or reconstructive) surgery* is used to restore a person's appearance or the function of an organ or body part after primary surgery. Examples include the use of tissue flaps, bone grafts or prosthetic materials after surgery.

Transoral laser microsurgery is a new trend for complete resection of tumours with preservation of function. Advanced reconstructive techniques that allow free transfer of soft tissue and bone from all over the body improve the functional and aesthetic outcomes following major ablative surgery. With successful surgical reconstruction, dental and prosthetic rehabilitation choices are enhanced. Neck dissection has also greatly advanced – from radical to function-preserving surgery, with sensory and spinal accessory nerve-preserving neck surgery resulting in a lower incidence and severity of neck and shoulder pain and loss of function compared to patients who have the nerve removed, and less depression and better quality of life scores with lower pain intensity.

Wound infection is a common complication after OSCC surgery and may result in significant functional morbidity, poor cosmetic results and prolonged hospitalization. The most important factors contributing to operative wound infections are male sex, tumour stage, reconstruction, tracheostomy, nasogastric tube or gastrostomy feeding and the extent of surgery.

RADIOTHERAPY

Radiation therapy is commonly used to treat OSCC (see http://www.oralcancerfoundation.org/facts/radiation.htm). Prior to therapy a planning session is required, including a computed tomography (CT) scan and measurements of the area to be treated, as well as skin markings to help with positioning during treatments. A porous mask is used in radiation treatment, to immobilize the patient's head so that radiation will only be delivered to the designated areas. The radiation therapy is given in small amounts (fractions) on a daily basis, usually 5 days in a row with a 2-day break each week. Normally, each daily treatment lasts about 10–15 min, with the majority of this time spent making sure the radiation blocking devices, which limit the radiation to the appropriate area, are properly in place, and the patient and machine are properly positioned. The daily dose must be great enough to destroy the cancer cells while sparing the normal tissues of excessive levels of radiation. Typically 2 Gy is delivered five times a week to a total dose of 64–70 Gy.

External beam radiotherapy

This is the use of machines to focus radiation on a cancer site. With modern radiation equipment, there is minimal scatter of X-ray energy outside the treatment beam.

X-rays were the first form of photon radiation to be used to treat cancer. Depending on the amount of energy they possess, the X-rays can be used to destroy cancer cells on the surface of an area, or penetrate to tissues deeper in the body. The higher the energy of the X-ray beam, the deeper the X-rays penetrate into the target tissue.

Linear accelerators produce X-rays of increasingly greater energy. Gamma rays are another form of photon radiation used and are produced spontaneously as certain elements (such as radium, uranium and cobalt 60) release radiation as they decompose, or decay.

Internal radiotherapy

Internal radiotherapy involves placing radioactive implants directly into a tumour or body cavity, resulting in less radiation exposure to other parts of the body. Brachytherapy, interstitial irradiation and intracavitary irradiation are types of internal radiotherapy.

Intraoperative irradiation

In intraoperative irradiation, a large dose of external radiation is directed at the tumour and surrounding tissue during surgery.

Intensity-modulated radiotherapy

Intensity-modulated radiotherapy (IMRT) uses a different software programme to administer the radiation from multiple angles in smaller doses, with a new shuttering device to limit the size of the radiation beams, thus sparing the salivary glands.

Particle beam radiation therapy

This involves the use of fast-moving subatomic particles to treat localized cancers. A sophisticated machine is needed to produce and accelerate the particles required for this procedure. Some particles (neutrons, pions and heavy ions) deposit more energy along the path they take through tissue than do X-rays or gamma rays, thus causing more damage to the cells they hit. This type of radiation is often referred to as high linear energy transfer (high LET) radiation.

The consensus is that patients with OSCC with involved margins or extracapsular spread (ECS) should have adjuvant radiotherapy. Techniques help: IMRT, three-dimensional (3-D) conformal radiotherapy, and conventional radiotherapy provide similar disease control but IMRT produces less xerostomia.

Chemoradiotherapy

Chemotherapeutic agents are increasingly used to enhance the effects of radiotherapy (chemo-radiation) (see below).

Dental aspects

Careful treatment planning, as well as close monitoring of the oral cavity with strict application of preventive measures, can reduce the incidence of complications significantly. Improved treatment techniques, such as the application of lower radiation

doses or IMRT, use of shielding, reduction in toxic drugs and improved oral hygiene can often reduce complications. Pain control is of paramount importance in patients with head and neck cancer. They may need potent analgesics, such as opioids, sedatives or antidepressants, particularly if they have terminal cancer. Completion of dental treatment before cancer care benefits the patient greatly.

Patients with advanced malignant disease in the head and neck have a high prevalence of oral complications, particularly xerostomia as a result of treatment. This is seen in nearly three-quarters, often also with soreness, taste disturbances and difficulties with wearing dentures. Candidosis is common. The most obvious oral importance of tumours involving other parts of the body is as a source of metastases. These can form in the jaws or occasionally in soft tissues, and can mimic a simple epulis clinically. Histological examination of all such swellings in a person with malignant disease elsewhere is therefore essential. Other oral manifestations of internal malignancy are summarized in Appendix 22.1.

Radiotherapy involving the oral cavity or salivary glands

External beam radiotherapy is often used to treat oral cancer (Table 22.9).

Radiotherapy used in the treatment of head and neck cancers, despite being targeted at cancerous cells, inevitably damages surrounding normal tissues, causing mucositis, and often salivary damage and xerostomia. (Table 22.10). Some complications such as xerostomia may be inevitable but permanent. Careful treatment planning before starting radiotherapy with precise dosimetry and careful shielding of the healthy tissues, as well as close monitoring of the oral cavity with strict application of preventive measures, can significantly reduce complications. Hair loss and skin erythema are common in the path of the radiation beam (Fig. 22.4). Carotid stenosis may arise.

Mucositis

Mucositis is virtually inevitable but can be mitigated by modifying the radiation schedule; protecting the mucosa with midline mucosa-sparing blocks; or theoretically by using amifostine, which, with its active metabolite, is a free-radical scavenger and is cytoprotective. It is rarely used in clinical practice because of fears that the free-radical scavenging action may reduce the effectiveness of radiotherapy on the cancer cell as well as protecting the normal cells.

Table 22.9 Types of external beam radiotherapy used to treat cancer in the head and neck

Type	Source	Used for
Electron beam	Electrical	Superficial lesions
Low voltage	X-ray	Superficial lesions
Orthovoltage	X-ray	Skin lesions
Supervoltage	Cobalt-60	Deeper lesions
Megavoltage	Linear accelerator	Larger lesions

Table 22.10 Oral complications of radiotherapy involving the mouth and salivary glands

Week 1	Week 2+	Week 3+	Later
Nausea Vomiting	Mucositis Taste changes	Dry mouth	Infections Caries Pulp pain and necrosis Tooth hypersensitivity Trismus Osteoradionecrosis Craniofacial defects

Table 22.11 Fall in salivary flow with different radiotherapy fields

Regimen	Approximate % fall in salivation
Mantle	30
Unilateral	50
Bilateral	75
Head and neck cancer	95
Nasopharynx	100

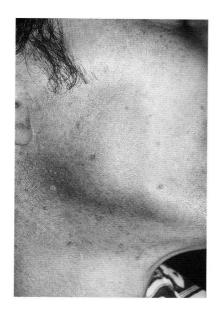

Fig. 22.4 Radiation erythema and hair loss

Xerostomia

Radiotherapy to tumours of the mouth, nasopharynx and oropharynx is especially liable to damage the salivary glands, depress salivary secretion and result in saliva of a higher viscosity but lower pH. The degree of xerostomia experienced depends on a number of factors but especially the volume of salivary tissue irradiated (Table 22.11) and dose. Doses greater than 30 Gy generally lead to a persistently if not permanently dry mouth.

Salivary secretion diminishes within a week of radiotherapy in virtually all patients and the saliva becomes thick and tenacious. Some salivary function may return after many months.

Both acute and long-term xerostomia can be reduced by using IMRT; sparing at least one parotid gland during irradiation of patients with head and neck cancer; or possibly by stimulating salivation pre-radiotherapy with pilocarpine, or by giving amifostine, which is a free-radical scavenger and protects acinar cells. Amifostine also reduces the risk of infection associated with neutropenia; however, it may cause severe nausea and vomiting, and is not used in clinical practice because of fears that the free-radical scavenging action may reduce the effectiveness of radiotherapy on the cancer cell as well as protecting the normal cells. Occasionally, submandibular gland transfer is used.

Infections

Infections (caries, oral candidosis and acute ascending sialadenitis) are predisposed to by xerostomia.

Loss of taste (hypoguesia)

Loss of taste follows radiation damage to the taste buds but xerostomia may contribute to disturb taste sensation. Taste may start to recover within 2–4 months and is typically complete by 6 months but, if more than 6000 cGy have been given, loss of taste may be permanent.

Radiation caries

Caries and dental hypersensitivity may follow radiotherapy. Patients frequently take a softer, more cariogenic diet because of dryness and soreness of the mouth and loss of taste. There is a change to a more cariogenic oral flora and the hypersensitive teeth make oral hygiene difficult. These factors combine to cause rampant dental caries, including areas such as incisal edges and cervical margins which are normally free from caries. Caries begins at any time between 2 and 10 months after radiotherapy, and may eventually result in the crown breaking off from the root. A complete dentition may be destroyed within a year of irradiation.

Caries may be minimized by controlling sugar intake, protecting salivary function as above and using fluorides.

Trismus

Trismus may result from replacement fibrosis of the masticatory muscles following progressive endarteritis of affected tissues, with reduction in their blood supply. Fibrosis becomes apparent 3–6 months after radiotherapy and can cause permanent limitation of opening. Fibrosis must be differentiated from recurrence of the tumour and from osteoradionecrosis.

Osteoradionecrosis

Radiation therapy induces endarteritis obliterans, which leads to progressive tissue fibrosis and capillary loss, leaving bone susceptible to avascular necrosis. The latter predisposes to the late and more severe complication of osteoradionecrosis (ORN), which may occur months to years later.

Osteoradionecrosis is a potentially serious complication of radiotherapy involving the jaws. Such infection often results from dental extractions carried out after radiotherapy because of diminished bone vascularity due to irradiation endarteritis. Oral sepsis, particularly from periodontal disease, may contribute.

The mandible, a compact bone with high density and poor vascularity, is more prone than the maxilla to ORN. ORN risk is greatest when radiation dose exceeds 60 Gy, when the floor of mouth is irradiated, from 10 days before to several years after radiotherapy (especially at 3–12 months after radiotherapy), and in patients who are malnourished or immunoincompetent. Osteoradionecrosis may follow months or years after radiotherapy but about 30% of cases develop within 6 months and are heralded by pain and swelling. The initiating factor is often trauma, such as tooth extraction, or oral infection or ulceration from an appliance. Presentation is of exposed bone in an irradiated mouth, with or without external sinuses, pain and pathological fracture.

In severe cases, the whole of the body of the mandible may become infected, both the overlying mucosa and skin may be destroyed, and the bone may become exposed internally and externally. ORN is a less frequent problem now, as megavoltage radiotherapy has less effect on bone than orthovoltage therapy.

The area involved is often small (less than 2 cm in diameter) and, with antibiotics, the signs and symptoms of inflammation may clear within a few weeks.

Osteoradionecrosis may be prevented by avoiding operations such as dental extractions after the jaws have been irradiated. This is achieved best by leaving only salvageable teeth and removing others, at least 2 weeks before starting radiotherapy.

New developments in radiotherapy, such as 3-D conformal radiotherapy and IMRT, have allowed radiation oncologists to escalate the dose of radiation delivered to tumours, while minimizing the dose delivered to surrounding normal tissue/ bone, contributing to the remarkable decline in the prevalence of ORN to < 4%. However, when ORN does occur, it is still associated with significant morbidity.

ORN may be prevented by removing teeth of dubious prognosis no less than 10 days before the start of radiotherapy. Local measures used to control the extent of ORN include meticulous oral hygiene, use of chlorhexidine mouthwash after meals, and wound care (irrigation of the wound, removal of loose sequestrae). Antibiotic therapy (tetracycline, clindamycin, metronidazole), ultrasound and hyperbaric oxygen (HBO) may help. The 'Marx protocol' consists of 20 HBO sessions prior to surgery and ten sessions afterwards. However, a high-quality trial has demonstrated that HBO alone is not effective in treating ORN of the mandible compared to placebo. There is a lack of evidence regarding the effect of HBO on dental implants/ORN risk. Complete resolution of ORN can, however, take two or more years despite intensive treatment with antimicrobials. HBO may be required.

Craniofacial defects

Craniofacial defects, tooth hypoplasia and retarded eruption can follow irradiation of developing teeth and growth centres in children. Children treated for neuroblastoma, therefore, are at particularly high risk for abnormal dental development.

Dental management of patients receiving radiotherapy to the head and neck

Before radiotherapy

Meticulous oral hygiene should be implemented, preventive dental care instituted and restorative procedures carried out. Neglected and unsalvageable teeth in the radiation path should be extracted. An interval of at least 2 weeks between extracting the teeth and starting radiotherapy is desirable, but the time interval permitted between extractions and radiotherapy is invariably a compromise because of the need to start radiotherapy as soon as possible. No bone should be left exposed in the mouth when radiotherapy begins since, once the blood supply is damaged by radiotherapy, wound healing is jeopardized.

During radiotherapy

During radiotherapy, mucosal and salivary gland protection with amifostine can minimize mucositis and xerostomia. Smoking and alcohol should be discouraged.

Mucositis may be relieved by using warm normal saline mouthwashes and benzydamine (which has anti-tumour necrosis factor activity) oral rinses, or lignocaine viscous 2%. Palifermin, transforming growth factor beta (TGF-beta), interleukin-1 (IL-1) and IL-11 show promise. A 0.2% chlorhexidine mouthwash improves oral hygiene. Antifungal drugs, such as nystatin suspension as a mouthwash used four times daily, may be required.

A saliva substitute, such as carboxymethylcellulose, may provide some symptomatic relief from xerostomia, as may salivary stimulants.

Trismus may be improved by jaw-opening exercises with tongue spatulas or wedges or *Therabite*, used three times a day.

After radiotherapy

Oral hygiene and preventive dental care should be continued. The dryness of the mouth is managed as for Sjögren syndrome (Ch. 18).

Radiation caries and dental hypersensitivity can be controlled with a non-cariogenic diet, high fluoride dentifrice and daily topical fluoride applications such as fluoride mouthwash. The standard of care for natural teeth is by daily application of fluoride by means of custom-fabricated carriers.

If extractions become unavoidable, trauma should be kept to a minimum, raising the periosteum as little as possible, ensuring that sharp bone edges are removed, suturing carefully and giving prophylactic antibiotics in adequate doses from 48 h pre-operatively and continued for 4 weeks at least. Clindamycin 600 mg three times daily is an appropriate antibiotic since it penetrates bone well.

If dentures are required, they should be fitted at about 4–6 weeks after radiotherapy, when initial mucositis subsides and there is only early fibrosis.

CHEMOTHERAPY

Chemotherapy alone is rarely appropriate in OSCC. Chemotherapeutic agents used include taxanes, cisplatin and 5-fluorouracil (TPF) as the most effective regimen, but carboplatin, methotrexate and bleomycin may be used. Mucositis may result.

Therapies that specifically target cell-signalling pathways dysregulated in tumours have focused mainly on epidermal growth factor receptor (EGFR or HER1) inhibitors, particularly cetuximab. EGFR inhibitors such as cetuximab appear not to exacerbate the common effects associated with radiotherapy, such as mucositis, xerostomia, dysphagia, pain, weight loss and quality of life. An acneiform rash is common, xerosis cutis and paronychia may be seen, and oral ulceration has been reported.

Cytotoxic chemotherapy drugs act mainly by interacting with the cancer cell DNA or RNA and affecting some phase of the cell's life cycle (http://www.oralcancerfoundation.org/facts/chemotherapy.htm). The first phase of the cell cycle (G1) is when the cell prepares to replicate its chromosomes. The second stage (S) is when DNA synthesis occurs and the DNA is duplicated. The next phase (G2) is when the RNA and protein duplicate. The final (M) stage is the stage of actual cell division: the duplicated DNA and RNA split and move to separate ends of the cell, and the cell actually divides into two identical, functional cells (mitosis).

Chemotherapy is used mainly for treating lympho proliferative neoplasms but increasingly also for solid tumours. Chemotherapeutic drugs used are divided into several broad categories, depending on their function (Table 22.12).

Chemotherapy is usually given orally or intravenously, then typically by catheter – a thin plastic tube – inserted into a central vein or artery and left in place throughout treatment, eliminating the need for multiple needle insertions every time treatment is needed. Chemotherapy results appear to be improving and the technique of continuous intra-arterial infusion therapy seems to be as effective as surgery or radiation therapy with an excellent cosmetic result, preservation of function and minimal side-effects.

Complications from cytotoxic chemotherapy

Most cytotoxic agents and other drugs used to treat cancer can cause complications, particularly if treatment is prolonged or in high dosage (Tables 22.12 and 22.13), especially alopecia, nausea and vomiting, anorexia, bone marrow suppression, hyperuricaemia, reproductive function damage, especially in males – and mucositis (Fig. 22.5). Some 90% of children and approximately 50% of adults develop oral lesions, more frequently when combined cytotoxic chemotherapy and radiotherapy is given.

Mucositis

Chemotherapy-induced mucositis typically appears from 7 to 14 days after the initiation of drug therapy. At least 90% of patients treated with fluorouracil and cisplatin develop mucositis (Table 22.14). Etoposide, melphalan, doxorubicin, vinblastine, taxanes and methotrexate are also particularly stomatotoxic. By contrast, mucositis is uncommon with asparaginase and carmustine.

Mucositis, if associated with neutropenia, predisposes to septicaemia. Potential pathogens include alpha-haemolytic streptococci especially *Streptococcus oralis* and *Strep. mitis*, *Candida albicans*, other *Candida* species, *Aspergillus* and *Mucor*. Mucositis may be a predictor of gastrointestinal toxicity and, after haematopoietic stem cell transplantation, may predict the onset of hepatic veno-occlusive disease.

General management

It is helpful to make an attempt to score the degree of mucositis in order to monitor progress and therapy. Several systems have been devised, but most lack standardization or validation, and none thus far has found universal acceptance; an example is shown in Table 22.15.

Despite the number of approaches tried for the prevention and treatment of chemotherapy-induced mucositis, virtually nothing works consistently or predictably. However, there is benefit from a soft diet (Table 22.16).

Ice chips sucked for 30 min before 5-fluorouracil administration may be beneficial. Mucosal cooling leads to constriction of mucosal vessels and consequent reduction in exposure of mucosal tissues to the chemotherapy agent. Ice chips may also benefit patients treated with methotrexate or melphalan. Folinic acid (as calcium folinate), levofolinic acid or disodium folinate can

	Actions	Administration route	Examples
Alkylating agents	Directly attack DNA	Orally or intravenously	Cyclophosphamide and mechlorethamine, cisplatin (Platinol), chlorambucil or melphalan
Nitrosoureas	Inhibit DNA repair	Orally or intravenously	Carmustine and lomustine
Anti-metabolites	Interfere with DNA synthesis	Orally or intravenously	6-Mercaptopurine, 5-fluorouracil, methotrexate, fludarabine and cytarabine
Antitumour antibiotics	Prevent RNA synthesis and DNA replication	Intravenously	Doxorubicin and mitomycin-C, daunorubicin, idarubicin and mitoxantrone
Plant (vinca) alkaloids	Prevent cell division	Intravenously	Vincristine and vinblastine
Taxanes	Stop microtubules from breaking down and thus prevent cancer cells growing and dividing	Intravenously	Paclitaxel and docetaxel
DNA-repair enzyme inhibitors	Attack DNA repair mechanisms	Orally or Intravenously	Etoposide or topotecan
Steroid hormones	Modify growth of hormone-dependent cancers	Orally	Tamoxifen and flutamide

Table 22.12 Chemotherapeutic drug groups

Table 22.13 Other drugs used in the treatment of malignant disease

Aromatase inhibitors	Aminoglutethimide Anastrozole Formestan Letrozole
Hormones	*For prostate carcinoma* 　Oestrogen 　Cyproterone 　Flutamide 　Bicalutamide 　Gonadotrophin-releasing hormone 　analogues (buserelin, goserelin, 　leuprorelin, triptorelin) *For breast carcinoma* 　Tamoxifen 　Toremifene 　Progestogens
Recombinant interleukin-2	Aldesleukin
Somatostatin analogues	Lanreotide Octreotide

reduce mucositis from methotrexate or fluorouracil. Palifermin, TGF-beta, IL-1 and IL-11 show promise.

Mucositis often necessitates the use of opioid analgesics for pain control, tube feeding and prophylaxis for infectious complications.

Infections

Cytotoxic agents predispose to infections with fungi, viruses, toxoplasma or bacteria. Oral candidosis is common, usually caused by *Candida albicans* or, less often, other *Candida* species. It is promoted especially by severe leukopenia and the use of antibiotics. Oral mucormycosis (phycomycosis) or aspergillosis is rare. Herpetic infections (herpes simplex or herpes zoster) are common and may cause chronic oral ulcers. Gram-negative oral infections may be caused by *Pseudomonas, Klebsiella, Escherichia, Enterobacter, Serratia* or *Proteus*, and dental

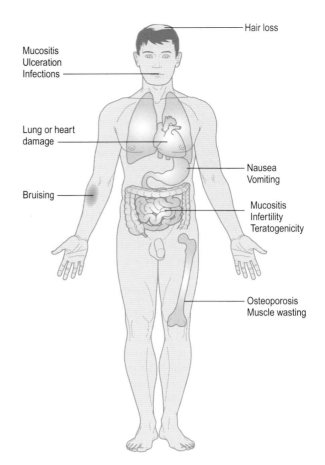

Fig. 22.5 Adverse effects from chemotherapy

infections may spread rapidly (Fig.). Gram-positive bacterial infections (staphylococci) are less common as patients usually receive antibiotics prophylactically.

Bleeding

Drug-induced thrombocytopenia may cause gingival bleeding, mucosal petechiae or ecchymoses.

Table 22.14 Main chemotherapeutic agents responsible for oral mucositis

Alkylating agents	Anthracyclines	Antibiotics	Anti-metabolites	Taxanes	Microtubule disassemblers
Busulfan	Daunorubicin	Actinomycin D	Cytosine arabinoside	Docetaxel	Etoposide
Cyclophosphamide	Doxorubicin	Amsacrine	5-Fluorouracil	Paclitaxel	Vinblastine
Mechlorethamine	Epirubicin	Bleomycin	Hydroxcarbamide		Vincristine
Melphalan		Dactinomycin	Methotrexate		Vinorelbine
Procarbazine		Daunorubicin	6-Mercaptopurine		
Thiotepa		Doxorubicin	Tioguanine		
		Mithromycin			
		Mitomycin			
		Mitoxantrone			

Note: Oral ulceration can be a complication of virtually any cancer chemotherapeutic agent but is most common in these groups. Most of these agents can also depress the bone marrow, leading to a tendency to infection and a bleeding state.

Table 22.15 Oral assessment guide (Eilers et al., 1988)

	1	2	3
Voice	Normal	Deeper or raspy	Difficulty talking
Swallow	Normal	Some pain	Unable
Lips	Smooth pink and moist	Dry or cracked	Ulcerated or bleeding
Tongue	Pink and moist	Coated and shiny ± red	Blistered or cracked
Saliva	Watery	Thick	Absent
Mucous membranes	Pink and moist	Red and coated without ulcers	Ulcers
Gingivae	Pink and firm	Oedematous ± redness	Spontaneous or pressure-induced bleeding
Teeth/denture areas	Clean, no debris	Plaque and localized debris	Generalized plaque or debris

Table 22.16 Diet in oral mucositis

Diet that is typically acceptable	Foods to avoid	Lifestyle habits to avoid
Liquids Purées Ice Custards Non-acidic fruits (banana, mango, melon, peach) Soft cheeses Eggs	Rough food (potato chips, crisps, toast) Spices Salt Acidic fruit (grapefruit, lemon, orange)	Smoking Alcohol

Xerostomia

Xerostomia can result from the use of cytotoxic agents (especially doxorubicin), and can lead to caries and other oral infections.

Craniofacial maldevelopment

Delayed and abnormal craniofacial, jaw and dentition development can follow prolonged chemotherapy.

Dental management of patients on cytotoxic chemotherapy

Before chemotherapy

Before chemotherapy, a careful oral assessment should be carried out to enable extractions and any other surgery to be completed before cytotoxic treatment (Table 22.17). Oral hygiene should be improved as far as possible.

During chemotherapy

During chemotherapy, it may be possible by using ice-cold water or sucking ice during infusion of the agent, to lessen the stomatitis. Oral ulceration caused by methotrexate can be reduced using systemic or topical folinic acid (leucovorin).

Established mucositis or oral ulceration is managed by maintaining good oral hygiene with twice-daily 0.2% aqueous chlorhexidine mouth rinses. Viscous 2% lidocaine or benzydamine rinse or spray can lessen discomfort. Nystatin suspension as a mouthwash, 4–6 times daily, may be given prophylactically. Fluconazole may be more appropriate for patients with candidosis who develop fever. Dentures should be carefully cleaned and stored overnight in 1% hypochlorite to reduce candidal carriage. Prophylactic aciclovir has lowered the incidence of herpes simplex and zoster and mortality from zoster. Oral herpetic infections should be treated with aciclovir suspension or systemic aciclovir or valaciclovir (tablets or infusion). Zoster immune globulin may help ameliorate varicella or zoster.

Although patients are frequently already on several antibiotics, Gram-negative infections may need treatment with gentamicin or carbenicillin as the oral lesions can act as portals for systemic spread. Possible drug interactions should be considered. Aspirin should not be given to patients on methotrexate as it may enhance its toxicity. Some cytotoxic drugs enhance the effects of suxamethonium (Ch. 23); others cause more serious complications that can influence dental management (Appendix 22.2, 22.3, 22.4 and 22.5).

After chemotherapy

After chemotherapy, there should still be close attention to oral hygiene and preventive dentistry, as many patients continue to have anaemia, bleeding tendencies and be susceptible to infection.

HAEMATOPOIETIC STEM CELL TRANSPLANTATION (BONE MARROW TRANSPLANTATION) (CH.35)

Haematopoietic stem cell transplantation (HSCT) involves harvesting bone marrow cells from a donor and transplanting them into the patient by injecting the cells intravenously. The donor cells are best from an identical twin or a close relative, as well HLA-matched as possible to minimize graft rejection (Table 22.18).

The recipient is prepared with a strong marrow-ablative treatment using cyclophosphamide and total body irradiation (TBI) to eradicate residual malignant disease and recipient leukocytes and is then highly susceptible to infection. Oral mucositis is experienced by up to 99% of patients receiving HSCT, typically beginning around 5 days

Table 22.17 Dental treatment for patients on cytotoxic chemotherapy

Blood cell type	Peripheral blood count	Precautions
Platelets	> 50×10^9/L	Routine management though desmopressin or platelets are needed to cover surgery
	< 50×10^9/L	Platelets needed for any invasive procedure[a]
Granulocytes	> 2×10^9/L	Routine management
	< 2×10^9/L	Prophylactic antimicrobials for surgery
Erythrocytes	> 5×10^{12}/L	Routine management
	< 5×10^{12}/L	Special care with general anaesthesia

[a]Any procedure where bleeding is possible.

Table 22.18 Donor cells used in haematopoietic stem cell transplantation (HSCT)

Donor	Comments
Autologous	Best for HSCT in non-malignant disease – no graft-versus-host disease (GVHD). In malignant disease, there is a risk of re-introducing malignant cells
Sibling: syngeneic (identical twin)	Best: no GVHD
Sibling: HLA-matched	Minimal GVHD
Unrelated donor: HLA-matched	Some GVHD

post-HSCT infusion and persisting for 2–3 weeks. A diagnosis of leukaemia, use of TBI, allogeneic transplantation and delayed neutrophil recovery are associated with worse mucositis, and the need for longer parenteral nutritional support.

Amifostine intravenously before each radiation treatment appears to have an impact upon short-term toxicity of combined radiochemotherapy.

Potent opioid analgesia is needed in up to 50% of patients because of mucositis. Oral hygiene should be maintained where possible: there are significantly increased plaque and gingival inflammation scores during the period of intense immunosuppression following allogeneic HSCT.

SALIVARY NEOPLASMS (SEE CH. 14)

CHILDHOOD NEOPLASMS

These include the following.

- Leukaemias, which are common in childhood (Ch. 8).
- Solid tumours – rare but most are treated with surgery plus radiotherapy and/or chemotherapy, which can damage

craniofacial and dental development. They include the following.

Brain tumours, especially gliomas, which are the most frequent solid tumours in childhood, and are usually low-grade astrocytomas or medulloblastomas found in the posterior cranial fossa.

Wilms tumour, which arises from the kidney, is often associated with aniridia, and may metastasize to the lungs, liver or bone.

Retinoblastomas, which have a strong hereditary basis, appear in pre-school children and cause blindness.

Neuroblastomas, which arise from neural crest cells, especially abdominally, and metastasize to lymph nodes, lungs, bone and liver.

END OF LIFE CARE

The quality of life is as important as, or more important than, its duration. Good communication with patient, partners, family and friends is essential. Many different people are involved, so that (providing the patient consents) all should be aware of: (a) the prognosis; (b) how much patients understand about their disease; (c) their psychological reactions to cancer; and (d) the side-effects of treatment.

PSYCHOLOGICAL CARE

Hope is all-important and management must include particular attention to psychological problems. Patients may or may not know, or may not want to know, that they have malignant disease, and, even if they are aware of it, may not appreciate, or be willing to accept, the prognosis.

PAIN CONTROL

Pain control is of paramount importance. Potent analgesics, such as opioids, sedatives or antidepressants, may be needed and are warranted in terminal cancer. The World Health Organization's three-step analgesic ladder (Ch. 3; Table 3.5) is a guideline for cancer pain management, and is effective in relieving pain for approximately 90% of patients with cancer and over 75% of cancer patients who are terminally ill. The five essential concepts in drug therapy for cancer pain are:

- By the mouth
- By the clock
- By the ladder
- For the individual
- With attention to detail,

Adjuvant drugs to enhance analgesic efficacy, treat concurrent symptoms that exacerbate pain, and provide independent analgesic activity for specific types of pain may be used at any step.

Step 1 in this approach is to give acetaminophen, aspirin or another non-steroidal anti-inflammatory drug (NSAID; orally) for mild to moderate pain.

Step 2: when pain persists or worsens, an opioid such as codeine or hydrocodone should be added (not substituted) to

Table 22.19 Analgesics; routes of administration

	Buccal	Intravenous	Per rectum	Subcutaneous	Sublingual	Transdermal
Fentanyl	+					+
Hydromorphone		+	+	+		
Morphine		+	+	+	+	
Oxycodone		+				

the NSAID. Opioids at this step are often administered in fixed-dose combinations with acetaminophen or aspirin because this combination provides additive analgesia. Fixed-combination products may be limited by the content of acetaminophen or NSAID, which may cause dose-related toxicity. When higher doses of opioid are necessary, the third step is taken.

Step 3, for pain that is still persistent, or moderate to severe, involves giving separate dosage forms of the opioid and non-opioid analgesic in order to avoid exceeding maximally recommended doses of acetaminophen or NSAID.

Patients who have moderate to severe pain when first seen should be started at the second or third step of the ladder. Pain that is severe at the outset should be treated by giving more potent opioids or using higher dosages. Drugs such as codeine or hydrocodone are replaced by more potent opioids (usually morphine, hydromorphone, methadone, fentanyl or levorphanol). Fentanyl transdermal patches can be helpful (Table 22.19).

Medications for persistent cancer-related pain should be administered on an around-the-clock basis, with additional 'as-needed' doses, because regularly scheduled dosing maintains a constant level of drug in the body and helps to prevent a recurrence of pain. Patient-controlled analgesia (PCA), usually delivered via continuous systemic intravenous infusion, allows patients to control the amount of analgesia they receive. PCA can also be accomplished by mouth, subcutaneously or epidurally. Patient-administered boluses are required to treat breakthrough pain, and to provide a basis for more accurate and rapid upward titration of the continuous infusion rate. Intravenous or subcutaneous PCA allows patients to accommodate transient changes in analgesic requirements (such as during dressing changes or positioning) and to tailor analgesic doses according to their own requirements. Intravenous and subcutaneous PCA is contraindicated for sedated and confused patients. Morphine and diamorphine, often by intravenous infusion, are the drugs of choice for severe pain in hospitalized patients. Phenazocine may be valuable in patients intolerant of, or allergic to, morphine. Pethidine has too short an action and the metabolite norpethidine can accumulate in renal failure and then cause convulsions. Buprenorphine is a partial agonist and should be avoided. Dextromoramide is only very short-acting but can be useful to 'cover' painful procedures. NSAIDs may help ease bone pain, while dexamethasone helps headaches associated with raised intracranial pressure. Carbamazepine or tricyclic antidepressants may relieve pain due to tumour infiltrating nerves. Transdermal fentanyl (skin patches) is increasingly used since it has an effect comparable with morphine and a duration of action of around 3 days. In the past, doctors have

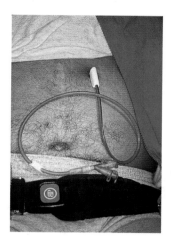

Fig. 22.6 Per endoscopic gastrostomy for feeding directly into the stomach

been anxious about giving sufficient opioids to terminally ill patients. However, if patients know that they can have opioids or other analgesics whenever they feel the need, the demand for these drugs falls.

QUALITY OF LIFE

Patients with any cancer may have severe psychological disturbances in view of the nature of the illness and these problems are compounded in oral cancer since there are additional disabilities, particularly interference with speech and swallowing, and disfigurement (e.g. 'Andy Gump' facies). Percutaneous endoscopic gastrostomy (PEG; Fig. 22.6) is a feasible and effective option when adequate oral nutrition is not possible. Patients are thus subject to considerable distress and up to a third have anxiety or depression, which occasionally leads to suicide. Counselling is especially important pre-operatively but should be continued post-operatively, and include family members and partners.

Most general QOL issues (emotional functioning, pain, insomnia, constipation) do not change after treatment or improve compared to baseline scores, and most head- and neck-specific QOL issues deteriorate after treatment but return to pre-treatment levels at 12 months, except for senses, opening mouth, sticky saliva and coughing, which remain deteriorated in the long term. Tumour site and stage, co-morbidity and extensive resections are significantly associated with adverse QOL outcomes, as are marital status and age.

PRESERVATION OF DIGNITY

Dignity is extremely important, and there are few other conditions that are as disfiguring as oral cancer. Patients are thus subject to considerable distress and up to a third have anxiety or depression, which may even lead to suicide. Pre-operative counselling is especially important but should be continued, and include family members and partners. Feeding can be difficult, especially if there is dysphagia, when nasogastric intubation may be needed, but PEG is a better long-term solution, as it avoids the fear of choking and aspiration pneumonia. In some cases, hospice care is preferable.

The type of oral health care must be planned in relation to the interest that the patient has in their oral state. Just because patients are dying does not mean that they should be allowed to suffer from pain or their appearance be neglected. Indeed, the provision of oral hygiene, attention to halitosis and dental attention (e.g. the construction of a new denture) may all help the patient's morale.

USEFUL WEBSITES

http://cis.nci.nih.gov/
http://www.nlm.nih.gov/medlineplus/encyclopedia.html
http://www.cancer.gov
http://www.sign.ac.uk/guidelines/fulltext/90/index.html
http://en.wikipedia.org/wiki/Cancer
http://www.cancerhelp.org.uk
http://www.cancerbackup.org.uk/headneck

FURTHER READING

Accortt, N.A., Waterbor, J.W., Beall, C., Howard, G., 2005. Cancer incidence among a cohort of smokeless tobacco users (United States). Cancer Causes Control 16, 1107–1115.

Annane, D., Depondt, J., Aubert, P., et al., 2004. Hyperbaric oxygen therapy for radionecrosis of the jaw: a randomized, placebo-controlled, double-blind trial from the ORN96 study group. J Clin Oncol 22, 4893–4900.

Annertz, K., Anderson, H., Biorklund, A., et al., 2002. Incidence and survival of squamous cell carcinoma of the tongue in Scandinavia, with special reference to young adults. Int J Cancer 101, 5–99.

Astsaturov, I., Cohen, R.B., Harari, P., 2007. EGFR-targeting monoclonal antibodies in head and neck cancer. Curr Cancer Drug Targets 7, 650–665.

Bagan, J.V., Jimenez, Y., Diaz, J.M., Murillo, J., Sanchis, J.M., Poveda, R., Carbonell, E., Gavalda, C., Scully, C., 2009. Osteonecrosis of the jaws in intravenous bisphosphonae use: Proposal for a modification of the clinical classification. Oral Oncology 45, 645–646 2008 Aug 18. [Epub ahead of print].

Bagan, J.V., Scully, C., 2009. Recent advances in Oral Oncology 2008; squamous cell carcinoma aetiopathogenesis and experimental studies. Oral Oncology 45 April 2 [Epub ahead of print].

Bagan, J.V., Scully, C., 2008. Recent advances in Oral Oncology 2007: epidemiology, aetiopathogenesis, diagnosis and prognostication. Oral Oncol 44, 103–108.

Bedi, R., Scully, C., 2008. Tobacco-debate on harm reduction enters new phase as India implements public smoking ban. Lancet Oncology 9, 1122–1123.

Belusic-Gobic, M., Car, M., Juretic, M., Cerovic, R., Gobic, D., Golubovic, V., 2007. Risk factors for wound infection after oral cancer surgery. Oral Oncol 43, 77–81.

Bennett, M.H., Feldmeier, J., Hampson, N., Smee, R., Milross, C., 2005. Hyperbaric oxygen therapy for late radiation tissue injury. Cochrane Database Syst Rev 3, CD005005.

Bernier, J., 2006. Cetuximab in the treatment of head and neck cancer. Expert Rev Anticancer Ther 6, 1539–1552.

Bernier, J., Schneider, D., 2007. Cetuximab combined with radiotherapy: an alternative to chemoradiotherapy for patients with locally advanced squamous cell carcinomas of the head and neck?. Eur J Cancer 43, 35–45.

Blackburn, T.K., Bakhtawar, S., Brown, J.S., Lowe, D., Vaughan, E.D., Rogers, S.N., 2007. A questionnaire survey of current UK practice for adjuvant radiotherapy following surgery for oral and oropharyngeal squamous cell carcinoma. Oral Oncol 43, 143–149.

Blick, S.K., Scott, L.J., 2007. Cetuximab: a review of its use in squamous cell carcinoma of the head and neck and metastatic colorectal cancer. Drugs 67, 2585–2607.

Borggreven, P.A., Aaronson, N.K., Verdonck-de Leeuw, I.M., Muller, M.J., Heiligers, M.L.C.H., de Bree, R., 2007. Quality of life after surgical treatment for oral and oropharyngeal cancer: a prospective longitudinal assessment of patients reconstructed by a microvascular flap. Oral Oncol 43, 1034–1042.

Boyle, P., Autier, P., Bartelink, H., et al., 2003. European Code Against Cancer and Scientific Justification: Third Version (2003). Ann Oncol 14, 973–1005.

Braakhuis, B.J., Brakenhoff, R.H., Leemans, C.R., 2005. Head and neck cancer: molecular carcinogenesis. Ann Oncol 16 (Suppl 2), ii249–50.

Brown, J.S., Blackburn, T.K., Woolgar, J.A., et al., 2007. A comparison of outcomes for patients with oral squamous cell carcinoma at intermediate risk of recurrence treated by surgery alone or with post-operative radiotherapy. Oral Oncol 43, 764–773.

Burtness, B., 2005. The role of cetuximab in the treatment of squamous cell cancer of the head and neck. Expert Opin Biol Ther 5, 1085–1093.

Dahlstrom, K.R., Little, J.A., Zafereo, M.E., Lung, M., Wei, Q., Sturgis, E.M., 2008. Squamous cell carcinoma of the head and neck in never smoker-never drinkers: a descriptive epidemiologic study. Head Neck 30, 75–84.

Derk, C.T., Rasheed, M., Spiegel, J.R., Jimenez, S.A., 2005. Increased incidence of carcinoma of the tongue in patients with systemic sclerosis. J Rheumatol 32, 637–641.

Downer, M.C., Moles, D.R., Palmer, S., Speight, P.M., 2006. A systematic review of measures of effectiveness in screening for oral cancer and precancer. Oral Oncol 42, 551–560.

D'Souza, G., Kreimer, A.R., Viscidi, R., et al., 2007. Case-control study of human papillomavirus and oropharyngeal cancer. N Engl J Med 356, 1944–1956.

Eilers, J., Berger, A.M., Petersen, M.C., 1988. Development, testing, and application of theoral assessment guide. Oncol Nurs Forum 15, 325–330.

Feng, F.Y., Lopez, C.A., Normolle, D.P., et al., 2007. Effect of epidermal growth factor receptor inhibitor class in the treatment of head and neck cancer with concurrent radiochemotherapy in vivo. Clin Cancer Res 13, 2512–2518.

Fuwa, N., Kodaira, T., Furutani, K., Tachibana, H., Nakamura, T., Daimon, T., 2007. Chemoradiation therapy using radiotherapy, systemic chemotherapy with 5-fluorouracil and nedaplatin, and intra-arterial infusion using carboplatin for locally advanced head and neck cancer – Phase II study. Oral Oncol 43, 1014–1020.

Galeone, C., Pelucchi, C., Talamini, R., et al., 2005. Role of fried foods and oral/pharyngeal and oesophageal cancers. Br J Cancer 92, 2065–2069.

Galimont-Collen, A.F., Vos, L.E., Lavrijsen, A.P., Ouwerkerk, J., Gelderblom, H., 2007. Classification and management of skin, hair, nail and mucosal side-effects of epidermal growth factor receptor (EGFR) inhibitors. Eur J Cancer 43, 845–851.

Gandolfo, S., Pentenero, M., Broccoletti, R., Pagano, M., Carrozzo, M., Scully, C., 2006. Toluidine blue uptake in potentially malignant oral lesions in vivo: clinical and histological assessment. Oral Oncol 42, 89–95.

Garavello, W., Spreafico, R., Gaini, R.M., 2007. Oral tongue cancer in young patients: a matched analysis. Oral Oncol 43, 894–897.

Gebbia, V., Giuliani, F., Valori, V.M., Agueli, R., Colucci, G., Maiello, E., 2007. Cetuximab in squamous cell head and neck carcinomas. Ann Oncol 18 (Suppl 6), vi5–vi7.

Goldwaser, B.R., Chuang, S.K., Kaban, L.B., 2007. Risk factor assessment for the development of osteoradionecrosis. J Oral Maxillofac Surg 65, 2311–2316.

Goutzanis, L., Vairaktaris, E., Yapijakis, C., et al., 2007. Diabetes may increase risk for oral cancer through the insulin receptor substrate-1 and focal adhesion kinase pathway. Oral Oncol 43, 165–173.

Grant, W.B.A., 2007. Meta-analysis of second cancers after a diagnosis of nonmelanoma skin cancer: additional evidence that solar ultraviolet-B irradiance reduces the risk of internal cancers. J Steroid Biochem Mol Biol 103, 668–674.

Hashibe, M., Ritz, B., Le, A.D., Li, G., Sankaranarayanan, R., Zhang, Z.F., 2005. Radiotherapy for oral cancer as a risk factor for second primary cancers. Cancer Lett 220, 185–195.

Ho, T., Li, G., Lu, J., Zhao, C., Wei, Q., Sturgis, E.M., 2007. X-ray repair cross-complementing group 1 (XRCC1) single-nucleotide polymorphisms and the risk of salivary gland carcinomas. Cancer 110, 318–325.

Karamouzis, M.V., Grandis, J.R., Argiris, A., 2007. Therapies directed against epidermal growth factor receptor in aerodigestive carcinomas. JAMA 4 (298), 70–82.

Klug, C., Berzaczy, D., Voracek, M., Millesi, W., 2008. Preoperative chemoradiotherapy in the management of oral cancer: a review. J Craniomaxillofac Surg 36, 75–88.

Koga, D.H., Salvajoli, J.V., Alves, F.A., 2008. Dental extractions and radiotherapy in head and neck oncology: review of the literature. Oral Dis 14, 40–44.

Kujan, O., Glenny, A.M., Oliver, R.J., Thakker, N., Sloan, P., 2006. Screening programmes for the early detection and prevention of oral cancer. Cochrane Database Syst Rev 3, CD004150.

Kujan, O., Glenny, A.M., Sloan, P., 2005. Screening for oral cancer. Lancet 366, 1265–1266; author reply 1266.

Le Tourneau, C., Faivre, S., Siu, L.L., 2007. Molecular targeted therapy of head and neck cancer: review and clinical development challenges. Eur J Cancer 43, 2457–2466.

McGurk, M.G., Fan, K.F.M., MacBean, A.D., Putcha, V., 2007. Complications encountered in a prospective series of 182 patients treated surgically for mouth cancer. Oral Oncol 43, 471–476.

Oliver, R.J., Clarkson, J.E., Conway, D.I., Glenny, A., Macluskey, M., Pavitt, S., Sloan, P., CSROC Expert Panel, Worthington, H.V., 2007. Interventions for the treatment of oral and oropharyngeal cancers: surgical treatment. Cochrane Database Syst Rev 4, CD006205.

Panikkar, R.P., Astsaturov, I., Langer, C.J., 2008. The emerging role of cetuximab in head and neck cancer: a 2007 perspective. Cancer Invest 26, 96–103.

Penel, N., Amela, E.Y., Mallet, Y., et al., 2007. A simple predictive model for postoperative mortality after head and neck cancer surgery with opening of mucosa. Oral Oncol 43, 174–180.

Perez-Ordoñez, B., Beauchemin, M., Jordan, R.C., 2006. Molecular biology of squamous cell carcinoma of the head and neck. J Clin Pathol 59, 445–453.

Petti, S., Scully, C., 2005. Oral cancer: the association between nation-based alcohol-drinking profiles and oral cancer mortality. Oral Oncol 41, 828–834.

Rades, D., Fehlauer, F., Wroblesky, J., Albers, D., Schild, S.E., Schmidt, R., 2007. Prognostic factors in head-and-neck cancer patients treated with surgery followed by intensity-modulated radiotherapy (IMRT), 3D-conformal radiotherapy, or conventional radiotherapy. Oral Oncol 43, 535–543.

Rapidis, A., Gullane, P., Langdon, J., Lefebure, J.L., Scully, C., Shah, J. 2009. Oral Cancer Management. Oral Oncology 45, 299–460.

Rapidis, A., Gullane, P., Langdon, J., Lefebvre, JL., Scully, C., Shah, J., 2009. Major advances in the knowledge and understanding of the epidemiology aetiopathogenesis, diagnosis, management and prognosis of oral cancer. Oral Oncology 45, 299–300.

Roh, J.L., Yoon, Y.H., Kim, S.Y., Park, C.I., 2007. Cervical sensory preservation during neck dissection. Oral Oncol 43, 491–498.

Ron, E., 2003. Cancer risks from medical radiation. Health Phys 85, 47–59.

Sciubba, J.J., Goldenberg, D., 2006. Oral complications of radiotherapy. Lancet Oncol 7, 175–183.

Sciubba, J.J., 2001. Oral cancer. The importance of early diagnosis and treatment. Am J Clin Dermatol 2, 239–251.

Scottish Intercollegiate Guidelines Network (SIGN), October 2006. Diagnosis and management of head and neck cancer. A national clinical guideline. Scottish Intercollegiate Guidelines Network (SIGN), Edinburgh.

Scully, C., Bagan, J.V., 2008. Recent advances in Oral Oncology 2007: imaging, treatment and treatment outcomes. Oral Oncol 44, 211–215.

Scully, C., Bagan, J.V., 2009. Recent advances in Oral Oncology 2008: squamous cell carcinoma imaging, treatment, prognostication and treatment outcomes. Oral Oncol 45, e25–30.

Scully, C., Bagan, J.V., 2009. Oral squamous cell carcinoma: overview of current understanding of aetiopathogenesis, and clinical implications. Oral Dis April 2. [Epub ahead of print].

Scully, C., Bagan, J.V., Newman, LN., 2005. The role of the dental team in preventing and diagnosing cancer;3. Oral cancer diagnosis and screening Dental Update 32, 326–337.

Scully, C., Bagan, J.V., Hopper, C., Epstein, JB., 2008. Oral cancer: current and future diagnostic techniques. American Journal Dentistry 21, 199–209.

Scully, C., Bagan, J.V., 2009. Oral squamous cell carcinoma overview. Oral Oncology 45, 301–308 Feb 25. [Epub ahead of print].

Scully, C., Bagan, J.V., (2009). Oral squamous cell carcinoma; overview of current understanding of aetiopathogenesis, and clinical implications Oral Diseases 15, 388–399 April 2 [Epus ahead of print].

Scully, C., Boyle, P., 2005. The role of the dental team in preventing and diagnosing cancer;1. Cancer in General Dental Update 32, 204–212.

Scully, C., Diz Dios, P., Shotts, R., 2004. Oral health care in patients with the most important medically compromising conditions; 6. patients undergoing radiotherapy. CPD Dentistry 6, 80–84.

Scully, C., Diz Dios, P., Shotts, R., 2005. Oral health care in patients with the most important medically compromising conditions; 7. patients undergoing chemotherapy. CPD Dentistry 6, 03–06.

Scully, C., Newman, L.N., Bagan, J.V., 2005. The role of the dental team in preventing and diagnosing cancer; 2. Oral cancer risk factors Dental Update 32, 261–274.

Scully, C., Bagan, J.V., Newman, L.N., 2005. The role of the dental team in preventing and diagnosing cancer; 3. Oral cancer diagnosis and screening Dental Update 32, 326–337.

Scully, C., Epstein, J., Sonis, S., 2003. Oral mucositis: a challenging complication of radiotherapy, chemotherapy, and radiochemotherapy: Part 1, pathogenesis and prophylaxis of mucositis. Head Neck 25, 1057–1070.

Scully, C., Epstein, J., Sonis, S., 2004. Oral mucositis: a challenging complication of radiotherapy, chemotherapy, and radiochemotherapy: Part 2, diagnosis and management of mucositis. Head and Neck 26, 77–84.

Scully, C., Sonis, S., Diz Dios, P., 2006. Oral mucositis. Oral Disease 12, 229–241.

Subramanian, S., Goldstein, D.P., Parlea, L., et al., 2007. Second primary malignancy risk in thyroid cancer survivors: a systematic review and meta-analysis. Thyroid 17, 1277–1288.

Tsantoulis, P.K., Kastrinakis, N.G., Tourvas, A.D., Laskaris, G., Gorgoulis, V.G., 2007. Advances in the biology of oral cancer. Oral Oncol 43, 523–534.

Warnakulasuriya, K.A.A.S., 2004. Smokeless tobacco and oral cancer. Oral Dis 10, 1–4.

Warnakulasuriya, S., Surtherland, G., Scully, C., 2005. Tobacco, oral cancer, and treatment of dependence. Oral Oncology 41, 244–260.

Whatley, W.S., Thompson, J.W., Rao, B., 2006. Salivary gland tumors in survivors of childhood cancer. Otolaryngol Head Neck Surg 134, 385–388.

Woolgar, J.A., Scott, J., Vaughan, E.D., Brown, J.S., West, C.R., Rogers, S., 1995. Survival, metastasis and recurrence of oral cancer in relation to pathological features. Ann R Coll Surg Engl 77, 325–331.

Worthington, H.V., Clarkson, J.E., Eden, O.B., 2007. Interventions for treating oral candidiasis for patients with cancer receiving treatment. Cochrane Database Syst Rev 2, CD001972.

Chih-Fung, Wu, Chung-Ming, Chen, Chung-Ho, Chen, Tien-Yu, Shieh, Maw-Chang, Sheen, 2007. Continuous intraarterial infusion chemotherapy for early lip cancer. Oral Oncol 43, 825–830.

Yao, M., Epstein, J.B., Modi, B.J., Pytynia, K.B., Mundt, A.J., Feldman, L.E., 2007. Current surgical treatment of squamous cell carcinoma of the head and neck. Oral Oncol 43, 213–223.

Appendix 22.1 Oral manifestations of internal cancer

METASTASES IN JAWS OR (RARELY) ORAL SOFT TISSUES, ESPECIALLY FROM CANCER OF

- Breast
- Lung
- Prostate
- Thyroid
- Kidney
- Stomach
- Colon

EFFECTS OF TUMOUR PRODUCTS

- Facial flushing (carcinoid syndrome)
- Pigmentations (ectopic adrenocorticotropic hormone-secreting tumours)
- Amyloidosis (multiple myeloma)
- Oral erosions (glucagonoma)
- Swellings (acanthosis nigricans)

CHANGES CAUSED BY OTHER FUNCTIONAL DISTURBANCES

- Purpura, anaemia, infections (leukaemia)
- Infections (lymphoma)
- Bleeding (liver cancer)
- Anaemia (bleeding from gastrointestinal tumours)

MUCOCUTANEOUS DISEASES

- Dermatomyositis (carcinoma)

- Acanthosis nigricans (abdominal carcinoma)
- Erythema multiforme (lymphoma, leukaemia or carcinoma, especially after radiotherapy)
- Paraneoplastic pemphigus (lymphomas or Castleman disease)
- Pemphigoid
- Dermatitis herpetiformis

INHERITED DISORDERS WITH PREDISPOSITION TO INTERNAL MALIGNANCY AND ORAL LESIONS

- Cowden syndrome
- Dyskeratosis congenita
- Gardner syndrome
- Gorlin–Goltz syndrome
- Maffuci syndrome
- Multiple endocrine neoplasia
- Neurofibromatosis (von Recklinghausen disease)
- Peutz–Jeghers syndrome
- Tuberous sclerosis
- Tylosis

Appendix 22.2 Chemotherapeutic agents: main uses and toxicities

	Main uses	Main toxicities			Main uses	Main toxicities
Alkylating agents[a,b]						Gynaecomastia Liver dysfunction
Busulfan	CML	Myelosuppression Hyperpigmentation Pulmonary fibrosis		Ifosfamide	CLL Lymphomas	Cystitis (avoid with mesna)
Carmustine	Multiple myeloma Lymphomas	Nephrotoxicity Pulmonary fibrosis		Lomustine	Hodgkin disease	Nausea and vomiting Delayed myelosuppression
Chlorambucil	CLL Lymphomas Ovarian cancer	Myelosuppression Erythema multiforme		Melphalan	Multiple myeloma	Delayed myelosuppression
				Mustine	Hodgkin disease	Severe vomiting
Cyclophospha-mide	CLL	Cystitis (avoid with mesna)		Thiotepa	Malignant effusions Bladder carcinoma	Enhances suxamethonium
	Lymphomas	Severe nausea and vomiting		Treosulfan	Ovarian carcinoma	Hyperpigmentation Pulmonary fibrosis Haemorrhagic cystitis
Estramustine	Prostatic carcinoma	Angina				

	Main uses	Main toxicities			Main uses	Main toxicities
Cytotoxic antibiotics[ac]				Vincristine	Acute leukaemias	Neurotoxicity
Aclarubicin	AML	Nausea and vomiting			Lymphomas	Inappropriate ADH secretion
Bleomycin	Squamous carcinomas	Pulmonary fibrosis		Vindesine	Acute leukaemias Lymphomas	Neurotoxicity Myelosuppression
Dactinomycin	Paediatric tumours	Similar to doxorubicin but no cardiotoxicity		Vinorelbine	Breast cancer Lung cancer	Neurotoxicity Myelosuppression
Daunorubicin	Kaposi sarcoma	Cardiotoxic		**Other anti-neoplastic drugs[a]**		
Doxorubicin (Adriamycin)	Acute leukaemias Lymphomas Ovarian cancer	Mucositis Nausea and vomiting Supraventricular tachycardia Cardiomyopathy Myelosuppression		Aldesleukin (interleukin-2)	Renal cancer	Capillary leak Marrow, liver, CNS, thyroid and kidney toxicity
Epirubicin	Breast carcinoma	Cardiotoxic		Alemtuzumab	CLL	Severe cytokine release syndrome (dyspnoea)
Idarubicin	Breast cancer Acute leukaemias	Cardiotoxic		Amsacrine	AML	Mucositis Myelosuppression Dysrhythmias
Mitomycin	Upper gastrointestinal and breast carcinomas	Myelosuppression Nephrotoxicity Lung fibrosis		Bexarotene	T-cell lymphoma	Hyperlipidaemia Hypothyroidism
Mitoxantrone (mitozantrone)	Breast carcinoma Lymphomas	Myelosuppression Cardiotoxicity		Carboplatin	Small oat cell carcinoma of lung	Myelosuppression Others like cisplatin
Plicamycin (mithramycin)	Hypercalcaemia in malignancy	Thrombo cytopenia		Cisplatin	Ovarian carcinoma Testicular carcinoma	Severe nausea and vomiting Ototoxicity Nephrotoxicity
Antimetabolites[a]				Crisantapase	ALL	Anaphylaxis Glucose intolerance CNS changes Liver dysfunction
Capecitabine	Colorectal cancer	Hand–foot syndrome (desquamation)		Dacarbazine	Hodgkin lymphoma	Severe nausea and vomiting Myelosuppression
Cladribine	Hairy cell leukaemia	Myelosuppression		Docetaxel	Breast cancer	Fluid retention
Cytarabine	Acute leukaemias	Myelosuppression		Hydroxycarbamide (hydroxyurea)	CML	Nausea Rashes Myelosuppression
Fludarabine	CLL	Myelosuppression Immunosuppression CNS and pulmonary toxicity		Irinotecan	Colorectal cancer	Acute cholinergic syndrome
Fluorouracil	Colon carcinoma Breast carcinoma	Mucositis Myelosuppression Cerebellar syndrome		Interferon-alpha	Kaposi sarcoma Hairy cell leukaemia Non-Hodgkin lymphoma	Flu-like symptoms Cardiotoxicity Hepatotoxicity Depression
Gemcitabine	Non small-cell lung carcinoma	Myelosuppression		Oxaplatin	Colorectal cancer	Neurotoxic Myelosuppression
Mercaptopurine	Acute leukaemias	Myelosuppression Hepatotoxicity		Paclitaxel	Ovarian cancer Breast cancer metastases	Hypersensitivity Myelosuppression Arrhythmias
Methotrexate	ALL Rheumatoid arthritis Psoriasis	Mucositis Myelosuppression (ameliorate with leucovorin)		Pentostatin	Hairy cell leukaemia	Myelosuppression Immunosuppression
Raltitrexed	Colorectal cancer	Fever cytokline release		Porfimer	Lung cancer	Photosensitivity
Tegafur	Colorectal cancer	Nausea and vomiting		Procarbazine	Hodgkin lymphoma	Myelosuppression Hypersensitivity Disulfiram reaction with alcohol
Tioguanine (thioguanine)	Acute leukaemias	myelosuppression				
Mitotic inhibitors[a]						
Etoposide	Small cell carcinoma or lung lymphomas	Nausea and vomiting Myelosuppression				
Vinblastine	Acute leukaemias Lymphomas	Myelosuppression Neurotoxicity				

(Continued)

Appendix 22.2 Chemotherapeutic agents: main uses and toxicities—cont'd

	Main uses	Main toxicities		Main uses	Main toxicities
Razoxane	Leukaemia	Myelosuppression	Trastuzumab	Breast cancer	Cardiotoxic if used with anthracyclines
Rituximab	Lymphoma	Severe cytokine release syndrome (dyspnoea)			
Temozolomide	Glioma	Myelosuppression	Tretinoin	Acute promyelocytic leukaemia	Dyspnoea Multiorgan failure
Topotecan	Ovarian cancer	Diarrhoea			

ADH, antidiuretic hormone; AML, acute myeloid leukaemia; CLL, chronic lymphocytic leukaemia; CML, chronic myeloid leukaemia; CNS, central nervous system.
[a]All can produce mucositis, nousea, vamiting, alopecia
[b]All can interfere with gametogenesis, and predispose to acute leukaemias.
[c]Should not be used with radiotherapy as they enhance radiation toxicity.

Appendix 22.3 Main chemotherapy complications and responsible agents

Early	Alopecia	Diarrhoea	Myelo Suppression	Mucositis	Nausea	Nephrotoxicity	Neurotoxicity	Ototoxicity	Urine dark
	Alkylating agents Anthracy clines Cisplatin	5-Fu Irontecan	Alkylating agents anthracyclines Taxanes	Etoposide 5-FU Methotrexate	All	Cisplatin	Cisplatin taxanes	Cisplatin	Anthracy clines
Late	Cardiotoxicity	Infertility	Menopause	Myelodysplasia	Pulmonary fibrosis				
	Anthracy clines	Akylating agents	Alkylating agents	Etoposide	Bleomycin mitomycin				

Appendix 22.4 Management of early adverse effects from chemotherapy

Adverse effect	Management
Anorexia	Megestrol acetate
Bladder damage (cystitis)	Mesna
Constipation	Docusate sodium, milk of magnesia
Diarrhoea	Loperamide, Lomotil
Dry skin, hair loss	Emollients, vitamin E, zinc supplements
Extravasation injury to soft tissue	DMSO topically
Heart injury	Dexrazoxane
Kidney injury	Sodium thiosulfate injection
Nausea and/or vomiting	Ondansetron, granisetron, dolasetron, metoclopramide, dexamethasone
Nerve injury	Amifostine

DMSO, dimethylsulfoxide.

Appendix 22.5 Colony stimutating factors

Colony-stimulating factors	
Marrow cell stimulated	Management
Erythrocytes	Erythropoietin alpha
Granulocytes	Filgrastim
Granulocytes and macrophages	Sargramostim
Platelets	Oprelvekin

METABOLIC SYNDROME

Metabolic syndrome (metabolic syndrome X, insulin resistance syndrome, dysmetabolic syndrome, hypertriglyceridaemic waist, obesity syndrome, Reaven syndrome) is the name for a group of risk factors that increase the risk for ischaemic heart disease (IHD), diabetes and stroke (Fig. 23.1). Whether the syndrome, which affects possibly 25% of the US population, is a specific syndrome, and nothing more than the sum of its parts, is controversial. The metabolic syndrome is diagnosed when at least three of the IHD risk factors listed in Table 23.1 are present.

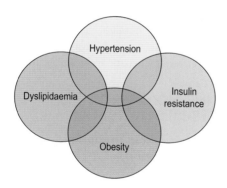

Fig. 23.1 Metabolic syndrome

Table 23.1 The metabolic syndrome	
Features	**Detail[a]**
Hypertension	Blood pressure 130/85 mmHg or higher
Hyperglycaemia	Fasting blood glucose of 5.6 mmol/L or higher
Dyslipidaemia	Triglycerides 150 mg/dl or higher
	HDL < 50 mg/dl for women and < 40 mg/dl for men
Abdominal obesity	Large waistline: women, 35 in or more; men, 40 in or more

[a]Figures given by various expert bodies differ.
HDL, high-density lipoprotein.

In general, a person with metabolic syndrome is twice as likely to develop IHD and five times as likely to develop diabetes as someone without it. The probability of developing metabolic syndrome is also closely linked to a lack of physical activity, and to being overweight or obese. Another cause is insulin resistance (also closely linked with overweight or obesity). Genetics (ethnicity and family history) and older age are other important underlying causes. Other groups at increased risk of developing metabolic syndrome are shown in Box 23.1.

Box 23.1 Groups at risk for metabolic syndrome

- People with a sibling or parent with diabetes
- People with a personal history of diabetes
- Certain ethnic groups (e.g. South Asians)
- Women with a personal history of polycystic ovarian syndrome
- People with sleep apnoea
- People with a prothrombotic state (e.g. high blood fibrinogen or plasminogen activator inhibitor-1)
- People with a pro-inflammatory state (raised blood C-reactive protein)

Associated diseases and signs are raised uric acid levels, hepatic steatosis, haemochromatosis and acanthosis nigricans.

The main emphasis in the treatment of metabolic syndrome is to reduce the effects of controllable underlying risk factors (overweight, lack of physical activity, unhealthy diet) with the goal to reduce the patient's risk for IHD by reducing low-density lipoprotein cholesterol, high blood pressure and diabetes (Chs 5 and 6).

Metabolic syndrome may be associated with inflammatory periodontal disease. Other dental aspects are discussed in the relevant chapters.

INBORN ERRORS OF METABOLISM

A vast number of rare metabolic disorders result from inherited enzyme defects. Some have a particularly high prevalence in certain racial groups (Table 23.2).

Most inborn errors of metabolism arise from recessive traits, and thus manifest only when both parents are heterozygous carriers. They affect one in four (in statistical terms) of the offspring of heterozygous parents, often as a result of first-cousin marriage.

Some inborn errors of metabolism, especially suxamethonium sensitivity, malignant hyperpyrexia, hyperlipoproteinaemias and porphyria, can seriously complicate management if general anaesthesia (GA) is required (Table 23.2 and Appendix 23.1). Many other inborn errors of metabolism are rare, but are often associated with learning impairment or neurological disease. Some, such as haemochromatosis, homocystinuria and glycogen storage diseases, can also be relevant occasionally, but others (e.g. hereditary pentosuria) are innocuous (see Appendix 23.1).

Most inborn errors of metabolism will be encountered rarely in general practice, but in certain situations – especially paediatric or special care clinics – they are more common.

Table 23.2 Inborn errors of metabolism

Defect in	Diseases
Structural proteins	Clotting factor defects Connective tissue proteins Oxygen-carrying proteins – sickle-cell anaemia and thalassaemias
Carbohydrate metabolism	Fructose, galactose and glycerol disorders, glycogen storage diseases
Cholesterol and lipoprotein metabolism	Hyperlipoproteinemias Hypolipoproteinemias
Mucopolysaccharide and glycolipid	Mucolipidoses Mucopolysaccharidoses (MPS) Oligosaccharidoses Sphingolipidoses
Lysosomal storage	These include: Lipid storage disorders (including Gaucher and Niemann–Pick diseases) Gangliosidosis (including Tay–Sachs disease) Leukodystrophies Mucopolysaccharidoses (including Hunter syndrome and Hurler disease) Glycoprotein storage disorders Mucolipidoses
Amino and organic acid metabolism	Amino-acid transport defects Specific amino acids Urea cycle defects
Haem and bilirubin	Bilirubin metabolism disorders Porphyrias
Fatty acid metabolism	Disorders of beta-oxidation Disorders of carnitine-mediated transport and carnitine uptake
Metal metabolism and transport	Copper transport disorders (Wilson disease) Haemochromatosis
Peroxisomes	Disorders of peroxisome biogenesis Adrenoleukodystrophies
Nucleotide metabolism	Defects in purine nucleotide metabolism [Lesch–Nyhan syndrome (HGPRT deficiency), severe combined immunodeficiency disease (SCID) – due to adenosine deaminase (ADA) deficiency; gout, renal lithiasis – due to adenine phosphoribosyltransferase (APRT) deficiency; xanthinuria – due to xanthine oxidase deficiency] Defects in pyrimidine nucleotide metabolism (Types I and II orotic aciduria, ornithine transcarbamylase deficiency)
DNA or repair	Ataxia telangiectasia (AT) Bloom syndrome Cockayne syndrome Fanconi anaemia Xeroderma pigmentosum (XP)
Drug-metabolizing enzymes	Glucose-6-phosphate dehydrogenase (G6PD) deficiency Malignant hyperthermia Neuroleptic malignant syndrome (NMS) Suxamethonium sensitivity

DEFECTS IN CARBOHYDRATE METABOLISM

Glycogen storage diseases

General aspects

Glycogen storage diseases (GSD) are rare disorders due to inherited defects in degradative enzymes. Glycogen cannot be mobilized to glucose, so glycogen accumulates and hypoglycaemia results.

Clinical features

Glycogen accumulates mainly in liver and muscle, resulting in hepatomegaly, muscle pain, weakness, respiratory muscle weakness and cardiac failure. Hypoglycaemia is common, as are infections.

Dental aspects

Enlarged tongue, periodontal breakdown and masticatory muscle pain may be complaints. Patients with GSD type 1b have a bleeding tendency which can be corrected pre-operatively by 24–48 hours' glucose infusion. Local anaesthesia (LA) appears to have no contraindications. Conscious sedation may be given if required. GA requires expert attention in hospital.

Defects in fructose metabolism

These disorders, which discourage the patient from ingesting sugar (sucrose) and are therefore associated with low caries rates, include hereditary fructose intolerance (aldolase B deficiency) and fructosuria – hepatic fructokinase deficiency.

DEFECTS IN CHOLESTEROL AND LIPOPROTEIN METABOLISM

Hyperlipoproteinaemia (hyperlipidaemia; hypercholesterolaemia)

General aspects

Cholesterol is found in every cell, as well as some hormones, and thus is an essential element. However, high cholesterol (hypercholesterolaemia), which is directly related to hyperlipoproteinaemia (Table 23.3), predisposes to atherosclerosis, but is largely preventable and treatable (Ch. 5). The lipoproteins consist of lipids (insoluble in plasma), phospholipids and apolipoproteins (apoproteins). Based on their density and electrophoretic mobility, the lipoproteins are divided into four groups.

Chylomicrons are large particles carrying mainly triglyceride to the liver, where lipoprotein lipase releases free fatty acids (Fig. 23.2). *Very low-density lipoproteins* (VLDL) carry triglycerides and cholesterol from the liver to the tissues and are hydrolysed by lipoprotein lipase to free fatty acids and intermediate-density and low-density lipoproteins. *Low-density lipoproteins* (LDL) are associated with a high risk of coronary heart disease. They contain a cholesterol core and are formed from intermediate-density lipoproteins by hepatic lipase. They bind to the LDL receptor and are taken up by cells, especially when there is inhibition of 3-hydroxy-3-methylglutaryl

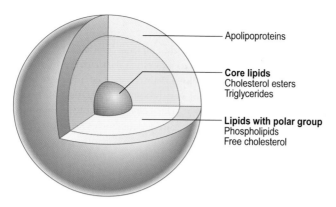

Fig. 23.2 Chylomicron structure

Image labels:
- Apolipoproteins
- **Core lipids**
  Cholesterol esters
  Triglycerides
- **Lipids with polar group**
  Phospholipids
  Free cholesterol

coenzyme A reductase (HMG-CoA reductase), which raises cellular cholesterol. An important form of LDL is lipoprotein-alpha, which inhibits fibrinolysis but promotes atherosclerosis. *High-density lipoproteins* (HDL), in contrast, are associated with a lowered risk of IHD. They are formed in liver and gut, and carry cholesterol from intracellular tissue pools back to the liver. The main plasma lipids transported are triglycerides, cholesterol ester and phospholipids (lecithin, sphingomyelin, etc.). Non-esterified fatty acids and cholesterol are also present.

In primary (familial) hyperlipidaemia (FH), genetic factors play a role with defects, for example, in the LDL receptor (*LDLR*) gene, apolipoprotein B-100 (*APOB*) and proprotein convertase subtilisin/kexin type 9 (*PCSK9*) genes. Hypercholesterolaemia can also be due to abnormalities in lipoprotein levels related to diet, or secondary to obesity, diabetes, hypothyroidism, nephrotic syndrome, chronic renal failure, liver disease, alcoholism, smoking (lowers HDL) and use of oral contraceptives.

Clinical features

Gout, arthralgias, arthritis and xanthomatous collections in soft tissue, tendons and subperiosteal and intraosseous locations are common. Premature coronary heart disease may result.

Cutaneous, slightly raised, yellowish plaques called xanthomas (xanthelasmas on the eyelids; Fig. 23.3) are associated with accelerated atherosclerosis and heart disease. Prominent xanthomas on the elbows and knees, especially with yellow to orange discoloration of the palmar creases, are unique to type II hyperlipoproteinaemia.

General management

Around 75% of FH is undiagnosed, so screening for *LDLR*, *APOB* and *PCSK9* genes may help. Dietary intervention and lipid-lowering drugs (particularly statins – HMG-CoA reductase inhibitors) are essential treatment (Ch **5**). Ezetimibe is an option for primary hypercholesterolaemia.

Table 23.3 Primary hyperlipoproteinaemias

Type	Name	Pathogenesis	Alternative name and lipid changes	Features in addition to atheroscelerosis
I	Hypertriglyceridaemia	AD. May occur as a secondary defect in diabetes mellitus, pancreatitis and alcoholism	Hyperchylomicronaemia Lipoprotein lipase deficiency Abnormality in chylomicron removal	Xanthomas Acute pancreatitis, hepato-splenomegaly
Ib	Hyperlipoproteinaemia	Apolipoprotein c-II deficiency	Reduced LDL and HDL; high triglycerdes	No xanthomas Acute pancreatitis
Ic	Hyperlipoproteinaemia	Circulating inhibitor of lipoprotein lipase	Chylomicronaemia	Xanthomas Acute pancreatitis
II	Hyperbetalipoprotein-aemia	AD. Also may be secondary to hypothyroidism, plasma cell myeloma, macroglobulinaemia and obstructive liver disease	Hypercholesterolaemia: increase in plasma beta-lipoproteins	Xanthomas and xanthelasmas (common) Premature coronary, cerebral, and peripheral vascular disease
IIa	Hyperlipoproteinaemia	AD. Also may be secondary to hypothyroidism, plasma cell myeloma, macroglobulinaemia and obstructive liver disease	Low-density lipoprotein (LDL) receptor disorder; increase in plasma LDLs	Xanthomas, corneal arcus Premature coronary, cerebral, and peripheral vascular disease
III	Dysbetalipoprotein-aemia	AR. Rarely secondary to severe diabetes and hypothyroidism	Broad-beta disease Apolipoprotein E deficiency	Peripheral vascular disease, hyperglycaemia, xanthomas (rare)
IV	Endogenous hyperlipo-proteinaemia	AR. Rarely secondary to diabetes mellitus, pancreatitis, alcoholism, hypothyroidism, glycogen storage disease, Gaucher disease, gout and hypercalcaemia	Carbohydrate-inducible hyperlipaemia	Mild glucose intolerance, hyper-uricaemia, atherosclerosis and IHD, xanthomas (common)
V	Mixed hyperlipidaemia	AD	–	Acute pancreatitis Xanthomas, hyperuricaemia, abdominal pain, hepatospleno-megaly, paraesthesias and lipaemia retinalis

AD, autosomal dominant; AR, autosomal recessive.
http://www.med.unibs.it/~marchesi/hyperlipoproteinemias.html

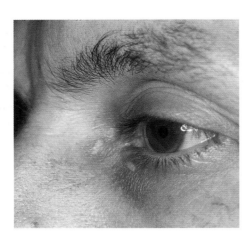

Fig. 23.3 Xanthelasma in familial hyperlipidaemia: such lesions may suggest a high risk of ischaemic heart disease

Dental aspects

Local anaesthetic is the safest method of pain control. Conscious sedation can be given if required. GA may be a risk because of IHD.

Facial xanthomas may help recognition of these potentially dangerous diseases. Type IV and V hyperlipoproteinaemias may be complicated by sicca syndrome.

Hypolipoproteinaemias

Pulpal calcifications and unusual odontomes, and orange deposits in the tonsils, may be found in high-density lipoprotein deficiency (Tangier disease).

ERRORS IN AMINO ACID AND ORGANIC ACID METABOLISM

Homocysteine (Hcy) is a sulfur amino acid formed in the methionine pathway. In blood, homocysteine can be present as the free form, two disulfide forms (homocystine, cysteine–homocysteine) or a form linked to proteins and peptides by disulfide bonds.

Hyperhomocysteinaemia

The amino acid homocysteine, an intermediate product in conversion of methionine to cysteine, participates in the re-methylation pathway enabling maintenance of adequate cellular levels of methionine, or is catabolized by trans-sulfuration. Several hereditary defects in the enzymes involved in homocysteine metabolism and acquired deficiencies in the vitamin cofactors of these enzymes can cause hyperhomocysteinaemia. This causes premature vascular thrombosis. Mild hyperhomocysteinaemia is an independent risk factor for arterial disease and venous thrombosis (Ch. 5). Homocysteine may also be a risk factor for Alzheimer disease.

Dietary folate supplementation may normalize homocysteine and modify the risk of vascular disease.

Homocystinuria

Homocystinuria is an autosomal recessive inborn error of methionine metabolism. Affected patients are tall with a Marfanoid appearance, joint hypermobility, ectopia lentis, and visual and mental deterioration. Blood vessel abnormalities together with excessive platelet adhesiveness predispose to thromboembolism, both spontaneously and post-operatively. Dextran 40 or 70 infusion intravenously peri-operatively may reduce the thromboembolic risk.

DEFECTS IN NON-AMINO-ACID NITROGEN METABOLISM

The porphyrias

General aspects

Porphyrias are rare inborn errors in enzymes involved in haem metabolism, which result in the accumulation of porphyrins, the intermediate compounds in haem (-oglobin) synthesis (Fig. 23.4). Porphyrias affect about 1 in 10 000 of the population, and are divided into two main groups according to the principal site of the enzyme defect, namely in liver (hepatic porphyrias) or erythrocytes (erythropoietic porphyrias; Table 23.4).

Table 23.4	**Porphyrias**		
Porphyrias	**Type**	**Alternative name**	**Particular features**
Acute	Acute intermittent porphyria[a]	Swedish porphyria	Acute, severe abdominal pain, cardiovascular disturbances, neuro-psychiatric disturbance, autonomic dysfunction
	Hereditary coproporphyria[a]	Coproporphyria	Acute, severe abdominal pain, cardiovascular disturbances, neuro-psychiatric disturbance, autonomic dysfunction
	Plumboporphyria	ALA dehydratase deficiency	Acute abdominal pain
	Variegate porphyria[a]	South African (Afrikaans) genetic porphyria	Acute, severe abdominal pain, cardiovascular disturbances, neuro-psychiatric disturbance, autonomic dysfunction, rashes
Chronic	Congenital porphyria[b]	Erythropoietic porphyria	Red teeth, hypertrichosis, severe mutilating photosensitivity rashes and haemolytic anaemia
	Porphyria cutanea tarda	Cutaneous hepatic porphyria	Photosensitivity and iron overload. Drugs do not precipitate acute attacks but the condition is aggravated by alcohol, oestrogens, iron and poly-chlorinated aromatic compounds

[a]Clinically significant.
[b]Erythropoietic.

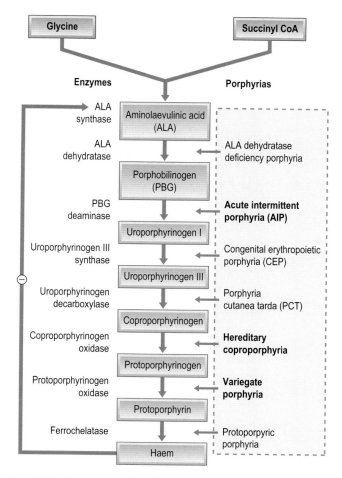

Fig. 23.4 Haem synthesis (bold disorders are most significant). Adapted from James MFM, Hift RI. 2000 Brit. J. Anaesth, 85.143

Generally, people with porphyrias enjoy entirely normal health; however, there are three porphyrias that are significant clinically, since drugs precipitate acute illness. *Variegate porphyria*, the commonest, is found mainly in South Africans of Afrikaans descent. *Acute intermittent porphyria* is seen less frequently but affects all population groups. *Hereditary coproporphyria* is rare and patients may appear normal apart from severe photosensitivity rashes. Patients may develop potentially fatal acute attacks of cardiovascular (hypertension and tachycardia) and gastrointestinal disturbances, accompanied by neuropsychiatric disturbance (porphyria in King George III of England probably explains his 'madness').

Most of the drugs that have been incriminated are enzyme inducers that also increase hepatic 5-aminolaevulinic acid (ALA) synthetase levels. Often a single dose of a drug of this type can precipitate an acute episode but, in some patients, repeated doses are necessary to provoke a reaction. Assessing drug safety in porphyria is an inexact science, for many drugs no such information is available and for some others, the data are of doubtful validity and often conflicting (Table 23.5). A wide array of other factors can cause exacerbations, including fasting, alcohol, infections and pregnancy.

Clinical features of attacks

Attacks are accompanied by cardiovascular disturbance (tachycardia and hypertension in the majority, sometimes followed

Table 23.5 Drug use in porphyria (list is not exhaustive)

	Contraindicated	Safer
Local anaesthetics	Articaine Mepivacaine	Bupivacaine Lidocaine (used with caution) Prilocaine (used with caution)
Conscious sedation	Diazepam	Flumazenil Midazolam
General anaesthetics	Barbiturates Enflurane Halothane	Nitrous oxide
Analgesics	Dextropropoxyphene Diclofenac Mefenamic acid Indometacin Pentazocine Opioids	Acetaminophen/paracetamol Aspirin
Antibiotics	Cephalosporins Clindamycin Co-trimoxazole Doxycycline Erythromycin Flucloxacillin Rifampicin Sulfonamides Tetracyclines	Metronidazole Penicillin
Antifungals	Fluconazole Griseofulvin Itraconazole Ketoconazole Miconazole Voriconazole	Nystatin
Psychoactive drugs	Amphetamines Antidepressants Antihistamines Barbiturates Calcium-channel blockers Carbamazepine Chlordiazepoxide Contraceptive pill Diazepam Dichloralphenazone Ergot Meprobamate Monoamine oxidase inhibitors Phenytoin Tricyclics	
Endocrine active drugs	Androgens Chlorpropamide Contraceptive pill Oestrogens Progestogens	
Others	Ethanol (alcohol) Clonidine Danazol Pentoxifylline Statins	

by postural hypotension). Respiratory embarrassment or major convulsions and neuropsychiatric disturbance (typically a peripheral sensory and motor neuropathy, but sometimes agitation, mania, depression, hallucinations and schizophrenic-like behaviour) may occur. Other manifestations may include autonomic dysfunction causing profuse sweating, pallor and pyrexia. Severe hyponatraemia, due to inappropriate secretion of antidiuretic hormone, sometimes causes convulsions or deterioration in consciousness.

General management

The diagnosis is confirmed by demonstrating ALA and porphobilinogen in urine, and attacks are accompanied by raised levels; the urine may turn red.

The essentials of treatment of attacks of porphyria are, if possible, to stop the administration of the triggering drug and to give an intravenous infusion of haem arginate, fluids, electrolytes and glucose.

Alcohol is sometimes an important trigger and, in some, the disease may be controlled simply by its withdrawal. Standard treatment aims at reducing hepatic iron overload by venesection, which is both safe and reliable.

Dental aspects

Anaesthetics, analgesics, antimicrobials and anxiolytics (benzodiazepines) liable to precipitate attacks are absolutely contraindicated (Table 23.5).

Congenital erythropoietic porphyria is characterized by red discoloration of the teeth (which fluoresce in ultraviolet light). Fewer than 100 cases have probably ever been reported, but it has been suggested that this disease might have been the source of the werewolf legend because of the red teeth (thought to be dripping with blood), the hairy distorted facial features and avoidance of daylight.

DISORDERS OF METAL METABOLISM AND TRANSPORT

Haemochromatosis

General aspects

Normally, about 10% of the iron contained in food is absorbed, and this meets the body's needs. Haemochromatosis is a disorder characterized by excessive absorption of iron: the body is unable to excrete the excess iron and the results are high serum ferritin levels and deposition of iron as haemosiderin, particularly in liver, abdominal lymph nodes, joints, skin, adrenals, pancreas, salivary glands, pituitary and heart (Fig. 23.5) which may thus be damaged. Males manifest problems earlier than females, who lose blood (and thus iron) in menstruation.

Hereditary haemochromatosis is one of the most common genetic disorders in the West, and most often affects male Caucasians of northern European descent. The defect in a gene on chromosome 6 called *HFE* affects more than 1 in 200 of the population and many cases remain undetected.

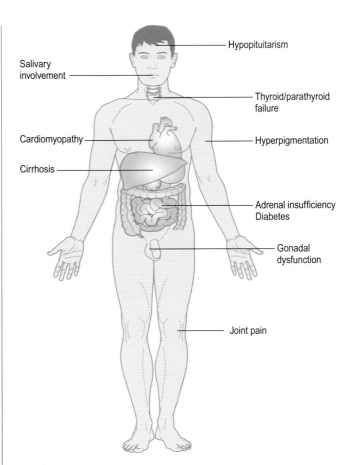

Fig. 23.5 Iron overload in haemochromatosis

Clinical features

Haemochromatosis mainly affects males but rarely before adolescence. The fibrotic reaction to haemosiderin deposits can eventually result in widespread disease including cirrhosis, skin pigmentation, adrenocortical insufficiency, cardiomyopathy or diabetes (bronze diabetes). The most common complaint is joint pain but other symptoms include fatigue, abdominal pain, and loss of libido due to hypopituitarism and hypogonadism. About 30% of patients with cirrhosis develop hepatocellular carcinoma.

General management

A sensitive and relatively inexpensive screening test for iron overload is the transferrin saturation test (serum iron divided by the total iron-binding capacity). High serum ferritin levels may also suggest the diagnosis. Treatment is iron removal by venesection and chelation using desferrioxamine. Liver transplantation is needed for end-stage haemochromatosis.

Dental aspects

Local anaesthesia is generally safe. Conscious sedation can be given. Cirrhosis, adrenocortical insufficiency, diabetes or cardiomyopathy may complicate care.

A sicca syndrome from salivary haemosiderin deposition may be a complication.

DISEASES ASSOCIATED WITH DEFECTIVE DNA REPAIR

Several inborn errors predispose to malignancy because of impaired DNA repair mechanisms (Table 23.6; Ch. 22).

Dental aspects

Bloom syndrome, dyskeratosis congenita and Fanconi anaemia have a higher than normal risk of oral carcinomas. Xeroderma pigmentosum produces a liability to skin and lip cancers.

ENZYME DEFECTS AFFECTING DRUG METABOLISM

Drug responses vary greatly between individuals, owing to genetic as well as environmental effects on drug absorption, distribution, metabolism or excretion (pharmacokinetics), and on receptor or post-receptor sensitivity (pharmacodynamics).

Genetic differences in drug metabolism can have profound effects on treatment in terms of genetically determined variation in the activity of enzymes involved in detoxification or of other abnormal proteins that render an individual especially susceptible to some adverse reaction.

Pharmacogenetic variation is sometimes due to the actions of a single mutant gene (as in genetic polymorphism, or Mendelian disorders that exhibit discontinuous variation), or polygenic influences. For example, some Asians metabolise carbamazepine poorly and can thus suffer from overdose. Some chinese metabolize carbamazepine poorly.

Drug-metabolizing enzymes include glucose-6-phosphate dehydrogenase, *N*-acetyltransferase, and the superfamily of cytochrome P450 (CYP) isoenzymes. Because CYP isoenzymes metabolize many structurally diverse drugs and chemicals, most of the variant genotypes of the CYP2D6, CYP2C9, CYP2C19 and CYP3A families have been identified and studied. Table 23.7 shows examples of major disorders that influence drug response.

Glucose-6-phosphate dehydrogenase deficiency

General aspects

Glucose-6-phosphate dehydrogenase (G6PD) is the enzyme responsible for maintaining the nicotinamide–adenine dinucleotide phosphate (NADPH) needed to keep glutathione in its reduced form to act as a scavenger for dangerous oxidative metabolites. Low G6PD activity (G6PD deficiency) results in methaemoglobinaemia and haemolysis when red blood cells are exposed to oxidizing agents such as various drugs, broad beans (*Vicia fava*) or naphthalene. Haemolysis can also be precipitated by intercurrent infection or, occasionally, it occurs spontaneously. Drugs that can be dangerous in G6PD deficiency are shown in Table 23.8.

Glucose-6-phosphate dehydrogenase deficiency is the most common enzyme deficiency, affecting 400 million people worldwide, and is seen mainly in people of Mediterranean, Middle Eastern, African or Asian descent. The high incidence in some areas is attributed to a balanced polymorphism – a selective advantage conferred on heterozygotes due to a protective effect of partial enzyme deficiency against falciparum malaria. Resistance may be due to malaria parasites surviving less well in G6PD-deficient cells, which are more rapidly removed from the circulation. G6PD deficiency is genetically heterogeneous, so individuals react differently to the above factors.

Several other enzymic defects in the glutathione-generating system also lead to haemolysis when oxidizing drugs are taken.

General management

The diagnosis is confirmed by G6PD enzyme assays. Haemolysis is self-limiting and splenectomy is rarely needed. Patients with G6PD deficiency who have to be treated with primaquine for acute malaria should spend at least the first few days in hospital under supervision. If there is acute severe haemolysis, the drug may have to be withdrawn and blood transfusion may be needed. Hydrocortisone is given intravenously and the urine alkalinized to reduce acid haematin deposition in renal tubules.

Table 23.6 Diseases associated with defective DNA repair

Disorder	Main genetics	Features
Ataxia telangiectasia (AT)	AR	Cerebellar ataxia, telangiectases, immune defects, neoplasms
Bloom syndrome	AR	Proportionate pre- and post-natal growth deficiency; sun-sensitive, telangiectatic, and hypo- and hyperpigmented skin
Cockayne syndrome	AR	Dwarfism, precociously senile, pigmentary retinal degeneration, optic atrophy, deafness, marble epiphyses in digits, photosensitivity and learning disability. Disproportionately long limbs with large hands and feet and flexion contractures of joints. Knee contractures result in a 'horseriding' stance
Dyskeratosis congenita	AR or AD	Abnormal skin pigmentation and nail growth, premature ageing and a high increased risk of malignancy (skin, gut and oral). Bone marrow failure (aplastic anaemia) affects 80%
Fanconi anaemia	AR	All bone marrow elements depressed with cardiac, renal and limb malformations, dermal pigmentary changes, oral cancer
Xeroderma pigmentosum (XP)	AR	Sensitivity to sunlight carcinomas at an early age. Starts with freckle-like lesions in exposed areas, usually in early years

AD, autosomal dominant; AR, autosomal recessive.

Dental aspects

It is vital to avoid oxidant drugs, which can precipitate haemolysis, particularly the sulfonamides. Aspirin up to at least 1 g a day is safe for most patients. Acetaminophen also appears to be safe, but doses should be limited. Codeine may also be used. LA with prilocaine may, in large doses, induce methaemoglobinaemia, and should be avoided (Table 23.8). Conscious sedation is usually safely given as relative analgesia. GA is given in hospital. Metabolic acidosis causes haemolysis and must be avoided.

Malignant hyperthermia (malignant hyperpyrexia)

General aspects

Malignant hyperthermia (MH) is a rare, potentially fatal, inherited condition, characterized by a rapid rise in temperature when the patient has a GA or other drugs that trigger an attack.

MH affects about 1 in 20 000, males predominantly, and 40% are children under 14. It is related to the ryanodine receptor (*RYR1*) gene (the muscle sarcoplasmic reticulum calcium release channel) on chromosome 19.

The most common trigger of an attack is the combination of a halogenated volatile GA, such as halothane or enflurane, together with muscle relaxants such as suxamethonium and curare-like (non-depolarizing) agents (Table 23.9).

Clinical features

Suxamethonium, unlike pancuronium or vecuronium, causes jaw stiffness in many normal children but the onset of MH may be detected by poor muscular relaxation after induction of GA or complete failure of the jaw to relax after suxamethonium has been given. However, it is controversial whether masseter spasm is a reliable early sign.

Table 23.7   Variations in drug response due to genetic polymorphism

Pharmacogenetic variation	Inheritance	Frequency	Drugs involved
G6PD deficiency	X-linked incomplete co-dominant	10 000 000 affected in the world	Many, including quinolines and most sulfonamides
Malignant hyperthermia	AD	1:20 000 of population	Anaesthetics especially halothane, suxamethonium
Methaemoglobinaemia	AR	1:100 are heterozygotes	Same drugs as for G6PD deficiency
Neuroleptic malignant syndrome	AD	Seen in from 0.02 to 3.23% of psychiatric patients receiving neuroleptics	Neuroleptics
Porphyria	AD	Acute intermittent type 15:1 000 000 in Sweden; porphyria cutanea tarda 1:100 in Afrikaaners	Barbiturates, chloral, chloroquine, ethanol, sulfonamides, phenytoin, griseofulvin (many others)
Suxamethonium sensitivity	AR	Most common in Europeans and rare in Asians	Suxamethonium, mivacurium

AD, autosomal dominant; AR, autosomal recessive; G6PD, glucose-6-phosphate dehydrogenase.

Table 23.8   Drugs that may precipitate haemolysis in glucose-6-phosphate dehydrogenase deficiency

Analgesic/antipyretic	Antimalarial	Cardiovascular	Cytotoxic/antibacterial	Miscellaneous	Sulfonamides/sulfones
Aspirin	Chloroquine	Procainamide	Chloramphenicol	Alpha-methyldopa	Dapsone
Phenacetin	Hydroxychloroquine	Quinidine	Ciprofloxacin	Ascorbic acid	Most sulfonamides including co-trimoxazole
Prilocaine	Mepacrine (quinacrine)		Furazolidone	Dimercaprol (BAL)	
	Pamaquine		Furmethonol	Hydralazine	
	Pentaquine		Moxifloxacin	Mestranol	
	Primaquine		Nalidixic acid	Methylene blue	
	Quinine		Neoarsphenamine	Naphthalene	
	Quinocide		Nitrofurantoin	Phenylhydrazine	
			Nitrofurazone	Pyridium	
			Norfloxacin	Toluidine blue	
			Ofloxacin	Trinitrotoluene	
			Para-aminosalicylic acid (PAS)	Urate oxidase	
				Vitamin K (water soluble) and menadione	

Table 23.9 Drugs contraindicated, and safer alternatives, in malignant hyperpyrexia in susceptible subjects

	Contraindicated	Safer
General anaesthetics	Halothane Ether Cyclopropane Ketamine Enflurane	Local anaesthetics Thiopental Nitrous oxide
Conscious sedation	Benzodiazepines	Nitrous oxide
Muscle relaxants	Suxamethonium Curare	Pancuronium
Antidepressants	Tricyclic antidepressants Monoamine oxidase inhibitors	SSRIs

The earliest signs of a MH reaction are rapid breathing and heart rate, and rising blood pressure.

There is also a temperature rise, with arrhythmias. Hyperkalaemia, cardiac arrhythmias and disseminated intravascular coagulation (DIC) may occur. The mortality rate of MH may approach 80% in the absence of treatment.

Two forms of MH are recognized: an autosomal dominant type, where patients are clinically normal between attacks; and a recessive type, which affects young boys with various congenital abnormalities such as myotonia congenita, myotonic dystrophy, central core disease and Evan syndrome (proximal wasting, short stature, kyphoscoliosis).

General management

The family history is important, as emphasized by the fact that a dental patient reported to the writer had had 14 relatives die under GA. Understandably, this patient was less than enthusiastic about the idea of a GA for dental purposes. Raised serum creatine kinase and pyrophosphate levels indicate susceptibility, but nearly one-third of patients have normal levels of creatine kinase. Muscle biopsy shows excessive *in vitro* response of muscle to halothane, suxamethonium or caffeine, and raised myophosphorylase A levels.

Malignant hyperthermia is a medical emergency with a high mortality rate. Management includes stopping the trigger, correcting respiratory acidosis and use of dantrolene.

All trigger agents (i.e. all anaesthetic vapours) should be withdrawn, dantrolene given and temperature, arterial blood gases, K$^+$ and creatine phosphokinase (CPK) measured. Surface cooling, avoiding vasoconstriction, is needed. Serious arrhythmias are treated with beta-blockers, and hyperkalaemia and metabolic acidosis corrected. A clotting screen is done to detect disseminated intravascular coagulation, urine sample for myoglobin estimation and output for developing renal failure. Diuresis is promoted with fluids/mannitol. The patient should also be referred to a MH unit.

Dental aspects

Infections should be quickly and effectively treated since they also may precipitate attacks of MH. LA is safe (amide LA agents, including lidocaine and prilocaine, were once thought to be weak triggering agents but this has been dismissed).

Adrenaline may cause signs similar to an attack of MH, confusing the diagnosis, and may enhance calcium release inside muscle cells and aggravate a MH episode. Endogenous adrenaline release should be minimized (avoid stress, anxiety, pain) and effective LA must be used (which may mean using an adrenaline-containing LA). Conscious sedation can usually be safely carried out using relative analgesia. MH has been reported after administration of nitrous oxide but this is rare. Benzodiazepines are contraindicated. Inquiry into the family history is essential before giving GA as there are no absolutely reliable predictive tests. Unfortunately, absence of reaction to a previous GA does not exclude the possibility of a reaction on the next occasion.

In the event of hyperthermia, surgery must be stopped and the patient cooled. Oxygen and a bicarbonate intravenous infusion to counteract the metabolic acidosis should also be given. Dantrolene sodium or procainamide are effective in controlling the reaction. Dantrolene given pre-operatively and postoperatively for about 3 days may prevent hyperthermia.

Methaemoglobinaemia

Haemoglobin can be oxidized to methaemoglobin (a nonfunctional form) by some drugs, including acetaminophen, anilines, chlorates, nitrates, nitrites, nitrobenzenes, nitrotoluenes, prilocaine, primaquine, sulfonamides and sulfones (e.g. dapsone). In certain haemoglobin variants (e.g. HbM, HbH), methaemoglobin is not readily converted back into reduced, functional haemoglobin and thus, in individuals with these variants, exposure to the above drugs causes methaemoglobinaemia. Drugs can also cause cyanosis in patients with a NADH–methaemoglobin reductase deficiency.

Rarely methaemoglobinaemia has been precipitated by injection of prilocaine. Sedation can be used but hypoxia must be avoided.

Neuroleptic malignant syndrome

Neuroleptic malignant syndrome (NMS) is a rare but potentially fatal complication of the use of certain non-anaesthetic drugs, especially the neuroleptics (Box 23.2).

Box 23.2 Precipitants of neuroleptic malignant syndrome

- Alcohol
- Amphetamines
- Antidepressants (tricyclic or monoamine oxidase inhibitors)
- Benzodiazepines
- Metoclopramide
- Neuroleptics (e.g. phenothiazines, haloperidol or flupentixol)
- Tetrabenazine
- Abrupt withdrawal of levodopa

The relationship of NMS to malignant hyperthermia is unknown.

There are disturbances in mental state, temperature regulation, and autonomic and extrapyramidal functions. Hyperthermia, muscle rigidity, fluctuating consciousness, obtundation, catatonia, pallor, sweating, tachycardia, labile blood pressure, incontinence, tremors, dysarthria, dysphagia and drooling result.

These features may develop dramatically within hours or insidiously over several days and may persist for several days, or death can result from renal failure.

Local anaesthesia can usually be safely given. Conscious sedation dentistry can usually be safely given using relative analgesia. Phenothiazines should be avoided for patients who have stopped their levodopa before a GA. Levodopa can be given before GA, apart from the fact that it may cause vomiting.

Suxamethonium sensitivity (pseudocholinesterase deficiency; scoline apnoea)

Suxamethonium (scoline) is a depolarizing neuromuscular blocker widely used for muscle relaxation during induction of GA. The usual response to a single intravenous dose of suxamethonium is muscular paralysis for about 6 min. The effect of suxamethonium is similar to that of acetylcholine and the drug usually has a brief action due to its rapid destruction by plasma cholinesterase.

About 1 in 2500 of the population have a defect in plasma cholinesterase (butyrylcholinesterase; pseudocholinesterase) and are abnormally sensitive to the action of suxamethonium, so that muscle paralysis and apnoea persist.

Suxamethonium sensitivity is an autosomal recessive trait due to mutant alleles of *CHE1* on chromosome 3. It is most common in Europeans and rare in Asians. Abnormal sensitivity to suxamethonium may also result from some other diseases (Box 23.3) or may be a type of hypersensitivity reaction.

When given suxamethonium, patients with suxamethonium sensitivity remain unable to breathe and will die unless artificially ventilated until the drug action abates after 2 h or more. Patients may also react similarly to other choline ester compounds, such as mivacurium, and can have severe reactions to cocaine.

Box 23.3 Conditions in which the action of suxamethonium may be prolonged

- Inherited suxamethonium sensitivity (scoline sensitivity)
- Myopathies
  - Malignant hyperpyrexia
  - Dystrophia myotonica
  - Myotonia congenita
  - Myasthenia gravis
- Liver disease
- Renal disease
- Burns
- Drugs
  - Cyclophosphamide
  - Cytotoxic drugs
  - Pancuronium
  - Phenothiazines
  - Procaine
  - Trasylol

Local anaesthetic action is occasionally prolonged. Nitrous oxide/oxygen sedation is preferable to GA.

ACQUIRED METABOLIC DISORDERS
AMYLOID DISEASE
General aspects

Amyloidosis is not a disease in itself, rather a manifestation of several diseases. Amyloid consists of deposits in tissues of an eosinophilic hyaline protein with a characteristic fibrillar structure on electron microscopy, in all secondary cases associated with amyloid – a non-fibrillar component derived from the acute-phase protein serum amyloid P (SAP; Fig. 23.6).

AA protein deposition is seen in conditions of excessive stimulation of the reticuloendothelial system – as in chronic suppurative or inflammatory disorders (*secondary amyloidosis*; Table 23.10). Amyloid is then deposited mainly in, and affects the functions of, the heart, skeletal muscle and gastrointestinal tract. Other secondary amyloid is of uncertain origin but affects mainly the spleen, liver, kidney and adrenals.

AL protein deposition is seen in conditions with immunoglobulin overproduction, as in benign monoclonal gammopathy (*primary amyloidosis*), or multiple myeloma and has a prominent immunoglobulin light-chain component (Table 23. 10) Localized amyloid may be seen in a range of disorders (Fig 23.6).

Clinical features

Amyloid is a great mimic in medicine. The widespread lesions, and the possible involvement of virtually any system, make amyloid disease protean in its manifestations. There may also be a bleeding tendency related to a factor X defect.

General management

The diagnosis is established by biopsy of lesional tissue, or by rectal or gingival biopsy examined with Congo Red and polarized light. An underlying cause must be sought and treated where possible. Combination therapy is used, with corticosteroids, melphalan and fluoxymesterone.

Dental aspects

Dental management may be influenced by the underlying disorder, or by cardiac, renal, adrenal or corticosteroid complications, or a bleeding tendency.

Local anaesthesia can safely be given. Conscious sedation can be given if required.

Macroglossia, gingival swellings, oral petechiae, bullae or, rarely, a sicca syndrome may result from amyloidosis, but virtually only in the primary type.

TRIMETHYLAMINURIA (TMA-URIA; FISH-ODOUR SYNDROME)

Trimethylaminuria is a rare autosomal recessive syndrome where there is abnormal trimethylamine (TMA) excretion.

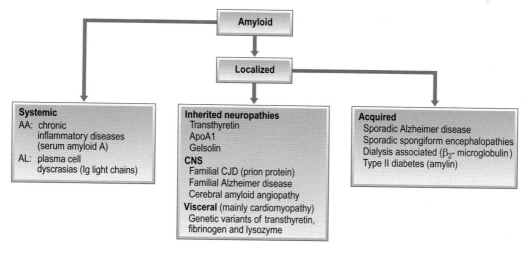

Fig. 23.6 Types of amyloid.

Amyloid type	Deposit	Comments
Idiopathic (primary) amyloidosis	AL	Derived from immunoglobulin light chains plus serum amyloid P
Myeloma-associated amyloidosis	AL	Derived from immunoglobulin light chains
Hereditary amyloidosis	AA	Derived from other proteins (lyosozyme, fibrinogen, apolipoproteins)
Secondary amyloidosis	AA	The most common form of amyloid disease. Derived from serum amyloid A protein, an acute-phase protein released by the liver in chronic infections or inflammatory states such as rheumatoid arthritis and ulcerative colitis, via interleukin-1 from activated mononuclear phagocytes
Other forms of amyloidosis	Range of proteins	Mainly pre-albumin. A heterogeneous group, some related to senility, to dialysis or drug abuse, and some localized to medullary carcinoma of thyroid or calcifying epithelial odontogenic tumour

Table 23.10   Amyloid types

TMA is found in some foods and is produced by gut bacteria from foods rich in TMA-oxide, choline, lecithin or carnitine.

TMA is found in milk from wheat-fed cows, TMA precursors in choline [eggs, liver, kidney, peas, beans, peanuts, soya and brassicas (Brussels sprouts, broccoli, cabbage, cauliflower)], lecithin and lecithin-containing fish oil supplements. TMA N-oxide is found in seafood (fish, cephalopods and crustaceans).

TMA is normally oxidized by liver flavin mono-oxygenase 3 (FMO3) to odourless trimethylamine N-oxide (TMAO). Trimethylaminuria is an inherited *FMO3* gene mutation leading to impaired TMA oxidation. Unoxidized TMA then appears in and causes odour from urine, sweat, genital secretions, saliva and breath. Other causes of excess TMA include:

- deficient nicotine *N*-oxidation
- disorders of carnitine and choline intake
- haematological anormalities
- Noonan syndrome
- Prader–Willi syndrome
- renal and hepatic disease
- Turner syndrome.

Similar symptoms may appear in some normal people under conditions such as fever, stress, exercise or menstruation. Trimethylaminuria is managed by diet (avoid eggs, fish, brassicas); antimicrobials (e.g. metronidazole); lactulose; activated charcoal and copper chlorophyllin; and riboflavin.

USEFUL WEBSITES

http://www.nlm.nih.gov/
http://themedicalbiochemistrypage.org
http://www.uq.edu.au/porphyria/
http://en.wikipedia.org/wiki/Metabolic_disorder
http://en.wikipedia.org/wiki/Metabolic_syndrome

FURTHER READING

Ayonrinde, O.T., Milward, E.A., Chua, A.C., Trinder, D., Olynyk, J.K., 2008. Clinical perspectives on hereditary hemochromatosis. Crit Rev Clin Lab Sci 45, 451–484.

Cappellini, M.D., Fiorelli, G., 2008. Glucose-6-phosphate dehydrogenase deficiency. Lancet 371, 64–74.

Cassiman, D., Vannoote, J., Roelandts, R., et al., 2008. Porphyria cutanea tarda and liver disease. A retrospective analysis of 17 cases from a single centre and review of the literature. Acta Gastroenterol Belg 71, 237–242.

Chen, M., Wang, J., 2008. Gaucher disease: review of the literature. Arch Pathol Lab Med 132, 851–853.

Cope, T.M., Hunter, J.M., 2003. Selecting neuromuscular-blocking drugs for elderly patients. Drugs Aging 20, 125–140.

Di Mauro, S., 2007. Muscle glycogenoses: an overview. Acta Myol 26, 35–41.

Dinauer, M.C., 2007. Disorders of neutrophil function: an overview. Methods Mol Biol 412, 489–504.

Friedlander, A.H., Golub, M.S., 2006. The significance of carotid artery atheromas on panoramic radiographs in the diagnosis of occult metabolic syndrome. Oral Surg Oral Med Oral Pathol Oral Radiol Endod 101, 95–101.

Friedlander, A.H., Weinreb, J., Friedlander, I., Yagiela, J.A., 2007. Metabolic syndrome: pathogenesis, medical care and dental implications. J Am Dent Assoc 138, 179–187, quiz 248.

Galley, H.F., Mahdy, A., Lowes, D.A., 2005. Pharmacogenetics and anesthesiologists. Pharmacogenomics 6, 849–856.

James, M.F.M, Hift, R.I, 2000. Porphyrias Brit J. Anaesth 85, 143–153.

Katzin, L.W., Amato, A.A., 2008. Pompe disease: a review of the current diagnosis and treatment recommendations in the era of enzyme replacement therapy. J Clin Neuromuscul Dis 9, 421–431.

Kopelman, P., 2004. The metabolic syndrome as a clinical problem. Nestle Nutr Workshop Ser Clin Perform Programme 9, 77–88; discussion 88–92.

Lajtman, Z., Surina, B., Bartolek, D., et al., 2002. 'Warning card' as a prevention of prolonged apnea in children. Coll Antropol 26 (Suppl), 129–137.

Lee, J.H., Berkowitz, R.J., Choi, B.J., 2002. Oral self-mutilation in the Lesch–Nyhan syndrome. ASDC J Dent Child 69, 66–69, 12.

Nishimura, F., Soga, Y., Iwamoto, Y., Kudo, C., Murayama, Y., 2005. Periodontal disease as part of the insulin resistance syndrome in diabetic patients. J Int Acad Periodontol 7, 16–20.

Olynyk, J.K., Trinder, D., Ramm, G.A., Britton, R.S., Bacon, B.R., 2008. Hereditary hemochromatosis in the post-HFE era. Hepatology 48, 991–1001.

Rosenberg, H., Davis, M., James, D., Pollock, N., Stowell, K., 2007. Malignant hyperthermia. Orphanet J Rare Dis 2, 21.

Sarkany, R.P., 2008. Making sense of the porphyrias. Photodermatol Photoimmunol Photomed 24 (2), 102–108.

Shimazaki, Y., Saito, T., Yonemoto, K., Kiyohara, Y., Iida, M., Yamashita, Y., 2007. Relationship of metabolic syndrome to periodontal disease in Japanese women: the Hisayama Study. J Dent Res 86, 271–275.

Taddei, T., Mistry, P., Schilsky, M.L., 2008. Inherited metabolic disease of the liver. Curr Opin Gastroenterol 24, 278–286.

Thomas, C.L., Badminton, M.N., Rendall, J.R., Anstey, A.V., 2008. Sclerodermatous changes of face, neck and scalp associated with familial porphyria cutanea tarda. Clin Exp Dermatol 33, 422–424.

Williams, D.S., 2007. Porphyria cutanea tarda. J Insur Med 39, 293–295.

Appendix 23.1 Inborn errors of metabolism

Disease	Management problems	Disease	Management problems
Abetalipoproteinaemia	Ataxia: haemorrhage	Fucosidosis	Learning impairment
Acatalasaemia	Gingival ulceration	Galactosaemia	Learning impairment;
Acid lipase deficiency	Learning impairment; anaemia		hepatic disease; cataracts; hypoglycaemia
Acrodermatitis enteropathica	Oral ulceration; neuropathies	Gilbert disease	Jaundice
Adenosine deaminase deficiency	Immunodeficiency	GM1 gangliosidosis	Learning impairment; epilepsy; blindness
Alpha$_1$-antitrypsin deficiency	Hepatic disease; emphysema		
Alkaptonuria	Arthritis; aortic valve disease	GM2 gangliosidosis	Learning impairment; epilepsy; blindness
Argininaemia	Spasticity; learning disability; epilepsy	Tay–Sachs disease	Learning impairment; epilepsy; blindness
Aspartylglucosaminuria	Learning impairment	Sandhoff disease	Learning impairment; epilepsy; blindness
Cerebrotendinous xanthomatosis	Dementia; ataxia; paresis; cataracts	Gaucher disease	Learning impairment; spasticity; thrombocytopenia; leukopenia
Cholinesterase deficiency	Suxamethonium sensitivity		
Chronic granulomatous disease	Lymph node abscesses (cervical, etc.); liability to severe bacterial infections	Glucose-6-phosphate dehydrogenase deficiency	Haemolytic anaemia, care with drugs
		Glutaric aciduria	Hypoglycaemia
Combined hyperlipidaemia	Atherosclerosis	Glycogen storage disease:	
Congenital adrenal hyperplasia	Hypoadrenocorticism	I	Hypoglycaemia; caries; bleeding tendency
Crigler–Najjar syndrome	Jaundice	II	Cardiomyopathy; respiratory infection; neurological abnormalities
Cystinosis	Renal disease		
Cystinuria	Renal disease		
Diphosphoglycerate mutase deficiency	Anaemia	III	Hypoglycaemia
Dubin–Johnson syndrome	Jaundice	IV	Hepatic disease; cardiac failure
Dysbetalipoproteinaemia	Atherosclerosis	VI	Mild hypoglycaemia
Fabry disease	Neuropathy; thromboses; renal failure; pulmonary failure	VIa	Mild hypoglycaemia
		O	Mild hypoglycaemia
Familial dysautonomia (Riley–Day syndrome)	Sensitive to barbiturates; dysphagia; sialorrhoea; insensitive to pain; learning impairment; epilepsy; labile BP	Gout	Renal disease; hypertension; atherosclerosis
		Haemochromatosis	Diabetes; hepatic disease; cardiomyopathy
Familial goitre	Hypothyroidism	Hereditary angioedema	Airways obstruction
Fanconi syndrome	Aminoaciduria; osteomalacia; oral cancer	Hereditary fructose intolerance	Hepatic disease; hypoglycaemia

Appendix 23.1   Inborn errors of metabolism—cont'd

Disease	Management problems		Disease	Management problems
Hereditary oroticaciduria	Severe anaemia; leukopenia		MPS V Ullrich–Scheie syndrome	Blindness; valvular heart disease
Hereditary spherocytosis	Haemolytic anaemia		MPS VI Maroteaux–Lamy syndrome	Learning impairment; blindness
Hexokinase deficiency	Anaemia		MPS VII	Learning impairment
Histidinaemia	Hearing deficit; speech deficit; infections; learning disability		Myeloperoxidase deficiency	Candidosis
Homocystinuria	Learning impairment; epilepsy; blindness; hepatic disease; chest deformities; thrombotic disease		Neuronal ceroid lipofuscinoses	Learning impairment; epilepsy; blindness
			Niemann–Pick disease	Learning impairment; epilepsy; pancytopenia
Hypercalcaemia	Renal disease; cardiac subaortic stenosis; learning disability (William syndrome)		Orotic aciduria	Megaloblastic anaemia
			Oxalosis	Renal disease; cardiac disease
			Phenylketonuria	Learning impairment; epilepsy
Hypercholesterolaemia	Atherosclerosis		Porphyrias	Drug sensitivities; neuropathies; hypertension
Hypercystinuria	Renal disease			
Hyperornithinaemia	Learning impairment		Primary hypophosphataemia (vitamin D-resistant rickets)	Dwarfism; rickets; dental abscesses
Hyperoxaluria	Renal disease			
Hypertriglyceridaemia	Atherosclerosis; pancreatitis		Prolinaemia	Epilepsy; deafness
Hypophosphatasia	Skeletal abnormalities; dental hypoplasia		Purine nucleoside phosphorylase deficiency	Immunodeficiency
Krabbe disease	Learning impairment; blindness		Pyruvate kinase deficiency	Anaemia
Lecithin/cholesterol/acetyltransferase deficiency	Haemolytic anaemia; atherosclerosis; renal disease		Renal glycosuria	Glycosuria (confusion with diabetes)
Lesch–Nyhan syndrome	Mutilation of tongue or lips; learning impairment; epilepsy; athetosis; renal failure		Refsum disease	Blindness; deafness
			Rotor syndrome	Jaundice
			Sandhoff disease	Learning impairment; epilepsy; blindness
Lipoprotein lipase deficiency	Pancreatitis		Tay–Sachs disease	Learning impairment; epilepsy; blindness
Lysinuria	Epilepsy			
Mannosidosis	Learning impairment		Transcobalamin II deficiency	Macrocytic anaemia; pancytopenia
Metachromatic leukodystrophy	Learning impairment; blindness; psychoses		Triosephosphate isomerase deficiency	Anaemia
Methionine malabsorption	Epilepsy		Tyrosinaemia	Hepatic disease
Mucolipidosis (I-cell disease)	Learning impairment; blindness; valvular heart disease		Tyrosinosis	Myasthenia; epilepsy
Mucopolysaccharidoses (MPS) I Hurler syndrome	Learning impairment; blindness; cardiac impairment; trismus		Wilson disease (hepatolenticular degeneration)	Hepatic disease; renal disease; spasticity; tremor; mental problems
MPS II Hunter syndrome	As in MPS I		Wolman disease	Learning impairment
MPS III Sanfilippo syndrome	Learning impairment		Xeroderma pigmentosum	Skin cancers
MPS IV Morquio syndrome	Blindness; chest deformity; aortic valve disease; enamel hypoplasia			

TRAUMA AND BURNS

This chapter deals with: trauma to the head, maxillofacial area and spine; burns; gunshot and stab wounds; and human bites. Animal bites, sports injuries and child abuse are discussed elsewhere (see Ch. 33).

GENERAL ASPECTS

It is males predominantly who are affected by trauma. Accidents are the most common cause of death in children and in men up to the age of 35. Up to a third of these deaths are, theoretically at least, preventable. Violence (assaults or fights; Figs 24.1–24.3) and road traffic accidents are the major causes of trauma, with alcohol or other drugs being a frequent cofactor. In the Western world, assaults are increasingly common but, in contrast, trauma from road accidents is less common since the institution of seat-belt wearing, although 3500 people are still

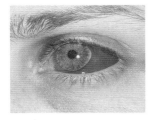

Fig. 24.1 Subconjunctival haemorrhage

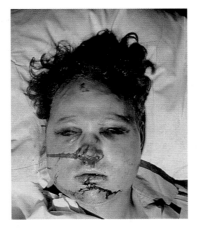

Fig. 24.2 Maxillofacial trauma

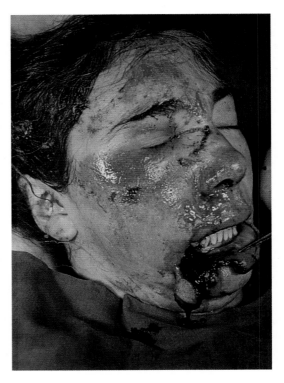

Fig. 24.3 Maxillofacial trauma

killed and 40 000 seriously injured each year from road accidents in Britain. Maxillofacial trauma is the single most common injury to occupants of vehicles involved in road accidents, even in seat-belted drivers. Airbags can act as a supplemental restraint system, but they themselves can cause injury – particularly if the person is of short stature, unrestrained or out of position within the vehicle.

Industrial accidents, sport, epilepsy and non-accidental injuries (child abuse) are other causes of trauma. Equine-related maxillofacial fractures mainly involve the young and predominantly females, and alcohol is rarely implicated.

Damage to the head, cervical spine, chest, liver or spleen can be life-threatening, and there can be additional damage to other bones and organs, such as kidneys or bladder. In war, assaults and road trauma, injuries often involve multiple organs. Death may result immediately from trauma, especially if there is head injury and brain damage, airway obstruction or damage to the spine and other vital organs (e.g. heart or liver). Head injuries are present in about 70% of patients admitted with multiple injuries and about 3% of multiply injured patients have intracranial haemorrhage.

HEAD INJURIES

Most head injuries are in previously fit young males, because of their risk behaviour. Road traffic accidents are a major cause (Fig. 24.4). Children and adolescents can sustain head injuries

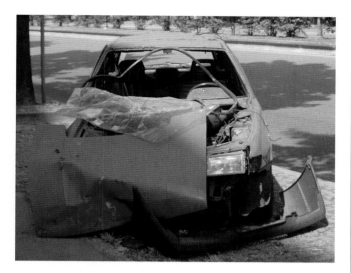

Fig. 24.4 Road traffic accident

In the case of bilateral mandibular body fractures, a traction suture through the tongue will hold it forward, but, frequently, medial displacement of the posterior fragments prevents the anterior fragment from falling backwards unless the bone is comminuted. Posterior displacement of the maxilla in middle third injuries may cause the soft palate to occlude the airway. Obstruction can then be overcome by manual disimpaction of the maxilla. In the unconscious patient, a cuffed endotracheal tube may be needed to maintain the airway.

Should these non-invasive manoeuvres fail to relieve obstruction immediately, a surgical airway, using endotracheal intubation or cricothyroidotomy, must be made. If there is supraglottic airway obstruction, a temporary airway can be established by laryngotomy using a wide-bore (2–3 mm) needle inserted through the cricothyroid membrane. In certain laryngotracheal crush injuries and other wounds that transect the trachea, it may be necessary to perform emergency tracheostomy (Fig. 24.5) or occasionally submental intubation. Indications for tracheostomy are summarized in Table 24.1.

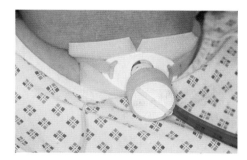

Fig. 24.5 Tracheostomy

during sports or fights, and young children, particularly before they have perfected their walking skills, are also uniquely susceptible to head trauma because of higher cranial mass to body ratio.

Head injuries are a major cause of death – almost 50% of which happen before the patient reaches hospital – and most of the remaining deaths follow within the first few hours. Of those with brain injury, 12% die within 2 days. The underlying mechanisms are unclear but brain injury may include tissue acidosis, free radical release, prostaglandin and electrolyte changes. It is important to appreciate that the brain can be fatally damaged without fracture of the skull or even a blemish on the scalp. Head injuries often are also associated with other bodily injuries that may be life-threatening, especially hazards to the airway, damage to the cervical spine, chest, liver, spleen, kidneys or long bones, and severe haemorrhage.

IMMEDIATE CARE

All life-threatening injuries must be urgently assessed using the ABC system: Airway and cervical spine, Breathing and bleeding, and Chest injuries.

Airway establishment and maintenance has the highest priority. Respiratory obstruction is the most important preventable cause of early death and may be due to several causes, such as those shown in Box 24.1.

Many patients have died from neglect of the airway before admission to hospital. Foreign bodies or the tongue can easily fall back to obstruct respiration, especially if there are bilateral fractures or comminution of the mandible, and the patient is unconscious. There is special danger to the airway if there has been trauma to and oedema of the tongue, fauces, pharynx or larynx, or uncontrollable nasoethmoidal haemorrhage.

Severely injured patients must have their airways (mouth and pharynx) cleared of debris and sucked out using direct vision and strong suction, and be laid semi-prone on their side, face towards the ground, to allow any potential obstruction to fall forwards. Great care must be taken to avoid further neurological damage if a cervical spine injury is suspected.

Chest injuries, particularly those causing tension pneumothorax or flail chest, or inhalation of toxic or hot gases, further impair respiration (see Burns). Flail chest can be recognized by extreme difficulty in breathing, associated with paradoxical movements of the chest and cyanosis. Intermittent positive-pressure ventilation must be given via a cuffed endotracheal tube.

Cervical spine stabilization is extremely important since injury is possible, especially in patients with injury above the clavicles or head injury resulting in an unconscious state, or any injury produced by high speed. Cervical spine injury is potentially fatal and may be symptomless whilst the patient is conscious due to protective muscle spasm which 'stabilizes' the spine. General anaesthesia (GA) is very dangerous, as this protective muscle spasm is abolished on induction. Features

Table 24.1 Indications for tracheostomy		
Obstruction of the airway by:	Where positive pressure ventilation is needed:	Where tracheobronchial suction is needed:
Gross retroposition of the middle third of the face	Crushed or flail chest	Chronic obstructive pulmonary disease
Pharyngeal oedema	Whenever prolonged mechanical ventilation is required	
Uncontrollable nasal haemorrhage		
Loss of tongue control		
Cancer surgery		

can include neurological deficit and neck pain. Avoid any movement of the spinal column, and establish and maintain proper immobilization with the use of an appropriate neck splint until vertebral fractures or spinal cord injuries have been carefully ruled out with lateral cervical spine radiographs and computed tomography (CT).

Haemorrhage must be controlled. External bleeding is controlled by direct pressure over any bleeding site until permanent control can be achieved by clamping and ligation. Shock because of bleeding leading to hypovolaemia should be prevented or controlled and an intravenous infusion established. The goal is to restore organ perfusion using intravenous fluid replacement (Ringer's lactate, normal saline or blood transfusion). Vital signs should be monitored closely.

Severe haemorrhage or shock only rarely results from isolated head injuries or maxillofacial trauma, unless caused by gunshot wounds. If a patient with such injuries is shocked, it is essential to look for other injuries such as damage to internal organs or fractures of the pelvis or limbs. Remember that bleeding may be concealed or occasionally aggravated by disseminated intravascular coagulation (Ch. 8) secondary to the head injury. Internal haemorrhage, for example into the abdomen from a ruptured viscus, or into the thigh from a fractured femur, can cause life-threatening hypotension. Haemorrhage into the pleural cavity from fractured ribs can also embarrass respiration. Severe haemorrhage can lead to cardiac or renal failure or cause fatal cerebral hypoxia.

Latent haemorrhage may be recognized by rising pulse rate, falling blood pressure, increasing pallor, air hunger or restlessness. If haemorrhage is suspected, a surgical opinion should be sought, a blood sample taken for grouping and cross-matching, and the following quarter- or half-hourly observations should be recorded:

- pulse rate
- blood pressure
- respiratory rate
- urine output and fluid balance (usually hourly).

Blood transfusion may be indicated but should be given only when genuinely warranted by the clinical condition, since there are risks, such as from transfusion reactions, fluid overload and infection. Blood may be needed to replace loss from

acute haemorrhage but is not needed to replace loss of less than 500 ml in an adult, unless there was pre-existing severe anaemia or deterioration of the general condition warrants transfusion. Since time is needed to obtain correctly cross-matched blood, normal saline, plasma or a plasma expander such as dextran 70 or 110 may be given initially. Dextrans or other plasma expanders together with tranexamic acid or desmopressin may be the only possibility for Jehovah's Witnesses. Dextran can interfere with blood-grouping and cross-matching so that blood samples should be collected before a dextran infusion is started (see Ch. 8).

Estimation of blood urea and electrolyte levels are needed in case there has been renal failure secondary to loss of blood, and as a baseline to monitor progress and the effects of intravenous fluid replacement. A full blood picture is also needed as a baseline for possible effects of transfusion and for any coincidental haematological disease. As described previously, early haemoglobin levels give no useful indication of the amount of blood lost as haemodilution will not have had time to develop.

Blood and urine samples should be collected for analysis for alcohol, drugs and metabolic disorders, particularly diabetes. However, transient glycosuria unrelated to diabetes may follow the stress of head injuries.

The initial management of patients with head injuries (Table 24.2) is thus maintenance of the airway, control of the cervical spine and haemorrhage, and care of chest and other life-threatening injuries. The reader should consult the Advanced Trauma Life Support Manual and similar guides for full details on this important topic.

Table 24.2 Head injuries: initial and early management			
Immediate care (ABC)	General assessment	Assessment of head injury	Assessment for other injuries
Airway and cervical spine Breathing and bleeding Chest injuries	State of consciousness Pulse Blood pressure Respiratory rate Pupil size and reaction	Skull examination Examination for cerebrospinal fluid leak Neurological assessment Skull radiography including CT Blood analyses	Neck Spine Abdomen Perineum Limbs

A detailed assessment of any maxillofacial injuries is only undertaken once the patient has been assessed as above and stabilized.

GENERAL ASSESSMENT

As good a history as possible must be obtained from the patient, if conscious, and witnesses. Reports of any loss of consciousness or any amnesia, nausea, vomiting or headache must be noted, as well as the medical history, especially use of drugs including anticoagulants, or any previous history of epilepsy. A description of the mechanism of injury is useful as it will give a clue as to what injuries to suspect. Family or friends may need to be questioned about the patient's medical background.

STATE OF CONSCIOUSNESS

Many patients brought in to the emergency department following head injury are confused, concussed or comatose, though 30% of patients with ultimately fatal head injuries may talk after injury and some are completely lucid for a time. However, the brain is invariably damaged in those who have lost consciousness for however brief a period, and sometimes in those who have not, and amnesia is common. Many are also suffering effects from alcohol or other drugs of misuse. Maintenance of consciousness does not therefore guarantee the absence of brain injury but the extent of retrograde amnesia is a rough measure of severity of brain injury.

Concussion, an immediate but transient loss of consciousness, is always associated with a short period of amnesia, and there is some brain damage even if after-effects are not detectable on neurological testing, cerebrospinal fluid (CSF) examination, CT or magnetic resonance imaging (MRI). Although the patient may lose consciousness only transiently, consciousness is almost invariably impaired after diffuse brain damage, and there is usually amnesia for the traumatic event, and afterwards (post-traumatic amnesia) for a period far exceeding that of coma. Consciousness may not be lost if brain damage is local, when, for example, the skull is penetrated by a sharp object.

Prolonged unconsciousness, when there are no complications such as brain haematomas and where there are no focal signs, is often caused by severe brain damage, but sometimes by drugs or other unrelated disease (Table 24.3).

Table 24.3 Main cerebral causes of coma (see also Appendix 24.1)

Brain lesions	Main causes
Cerebral cortex damage	Trauma, haemorrhage, hypoglycaemia, hypoxia, infection
Brainstem compression	Various
Brainstem localized pressure	Cerebellar haemorrhage, abscess, neoplasm
Brainstem reticular activating substance suppression	Drugs (alcohol and others)

The most essential examination is immediately to assess, record and monitor the level of consciousness using the Glasgow coma scale (GCS), which scores points (EMV score) derived from three features: eye opening (E); motor response (M); and verbal response (V; Table 24.4). The degree of brain damage is initially assessed by the level of consciousness assessed by the GCS and, later, by the duration of coma and of post-traumatic amnesia. It is important to consider causes of coma other than acute head injury (see Appendix 24.1).

The EMV score or responsiveness sum can range from 3 to 15. A fully alert and otherwise well patient with a full and unchanging score of 15 and no neurological signs or

Table 24.4 Glasgow coma or responsiveness scale (GCS)

Eye opening	E	Motor response	M	Verbal response	V
Spontaneous	4	Obeys	6	Orientated	5
To speech	3	Localizes	5	Confused conversation	4
To pain	2	Withdraws	4	Inappropriate words	3
Nil	1	Abnormal flexion	3	Incomprehensible sounds	2
		Extends	2	Nil	1
		Nil	1		

symptoms and no skull fracture or intracranial haemorrhage on CT or MRI scan does not need hospital admission for observation unless for other reasons.

All patients who score less than the full 15 points should be admitted to hospital for observation, even if drugs or alcohol are the suspected causes of depressed consciousness (Table 24.4). Patients with a GCS score of less than 8 require immediate neurosurgical attention (Table 24.5). A score of 7 or less indicates coma in 100%; 9 or more indicates absence of coma. About 85% of patients with a score of 3 or 4 succumb within 24 h. It is important also to recognize and to treat other factors that can contribute to the morbidity and mortality, which can include airway obstruction, hypotension, meningitis, uncontrolled epilepsy, stress-induced gastric bleeding or diabetic ketoacidosis.

Patients who survive with head injuries fall into three main groups. Most are stable neurologically with gradual improvement in consciousness. Some progressively deteriorate in the level of consciousness with localizing signs, often because of intracranial bleeding with or without cerebral oedema, when the bleeding usually needs to be evacuated by craniotomy. Some have rising intracranial pressure causing progressive deterioration in the level of consciousness in the absence of localizing signs. Cerebral oedema may be reduced by ensuring adequate oxygenation and by giving mannitol, fluid restriction and furosemide and/or dexamethasone. The management of cerebral oedema remains controversial.

Patients must be carefully and regularly observed to detect the development of complications, especially intracranial haematomas, which need immediate neurosurgical attention, so the level of consciousness should be charted as assessed by the GCS and, later, by the duration of coma and of post-traumatic amnesia, regularly half-hourly, or even more frequently, along with the pulse, blood pressure, respiration and pupil reactivity, and temperature.

Deterioration of consciousness is the most important sign, sometimes with worsening restlessness, headache and vomiting. Fixed dilatation of the pupil on the side of the fracture and decerebrate rigidity – late signs caused by raised intracranial pressure and brain shift – are soon followed by bilateral pupil dilatation, periodic respiration, respiratory arrest and death, unless there is immediate neurosurgical intervention. Focal signs such as hemiparesis, dysphasia or focal epilepsy are uncommon.

In deep coma there are no verbal or motor responses, but in less severe cases the eyes may open transiently from time to time and there may be vague or weak responses to stimuli.

Up to 60% of all patients admitted in coma are alcoholics or other drug users who have often had a head injury. Toxic and metabolic disorders cause no focal or localizing neurological signs, although some drug misuse (opiates) can affect pupil reactivity. When there is disease of the central nervous system (CNS) itself, sensory or motor disturbances may indicate the site of the lesion. In some of these diseases, white cells, bacteria or blood may also appear in the CSF. Intoxications, whether the result of exogenous agents or disorders of metabolism and severe infections, all have essentially similar effects and will not be discussed further here.

The level of consciousness is depressed further by sedatives and many analgesics, especially morphine and its analogues, which not only depress respiration but also disguise eye signs of rising intracranial pressure, by causing pupillary constriction. Pentazocine is also contraindicated. If analgesia is essential, codeine, diclofenac or buprenorphine can be used. Benzodiazepines should not be given for purposes such as controlling fits or to allow suturing of head wounds, since they cause respiratory depression, which can be fatal unless ventilation is given. If there are repeated fits, phenytoin by intravenous infusion is less likely to depress respiration. Alcohol must be prohibited.

Pupil size and reaction must be checked for localizing signs of neurological damage. A dilated fixed (unreactive to light) pupil often indicates rising intracranial pressure and is usually a serious sign. Severe facial oedema may make examination of the eyes difficult and the eyelids should then be prised open. A fixed dilated pupil may also be caused by local damage to the optic or oculomotor nerves, and must be differentiated by clinical examination, radiographs (usually CT), MRI and by the absence of signs associated with brain damage or of rising intracranial pressure. Limb reflexes should be tested.

Regular monitoring of blood pressure (BP) and pulse rate is essential. A low or falling BP with rising pulse rate is indicative of haemorrhage or shock, which can lead to fatal cerebral anoxia or renal failure. A systolic BP lower than 60 mmHg brings with it a risk of brain damage. A high or rising BP with bradycardia, by contrast, is indicative of raised intracranial pressure secondary to cerebral oedema or haemorrhage as a result of the injury. Respiratory rate, urine output and fluid balance must also be monitored.

ASSESSMENT OF HEAD INJURY

Skull examination

Lacerations of the scalp may be associated with a fracture and can cause severe loss of blood, and can provide a pathway for infection into the cranial cavity. The presence of a skull fracture greatly increases the risk of brain damage and an intracranial haematoma; significant intracranial lesions are found in two-thirds. A depressed skull fracture may be palpable, although it is often concealed by overlying oedema of the soft tissues. About 80% of skull fractures are linear, and many are associated with subepidural or epidural haematomas. Basal skull fractures are usually uncomplicated; they may not show on routine radiography but may be revealed by bleeding, which may show as haemotympanum (blood behind the ear drum), as ecchymosis over the mastoid process (Battle's sign), as periorbital ecchymosis (raccoon sign), by CSF rhinorrhoea or otorrhoea. Alternatively they may be suggested by cranial nerve lesions involving the olfactory nerve (cribriform plate fracture), optic nerve (sphenoid), facial nerve (petrous) or abducens and facial nerve (sella fracture).

Skull fractures can also cause cranial nerve damage, and provide an entry to the CSF for infection or air (pneumocephalus).

Examination for leak of cerebrospinal fluid

Particular care must be taken to examine for CSF leaks – rhinorrhoea or otorrhoea – and signs of orbital or retromastoid haematomas (which may indicate fractures with dural tears). In these instances there is the risk of meningitis and an early neurosurgical opinion should therefore be obtained. In the early stages, leakage of CSF may be obscured by haemorrhage,

---

Table 24.5 Indications for neurosurgical attention after head injury

Immediate neurological attention indicated	Early neurological attention indicated	Admit to hospital for neurological observation
GCS < 8	GCS 8–14	GCS < 15
Deteriorating consciousness	Convulsions	Minor skull fracture[a]
Neurological lateralization (pupillary inequality and hemiparesis)	Cerebrospinal rhinorrhoea or otorrhoea	Post-traumatic amnesia
Dilated fixed (unreactive to light) pupil	Orbital or retromastoid haematomas	Other serious injuries
Major skull fractures (depressed or compound)	Pneumoencephalocoele	Children
CT signs of compression or obliteration of mesencephalic cisterns, midline hemisphere shift, or one or more surgical masses	Worsening restlessness, headache and vomiting	Patients with psychiatric disease, drug abuse or learning impairment
Uncontrollable bleeding		Patients living alone or without a responsible adult companion
Rising blood pressure with bradycardia		

[a]There is some controversy among neurosurgeons about whether patients with skull fractures with *no* evidence of cerebrospinal fluid leak, cerebral haemorrhage, or pneumoencephalocoele should receive observation or operative treatment.
GCS, Glasgow coma scale.

but any clear watery discharge from the nose is suspect and should be tested for sugar and protein. CSF, unlike a serous nasal discharge, contains sugar but little protein. However, lacrimal fluid also contains small amounts of glucose, and CSF must therefore be positively identified by protein electrophoresis and accurate measurement of the glucose.

Cerebrospinal fluid rhinorrhoea is found in about 2% of all head injuries, but in 25% of fractures of the middle third of face and nasoethmoidal complex. CSF leaks usually persist for about a week and the risk of meningitis is greatest within the first fortnight. Occasionally the fistula may be occluded by herniated brain but the dural tear fails to heal. If there is a dural tear, meningitis may follow after some months or years and therefore dural repair is desirable.

In all patients with ocular or orbital injuries, the orbit should be examined radiologically usually by CT for fracture and, if suspected, should undergo exploration and receive prophylaxis as recommended for penetrating intracranial wounds.

Prophylactic antimicrobials are needed if there is a meningitis risk and should therefore be given to all patients with a penetrating brain injury (PBI). The risk of intracranial infection among patients with PBIs is high because of the presence of contaminated foreign objects, skin, hair and bone fragments driven into the brain along the missile track. Antimicrobials are also indicated in compound depressed skull fractures, CSF leaks or fractures of the middle third.

Many bacteria causing post-traumatic meningitis, such as meningococci, *Staphylococcus aureus* or *Streptococcus pneumoniae,* are resistant to the traditional treatment with sulfonamides. Recommended antimicrobials that readily reach the CSF and are well absorbed when given orally include co-amoxiclav, or cefuroxime with metronidazole, or vancomycin and ceftazidime. Effective alternatives are rifampicin or minocycline.

Intracranial bleeding

Intracranial haematomas may be of three types. Intracerebral (subarachnoid) haematomas are usually not amenable to surgical intervention. Epidural or extradural (between dura mater and skull) haematomas are usually due to tearing of the middle meningeal artery after a fracture of the temporal bone. They evolve rapidly and are neurosurgical emergencies requiring burr holes through the skull to drain the clot and ligate the bleeding vessel. The haematoma forms a tumour-like mass, which compresses part of the brain and raises intracranial pressure as it expands. Clinically, the typical story is of a heavy blow followed by loss of consciousness. There is usually then a period of apparent recovery (lucid interval) followed by signs of rising intracranial pressure. If the clot is not removed, death from respiratory arrest follows. A radiograph showing a fracture line crossing the line of the middle meningeal artery strongly suggests extradural haemorrhage and CT scanning will confirm the diagnosis.

Subdural haematomas – between the dura and leptomeninges – are venous and associated with contusion of the underlying brain. Early operation to evacuate the clot through burr holes improves survival. They may be acute or chronic. Acute subdural haematoma is often the result of an injury causing a tear in the arachnoid and may be associated with laceration or contusion of the brain. Clinically, there is a latent interval after the injury, followed by progressive deterioration of consciousness and development of symptoms somewhat similar to those of an extradural haematoma. Once coma has developed, up to 50% die. Chronic subdural haematoma can be caused by a very mild injury. Nevertheless, the veins between the pia and the dura mater are torn. Leakage of blood into the subdural space is very slow. There is a fibroblastic response and eventually the haematoma becomes enclosed in scar tissue or, occasionally, resorbed. Clinically, the head injury, especially in an elderly person, may be so slight as to have been forgotten but, after several weeks, or even months, symptoms such as headache, dizziness, slowness of thinking, or confusion and disturbance of consciousness develop. There may be localizing signs such as hemiparesis or aphasia; the patient may have ptosis and be unable to look upwards (pressure on the IIIrd nerve).

Neurological assessment

After head injury, approximately 50% of patients have permanent after-effects such as paralyses, loss of speech, impaired vision, epilepsy, disturbances of personality or severe mental defects, rendering them disabled for life. Delayed effects may result from ischaemia, hypoxia, cerebral oedema, intracranial hypertension and/or abnormalities of cerebral blood flow.

The goals of head injury treatment are therefore to detect any damage and prevent or reverse secondary insults to the damaged brain, such as from hypoxaemia, hypotension and intracranial bleeding or haematoma, and to allow recovery of as much damaged brain tissue as possible.

Cranial nerve injuries in patients with head injuries may indicate a basal skull fracture or other lesion: cranial nerves I, II, III, V, VII and VIII are most vulnerable (Table 24.6 and Ch. 13). Sense of smell is disturbed or lost (anosmia) in 5–10% of head injuries since the olfactory nerves are damaged in frontal bone injuries and fractures involving the ethmoid cribriform plate. Cerebrospinal fluid rhinorrhoea is often associated. Traumatic anosmia improves in only about 10% and perversion of the sense of smell may develop during recovery, effects that are remarkably troublesome or even disabling, but untreatable.

Skull radiography including computed tomography

Radiography should be carried out early before infection can reach the cranial cavity (typically anteroposterior, lateral and Towne's views). CT scans are essential to exclude skull fractures and brain lesions. MRI can provide better brain images but cannot always be used. Imaging may also reveal a depressed fracture involving the paranasal sinuses; this suggests a meningeal tear which is occasionally confirmed by seeing intracranial air (aerocoele). A linear fracture indicates the possibility of intracranial haematoma but even normal radiographs do not exclude brain damage. About 50% of patients with intracranial injuries have no skull fracture, and approximately 90% of patients with fractures of the skull have no resulting intracranial injury. CT signs such as compression or obliteration of mesencephalic cisterns,

Table 24.6 Cranial nerve lesions complicating head injuries

Nerve lesion	Usual site of injury	Comments
I (olfactory)	Ethmoidal complex (may be no fracture)	Anosmia (usually permanent); apparent loss of taste
II (optic)	Orbit[a] or sphenoid	Pupil dilated, unreactive to light, but consensual reflex retained[b]; partial or complete blindness
III (oculomotor)	Orbit[a]	Affected eye looks down and out. Pupil dilated, unreactive to light. No consensual reflex. Loss of medial and vertical movement of eye. Divergent squint
IV (trochlear)	Orbit[a]	Diplopia only on looking down. Similar features result if superior oblique muscle is entrapped. Pupil – normal reactivity
V (trigeminal)	Middle fossa, orbit,[a] maxilla or mandible	Commonly extracranially. Anaesthesia or paraesthesia in sensory area
VI (abducens)	Orbit[a] or petrous temporal	Diplopia. Loss or lateral movement of eye. Convergent squint. Pupil reacts normally
VII (facial)	Direct trauma to nerve or basal skull fracture (see Facial paralysis)	Facial paralysis, which may be delayed for a few days
VIII (vestibulocochlear)	Petrous temporal	Deafness, vertigo and nystagmus alone or together. Deafness after head injury may also be caused by ruptured ear drum or blood in middle ear
IX–XII	Corticobulbar	Uncommon as a result of head injuries

[a]May be damage to orbital contents with or without fracture. These nerves are often injured together and urgent neurosurgery may be indicated since nerve dysfunction, if caused by haemorrhage or oedema within the optic canal or other confined space, may be reversible. In the superior orbital fissure syndrome there may be damage to the lacrimal, frontal, trochlear, abducens and oculomotor nerves with minimal damage to the globe.
[b]Consensual reflex is the constriction of the pupil as a normal response when a light is shone into the other eye.

midline hemisphere shift, or one or more surgical masses correlate with raised intracranial pressure and shortened survival.

Blood analyses

Up to 60% of all patients admitted in coma are drug users or alcoholics who have often had a head injury.

ASSESSMENT FOR OTHER INJURIES

Multiply injured patients can be assessed using the revised trauma score (RTS), calculated mainly from the GCS, the BP and the respiratory rate. Injuries can be categorized using the Abbreviated Injury Scale (AIS), which scores from minor (1) to fatal (6) injuries; the injury severity score (ISS) is calculated by the addition of the AIS for the three most severely injured areas of the body.

MEDICAL COMPLICATIONS OF HEAD INJURIES

Tetanus can be an issue in some head injuries (Ch. 21). Medical complications can arise since the brain controls many organs and processes via neurological and hormonal influences and can include: cardiovascular (neurogenic hypertension, myocardial dysfunction, arrhythmias or deep vein thrombosis); respiratory (neurogenic pulmonary oedema – a form of adult respiratory distress syndrome – infections, embolism); coagulopathy (disseminated intravascular coagulopathy); electrolyte imbalance (hyponatraemia, hypernatraemia or hypokalaemia); endocrine (inadequate or inappropriate secretion of ADH; Ch. 6); gastrointestinal (stress gastritis and haemorrhage); fat embolism (mainly where there have been long bone fractures); or infections (of wounds, foreign bodies, CSF, intravenous lines, intracranial pressure monitoring devices, sinuses and lungs).

LATE SEQUELAE OF HEAD INJURY

Late sequelae may include: chronic extradural or subdural haematomas; epilepsy (Ch. 13); infection (see earlier); mental or physical disability; compensation neurosis (Ch. 10); or post-traumatic syndrome (which may result from mild brain damage or damage to the cochlear–vestibular apparatus). Complaints include temporary headache, irritability, inability to concentrate, short temper, loss of confidence, vertigo and hyperacusis. If symptoms persist, psychiatric advice should be sought.

MAXILLOFACIAL INJURIES

Most maxillofacial injuries in the UK are due to interpersonal violence and most are in previously fit young men; alcohol or other drugs are frequently factors. Road traffic accidents are also a major cause and produce fractures that often involve the midface, especially in patients who were not wearing their seatbelts. Industrial accidents, sport and epilepsy are other causes. Other important causes of facial trauma include penetrating trauma and abuse (children and older individuals).

High-impact maxillofacial fractures often are associated with head and other bodily injuries that may be life-threatening. Patients are often multiply injured and may have hazards to the airway, head, cervical or thoracolumbar spine, eye, chest, liver, spleen, kidneys, long bones or bladder, and severe haemorrhage from massive midface injuries. Extensive soft tissue injuries or avulsions and comminuted fractures are difficult to treat and may have poor outcomes.

Low-impact maxillofacial fractures rarely result in mortality if proper treatment is administered.

The bones most commonly fractured are the nasal, zygoma, mandible and maxilla. Trauma to the maxillofacial area demands special attention since it may damage specialized functions including breathing, sight, hearing, smelling, eating and speech. This is especially the case with middle third facial fractures (particularly Le Fort III fractures). Also, the vital structures in the head and neck region are intimately associated. The psychological impact of disfigurement can be devastating.

Many fractures are reduced and fixed with mini-plates (Champy plates are almost never used currently) and/or intermaxillary fixation. Closed reduction, open reduction and endoscopic techniques may be employed (see textbooks of maxillofacial surgery).

The management of patients with maxillofacial injuries is similar to that of head and other severe injuries (Box 24.2).

Box 24.2 Initial management of maxillofacial trauma

- Maintain the airway
- Control haemorrhage
- Reduce fractures
- Prevent infection
- Maintain fluid balance

Special problems also arise because of mechanical interference with breathing and swallowing. Shock is most unusual in uncomplicated maxillofacial injuries or head injuries, and its presence is often an indication of internal haemorrhage. The possibility of pre-existing disease must always also be considered. The management is divided into: emergency, immediate or initial care; early primary care; and reconstructive phases (definitive care and secondary care or revision).

EMERGENCY CARE

As in any trauma situation, life-threatening injuries must immediately be addressed – airway establishment and maintenance, and control of haemorrhage have highest priority. A patent airway and an adequate fluid and nutritional intake can be difficult to achieve in maxillofacial injuries because of partial or complete obstruction of the respiratory or alimentary orifices. Altered level of consciousness is the most common cause of upper airway obstruction. Stabilize the cervical spine, which may be fractured, especially in any patient with injury above clavicle or head injury resulting in unconsciousness, or any injury produced by high speed. Despite the extensive vascularity of the head and neck, massive blood loss due to maxillofacial injuries is uncommon. Penetrating injuries need to be explored. A nasogastric tube may be needed for feeding in the immediate post-operative period if there are extensive intraoral wounds. Immediate and early assessment of maxillofacial trauma is summarized in Table 24.7. The reader should consult The Advanced Trauma Life Support Manual and similar guides for full details on this important topic.

EARLY CARE

The priorities of early management of a patient with maxillofacial and other injuries, especially if in coma, are as follows.

- Maintain a clear airway.
- Establish a neurological baseline from the history, consciousness level, examination and pupil reactions for future reference.
- Establish baseline BP, pulse and respiratory rates

Table 24.7 Maxillofacial trauma: immediate and early assessment

Step	Assess
Immediate care (ABC)	Airway and cervical spine Breathing and bleeding Chest injuries
General assessment	State of consciousness Pulse Blood pressure Respiratory rate Pupil size and reaction
Assessment of head injury	Skull examination Examination for cerebrospinal fluid leak Neurological assessment Skull radiography including CT Blood analyses
Assessment for other injuries	Chest Neck Spine Abdomen Perineum Limbs

---

- Exclude other serious injuries, head and neck, thorax and abdomen, other bones, CSF leak and eye injuries. The force necessary to create severe maxillofacial injuries is often significant enough to cause concomitant injury to CNS, spine, chest, abdomen, pelvis and/or extremities.
- Reduce and immobilize maxillofacial fractures only if they threaten the airway or there is severe haemorrhage. Definitive treatment must usually be delayed until the patient is out of danger, but early stabilization of grossly displaced or comminuted facial bone fragments may facilitate later management and lessen facial deformity. Avoid nasotracheal intubation in patients with upper face or upper midface fractures as it can result in nasocranial intubation or severe nasal haemorrhage. Avoid clamping blind in order to prevent injuries to vital structures.
- Treat soft tissue injuries early: large open wounds should be debrided and closed in a layered fashion promptly. Wounds that are to be used later for access to repair fractures, or are not a priority, may be closed in a temporary manner. Burns may be chemical or thermal, and their effect may be full or partial thickness. Lacerations result from the compression of the skin between the underlying bone (or teeth) and another object. The skin is crushed and or torn leading to an irregular skin edge injury. Incised wounds, in comparison to lacerations, are the result of cutting the skin with a knife or blade. In general the skin edges are less irregular than with lacerations; however, combinations of the two may coexist in the same injury. Nerve injuries in the maxillofacial region primarily affect the sensory (trigeminal) or motor (facial) nerves. In addition the nerves of the orbit (ophthalmic, oculomotor, trochlear and abducent) may also be injured. Rarely the other nerves of the head and neck may be injured. Facial fractures may compress or indirectly injure sensory nerves; typically zygomatico-orbital injuries lead to infraorbital and/or zygomatico-temporal or zygomatico-facial nerve

neuropraxias. Mandibular fractures often injure the inferior alveolar nerve along its course manifesting as mental nerve altered sensation. Facial nerve injuries manifest as weakness or paralysis of the muscles of facial expression. For those injuries that result from transections of the nerve between the facial canal and a line drawn between the lateral canthus and angle of the mouth, early microneural repair is indicated. Salivary gland injuries can lead to fistulas or sialoceles.

- Prevent infection. Because of the contiguity of the naso-oral passages and the perforating nature of these wounds, maxillofacial wounds are doubly exposed to contamination. Except for fractures of the ascending ramus, all fractures in which the periosteum is torn are compound and usually communicate with an internal mucous membrane wound and/or the external skin wound. Antibiotic therapy must be started early and maintained until fractures are immobilized (Table 24.8).

Table 24.8 Antimicrobial prophylaxis in facial injuries

Injuries	Antimicrobial if indicated
Compound fractures	Penicillin or, in penicillin allergy, clindamycin
Contaminated skin lacerations	Cefazolin
Contaminated oral lacerations	Clindamycin
Fractures communicating with antrum	Amoxicillin
Fractures with dural tears or CSF leaks	Co-amoxiclav, or cefuroxime with metronidazole or vancomycin and ceftazidime

CSF, cerebrospinal fluid.

- Oral hygiene, with particular attention to the teeth, is also necessary. Appropriate protective dressings are applied and hydration is maintained.
- Reconstruct. The reconstructive phase of care of maxillofacial injuries is discussed in textbooks of maxillofacial surgery; a few comments are included here. The maxillofacial region is divided into three parts: the upper face, where fractures involve the nasoethmoidal structures, frontal bone and sinus; the midface; the lower face, where fractures are isolated to the mandible. The upper midface is where Le Fort II and Le Fort III fractures occur and/or where fractures of the nasal bones, nasoethmoidal or zygomaticomaxillary complex, and the orbital floor occur. Le Fort I fractures are in the lower midface.
- A high-impact force is usually required to damage the supraorbital rim, mandible (symphysis and angle) and frontal bones. A low-impact force is all that is required to damage the zygoma and nasal bone.
- Pan-facial injuries management is usually by internal rigid fixation using plates-and-screws.

COMPLICATIONS OF MAXILLOFACIAL INJURIES

Infective problems

Meningitis is an important complication of opening the cranial cavity (shown by leakage of CSF), as discussed above. It is by far the most important infective complication of maxillofacial injuries and can also result from lacerations of the scalp when infection can reach the brain via the emissary veins.

Local wound infection and osteomyelitis risk is greater when there is inadequate wound toilet, foreign bodies in the wound, teeth in the fracture line, gross delay in treatment or systemic disease with diminished resistance to infection, particularly alcoholism. Extreme care must be taken to identify foreign material within the tissues; some types of glass and plastic, and all wood, are radiolucent and may be missed unless the wound is systematically probed. They may be identified on MRI. Gross debris, broken teeth, detached bone and foreign bodies should be removed. After preliminary wound toilet, lacerations can usually be sutured under LA. Larger lacerations can be covered with tulle gras and dry dressings for closure as soon as possible under GA. Teeth in the fracture line may need to be extracted unless required for stabilization of a bone fragment. Intramuscular benzyl penicillin or cefazolin are usually effective antimicrobial prophylaxis.

Tetanus (Ch. 21)

Actinomycosis (Ch. 21)

Ocular or orbital injuries

Zygomatic fractures or isolated orbital injuries may hazard vision. Diplopia (double vision) is common, often because of oedema and haemorrhage within the confined space of the orbit; circumorbital and subconjunctival ecchymoses are usually associated. Occasionally periorbital emphysema is present. Diplopia sometimes arises from enophthalmos associated with orbital floor or wall fractures, from muscle or nerve injury, or from muscle entrapment. Untreated orbital blowout fractures also depress the level of the eye (this may be concealed initially as intraorbital oedema maintains the level of the globe) and limit ocular movement, especially upwards.

The superior orbital fissure syndrome of ophthalmoplegia, ptosis, exophthalmos, a fixed dilated pupil or absence of consensual reflex, and some sensory loss over the distribution of the ophthalmic division of the trigeminal nerve, is caused by injury to cranial nerves III, IV, V and VI, where they pass through the orbital fissure. The syndrome may be caused by disruption of the bony margins of the superior orbital fissure, haematoma or traumatic aneurysm at this site.

In all patients with ocular or orbital injuries, the orbit should be imaged by CT for fracture and, if suspected, should undergo exploration and receive prophylaxis as recommended for penetrating intracranial wounds. If there are ocular injuries, an ophthalmological opinion should be sought as the eye can be lost or vision impaired.

BURNS

Burns can be serious injuries, especially where more than 10% of the body surface area is involved. First-aid care includes airway maintenance, oxygen administration if there has been exposure to hot air or smoke, and pain reduction by cooling the burn and giving analgesics such as morphine (5–15 mg for an adult). Subsequent treatment should be in a burns or plastic surgery unit.

After receiving burns in a closed or confined space, a change in voice, hoarseness, dysphonia, stridor or the coughing of sooty sputum are all signs suggesting inhalation injury; endotracheal intubation or tracheostomy may be indicated. Adult respiratory distress syndrome (ARDS), sometimes a sequel to burns and other pulmonary injury, is characterized by diffuse alveolar damage, pulmonary oedema and hyaline membrane formation, and may culminate in respiratory failure; mortality is high. Patients with a raised respiratory rate, abnormal breath sounds (rales) with bilateral diffuse interstitial and intra-alveolar oedema on radiography, should be admitted to an intensive care unit.

STAB AND OTHER PENETRATING WOUNDS

Stab wounds should always be treated with suspicion as a small entrance wound can hide injuries to deeper structures. Thus the wound may need to be explored carefully before closure, especially if in the chest, neck, back or abdomen. Radiographs are indicated especially where the wound is caused by glass, remembering that some glass is radiolucent.

Computed tomographic angiography (CTA) has altered the management of patients with penetrating injuries in the neck, with fewer formal neck explorations and virtual elimination of negative exploratory surgery.

GUNSHOT AND EXPLOSIVE WOUNDS

The management of gunshot wounds to the head and neck is covered in surgical texts (Fig. 24.6).

Traditionally, civilian injuries were inflicted with low-velocity weapons (90–210 m/s), while military wounds typically were caused by high-velocity weapons (610 m/s and up; Table 24.9).

Table 24.9 Gunshot wounds

Type of gun	Comment
Airgun	Can be left *in situ* if deep and not in orbit or causing damage
0.22 rifle	Can be left *in situ* if deep and not in orbit or causing damage
0.410 shotgun	May cause considerable damage at close range
Twelve-bore shotgun	Dangerous even from a distance; widespread damage
High-velocity bullets	Cause damage more extensive than initially evident
Explosive bullets	Cause damage more extensive than initially evident

Hand guns usually inflict low-velocity bullet wounds that damage only the tissues they hit. Such wounds can be managed by conventional surgical methods. Owing to medium- to high-velocity weapons appearing on the streets, more civilians are suffering from military-type injuries. High-velocity missiles (from rifles or explosive blast fragments) can cause extensive tissue damage and contamination, and have a mortality rate 4–5 times higher and thus require specialized attention. Though the entrance wounds may be minute, they can hide extremely severe wounds caused by the cavitation effect of rapid compression and expansion with extensive necrotic tissue contaminated with clostridia spores, other bacteria, clothing and debris. The kinetic energy is directly proportional to the mass of the projectile and proportional to the square of the velocity at which the bullet is travelling. The most efficient missile enters tissues and imparts the majority of its kinetic energy to surrounding structures without exiting the victim.

All patients with gunshot wounds should be imaged to locate the missiles. To avoid gas gangrene, high-velocity wounds must be treated by excision of the damaged tissue, and antibiotics, followed 4–5 days later by delayed primary closure and, if necessary, skin grafts. Consider tetanus risk (Ch. 21).

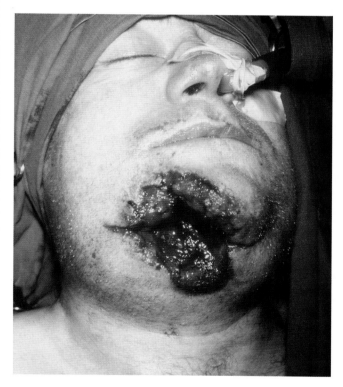

Fig. 24.6 Gunshot wound

HUMAN BITES

Human bites are more likely to cause infections than are animal bites (Ch. 33) since the oral flora contains many potentially pathogenic aerobic and anaerobic bacteria, among which are

Staphylococcus, *Streptococcus*, *Clostridia* (and other anaerobes), and fusiform species, as well as viruses. Tetanus is rarely a concern unless the wound is contaminated by soil. Hepatitis B, C and human immunodeficiency virus (HIV) are a concern, since they can be transmitted by bites both from biter to victim and the converse (see http://www.dh.gov.uk/en/Publicationsandstatistics/Publications/PublicationsPolicyAndGuidance/Browsable/DH_5368137).

Staff working in areas posing a significant risk of biting should not be treated as performing exposure-prone procedures (EPPs). In October 2003, the UK Advisory Panel considered a review of the available literature on the risk of onward transmission from health care workers infected with blood-borne viruses to patients. The review showed that the published literature on this subject is very scarce. In follow-up studies of incidents involving infected health care workers working with patients known to be 'regular and predictable' biters, there were no documented cases of transmission from the health care worker to the biter. However, where biters were infected, there were documented cases of seroconversion in their victims and the risk of infection was increased in the presence of:

- blood in the oral cavity – risk proportionate to the volume of blood
- broken skin due to the bite
- bite associated with previous injury (i.e. non-intact skin)
- biter deficient in anti-HIV salivary elements (IgA deficient).

Based on the available information, it can only be tentatively concluded that, even though there is a theoretical risk of transmission of a blood-borne virus from an infected health care worker to a biting patient, the risk remains negligible. The lack of information may suggest that this has not been perceived to be a problem to date, rather than that there is an absence of risk. UKAP has advised that, despite the theoretical risk, since there is no documented case of transmission from an infected health care worker to a biting patient, individuals infected with blood-borne viruses should not be prevented from working in or training for specialties where there is a risk of being bitten.

The evidence is dynamic and the area will be kept under review and updated in the light of any new evidence that subsequently emerges suggesting there is a risk. However, it is important for biting incidents to be reported and risk assessments conducted in accordance with NHS procedures. Biting poses a much greater risk to health care workers than to patients. Therefore employers should take measures to prevent injury to staff, and health care workers bitten by patients should seek advice and treatment, in the same way as after a needlestick injury.

Patients with hand infections from bite wounds may require hospital admission, antibiotics (co-amoxiclav most commonly), wound incision and drainage.

Any human bite could be abusive and therefore should be assessed, preferably by a forensic dentist (http://www.bafo.org.uk/). DNA should where possible be retrieved, and serial photographs and casts taken (Ch. 25).

SPINAL CORD INJURIES

Spinal cord injuries are a common result of road traffic or sports injuries. Cord injury is usually the result of vertical compression, sometimes with flexion or extension of the neck, or violent sudden extension of the neck (whiplash injury), as when a vehicle is hit from behind. The possibility of such damage should always be considered in patients involved in road traffic or contact sport accidents, since movement of the neck may then cause serious cord damage, spastic quadriplegia or death. The neck must therefore not be extended or rotated, and a support collar should be fitted prophylactically. Decompression by reduction of any vertebral dislocations should be carried out by the neurosurgeon within 2 h of injury. Spinal cord damage can be most incapacitating (Table 24.10).

Table 24.10 Effects of spinal cord damage	
Early (spinal shock): losses of	**Delayed (after 2–3 weeks):**
Motor function: quadriplegia if damage in cervical cord, paraplegia if damage in thoracic cord	Motor function may improve if cord not completely transected
Sensation below lesion, leading to skin pressure ulcers	Sensation may improve if cord not completely transected
Reflexes below lesion, with muscle flaccidity	Reflexes: involuntary flexor, then extensor spasms below level of lesion
Bladder and bowel sphincter control leading to urinary or faecal retention	Bladder and bowel sphincter control impaired causing irregular reflex micturition and defaecation

Most vertebral injuries affect the C1–2, C4–7 and T11–L2 vertebrae, the clinical sequelae being determined largely by the level of spinal cord damage, but the result can be fatal or appallingly severe disability (Table 24.11).

Traumatic atlanto-axial dislocation may be fatal. If not, there may only be weakness of the legs or even no immediate neurological sequelae. Transient blackouts, weakness of the limbs, sensory loss, facial paraesthesia, nystagmus, ataxia and dysarthria may be complaints. Atlanto-axial subluxation, or dislocation or fracture of the odontoid peg, may occur in other conditions such as congenital anomalies of the odontoid process (as in Down syndrome), rheumatoid arthritis or ankylosing spondylitis.

The clinical effects of spinal cord injury (SCI) develop in two main stages: spinal shock and reflex activity (Table 24.10). If movement can be elicited or any sensation is retained during the first 2–3 days, the prognosis is more favourable. Paraplegia is common but high doses of methylprednisolone given within 8 h of the injury may minimize cord damage. Any symptoms persisting after 6 months are likely to be permanent.

Most patients with thoracic cord injuries need wheelchairs. Mechanical bracing systems can restore upright mobility following SCI, and can improve bone density, urinary drainage, bowel function, spasticity, respiratory mechanics, contractures,

Table 24.11 Effects of spinal cord injuries at different levels

Level of spinal cord damage	Features
C1–C5	Quadriplegia (tetraplegia) or death
C5–C6	Paraplegia. Hands paralysed. Arms paralysed except for abduction and flexion
C6–C7	Paraplegia. Hands, but not arms, paralysed
T1	Paraplegia. Normal hand function. Patients can perform all functions of a non-injured person, with the exception of standing and walking
T2–T5	Paraplegia. Patients have partial trunk movement and may be able to stand, with long leg braces and a walker, and may be able to walk short distances with assistance
T6–T12	Paraplegia. Patients have partial abdominal muscle strength, and may be able to walk independently for short distances with long leg braces and a walker or crutches
T11–T12	Paraplegia. Sensory loss T12 and below
T12–L1	Legs paralysed below knees
L2	Patients have all movement in the trunk and hips
L3	Patients have knee extension
L4	Patients have ankle dorsiflexion
L5	Patients have extensor hallucis longus function. They are able to walk independently with ankle braces and canes, and may use wheelchairs for long distances
S1–S2	Patients have function of the gastrocnemius and soleus muscles and walk independently on all surfaces, usually without bracing

and psychological health, but are perceived by some to be less safe and more difficult to use than wheelchairs.

Most patients with injuries at or below the lumbar level are wheelchair-independent and may be able to walk independently with long leg braces and crutches.

GENERAL MANAGEMENT OF PARAPLEGICS

Treatment in general is supportive and symptomatic, and mainly directed toward the prevention of complications such as muscle wasting or contractures, pressure sores (bed sores), postural hypotension, urinary infections, constipation or psychological problems.

Physiotherapy is essential to limit muscle wasting and to maintain function in un-paralysed or partly paralysed muscles. Joints must be regularly passively moved and the position of the patient carefully checked to prevent soft tissue contractures and pressure sores.

Postural hypotension and autonomic dysreflexia can complicate high-level spinal cord lesions. Intense vasoconstriction below the level of the cord injury follows certain stimuli such as bladder contraction. The vasoconstriction is associated with rapid onset of hypertension, facial sweating and headache.

Urinary retention invariably complicates acute spinal cord lesions, and aseptic catheterization is needed. Infections must be treated promptly. Recurrent urinary infections were previously the main factor in renal disease and amyloidosis complicating paraplegia. Latex allergy commonly develops in such patients.

Dental aspects

Access to health care is a major problem since patients are at least chairbound. Dental management may be uncomplicated, although postural hypotension in the early stages may necessitate treatment in the upright position and latex allergy should be considered (Ch. 17). Quadriplegics are at risk from respiratory infections, so that GA should be avoided if possible. Other problems are dealt with in Ch. 13.

PREVENTION OF TRAUMA

Many of the problems caused by trauma could be avoided by abstention from drug and alcohol use and risky behaviour, and the use of body protection and application of health and safety laws and regulations in dangerous occupations, sports and other activities (Fig. 24.7).

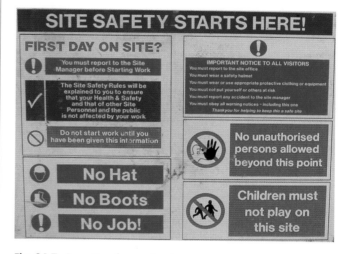

Fig. 24.7 Prevention of occupational trauma

USEFUL WEBSITES

http://www.cmsllc.com/toptrm.html
http://www.merck.com/mmpe/index.html
http://calder.med.miami.edu/providers/MEDICINE/parap.html
http://en.wikipedia.org/wiki/Stabbing

FURTHER READING

Andreasen, J.O., Storgård Jensen, S., Kofod, T., Schwartz, O., Hillerup, S., 2008. Open or closed repositioning of mandibular fractures: is there a difference in healing outcome? A systematic review. Dent Traumatol 24, 17–21.

Assael, L.A., 2003. Managing the trauma pandemic: learning from the past. J Oral Maxillofac Surg 61, 859–860.

Bagheri, S.C., Khan, H.A., Bell, R.B., 2008. Penetrating neck injuries. Oral Maxillofac Surg Clin North Am 20, 393–414.

Bell, R.B., Verschueren, D.S., Dierks, E.J., 2008. Management of laryngeal trauma. Oral Maxillofac Surg Clin North Am 20, 415–430.

Bellander, B.M., Sollid, S., Kock-Jensen, C., et al., 2008. Prehospital management of patients with severe head injuries. Scandinavian guidelines according to Brain Trauma Foundation Lakartidningen 105, 1834–1838 [In Swedish].

Ben-Galim, P.J., Sibai, T.A., Hipp, J.A., Heggeness, M.H., Reitman, C.A., 2008. Internal decapitation: survival after head to neck dissociation injuries. Spine 33, 1744–1749.

Bissada, E., Chacra, Z.A., Ahmarani, C., Poirier, J., Rahal, A., 2008. Orbito-zygomatic complex fracture reduction under local anesthesia and light oral sedation. J Oral Maxillofac Surg 66, 1378–1382.

Boyd, B.C., 2002. Automobile supplemental restraint system-induced injuries. Oral Surg Oral Med Oral Pathol Oral Radiol Endod 94, 143–148.

Brookes, C.N., 2004. Maxillofacial and ocular injuries in motor vehicle crashes. Ann R Coll Surg Engl 86, 149–155.

Brookes, C., Wang, S., McWilliams, J., 2003. Maxillofacial injuries in North American vehicle crashes. Eur J Emerg Med 10, 30–34.

Cavalcanti, A.L., Melo, T.R., 2008. Facial and oral injuries in Brazilian children aged 5–17 years: 5-year review. Eur Arch Paediatr Dent 9, 102–104.

Chen, C.H., Wang, T.Y., Tsay, P.K., et al., 2008. A 162-case review of palatal fracture: management strategy from a 10-year experience. Plast Reconstr Surg 121 (6), 2065–2073.

Cox, D., Vincent, D.G., McGwin, G., MacLennan, P.A., Holmes, J.D., Rue 3rd, L.W., 2004. Effect of restraint systems on maxillofacial injury in frontal motor vehicle collisions. J Oral Maxillofac Surg 62, 571–575.

Cunningham, L.L., Haug, R.H., Ford, J., 2003. Firearm injuries to the maxillofacial region: an overview of current thoughts regarding demographics, pathophysiology, and management. J Oral Maxillofac Surg 61, 932–942.

Ducic, Y., 2008. Endoscopic treatment of subcondylar fractures. Laryngoscope 118, 1164–1167.

Ellis 3rd, E., Miles, B.A., 2007. Fractures of the mandible: a technical perspective. Plast Reconstr Surg 120 (7 Suppl 2), 76S–89S.

Ellis 3rd, E., Muniz, O., Anand, K., 2003. Treatment considerations for comminuted mandibular fractures. J Oral Maxillofac Surg 61, 861–870.

Espinosa-Aguilar, A., Reyes-Morales, H., Huerta-Posada, C.E., et al., 2008. Design and validation of a critical pathway for hospital management of patients with severe traumatic brain injury. J Trauma. 64, 1327–1341.

Ferreira, P., Marques, M., Pinho, C., Rodrigues, J., Reis, J., Amarante, J., 2004. Midfacial fractures in children and adolescents: a review of 492 cases. Br J Oral Maxillofac Surg 42, 501–505.

Fraioli, R.E., Branstetter 4th, B.F., Deleyiannis, F.W., 2004. Facial factures: beyond Le Fort. Otolaryngol Clin North Am 41, 51–76, vi.

Francis, D.O., Kaufman, R., Yueh, B., Mock, C., Nathens, A.B., 2006. Air bag-induced orbital blow-out fractures. Laryngoscope 116, 1966–1972.

Frodel Jr, J.L., 2008. Dealing with the difficult trauma and reconstructive surgery patient. Facial Plast Surg Clin North Am 16, 225–231, vii–viii.

Gasparini, G., Brunelli, A., Rivaroli, A., Lattanzi, A., De Ponte, F.S., 2002. Maxillofacial traumas. J Craniofac Surg 13, 645–649.

Gibbons, A.J., Patton, D.W., 2003. Ballistic injuries of the face and mouth in war and civil conflict. Dent Update 30, 272–278.

Haug, R.H., Brandt, M.T., 2007. Closed reduction, open reduction, and endoscopic assistance: current thoughts on the management of mandibular condyle fractures. Plast Reconstr Surg 120 (7 Suppl 2), 90S–102S.

Haug, R.H., Foss, J., 2000. Maxillofacial injuries in the pediatric patient. Oral Surg 90, 126–134.

Hawkins, S.C., 2003. Saving face: identification and management of facial fractures. J Emerg Med Serv JEMS 28, 72–87.

Hermund, N.U., Hillerup, S., Kofod, T., Schwartz, O., Andreasen, J.O., 2008. Effect of early or delayed treatment upon healing of mandibular fractures: a systematic literature review. Dent Traumatol 24, 22–26.

Kim, J.M., Kim, K.O., Kim, Y.D., Choi, G.J., 2004. A case of air-bag associated severe ocular injury. Korean J Ophthalmol 18, 84–88.

Krishnan, B., El Sheikh, M.H., 2008. Dental forceps reduction of depressed zygomatic arch fractures. J Craniofac Surg 19, 782–784.

Krohner, R.G., 2003. Anesthetic considerations and techniques for oral and maxillofacial surgery. Int Anesthesiol Clin 41, 67–89.

Landes, C.A., Day, K., Glasl, B., Ludwig, B., Sader, R., Kovács, A.F., 2008. Prospective evaluation of closed treatment of nondisplaced and nondislocated mandibular condyle fractures versus open reposition and rigid fixation of displaced and dislocated fractures in children. J Oral Maxillofac Surg 66, 1184–1193.

Levin, L., Zadik, Y., Peleg, K., Bigman, G., Givon, A., Lin, S., 2008. Incidence and severity of maxillofacial injuries during the Second Lebanon Waramong Israeli soldiers and civilians. J Oral Maxillofac Surg 66, 1630–1633.

Lin, K.C., Chou, C.H., Chang, W.L., Ke, D.S., Kuo, J.R., 2008. The early response of mannitol infusion in traumatic brain injury. Acta Neurol Taiwan 17, 26–32.

Macciocchi, S., Seel, R.T., Thompson, N., Byams, R., Bowman, B., 2008. Spinal cord injury and co-occurring traumatic brain injury: assessment and incidence. Arch Phys Med Rehabil 89, 1350–1357.

Major, M.S., MacGregor, A., Bumpous, J.M., 2000. Patterns of maxillofacial injuries as a function of automobile restraint use. Laryngoscope 110, 608–611.

Mitchener, T.A., Hauret, K.G., Hoedebecke, E.L., Darakjy, S., Jones, B.H., 2008. Air medical evacuations of soldiers due to oral-facial disease and injuries. Operations Enduring Freedom/Iraqi Freedom. Mil Med 173, 465–473.

Mitra, B., Cameron, P.A., Gabbe, B.J., Rosenfeld, J.V., Kavar, B., 2008. Management and hospital outcome of the severely head injured elderly patient. ANZ J Surg 78, 588–592.

Moos, K.F., 2002. Diagnosis of facial bone fractures. Ann R Coll Surg Engl 84, 429–431.

Mouzakes, J., Koltai, P.J., Kuhar, S., Bernstein, D.S., Wing, P., Salsberg, E., 2001. The impact of airbags and seat belts on the incidence and severity of maxillofacial injuries in automobile accidents in New York State. Arch Otolaryngol Head Neck Surg 127, 1189–1193.

Newlands, S.D., Samudrala, S., Katzenmeyer, W.K., 2003. Surgical treatment of gunshot injuries to the mandible. Otolaryngol Head Neck Surg 129, 239–244.

Nussbaum, M.L., Laskin, D.M., Best, A.M., 2008. Closed versus open reduction of mandibular condylar fractures in adults: a meta-analysis. J Oral Maxillofac Surg 66, 1087–1092.

Ocak, G., Sturms, L.M., Hoogeveen, J.M., Le Cessie, S., Jukema, G.N., 2009. Prehospital identification of major trauma patients. Langenbecks Arch Surg 394, 285–292.

Osborn, T.M., Bell, R.B., Qaisi, W., Long, W.B., 2008. Computed tomographic angiography as an aid to clinical decision making in the selective management of penetrating injuries to the neck: a reduction in the need for operative exploration. J Trauma 64, 1466–1471.

Plurad, D., Demetriades, D., Gruzinski, G., et al., 2008. Motor vehicle crashes: the association of alcohol consumption with the type and severity of injuries and outcomes. J Emerg Med Jun 10 [Epub ahead of print].

Ramesh, V.G., Thirumaran, K.P., Raja, M.C., 2008. A new scale for prognostication in head injury. J Clin Neurosci 15, 1110–1114.

Rezende-Neto, J., Marques, A.C., Guedes, L.J., Teixeira, L.C., 2008. Damage control principles applied to penetrating neck and mandibular injury. J Trauma 64, 1142–1143.

Rodriguez, E.D., Martin, M., Bluebond-Langner, R., Khalifeh, M., Singh, N., Manson, P.N., 2007. Microsurgical reconstruction of posttraumatic high-energy maxillary defects: establishing the effectiveness of early reconstruction. Plast Reconstr Surg 120 (7 Suppl 2), 103S–117S.

Schütz, P., Hamed, H.H., 2008. Submental intubation versus tracheostomy in maxillofacial trauma patients. J Oral Maxillofac Surg 66, 1404–1409.

Strauss, E., Slick, D.J., Levy-Bencheton, J., Hunter, M., MacDonald, S.W., Hultsch, D.F., 2002. Intraindividual variability as an indicator of malingering in head injury. Arch Clin Neuropsychol 17, 423–444.

Thomas, J., Rideau, A.M., Paulson, E.K., Bisset 3rd, G.S., 2008. Emergency department imaging: current practice. J Am Coll Radiol 5, 811–816e2.

Undén, J., Ingebrigtsen, T., Romner, B., 2008. Management of minor head injuries with the help of a blood test. S100B analysis can reduce the number of CT examinations and patient admissions Lakartidningen. 105, 1846–1848 [In Swedish].

von Elm, E., Osterwalder, J.J., Graber, C., et al., 2008. Severe traumatic brain injury in Switzerland – feasibility and first results of a cohort study. Swiss Med Wkly 138, 327–334.

Yokoyama, T., Motozawa, Y., Sasaki, T., Hitosugi, M., 2006. A retrospective analysis of oral and maxillofacial injuries in motor vehicle accidents. J Oral Maxillofac Surg 64, 1731–1735.

Zaglia, E., De Leo, D., Lanzara, G., Urbani, U., Dolci, M., 2007. Occipital condyle fracture: an unusual airbag injury. J Forensic Leg Med 14, 231–234.

Appendix 24.1 Causes of coma

- Acute disseminated encephalomyelitis
- Addison disease
- African sleeping sickness
- Alcohol poisoning
- Asphyxia
- Brain compression
- Brain infection
- Brain inflammation
- Chagas disease
- Concussion
- Creutzfeldt–Jakob disease
- Diabetic ketoacidosis
- Eclampsia
- Ehrlichiosis
- Encephalitis
- Head trauma
- Heatstroke
- Hepatitis
- High-altitude cerebral oedema
- HIV/AIDS
- Hyperparathyroidism
- Hypothermia
- Japanese encephalitis
- Kidney failure
- Lead poisoning
- Liver failure
- Melioidosis
- Meningitis
- Mountain sickness
- Poisoning
- Progressive multifocal leukoencephalopathy
- Pulmonary embolism
- Reye syndrome
- Rift Valley fever
- Rocky Mountain spotted fever
- Shock
- Streptococcal toxic shock syndrome
- Stroke
- Subarachnoid haemorrhage
- Toxoplasmosis
- Typhoid fever
- Viral haemorrhagic fevers
- Yellow fever

SECTION D

OTHER HEALTH ISSUES

CHILDREN

GENERAL ASPECTS

In the UK, people up to the age of 16 years are regarded as children. At birth they are classified as premature or preterm (less than 37 weeks' gestation), full-term (37–42 weeks' gestation), or post-dates (born after 42 weeks' gestation).

PREMATURE BABIES

About 5–10% of all births are preterm. In about 40% of cases the cause is unknown, but it may be iatrogenic, that is, elective delivery due to pregnancy complications such as pre-eclampsia (maternal hypertension, fluid retention and proteinuria) or placenta praevia (low-lying placenta). Predictors are shown in Table 25.1. Maternal periodontal infection may possibly also be a risk factor.

Table 25.1   Predictors of preterm birth

Primary predictors	Secondary predictors
Black race	Anaemia
Chronic kidney disease	Bacterial vaginosis
Chronic respiratory disease	Chorioamnionitis
Cigarette smoking	Hydramnios
Depression	Inadequate pre-natal care
Diabetes mellitus	IVF
Domestic violence	Low maternal weight gain
Family history	Multiple fetuses
Hypertension	Pre-eclampsia
Inflammatory gene polymorphism	Raised fibronectin,
Low BMI	alpha-fetoprotein, alkaline
Low SES	phosphatase or granulocyte
Previous pre-term birth or abortion	colony-stimulating factor
Stress	Vaginal bleeding
Substance abuse	
Young mother	

BMI, body mass index, IVF, *in vitro* fertilization; SES, socioeconomic status.

Pre-term babies usually have a low birthweight (< 2500 g). Dependent on their degree of prematurity, they may suffer apnoea or irregular breathing, a weak cry, inactivity, ineffective sucking and swallowing (with poor feeding), shiny wrinkled skin with fine body hair (lanugo), soft, flexible ear cartilage, enlarged clitoris (female) or a small scrotum (male). Preterm babies are less able to maintain body temperature and haemostasis, and are prone to several health consequences (Table 25.2). Up to a half suffer long-term sequelae including low IQ, behavioural disorders, coordination problems, respiratory and feeding problems.

Low birthweight may also result from intrauterine growth retardation. Causes include multiple pregnancy, infection, maternal smoking, pre-eclampsia, severe anaemia, and heart and renal disease; these babies may go on to have lower IQs and smaller stature.

Table 25.2   Possible consequences of preterm birth

Early	Long-term
Bronchopulmonary dysplasia (BPD)	Attention deficit disorder
Hypocalcaemia	Cerebral palsy
Hypoglycaemia	Hearing impairment
Intraventricular brain haemorrhage or	Learning impairment
periventricular infarction	Retinopathy
Necrotizing enterocolitis	
Neonatal jaundice	
Patent ductus arteriosus	
Respiratory distress syndrome	
(RDS; hyaline membrane disease)	
Sepsis	

NEONATES

A neonate is a newborn infant up to 1 month old. Neonate behaviour is characterized by six states of consciousness: quiet sleep, active sleep, drowsy waking, quiet alert, fussing and active crying. The amount a healthy infant cries in the first 3 months varies from 1 to 3 hours a day. Periodic breathing is normal. Temperature control, skin colour, stooling, yawning, gagging, hiccoughing, vomiting and sleep are easily affected by stress and stimulation. Sleep/wake cycles occur in random intervals of 30–50 min and gradually increase as the child matures. By 4 months old, most infants will have one long period of uninterrupted sleep and breathing stabilizes. The neonate can see objects within a range of 8–12 inches, has excellent colour vision, can track moving objects up to 180 degrees, and sees faces. Infants prefer the frequencies of the human voice. Senses of hearing, touch, taste and smell are mature at birth. Vestibular senses are also mature and the infant responds to rocking and changes of position.

During the neonatal period, most congenital defects (e.g. congenital heart disease) are detected. Congenital infections (e.g. rubella, herpesviruses, toxoplasmosis) may manifest. Immunological immaturity predisposes to candidosis: infections may be transmitted by parents or carers, or from the environment; even tongue spatulas can be a source of infection.

This is a period of rapid growth and development. Facial, skull, jaw and tooth development can be impaired by radiotherapy, by chemotherapy, and by some immunosuppressants during this period. Oropharyngeal or orogastric intubation may result in palatal grooving, acquired cleft palate and damage to the deciduous dentition. Appliances can be constructed to protect against this damage.

INFANTS

The first year of life is infancy. The healthy infant possesses a number of primitive reflexes (Table 25.3).

Physical development begins at the head, then progresses to other parts (sucking precedes sitting, which precedes walking). Mental and neurological functions develop, with gross motor (e.g. head control, sitting, walking), fine motor (e.g. holding a spoon, pincer grasp), sensory, language and social development. There are several recognised 'milestones' in development, recognized as shown in Table 25.4.

Table 25.3 Infant normal reflexes

Reflexes	Composition
Babinski reflex	Toes fan when sole of foot is stroked
Moro reflex	On momentarily releasing the head from a supported sitting position, the arms abduct, the hands open and then the arms adduct
Palmar hand grasp	Closure over finger
Plantar grasp	Flexion of toe and forefoot
Rooting and sucking	Turns head in search for nipple when cheek is touched and begins to suck when nipple touches lips
Stepping and walking	Takes brisk steps when both feet placed on a surface, with body supported
Tonic neck response	Leg extends on side of head direction, flexion occurs in opposite arm and leg

THE CHILD FROM 1 YEAR (PRE-SCHOOL CHILD)

Development proceeds with gross motor development shown by milestones (see Table 25.5), as the child becomes able to stand alone, stoop, pick something up and recover to standing (toddler). Young children strive constantly for independence, creating not only special safety concerns, but also discipline challenges.

CHILDREN AGED 5–12 YEARS (SCHOOLCHILD)

School-age children typically have fairly good gross motor skills, but there is wide variance in coordination, endurance, balance, physical tolerance and fine motor skills. They are usually able to use simple, complete, short sentences consistently. Receptive language skills necessary to understand long or complex instructions and the use of increasingly complex sentences develop. Delayed language development may indicate hearing or learning impairment.

The attention span increases from about 15 min in 5-year-olds to about an hour by the age of 10. By about 10 years old, most children can follow five commands in a row.

PUBERTY

Puberty refers to the physical and psychological changes by which a child matures into an adult capable of reproduction, manifest by the development of secondary sexual characteristics. It begins between 9 and 16 years of age, but children vary as to when. On average, girls enter puberty 2 years earlier than boys.

The hypothalamus and pituitary gland hormones that control growth and maturation at puberty trigger rapid growth, with increases in height and weight, and the appearance of secondary sexual characteristics and increased sexual interest ('sex drive').

Table 25.4 Developmental milestones in infancy

Months	Milestones		
0–2	Infant can lift and turn its head when lying on its back	Cannot support the head upright when held in a sitting position	Has fisted hands and flexed arms
3–4	Can track objects and discriminate objects from backgrounds with minimal contrast	Can sit, with support, and keep the head up. Can raise upper torso and head when prone	Hand and feet actions start to come under willed control and reflexes have disappeared, or are in the process of so doing
5–6	Begins to grasp objects using ulnar–palmar grasp	Rolls from supine to prone position and starts to sit alone, without support, for short periods	
6–9	May pull self into standing position while holding on to furniture; can walk while holding the hand of an adult	Able to sit steadily without support, for long periods	Learns to sit down from standing position
9–12	Begins to balance while standing alone	Takes steps and begins to walk alone	Says mum and dad

Table 25.5 Developmental milestones in early (pre-school) childhood

Months	Milestones		
14–15	Child is walking well by 14 months and learns to walk backwards and up steps	Begins to scribble and can place a block in a cup and begin to stack blocks	Can use 2–3 words (other than mum or dad)
16–18	Able to kick a ball forward; at about 18–24 months is able to throw ball overhand	Can combine two words	
22–24	Can jump	Can often state their name	Able to point to named body parts and to name pictures of items and animals

The sweat glands become more active and produce sweat with more of an odour. Oil glands become more active and acne may appear.

In girls, the ovaries begin to increase oestrogen production (along with other 'female' hormones). Girls experience rapid growth in height and increased hip width, breast enlargement, pubic, axillary and leg hair growth and vaginal secretions followed by the onset of menstrual periods (menarche). The ovaries begin to release ova that, over 3 or 4 days, travel along the Fallopian tubes to the uterus. Meanwhile, the endometrium (uterine lining) thickens by filling with blood and fluid. If the ovum is not fertilized, it dissolves and the endometrium sloughs, causing menstruation (mexses). Menstrual cycles occur over about 1 month (28–32 days) and may be irregular initially. There may also be cyclical hormonal and physical changes such as emotional or depressive reactions – the premenstrual syndrome (PMS) – and cramping menstrual pain. In girls, full physical maturation is usually complete by age 17, but educational and emotional maturity is ongoing.

In boys, the testicles increase testosterone production so that puberty usually occurs between 13 and 15 years of age. The pubescent boy experiences accelerated growth, especially in height, shoulder width and growth of penis and testicles, and voice changes along with growth of pubic, beard and axillary hair. Sperm is manufactured constantly in the testes (a process termed spermatogenesis) and is stored in the epididymis. This is released following masturbation or sexual intercourse or during sleep, when it is known as a nocturnal emission or a 'wet dream'.

ADOLESCENCE

Adolescence refers to the transition from child to adult, between 13 and 19 years of age. As well as sexual maturation, there are psychological changes resulting in emotional, behavioural and social changes. Specific health concerns for this age group are shown in Box 25.1.

Box 25.1 Adolescents: health concerns

- Accidental injuries [leading cause of death (70%) from motor vehicle accidents, drowning or poisoning (usually drug or alcohol related)]
- Unlawful killing, often gang related (second leading cause of death)
- Suicide (third leading cause of death)
- Substance abuse
- Stress, depression, eating disorders
- Sexually transmitted diseases
- Pregnancy
- Assaults (gang related)

GENERAL MANAGEMENT

Children rely on parents for protection from harm. Accidents are the major cause of morbidity and mortality: children are at increased risk because of a need for strenuous physical activity, a desire for peer approval and increased adventurous behaviour. Continued emphasis upon wearing seat-belts remains the single intervention most capable of preventing major injury

or death due to a motor vehicle accident. Children should be taught to play sports in appropriate, safe, supervised areas, with proper equipment and rules, and with safety equipment (such as a bicycle and other safety helmets, knee, elbow, wrist pads/braces, etc.). Safety instruction regarding contact sports, vehicle use, swimming and water sports, matches, fires, lighters and cooking are important to prevent accidents.

DENTAL ASPECTS

Care of children is discussed fully in textbooks of paediatric dentistry. Important issues include consent; the treatment of trauma, caries and malocclusion; and issues related to anaesthesia and sedation.

Informed consent can be difficult to ensure in children too young to understand but conversely may be possible in some children under age 16 (Gillick competence). Children may present behavioural challenges in dental treatment: relative analgesia and local anaesthesia (LA) may be difficult or impossible to administer to some. Some drugs are contraindicated in childhood (Table 25.6). Children may also have some unusual reactions to drugs, such as diazepam and intravenous anaesthetics.

Drug doses should be checked in the paediatric British National Formulary and adjusted for weight as necessary. All drug doses must be lowered for children and sugar-free preparations used.

After the eruption of the teeth, drugs that cause xerostomia and procedures such as radiotherapy involving the salivary glands predispose to caries, especially in children. Preventive dental care and dietary counselling are of crucial importance.

Lengthening survival rates of premature infants have revealed several long-term sequelae, including orofacial defects. Some 20–55% have enamel hypoplasia, compared with 2% of controls, caused by birth trauma, infections, metabolic or nutritional disorders. Calcium disturbances are also common. Laryngoscopy can damage the unerupted maxillary anterior teeth and intubation with an oropharyngeal tube can cause grooving of the anterior maxillary ridge. The latter has few serious consequences.

Disturbed orofacial development can result from a range of causes in childhood, including radiotherapy, chemotherapy, drugs, infections or toxins. Disturbed odontogenesis can

Table 25.6 Drugs that may be contraindicated in children

Drug contraindicated	Possibility of
Antidepressants	Suicide attempts
Aspirin (salicylates)	Reye syndrome
Diazepam	Paradoxical reactions
Kaopectate	Reye syndrome
Promethazine	Drowsiness and respiratory depression
Propofol	Propofol syndrome
Tetracyclines	Tooth discoloration

have similar causes. Children may also be the subjects of abuse resulting in orofacial and other injuries.

CHILD ABUSE (BATTERED CHILD SYNDROME; NON-ACCIDENTAL INJURY; NAI)

General aspects

Up to 50% of children sustain injuries to their mouth by the time they leave school – mostly from accidents. The head and face are also the areas, however, most commonly affected in physical abuse: they are involved in 65% of cases.

Child abuse is any act of omission or commission that endangers or impairs the physical or emotional health or development of a child. The threshold beyond which actions or omissions become abusive or neglectful is, to a certain extent, socially and culturally defined. A child is considered to be abused if he or she is treated in a way that is unacceptable in a given culture at a given time. For example, physical punishment of children has become progressively less acceptable in the UK in recent years.

Abuse and neglect are described in four categories, as defined in the Department of Health's document 'Working Together to Safeguard Children' – physical, emotional, sexual abuse and neglect. Some level of emotional abuse is involved in all types of ill-treatment of a child, though it may occur alone. Physical abuse may involve hitting, shaking, throwing, poisoning, burning or scalding, drowning, suffocating or otherwise causing physical harm to a child. Physical harm may also be caused when a parent or carer fabricates the symptoms of, or deliberately causes illness in a child.

Children affected are usually < 1 year; most are under 3 years of age. The injuries are usually inflicted by an adult, often a parent or parent's partner or an older sibling, and affected families are predominantly of socioeconomic classes IV and V. Causal factors may be related either to the parent, social factors or the child – often all (Table 25.7).

Table 25.7 Non-accidental injury: associated factors

Parental	Social	Child
Marital disharmony	Poor housing	Abnormal pregnancy or delivery
Emotionally deprived, abused themselves	Poverty	Neonatal separation
Chronic physical illness		Unwanted
Low intelligence	Social isolation	Hyperactive, ill or aggressive
Young age or single parents		Stepchild
Drug/alcohol dependence		< 1 year of age
Mental disorders		

Young or single parents, parents with learning difficulties, those who themselves have experienced adverse childhoods and those with mental health problems (including drug or alcohol abuse) are all more at risk of abusing their children. The assaulter may be supported by an inactive partner. Families living in adverse social environments, for example due to poverty, social isolation or poor housing, may also find it both materially and socially harder to care for their children. Children with disabilities are much more at risk of experiencing abuse of all kinds.

Clinical features

Recognition of child abuse is important since there is a very high risk of further assaults on, or death of, the child and of siblings: some 35–60% of physically abused children suffer further injury, with a 5–10% mortality rate. The child who has been subjected to abuse is often cowed, may also be malnourished and generally neglected, and there may be evidence of previous trauma. Some suffer significant neurological, intellectual or emotional damage. There may be delay in seeking care (Box 25.2).

Box 25.2 Findings suggestive of non-accidental injury

- Cowed child
- Long interval before attendance for treatment
- Evidence of previous injury (or a previous history of injury)
- Injuries often committed at night
- Multiple injuries incompatible with history at unusual sites

---

The injuries in child abuse can be varied and are often multiple, including bite marks (Ch. 24), bruises, black eyes, torn frenulum, hair loss, laceration, weals, ligature marks, marks from a gag, burns and scalds often from cigarettes or demarcated from other objects. Lacerations of the upper labial mucosa and tearing of the lip from the gingiva are found in about 45% of victims but are not diagnostic of child abuse.

Teeth may be devitalized, broken or lost. Bone fractures are common – mainly affecting ribs or long bones – but the skull and jaws can also be fractured. Head injuries are the commonest cause of death in abused children.

General management

After genuine accidents, children are usually immediately taken for medical or dental attention but, when children are abused, there is often considerable delay. Child abuse should also be suspected if any injuries are incompatible with the history and if any of the features in Box 25.2 are noted. Health care professionals are obliged to know and follow the local child protection procedures (see http://www.cpdt.org.uk/). Full records must be kept. The child must be fully and immediately examined to exclude serious injury, especially subdural haematomas or intraocular bleeding, and must therefore be admitted to hospital. A skeletal radiographic survey should be undertaken to reveal both new and old injuries (osteogenesis imperfecta may need to be excluded). All injuries including facial and oral tissues must be carefully recorded, preferably with photographs.

Patients should be kept in hospital until the diagnosis is confirmed, since there is a high risk of further injury which may be fatal. A paediatrician should be consulted and the general medical practitioner, social services and a child protection agency must be involved early on, but strict confidentiality must be observed. Social services departments keep registers of non-accidental injuries, which help identify known offenders. The child may already be on the 'at-risk' register. The dentist should also inform their Medical Defence Society as there may later be legal involvement.

Dental aspects

Orofacial lesions are common. Abuse or neglect may present in a number of different ways, such as through a direct allegation (sometimes termed a 'disclosure') made by the child, a parent or some other person; signs and symptoms that are suggestive of physical abuse or neglect; or through observations of child behaviour or parent–child interaction.

SEXUAL ABUSE

Sexual abuse can take many forms but, in addition to physical and psychological injury, the victim may also acquire one or more sexually transmitted infection, including human immunodeficiency virus (HIV).

EMOTIONAL ABUSE

Emotional abuse is more difficult to define and prove, but can manifest as development delay, failure to thrive, a watchful 'radar' gaze, behavioural problems and limited attention span.

SELF-INFLICTED (FACTITIOUS) ORAL LESIONS (CH. 10)

OLDER PEOPLE
GENERAL ASPECTS

Older people now account for some 15% of the UK population and this is set to increase. A growing proportion of the population, especially in developed countries, is over the age of 65 (a chronological criterion of 'elderly'), with a rise in the proportion of older females, a significant number of whom are single (Fig. 25.1).

Many older people enjoy *la troisième age* but, over the years, they are increasingly likely to need health care (Table 25.8). Up to 75% have one or more chronic diseases (30% have more than three), 11% are housebound, 8% walk with difficulty and some 3% are bedridden. Problems may be compounded if they are from non-dominant populations (Fig. 25.2: Ch. 30).

MEDICAL PROBLEMS

Many older patients have difficulty in accessing health care and some are reluctant to seek attention, especially if they fear consequent hospitalization. There is a greater incidence and severity of many diseases, especially arthritis, and cerebrovascular disease, and these may cause ataxia and falls (Table 25.9). Fractures and bruising may result, and senile purpura is common in many older people (Fig. 25.3). Defects of hearing or sight increase the liability to accidents, feeling of isolation and

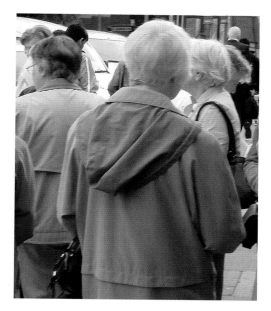

Fig. 25.1 The grey age

Table 25.8 Approximate number of years that older people are likely to be free from disability		
Age group	Men	Women
65–69	9	11
70–74	7	9
75–79	5	7
80–84	3	5
85+	1	3

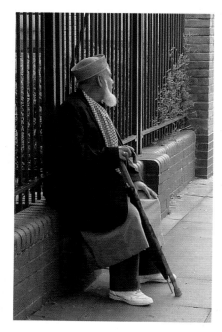

Fig. 25.2 Old age and culture

Table 25.9   Diseases especially affecting the older person^a

Blood and others	Cardiorespiratory	Genitourinary	Musculoskeletal	Neurological and psychiatric	Oral or predominantly oral
Accidents Anaemia (especially pernicious anaemia) Cancer Chronic leukaemia Myelodysplasia Nutritional deficiencies	Cardiac failure Chronic bronchitis, and emphysema Hypertension Ischaemic heart disease Pneumonia Temporal arteritis	Prostatic hypertrophy and cancer Renal failure Urinary retention or incontinence	Osteoarthritis Osteoporosis Paget disease	Acute confusional states Alzheimer disease Ataxia Dependence on hypnotics Insomnia Loneliness and depression Multi-infarct (cerebrovascular) dementia Paranoia Parkinson disease or parkinsonism Strokes Visual impairment	Atypical facial pain Candidiosis (denture-induced stomatitis and angular stomatitis) Carcinoma Herpes zoster and post-herpetic neuralgia Lichen planus Mucous membrane pemphigoid Pre-malignant lesions Sjögren syndrome Sore tongue Trigeminal neuralgia

^{a}Multiple conditions are common.

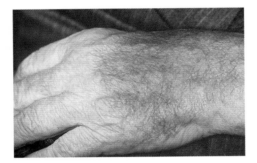

Fig. 25.3   Senile purpura

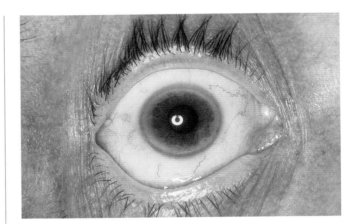

Fig. 25.4   Arcus senilis

reducing independence. The eyes may also show an arcus senilis (Fig. 25.4). Common causes of ataxia, faints and falls are visual impairment, transient cerebral ischaemic attacks, parkinsonism, postural hypotension (often drug-related), cardiac arrhythmias or ischaemic heart disease.

Atypical symptomatology is common: physical disease may present in a less florid and dramatic way in older people. Temperature regulation may be so disturbed that respiratory, urinary or even more serious infections often fail to cause fever. Older patients also readily become hypothermic, especially if thyroid function is poor. Many disorders in older patients also present with non-specific features such as general malaise, social incompetence, a tendency to fall and mild amnesia.

Dementia becomes increasingly common with age. If responses are slow, it may be caused by underlying physical disease, especially if the symptoms are of acute onset. A confusional state may result acutely from disorders as widely different as minor cerebrovascular accidents, respiratory or urinary tract infections, or left ventricular failure. Confusional states may be more chronic when caused by poorly controlled diabetes mellitus, hypothyroidism, carcinomatosis, anaemia, uraemia or drug therapy.

Social disabilities are common as a result of such causes as loss of the spouse, isolation from family, poverty, and lack of mobility and independence. Old people may need to be thrifty, careful with food purchasing and the heating of their accommodation, contributing to overall self-neglect. Nutrition may also be defective due to apathy, mental disease or dental defects. Malnutrition may in turn lead to poor tissue healing and predispose to ill-health. Deterioration in sense of smell and taste may also result in a poor or unhealthy diet. Psychological disorders such as loneliness and depression may follow. Depression may also be a feature in hypothyroidism or a side-effect of medications.

Older people are more likely to be given medication and complications account for about 10% of admissions to geriatric units. Polypharmacy, abnormal reactivity towards many drugs, poor compliance, inappropriate treatment and deteriorating renal and other metabolic pathways affecting drug metabolism can result in toxicity and serious interactions. Older people tend to be more liable to adverse drug reactions, and the reactions tend to be more serious and last longer than in younger people.

Drugs may also precipitate or aggravate physical disorders that are more frequent in the older person. For example, drugs with anti-muscarinic activity, such as atropine or antidepressants,

Table 25.10 Drug use in the older person		
	Problems	**Possible solutions**
Analgesics	Sensitivity to their effects	Restrict dose
Dosage regimens	Difficulties remembering regimens	Simplify regimens and write clear instructions; use dossett boxes
Drug dose	Overdose from sensitivity to agents	Restrict dose
Form of medicine	Difficulty swallowing tablets	Take with water, or use liquid preparations
Non-prescribed drugs	Self-medication without medical advice	Restrict drug availability
Psychotropics	Sensitivity to their effects	Restrict dose

may precipitate glaucoma, may cause dry mouth or, if there is prostatic enlargement, urinary retention. Phenothiazines may precipitate or aggravate parkinsonism or hypotension, or may cause apathy, hypothermia, excessive sedation or confusion. Drowsiness, excessive sedation or confusional states may also be caused by the benzodiazepines or tricyclic antidepressants, while depression and postural hypotension not uncommonly follow the use of hypotensive agents. Drugs should therefore be used cautiously (Table 25.10).

Based on the capacity to carry out activities of ordinary life (to dress, to eat, to bathe, etc.), which is assessed with specific tests, for example the activities of daily living scale (ADLS) or Katz, the older person is classified as functionally independent or dependent.

GENERAL MANAGEMENT

Social support is crucial, preserving as much independence and dignity as possible.

DENTAL ASPECTS

Many older people receive no dental attention whatsoever, despite much evidence of their need. It has been found, for example, that in one study 81% had oral lesions and 20% needed further investigation to exclude serious oral disease. Access to dental care can be a major difficulty for the person who is frail or has limited mobility. Handling of older patients may demand immense patience, but remember always to treat the older patient with sympathy and respect. It can take a long time for a patient in a wheelchair, or using a Zimmer frame, to get into the surgery and on to the dental chair. Domiciliary care may be more appropriate and avoids the physical and psychological problems of a hospital or clinic visit. Older people are often extremely anxious about treatment and should therefore be sympathetically reassured and, if necessary, sedated.

Mucosal lesions may be present in up to 40% of older people. Most of these are fibrous lumps or ulcers, but a minority are potentially or actually malignant lesions. Oral cancer is mainly a problem of older people and is a further reason for regular oral examination (Ch. 22). Atypical facial pain (often related to depressive illness), migraine, trigeminal neuralgia, zoster and oral dysaesthesias are more common as age advances.

Many older people with remaining teeth have periodontal disease. Dental caries are usually less acute but root caries are more common. Caries may become active if there is xerostomia, especially if there is overindulgence in sweet foods. Xerostomia is even more likely with medications such as neuroleptics or antidepressants (Ch. 10). Poor salivation may contribute to a high prevalence of root caries and oral candidiasis, which especially affect hospitalized patients.

Very many older patients are edentulous and some problems of dental management are thereby greatly reduced. It seems, however, that the proportion of edentulous older patients is gradually falling and, as a consequence, more of them need restorative dentistry or surgery of various types. Many edentulous older people have little alveolar bone to support dentures, and have a dry mouth as well as frail, atrophic mucosa. Implants may be helpful inability to cope with dentures, or a sore mouth for any reason, or to afford appropriate care, readily demoralizes the older patient, and may tip the balance between health and disease.

Food can become tasteless and unappetizing as the result of declining taste and smell perception. Older patients should be encouraged to add seasonings to their food instead of relying on excessive consumption of salt and sugar to give their food flavour.

The dentist therefore has an important role in supporting morale and contributing to adequate nutrition. Handling of older patients may demand increased time and patience.

Sound teeth should be conserved if they can serve, at least for a few years, as abutments or retainers for prostheses. It may also be unwise to alter radically the shape or occlusion of dentures where they have been worn for years. It is wise to label the dentures with the name of the patient, particularly for those living in sheltered or other residential accommodation, as dentures can easily be mislaid or mixed up between patients.

Attrition and brittleness of the teeth may complicate treatment, and it may be necessary to provide cuspal coverage in complex or large restorations. Endodontic therapy may be more difficult in view of secondary dentine deposition. Hypercementosis, brittle dentine, low bone elasticity and impaired tissue healing may also complicate surgical procedures.

The major goals of oral health care are preventive and conservative treatment for conditions such as xerostomia, root caries, secondary caries, periodontal disease and gingival recession, and the elimination/avoidance of pain and oral infections.

Independent people with no serious medical problems may be treated in primary dental care. Dependent people may need domiciliary dental care with portable dental equipment. When significant medical problems are present, the older person may be best seen in a hospital environment, though this raises issues of adequate transportation and availability of escorts.

Prevention is of paramount importance in caring for older adults. Therefore, the most important considerations for dental professionals are how well the patient has compensated for his or her medical problem and the exact dental intervention needed. Non-invasive procedures in patients with minimal incapacity carry less risk than do surgical procedures. Older people tend to be more sensitive to drugs and to trauma. Dental treatment planning may be conditioned by factors such as oral health status, capacity to move, motor and mental skills to follow a preventive programme, survival prognosis and economical resources. The whole range of dental treatments may be considered. Dental implants are not at all contraindicated, and they may help to maintain the remaining alveolar bone.

Appointment times may be conditioned by systemic diseases. Sympathetic reassurance is indicated and, if necessary, sedation, with short-acting benzodiazepines. Treatment is often best carried out with the patient sitting upright, as few like reclining for treatment, and some may become breathless and panic. Dentists should recognize that older people, especially women, also heal slowly and bruise readily if tissues are not handled carefully.

To control pain and anxiety, dentists should use LA whenever possible, since the risks of using general anaesthesia (GA) are greater than in younger patients. LA used in recommended dosages has no effect on cardiac arrhythmias in the ambulatory older patient. Intravenous sedation in the dental chair is best avoided if there is any evidence of cerebrovascular disease, as a hypotensive episode may cause cerebral ischaemia. The risks of conscious sedation or GA are greater than in the young patient, not least because of associated medical problems. Relative analgesia is preferable to benzodazepines for sedation and benzodiazepines are preferable to opioids. GA may be necessary for patients unable to cooperate and those with dementia. After long operations, older patients are prone to pulmonary complications, such as atelectasis, deep vein thrombosis and pulmonary embolism; they may also become confused in an unfamiliar environment.

Polypharmacy should be avoided, not only because of the danger of drug interactions but also because of the practical difficulties that the patient may have in taking the correct doses at the correct times. Older people frequently have difficulties in understanding the medication and in remembering to keep to a regimen. Compliance may therefore be lacking. If there is hepatic or renal disease likely to impair drug metabolism or excretion, drug dosage must be reduced appropriately.

ABUSE OF OLDER PEOPLE

Elder abuse occurs when an older person is harmed, mistreated or neglected. There are five types of elder abuse: psychological, physical, financial, sexual and neglect (Box 25.3).

Box 25.3 Elder abuse

- 500 000 are abused at any one time in the UK
- Most abuse is perpetrated against people who are over the age of 70
- Two-thirds of abuse is committed at home
- In nearly a half, two types of abuse occur simultaneously
- In one-third of cases, the abuse is perpetrated by more than one person
- Only rarely is the abuser the main family carer
- 46% of abusers are related to the person they are abusing: a quarter of those who abuse are sons or daughters
- Staff in care homes or visiting carers may also abuse

People who are being abused are often scared that they will not be believed. Those who witness or suspect abuse may not want to be seen as 'interfering' or may be scared of 'getting it wrong'. If abuse is suspected, always talk to the "victim" first and tell them what you want to do. The main charitable and government-sponsored organizations that can offer support to those affected include police, hospitals, general medical practitioners, carer organizations, social services/social work departments, and social care inspection bodies. Be clear about whether the person knows you are reporting your concerns; whether the older person is confused or lacks the capacity to make informed decisions about his/her life; who you think is being abused (name, address, age); what you think is happening to that person; and give reasons/examples to illustrate why you think abuse is occurring. It helps if you can provide dates and times of incidents; what has been said; who you believe is responsible; and the relationship of that person with the older person.

See http://www.helptheaged.org.uk/

MEN'S HEALTH
MALES

The male genitals include the testes, the vas deferens, epididymis and the penis, together with accessory structures – the prostate and bulbourethral glands. The testes, located in the scrotum, produce sperm cells and the hormone testosterone, which influences development of body shape and hair, and regulates spermatogenesis. Disorders of the gonads are outside the remit of this text.

There are some conditions that affect only men and there are gender differences in regard to patterns of many diseases (Box 25.4). Men generally also access and use health care differently from women (typically less): generally they are less likely to react to health promotion and are more likely to have lifestyle habits that are detrimental to their health (e.g. alcohol or drug abuse).

Box 25.4 Health problems more common in men

- Alcoholism
- Balanitis
- Bladder
  - Stones
  - Cancer
- Drug abuse and addiction
- Hydrocele and varicocele
- Orchitis and epididymitis
- Peyronie disease
- Phimosis and paraphimosis
- Prostate
  - Prostatitis
  - Benign prostatic hyperplasia
  - Cancer
- Snoring and obstructive sleep apnoea
- Testicular
  - Torsion
  - Cancer
- Tinea
- Trauma

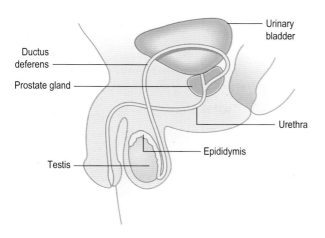

Fig. 25.5 Male genital anatomy

Labels: Ductus deferens, Prostate gland, Testis, Urinary bladder, Urethra, Epididymis

---

PENIS AND SCROTUM

The anatomy of the male genital system is shown in Fig. 25.5.

BALANITIS (BALANOPOSTHITIS)

Balanitis is inflammation of the skin covering the glans penis. The most common cause is neglected hygiene and tight foreskin (phimosis) leading to irritation by smegma, but less common causes are shown in Box 25.5. Treatment depends on the underlying cause.

CIRCUMCISION

Circumcision, a surgical procedure that involves partial or complete removal of the foreskin (prepuce), is a feature of both Judaism and Islam, and many African and New World cultures. About one-fifth of men worldwide have been circumcised, commonly soon after birth or at puberty. Circumcision may also be carried out for medical reasons such as balanitis, phimosis or paraphimosis (the foreskin forms a tight tourniquet around the glans, causing pain). Sexually transmitted infections that cause genital ulcers (syphilis, chancroid, herpes simplex) are more common in uncircumcised men. However, penile warts and urethritis are more common in circumcised men. Poor personal hygiene, smoking and exposure to human papillomavirus (HPV) are risk factors for penile cancer and that risk is not reduced by circumcision, but it does appear to reduce

the risk of cervical cancer in women. Candidosis is equally common in circumcised and uncircumcised men. Views conflict as to whether circumcision can significantly reduce HIV transmission.

PEYRONIE DISEASE

This is the slowly progressive development of fibrous plaques around the corpora cavernosa of the penis, which mainly affects young adults and is of unknown aetiology. It causes bending to the affected side on erection. The condition may resolve but otherwise may require surgery.

HYDROCELE

A hydrocele is accumulation of fluid around the testis. Diagnosis is confirmed by transillumination and ultrasound. Most hydroceles in children resolve spontaneously and rarely cause discomfort. Most hydroceles in adults are persistent and therefore usually managed by draining the fluid under LA, introducing a sclerosing agent to prevent recurrence. Alternatively, the hydrocele can be removed surgically.

VARICOCELE

A varicocele is enlargement of the veins in the scrotum. It is most common on the left-hand side and may result in scrotal heaviness or pain and impaired fertility. In some cases, an operation can increase fertility.

ORCHITIS AND EPIDIDYMITIS

Sperm and hormones are produced in the testes and stored in the epididymis before being conveyed to the spermatic ducts (Fig. 25.5).

Orchitis is an inflammation of testicular tissue. The mumps virus is a common cause. Orchitis causes pain in the scrotum (which may become hot and swollen) and fever; it can also result in infertility. Treatment is bed rest, a suspensory bandage and analgesics. All children are offered mumps vaccination when they are 12–15 months old.

Epididymitis is far more common than orchitis and usually arises from a bacterial urinary infection. Coliforms, pyogenic staphylococci and faecal streptococci are most often responsible, but it may also be caused by *Chlamydia* or gonorrhoea; in many cases, no organism is identifiable. Symptoms may include fever, a hot, red and painful scrotal swelling, and dysuria and frequency may be present. Bed rest, analgesics and antibiotics are indicated.

TESTICULAR PROBLEMS

Torsion

Testicular torsion usually appears in teenage boys. The testicles hang loose in the scrotum and in rare cases they are twisted, obstructing their blood flow. Torsion presents with sudden pain and swelling of the scrotum. Urgent surgery is indicated and, to prevent recurrence, testicular fixation is performed.

Testicular cancer

Testicular cancer affects younger men, particularly those between ages 20 and 40, and is more common in Caucasians than those of African heritage. Most are seminoma, others are non-seminoma – a group which includes choriocarcinoma, embryonal carcinoma, teratoma and yolk sac tumours. Risk factors may include undescended testicle and age.

Clinical features

Testicular cancer usually affects only one testicle, presenting as a swelling, discomfort or feeling of heaviness in the scrotum/testicle, dull ache in the abdomen or groin, sudden collection of fluid in the scrotum, breast enlargement or tenderness or unexplained fatigue.

General management

Diagnosis is confirmed with ultrasound and biopsy, staging by computed tomography (CT) scanning. Treatments include radical inguinal orchidectomy, radiotherapy (seminomas respond well) or chemotherapy (the treatment of choice for widespread disease). Chemotherapy may affect sperm production, but sperm can be frozen and preserved (cryopreservation) beforehand.

BLADDER PROBLEMS

Urine passes from each kidney through the ureter to be stored in the bladder (Ch. 12). An outer muscle layer surrounds the bladder inner lining, which is made up of a uniform transitional epithelium resting on a thin basal lamina When the bladder is full, the muscles can tighten to allow urination via the urethra.

Stones

General aspects

Bladder stones are common in men, especially in those over 45. They can form in healthy individuals for no apparent reason. Bladder stones can also develop in gout or urinary infections, or if urine stagnates in the bladder as in prostatic hypertrophy. Most are formed of calcium, from excess salt in the urine (or too little water). Most bladder stones form within the bladder, but a few form in the kidneys and then travel to the bladder causing acute pain or colic en route in the ureter.

Clinical features

Bladder stones may be symptomless, or cause frequency and urgency of micturition, pain when urinating or blood in the urine (haematuria). Problems arise when stones become too large to be flushed out during urination, particularly if they trap in the urethra when they cause pain (dysuria) and difficulty passing urine. If left untreated, bladder stones can irritate the muscles of the bladder wall and lead to incontinence.

General management

Diagnosis is confirmed by ultrasound, intravenous urography or cystoscopy. Bladder stones usually need to be broken down during cystoscopy, or by lithotripsy in order to flush them out.

Bladder cancer

General aspects

Bladder cancer is the fourth most common cancer in males: 90% are transitional cell and 8% are squamous cell carcinomas. Incidence is increasing. Risk factors for bladder cancer include older age, male sex (men are 2–3 times more predisposed than women), a positive family history, and race (Caucasians are twice as frequently affected as Africans, with lowest rates in Asians). Important causes are carcinogens concentrated in the bladder – from cigarette smoking (raises risk by 2–3 times) or occupation (e.g. workers in rubber, chemical, leather, metal, print, and textile industries, or hairdressers, machinists, painters, or truck drivers), or treatment with cyclophosphamide or arsenic. Infections – particularly schistosomiasis – may occasionally be implicated (Ch. 21). Factors *not proven* in aetiology include coffee, chlorine in drinking water, nor saccharine, the sweetener that, in large doses, causes bladder cancer in animals.

Clinical features

The most common presentation is painless haematuria but dysuria, urgency, polyuria and/or urinary obstruction may be seen. Such symptoms are also common in prostatic hyperplasia and carcinoma. Bladder cancer can invade to involve nearby organs such as the prostate (or uterus/vagina) and can metastasize to regional lymph nodes and to lungs, liver or bones.

General management

Malignant cells may be seen on urine cytology; intravenous urography may show a filling defect, but cystoscopy and biopsy give the definitive diagnosis. Surgery is the common treatment; other treatments include transurethral resection (TUR) for superficial cancer, segmental cystectomy for localized cancer and radical cystectomy for more widespread disease Radiation, intravesical chemotherapy or immunotherapy using intravesical BCG may also be used.

Dental aspects

Metastases may involve the jaws; chemotherapy may cause mucositis.

PROSTATE DISORDERS

Prostatitis

Prostatitis is the most common prostate disease and accounts for up to 25% of all visits to general practitioners by young and middle-aged men with genitourinary symptoms. The types are shown in Table 25.11.

Table 25.11   Prostatitis

Type	Comments	Therapy
Acute bacterial prostatitis	Fever, pain in the lower back and genital area, urinary frequency and urgency often at night, burning or painful urination, and urinary infection	Antibiotics
Chronic bacterial prostatitis	Uncommon. Associated with an underlying prostatic defect, forming a focus for infection	Removing the defect and using antibiotics
Chronic prostatitis/chronic pelvic pain syndrome	In the inflammatory form, urine and semen contain leukocytes but no bacteria; in the non-inflammatory form, no evidence of inflammation is found	Antibiotics
Asymptomatic inflammatory prostatitis	Semen contains leukocytes	-

Prostatic hyperplasia

General aspects

The prostate almost invariably enlarges with age (benign prostatic hyperplasia or hypertrophy; BPH) possibly related to oestrogen or dihydrotestosterone (DHT) production, so that at least 50% of men in their sixties and as many as 90% in their seventies and above have symptoms.

Clinical features

An enlarging prostate constricts the urethra causing a hesitant, interrupted or weak urine stream. The bladder hypertrophies and then begins to contract even when it contains little urine, causing urgency, frequency, nocturia and leaking or dribbling. Urinary infections are also more common. The bladder may become distended and atonic leading to overflow incontinence. Sustained raised intravesical pressure can cause hydronephrosis and renal damage. Acute urinary retention can be precipitated by alcohol, cold temperatures or immobility, and is an emergency.

General management

Investigations indicated may include prostate-specific antigen (PSA) blood test and digital rectal examination (DRE), MSU (mid-stream urine), urine flow study and blood urea and electrolytes. Cystoscopy should identify the location and degree of any obstruction – and rectal ultrasound with biopsies may be indicated.

The level of PSA can rise in BPH, infection or prostate cancer, so the result should be interpreted with caution as there is also a high rate of false positives and false negatives. PCA3 is probably a more specific marker for prostate cancer (Ch. 22).

The symptoms of BPH may resolve without treatment in as many as one-third of mild cases but, if it causes major inconvenience or complications, treatment is recommended. Drug therapy includes finasteride or dutasteride (5-alpha-reductase inhibitors inhibit DHT production and shrink the prostate), saw palmetto (a herbal remedy possibly as effective as finasteride) or alpha-blockers (e.g. alfuzosin, doxazosin, indoramin, prazosin, tamsulosin or terazosin, which relax the prostate and bladder neck smooth muscle). Surgical treatment includes: transurethral resection of the prostate (TURP); transurethral microwave thermotherapy (TUMT); transurethral needle ablation (TUNA; which delivers low-level radiofrequency energy with fewer side-effects compared with TURP); transurethral laser surgery (Nd:YAG lasers); transurethral incision of the prostate (TUIP); or open excisional surgery (prostatectomy).

Prostatic cancer

General aspects

Risk factors for prostate cancer include age (mainly age > 55), family history of prostate cancer, ethnicity (more common in those of African descent), and diet and dietary factors (animal fat may possibly increase the risk, and diets high in fruits and vegetables may lower it) (Ch. 22). BPH does *not* seem to raise the chance of getting prostate cancer.

Clinical features

Early prostate cancer usually causes no symptoms, but later features can mimic BPH or infection. These can include: urinary frequency, especially at night; difficulty starting urination or holding back urine; inability to urinate; weak or interrupted urine flow; painful or burning urination; difficulty in having an erection; painful ejaculation; blood in urine or semen; or frequent pain or stiffness in the lower back, hips or upper thighs.

General management

Investigations may include PSA, urinalysis for blood or infection and a DRE. In some cases, blood prostatic acid phosphatase or PCA3 is helpful, especially if PSA results are positive. All men over 40 should have a DRE once a year to screen for prostate cancer. If results suggest cancer, a prostate biopsy is needed.

Prostate cancer can be managed by watchful waiting, surgery, radiation, chemotherapy or hormone therapy [androgen deprivation therapy (ADT) or androgen suppression therapy]. ADT aims to reduce androgens (testosterone and dihydrotestosterone) by: orchidectomy (removal of the testes – the main androgen source); luteinizing hormone-releasing hormone (LHRH) agonists (leuprolide, goserelin, buserelin, triptorelin), which prevent the testicles from producing testosterone; LHRH antagonists (abarelix); anti-androgens (e.g. flutamide, nilutamide or bicalutamide); or drugs to inhibit adrenal androgen production (e,g. ketoconazole and aminoglutethimide).

Dental aspects

Metastases occasionally involve the jaws and are typically osteosclerotic. Cancer chemotherapy may cause mucositis and immunosuppression.

WOMEN'S HEALTH

GENERAL ASPECTS

Females

The ovaries are a pair of female reproductive organs located in the pelvis, alongside the uterus. They produce ova (eggs) and female hormones (oestrogen and progesterone) which influence the development of breasts, body shape and body hair, and regulate the menstrual cycle and pregnancy. Oestrogen stimulates uterine growth and development at puberty, thickens the endometrium during the first half of the menstrual cycle, and stimulates changes in breast tissue at puberty and childbirth. Progesterone, produced during the last half of the menstrual cycle, prepares the endometrium to receive the ovum. Every month, during the menstrual cycle, an ovum is released from one ovary (ovulation) and travels through the Fallopian tube to the uterus. If the egg is fertilized, progesterone secretion continues, preventing release of additional eggs.

Women generally live longer than men, there are gender differences in regard to patterns of many diseases and some conditions that affect only women (Box 25.6).

Box 25.6 Some of the more common problems in women

- Bacterial vaginosis
- Cancer
  - Breast
  - Cervical
  - Ovarian
- Cystitis
- Eating disorders
- Endometriosis
- Female genital cutting
- Fibroids
- Osteoporosis
- Pregnancy-related disorders
- Menopausal disorders

Women generally access and use health care differently from men (typically more) and generally react positively to health promotion. There has also been discrimination against women across cultures, and subordination and compromised dignity, and women more frequently suffer the consequences of domestic violence and/or sexual abuse than men.

Certain diseases that can have orofacial manifestations are especially common in women [e.g. anorexia nervosa/bulimia, atypical facial pain, burning mouth syndrome, facial arthromyalgia (temporomandibular joint dysfunction), pemphigus and pemphigoid, rheumatoid arthritis and Sjögren syndrome].

BACTERIAL VAGINOSIS

Bacterial vaginosis (BV) is a common condition due to an imbalance in the normal vaginal bacteria. It is not a sexually transmitted infection. BV may be symptomless or characterized by a discharge with a fishy smell. It is diagnosed by microbiology and treated with oral metronidazole, or with clindamycin vaginal cream.

CANCER

Breast cancer

General aspects

Other than skin cancer, breast cancer is the most common cancer among women and is more common in white women than in those of African or Asian descent. The causes are not clear but most cases are seen over the age of 50, and the risk is especially high over age 60. Risk factors are shown in Box 25.7.

Box 25.7 Risk factors for breast cancer

- Personal history of breast cancer
- A positive family history: the risk doubles if a woman's mother or sister has had breast cancer, especially at a young age. Changes in certain genes (BRCA1, BRCA2 and others) increase risk
- Having a diagnosis of atypical hyperplasia or lobular carcinoma in situ (LCIS)
- Oestrogen exposure
- Late childbearing (after about age 30)
- Early menarche
- Breast density
- Radiation therapy
- Alcohol
- A fatty diet
- Long-term use of combined oral contraceptives or hormone replacement therapy (HRT)
- High body mass index (BMI) and taller stature
- Higher social class

Clinical features

Early breast cancer rarely causes pain; more commonly it may be detected on self-examination as a lump or thickening. Later, cancer may result in a change in breast size or shape, nipple discharge, tenderness or inversion, ridging or pitting (the skin looks like orange skin – *peau d'orange*), or a change in the way the skin of the breast, areola or nipple looks or feels (e.g. warm, swollen, red or scaly; Fig. 25.6).

General management

Current recommendation is 3-yearly screening from the age of 50 but, in cases of increased risk such as positive family history, screening may start earlier, with mammograms (Fig. 25.7). If an area of the breast looks suspicious on screening mammogram, diagnostic mammograms may be needed. Ultrasonography can often then help. Biopsy is generally needed – by needle or open biopsy.

Lobular carcinoma in situ (LCIS) refers to abnormal cells in the lining of a lobule, which seldom become invasive cancer. Tamoxifen, a hormone receptor blocker, is the usual therapy. Occasionally women with LCIS may decide to have bilateral mastectomy to try to prevent cancer, but most just have regular screening.

Ductal carcinoma in situ (DCIS or intraductal carcinoma) refers to abnormal cells in the lining of a duct which are at greater risk of invasive breast cancer. Treatments include breast-sparing surgery followed by radiation therapy or mastectomy,

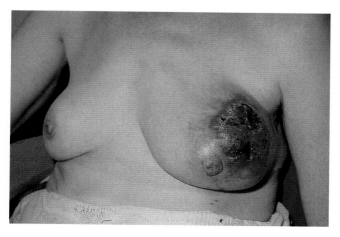

Fig. 25.6 Advanced cancer of the breast

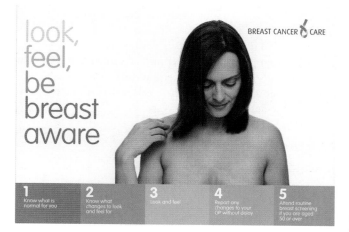

look,
feel,
be
breast
aware

BREAST CANCER CARE

| 1 | 2 | 3 | 4 | 5 |
| Know what is normal for you | Know what changes to look and feel for | Look and feel | Report any changes to your GP without delay | Attend routine breast screening if you are aged 50 or over |

Fig. 25.7 Breast self-awareness

with or without breast reconstruction. Tamoxifen may reduce the risk of developing invasive breast cancer.

Breast carcinoma treatment most commonly involves surgery – usually a wide local excision with axillary node sampling or sentinel node biopsy. Histopathology results then dictate further treatment, which may be more radical surgery, or adjuvant radiotherapy plus or minus chemotherapy. Treatment may include biological therapy. Hormone (oestrogen and progesterone) receptor tests can help determine whether a tumour is hormone-dependent. ER (oestrogen receptors) and PR (progesterone receptors) tests help predict response to hormone therapy after surgery. Tamoxifen is the most common hormonal treatment used, usually for 5 years following the main treatment, and may cause hot flushes, vaginal discharge or irritation, nausea and irregular periods. Serious adverse effects are rare but tamoxifen can cause deep vein thrombosis and, in a few women, it can increase the risk of uterine cancer or stroke. Anastrozole is a safer alternative in respect of stroke risk.

Human epidermal growth factor receptor-2 or *HER-2* gene may be associated with a higher risk for cancer recurrence. Trastuzumab – a monoclonal antibody that targets breast cancer cells having excess HER-2 – may be given alone or along with chemotherapy. HER-2 test results help predict response to trastuzumab and other anti-HER-2 treatments and some types of chemotherapy (Table 25.12). Advanced breast cancer may be treated with vinorelbine; capecitabine may be used for locally advanced or metastatic cancer.

Dental aspects

Metastases occasionally affect the jaws.

Cervical cancer

General aspects

Cancer of the uterine cervix is the most common genitourinary neoplasm and most often affects women > 40 years. It is most common in sexually active persons and recognized to be associated with human papillomaviruses, particularly HPV-16 and HPV-18. Smoking, lower socioeconomic class and HIV disease increase the risk.

A vaccine for HPV-16 and HPV-18 has now been added to the immunization schedule and is given to girls of 12–13 years of age; there will be a catch-up programme for older girls.

Table 25.12 Oestrogen receptors/progesterone receptors and breast cancer	
Breast cancer	**Receptor relevance**
Newly diagnosed invasive	The cancer is classified as ER-positive (if the tumour has oestrogen receptors) or ER-negative (if the tumour does *not* have oestrogen receptors); PR-positive (if the tumour has progesterone receptors) or PR-negative (if the tumour does *not* have progesterone receptors); and HER-2-positive (if the tumour does have HER-2) or HER-2-negative (if the tumour does *not* have HER-2)
Node-negative	Patients with tumours that do not have uPA (urokinase plasminogen activator) and PAI-1 (plasminogen activator inhibitor 1) have a good prognosis and may not need chemotherapy
Node-negative and ER-positive and/or PR-positive	Oncotype DX test identifies patients who may be successfully treated with tamoxifen alone and may not need chemotherapy
Metastatic	ER and PR tests help predict response to hormone therapy. HER-2 test helps predict response to trastuzumab and other anti-HER-2 treatments. CA 15-3, CA 27.29 and CEA (carcinoembryonic antigen) help monitor patients; these should be used along with the patient's health history, a physical examination, and diagnostic imaging tests such as radiography, bone scans, MRI (magnetic resonance imaging) and CT (computed tomography)
Recurrent	HER-2 test helps predict the response to trastuzumab and other anti-HER-2 treatments, and guides the use of specific chemotherapy

Screening for pre-cancerous cells is carried out by a 'cervical smear' test – 3-yearly on women aged 25–50 and then 5-yearly until 64 years of age. The cells from the squamocolumnar junction in the cervical canal are then described as normal; mild dyskaryosis (CIN 1; this may resolve spontaneously), moderate dyskaryosis (CIN 2) or severe dyskaryosis (CIN 3), sometimes referred to as carcinoma *in situ*.

Clinical features

Pre-cancerous changes of the cervix rarely cause pain. When cancer develops and invades, the most common manifestations are abnormal vaginal bleeding or abnormal vaginal discharge.

General management

Following pelvic examination and liquid-based cytology from brushings at routine screening, women with CIN 2 or 3 then undergo colposcopy and biopsy. LLETZ (large loop excision of the transformation zone) may be carried out using diathermy, laser ablation or cold coagulation. A cone biopsy removing the entire transformation zone may be carried out and often the entire pre-cancerous area is removed in this way. Staging for cervical cancer includes a pelvic examination, cystoscopy and proctosigmoidoscopy. Other investigations include intravenous pyelography, barium enema, CT scan, ultrasonography and magnetic resonance imaging (MRI). Treatment for a pre-cancerous lesion depends on several factors, such as whether the lesion is low or high grade, whether the woman wants to have children, her age and general health, and her preferences. Treatment may be surgery, radiotherapy or chemotherapy or a combination depending on the stage. Simple local excision may be all that is required for early disease, whereas for more advanced disease a radical hysterectomy and excision of other involved tissues may be necessary. Radiotherapy may be given alone or with concurrent chemotherapy (e.g. cisplatin).

Dental aspects

Other than the fact that consorts and sometimes the patient can have a higher risk of oral cancer, cervical cancer is rarely of direct relevance to oral health. Metastases occasionally involve the jaws and cancer chemotherapy may cause mucositis.

Ovarian cancer

Most ovarian cancer is carcinoma, but there are rare germ-cell tumours and cancers that begin in the stroma. The causes are unclear but risk factors are shown in Box 25.8.

Factors that reduce the risk include breast-feeding, use of combined oral contraceptives, a low-fat diet and childbearing (the more children a woman has had, the less likely she is to develop ovarian cancer).

Clinical features

Ovarian cancer often causes no symptoms or only mild symptoms until the disease is advanced but may include abdominal

---

Box 25.8 Risk factors for ovarian cancer

- Family history of ovarian, breast or colon cancer
- Personal history of breast or colon cancer
- Age: risk grows as a woman gets older, with the highest risk over 60
- Fertility drugs
- Talc
- Hormone replacement therapy (HRT)
- Endometriosis

---

discomfort and/or pain; nausea, diarrhoea, constipation or frequent urination; anorexia; weight gain or loss; and abnormal vaginal bleeding. Fluid in the abdomen (ascites) may be seen when it metastasizes to the peritoneum.

General management

Diagnosis is from pelvic examination together with ultrasound, CA-125 assay, radiography of the lower gastrointestinal tract, or barium enema, CT or MRI and biopsy.

Women at high risk due to a positive family history may consider prophylactic oophorectomy. Treatments for ovarian cancer include surgery (hysterectomy with bilateral salpingo-oophorectomy), chemotherapy or external or intraperitoneal radiation therapy.

Dental aspects

Metastases occasionally affect the jaws.

CYSTITIS

Genitourinary tract infections are particularly common in females, often ascending the short urethra from the vulva frequently as a consequence of intercourse ('honeymoon cystitis'). Cystitis can ascend the ureter to cause pyelonephritis.

Bladder infections usually have little relevance for dental care, although the symptoms of cystitis may cause the patient to defer treatment for a few days. Such infections often suggest that the patient is sexually active and at risk from sexually transmitted diseases (Ch. 32). Cranberry juice (*Vaccinium macrocarpon*), popularly used to prevent cystitis, may enhance warfarin activity.

ENDOMETRIOSIS

General and clinical aspects

Endometriosis is an enigmatic disease affecting women in their reproductive years, in which endometrium-like tissue is found outside the uterus, where it develops into nodules. Like the endometrium, the nodules usually respond to the menstrual cycle hormones. Tissue accumulates each month, breaks down, and causes bleeding, pain, infertility and other problems. Prostaglandins may cause many of the symptoms. Pregnancy often causes a temporary remission of symptoms, and mild or moderate endometriosis generally ceases after the menopause. About one-third of women with endometriosis are infertile and there is an increased frequency of malignancy in people with endometriosis.

Endometrial nodules occur typically in the abdomen, usually involving the ovaries, Fallopian tubes, outer uterine surface and pelvic lining.

General management

Diagnosis is generally confirmed by laparoscopy. Treatment has varied, with no certain cure. Hormonal treatments for endometriosis aim to suppress ovulation [oestrogen and progestogen, progestogen alone, a testosterone derivative (danazol) and GnRH (gonadotropin-releasing hormone)]. Hysterectomy with oophorectomy has been considered a cure, but there can be continuation/recurrence. Conservative surgery, either major or laparoscopic, involving removal or destruction of the nodules, can relieve symptoms and allow pregnancy to occur in some cases. Again, recurrences are common.

FEMALE GENITAL CUTTING

Female genital cutting (FGC) is the collective name given to traditional practices involving the partial or total cutting away of, or other injury to, female external genitalia, whether for cultural or other non-therapeutic reasons. FGC is practised predominantly in Africa, and also in some Middle Eastern countries, typically being performed on girls between 4 and 12 years old.

FIBROIDS

Fibroids are benign tumours of uterine muscle fibres. Probably 20–50% of women have, or will have, fibroids but they are rare at age < 20. Fibroids occur up to nine times more often in black than in white women. The cause is unknown but fibroids seem to be influenced by oestrogen (which might explain why they appear during a woman's middle years when oestrogen levels are high, and stop growing after the menopause, when oestrogen levels fall). Fibroids are often symptomless but the most common symptom is heavy menstrual bleeding. Other symptoms include abdominal pain or pressure, changes in bladder and bowel function and, in some cases, infertility.

MENSTRUATION

Menstruation is the shedding of the endometrium that occurs on a regular basis in females of reproductive age (Fig. 25.8). Plasmin in the endometrium tends to inhibit blood clotting. Normal, regular menstruation lasts for about 3–5 days. The average blood loss during menstruation ranges from 10 to 80 ml and many women experience cramps (dysmenorrhoea) during this time.

PREGNANCY

Sex hormones, prolactin and thyroid hormones rise in pregnancy, but levels of luteinizing hormone (LH) and follicle-stimulating hormone (FSH) fall. Consequences may include deepened pigmentation, particularly of the nipples and sometimes the face (chloasma), and a rise in both blood volume and cardiac output associated with tachycardia. Endocrine,

cardiovascular, haematological and often mental (attitude, mood or behaviour) changes can be seen.

General aspects

The mother

Variations in hormone levels result in changes that may include those shown in Fig. 25.8.

Pregnancy may be accompanied by a range of complaints (Table 25.13). Medical complications can include glycosuria and impaired glucose tolerance, which occasionally cause gestational diabetes. Disturbances of carbohydrate metabolism usually resolve after pregnancy. Diabetic control can be difficult, since insulin requirements rise, pregnant diabetics need specialist monitoring and care.

Hypertension may be asymptomatic but, when associated with oedema and proteinuria (pre-eclampsia), may culminate in eclampsia (hypertension, oedema, proteinuria and convulsions) leading to greater morbidity and mortality in both fetus and mother. Pre-eclampsia or PET (pre-eclamptic toxaemia) may cause intrauterine growth retardation (IUGR), fetal death and extreme prematurity. It rarely occurs before 28 weeks and affects 5–10% of pregnancies. In the mother it can cause haemorrhagic stroke, eclamptic fits, renal or liver failure, or abruption, where the placenta separates from the uterus, which can result in intrauterine death of the fetus. Treatment involves bed rest, antihypertensives and close monitoring of both the mother and fetus and possible early delivery.

In later pregnancy, up to 10% of patients may become hypotensive if laid supine, when the gravid uterus compresses the

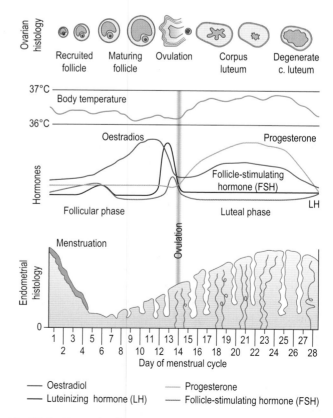

Fig. 25.8 Menstrual cycle, with hormonal and other changes

Table 25.13 Common complaints in pregnancy

	MAIN TRIMESTER IN WHICH COMPLAINT OCCURS		
First	**Second**	**Third**
Breast tenderness Dizziness Frequency of urination Haemorrhoids Leg cramps Nausea and vomiting Nosebleeds, nasal stuffiness Tiredness Deepened pigmentation, particularly of the nipples and sometimes the face (chloasma)	Aches and pains Stretch marks Weight gain	Haemorrhoids Heartburn Swelling Varicose veins Dizziness/fainting Itching (pruritus of pregnancy, or cho- lestasis of pregnancy) Shortness of breath Urinary incontinence Backache Pubic symphysis dysfunction

Table 25.14 Drugs to avoid in pregnant mothers[a]

Drug	Potential effects on the fetus
Alcohol	Fetal alcohol syndrome (Box 25.9)
Aminoglycosides	Deafness
Aspirin	Possible abortion; premature closure of ductus arteriosus Persistent pulmonary hypertension; bleeding tendency
Carbamazepine	Neural tube defects; vitamin K impairment and bleeding tendency
Carbimazole	Goitre
Cocaine	Ankyloglossia
Codeine	Respiratory depression
Corticosteroids	Adrenal suppression Growth retardation
Cotrimoxazole	Haemolysis, teratogenicity, methaemoglobinaemia
Dapsone	Haemolysis
Diazepam	Cleft lip/palate
Ephedrine	*
Epsilon-aminocaproic acid	Possible fibrinolysis
Etretinate	Teratogenicity,
Felypressin	Oxytocic
Fluconazole	Congenital anomalies
Flumazenil	*
Gabapentin	*
Gentamicin	Deafness
Itraconazole	*
Ketoconazole	*
Lithium	Cardiac abnormalities
Mefenamic acid	*
Methotrexate	Foetal methotrexate syndrome
Metronidazole	Reduce birth weight
Midazolam	*
Nitrous oxide (repeated large doses)	Congenital anomalies
Non-steroidal anti-inflammatory drugs	Persistent pulmonary hypertension; bleeding tendency Premature closure of ductus arteriosus
Opioids	Possible bradycardia
Oxcarbazepine	*
Pentazepine	Fetal addiction and withdrawal symptoms
Phenytoin	Fetal phenytoin syndrome
Prilocaine	Methaemoglobinaemia
Retinoids	Neural tube defects
Sulfonamides	* Growth retardation
Teicoplanin	*

inferior vena cava and impedes venous return to the heart (supine hypotension syndrome).

Blood hypercoagulability can lead to venous thrombosis, particularly post-operatively, or occasionally to disseminated intravascular coagulopathy.

Pregnancy may worsen pre-existing anaemias, especially sickle cell anaemia. Deficiency anaemias may develop in about 20%, mainly because of fetal demands for iron and folate. Most pregnant patients are given both of these haematinics. Expansion of the blood volume may cause an apparent anaemia.

The fetus

Fetal development during the first 3 months (trimester) of pregnancy is a complex process of organogenesis and the fetus is then especially at risk from developmental defects. The most critical period is the third to eighth week. Most fetal developmental defects are of unknown aetiology but, in addition to hereditary influences, infections, alcohol, smoking, drugs, deficiencies and irradiation can be implicated in some cases (Table 25.14). Folic acid supplements taken pre-conception and for the first trimester may minimize the risk of neural tube defects, such as spina bifida, and of facial clefts.

All drugs should be avoided in pregnancy unless potential benefit outweighs potential risks. Any woman of childbearing age is a potential candidate for pregnancy and may not be aware of pregnancy for 2 months or more, when the fetus is most vulnerable to damage. A total of 10–20% of all pregnancies abort at this time, often because of fetal defects. Alcohol, anticonvulsants, thalidomide and isotretinoin can be teratogenic. Even a single exposure to high alcohol intake can cause significant brain damage; more than 10% of children have been exposed to high levels of alcohol *in utero* and many suffer effects ranging from mild learning disabilities to major physical, mental and intellectual impairment (fetal alcohol syndrome; FAS; Box 25.9).

Nevertheless, very few therapeutic drugs have been proved to be teratogenic. Aspirin and other NSAIDs may cause closure of the ductus arteriosus *in utero*, and fetal pulmonary hypertension, as well as delaying or prolonging labour, and therefore

Table 25.14 Drugs to avoid in pregnant mothers^a—cont'd

Drug	Potential effects on the fetus
Tetracyclines	Discoloured teeth and bones
Thalidomide	Phocomelia
Tranexamic acid	Possible fibrinolysis
Valproate	Neural tube defects
Vancomycin	Toxicity (monitor levels)
Voriconazole	*
Warfarin	Long bone and cartilage abnormalities; bleeding tendency

^aDrugs of abuse cause neonatal addiction.

*In animals damages the foetus.

Box 25.9 *In utero* alcohol damage and later possible sequelae

- Asthma
- Attention deficit disorder/attention deficit hyperactivity disorder (ADD/ADHD)
- Autistic traits
- Behavioural problems
- Central auditory processing disorder
- Cerebral palsy
- Cleft palate
- Cognitive perseveration
- Complex seizure disorder
- Deafness
- Death
- Dental abnormalities
- Depression
- Developmental coordination disorder
- Developmental delay
- Developmental speech and language disorder
- Dyslexia
- Echolalia
- Epilepsy
- Extreme impulsiveness
- Heart defects
- Heart failure
- Height and weight deficiencies
- Higher than normal pain tolerance
- Immune defect
- Learning disability
- Little or no capacity for interpersonal empathy
- Little or no capacity for moral judgement
- Little or no retained memory
- Loss of intellectual functioning (IQ)
- Mild to severe vision problems
- Night terrors
- Poor judgement
- Precocious puberty
- Reactive outbursts
- Renal failure
- Rigidity
- Serious maxillofacial deformities
- Severe loss of intellectual potential
- Sleep disorder
- Social problems
- Sociopathic behaviour
- Suicide
- Tourette's traits
- Tremors

---

are contraindicated in the third trimester. Aspirin, in addition, causes a platelet defect and may induce abortion and is best avoided throughout pregnancy. Corticosteroids can suppress the fetal adrenals and, if given, steroid cover is needed for labour. Tetracyclines stain developing teeth.

Serious damage to the fetus or child can also be caused by maternal tobacco smoking during or after pregnancy. Smoking increases the risk of stillbirth, low birthweight, and impaired mental and physical development. Smoking by either parent after the child's birth increases the child's risk of respiratory tract infection, asthma and sudden death.

Dental aspects

Pregnancy is the ideal opportunity to begin preventive dental education and to advise on fluoride administration to the infant. Prenatal fluorides are not indicated as there is little evidence of benefit to the fetus. The teeth do not, of course, lose calcium as a result of fetal demands and there is no reason to expect caries to become more active unless the mother develops a capricious desire for sweets.

As much treatment as possible should be postponed until after parturition in those with a history of abortions and those who have achieved pregnancy after years of failure to conceive. During the first trimester, the only safe course of action is to protect the patient as far as possible from infections and to avoid the use of drugs (particularly GA) and radiography.

In the second and third trimesters, the fetus is growing and maturing but can still be affected by infections, drugs and possibly other factors. Nevertheless, dental treatment is best carried out during the second trimester, though advanced restorative procedures are probably best postponed until the periodontal state improves after parturition and prolonged sessions of treatment are better tolerated. In the third trimester, the supine hypotension syndrome may result if the patient is laid flat. The patient should therefore be put on one side to allow venous return to recover. Some pregnant women also have a hypersensitive gag reflex.

Elective dental care should be avoided in the last month of pregnancy, as it is often uncomfortable for the patient. Moreover, premature labour or even abortion may also be ascribed, without justification, to dental treatment.

Routine dental treatment of pregnant women under LA is safe but unnecessary drugs should be avoided (Table 25.15). Because of the risk of coincidental mishaps, it is wise to try to avoid giving any drugs, possibly even LA. GA, and sedation with midazolam or diazepam, are particular hazards and should be avoided in the first trimester and in the last month of the third trimester of pregnancy. Nitrous oxide, though able to interfere with vitamin B_{12} and folate metabolism, does not appear to be teratogenic, though it is advisable to restrict use to the second or third trimester, limit the duration of exposure to < 30 min, use 50% oxygen, avoid repeated exposures, and use scavenging in the dental surgery to minimize staff exposure.

When GA is unavoidable and there is a mishap to the fetus, the mother is likely to blame the anaesthetist, even though this may be quite unjustifiable. Yet another hazard is a greater tendency to vomit during induction in the third trimester.

Table 25.15 Known risks to the fetus of some drugs used systemically in dentistry

Category[a]	A	B	C	D and X
	No risk to fetus in animal model or human studies	Either safe to fetus in animal models without human data, or risk in animal models but safe in human studies	Risk to fetus in animal models but no human studies available, or no human studies support safety	Definitive human data demonstrating risk to fetus
Use in dentistry	When desired (completely safe)	Where necessary	Only if really essential and after consulting physician	Never
Analgesics	–	Meperidine Paracetamol/acetaminophen	Codeine Diflunisal Rofecoxib	Aspirin NSAIDs[b]
Antimicrobials	–	Azithromycin Cefadroxil Cefuroxime Cephalexin Clindamycin Erythromycin Loracarbef Metronidazole Penciclovir (cream) Penicillins	Aciclovir Ciprofloxacin Clarithromycin Fluconazole	Doxycycline Minocycline Tetracyclines
Local anaesthetics	–	Lidocaine Prilocaine*	Articaine[c] Bupivacaine Mepivacaine	–
Sedatives	–	Promethazine		Benzodiazepines[c] Nitrous oxide[d]
Others	–	–	Corticosteroids (even topical)	Antidepressants Carbamazepine Colchicine Danazol Phenytoin Povidone–iodine Retinoids Thalidomide Warfarin

[a]US Federal Drug Agency (FDA) pregnancy categories.
[b]May be safer in first and second trimesters.
[c]Sometimes categorized as B.
[d]Nitrous oxide, though able to interfere with vitamin B_{12} and folate metabolism, does not appear to be teratogenic in normal use, though it is advisable to restrict use to the second or third trimester.
*Prilocaine, at least in theory, can cause methaemoglobinaemia.
NSAIDs, non-steroidal anti-inflammatory drugs.

Despite such considerations, there is scanty evidence of teratogenic effects in humans from exposure to GA agents. The greater risk is late in pregnancy when GA may induce respiratory depression in the fetus. As always, GA must be given in hospital.

Dental amalgam restorations release mercury vapour when teeth are chewed on or brushed, or the restorations are removed, some of which is inhaled, and some may dissolve in saliva and be swallowed. Most mercury entering the body is excreted, a small amount accumulates in the kidneys and, to a very much lesser extent, in brain, lungs, liver and gastrointestinal tract. Mercury can cross the placenta to the fetus and can also be detected in breast milk. However, there is no evidence of any link between amalgam use and birth defects or stillbirths. Generally, it is wise to minimize any health interventions during pregnancy and, though there is no reason to think that the placement or removal of amalgam during pregnancy

is harmful, it may be prudent, where clinically reasonable, to avoid this during pregnancy.

Radiography should be avoided, especially in the first trimester, even though dental radiography is unlikely to be a significant risk. Current guidelines are that exposure must be minimal but a lead apron is unnecessary unless the beam is directed at the fetus such as in vertex-occlusal radiography. It has been estimated that two periapical dental x-rays give an exposure less than that due to natural radiation for 1 day. MRI is best avoided during the first trimester.

In some pregnant women, gingivitis is aggravated (pregnancy gingivitis) or may even result in a pyogenic granuloma at the gingival margin (pregnancy epulis). These conditions typically arise after the second month and resolve on parturition. Pyogenic granulomas elsewhere may grow rapidly during pregnancy. Chronic periodontal disease in the mother has been linked with low-birthweight babies. In a few women subject

Box 25.10 Drugs that may be contraindicated in breast-feeding

- Aciclovir
- Alcohol
- Antidepressants
- Aspirin
- Azithromycin
- Benzodiazepines
- Buspirone
- Clarithromycin
- Corticosteroids
- Co-trimoxazole
- Dapsone
- Dihydrocodeine
- Famciclovir
- Indometacin
- Iodides
- Itraconazole
- Ketoconazole
- Oxcarbazepine
- Pentazocine
- Phenytoin
- Povidone–iodine
- Sulfonamides
- Sumatriptan
- Tetracyclines
- Voriconazole
- Warfarin

Table 25.16 Drugs that may be used in dentistry but are contraindicated in breast-feeding mothers, and alternatives

	May be contraindicated	Use alternative
Analgesics	Aspirin (high dose)	Aspirin (low dose)
	Dextropropoxyphene	Codeine
	Diflunisal	Diclofenac
	Indometacin	Mefenamic acid
		Acetaminophen
Anti-microbials	Tetracyclines	Erythromycin
	Aminoglycosides	Cephalosporins
	Co-trimoxazole	Penicillins
	Fluconazole	Rifampicin
		Ganciclovir
		Metronidazole
		Sulfonamides
Pre-medication	Atropine	Benzodiazepines (low dose)
	Chloral hydrate	Phenothiazines (low dose)
		Beta-blockers
Others	Antidepressants	
	Barbiturates	
	Etretinate	
	Carbamazepine	
	Corticosteroids (high dose)	
	Povidone–iodine	

to recurrent aphthae, ulcers may stop (or occasionally become more severe) during pregnancy.

Hazards to pregnant dental staff

Exposure to infections such as rubella or herpesviruses should be minimized or avoided.

Nitrous oxide scavenging must always be used and some pregnant staff exempt themselves from work involving GA or sedation.

Concern has been expressed, particularly in Sweden, about the risk of placental transfer of mercury as a result of exposure to the metal during pregnancy. However, measurements on female dental personnel and their newborn babies and non-exposed controls have shown no significant differences in the plasma mercury levels or in the fetal/maternal ratios of mercury levels. Experimental and clinical data do not suggest that there should be any restriction on use of amalgams or work restriction of dental professionals, provided that work practices are up to accepted standards.

Lactation and breast-feeding

Drugs may pass in the breast milk from mother to fetus, and thus care should be taken in their use (Box 25.10 and Table 25.16).

Various drugs can affect infants (Table 25.17). Drugs, if essential, should preferably be taken by the mother immediately after breast-feeding, so the milk levels of the drug are as low as possible at the next feed. Cephalexin is a useful antimicrobial as it is not secreted in the milk.

Fluoride passes into breast milk and, if the local water supply contains more than 1 mg/L fluoride, supplements are not indicated for the breast-fed infant.

THE MENOPAUSE

General and clinical aspects

The menopause – marked by cessation of menstrual periods – can start at any age between 40 and 55 years. It is the end of a woman's reproductive life. Although rarely associated with serious physical or other complications, some women in the menopause gain weight, lose muscle tone, develop a few hairs on the chin or upper lip or have hot flushes. These appear to be caused by vasomotor instability, and may sometimes be controlled by hormone replacement therapy (HRT). The menopause is frequently associated with emotional disturbances and stresses, often due to the changes in the pattern of family life around that time. Psychological disorders are not uncommon and are usually mild (e.g. dizziness and insomnia), but depression or paranoia may develop.

Osteoporosis is more common (Ch. 16); HRT slows its development, and reduces the risk of fractures.

General management

Hormone replacement therapy is replacement of reduced oestrogen secretion after menopause or oophorectomy, with

Table 25.17 Drug effects on breast-feeding infants

Drug	Reported outcomes of use
Alcohol (ethanol)	With large amounts, drowsiness, weakness, decrease in linear growth, abnormal weight gain
Aspirin (salicylates)	Metabolic acidosis (rare)
Atenolol	Cyanosis; bradycardia
Bendroflumethiazide	Suppresses lactation
Caffeine	Irritability, poor sleeping pattern, excreted slowly; no effect with moderate intake of caffeinated beverages (2–3 cups per day)
Carbimazole	Goitre
Chloral hydrate	Sleepiness
Contraceptive pill with oestrogen/progestogen	Rare breast enlargement; decrease in milk production and protein content
Danthron	Increased bowel activity
Dexbrompheniramine maleate with D-isoephedrine	Crying, poor sleeping patterns, irritability
Ethosuximide	Drug appears in infant blood
Indometacin	Seizure (rare)
Iodides	May affect thyroid activity; goitre
Iodine	Goitre
Iodine (povidone–iodine)	Elevated iodine levels in breast milk, odour of iodine on infant's skin
Nalidixic acid	Haemolysis in glucose-6-phosphate dehydrogenase (G6PD) deficiency
Nitrofurantoin	Haemolysis in infant with G6PD deficiency
Phenobarbital	Sedation; infantile spasms after weaning, methaemoglobinaemia (rare)
Phenytoin	Methaemoglobinaemia (rare)
Sulfapyridine	Caution in jaundice or G6PD deficiency and ill, stressed or premature infant
Sulfisoxazole	Caution in jaundice or G6PD deficiency and ill, stressed or premature infant
Tetracyclines	Tooth discolouration
Theophylline	Irritability
Tolbutamide	Possible jaundice

Table 25.18 Marketed herbal alternatives to hormone replacement therapy

REPORTED POSSIBLE BENEFIT		NO REPORTED BENEFIT FROM THESE HERBAL ALTERNATIVES
Herbal alternatives	Comments	
Soy and isoflavones (plant oestrogens in beans, particularly soybeans)	Helpful in short term to relieve hot flushes and night sweats, but may be harmful to women with oestrogen-dependent breast cancer	Chasteberry (monk's pepper, Indian spice, sage tree hemp or tree wild pepper), dong quai, evening primrose, ginseng, valerian root, wild and Mexican yam
St John's wort	Helpful in short term for mild to moderate depression	
Black cohosh	Helpful in short term (6 months or less) for hot flushes and night sweats	

plus progestogen may cause more harm than good. Alternatives to HRT are shown in Table 25.18. Bisphosphonates along with calcium and vitamin D supplements can also be used to minimize osteoporosis (Ch. 16).

Dental aspects

Local anaesthesia is satisfactory. Conscious sedation can be given if required. GA must as always be carried out in hospital.

Hormone replacement therapy appears to lessen alveolar bone and tooth loss as well as gingival bleeding in older women, and improves salivary flow and buffering capacity. Overall, however, HRT appears not to improve complaints such as oral discomfort. Adverse effects from bisphosphonates are discussed in Ch. 16.

Atypical facial pain and oral dysaesthesias are particularly common, but there is little evidence of benefit from use of steroid sex hormones.

Dryness of the mouth and desquamative gingivitis are more common in the middle-aged or older, and particularly in females, but are not hormonal – rather immunological – in origin. Sjögren syndrome, lichen planus and mucous membrane pemphigoid are simply more common at this age.

FACIAL COSMETIC PROCEDURES

Cosmetic facial procedures include orthognathic surgery; removal or unsightly skin lesions; laser resurfacing; chemical peeling; or injections of botulinum toxoid (Ch. 13)- and a range of other procedures some of which are shown in Table 25.19. Often performed as outpatient procedures under local anesthesia with or without sedation but general anaesthesia may be used. Outcomes may include pain, swelling, bleeding and bruising and infection. The resultant changes in appearance typically persist for months or sometimes years, notably where non-resorbable materials have been used.

oestrogens taken orally, via a patch on the skin or implanted; or with oestrogens plus progestogens (progestin). Tibolone, a steroid with oestrogenic, progestogenic and androgenic activities, has the same licensed applications. HRT is used mainly for the benefits from short-term relief of menopausal symptoms and prevention of osteoporosis. There may also be benefits from reduced colorectal cancer. Adverse effects of HRT may include a predisposition to deep vein thrombosis, stroke and coronary heart disease, and an increase in breast, and possibly ovarian and endometrial cancers.

Consideration of the risks and benefits of HRT has concluded it is beneficial but that the combined HRT of oestrogen

Table 25.19 Facial cosmetic procedures other than use of orthognathic surgery or botulinum toxoid

Common terminology	Alternative terminology	Intended outcomes	Comments
Brow lift	Forehead lift	Eliminate stern or furrowed brows	Multiple incisions within hairline or single incision in upper eyelids. Alternatively a wide incision across top of the scalp
Ear surgery	Ear pinning or otoplasty	Correct protruding or deformed ears	–
Eyelid surgery	Blepharoplasty	Eliminate tired or droopy eyelids	Incision within upper eyelid
Facial augmentation	Injectable fillers (see Table 25.20)	Change facial contours, lines and creases	Pharmaceutical filler or patients own fat is injected below skin
Face lift	Rhytidectomy	Eliminate facial signs of aging, including wrinkles and sagging skin	Incisions within hairline, above the temple and continue along or just inside ear, ending behind the ear, A second incision beneath the chin is sometimes necessary
Facial implants	Used most commonly in the cheek, chin, jaw or nasal region	Change facial contours	Polyethylene*, e-PTFE*, silicone*, hydroxyapatite*, collagen, or injectables are used. Incisions if needed are placed inside mouth or discreetly externally
Rhinoplasty	Nasal reshaping or nose job	Correct deviated septum, bump on the bridge, wide nostrils, bulbous tip, or hooked nose	Incisions at the nostril base and/or inside nose

*usually non-resorbable

Fillers

Injectable fillers are an increasingly popular cosmetic procedure. Results are temporary, lasting a few months with natural products to several years when synthetic materials are used. Complications may include temporary pain, bleeding, bruising, swelling, seromas (fluid collections), infection or allergy or mainly with synthetic materials such as silicone – long-term granulomas/disfigurement. However, the existence of a so-called Silicone immune Toxicity Syndrome is controversial.

The U.S. Food and Drug Administration (FDA) reviews and approves pharmaceutical fillers in the same manner as medical devices. However, some fillers may be used on an off-label basis and injection of permanent substances (e.g. sillicone) in particular poses safety issues such as granuloma formation (Table 25.20).

Table 25.20 Fillers used include those shown

Origin	Material	Source
Natural	Collagen	Human or bovine natural skin protein
	Fat (free fat transfer, autologous fat transfer/transplantation, lipos-culture, lipostructure micro-lipoinjection)	Human-typically from inner thigh or abdomen
	Hyaluronic Acid	Human or animal
	Hydroxyapatite	Mineral suspended in a gel-like formulation
Synthetic*	Polyacrylamide	Hydrophilic polyacrylamide gel (HPG)
	Poly-L-lactic acid	
	Polymethylmethacrylate	20-25% PMMA microspheres in collagen gel
	Silicone	Dimethylsiloxane

*usually non-resorbable

TRANSGENDER

Transgender is the state of gender identity (self-identification) not matching one's "assigned sex" (identification by others as male or female based on physical features or genetic make-up) and does not imply any specific form of sexual orientation (see http://en.wikipedia.org/wikii/Transgender).

USEFUL WEBSITES

http://www.2niddk.nih.gov/pubs/pregnancy
http://www.cancer.gov/cancertopics/types/prostate
http://bmj.bmjjournals.com/cgi/collection/pregnancy
http://health.yahoo.com/children
http://www.bafo.org.uk/
http://www.womenshealth.gov/
http://www.womens-health.co.uk/
http://www.cpdt.org.uk/
http://www.nice.org.uk/CG89
http://www.uihealthcare.com/topics
http://news.bbc.co.uk/2/hi/health/2772263.stm
http://www.plasticsurgery.org/news_room/press_releases/A-Party-May-Not-Be-Best-Setting-for-Botox-Injections.cfm
http://www/lipaugmentation.com/microimplants.htm#Injectable%20Silicone%20gel:
http://www.lipaugmentation.com/microimplants.htm#Artecoll™.
http://www.canderm.com/page.asp?intNodeID=8035.
http://www.talksurgery.com/
http://www.drbader.com/
http://www.surgery.org/public/consumer/fag/glossary_of_injectables_and_ermal_fillers_terms
http://www.center4research.org/Injectables.html
http://dermnetnz.org/procedures.html

FURTHER READING

Allen, P.F., Whitworth, J.M., 2004. Endodontic considerations in the elderly. Gerodontology 21, 185–194.

Chalmers, J.M., 2006. Minimal intervention dentistry, part 2: strategies for addressing restorative challenges in older adults. J Can Dent Assoc 72, 435–440.

Durso, S.C., 2005. Interaction with other health team members in caring for elderly patients. Dent Clin North Am 49, 377–388.

Epstein, J.B., Parker, I.R., Epstein, M.S., Gupta, A., Kutis, S., Witkowski, D.M., 2007. A survey of National Cancer Institute-designated comprehensive cancer centers' oral health supportive care practices and resources in the United States. Support Care Cancer 15, 357–362.

Ettinger, R.L., 2007. Oral health and older adults. J Am Dent Assoc 138, 1S–56S.

Fatahzadeh, M., Glick, M., 2006. Stroke: epidemiology, classification, risk factors, complications, diagnosis, prevention, and medical and dental management. Oral Surg Oral Med Oral Pathol Oral Radiol Endod 102, 180–191.

Fiske, J., Frenkel, H., Griffiths, J., Jones, V., 2006. Guidelines for the development of local standards of oral health care for people with dementia. Gerodontology 23 (Suppl 1), 5–32.

Frutos, R., Rodriguez, S., Miralles-Jorda, L., Machuca, G., 2002. Oral manifestations and dental treatment in menopause. Med Oral 7, 26–30, 31–5.

Gupta, A., Epstein, J.B., Sroussi, H., 2006. Hyposalivation in elderly patients. J Can Dent Assoc 72, 841–846.

Herman, W.W., Konzelman Jr., J.L., Prisant, L.M., 2004. Joint National Committee on Prevention, Detection, Evaluation, and Treatment of High Blood Pressure. New national guidelines on hypertension: a summary for dentistry. J Am Dent Assoc 135, 576–584.

Hupp, J.R., 2006. Ischemic heart disease: dental management considerations. Dent Clin North Am 50, 483–491.

Marx, R.E., 2006. Oral and intravenous bisphosphonate-induced osteonecrosis of the jaws: history, etiology, prevention and treatment. Quintessence Publishing, Chicago.

McKenna, S.J., 2006. Dental management of patients with diabetes. Dent Clin North Am 50, 591–606.

Montandon, A.A., Pinelli, L.A., Fais, L.M., 2006. Quality of life and oral hygiene in older people with manual functional imitations. J Dent Educ 70, 1261–1262.

Muller, F., Schimmel, M., 2007. Management of preventive care for an ageing population. Int Dent J 57, 215–220.

Sacco, D., Frost, D.E., 2006. Dental management of patients with stroke or Alzheimer's disease. Dent Clin North Am 50, 625–633.

Scully, C., Diz Dios, P., Kumar, N., 2007. Special care in dentistry: handbook of oral healthcare. Elsevier Churchill Livingstone, Edinburgh.

Scully, C., Ettinger, R.L., 2007. The influence of systemic diseases on oral health care in older adults. J Am Dent Assoc 138, 7S–13S.

Scully, C., Wolff, A., 2004. Oral surgery in patients on anticoagulant therapy. Oral Surg Oral Med Oral Pathol Oral Radiol Endod 94, 57–64.

Shay, K., 2004. The evolving impact of aging America on dental practice. J Contemp Dent Pract 5, 101–110.

The Gerodontology Association, 2005. Meeting the challenges of oral health for older people; a strategic review. Gerodontology 22 (Suppl 1), 2–48.

Yagiela, J.A., Haymore, T.L., 2007. Management of the hypertensive dental patient. J Calif Dent Assoc 35, 51–59.

ALTERNATIVE AND COMPLEMENTARY MEDICINE

Therapies that are not currently considered an integral part of conventional allopathic medical practice are termed *complementary* when used in addition to, and *alternative* when used instead of, conventional treatments. Such therapies include, but are not limited to, acupuncture, chiropractic, diet fads (Ch. 27), faith healing, folk medicine, herbal (natural) medicine, homoeopathy, naturopathy, new age healing, massage and music therapy.

This section focuses on acupuncture and herbal medicines, since there is some evidence of efficacy, and increasing use of them by the public.

ACUPUNCTURE

A limited number of randomized controlled trials (RCTs) have given some support to acupuncture as a possible effective treatment for a range of conditions including anxiety, cancer and chemotherapy-induced nausea, depression, insomnia, migraine, musculoskeletal pain and post-operative pain. However, there is inadequate evidence of benefit for acupuncture in other conditions such as asthma, dysphagia, epilepsy, schizophrenia, smoking cessation or stroke.

There are very few published RCTs of acupuncture used for orofacial conditions (Table 26.1). A recent study showed that 15 of 48 papers on the treatment of temporomandibular dysfunction met the inclusion criteria for analysis; acupuncture in the majority proved effective but four studies showed no effect. Another author found 16 controlled studies showing relief of dental pain, concluding that most trials suggest acupuncture can be effective in analgesia.

Early studies suggested a relationship between acupuncture and release of endogenous opiates (beta-endorphin, enkephalin, endomorphin and dynorphin) (Ch. 10). The serotoninergic

descending inhibitory pathway is also suggested to be a mechanism of acupuncture analgesia. The autonomic nervous system (ANS) may also have a connection with acupuncture: the inflammatory reflex (via the ANS) might be part of anti-hyperalgesia elicited by acupuncture. Many efforts have been made to clarify these mechanisms, but satisfactory consensus has yet to be reached.

HERBAL MEDICINES

Many conventional and proven effective drugs have originated from plant sources. Examples include aspirin (from willow bark), digoxin (foxglove), morphine (opium poppy) and quinine (cinchona bark). However, not all natural medicines are safe. Some plant products such as opioids and cocaine are addictive (Ch. 35); many are highly toxic, for example some Chinese herbs prescribed for weight loss are nephrotoxic, and kava-kava (*Piper methysticum*) is hepatotoxic. Some herbal products may cause problems in surgery by, for example, impairing platelet aggregation, thus prolonging bleeding (Table 26.2).

However, research into safety and efficacy of herbal drugs has been limited because of product variability, lack of controlled studies and few legal controls. Some herbal drugs appear to be effective and fairly safe. Reliable published data support a potential medicinal role for saw palmetto, melatonin and St John's wort (Table 26.3). Reliable published data on efficacy

Table 26.1 Acupuncture in orofacial conditions

BENEFIT PROVED		
Probably	**Short term possibly**	**Inconclusive at best**
Dental pain	Dental LA reduced time to onset	Bell palsy
Post-operative or chemotherapy-induced nausea/vomiting	Gag reflex	Mouth ulceration
Post-operative pain	Neck pain	Sensory loss
TMJ pain		Sinusitis
		Xerostomia

LA, local anaesthesia; TMJ, temporomandibular joint.

Table 26.2 Herbal products that may interfere with haemostasis

Bilberry	Vaccinium myrtillus
Bromelain	Anas comosus
Cat's claw	Uncaria tomentosa
Devil's claw	Harpagophytum procumbens
Dong quai	Angelica sinensis
Evening primrose	Oenothera biennis
Feverfew	Tanacetum parthenium
Garlic	Allium savitum
Ginger	Zingiber officinale
Ginkgo biloba	Ginkgo biloba
Ginseng	Panax ginseng
Grape seed	Vitis vinifera
Green tea	Camellia sinensis
Horse chestnut	Aesculus hippocastanum
Turmeric	Curcuma longa

are weaker for gingko biloba, and are contradictory for valerian and echinacea.

Saw palmetto, from *Serenoa repens* fruit, can be effective treatment for benign prostatic hypertrophy (BPH), producing similar improvement in urinary symptoms and flow as finasteride and with fewer adverse effects. However, the long-term effectiveness, safety and ability to prevent BPH complications are unknown.

Melatonin taken in the evening in the new time zone will reset the biological clock and alleviate (or prevent) the symptoms of jet lag. The incidence of adverse effects is low. The effects of melatonin in people with epilepsy, and a possible interaction with warfarin, however, need investigation.

St John's wort (*Hypericum perforatum*; SJW) provides effective treatment for mild to moderate major depression. SJW also induces various drug-metabolizing enzymes (cytochrome P450 isoenzymes, CYP3A4, CYP2C9, CYP1A2, and the transport protein P-glycoprotein), which results in lower blood levels and therapeutic effect of some drugs. Because levels of active SJW ingredients vary from one preparation to the other, and patients may switch between preparations, the degree of induction is likely to vary. It is important also to note that, when patients stop taking SJW, blood levels of interacting medicines may rise, resulting in toxicity.

St John's wort affects brain neurotransmitters and may interact with psychotropic medicines including antidepressants such as selective serotonin reuptake inhibitors (SSRIs) and serotonin (5HT$_{1D}$) receptor agonists such as triptans; it should not be used with several other drugs (Box 26.1). SJW may interact with anticonvulsants and is therefore contraindicated in patients with epilepsy.

Although there is no direct evidence, clinically important interactions are also likely between SJW and anti-HIV drugs [particularly protease inhibitors (saquinavir, ritonavir, nelfinavir) and non-nucleoside reverse transcriptase inhibitors (efavirena, nevirapine)].

Dehydroepiandrosterone (DHEA), an adrenal androgen and neurosteroid, may also be an effective treatment of midlife-onset minor and major depression.

Gingko biloba appears to improve memory and serial arithmetic tasks in young healthy adults and, in cognitively intact older adults, appears to enhance certain neuropsychological/memory processes. Ginkgo appears effective in Alzheimer disease, improving cognitive performance, global function and activities of daily living and, at least *in vitro*, appears to inhibit the amyloid-beta aggregation and caspase-3 activation implicated in its pathogenesis (Ch. 13). Meta-analyses comparing ginkgo with acetylcholinesterase inhibitors have shown similar clinical efficacy, with an additional safety benefit for ginkgo.

DENTAL ASPECTS

Various herbal preparations have a potential for effects on oral disease (Table 26.4) and treatment, especially when benzodiazepine sedation is used (Table 26.5).

Box 26.1 Drugs to be avoided with St John's wort

- Anticonvulsants (including carbamazepine)
- Ciclosporin
- Cytotoxic drugs
- Digoxin
- Indinavir and other protease inhibitors
- Oral contraceptives
- Selective serotonin reuptake inhibitors
- Serotonin receptor agonists such as triptans
- Theophylline
- Warfarin

Table 26.3 Herbal preparations and supplements of proven efficacy

Herbal preparation	Effective for treating	Derived from	Interactions	Adverse effects
Saw palmetto	Benign prostatic hyperplasia	*Serenoa repens*	–	Minimal
Melatonin	Jet lag	Synthetic	Warfarin	–
St John's wort (SJW)	Mild to moderate depression	A yellow-flowered weed *Hypericum perforatum*	Induces cytochrome P450 hepatic enzyme system, specifically CYP3A4 isoform, and thus interacts with drugs such as indinavir, irinotecan, ciclosporin, digoxin, warfarin, oral contraceptives, antidepressants, phenprocoumon, theophylline, loperamide, vinca alkaloids, etoposide, teniposide, anthracycline, paclitaxel, docetaxel and tamoxifen. SJW may also intensify or prolong the effects of some narcotic drugs and anaesthetic agents	Dry mouth, dizziness, gastrointestinal symptoms, increased sensitivity to sunlight and fatigue
Gingko biloba	Improved memory; stable or slowed deterioration in Alzheimer disease	A flowering tree native to China	Anticoagulant and antiplatelet medicines	Minimal
Echinacea	Increases the 'non-specific' activity of the immune system Contradictory reports of efficacy in prevention of upper respiratory infections	*Echinacea purpurea*	Anabolic steroids	Should not be used in progressive systemic and autoimmune disorders such as tuberculosis, or connective tissue disorders

Table 26.4 Herbals and other preparations and oral disease

Preparation	Effects
Pilocarpine	Brazilian 'slobber plant' (*Pilocarpus jaborandi*) helps xerostomia
Aloe vera	Reportedly provides relief in oral lichen planus
B vitamins *Eupatorium laevigatum* Lam. Liquorice with glycyrrhizic acid removed (deglycyrrhizinated liquorice; DGL) Acemannon (an aloe polysaccharide) Tannins (in agrimony, cranesbill, tormentil, oak, periwinkle and witch hazel) Zinc *Lactobacillus acidophilus* and *L. bulgaricus* LongoVita	Reportedly provide relief in aphthae
Coenzyme Q	Not demonstrated reliably to control periodontal disease

Table 26.5 Potential interactions of herbal preparations with benzodiazepines

Herbal preparation	Potential effect on sedation
Dong quai	Increased
Houpu	Increased
Kava kava	Increased
Passion flower	Increased
St John's wort	Reduced
Tan shen	Increased
Valerian	Reduced

PROBIOTICS

Probiotics are living micro-organisms added to food which beneficially affect the host by improving intestinal microbial balance and thus exert positive health effects. The main probiotics used include *Lactobacillus rhamnosus* GG, *L. reuteri*, bifidobacteria, certain strains of *L. casei* or the *L. acidophilus* group, *Escherichia coli* strain Nissle 1917, and certain enterococci (*Enterococcus faecium* SF68) and the probiotic yeast *Saccharomyces boulardii*.

The underlying mechanisms of probiotic action are unclear, but may include strengthening of the non-immunological gut barrier, pathogen growth inhibition and interference with adhesion, and enhancement of local mucosal immune systems, as well as of the systemic immune response. Probiotics appear effective in preventing and reducing the severity of a number of conditions shown in Box 26.2.

There is insufficient, or at most preliminary, evidence with respect to suggested benefits from probiotics in prevention or therapy of ischaemic heart diseases, amelioration of auto-immune disease, or prevention of cancer.

Oral instillation of probiotic bacteria produces detectable levels in saliva shortly after, but much longer-term instillation has not been shown. Randomized controlled trials on probiotics in oral health are few. Lactic acid-producing bacteria can produce antimicrobial factors (e.g. organic acids, hydrogen peroxide, carbon peroxide, diacetyl, low-molecular-weight antimicrobial substances, bacteriocins and adhesion inhibitors). *Lactobacillus* and *Bifidobacterium* may have beneficial effects by inhibiting cariogenic streptococci and *Candida* species. Six of seven placebo-controlled studies on the effect of probiotics from these bacteria reported reduced salivary *Streptococcus mutans* and/or yeasts. A study carried out in 3–4-year-old children reported significant caries reduction after 7 months of daily consumption of probiotic milk. The bacteriocin producer *Streptococcus salivarius* K12 may reduce halitosis.

A prebiotic is a selectively fermented ingredient that allows specific changes in the composition and/or activity of the gastrointestinal microflora that confer benefits upon host well-being and health. Only bifidogenic, non-digestible oligosaccharides [particularly inulin, its hydrolysis product oligofructose, and (trans) galacto-oligosaccharides] fulfil criteria to be classed as prebiotic. Prebiotics are thus dietary fibres with a well-established positive impact on the intestinal microflora, which may help prevent diarrhoea or constipation, modulate intestinal flora metabolism, and may have positive effects on cancer prevention lipid metabolism, mineral adsorption and immunity.

Synergistic combinations of probiotics and prebiotics are called *synbiotics*.

Box 26.2 Conditions benefiting from use of probiotics

- Acute diarrhoea in children
- Antibiotic-associated diarrhoea
- Inflammatory bowel disease, especially ulcerative colitis
- Prevention of urogenital tract infection
- Reduction of atopy in children
- Reduction of lactose intolerance
- Reduction of the concentration of cancer-promoting enzymes and/or gut putrefactive (bacterial) metabolites
- Normalization of passing stool and stool consistency in subjects suffering from irritable bowel syndrome
- Prevention of respiratory tract infections (common cold, influenza)

USEFUL WEBSITES

http://altmedicine.about.com/
http://nccam.nih.gov/
http://www.dh.gov.uk/en/Publichealth/Healthimprovement/Complementaryandalternativemedicine/index.htm
http://www.gdc-uk.org/search?text=cosmetic

FURTHER READING

Ang-Lee, M.K., Moss, J., Yuan, C.S., 2001. Herbal medicines and perioperative care. JAMA 286, 208–216.

Bardia, A., Barton, D.L., Prokop, L.J., Bauer, B.A., Moynihan, T.J., 2006. Efficacy of complementary and alternative medicine therapies in relieving cancer pain: a systematic review. J Clin Oncol 24, 5457–5464.

Bergström, I., List, T., Magnusson, T., 2008. A follow-up study of subjective symptoms of temporomandibular disorders in patients who received acupuncture and/or interocclusal appliance therapy 18–20 years earlier. Acta Odontol Scand 66, 88–92.

Birch, S., Hesselink, J.K., Jonkman, F.A., Hekker, T.A., Bos, A., 2004. Clinical research on acupuncture. Part 1. What have reviews of the efficacy and safety of acupuncture told us so far? J Altern Complement Med 10, 468–480.

Caglar, E., Kargul, B., Tanboga, I., 2005. Bacteriotherapy and probiotics' role on oral health. Oral Dis 11, 131–137.

Chen, H.Y., Shi, Y., Ng, C.S., Chan, S.M., Yung, K.K., Zhang, Q.L., 2007. Auricular acupuncture treatment for insomnia: a systematic review. J Altern Complement Med 13, 669–676.

Cheuk, D.K., Wong, V., 2006. Acupuncture for epilepsy. Cochrane Database Syst Rev (2), CD005062.

Cheuk, D.K., Yeung, W.F., Chung, K.F., Wong, V., 2007. Acupuncture for insomnia. Cochrane Database Syst Rev (3), CD005472.

Eitner, S., Wichmann, M., Holst, S., 2005. A long-term therapeutic treatment for patients with a severe gag reflex. Int J Clin Exp Hypn 53, 74–86.

Endres, H.G., Diener, H.C., Molsberger, A., 2007. Role of acupuncture in the treatment of migraine. Expert Rev Neurother 7, 1121–1134.

Ernst, E., Pittler, M.H., 2001. The desktop guide to complementary and alternative Medicine. Mosby, Edinburgh.

Ernst, E., Pittler, M.H., 1998. The effectiveness of acupuncture in treating acute dental pain: a systematic review. Br Dent J 184, 443–447.

Ezzo, J.M., Richardson, M.A., Vickers, A., et al., 2006 Apr 19. Acupuncture-point stimulation for chemotherapy-induced nausea or vomiting. Cochrane Database Syst Rev (2) CD002285.

Goddard, G., Karibe, H., McNeill, C., Villafuerte, E., 2002. Acupuncture and sham acupuncture reduce muscle pain in myofascial pain patients. J Orofac Pain 16, 71–76.

Goddard, G., 2005. Short term pain reduction with acupuncture treatment for chronic orofacial pain patients. Med Sci Monit 11, CR71–CR74.

Hammerschlag, R., 2003. Acupuncture: on what should its evidence base be based? Altern Ther Health Med 9, 34–35.

He, L., Zhou, M.K., Zhou, D., et al., 2007. Acupuncture for Bell's palsy. Cochrane Database Syst Rev (4), CD002914.

Henney, J.E., 2000. Risk of drug interactions with St. John's wort. From the Food and Drug Administration. JAMA 283, 1679.

Jedel, E., 2005. Acupuncture in xerostomia – a systematic review. J Oral Rehabil 32, 392–396.

Jorm, A.F., Christensen, H., Griffiths, K.M., Parslow, R.A., Rodgers, B., Blewitt, K.A., 2004. Effectiveness of complementary and self-help treatments for anxiety disorders. Med J Aust 181 (7 Suppl), S29–S46.

Ka, L., Hirata, Y., Kobayashi, A., Wake, H., Kino, K., Amagasa, T., 2006. [Treatment results of acupuncture in inferior alveolar and lingual nerves sensory paralysis after oral surgery]. Kokubyo Gakkai Zasshi 73, 40–46.

Kaye, A.D., Baluch, A., Kaye, A.J., Frass, M., Hofbauer, R., 2007. Pharmacology of herbals and their impact in anesthesia. Curr Opin Anaesthesiol 20, 294–299.

Leo, R.J., Ligot Jr., J.S., 2007. A systematic review of randomized controlled trials of acupuncture in the treatment of depression. J. Affect Disord 97, 13–22.

Lin, J.G., Chen, W.L., 2008. Acupuncture analgesia: a review of its mechanisms of actions. Am J Chin Med 36, 635–645.

Linde, K., Hondras, M., Vickers, A., Riet Gt, G., Melchart, D., 2001. Systematic reviews of complementary therapies – an annotated bibliography. Part 3: Homeopathy. BMC Complement Altern Med 1, 4.

Linde, K., ter Riet, G., Hondras, M., Vickers, A., Saller, R., Melchart, D., 2001. Systematic reviews of complementary therapies – an annotated bibliography. Part 2: Herbal medicine. BMC Complement Altern Med 1, 5.

Linde, K., Vickers, A., Hondras, M., et al., 2001. Systematic reviews of complementary therapies – an annotated bibliography. Part 1: Acupuncture. BMC Complement Altern Med 1, 3.

Little, J.W., 2004. Complementary and alternative medicine: impact on dentistry. Oral Surg Oral Med Oral Pathol Oral Radiol Endod 98, 137–145.

Lu, D.P., Lu, G.P., 2003. Anatomical relevance of some acupuncture points in the head and neck region that dictate medical or dental application depending on depth of needle insertion. Acupunct Electrother Res 28, 145–156.

McCarney, R.W., Lasserson, T.J., Linde, K., Brinkhaus, B., 2004. An overview of two Cochrane systematic reviews of complementary treatments for chronic asthma: acupuncture and homeopathy. Respir Med 98, 687–696.

Meurman, J.H., 2005. Probiotics: do they have a role in oral medicine and dentistry? Eur J Oral Sci 113, 188–196.

Morganstein, W.M., 2005. Acupuncture in the treatment of xerostomia: clinical report. Gen Dent 53, 223–226, quiz 227.

Myers, C.D., White, B.A., Heft, M.W., 2002. A review of complementary and alternative medicine use for treating chronic facial pain. J Am Dent Assoc 133, 1189–1196, quiz 1259–60.

Nieuw Amerongen, A.V., Veerman, E.C., 2003. Current therapies for xerostomia and salivary gland hypofunction associated with cancer therapies. Support Care Cancer 11, 226–231.

Pilkington, K., Kirkwood, G., Rampes, H., Cummings, M., Richardson, J., 2007. Acupuncture for anxiety and anxiety disorders – a systematic literature review. Acupunct Med 25, 1–10.

Pirotta, M., 2007. Acupuncture in musculoskeletal disorders – is there a point? Aust Fam Physician 36, 447–448.

Pohodenko-Chudakova, I.O., 2005. Acupuncture analgesia and its application in cranio-maxillofacial surgical procedures. J Craniomaxillofac Surg 33, 118–122.

Rathbone, J., Xia, J., 2005. Acupuncture for schizophrenia. Cochrane Database Syst Rev (4), CD005475.

Robb, K.A., Bennett, M.I., Johnson, M.I., Simpson, K.J., Oxberry, S.G., 2008. Transcutaneous electric nerve stimulation (TENS) for cancer pain in adults. Cochrane Database Syst Rev (3), CD006276.

Rosted, P., Bundgaard, M., Fiske, J., Pedersen, A.M., 2006. The use of acupuncture in controlling the gag reflex in patients requiring an upper alginate impression: an audit. Br Dent J 201, 721–725, discussion 715.

Rosted, P., Bundgaard, M., Pedersen, A.M., 2006. The use of acupuncture in the treatment of temporomandibular dysfunction-an audit. Acupunct Med 24, 16–22.

Rosted, P., Bundgaard, M., 2003. Can acupuncture reduce the induction time of a local anaesthetic? A pilot study. Acupunct Med 21, 92–99.

Rosted, P., 1998. The use of acupuncture in dentistry: a review of the scientific validity of published papers. Oral Dis 4, 100–104.

Smith, C.A., Hay, P.P., 2005. Acupuncture for depression. Cochrane Database Syst Rev (2), CD004046.

Snyder, M., Wieland, J., 2003. Complementary and alternative therapies: what is their place in the management of chronic pain? Nurs Clin North Am 38, 495–508.

Stavem, K., Rossberg, E., Larsson, P.G., 2008. Health-related quality of life outcomes in a trial of acupuncture, sham acupuncture and conventional treatment for chronic sinusitis. BMC Res Notes 1, 37.

Sun, Y., Gan, T.J., Dubose, J.W., Habib, A.S., 2008. Acupuncture and related techniques for postoperative pain: a systematic review of randomized controlled trials. Br J Anaesth 101, 151–160.

Thayer, M.L., 2007. The use of acupuncture in dentistry. Dent Update 34, 244–246, 249–50.

Tweddell, P., Boyle, C., 2009. Potential interactions with herbal medications and midazolam. Dent Update 36, 175–178.

Vachiramon, A., Wang, W.C., Vachiramon, T., 2004. The use of acupuncture in implant dentistry. Implant Dent 13, 58–64.

Wang, H., Qi, H., Wang, B.S., et al., 2008. Is acupuncture beneficial in depression: a meta-analysis of 8 randomized controlled trials? J Affect Disord 111, 125–134.

Wang, S.M., Caldwell-Andrews, A.A., Kain, Z.N., 2003. The use of complementary and alternative medicines by surgical patients: a follow-up survey study. Anesth Analg 97, 1010–1015.

Wang, S.M., Kain, Z.N., White, P.F., 2008. Acupuncture analgesia: II. Clinical considerations. Anesth Analg 106, 611–621.

White, A.R., Filshie, J., Cummings, T.M., 2001. International Acupuncture Research Forum. Clinical trials of acupuncture: consensus recommendations for optimal treatment, sham controls and blinding. Complement Ther Med 9, 237–245.

White, A.R., Rampes, H., Campbell, J.L., 2006. Acupuncture and related interventions for smoking cessation. Cochrane Database Syst Rev (1), CD000009.

Wong, Y.K., Cheng, J., 2003. A case series of temporomandibular disorders treated with acupuncture, occlusal splint and point injection therapy. Acupunct Med 21, 138–149.

Yukizaki, H., Nakajima, S., Nakashima, K., Yamada, Y., Sato, T., 1986. Electroacupuncture increases ipsilaterally tooth pain threshold in man. Am J Chin Med 14, 68–72.

Zhang, S.H., Liu, M., Asplund, K., Li, L., 2005. Acupuncture for acute stroke. Cochrane Database Syst Rev (2), CD003317.

Zollman, C., Vickers, A., 2000. ABC of complementary Medicine. BMJ Books, London.

Appendix 26.1 Herbal preparations and supplements of unproven efficacy

Herbal preparation	Purported used for 'treating'	Interactions possible with	Comments
Agnus castus fruit extract	Premenstrual syndrome	–	–
Butterbur (*Petasites hybridus*)	Allergic rhinitis	–	–
Coenzyme Q_{10} (CoQ_{10}, Q_{10}, vitamin Q_{10}, ubiquinone or ubidecarenone)	Breast and other cancer control Periodontal disease (no proven benefit)	Warfarin Insulin	–
Cranberry–lingonberry juice	Recurrent urinary tract infections	–	Possibly effective
Feverfew (*Chrysanthemum parthenium*)	Migraine prophylaxis	Anticoagulants	–
Garlic	Mildly elevated cholesterol and blood pressure and to help arteries remain elastic. Also has antibacterial properties	Anticoagulants Saquinavir	Has antiplatelet activity
Ginger	Nausea and vomiting	–	May impair platelet activity
Ginseng	Aphrodisiac, antidepressant, increases resistance, and improves both physical and mental performance	–	Possibly effective. Can cause bleeding, hypertension and tachycardia
Glucosamine	Pain control and for improving function in osteoarthritis	–	Possibly effective
Senna	Constipation	–	Possibly effective
Valerian (*Valeriana officinalis*)	Sleep disturbance	Barbiturates	–

Appendix 26.2 Herbal preparations and supplements of unproven efficacy, but possible adverse effects

Herbal medicine	May also contain	Possible health hazard
Aristolochia plantain	Digitalis lanata	Cardiac
Arthrin	Indometacin and alprazolam	Sedation
Chaparral (a traditional American Indian medicine)		Liver disease
Comfrey (*Symphytum* species)		Hepatic blood flow obstruction
Ephedra, Ma huang, Chinese ephedra and epitonin		Hypertension, arrhythmia. Nerve damage, insomnia, tremors, headaches, seizures, stroke and death
Germander (*Teucrium* species)		Liver disease
Germanium		Kidney damage, possibly death
Green leaf tobacco		Nicotine poisoning
Hepastat, neutralis, poena, osporo	Indometacin	–
Hua fo	Sildenafil	–
Jin bu huan		Liver disease
Kava		Liver damage
Lobelia (also known as Indian tobacco)		Breathing problems. Sweating, hypotension, tachycardia, and possibly coma and death at higher doses
L-Tryptophan		Eosinophilia myalgia syndrome
Magnolia-stephania		Renal disease

Appendix 26.2 Herbal preparations and supplements of unproven efficacy, but possible adverse effects—cont'd

Herbal medicine	May also contain	Possible health hazard
Neo-melubrina	Dipyrone	–
Niacin		Stomach pain, vomiting, bloating, nausea, cramping, diarrhoea, liver disease, muscle disease, cardiac and eye damage
PC SPES (a formula consisting of a combination of eight herbs which contain a range of plant chemicals including flavonoids, alkanoids, polysaccharides)	Warfarin	Bleeding
Pennyroyal		Liver disease
RA Spes	Alprazolam	Sedation
5OA Plus	Indometacin	–
Selenium		Tissue damage
Slimming/dieter's teas		Nausea, diarrhoea, vomiting, stomach cramps, constipation, fainting
SPES	Alprazolam	Sedation
Vitamin A		Birth defects, bone abnormalities, and severe liver disease
Vitamin B$_6$		Ataxia, nerve injury
Willow bark	Salicylates	Reye syndrome
Wormwood		Hypoaesthesia of legs and arms, loss of intellect, delirium and paralyses

NSAIDs, non-steroidal anti-inflammatory drugs.

It is widely believed that a diet such as that discussed in Ch. 36 may be beneficial to health. There is also some evidence available to support this.

DIET AND HEALTH

Dietary factors have been implicated as influencing a range of conditions (Box 27.1).

Minimizing the intake of saturated fats (especially those from dairy sources) and partially hydrogenated vegetable fats has long been believed to lower the risk of coronary artery disease and some cancers (Chs. 5 and 22). In contrast, consumption of monounsaturated fats, such as olive oil, are alleged to be beneficial.

Generous amounts of vegetables and fruit daily appear to offer some protection against cancers of the stomach, colon and lung, and possibly against cancers of the mouth, larynx, cervix, bladder and breast (Ch. 22). Citrus fruits and juices in excess, however, may cause tooth erosion.

A high-fibre diet may also offer some protection against hypertension and coronary heart disease (Ch. 5). Carbohydrates as whole-grain unrefined products may offer some protection against colon cancer, diverticulitis and dental caries.

Box 27.1 Conditions that may be influenced by diet

- Alzheimer disease
- Birth defects such as facial clefts and spina bifida
- Cancer
- Cardiovascular disease (arteriosclerosis, hypertension and coronary artery disease
- Dental caries and erosion
- Diabetes and the 'metabolic syndrome'
- Drug absorption and metabolism

MALNUTRITION

Malnutrition is mainly a consequence of poverty or ignorance, and results from imbalance between the body's needs and the intake of nutrients, which can lead to obesity, or syndromes of deficiency, dependence or toxicity.

Overnutrition develops over time from overeating; insufficient exercise; overprescription of therapeutic diets, including parenteral nutrition; excess intake of vitamins, particularly pyridoxine (vitamin B_6), niacin, and vitamins A and D; and excess intake of trace minerals.

Undernutrition usually results from inadequate intake; malabsorption; abnormal systemic loss of nutrients due to diarrhoea, haemorrhage, renal failure, cancer, or excessive sweating; infection or addiction to drugs. Undernutrition (starvation) can develop rapidly.

OBESITY

General aspects

Obesity is the main nutritional problem in developed countries (Fig. 27.1) though some body fat is needed for stored energy, heat insulation, shock absorption and other functions. As a rule, women have more body fat than men.

To most people, the term 'obesity' means to be very overweight but 'overweight' is sometimes defined as an excess amount of body weight that includes muscle, bone, fat and water, while 'obesity' specifically refers to excessive body fat. Some people, such as bodybuilders or other athletes with a lot of muscle, can be overweight without being obese.

Men with more than 25% body fat and women with more than 30% body fat are obese. Almost 25% of North American adults are now clinically obese, and obesity is growing in children. More than 60% of Americans aged 20 years and older are overweight. Europe and Japan follow similar patterns. The National Health Service (NHS) survey in England showed male obesity rising from 13% (in 1993) to 24% (in 2006), and in females rising from 16% to 24% in the same period.

Obesity results from eating more than the body needs – an imbalance between calories in and calories out. Control of eating and weight regulation is complex, and involves a range of endocrine and nervous signals, especially peptide YY, ghrelin, insulin, cholecystokinin and leptin (Table 27.1).

The body monitors blood glucose concentration which contributes to the overall regulation of food intake, via GLUT2 transporters mediating glucose entry to the cells and the glucokinase enzyme. This makes their intracellular ATP supply exquisitely sensitive to glucose availability, and forms the basis for their signalling systems by pancreatic beta cells; portal vein glucose sensor; carotid bodies; the nucleus of the solitary tract; and the hypothalamus – which triggers a massive sympathetic response to hypoglycaemia, with pounding heart, trembling, anxiety, sweating and hunger. However, the effects of hyperglycaemia on feeding and satiation are less obvious, and may even lead to paradoxical overeating.

Leptin (from the Greek *leptos*, meaning thin) is a protein hormone released by fat cells that counteracts the effects of neuropeptide Y, a potent feeding stimulant secreted by cells

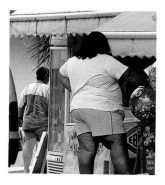

Fig. 27.1 Obesity – the main nutritional problem today

Table 27.1 Complications of obesity (plus various cancers)

Cardiovascular	Orthopaedic	Psychosocial	Gastrointestinal	Respiratory	Metabolic and endocrine	Gynaecological
Hypertension Ischaemic heart disease Stroke Varicose veins	Accidents Gout Osteoarthritis	Depression Social effects	Diverticulitis Gallstones Hiatus hernia (and other hernias) Liver disease	Cor pulmonale Sleep apnoea	Diabetes mellitus Hyperlipoproteinaemias (type II, III and IV)	Amenorrhoea Menstrual irregularities and infertility Polycystic ovaries Uterine prolapse

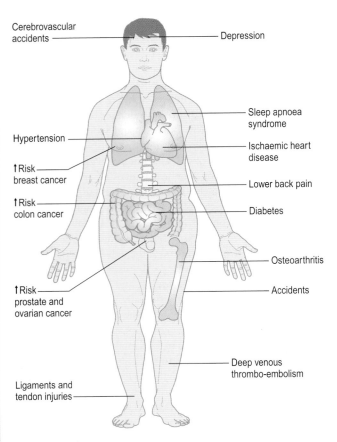

Fig. 27.2 Obesity outcomes

in the gut, and has important effects in regulating metabolism, reproductive function and body weight, acting on the hypothalamic arcuate nucleus to suppress eating behaviour and also increase energy expenditure. Leptin also acts directly on the liver and skeletal muscle where it stimulates the oxidation of fatty acids in the mitochondria, reducing the storage of fat in those tissues (but not in adipose tissue). The absence of functional leptin (or its receptor) leads to uncontrolled food intake and resulting obesity. Rarely, mutations in the leptin gene or its receptor are found in obese people, but these are only a very uncommon cause of morbid obesity. Recombinant human leptin trials are under way in the hope of reducing obesity in humans but the results so far have not shown any great benefit.

Many other factors that appear to affect appetite, satiation and obesity include pro-inflammatory cytokines [tumour necrosis factor-alpha (TNF-alpha), interleukin-6 (IL-6) and IL-1], incretins [cholecystokinin, gastric inhibitory peptide (GIP), glucagon-like peptide 1 and glucagon-like peptide 2],

the melanocortin receptor system (MCR), CART (cocaine and amphetamine-regulated transcript), thyrotropin-releasing hormone, corticosteroids and growth hormone (see http://www.bmb.leeds.ac.uk/teaching/icu3/lecture/26).

Environmental factors affecting body weight include lifestyle behaviours, such as what a person eats and his or her level of physical activity. Psychological factors may play a role; many people eat in response to negative emotions such as boredom, sadness or anger. Some antidepressants can cause weight gain. Genetic factors, hormonal, hypothalamic disease (Frohlich, Laurence–Moon–Biedl or Prader–Willi syndromes), endocrinopathies (hypothyroidism, Cushing disease or insulinoma) or drugs (e.g. steroids) can rarely be implicated.

Clinical features

Obese patients have about a threefold increase in premature deaths because of chronic diseases such as heart disease, type 2 diabetes, hypertension, stroke and cancer (Table 27.1; Fig. 27.2). Obese men are more likely than non-obese men to die from cancer of the colon, rectum or prostate. Obese women are more likely to die from cancer of the gall bladder, breast, uterus, cervix or ovaries.

General management

Measuring body fat is not easy. A simple method to estimate body fat is to measure the thickness of the subcutaneous layer of fat in several parts of the body with skin calipers. The most accurate methods are to weigh the person under water or to use dual-energy X-ray absorptiometry (DEXA).

Body mass index (BMI), now the standard for measuring overweight and obesity, uses a mathematical formula based on height and weight. BMI equals weight in kilograms divided by height in metres squared (BMI = kg/m^2; Table 27.2).

Table 27.2 Body mass index (BMI) and definitions

BMI (kg/mm²)	Classification
< 18.5	Underweight
18.5–24.9	Normal
25.0–29.9	Overweight
30.0–34.9	Obesity class I
35.0–39.9	Obesity class II
≥ 40	Obesity class III

Table 27.3 Drugs used in treatment of obesity

Drug	Mechanism	Possible adverse effects	Comments
Butabindide	Blocks cholecystokinin breakdown	Not yet in clinical use	Inhibits tripeptidylpeptidase
Cholecystokinin promoters	Increase cholecystokinin receptors		
Glucagon-like peptide 1	Delays gastric emptying, more insulin	—	Used in type 2 diabetes
Orlistat	Blocks pancreatic lipase	Anal leakage	Fatty stools
Sibutramine	Blocks 5-hydroxytryptamine (5HT) uptake/sympathomimetic	Dry mouth, headache	May cause hypertension and tachycardia
(Dex)fenfluramine	Blocks 5HT uptake	Cardiac valve defects	Withdrawn because of adverse effects
Troglitazone	Activates peroxisome proliferator-activated receptor gamma (PPARγ)	Liver damage	Withdrawn because of adverse effects
Topiramate	CNS effects	CNS effects	Poor compliance

Bariatric medicine [from the Greek *baros* (weight) and *-iatrics* (medical treatment)] is the term for the specialty of caring for obese patients. These people can encounter many problems apart from morbidity and mortality – most relating to access for health care. Because measuring body fat is difficult, health care providers often rely on weight-for-height tables – a range of acceptable weights for a person of a given height. However, these tables do not distinguish between muscle and excess fat.

Weight loss is recommended, particularly if there are two or more of the following:

- family history of certain chronic diseases (heart disease or diabetes)
- pre-existing disorders, such as hypertension, hyperglycaemia or hypercholesterolaemia
- 'apple' body shape.

The method of treatment depends on the degree of obesity, overall health condition and motivation to lose weight. It may include a combination of diet, exercise, behaviour modification and sometimes weight-loss drugs (Table 27.3). People who have a BMI of 30 or more can improve their health by weight loss. This is especially true for those who are severely obese. A weight loss of 5–10% can do much to improve health by lowering blood pressure and cholesterol levels, and preventing type 2 diabetes in people at high risk for it. Sympathomimetic appetite suppressants are used only in the short-term treatment of obesity since their effect tends to decrease after a few weeks. Tesofensine is a new agent of possible benefit.

In severe obesity, surgery that may be rarely recommended aims at:

- reducing stomach size
  vertical banded gastroplasty (Mason procedure, stomach stapling)
  laparoscopic adjustable gastric band (LAGB; REALIZE band – lap band)
  sleeve gastrectomy
  transoral gastroplasty
- reducing food absorption
  biliopancreatic diversion (Scopinaro procedure – rare)
- or mixed procedures
  gastric bypass

sleeve gastrectomy with duodenal switch
implantable gastric stimulation.

Dental aspects

Jaw wiring of obese patients appears to be an effective and safe way of substantially reducing weight in those in whom simpler methods fail, but relapse frequently follows.

Dental treatment of obese patients may be complicated mainly by the sheer size of the patient and difficulties in accessing the dental chair.

Respiration is impaired if the patient is laid supine. The total work of breathing is greater and, even at rest, obese patients need to ventilate more than normal. Some 10% of the grossly obese have hypoventilation, cor pulmonale and episodic somnolence (Pickwickian syndrome).

Local anaesthetic is satisfactory but may be more difficult because of the thickness of the tissues. Conscious sedation may be given if required.

Treatment may also be complicated by diabetes or cardiovascular disease, or, very rarely, by an organic cause of the obesity. Sympathomimetic appetite suppressants may interact with a range of drugs (Box 27.2). Cardiac arrhythmias may be produced by the interaction of halogenated anaesthetics and large doses of amphetamines or amphetamine-like appetite suppressants (all controlled drugs), which should be discontinued a week before general anaesthesia (GA).

Appetite suppressants, including sibutramine and phentermine, and the herbal supplements ma huang and kola nut (containing ephedrine alkaloids/caffeine), can produce dry mouth.

Box 27.2 Drugs that can interact with sympathomimetic appetite suppressants

- Antidepressants
- Amantadine
- Amphetamines
- Caffeine
- Chlophedianol
- Cocaine
- Methylphenidate
- Nabilone
- Pemoline

EATING HABITS

Vegetarianism

Vegetarianism includes a range of habits (Table 27.4). *Semi-vegetarians* eat a little poultry along with fish, as well as dairy products and eggs. *Vegans*, strict vegetarians, avoid all foods of animal origin, including meat, poultry, fish, dairy products and eggs. This can lead to vitamin B_{12} deficiency (Ch. 8), though the latter is surprisingly uncommon, as vegans typically use yeast extracts and oriental-style fermented foods to provide this vitamin. Intakes of calcium, iron and zinc also tend to be low. *Lacto-vegetarians* include dairy products in their diet. The most common form of vegetarianism is lacto-ovo-vegetarianism – vegetarians who also eat dairy products and eggs. *Pesco-vegetarians* eat fish, dairy products and eggs along with plant foods. *Fruitarians* eat only fruit and their diet is thus deficient in protein, salt and many micronutrients, and is not recommended.

Table 27.4 Vegetarianism

Type of vegetarianism	Dietary habits
Fruitarianism	Fruit products only eaten
Veganism	Abstain from all foods from animals, including dairy products
Lacto-vegetarianism	Like vegans, but eat dairy products
Lacto-ovo-vegetarianism	Like vegans, but eat dairy products and eggs
Pesco-vegetarianism	Like vegans, but eat dairy products, eggs and fish
Semi-vegetarianism	Like vegans, but eat dairy products, eggs, fish and poultry

Vegetarians tend to live longer and to develop fewer chronic disabling conditions than their meat-eating peers. However, their lifestyle usually also includes regular exercise and abstention from alcohol and tobacco, which may contribute to this improved health. Iron deficiency is the main risk. Vegetarians may have fewer caries than others. A fruitarian or prolonged lacto-vegetarian diet may result in dental erosion: citrus fruits, vinegar and acidic berries are especially responsible, particularly if ingested just before retiring to sleep.

Fad diets

Many commercial diets claim to enhance well-being or reduce weight but some such diets have resulted in frank vitamin, mineral and protein deficiency states. Cardiac, renal and metabolic disorders as well as some deaths have resulted.

EATING DISORDERS

Eating is controlled by many factors, including appetite, food availability, family, peer and cultural practices, and attempts at voluntary control. Dieting is a common practice in the developed world and dieting to a body weight lower than needed for health is common and heavily promoted by fashion trends, sales campaigns and in some activities (e.g. fashion models).

Food fads, selective eating (extreme fussiness), and food avoidance (food avoidance but without any fear of weight gain) are relatively common and usually fairly inconsequential in medical terms. Eating disorders, however, are of concern and are frequent among models and elite performers of certain sports or physical activities, and among ballet dancers, gymnasium users and body builders. Eating disorders usually develop during adolescence or early adulthood and most often in females. They often coexist with other psychiatric problems, such as depression, substance abuse and anxiety disorders, and can disturb growth and lead to endocrine problems, cardiac disease and renal failure, and can be fatal. Eating disorders are common; there are probably 90,000 people in UK receiving treatment.

Eating disorders include the two well-recognized conditions of anorexia nervosa (self-imposed starvation) and bulimia nervosa (binge-eating and dieting), but two others – binge-eating disorder and eating disorder not otherwise specified (EDNOS) – are probably more common (Table 27.5). Night-eating syndrome (NES) is also reportedly common – especially in obese people. Nocturnal sleep-related eating disorder (NS-RED) is not strictly an eating disorder, rather it is a type of sleep disorder in which people eat while 'sleep walking', seeming to be sound asleep. Most people are concerned about their weight, so the early signs of eating disorders may easily be overlooked (Box 27.3).

The main disorders that can have life-threatening health complications include mainly anorexia nervosa (self-imposed starvation) and bulimia nervosa (binge-eating and dieting).

Anorexia nervosa

General aspects and features

Anorexia nervosa is failure to eat, in the absence of any physical cause, to the extent that > 15% of body weight is lost. It may become life-threatening and has several complications (Fig. 27.3). Body image may be distorted, so the emaciated patients consider themselves normal or even fat. Intense fear of gaining weight or becoming fat, even though underweight, with resistance to maintaining body weight at or above a minimally normal weight for age and height are prominent (Box 27.4).

Anorectics may repeatedly check their body weight. Disturbance in body image, the way in which the body weight or shape is perceived, undue influences of body weight or shape on self-evaluation, denial of the seriousness of the current low body weight or obsession in the process of eating and development of unusual habits are common. Examples include avoiding food and meals, picking out a few foods and eating these in small amounts, pushing food around the plate instead of eating, or carefully weighing and portioning food. Engaging in techniques to control their weight such as intense and compulsive exercise, or purging by means of vomiting, or abuse of laxatives, enemas, appetite suppressants, diuretics and thyroid hormones are common. Girls with anorexia often experience a delayed onset of the first menstrual period, since gonadotropin release is impaired. In others menstrual periods may become infrequent or cease. Depression, anxiety, obsessive–compulsive disorder and self-harming are common. Growth may be impaired.

Table 27.5 The eating disorders[a]

	Anorexia nervosa	Bulimia nervosa	Binge-eating disorder	Night-eating syndrome	Eating disorder not otherwise specified[b]
Food intake	Refusal to maintain body weight over a minimal normal for age and height	Recurrent episodes of binge-eating including eating more than most people in a discrete period of time, and sense of loss of control	Recurrent episodes of binge-eating, including eating more than most people in a discrete period of time, and sense of loss of control	Eating excessively (hyperphagia) at night after retiring to bed	
Behaviour	Intense fear of gaining weight or of becoming fat, even though underweight Disturbance in body perception	Regularly engage in inappropriate compensatory behaviours Minimum of at least two bingeing episodes each week for at least 3 months Persistent overconcern about body shape and weight	At least three behavioural measures of loss of control during bingeing Rapid eating Eating until uncomfortably full Eating large amounts when not hungry Eating large amounts outside meal times Eating alone because of embarrassment at how much eating Negative feelings about oneself because of eating Minimum of at least two bingeing episodes each week for at least 6 months Marked distress at bingeing	Obesity Insomnia, anorexia in the mornings Minimum of at least 2 months Eating produces guilt and shame, not enjoyment	
Others	Amenorrhoea	May be abuse of medications in order to lose weight	No abuse of medications in order to lose weight	Mood lower in mornings Depression common	

[a]Modified from Diagnostic and Statistical Manual of Disease version 4 (DSM-IV).
[b]Disorders of eating that do not fit criteria for other categories.

Box 27.3 Early signs of eating disorders

- Changes in habits or activities
- Secretive behaviour
- Withdrawal from family or friends
- Weight loss
- Irregular menstruation or amenorrhoea
- Signs of vomiting
- Sudden disappearance of food from kitchen
- Finding of laxatives or diuretics

Anorexia nervosa may be complicated by anaemia, endocrine disturbances, peripheral oedema and electrolyte depletion (hypokalaemia), peripheral cyanosis and coldness with bradycardia (Table 27.7).

The course and outcome of anorexia nervosa vary. Some sufferers recover fully after a single episode, some have a fluctuating pattern of weight gain and relapse; others experience a chronically deteriorating course of illness over many years. The morbidity is high (Table 27. 6) and mortality rate is about 12 times higher than normal. Cardiac arrest, electrolyte imbalance or suicide are the main causes.

Bulimia nervosa

General aspects

Bulimia nervosa is recurrent episodes of binge-eating, which may be associated with compensatory behaviours such as self-induced vomiting and purgative abuse. The binge-eating and inappropriate compensatory behaviours are both practised, on average, at least twice a week for 3 months.

Features include irresistible craving for food, characterized by eating an excessive amount of food within a discrete period of time and by a sense of lack of control over eating during the episode. Recurrent inappropriate compensatory behaviour in order to prevent weight gain is common – such as self-induced vomiting or misuse of laxatives, diuretics, enemas or other medications (purging), fasting or excessive exercise. Bulimics often perform their behaviours in secrecy, feeling disgusted and ashamed when they binge, and relieved once they purge.

Clinical features

These can be similar to anorexia nervosa (Box 27.5). Bulimics usually weigh within the normal range for their age and height, but, like individuals with anorexia, may fear gaining weight, desire to lose weight and feel intensely dissatisfied with their bodies.

General management of eating disorders

Eating disorders are serious conditions with a high co-morbidity and a poor prognosis: only 30–50% make a full recovery. Acute management of severe weight loss (BMI < 13) is usually provided in hospital, where feeding plans address the patient's medical and nutritional needs.

Medical care and monitoring are needed to try to restore healthy eating and deal with the underlying emotional/psychological issues. Patients with eating disorders require a comprehensive treatment plan involving psychosocial interventions (cognitive behavioural or interpersonal psychotherapy), nutritional counselling and, when appropriate, medication. Selective

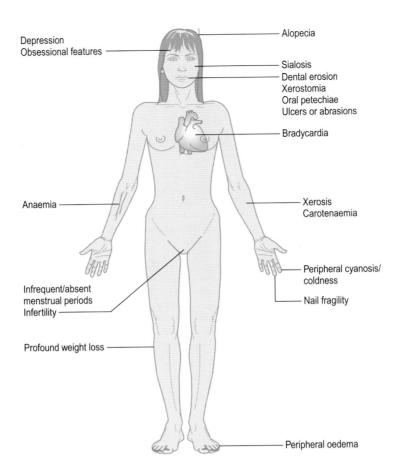

Depression
Obsessional features

Alopecia

Sialosis
Dental erosion
Xerostomia
Oral petechiae
Ulcers or abrasions

Bradycardia

Anaemia

Xerosis
Carotenaemia

Infrequent/absent
menstrual periods
Infertility

Peripheral cyanosis/
coldness

Nail fragility

Profound weight loss

Peripheral oedema

Fig. 27.3 Anorexia nervosa

Box 27.4 Features of anorexia nervosa

- Low body weight
- Intense fear of gaining weight
- Disturbance in body image
- Attempting to control their weight
- Peripheral cyanosis and coldness with bradycardia
- Females under 25 years, mainly
- Severe anorexia overriding hunger
- Sometimes self-induced vomiting (especially after orgies of eating)
- No other causal organic or mental disease
- Amenorrhoea

Box 27.5 Features of bulimia nervosa

- Recurrent episodes of binge-eating
- Recurrent inappropriate compensatory behaviour in order to prevent weight gain, for example self-induced vomiting or misuse of laxatives, diuretics, enemas or other medications (purging)

---

serotonin reuptake inhibitors (SSRIs) may be helpful for weight maintenance, and resolving mood and anxiety symptoms.

Dental aspects of eating disorders

Anaemia and the possibility of hypokalaemia and consequent arrhythmias must be kept in mind if GA is considered necessary. Repeated doses of acetaminophen may be hepatotoxic in anorexia nervosa: doses should be kept to the minimum.

Oral manifestations can cause discomfort and impair oral function (Table 27.6). Erosion of teeth (perimylolsysis) may result from repeated vomiting and is the prominent oral problem. The erosion is usually most severe on lingual, palatal and occlusal surfaces. The patient should be counselled about diet and oral hygiene, and what drinks and foods to avoid (Table 27.7) and how to reduce erosion (e.g. by drinking through a straw).

There is no evidence that toothbrushing is harmful to eroded teeth, even soon after taking a drink of low pH. Topical daily sodium fluoride gel applications or a 0.05% sodium fluoride mouthwash, combined with bicarbonate after each vomiting incident, may lessen dental damage. A specific desensitizing toothpaste may also be indicated. Full-coverage plastic splints may be needed to protect the teeth and it may help to fill these splints with magnesium hydroxide. Restorative care may include dentine-bonded resins or composites, crowns or use of a Dahl appliance.

Parotid enlargement (sialosis) and angular stomatitis may develop as in other forms of starvation. The parotid swellings tend to subside if the patient resumes a normal diet. Oral ulcers or abrasions, particularly in the soft palate, may be caused by fingers or other objects used to induce vomiting.

Table 27.6 Medical and oral complications of anorexia nervosa

Cardiovascular	Bradycardia Hypotension Arrhythmias Cardiac failure
Endocrinological	Raised cortisol Reduced gonadotropins, thyroid and sex hormones
Gastrointestinal	Oesophagitis Oesophageal rupture Duodenal dilatation Constipation
Haematological	Bone marrow hypoplasia Pancytopenia Lowered plasma protein levels
Metabolic	Dehydration Hypothermia Hypokalaemia Hypercholesterolaemia Hypoglycaemia Abnormal liver function
Musculoskeletal	Osteoporosis Pathological fractures Impaired growth Myopathies Tetany
Neurological	Brain atrophy Seizures
Oral	Mucosal atrophy, glossitis and glossodynia Dental erosion Sialosis Xerostomia
Renal	Low glomerular filtration rate (GFR) Hypokalaemic nephropathy

Table 27.7 Management of patients with tooth erosion

Minimize tooth exposure to dietary acids	Increase oral pH	Caries protection
Reduce carbonated drinks, fruit juices, vinegar, alcohol Use a straw to drink low-pH fluids where feasible	Mouth rinses of water, milk or bicarbonate Chewing gum	Non-cariogenic diet Fluorides Plaque control

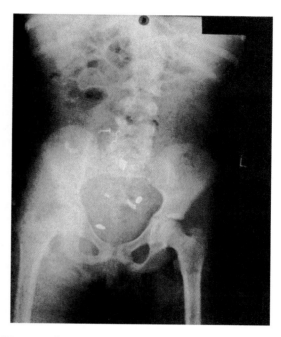

Fig. 27.4 Pica showing intraabdominal opacities

Pica

Pica is a condition in which the appetite is perverted; it seen mainly in persons with learning disability or psychiatric disease, but is sometimes due to pregnancy or iron deficiency. Many unusual objects and substances may be ingested. Objects such as buttons, screws, pins, nails, etc. may cause gastrointestinal obstruction or perforation (Fig. 27.4). In the past children sometimes chewed painted objects and succumbed to lead poisoning; this still occurs in the developing world.

UNDERNUTRITION

General aspects

Severe undernutrition results mainly from poverty, especially in children and the elderly, in the developing world or in war zones. Other causes include eating disorders, abuse (food restriction), oral problems or obstruction to the pharynx or oesophagus, malabsorption and in cachexia of malignant disease.

Infants and children are at particular risk of undernutrition because of a high demand for energy and essential nutrients. Protein-energy malnutrition in children consuming inadequate amounts of protein, calories and other nutrients is a particularly severe form of undernutrition. It retards growth and development. Deficiencies of iron, folic acid, vitamin C, copper, zinc and vitamin A may develop in inadequately fed infants and children. An exclusively breast-fed infant can develop vitamin B_{12} deficiency if the mother is a vegan.

Adolescents are at risk since nutritional requirements increase as the growth rate increases. Requirements for all nutrients rise during pregnancy and lactation. Anaemia due to folic acid deficiency is common in pregnant women, especially those who have taken oral contraceptives, so folic acid supplements are now recommended for pregnant women to prevent neural tube defects (spina bifida) in their children. Aberrations of diet (rarely including pica) are common in pregnancy. An alcoholic mother may have a handicapped and stunted child with fetal alcohol syndrome. Caffeine has been implicated in miscarriages and underweight babies.

Older people, despite a reduction in physical activity lowering their energy and protein requirements, are at risk of malnutrition because of poverty, apathy or dementia. Diminished senses of taste and smell, poverty (real or perceived), loneliness, physical and mental impairments, immobility, and chronic illness can also militate against adequate dietary intake.

Furthermore, absorption may be impaired, contributing to iron deficiency, osteoporosis (also related to calcium deficiency), and osteomalacia due to lack of vitamin D and absence of exposure to sunshine (Ch. 25).

Clinical features

Features of undernutrition may include listlessness, emaciation, skin dryness, scaliness, atrophy, petechiae, ecchymoses, spooned nails, depigmentation and loss of hair, and orofacial problems (angular stomatitis, glossitis, ulcers and sialosis).

General management

The history may reveal food faddism, lack of variety or inadequate intake of energy-rich and essential nutrients, poor appetite, gastrointestinal disturbance and recent weight loss. Anaemia may indicate iron deficiency. Chronic use of alcohol, cocaine, heroin, immunosuppressants or some antibiotics and anticonvulsants raises questions about the adequacy of vitamin and mineral nutrition.

The musculature should be examined for size, strength and tenderness. Neurological examination may detect disorientation, an abnormal gait, altered reflexes, and sensory or motor neuron abnormalities. Painful bones and joints, osteopenia and distortions in the shape or size of bones (e.g. rachitic rosary) may indicate current or past malnutrition.

Anthropometric measurements are essential to diagnosis. Nutritional status can be classified on the basis of body mass index. The triceps skinfold estimates the amount of body fat within 20% and is therefore useful in determining the body's energy stores. Based on the mid-arm muscle area, muscle mass may be classified as adequate, marginal, depleted or wasted.

A full blood count and measurement of plasma proteins reflect the adequacy of amino acid nutrition (albumin, prealbumin and transferrin). Electrolyte assays may point to a mineral deficiency. Lipids and related lipoproteins should be assayed. Various imaging techniques (radiography, computed tomography and magnetic resonance imaging) may be helpful.

The patient may need hospital treatment including nasogastric feeding.

Dental aspects

Local anaesthesia is satisfactory. Conscious sedation may be given in hospital. GA should, as always, be given in hospital.

Undernutrition in children can result in retarded tooth eruption. Latent undernutrition may predispose to burning mouth syndrome, mouth ulcers, glossitis and angular stomatitis. Resulting immunodeficiencies predispose to oral ulceration, angular stomatitis, necrotizing gingivitis and, rarely, gangrenous stomatitis (noma; cancrum oris) or sialosis (Ch. 20).

Whether chronic undernutrition is a significant factor that underlies many oral cancers is unclear, but there is a protective effect of diets rich in fresh fruits and vegetables, and in vitamins A and C. Iron deficiency is seen in the Paterson–Brown-Kelly (Plummer–Vinson) syndrome.

PROTEIN-ENERGY MALNUTRITION

General aspects

Protein-energy malnutrition (PEM), or protein-calorie malnutrition, is seen mainly in infants and children of some developing nations but it can affect persons of any age in any country. Characterized not only by an energy deficit due to a reduction in all macronutrients and a deficit in many micronutrients, this syndrome is an example of the various levels of inadequate protein and/or energy intake between starvation (no food intake) and adequate nourishment.

Clinical features

Clinically, PEM has three forms, which depend on the balance of non-protein and protein sources of energy. Each of the three forms of PEM can be graded as mild, moderate or severe by calculating weight as a percentage of expected weight for length using international standards (normal, 90–110%; mild, 85–90%; moderate, 75–85%; severe, < 75%).

Marasmus (dry, thin, desiccated) is the predominant form of PEM in most developing countries, and results from near starvation with deficiency of protein and non-protein nutrients. The consequence is emaciation due to loss of muscle and body fat. Marasmic infants have hunger, gross weight loss, growth retardation, and wasting of subcutaneous fat and muscle. Marasmus is associated with the early abandonment or failure of breast-feeding and with consequent infections, most notably those causing infantile gastroenteritis.

Kwashiorkor (an African word for 'first child–second child') is characterized by protein deficiency more severe than energy deficiency, and by oedema. It refers to the observation that the first child develops PEM when the second child is born and replaces the first child at the breast. Kwashiorkor is confined to parts of the world where staple and weaning foods – such as yam, cassava, sweet potato and green banana – are protein deficient and excessively starchy (rural Africa, the Caribbean and Pacific islands). Generalized oedema, 'flaky paint' skin, thinning, decoloration and reddening of the hair, enlarged fatty liver and apathy are seen in addition to retarded growth. Pneumonia, diarrhoea, otitis media, genitourinary disease and sepsis are almost invariable because of depressed immunity.

Marasmic kwashiorkor is a combined form of undernutrition between the two extremes.

General management

Differential diagnosis includes consideration of secondary growth failure due to malabsorption, congenital defects, renal failure, endocrine disease or emotional deprivation.

In children, mortality varies between 5% and 40%, the lower mortality rates being seen in those receiving intensive care. Fluid and electrolyte abnormalities (hypokalaemia, hypocalcaemia, hypophosphataemia and hypomagnesaemia) must be corrected and infections treated. Macronutrients should be supplied by milk-based formulas. A full-fat desiccated milk product can be fortified with additional corn oil and maltodextrin. After 4 weeks, the formula can be replaced with whole milk plus solid foods, including eggs, fruit, meats, cod liver oil and yeast.

Dental aspects

Noma (maxillofacial gangrene; cancrum oris) is a severe, potentially fatal infection common in starving children, particularly in Africa.

STARVATION

General aspects

Starvation is the most severe form of malnutrition and may result from famine, fasting, anorexia nervosa, disease of the gastrointestinal tract, stroke, cancer or coma. The basic metabolic response to starvation is conservation of energy and body tissues, but the body will mobilize its own tissues, resulting in destruction of visceral organs and muscle and extreme shrinkage of adipose tissue. Loss of organ weight is greatest in the liver and intestine, moderate in the heart and kidneys, and least in the nervous system.

Clinical features

Emaciation is most obvious in areas where prominent fat depots normally exist. Muscle mass shrinks and bones protrude. The skin becomes thin, dry, inelastic, pale and cold. The hair is dry and sparse and falls out easily. Most body systems are affected (Box 27.6).

Box 27.6 Features of emaciation

- Achlorhydria and diarrhoea
- Anaemia
- Apathy and irritability
- Body temperature fall
- Cell-mediated immunity compromised
- Wound-healing impaired
- Fat and muscle loss
- Gonadal atrophy, loss of libido and amenorrhoea
- Heart size and cardiac output fall
- Respiratory rate and vital capacity fall
- Weakness

General management

Total starvation is fatal in 8–12 weeks. At first, food repletion must be limited until gastrointestinal function is restored. Food intake is then gradually increased until it is about 5000 kcal/day and weekly weight gain is 1.5–2.0 kg. Non-responsive patients may require nasogastric feeding, and parenteral nutrition is indicated if malabsorption is severe.

ALCOHOL OR DRUG DEPENDENCY

Patients with alcohol or drug dependency often have lifestyles in which nourishment is neglected. Nutrient absorption and metabolism are also impaired. For example, alcoholics who consume ≥ 1 litre of spirits per day usually lose weight and become undernourished. Alcoholism is the most common cause of thiamine deficiency in the developed world and may also lead to deficiencies of magnesium, zinc, folic acid and other vitamins.

CACHEXIA

Cachexia is the weakness and emaciation commonly associated with serious illness, such as cancer, HIV/AIDS ('slim disease') and tuberculosis, and after burns, major surgery or trauma. Cachexia is mediated by pro-inflammatory cytokines, such as tumour necrosis factor-alpha (TNF-alpha; originally termed cachexin), interleukin-6 (IL-6) and IL-1.

CARNITINE DEFICIENCY

Carnitine is an amino acid required for the transport of long-chain fatty acyl coenzyme A (CoA) esters into mitochondria. Carnitine requirements are met by a combination of dietary intake (mainly animal products) and endogenous biosynthesis. Carnitine deficiency can result from inadequate intake during long-term total parenteral nutrition (TPN), impaired biosynthesis caused by liver disease, increased requirements for carnitine in states of ketosis and high demand for fat oxidation or excess loss of carnitine due to diarrhoea, diuresis or haemodialysis. Although uncommon, carnitine deficiency may cause muscle necrosis, myoglobinuria, lipid-storage myopathy, hypoglycaemia, fatty liver and hyperammonaemia – with muscle aches, fatigue and confusion.

CHRONIC DISEASES

In patients with chronic diseases (including major surgery), there may be impaired absorption of fat-soluble vitamins, vitamin B_{12}, calcium and iron. Liver disease impairs the storage of vitamins A and B_{12}, and interferes with protein and energy metabolism. Chronic kidney disease and dialysis lead to deficiencies of protein, iron and vitamin D. Patients receiving long-term home parenteral nutrition, most commonly after total or near-total resection of the gut, tend to develop vitamin and trace mineral deficiencies. Biotin, vitamin K, selenium, molybdenum, manganese and zinc must be adequately supplied.

ESSENTIAL FATTY ACID DEFICIENCY

Essential fatty acids (EFAs) are those that must be taken in the diet. EFAs are needed for many physiological processes, including maintaining the structure of cell membranes and synthesizing prostaglandins and leukotrienes, and the integrity of skin. They include linolenic acid, eicosapentaenoic acid and docosahexaenoic acid (omega-3 fatty acids and largely from fish oils), and linoleic acid and arachidonic acid (omega-6 fatty acids and largely from vegetable oils, such as corn oil, cottonseed oil and soybean oil). Omega-3 fatty acids are needed for synthesis of prostaglandins and leukotrienes, and tend to reduce inflammation. Eicosapentaenoic acid and docosahexaenoic acid are important components of the brain and retina. Omega-6 fatty acids tend to promote inflammation and cancer, and autoimmune and inflammatory disease. A diet with a high omega-3:omega-6 ratio appears to be most healthy (Ch. 5).

Deficiency in EFAs may occur in patients with fat malabsorption, serious trauma and burns. EFA deficiency used to be a hazard of long-term fat-free TPN, but fat emulsions now prevent this.

LIPODYSTROPHY

Lipodystrophy is a rare condition in which adipose tissue cannot be produced and, in the absence of fat cells, leptin is not produced; as a result, patients cannot become obese but often develop type 2 diabetes. Treatment with recombinant leptin helps.

A rare form of lipodystrophy is facial hemiatrophy of Romberg, starting typically in adolescence and females, in which there is progressive disappearance of facial fat unilaterally, mimicking facial paralysis. Patients appear to be otherwise well. Plastic surgery is the only treatment.

Lipodystrophy may also follow active antiretroviral therapy (ART) with protease inhibitors for HIV disease. Clinically there may be peripheral fat-wasting but central adiposity, with expanding abdominal girth ('protease paunch' or 'Crix belly'), growing dorsicervical fat pads ('buffalo hump'), loss of subcutaneous fat over cheeks and temples (facial thinning), and arm, buttock and leg wasting and growing prominence of leg veins. Persons with raised blood cholesterol are at greater risk of developing lipodystrophy. Age, use of anabolic steroids, and use of psychotropic medications (including antidepressants and benzodiazepines) are also associated with lipodystrophy. Associated adverse metabolic effects include hyperlipidaemia, hypercholesterolaemia, hypertriglyceridaemia, hyperglycaemia, insulin resistance and late-onset diabetes, increasing the risk of cardiovascular and other complications. Parotid lipomatosis can be a complication of ART.

VITAMINS AND THEIR DISORDERS

Vitamins are essential organic dietary factors that cannot be synthesized within the body (Table 27.8). They are required in only small amounts but absence can result in disease (Table 27.9).

Sometimes, vitamin excess can be dangerous (Table 27.10). Vitamin A supplementation has been linked to birth defects and irreversible bone and liver damage. Vitamin D supplementation can cause hypercalcaemia. Other adverse effects include diarrhoea (from vitamin C), neuropathies (long-term use of high doses of vitamin B_6) and flushing (niacin) during treatment.

Vitamin A (retinol)

Vitamin A is fat-soluble and found in animal fats, milk and liver. It can also be derived from precursors (carotenes or carotenoids) found in plants, particularly green leafy vegetables. Vitamin A is stored in the liver; reserves can last about 1 year.

Vitamin A deficiency is usually dietary in origin and the eyes are first affected with night blindness, xerophthalmia and

Table 27.8 Vitamins

Fat-soluble	Water-soluble
Vitamin A	Vitamin B_1 (thiamine)
Vitamin D	Vitamin B_2 (riboflavine)
Vitamin E	Vitamin B_6 (pyridoxine)
Vitamin K	Vitamin B_{12}
	Vitamin C (ascorbic acid)
	Folic acid
	Pantothenic acid
	Biotin
	Nicotinic acid (niacin)

Table 27.9 Vitamin deficiency syndromes

Vitamin	Deficiency syndrome	Usual causes
A	Night blindness, xerophthalmia	Malabsorption, inadequate diet, PEM
Thiamin (B_1)	Beri-beri, Wernicke encephalopathy	Inadequate diet, alcoholism
Riboflavin (B_2)	Mucosal lesions, corneal opacities	Inadequate diet, drugs, alcoholism
Niacin (nicotinic acid)	Pellagra (dementia, dermatitis, diarrhoea)	Alcoholism, inadequate diet, carcinoid syndrome
Pyridoxine (B_6)	Glossitis, neuropathy, dermatitis	Inadequate diet, drugs (isoniazid, hydralazine)
Folate	Megaloblastosis; villous atrophy; mucosal lesions	Inadequate diet, alcoholism, pregnancy, haemolytic anaemia, drugs
B_{12}	Megaloblastosis; villous atrophy; neuropathies, mucosal lesions	Inadequate diet, pernicious anaemia, Crohn disease
C (ascorbic acid)	Scurvy	Inadequate diet
D	Rickets; osteomalacia	Inadequate exposure to sunlight, malabsorption
E	Spinocerebellar degeneration	Severe fat malabsorption, abetalipoproteinaemia
K	Hypoprothrombinaemia, bleeding	Warfarin, oral antibiotics, biliary obstruction

PEM, protein-energy malnutrition.

Table 27.10	Main consequences of vitamin overdose
Vitamin	**Toxicity**
A	Headache, convulsions, hepatotoxicity, bone damage, teratogenicity
Thiamine (B₁)	?
Riboflavin (B₂)	?
Nicotinic acid (niacin)	Vasodilatation
Pyridoxine (B₆)	Peripheral neuropathy
Folate	?
Vitamin B₁₂	?
Ascorbic acid (C)	Increased urinary oxalate
D	Hypercalcaemia, renal failure
E	Nausea
K	Hyperbilirubinaemia

conjunctival ulceration. The skin becomes dry and scaly (follicular hyperkeratosis) and the oral mucosa becomes hyperkeratinized.

Natural derivatives of vitamin A (carotenoids) and synthetic analogues of vitamin A (retinoids) can modulate epithelial cell differentiation, possibly by regulating gene expression, and may have some protective effect against cancers.

In hypervitaminosis A there is alopecia, peeling of the skin, coarsening of the hair and bone pain.

Vitamin B

There are several B vitamins; all are water-soluble and the most widely recognized deficiencies are of vitamin B₁₂ and folic acid.

Vitamin B₁₂

Vitamin B₁₂ is found mainly in liver, eggs, meat and milk; liver stores last for up to 3 years and thus deficiency is rarely of dietary origin, except in vegans.

Vitamin B₁₂ deficiency is typically seen in pernicious anaemia, where there is deficiency of the gastric intrinsic factor required for its absorption. Vitamin B₁₂ deficiency causes defective cellular uptake of 5-methyltetrahydrofolate, and its impaired conversion by the homocysteine methyl transferase reaction, and thus vitamin B₁₂ deficiency interferes with development of rapidly dividing cells including mucosae, erythrocytes, granulocytes and platelets. Impaired erythrocyte production leads to a macrocytic anaemia; haemoglobin synthesis continues relatively normally but cell size remains large, and condensation and extrusion of the nucleus are delayed (megaloblastosis).

Neuropathies (subacute combined degeneration of the cord), glossitis and stomatitis may result from vitamin B₁₂ deficiency.

Vitamin B₁ (thiamine, aneurine)

Vitamin B₁ is widely distributed in foods and is necessary in the formation of the coenzyme thiamine pyrophosphate required for oxidative decarboxylation of pyruvate and alpha-ketoglutarate, and utilization of pentoses.

In vitamin B₁ deficiency, therefore, there is a build-up of lactate and pyruvate that interferes with carbohydrate metabolism. Deficiency of vitamin B₁ is common in alcoholism and leads to beriberi. This is characterized by polyneuritis, muscular weakness, cardiac failure, mental changes and, in children, growth retardation. Thiamine given intravenously may precipitate anaphylaxis, so caution is advised.

Riboflavine (vitamin B₂)

Riboflavine is found in leafy vegetables, meat, milk and fish. It acts in the formation of two coenzymes, flavine–adenine dinucleotide and flavine mononucleotide, involved in oxidative metabolism. Deficiency of vitamin B₂ is commonly dietary, seen especially in alcoholics. This leads to seborrhoeic dermatitis, corneal vascularization and anaemia, and oral mucosal manifestations similar to those of vitamin B₁₂ deficiency.

Vitamin B₆ (pyridoxine)

Vitamin B₆ is found in meat and vegetables, and is involved in the formation of pyridoxal phosphate and pyridoxamine phosphate, coenzymes in amino acid metabolism. Vitamin B₆ deficiency is found particularly in alcoholism, pregnancy and the use of some drugs (e.g. isoniazid). Deficiency of vitamin B₆ leads to dermatitis and peripheral neuropathy, and oral mucosal manifestations similar to those of vitamin B₁₂ deficiency.

Pantothenic acid

Pantothenic acid is needed for the synthesis of coenzyme A, which is necessary for several metabolic pathways.

Biotin

Biotin is a coenzyme in carboxylation reactions. Deficiency is rare.

Nicotinic acid (niacin; nicotinamide)

The active derivative of nicotinic acid, nicotinamide, is necessary for the production of NAD and NADP for oxidative metabolism. Wheat, nuts, meat and fish are rich sources of nicotinic acid. Deficiency of nicotinic acid is seen mainly in alcoholics, and causes pellagra (dermatitis and neurological disturbances), oral mucosal erythema and papillary atrophy of the tongue.

Folic acid

Folic acid (pteroylglutamic acid) is biologically inactive; folates are the active forms. Folate, present in green vegetables, liver and yeast, is converted, after small intestinal absorption, to the active tetrahydrofolate, which is involved in synthesis of purine and pyrimidine bases.

Folate deficiency typically results from a diet deficient in green vegetables and can arise within a relatively short period of time, since body stores last less than 3 months. Alcoholism, some cytotoxic drugs such as methotrexate, and phenytoin are other relatively common causes of folate deficiency.

Folate deficiency leads to impaired synthesis and repair of DNA with megaloblastic change in haemopoietic and other cells. The oral effects of folate deficiency in humans are virtually indistinguishable from those of vitamin B$_{12}$ deficiency.

Vitamin C (ascorbic acid)

Vitamin C is water-soluble, and found especially in fresh fruits (mainly in citrus fruits) and vegetables, including potatoes. It is involved in the hydroxylation of proline in collagen synthesis. Deficiency results from a dietary lack of vitamin C, and leads to defective collagen with capillary fragility, a haemorrhagic state, anaemia, and follicular hyperkeratosis and gingival changes (scurvy) of swelling and haemorrhage.

Vitamin D

Vitamin D is the general name for a group of fat-soluble sterols (cholecalciferol) found in fish, eggs and milk products. Cholecalciferol from the diet is converted into 25-hydroxycholecalciferol in the liver and this is converted in the kidneys to the active form, 1,25-dihydroxycholecalciferol. Ultraviolet light converts a skin precursor 7-dehydrocholesterol to vitamin D. Vitamin D affects calcium and phosphate metabolism; deficiency leads to rickets or osteomalacia.

Vitamin E

Vitamin E is the general name for a group of fat-soluble tocopherols that are found particularly in asparagus, avocado, nuts, olives and vegetable oils. Vitamin E is important in erythropoiesis and helps the body to use vitamin K. It has been claimed that alpha-tocopherol is the most important lipid-soluble antioxidant. It may have some protective effect against some leukoplakias and carcinomas. Deficiency is rare except in premature infants, people with fat malabsorption and rare genetic abnormalities in the alpha-tocopherol transfer protein (ataxia and vitamin E deficiency; AVED). Neuropathies may result. There is no good evidence that vitamin E is cardioprotective.

Vitamin K

Vitamin K is a fat-soluble naphthaquinone derivative found in green vegetables. Malabsorption, parenteral nutrition and warfarin cause deficiency, the manifestations of which can include gingival bleeding and post-operative haemorrhage.

OXIDATIVE DAMAGE AND ANTIOXIDANTS

In fats and oils, oxidation is the prime cause of rancidity, causing them to become unpleasant to eat and potentially dangerous. All fats and oils will become rancid given enough exposure to air, sunlight and heat, but antioxidants will combat this, and confer huge economic and environmental benefits in preventing wastage of food. In humans, oxidation by oxides and peroxides from atmospheric pollution, cigarette smoke and in some normal bodily processes can cause DNA breaks (and hence the risk of cancer), can oxidize polyunsaturated fatty acids (and thus contribute towards heart disease and strokes), and can

Table 27.11 Antioxidant-containing foods

Food	High in antioxidants	Very high in antioxidants
Beans	Various beans	Cacao (including chocolate)
Beverages	Beer, cider, coffee, tea	Green tea, red wine
Cereals	Barley, hops, maize, millet	–
Fruits	Apples, cherries, lemons, mangos, melons, oranges, peaches, pineapples, plums, tangerines	Blackberries, blackcurrants, blueberries, cranberries, elderberries, pomegranates, raspberries, strawberries
Nuts	Almonds, pistachios	Hazelnuts, pecans, walnuts
Vegetables	Artichokes, mushrooms, onions, parsley, peppers, spinach	–

damage proteins (e.g. eye proteins are particularly vulnerable because light also assists oxidation). Considerable evidence indicates that increased oxidative damage is associated with and may contribute to the development of most major age-related degenerative diseases (e.g. cancer, heart disease, strokes, diabetes, cataracts, Parkinson disease and Alzheimer disease).

Antioxidants are chemicals that slow oxidation reactions, which can otherwise produce the damaging 'free radicals' or 'reactive oxygen species'. It is not clear which antioxidants are the most effective. Many foods, particularly pecan nuts, walnuts and various beans, contain high levels of various antioxidants (Table 27.11).

Vitamins A, C and E, and plant polyphenols (including flavonoids) and carotenoids (including beta-carotene and lycopene) are amongst the most powerful antioxidants. Flavonoids, typical examples of which are quercetin in onions and apples, and epigallocatechin in tea, are other antioxidants.

Fruits are high in antioxidants, the purple, blue, red and orange fruits being the most antioxidant-rich. Good sources of flavonoids include citrus fruits (*hesperidin*, *quercetin*, *rutin*) and berries (purple berries due to their dark colour are as much as 50% higher in antioxidants than some of the more common berry varieties). Both red and white wine contain flavonoids but, since red wine is produced by fermentation in the presence of grape skins, red wine has higher levels of flavonoids, and other polyphenolics such as resveratol. Green plants or herbs contain antioxidants, as do green tea (contains catechins), jiaogulan (southern ginseng or xiancao – the 'immortality herb'– contains gypenosides), tomatoes (lycopene), chocolate (relatively high amounts of epicatechin) and grape seeds (resveratol). 'ACES' products contain pro-vitamin **A** (beta-carotene), vitamin **C**, vitamin **E** and **S**elenium. Vitamin C (E300) and vitamin E (E306) are antioxidants found in fruit and vegetables, and also widely used as supplementary additives, and are amongst the safest chemicals known. A recent survey concluded 'vitamin C inhibits the formation of carcinogenic nitrosamines, stimulates the immune system, protects against chromosome breakage, and regenerates vitamin E as part of the antioxidant defence system'.

Some dietary antioxidant vitamins are required for good health, and antioxidant-containing foods are recommended.

However, although some foods have a high antioxidant content, not all are absorbed because of variable absorption or metabolism (bioavailability) in the gut. In one study, increasing vegetable intake by at least 400 g per day resulted in a 42% reduction in the risk of coronary heart disease and this has been attributed largely to antioxidants.

Heart disease, strokes, diabetes, cataracts, Parkinson disease and Alzheimer disease seem to occur less frequently in people who eat antioxidant-rich diets, but it is a moot point whether or not the effect is due to some other lifestyle factor.

There is considerable doubt, however, as to whether anti-oxidant *supplementation* is beneficial. Some studies have suggested antioxidant supplementation benefits health, but several large clinical trials have failed to demonstrate definite benefit, and excess supplementation may even be harmful. The most common synthetic antioxidants are butylated hydroxyanisole (E320) and butylated hydroxytoluene (BHT; E321). BHT has been controversial; it has produced adverse reactions in dogs but, like all antioxidants, it is anticarcinogenic.

POLYPHENOLS

Polyphenols (PPs) are derived from L-phenylalanine and have several phenol groups (i.e. aromatic rings with hydroxyls). The most important PP classes are phenolic acids, flavonoids, lignans and stilbenes. Flavonoids are divided into flavonols (such as quercetin and kaempferol, the most ubiquitous flavonoids in foods), flavones, isoflavones, flavanones, anthocyanidins (pigments responsible for the colour of most fruits) and flavanols (catechins, monomers and proanthocyanidins – polymers known as condensed tannins).

The PPs that are best absorbed in humans are isoflavones and gallic acid (a phenolic acid), followed by flavanones, catechins and quercetin glucosides. The least well absorbed are proanthocyanidins, anthocyanins and galloylated catechins. All PPs are excreted chiefly in the urine and bile.

Polyphenols have powerful antioxidant activities *in vitro*, capable of scavenging a range of reactive oxygen, nitrogen and chlorine species, such as superoxide, hydroxyl radical, peroxyl radicals, hypochlorous acid and peroxynitrous acid. PPs have some activity *in vitro* and in animal studies, but this has generally not been confirmed by human studies. PPs have been proposed to exert beneficial effects in a number of disease states, especially cancers, cardiovascular diseases and neurodegenerative disorders, but, although there are many epidemiological studies, comprehensive data are available only for flavonoids, specifically flavonols, flavones and catechins, indicating that flavonoids reduce the risk of coronary artery disease. In contrast, the association between flavonoid intake and cancer protection is controversial.

There is also some alleged antimicrobial activity of PPs against some infectious diseases. It is unclear whether the data from experimental studies are relevant for human disease outcomes. In fact, the classical antioxidant activity of PPs is unlikely to be the principal explanation for cellular effects in humans; rather, non-specific protein/enzyme-modulating mechanisms may be involved. Indeed, dietary PPs exert pharmacological activity against a wide range of receptors, enzymes and transcription molecules, and are likely to affect cell functions profoundly by altering the phosphorylation state of target molecules and/or by modulating gene expression. Interestingly, some oxidized PP metabolites act as pro-oxidants, which suggests that high dietary PP intake could be potentially more of an oxidative risk than a benefit – a concern corroborated by an epidemiological study reporting an association between flavonoid intake and colon cancer. This suggests that dietary supplementation with large amounts of a single antioxidant might be *deleterious* to human health.

FOOD ADDITIVES

The main reasons for adding chemicals to foods include the following: to improve shelf-life or storage time; make food convenient and easy to prepare; increase the nutritional value; improve the flavour and enhance the attractiveness; and improve consumer acceptance. For decades, the food industry has created new chemicals to manipulate, preserve and transform food, and has created altered versions of breads, fruits, vegetables, meats, dairy products and many more commonly used foods. Several foods contain large numbers of additives and now there are even 'foods', such as coffee creamers, sugar substitutes and confectionery, that consist almost entirely of artificial ingredients.

Some additives have undoubted health benefits, such as the antioxidants. Other food additives may actually cause disease such as benzoates, tartrazine and cinnamonaldehyde, which is implicated, for example, in orofacial granulomatosis. Some are dangerous: the recent adulteration of milk in China with melamine and the subsequent renal or bladder stones, or cancer, is a prime example. Additives known to have health risks are shown in Table 27.12.

NUTRITIONAL INTERVENTIONS

Most conventional diets recommend recognized 'healthy' patterns of eating (reduction or elimination of fat, sugar, alcohol and coffee, and an increase in fresh vegetables and fibre) that most people with normal digestion can tolerate without adverse effects. Unconventional nutritional interventions can be divided into nutritional supplements, dietary modification and therapeutic systems. Some supplements are taken to improve general health and performance, whereas others are purported to be for specific clinical indications, not always with evidence for efficacy. Very low-calorie diets (< 400 kcal/day) cannot sustain health for long, and high-dose nutritional supplementation can sometimes lead to adverse effects. Vitamin D supplementation is discussed above. High doses of single minerals or amino acids may induce deficiencies in nutrients that share similar metabolic pathways. Some trace mineral supplements have had toxic effects; excessive doses of zinc and selenium can cause immune suppression, and evening primrose oil may exacerbate temporal lobe epilepsy.

Many commercial fad diets are claimed to enhance well-being or reduce weight but some such diets have resulted in frank vitamin, mineral and protein deficiency states. Cardiac, renal and metabolic disorders as well as some deaths have resulted. Many diets, such as vegetarianism and veganism, originated as 'movements' characterized by political and/or ecological

Table 27.12 Food additives that may present health risks

Additive[a]	Possible associations	Possible carcinogenicity
Aluminium sulfide, aluminium phosphate, sodium phosphate, aluminium chloride – common leavening agents in baked goods	Possible link to Alzheimer disease	–
Artificial sweeteners (aspartame, acesulfame K and saccharin)	Behavioural problems, hyperactivity, allergies	+
Artificial food colours	Allergies, asthma, hyperactivity	+
Artificial flavours	Allergic or behavioural reactions	–
Bromates (usually potassium bromate)	?	Carcinogenic in animals
Caffeine	Promotes stomach acid secretion, temporarily raises blood pressure, and dilates some blood vessels while constricting others. Excessive caffeine intake results in 'caffeinism', with symptoms ranging from nervousness to insomnia	–
Carbonated beverages	Tooth erosion; obesity, metabolic syndrome, chronic kidney disease, pancreatic carcinoma; rarely, hyponatraemia	–
Food waxes (protective coating of produce, as in cucumbers, peppers and apples)	May trigger allergies, can contain pesticides, fungicide sprays or animal by-products	–
Hydrogenated fats	Cardiovascular disease, obesity	–
MSG (monosodium glutamate)	Common allergic and behavioural reactions, including headaches, dizziness, chest pains, depression and mood swings; also a possible neurotoxin	–
Nitrites and nitrates	Headaches	Can develop into nitrosamines in body, which can be carcinogenic
Olestra (an artificial fat)	Diarrhoea and digestive disturbances. Olestra inhibits the absorption of some vitamins and other nutrients	–
Phosphorous compounds, which make soft drinks bubbly (phosphoric acid), as well as keeping canned vegetables firm (calcium phosphate) and dried instant oatmeals and soup mixes easy to hydrate (sodium phosphate)	Might possibly interfere with calcium absorption and predispose to osteoporosis	–
Plastic packaging	Immune reactions, lung shock	+ (vinyl chloride)
Preservatives – butylated hydroxyanisole (BHA) and butylated hydroxytoluene (BHT), etc.	Allergic reactions, hyperactivity; BHT may be toxic to the nervous system and the liver	+
Refined flour	Low-nutrient calories, carbohydrate imbalances, altered insulin production	–
Salt (excessive)	Fluid retention and blood pressure increases	–
Sugar and sweeteners	Obesity, dental caries, diabetes and hypoglycaemia, increased triglycerides or candidiasis	–
Sulfites (sulfur dioxide, metabisulfites and others) can keep cut fruits and vegetables looking fresh – they also prevent discoloration in apricots, raisins and other dried fruits; control 'black spot' in freshly caught shrimp; and prevent discoloration, bacterial growth and fermentation in wine	Allergic and asthmatic reactions	–

[a]Some are naturally present in some foods.

concerns, a moral stance toward food, and a view of diet as inseparable from lifestyle. Many diets are based on theoretical considerations rather than empirical data. For example, the rationale for the principle in the Hay diet that starch and protein should not be eaten together is that each type of food requires a different pH for optimum digestion. The principle of the Stone Age diet is that humans are not adapted by evolution to eat grains and legumes.

'Therapeutic' systems include techniques such as elimination dieting and naturopathy. Elimination dieting is based on the principle that foods particular to each patient may contribute to chronic symptoms or disease when eaten in normal quantities. Exclusion dieting appears to benefit conditions including coeliac disease, orofacial granulomatosis, rheumatoid arthritis, hyperactivity and migraine. Unlike classic allergies, these 'food intolerances' do not involve a conventionally understood immune mechanism or have a rapid onset. Diagnosis consists of eliminating all but a few foods from the diet and then reintroducing foods one by one to see if they provoke symptoms. After a period of complete exclusion, the problem substances can usually be reintroduced gradually without recurrence of symptoms. Although practitioners commonly diagnose wheat and dairy 'intolerance', each patient is said to be sensitive to a different set of foods.

Less evidence-based therapeutic diets are also promoted. In 'Vega' or electrodermal testing, an electrical circuit is made that includes both the patient and the food suspected of causing disease. In applied kinesiology, practitioners claim to be able to diagnose allergy or deficiency on the basis of changes in muscle function. Naturopathy is a therapeutic system emphasizing the philosophy of 'nature cure' and incorporating dietary intervention among other practices such as hydrotherapy and exercise. For example, a naturopath might advise a patient with recurrent vaginal candidosis to undertake a limited fast, reduce intake of foods containing sugar and yeast, and take herbal and probiotic preparations. Another therapeutic system tests patients for 'subclinical' nutritional deficiencies – thought to arise where systems of food intake, digestion or absorption are not fully functional – and gives appropriate supplementation. Tests include biochemical assays of the vitamin and mineral content of blood or hair. The evidence for the effectiveness of many of these unconventional nutritional interventions in treating disease is often doubtful.

EFFECTS OF FOODS ON DRUG ABSORPTION

Foods and drugs can affect the absorption or activity of various drugs (Box 27.7). *Antacids* can cause early release of drugs from enteric-coated capsules, and can reduce absorption of antimicrobials and several drugs such as in Box 27.8. *Citrus fruit acids* may cause some medications to dissolve prema-

> **Box 27.7 Foods that might influence drug absorption**
>
> - Antacids
> - Citrus fruits (mainly grapefruit)
> - Garlic
> - Minerals (mainly calcium and iron)
> - Phytates
> - Vitamin K

> **Box 27.8 Drugs whose absorption is reduced by antacids**
>
> - Angiotensin-converting enzyme (ACE) inhibitors
> - Antimicrobials – azithromycin, ciprofloxacin, isoniazid, nitrofurantoin, norfloxacin, pivampicillin, rifampicin, some tetracyclines (doxycycline, lymeclocycline), antimalarials, itraconazole, ketoconazole
> - Bisphosphonates
> - Digoxin
> - Gabapentin
> - Lithium
> - Penicillamine
> - Phenothiazines
> - Phenytoin

turely in the stomach rather than in the intestine as intended. Therefore, taking drugs with acid fruit juices (and carbonated sodas) is usually not recommended. Citrus juice, however, improves the absorption of iron. *Grapefruit juice*, and drinks

> **Box 27.9 Drugs affected by grapefruit juice**
>
> - Amlodipine
> - Astemizole
> - Atorvastatin
> - Buspirone
> - Caffeine
> - Calcium-channel blockers
> - Carbamazepine
> - Ciclosporin
> - Cisapride
> - Diazepam
> - Dihydropyridine calcium antagonists
> - Diltiazem
> - Felodipine
> - HIV-protease inhibitors (e.g. saquinavir)
> - HMG-CoA reductase inhibitors
> - Lovastatin
> - Methadone
> - Midazolam
> - Nifedipine
> - Nisoldipine
> - Sertraline, a selective serotonin reuptake inhibitor
> - Tacrolimus
> - Terfenadine
> - Triazolam
> - Verapamil

that contain grapefruit juice or fresh, canned or frozen grapefruit, can affect the metabolism of several drugs (Box 27.9 and Table 27.13). The effect of grapefruit juice on drugs appears primarily to result from inhibition of intestinal cytochrome P450 3A4 (CYP3A4), drug-metabolizing enzymes that would otherwise break drugs down. Medications such as itraconazole, ketoconazole, ciclosporin, diltiazem and erythromycin may have a similar effect – inhibiting both intestinal CYNA4 and hepatic CYP3A4. Grapefruit juice constituents, including flavonoids (naringin and naringenin, along with the furanocoumarins, bergapten and 6,7-dihydroxybergamottin), have also been implicated in activating P-glycoprotein, an intestinal-wall drug efflux mechanism. The grapefruit juice effect appears to last for at least 3 days but may vary depending on brand, juice fraction and time of year.

In dentistry, the main problem is with benzodiazepines: one glass of grapefruit juice more than triples the bioavailability of diazepam, with more drowsiness. The bioavailability of oral midazolam and triazolam is also increased. Patients about to be given benzodiazepines, therefore, should avoid drinking grapefruit juice (Table 27.13).

Sour orange juice (e.g. Seville oranges), real lime juice, cranberry and tangelos (a hybrid of grapefruit) may possibly also have this effect. Most other citrus fruits, such as lemons, naturally sweet oranges and tangerines, are considered safe.

Garlic supplements appear to enhance anticoagulants. Cranberry juice (*Vaccinium macrocarpon*), popularly used to prevent cystitis, may also enhance warfarin. Vitamin K in foods (e.g. liver, cabbage, spinach, cauliflower, green tea and broccoli), in contrast, can substantially reduce the effectiveness of warfarin.

Minerals may influence drug absorption. Iron can reduce absorption of quinolones (e.g. ciprofloxacin). Calcium in dairy

Table 27.13 Effects of grapefruit juice on some relevant drugs

Drug(s)	Effect of grapefruit juice	Implications
Benzodiazepines	Increases blood drug concentrations	Increased sedation. Clinical significance of effect on cognitive function unclear
Carbamazepine	Increases blood drug concentrations	Toxicity (e.g. dizziness, poor balance and coordination, drowsiness, nausea, vomiting, tremor and agitation)
Ciclosporin	Increases blood drug concentrations	Toxicity, such as kidney and liver damage, and immune suppression
Corticosteroids	Increases blood drug concentrations	Consumption of large amounts of grapefruit might increase the risk of adverse effects
Itraconazole	Impairs drug absorption	The clinical significance of this interaction is unclear; theoretically, it could decrease efficacy of itraconazole

foods and in supplements chelates tetracylines. Avoiding high-calcium foods within 2 h of taking the medication minimizes this problem.

Phytates in chapattis bind calcium and impair its absorption.

USEFUL WEBSITES

http://www.food.gov.uk/healthiereating/
http://www.obesity.org/education/
http://www.edr.org.uk/
http://www.b-eat.co.uk/
http://www.nimh.nih.gov/health/topics/eating-disorders/index.shtml
http://www.nice.org.uk/CG9

FURTHER READING

Ashcroft, A., Milosevic, A., 2007. The eating disorders; 1. Current scientific understanding and dental implications. Dent Update 34, 544–554.

Ashcroft, A., Milosevic, A., 2007. The eating disorders; 2. Behavioural and dental management. Dent Update 34, 612–620.

Dhingra, R., Sullivan, L., Jacques, P.F., et al., 2007. Soft drink consumption and risk of developing cardiometabolic risk factors and the metabolic syndrome in middle-aged adults in the community. Circulation 116, 480–488 [Erratum in Circulation 2007;116:e557].

Dubois, L., Farmer, A., Girard, M., Peterson, K., 2007. Regular sugar-sweetened beverage consumption between meals increases risk of overweight among preschool-aged children. J Am Diet Assoc 107, 924–934, discussion 934–5.

Faine, M.P., 2007. Recognition and management of eating disorders in the dental office. Dent Clin North Am 47, 395–410.

Harris, R., Jang, G., Tsunoda, S., 2003. Dietary effects on drug metabolism and transport. Clin Pharmacokinet 42, 1071–1088.

Hoek, H.W., Van Hoeken, D., 2003. Review of the prevalence and incidence of eating disorders. Int J Eat Disord 34, 383–396.

Kitchens, M., Owens, B.M., 2007. Effect of carbonated beverages, coffee, sports and high energy drinks, and bottled water on the in vitro erosion characteristics of dental enamel. J Clin Pediatr Dent 31, 153–159.

Larsson, S.C., Bergkvist, L., Wolk, A., 2006. Consumption of sugar and sugar-sweetened foods and the risk of pancreatic cancer in a prospective study. Am J Clin Nutr 84, 1171–1176.

Lo Russo, L., Campisi, G., Di Fede, O., Di Liberto, C., Panzarella, V., Lo Muzio, L., 2008. Oral manifestations of eating disorders: a critical review. Oral Dis 14, 479–484.

Milosevic, A., Thomas, J., Mitzman, S., 2003. Satisfaction with dento-facial appearance in the eating disorders. Eur J Prosthodont Restor Dent 11, 125–128.

Mortelmans, L.J., Van Loo, M., De Cauwer, H.G., Merlevede, K., 2008. Seizures and hyponatremia after excessive intake of diet coke. Eur J Emerg Med 15, 51.

Petti, S., Scully C. 2009. Polyphenols, oral health and disease. J Dent. 37, 413–423.

Ravaldi, C., Vannacci, A., Zucchi, T., et al., 2003. Eating disorders and body image disturbances among ballet dancers, gymnasium users and body builders. Psychopathology 36, 247–254.

Saldana, T.M., Basso, O., Darden, R., Sandler, D.P., 2007. Carbonated beverages and chronic kidney disease. Epidemiology 18, 501–506.

Yellowlees, W., 2002. Marine fat and human health. Nutr Health 16, 345–346.

The International Classification (ICIDH) system, distinguishes impairment (I) from disability (D) and handicap (H; Table 28.1).

Table 28.1	International Classification system
	Definition
Impairment	The functional limitation caused by physical, mental or sensory impairment (i.e. it is organ-based)
Disability	The loss or limitations of opportunities to participate in the normal life of the community on an equal level with others, due to physical or social barriers (i.e. it is person-based)
Handicap	The disadvantage suffered as a consequence of impairment and disability (i.e. it is socially based)

There are significant differences in terminology related to disability in different countries. For example, the term 'mental retardation' as used in the USA is not used in the UK, where 'learning disability' or 'learning, intellectual or cognitive impairment' are among the terms accepted. The Disability Discrimination Act 1995 (DDA) in the UK considers a persons as disabled if they have a mental or physical impairment that interferes with their ability to carry out everyday activities. The DDA, the Americans with Disabilities Act 1990, and similar Acts in Canada, Australia and other countries make it unlawful to treat disabled people less favourably for reasons related to their disability.

Service providers particularly need to make adjustments to physical features of their premises to overcome physical barriers to access. The activity limitation has more to do with an unaccommodating environment than the impairment itself; no access except via stairs is a good example of the type of barrier people may face, but there can be many (Table 28.2).

The main conditions causing disability are shown in Table 28.3. Only patients with physical or mental impairment and some specific conditions will be considered here. Patients with other important specific diseases, such as haemophilia, neurological disorders and muscular dystrophies, children and older people are discussed in other chapters.

PHYSICAL IMPAIRMENTS
GENERAL AND CLINICAL ASPECTS

Physical disabilities include orthopaedic, neuromuscular, cardiovascular and pulmonary disorders. The disability may be either congenital or acquired – typically the result of injury, or disease. People with disabilities often must rely for mobility upon devices such as wheelchairs, crutches, frames (e.g. Zimmer), walking sticks and artificial limbs. Some people may have hidden (non-visible) disabilities, which include epilepsy, respiratory and other disorders. Limited access to transport, buildings or reluctance of staff to provide care are their major barriers to health care.

GENERAL MANAGEMENT

Decreased physical stamina and endurance, impaired eye–hand coordination or impaired verbal communication may complicate care. Assistance, if requested, should be provided. When it appears that a person needs assistance, ask if help can be given. Accept the fact that a disability exists. Sensitivity to using words like 'walking' or 'running' is inappropriate; people who are handicapped use these words. Always ask first while facing a person who uses a wheelchair; never come up from behind and push them. Try to have conversations at the same eye level by sitting, kneeling or squatting where appropriate. However, a wheelchair is part of the person's body space, so do not automatically hang or lean on it. Some who use wheelchairs can achieve amazing feats, such as performing in the Para-Olympics (Fig. 28.1), and can walk with the aid of canes, braces, crutches or walkers. Others cope with extraordinary impairments. If a person's speech is difficult to understand, do not hesitate to ask them to repeat.

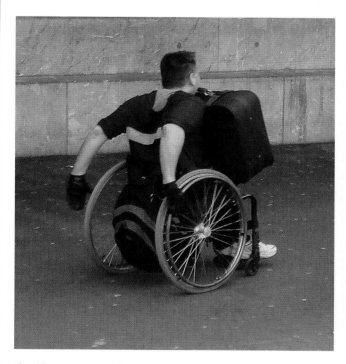

Fig. 28.1 A person with paraplegia showing impressive independence

DENTAL ASPECTS

Guidelines for care are available at http://www.bsdh.org.uk/guidelines/physical.pdf.

CEREBRAL PALSY

Cerebral palsy (CP) is the most common congenital physical handicap, with abnormalities of motor control caused by brain damage early in development, either during fetal life, during

Table 28.2   Barriers that can create disability from impairment.

Barriers	Main problems	Possible consequences
Discrimination	Access to: • premises • facilities • health care • education • employment • recreation	Difficulties with stairs Inappropriate toilets Inadequately trained staff Often lower wages
Prejudice	Denied anonymity Denied respect Hostility Patronization Lowered expectations of achievements	Stared at Regarded as a 'burden' Intolerance
Ignorance	Fear of people with disabilities Inadequate education of carers or professionals	Fear of aggression or being bitten Undergraduate training lacking or scarce

(Reproduced from Scully C, Diz Dios P, Kumar N. Special care in dentistry: handbook of oral healthcare. Churchill Livingstone Elsevier, Edinburgh, 2007).

Table 28.3   Important conditions with impairments

Mental impairment	Visual defects and hearing defects	Physical disorders
Autism disorders Chromosomal anomalies, especially Down syndrome Dyslexia Learning impairments	Various	Cardiac disease Cerebral palsy Cleft deformities Cystic fibrosis Hydrocephalus Juvenile arthritis Muscle diseases Spinal cord damage (especially paraplegia) and spina bifida Thalidomide deformities

the birth process or during the first few months of infancy. Brain damage is caused mainly by hypoxia, trauma, infection or hyperbilirubinaemia, but genetic or other biochemical factors may be involved. Risk factors are shown in Box 28.1.

Clinical features

Cerebral palsy can cause abnormalities of movement and posture in various parts of the body, but there is no uniform pattern because of the many variations in brain damage. CP features depend on the type (Table 28.4), but may include delays in motor skills development, poor control over hand and arm movement, weakness, abnormal walking, with one foot or leg dragging, and excessive drooling or difficulties in swallowing. Up to 50% have additional challenges such as epilepsy, defects of hearing, vision or speech, learning impairment or emotional disturbances. Many patients are highly intelligent but may have such severely impaired speech as to *appear* to have learning impairment.

Box 28.1   Risk factors for cerebral palsy

- Breech presentation
- Low birthweight
- Maternal infection
- Meconium staining of amniotic fluid – caused by stool passed by the fetus *in utero*
- Vaginal bleeding during pregnancy

Table 28.4   Types of cerebral palsy

Type	Subtype	Involves
Spastic	Monoplegic	Only one limb
	Paraplegic	Lower extremities
	Hemiplegic	One upper and lower limb on same side
	Double hemiplegic	All limbs but mainly the arms
	Diplegic	All limbs but mainly the legs
	Quadriplegic (tetraplegic)	All limbs equally
Athetoid	Athetosis	All limbs equally
	Chorea	
	Choreoathetosis	
Ataxic		
Rigid		
Mixed		

Spastic cerebral palsy is the most common type, and CP patients are therefore sometimes loosely referred to as 'spastics'. It manifests with excessive muscle tone and contractures, pathological reflexes and hyperactive tendon reflexes. It is an upper motor neuron lesion, and affects 50% of CP patients (Fig. 28.2). Hemiplegia is the most common subtype, often associated with neurological disorders such as epilepsy, or sensory or visual field defects. Quadriplegics may more frequently have learning impairment but are less often epileptic. Paraplegics and diplegics have an IQ intermediate in level between quadriplegics and hemiplegics, but are the least likely to have epilepsy.

Athetoid cerebral palsy accounts for 15–20% of CP, is caused by extrapyramidal damage, usually in the basal ganglia, and causes smooth worm-like movements, which become exaggerated if the patient is anxious. There is excessive muscle tone of the 'lead-pipe' type: the limb when flexed moves like a lead pipe being bent, but there are normal tendon reflexes and no contractures. Athetoid CP is mainly caused by intrauterine rubella and by hyperbilirubinaemia (kernicterus as in rhesus incompatibility). It usually involves the arms especially but all four limbs are affected, and is often accompanied by high-tone deafness. Epilepsy can be associated but learning impairment is less common than in spastic CP.

Ataxic cerebral palsy accounts for about 10% of all CP, is caused by a cerebellar lesion and characterized by disturbed balance.

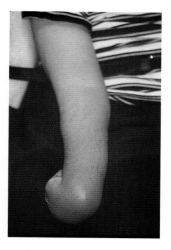

Fig. 28.2 Cerebral palsy showing contractures in spasticity

General management

The brain damage in CP is irreversible. However, muscle training and exercises help the child's strength, balance and mobility, and increase independence. Muscle relaxants ease stiffness and anticonvulsants reduce seizures. Support from occupational therapy, speech therapy, audiologists, ophthalmics, orthopaedics and dieticians can be invaluable.

Dental aspects

Dental management may be difficult because of access problems. Patients restricted to wheelchairs can sometimes be treated in their chair but it is often better to transfer them to the dental chair by carrying them or by sliding them across a board placed between the wheelchair and dental chair. Manual support is often required and ataxic patients may need the chair to be tilted backwards. Many, however, become apprehensive when this is done. Uncontrollable movements, especially in athetosis, bruxism, abnormal attrition and spontaneous dislocation or subluxation of the temporomandibular joint (TMJ), are common.

Communication difficulties, along with concentration, which is often poor, may give a misleading impression of low intelligence. Epilepsy may be seen. Abnormal swallowing and drooling are common due to poor control of the oral tissues and head posture. Anxiety may worsen athetosis or spasticity, so that anxiolytic drugs such as diazepam are useful as pre-medication.

Preventive dental care is important. Parental counselling about diet, oral hygiene procedures and the use of fluorides should be started early. Manual dexterity is usually poor but favourable results are often achievable with an electric toothbrush or a modified handle to a normal brush. Most dental disease is more common when the arms are severely affected. Periodontal disease is common, especially in the older child because soft tissue movement is abnormal and oral cleansing is impaired. Mouth-breathing worsens the periodontal state, and papillary hyperplastic gingivitis may be seen, even in the absence of treatment with phenytoin.

There may be delayed eruption of the primary dentition and enamel hypoplasia is common. Caries activity appears normal, unless there is overindulgence by parents, but lack of treatment frequently leads to premature loss of primary teeth, and earlier eruption of premolars and permanent canines. Malocclusion is common and thought to be caused by abnormal muscle behaviour. The maxillary arch is frequently tapered or ovoid, with a high palate. The upper teeth are often labially inclined, due to the pressure of the tongue against the anterior teeth during abnormal swallowing. Most, however, have skeletal patterns within normal limits.

CLEFT LIP AND PALATE (SEE CH. 14)

HYDROCEPHALUS

General aspects

Hydrocephalus (Greek *hydro* meaning water and *cephalus* meaning head) is a neurological disorder that affects approximately one out of every 1000 children and is caused by raised intracranial pressure (ICP), usually due to an abnormal accumulation of cerebrospinal fluid (CSF) within the ventricles and/or subarachnoid space. CSF is overproduced, its flow is obstructed, or there is a failure to reabsorb it. In *normal pressure* hydrocephalus, the ventricles are enlarged, but there is little or no rise in intracranial pressure.

Hydrocephalus is considered *congenital* when it is X-linked, or its origin can be traced to a birth defect or brain malformation that causes a raised resistance to the drainage of CSF. It can be caused by TORCH syndrome from intrauterine infection. Congenital hydrocephalus is often a part of other neurological conditions and congenital malformations (e.g. Dandy–Walker syndrome, neural tube defects, spina bifida, Chiari malformations, vein of Galen malformations, hydranencephaly, craniosynostosis, schizencephaly and tracheoesophageal fistula).

Hydrocephalus can be *acquired* later in life if there is a rise in the resistance to the drainage of CSF, such as an obstruction by brain tumour, arachnoid cyst, intracranial or intraventricular haemorrhage (IVH), trauma to the head, or by infections such as meningitis. The term 'communicating hydrocephalus' means that the site of raised resistance to CSF drainage resides outside of the ventricular system in the subarachnoid space. Non-communicating, or *obstructive*, hydrocephalus is caused by an obstruction in the flow of CSF within the ventricular system of the brain, especially in the aqueduct of Sylvius, or at the outlets of the fourth ventricle (the foramina of Luschke and Magendie) and from the lateral ventricles into the third ventricle at the foramina of Monro.

Clinical features

The main features of hydrocephalus are outlined in Table 28.5.

Table 28.5 Hydrocephalus

Signs	Complications
Large head and bulging fontanelles in children Headache, vomiting, mental changes, papilloedema	Epilepsy
	Spasticity
	Learning impairment, or dementia
	Visual impairment

General management

Hydrocephalus can be treated directly, by removing the cause of CSF obstruction or overproduction if one can be found, or indirectly, by diverting the fluid build-up to somewhere else, typically into another body cavity – usually into the peritoneal cavity (ventriculo-peritoneal shunt; VP shunt) by implanting a silastic device that can divert the excess CSF away from the brain (Fig. 28.3). An older shunt, into the right atrium (Spitz–Holter shunt, a ventriculo-atrial shunt; VA shunt) is shown in Fig. 28.4. Shunt lengthening surgery may be needed as the child grows.

Diuretics (acetazolamide and furosemide) may help reduce CSF production.

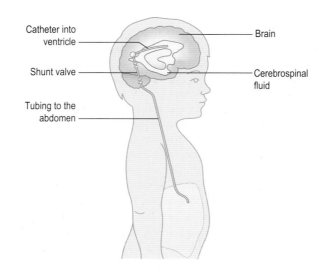

Fig. 28.3 Hydrocephalic shunt

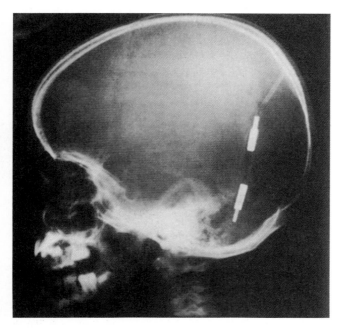

Fig. 28.4 Hydrocephalic shunt

Dental aspects

The weight of the hydrocephalic head may cause difficulties, especially in the anaesthetized patient, and there may be other management difficulties, including infection of shunt, spina bifida (frequently associated), latex allergy, epilepsy, and learning and visual impairment.

The consequences of infection can be so devastating that antibiotic cover may occasionally need to be given before oral procedures that might produce bacteraemia in patients with a VA shunt. There is probably no indication for patients with a VP shunt; the neurosurgeon should be consulted.

SPINA BIFIDA

General aspects

Spina bifida is failure of fusion of vertebral arches, an important cause of spinal cord disease and severe physical handicap. Deficiency of folic acid in pregnancy may predispose but most cases are of unknown aetiology.

Clinical features

There is a range of impairments in spina bifida (Table 28.6). Patients with myelomeningocoele tend also to suffer from inability to walk, liability to develop pressure sores, urinary incontinence, faecal retention and other problems, such as hydrocephalus, cerebral complications (epilepsy or learning impairment), and other vertebral or renal anomalies.

Table 28.6 Types of spina bifida	
Type	Features
Spina bifida occulta	Rarely any obvious clinical or neurological disorder but may be detected by a small naevus or tuft of hair over the lumbar spine in some patients, and radiographically in about 50% of apparently healthy children
Spina bifida cystica	Extensive vertebral defect through which the spinal cord or its coverings protrude
Meningocele	Protrusion of the meninges as a sac covered by skin, rarely causing neurological defect but 20% have hydrocephalus
Myelomeningocele	Characterized by meninges and nerve tissue protruded and exposed, and liable to infection, particularly meningitis. Causes severe neurological defects, typically complete paralysis of, and loss of sensation and reflexes in, the lower limbs (paraplegia)

General management

Patients with myelomeningocele are severely handicapped and require specialist paediatric attention to manage urinary tract, bowel and locomotion disabilities. Surgical closure of myelomeningocele and decompression of hydrocephalus is often carried out in early infancy.

Dental aspects

Bowel and bladder are best emptied before dental treatment. Postural hypotension is likely, and thus the patient is best not treated supine. In any event, many are chairbound, and it is better just to tilt the wheelchair back slightly if there are facilities for this, or transfer the patient to the dental chair using a board between wheelchair and dental chair, and then treat the patient in the semi-reclined position.

Care must be taken not to traumatize the patient who is unable to respond protectively. Some patients are on anti-coagulants or other medication. There is a very high prevalence of latex allergy in these people (Ch. 17).

THALIDOMIDE SYNDROME

General aspects

In 1957, the hypnotic thalidomide was marketed for morning sickness and nausea and soon became the 'drug of choice to help pregnant women. It went into general use, and was widely prescribed. The years that followed witnessed a dramatic increase in babies born with birth defects which included deafness, blindness, cleft palate, malformed internal organs and phocomelia (seal-like limbs). Thalidomide did not affect normal intelligence. Since the withdrawal of thalidomide, those affected are now adults.

Thalidomide has activity against tumour necrosis factor (TNF) and is therefore now being used to treat leprosy, some cancers, Behçet disease and major aphthae, on a named-patient basis.

Clinical features

The severe deformity of the limbs (phocomelia) included trunks lacking either arms or legs or both, or sometimes flippers extended from the shoulders, or toes extended directly from the hips (Fig. 28.5).

Dental aspects

Many thalidomide victims have a globular head with hypertelorism (widely spaced eyes), depressed nasal bridge and a central facial naevus extending from the forehead down to the

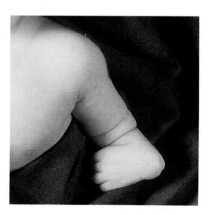

Fig. 28.5 Thalidomide phocomelia

nose. Oral effects include enamel hypoplasia, cleft palate and abnormalities in tongue morphology.

LEARNING IMPAIRMENT

GENERAL ASPECTS

Learning impairment or disability is a term used for limitations in mental functioning and in skills such as communicating, self-care and social skills. In the USA, this same term is usually used to denote specific learning impairments, such as dyslexia, rather than impaired cognition.

An IQ of < 70 is the arbitrary dividing line that defines learning disability. The average score in the population is 100. Learning impairment affects as many as three out of every 100 people and is frequently the result of brain damage, often of unknown reason, but defined causes are shown in Table 28.7.

CLINICAL FEATURES

The limitations will cause children to learn and develop more slowly than normal children. Most patients have an IQ between 50 and 75, and often live at home. However, patients with severe learning impairment (IQ < 50) are often totally dependent on others. Brain damage may cause not only mental but also physical impairment and epilepsy; visual defects, hearing, speech or behavioural disorders, facial deformities or cardiac defects are often associated.

Children with learning disability typically take longer to learn to speak, walk and take care of their personal needs, such as dressing or eating, and they typically have trouble learning. They may sit up, crawl, walk or talk late, or have trouble speaking. They may find it hard to remember things, have trouble solving problems or thinking logically. They may also have trouble understanding social rules, may not understand how to pay for things and can have trouble seeing the consequences of their actions.

Other problems may include psychiatric disorders (symptoms are often modified by poor language development and other defects), hyperkinesis and stereotyped movements (body-rocking and self-mutilation are common; Fig. 28.6).

Feeding difficulties may be present. Pica (the ingestion of inedible substances) is also fairly common.

GENERAL MANAGEMENT

Learning impairment is diagnosed by the ability to learn, think, solve problems and make sense of the world (called IQ or intellectual functioning), and whether the person has the skills needed to live independently (adaptive behaviour or adaptive functioning). Adaptive behaviour skills include daily living skills (getting dressed, going to the bathroom and feeding), communication skills (understanding what is said and being able to answer) and social skills (with peers, family members, adults and others).

Learning impairment is so varied in severity and character that generalizations about care cannot be made. Many people learn to live independently as adults in community housing. Others can be cared for adequately by committed parents or guardians.

28

LEARNING IMPAIRMENT

617

Table 28.7 Causes of learning impairment

	Cause	Examples
Genetic conditions	Chromosomal anomalies	Autosomal trisomies (Edward, Patau and Down syndromes). Deletions (chromosome 5, short arm – *cri du chat* syndrome; chromosome 4, short arm – Wolf syndrome) Sex chromosome anomalies (XO Turner syndrome; XXX superfemale; XXY Klinefelter syndrome; XYY syndromes). Fragile X syndrome
	Inborn errors of metabolism	Hypothyroidism (cretinism), phenylketonuria, homocystinuria, Wilson disease, galactosaemia, mucopolysaccharidosis, Tay–Sachs disease, Gaucher disease, Lesch–Nyhan syndrome
	Phakomatoses	Neurofibromatosis (von Recklinghausen disease), encephalofacial angiomatosis (Sturge–Weber syndrome), tuberous sclerosis (epiloia)
	Microcephaly	Angelman syndrome
Pregnancy problems	Drugs	Fetal alcohol syndrome Fetal anticonvulsant syndrome
	Infections	HSV, CMV, HIV, rubella, syphilis, toxoplasmosis
	Hypoxia	
	Prematurity	
Birth problems	Hypoxia	
	Metabolic/toxins	Rhesus incompatibility, kernicterus, hypoglycaemia
Post-natal problems	Infections	Pertussis, measles, meningitis, encephalitis, HIV
	Metabolic/toxins	Hypoglycaemia, extreme malnutrition, lead or mercury
	Trauma	Accidents or assaults with head trauma
	Hypoxia	
	Radiation	
	Alzheimer disease	

CMV, cytomegalovirus; HIV, human immunodeficiency virus; HSV, herpes simplex virus.

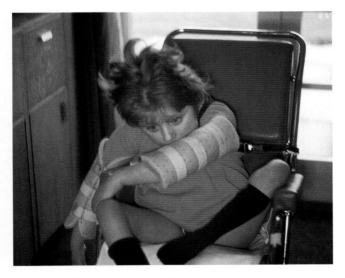

Fig. 28.6 Self-harm in a person with learning impairment

Limited access to buildings or reluctance of staff to provide care are the major barriers. Complications may result from prolonged medication (e.g. sedatives, tranquillizers or anticonvulsants); overindulgence (with consequent obesity and its sequelae); or infections (viral hepatitis, gastrointestinal infections or infestations, and tuberculosis – particularly a problem in institutionalized persons in the past).

Access and informed consent to treatment can be difficult issues for people with learning impairment. Some people may not themselves be able to give informed consent and, in many countries, relatives and staff have no legal right to give consent on the patient's behalf. If a person is not capable of giving or refusing consent, and has not validly refused such care in advance, treatment may often still be given lawfully if it is deemed to be in the patient's best interests. However, this should happen only after full consideration of its potential benefits and unwanted effects and after consultation with the carer(s), relatives and other people close to the patient.

DENTAL ASPECTS

Diet make-up, maintenance of good oral hygiene and prevention of caries and periodontal disease can be significant challenges. People with learning disability tend to have the same pattern of caries but more teeth decayed and missing, and fewer filled teeth than in the national population of similar age. Age-adjusted CPITN (community periodontal index of treatment need) scores significantly differ by behavioural group. Those people with severe physical and learning disability have the highest CPITN 3 category mean score.

It is frequently impossible, because of impaired cognition, mobility and manual dexterity, for these patients to improve their level of plaque control. Electric toothbrushes may be easier and more effective for these people to use or they may need help.

Many people with learning disability are amenable to treatment in the dental surgery, but more time may be required, and they may require special facilities or an escort. Regular, routine scaling usually improves the gingival state considerably but there is no indication for sophisticated periodontal surgery.

Routine conservative dental treatment should be carried out wherever possible to preserve the teeth. Local anaesthesia (LA; if necessary with inhalational or intravenous sedation) is preferable and usually satisfactory. Up to one-third require sedation or general anaesthesia (GA) for dental treatment, sometimes because they are unable to understand and cooperate. GA may also be used to carry out more complex procedures and, by saving time, may enable more patients to be treated. This must be carried out in hospital with advanced life support facilities. Intraoperative complications are uncommon, but may include non-fatal ventricular arrhythmias, slight falls in blood pressure or hypertension (greater than 20% of pre-operative value), laryngospasm and minor airway problems resulting in a desaturation of oxygen to a level below 85%.

Restoring the dentition and preventing further dental disease avoids the situation of loss of teeth and the need to manage dentures. Clinical prosthetic work can be very difficult. Impression-taking is facilitated by using a viscous composition or a putty-type material. If the patient objects violently, it can be readily removed without leaving unset material in the oropharynx. If patients will not keep their mouths open, a mouth prop on alternate sides and sectional impressions may overcome the difficulty. In severely handicapped patients with severe cerebral palsy, stridor can be caused by a bite block. Those people who are more severely handicapped tend to have a deterioration of breathing function when using a bite block. Registration of occlusal records can be very difficult.

Prostheses may also be contraindicated in severe epileptics, who may inhale foreign bodies during a convulsion. Any prosthesis for an epileptic should be constructed of radio-opaque material and marked with the patient's name typed on to a paper strip. This can be added to the fitting surface at flasking and covered with clear acrylic before processing. Those patients who are incapable of managing full dentures become dental cripples in addition to their other disabilities.

Self-mutilation may involve the oral or orofacial tissues, as in Lesch–Nyhan syndrome (see Ch. 23) where the lips or tongue may be chewed severely. Rarely, oral self-mutilation is accidental in patients with congenital indifference to pain, including Riley–Day syndrome (familial dysautonomia; see Ch. 23).

AUTISM SPECTRUM DISORDERS (ASD)

Autism

General aspects

Autism is a spectrum of disorders with three cardinal clinical features: onset within the first 2–3 years of life, autism (profound aloneness) and obsessional desire for maintaining an unchanging environment. Autism affects about one or two people in every thousand and is 3–4 times more common in boys, is seen mainly in first-born males and a genetic basis is possible. Implicated are genes on chromosomes 5 and 7, which affect synapses. Genes involved appear to include: *NLGN1*, *ASTN2*, *CDH9* and *CDH10* – genes which code for nerve cell surface proteins that facilitate adhesion between neurons; and *DOCK4* and *IMMP2L*, which affect dendrite development.

Clinical features

Autists live in isolated worlds of their own (Table 28.8). They are apparently indifferent and remote, unable to form emotional bonds with others, and incapable of understanding other people's thoughts, feelings and needs.

Children with autism reject people, act strangely, and lose language and social skills already acquired. They seem to have difficulty learning to engage in the give-and-take of everyday human interaction. These children appear to be isolated from everyone around them and fail to respond to any stimuli, even to being lifted by the parents. They show complete lack of interest in others but are often fascinated by inanimate objects. They seem to prefer being alone, and may resist attention and affection or passively accept hugs and cuddling. Later, they seldom seek comfort or respond to anger or affection. They rarely become upset when the parent leaves or show pleasure when the parent returns. There is ritualistic or compulsive behaviour. Autists typically demand consistency in their environment – eating the same foods, at the same time, sitting at precisely the same place. They may get annoyed with any minor change in their routine (e.g. if their toothbrush has been moved). Many autists engage in repetitive activities, such as rocking or banging their heads, or rigidly following familiar patterns in their routines. Most characteristic are finger-flicking near the eyes, hand-flapping, facial grimaces, jumping and toe walking, and all such mannerisms are exaggerated if the

Table 28.8 Difference in behaviour of young children with and without autism

Autism	Non-autism
Avoid eye contact	Study mother's face
May appear deaf	Easily stimulated by sounds
Start developing language, then abruptly stop talking altogether	Keep adding to vocabulary and expanding grammatical usage
Social relationships	
Act as if unaware of others	Recognize familiar faces and smile
Physically attack and injure others without provocation	Cry when mother leaves room
Inaccessible	Anxious with strangers
	Upset when hungry or frustrated
Exploration of environment	
Remain fixated on single item or activity	Move from one object or activity to another
Habitual rocking or hand-flapping	Reach out to acquire objects
Sniff or lick toys	Explore and play with toys
Appear to have no sensitivity to burns or bruises	Seek pleasure
May engage in self-mutilation	Avoid pain

person becomes anxious or excited. Some autistics are especially sensitive to sound, touch, sight or smell, but some seem oblivious to cold or pain. Rages, tantrums and self-directed aggression are common.

The autistic child rarely uses the pronoun 'I' and frequently uses meaningless words or phrases in a generally immature speech. Language and intelligence often fail to develop fully, making communication and social relationships difficult; delayed or immediate echolalia (repetition of words heard) may develop. Some autistics are highly intelligent but 70% have an IQ < 70. Temporal lobe epilepsy develops in about 30%.

It is essential to rule out other disorders, including hearing loss, speech problems, learning disability, neurological problems and Rett syndrome (a progressive brain disease that affects only girls and causes repetitive hand movements, bruxism and loss of language and social skills).

General management

Medications used to treat certain symptoms of autism include clomipramine and selective serotonin reuptake inhibitors (SSRIs).

Dental aspects

It is essential to ensure the child is not kept waiting and has a short quiet visit with a routine that includes always seeing the same dental staff. Patients with autism may be disturbed by noise, such as a high-speed aspirator or air rotor, and it may be necessary to avoid their use. Autists may be unable to accept dental treatment under LA. GA may be needed, but some may be on medication, such as antidepressants, which can complicate treatment.

Asperger syndrome

Asperger syndrome (AS) is a type of autism that is considerably more common than classic autism; however, AS differs from classic autism in that language is usually intact and features typically appear later in childhood. Indeed, the diagnosis is not usually suspected or made until school age, and patients often go on to have the capacity to live an independent adult life. The sex ratio of AS is about eight boys to one girl and the prevalence among schoolboys is about 0.3%.

Positron emission tomography (PET) scan studies in AS have shown an absence of the normal task-related activity in the left medial prefrontal cortex region, although normal activity is observed in the areas immediately adjacent.

Repetitive behaviours, severe social problems and clumsy movements are seen in AS. There are qualitative abnormalities in reciprocal social interaction, restricted and repetitive patterns of behaviour and interests, and often motor clumsiness and difficulties with non-verbal and social aspects of communication.

CHROMOSOMAL ANOMALIES

Most human cells contain 46 chromosomes (23 pairs), half of which are inherited from each parent. Only the reproductive cells (the sperm cells in males and the ova in females) have 23 *individual* chromosomes, not pairs. When the sperm and ovum combine at fertilization, the fertilized egg that results contains 23 chromosome pairs. A fertilized egg that will develop into a female contains chromosome pairs 1–22 and the XX pair. A fertilized egg that will develop into a male contains chromosome pairs 1–22 and the XY pair.

Chromosomal anomalies affect sex chromosomes and autosomes equally. Sex chromosome anomalies are usually compatible with life and are rarely associated with severe physical disability. Autosomal anomalies affecting the larger chromosomes commonly cause spontaneous abortions and natal and early neonatal deaths. However, anomalies of the smaller chromosomes may be compatible with life, though they can cause multiple impairments, as in Down syndrome.

The most common source of major chromosomal anomalies is an error in meiosis (non-disjunction). One chromosome too few, or one too many, enters a gamete and subsequently the zygote. Most of the chromosomal anomalies are rare and many affected individuals survive for only a few years. Chromosomal deletions may also cause learning disability.

The most common chromosomal anomalies of significance in dentistry are Down syndrome and fragile X syndrome. Medical problems and the main oral manifestations of other chromosomal anomalies are summarized in Appendix 28.1.

Down syndrome (mongolism or trisomy 21)

General aspects

Named after John Langdon Down, who identified it, Down syndrome is the most frequent genetic cause of learning impairment, appearing in one in 800 live births, in all races and economic groups. It is caused by an error in cell division that results in the presence of an additional third chromosome 21 (trisomy 21), in 88% derived from the mother. The resultant range of physical disabilities varies, depending on the proportion of cells carrying the additional chromosome 21.

Down syndrome is usually due to a random event during formation of the ovum or sperm causing one of three genetic variants. In 92%, there is an extra chromosome 21 in all cells (*trisomy 21*). In 2–4% there is a *mosaic trisomy 21* – the extra chromosome 21 is present only in some cells. In approximately 3–4%, material from one chromosome 21 is translocated on to another chromosome (*translocation trisomy 21*); cells then have two normal chromosomes 21, but also have additional chromosome 21 material on the translocated chromosome, usually chromosome 14 or 15. There may be an increased likelihood of Down syndrome in future pregnancies where the mother has had a child with translocation trisomy 21.

An older mother is more likely to have a baby with Down syndrome but, since older mothers have fewer babies, about 75% of babies with Down syndrome are born to younger women.

A range of chromosome 21 genes is implicated in Down syndrome features (Table 28.9).

Clinical features

The characteristic features are short stature, learning disability, and a typical facies with brachycephaly, widely spaced eyes, Brushfield's spots in the iris and epicanthic folds (Fig. 28.7).

Table 28.9 Genes implicated in Down syndrome

Gene	Gene product	Possible sequelae
APP	Amyloid beta A4 precursor protein	Cognitive difficulties
COL6A1	Collagen type 1	Cardiac defects
CRYA1	Crystallin, Alpha-A	Cataracts
DSCR1	Down syndrome critical region gene 1	Defect in signal transduction pathway involving both heart and brain
DYRK	Tyrosine phosphorylation-regulated kinase 1A	Poor mental development
ETS2	Avian erythroblastosis virus E26 oncogene homologue 2	Lymphocyte and thymus abnormalities
IFNAR	Interferon receptor	Impaired interferon expression; immune defect
SOD1	Superoxide dismutase	Dementia; immune defect

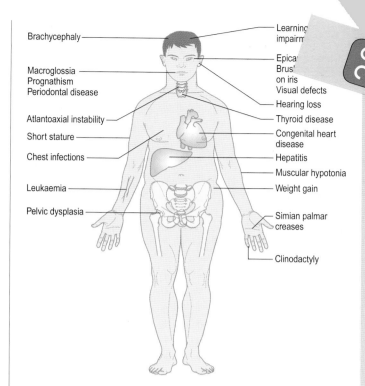

Fig. 28.8 Down syndrome

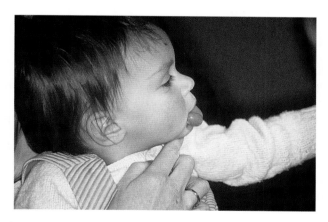

Fig. 28.7 Down syndrome facies

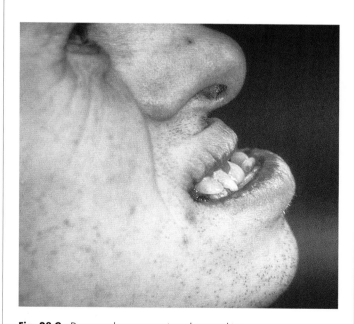

Fig. 28.9 Down syndrome cyanosis and prognathism

The hands show clinodactyly (short fifth finger) and simian (single) palmar creases. However, Down syndrome affects many, if not most, organs and may result in multiple impairments, and about one-third succumb in the first few years (Fig. 28.8).

Approximately 50% have congenital cardiac disorders (atrial septal defect, mitral valve prolapse or, less often, atrioventricular and ventricular septal defect) and associated early onset of pulmonary hypertension (Fig. 28.9). Mitral valve prolapse can lead to arrhythmias, embolism or sudden death. If it causes a systolic murmur, it can predispose to infective endocarditis, particularly in older persons.

Seizure disorders affect between 5% and 13%, a tenfold greater incidence than in the general population. Dementia, or memory loss and impaired judgement similar to that in Alzheimer disease patients may develop. There is susceptibility to transient myelodysplasia or defective development of the spinal cord. Atlantoaxial instability can cause spinal cord compression if the neck is not handled gently. The external ear and the bones of the middle and inner ear may develop differently and thus up

to 90% have hearing loss of greater than 15–20 decibels in at least one ear. Cataracts appear in approximately 3%. Children with Down syndrome are 10–15 times more likely than other children to develop leukaemia.

Multiple immune defects mean that infections of the skin, gastrointestinal and respiratory tracts, and periodontal disease, are common; superoxide dismutase has been shown to increase in Down syndrome and may be implicated in the immune defect. Chronic respiratory infections include tuberculosis and recurrent middle ear, tonsil, nasal and sinus infections.

Institutionalized patients are also liable to be hepatitis B carriers. There is a 12-fold higher mortality rate from infectious diseases, particularly pneumonia.

The life expectancy for people with Down syndrome, though low, has increased substantially to age 50 and beyond, particularly because infections are now more readily controlled.

General management

Many specialists recommend that women who become pregnant at age 35 or older undergo pre-natal testing for Down syndrome (DS). After counselling, this includes the following.

- Blood screening for maternal serum alpha-fetoprotein (MSAFP – low in DS), human chorionic gonadotropin (hCG – raised in DS) and unconjugated oestriol (uE3 – low in DS).
- Amniocentesis – removal and analysis of a small sample of fetal cells from the amniotic fluid (generally safe but cannot be done until the 14–18th week of pregnancy, and it usually takes more time to determine whether the cells contain extra material from chromosome 21).
- Chorionic villus sampling (CVS), conducted at 9–11 weeks of pregnancy, involves testing a tiny amount of chorionic villi that are obtained through the abdomen or cervix for extra material from chromosome 21.
- Percutaneous umbilical blood sampling (PUBS), the most accurate method and used to confirm the results of CVS or amniocentesis, cannot be performed until later in the pregnancy (during the 8th to 22nd weeks) and carries the greatest risk of miscarriage.

With assistance from family and carers, many adults with Down syndrome develop the skills required to hold jobs and to live semi-independently.

Dental aspects

People with Down syndrome are usually amiable and cooperative, and generally more easily managed than many other types of patient with learning disability.

Most can be treated under LA with sedation if necessary. GA must be administered by a specialist anaesthetist in hospital or is best avoided where possible, in view of other management difficulties which may include cardiac defects, anaemia, possible atlantoaxial subluxation (care needed when extending neck) or respiratory disease. There may also be difficulty in intubation because of the hypoplastic mid-face, congenital anomalies of the respiratory tract may be present and there is increased susceptibility to chest infections.

The tongue may be absolutely or relatively large and is often scrotal, more especially after the age of about 4 years (Table 28.10). The circumvallate papillae enlarge but the filiform papillae may be absent. The lips tend to be thick, dry and fissured. Poor anterior oral seal and also a strong tongue thrust may be seen. Anterior open bite, posterior cross-bite and other types of malocclusion are common.

The maxillae and molars are small and the mandible is somewhat relatively protrusive. Class III malocclusion is common,

Table 28.10 Orofacial abnormalities in Down syndrome

Hard tissue	Soft tissue
Omega-shaped palate	Macroglossia
Midface hypoplasia	Tongue fissuring
Hypodontia	Lip fissuring
Microdontia	Cheilitis
Delayed eruption in both dentitions	Drooling
Bruxism	

but 46% are class I. The orthodontic prognosis is often poor because of learning disability, parafunctional habits and severe periodontal disease. The palate often appears to be high, with horizontal palatal shelves (the omega palate), but a short palate is more characteristic. There is also a higher incidence of bifid uvula, cleft lip and cleft palate.

The first dentition may begin to appear only after 9 months and may take 5 years to complete, if ever. The deciduous molars may erupt before the deciduous incisors and deciduous lateral incisors are absent in about 15%. The eruption of the permanent teeth is often also irregular. Missing teeth are common: the third molars and lateral incisors are most often absent. Up to 30% have morphological abnormalities in both dentitions, particularly teeth with short small crowns and roots. The occlusal surfaces of the deciduous molars may be hypoplastic and both dentitions may be hypocalcified. Caries activity is usually low in both dentitions.

Severe early-onset periodontal disease may be partly due to poor oral hygiene, but may be the result of impaired cell-mediated and humoral immunity and a deficient phagocytic system. Acute ulcerative gingivitis may also be seen.

Short roots and poor manual dexterity and oral hygiene often complicate the situation. A well-planned preventive dental health programme, started early, can lead to a high degree of success in the prevention of dental diseases.

Fragile X syndrome

General aspects

Fragile X syndrome affects one in 1000 to one in 1500 of the population and is the second most common chromosomal defect associated with learning impairment, after Down syndrome. Fragile X syndrome is so named because the tip of the X chromosome is susceptible to breakage. Fragile X syndrome is a sex-linked dominant trinucleotide repeat disorder (other trinucleotide repeat disorders include Huntington chorea, spinocerebellar ataxia, myotonic dystrophy and Friedreich ataxia).

Clinical features

Fragile X syndrome affects males and manifests with learning impairment, long face, prominent ears, large testes and seizures.

Dental aspects

Hyperactivity, a short attention span and behavioural disorders similar to those of autism make dental management difficult. Cross-bite and open bite are abnormally frequent.

SPECIFIC TYPES OF LIMITED LEARNING DISABILITY

Dyslexia (reading disability)

Dyslexia is perhaps the most commonly known learning disability: an impairment in the brain's ability to translate written images into meaningful language. It is primarily used to describe difficulty with language processing and its impact on reading, writing and spelling. People with dyslexia have normal intelligence and normal speech, but often have difficulty interpreting spoken language and writing, and they read at levels significantly lower than expected. There is often a family history.

Clinical features

Common signs are delay in speaking, delay in learning the alphabet, numbers, days of the week, months, colours and shapes, reduced reading achievement, lack of awareness of phonemes (sounds that make up words), difficulty in spelling and difficulty with sequences of letters in words and in understanding language subtleties (such as jokes). Inability to recognize words and letters on a printed page; reading ability level much below that expected; problems processing and understanding; difficulty with rapid instructions, more than one command at a time or remembering the sequence of things; and reversals of letters (e.g. b for d) and words (e.g. saw for was) are common. Untreated, dyslexia may lead to low self-esteem, behavioural problems, delinquency, aggression, and withdrawal or alienation from friends, parents and teachers.

General management

Treatment is by remedial education.

Dysgraphia

Dysgraphia involves difficulty with writing, but there are also difficulties with spelling and the formulation of written composition. The common signs include problems involving the steps of putting together a written document, bad handwriting, awkward pen grip, avoidance of tasks that involve writing, difficulty fleshing out ideas on paper in contrast to the ability to discuss such ideas verbally, and inconsistency in the way letters and words look. People with dysgraphia can benefit from explicit instruction in the skills required to produce written work. Computers can help enormously.

Dyscalculia

Dyscalculia involves difficulty with mathematics skills (addition, subtraction, multiplication) and concepts (sequencing of numbers). Memory of maths facts, concepts of time, money and musical concepts can be impacted. Language and other skills, however, may be advanced, and visual memory for the printed word is good. There may be poor sense of direction, as well as trouble reading maps, telling time, grappling with mechanical processes, difficulty with abstract concepts of time and direction, schedules, keeping track of time, and the sequence of past and future events. Individuals with dyscalculia need help in organizing and processing information related to numbers and mathematical concepts. Again, computers can help.

Dyspraxia

Dyspraxia (apraxia) is difficulty with motor planning, affecting a person's ability to coordinate appropriate body movements, resulting in various problems such as:

- *ideomotor dyspraxia* (inability to perform single motor tasks, such as combing hair or waving goodbye)
- *ideational dyspraxia* (difficulty with multilevel tasks, such as taking the proper sequence of steps for brushing teeth)
- *dressing dyspraxia* (difficulty with dressing and putting clothes on in order)
- *oromotor dyspraxia* (difficulty with speech)
- *constructional dyspraxia* (difficulty with spatial relations).

Features may be: coordination problems, including awkwardness in walking, clumsiness or trouble with hopping, skipping, throwing and catching a ball, or riding a bicycle; confusion about which hand to use for tasks; inability to hold a pen or pencil properly; sensitivity to touch; poor short-term memory; trouble with reading and writing; poor sense of direction; speech problems; phobias or obsessive behaviour; and impatience.

ATTENTION DEFICIT (HYPERACTIVITY) DISORDER

Attention deficit (hyperactivity) disorder (ADD/ADHD) may be associated with learning difficulties (see Ch. 10).

OTHER HANDICAPPING SYNDROMES

See Appendix to this chapter, and Appendix to Ch. 23 for inborn errors of metabolism.

USEFUL WEBSITES

http://www.ada.gov/
http://www.patientcenters.com/hydrocephalus
http://www.faces-cranio.org/
http://www.bsdh.org.uk/guidelines/physical.pdf
http://www.csun.edu/~sp20558/dis/emcontents.html
http://health.nih.gov/topic/DownSyndrome
http://health.nih.gov/topic/cleftlipandpalate.html
http://www.ninds.nih.gov/disorders/cerebral_palsy/cerebral_palsy.htm

---

FURTHER READING

Acs, N., Bánhidy, F., Horváth-Puhó, E., Czeizel, A.E., 2006. Population-based case-control study of the common cold during pregnancy and congenital abnormalities. Eur J Epidemiol 21, 65–75.

Mahoney, E.K., Kumar, N., Porter, S.R., 2008. Effect of visual impairment upon oral health care: a review. Br Dent J 204, 63–67.

Proctor, R., Kumar, N., Davies, R., et al., 2004. Cerebrospinal fluid shunts and dentistry: a short review of relevant literature. J Disabil Oral Health 5, 27–30.

Scully, C., van Bruggen, W., Diz Dios, P., Casal, B., Porter, S., Davison, M.F., 2002. Down syndrome: lip lesions (angular stomatitis and fissures) and *Candida albicans*. Br J Dermatol 147, 37–40.

Scully, C., Diz Dios, P., Kumar, N., 2007. Special care in dentistry: handbook of oral healthcare. Churchill Livingstone Elsevier, Edinburgh.

Stanfield, M., Scully, C., Davison, M.F., Porter, S.R., 2003. The oral health of clients with learning disability: changes following relocation from hospital to community. Br Dent J 194, 271–277.

Appendix 28.1   Chromosomal anomalies not discussed in text

Syndrome	Anomaly	Features and possible management problems	Orofacial manifestations
Angelman syndrome	Chromosome 15 deletion	'Happy puppet' – laughs and claps, learning impairment, ataxia, seizures	Microcephaly
Cri du chat syndrome	Chromosome 5 short arm deletion	Learning impairment, cardiac defects, respiratory infections	Cranial abnormalities Malocclusions
DiGeorge syndrome	Chromosome 22 microdeletion	Hypoparathyroidism, thymic hypoplasia, T-cell defect, major cardiac anomalies, learning disability	Cleft palate Candidosis Dental hypoplasia
Edwards syndrome	Trisomy 18	Learning impairment, cardiac defects, renal disease	Cranial abnormalities Microstomia Hypoplastic parotids Gingival cysts
Klinefelter syndrome	47,XXY	Tall stature, personality defects, diabetes, asthma	Taurodontism
Patau syndrome	Trisomy 13	Rarely survive infancy, learning impairment, cardiac defects in 80%, deafness, epilepsy	Cranial abnormalities Cleft lip or palate in 75%
Superfemale	Trisomy X (47,XXX)	Tall females, learning impairment, early menopause	–
Turner syndrome	Monosomy X (45,X)	Females only, normal intelligence, infertility, short stature, webbed neck, renal anomalies, cardiac defects, diabetes, keloid formation, lymphoedema	Small mandible Malocclusions
Williams syndrome	Microdeletion of elastin gene on chromosome 7	Supravalvular aortic stenosis, hypercalcaemia, learning impairment	Elfin facies Dental anomalies
Wolf syndrome	Short arm of chromosome 4 deletion	Learning impairment	Hypodontia
XYY	47,XYY	Tall males, normal intelligence, behavioural abnormalities	–

Few of the dental materials or drugs commonly used in general practice cause significant interactions or adverse reactions (Appendices Ch. 29). The main concern is allergies (e.g. to latex, iodides, Elastoplast and drugs (Ch. 17). Other concerns include dental materials (especially mercury), other drug adverse effects, oral side-effects, interactions and the effects of foods on drugs.

DENTAL MATERIALS

Possible toxic effects of mercury on the nervous system are discussed below and in Ch. 13; some effects of dental materials have been discussed in Ch. 17.

MERCURY CONCERNS

There has long been concern about the possible toxicity of mercury. One suggested relationship – between autism and vaccines containing the mercury-containing preservative, thimerosal – has been disproved. Mercury, however, is a well-known neurotoxin and nephrotoxin.

There are three kinds of mercury exposure: elemental (metallic) mercury poisoning, inorganic mercury poisoning and organomercury poisoning. Metallic mercury can be absorbed by inhalation of its vapour or through the skin and mucous membranes, and mercury salts can be absorbed after their ingestion. Mercury is highly lipid-soluble, rapidly penetrates the blood–brain barrier and infiltrates neurons.

Acute poisoning by massive inhalation of mercury vapour is rare but can cause potentially fatal pneumonitis and neurological symptoms, particularly tremor and excitability. Chronic poisoning by inhalation of mercury vapour primarily causes lassitude, gastrointestinal disturbances, anorexia and weight loss, and affects the central nervous system with tremor, memory loss, timidity and excitability (erethism). Poisoning was well recognized in the past among people working with metallic mercury (e.g. thermometer makers and makers of felt hats – hence, 'mad as a hatter'). Other effects include hypersalivation, accelerated periodontitis and a characteristic black gingival line due to deposition of mercury sulfides. Rarely, jaw necrosis could follow. Although such manifestations are mainly of historical interest, accidents continue to be reported, since metallic mercury is still found in equipment such as thermometers, fluorescent lights and personal computers. There are even some who inject it intravenously in suicide attempts!

Poisoning with mercury salts caused acrodynia (pink disease), a condition seen mainly at the end of the nineteenth century in children and others who used calomel (a mercury salt) in teething powders and gastrointestinal medications. Mercury poisoning is still occasionally seen in people using mercuric chloride in skin creams available in the developing world, in some traditional Chinese and herbal preparations, in some ritual spiritual or 'medical' practices, in suicide attempts and in forensic science, as well as in bizarre accidents.

Environmental poisoning from methyl mercury is also well recognized and was widespread in Minimata Bay and Nigata, Japan, in the 1950s, as a result of eating fish contaminated by mercury from industrial discharge into the sea. Many people suffered neurological damage, some died and later there was a high incidence of cerebral palsy in newborn children. Mercury poisoning of this type was seen in Iraq in the 1970s, and continues as a problem in parts of China, Brazil, Venezuela, Suriname and the Philippines, associated with occupations such as mining activities.

METALLIC MERCURY

Mercury can be an occupational hazard since dental staff who fail to follow good work practices can be exposed to mercury. On average up to 1.5 kg of mercury are used by a dental practice annually and, in the past, when little attention was paid to mercury hygiene, mercury vapour in the surgery atmosphere and its levels in the blood, hair, nails and urine in dental professionals were frequently above controls. Droplets of mercury could also accumulate in significant amounts in surgery carpeting or crevices in the floor. Mercury is also absorbed during hand trituration of amalgam or other skin contact. In the past, after decades of practice, a few dental professionals suffered from chronic mercury toxicity with tremor, incoordination, polyneuropathies and accelerated senility. Autopsy studies have also shown mercury deposits, particularly in the pituitary glands and occipital lobes. Rarely, deaths have been reported after prolonged heavy exposure.

In a study of female dental professionals, a history of reproductive failures, menstrual disorders and spina bifida in their children was suggested to be related to mercury levels in hair, but this has not been widely confirmed and other larger studies have shown no such correlation. Indeed, the perinatal death and birth defect rate for infants born of dentists is lower than average.

Urinary mercury levels also appeared to be lower in studies of dentists in 1996 than in 1983, and more recent studies of dental professionals have not shown excessively high urinary mercury levels where good mercury hygiene was practised. A recent study found no consistent association between either urinary mercury or chronic mercury exposure and any category of self-reported symptoms of depression, anxiety and memory, but both significant and consistent associations were found between increased symptoms and polymorphism of the serotonin transporter gene *5-HTTLPR* in a gene–dose relationship, suggesting these symptoms were associated with *5-HTTLPR* polymorphism in both genders.

It seems unlikely therefore that there is now a significant risk to dental professionals who apply adequate standards of mercury hygiene. The greatest hazard is from inhalation of mercury vapour as a result of any spillage, particularly when in proximity to an autoclave or other source of heat.

Indeed, mercury levels in dental professionals are highest in those who eat fish, indicating that at least part of the mercury burden was from diet and not from dental sources.

AMALGAMS

Dental amalgam restorative materials generally contain 50% mercury (Hg) in a complex mixture of copper, tin, silver and zinc which continually emits mercury vapour, which is increased by chewing, eating, brushing and drinking hot liquids. Removal of old amalgams from teeth with an air-rotor produces traces of mercury vapour – but not if adequate water-cooling and aspiration are used.

Because of the concerns about mercury toxicity, the American Dental Association carried out extensive investigation of the data available and, in 1989, their Council on Dental Therapeutics concluded 'there is insufficient evidence to justify claims that mercury from dental amalgams has an adverse effect on the health of patients'.

In one more recent study, children who received dental restorative treatment with amalgam did not, on average, have statistically significant differences in neurobehavioural assessments or in nerve conduction velocity compared with children who received resin composite materials only. In the New England Children's Amalgam Trial, a randomized trial involving children, the hypothesis that restorations using amalgam resulted in worse psychosocial outcomes than restorations using composite resin over a 5-year period following initial placement was not supported by the results. These findings, combined with the trend of higher treatment need later among those receiving composite restorations, suggested that amalgam should remain a viable dental restorative option for children. The situation has been summarized as follows:

> "Amalgam fillings release mercury (mercury vapour or inorganic ions) at a low level (about 2–5 micrograms/ day in an adult). Evidence on the health effect of dental amalgams comes from studies of the association between their presence and signs or symptoms of adverse effects or health changes after removal of dental amalgam fillings. More formal risk assessment studies focus on occupational exposure to mercury and health effects. Numerous methodological issues make their interpretation difficult but new research will continue to challenge policymakers. Policy will also reflect prudent and cautious approaches, encouraging minimization of exposure to mercury in potentially more sensitive population groups. Wider environmental concerns and decreasing tolerance of exposure to other mercury compounds (for example, methylmercury in seafoods) will ensure the use of mercury in dentistry remains an issue, necessitating dentists keep their patients informed of health risks and respect their choices". (Spencer AJ. Dental amalgam and mercury in dentistry. Aust Dent J 2000;45:224–34.)

Thus, according to present scientific evidence, the use of amalgam is not a proven health hazard and, to date, there is no dental material that can fully substitute amalgam as a restorative material. More recent studies and reviews have also found little to no correlation between systemic or local diseases and amalgam restorations, although extensive amalgam restorations in pregnant or nursing women are not recommended.

Nevertheless, the state governments of California, Connecticut, Maine and Vermont, and the federal governments of Denmark, Finland, Norway and Sweden, have legislation requiring that dental patients receive informed consent information about the restorative material that will be used.

'MERCURY ALLERGY'

Mercury and its salts are potential sensitizing agents: exposure to them can occasionally lead to contact dermatitis and the frequency of positive patch tests increases as dental students progress through their course. Also, a few patients have genuine contact sensitivity to mercury though they can generally tolerate the placement of amalgam restorations, provided that none is spilt on to the skin. 'Baboon syndrome' is a special form of systemic contact-type dermatitis (SCTD) manifesting with bright red buttocks and flexural eczema that occurs after ingestion or systemic absorption of a contact allergen in individuals previously sensitized by topical exposure to the same allergen in the same areas, and has been reported as a reaction to mercury. Occasionally, oral lichenoid lesions arise as a reaction to amalgam or other restorations.

Another group of patients have symptoms such as headache, lassitude or a general feeling of ill-health they ascribe to mercury, although there is no reliable evidence that mercury underlies these problems. Unfortunately this belief has been encouraged by a few practitioners who carry out spurious tests to detect alleged effects of dental amalgams. It has also been shown that patients who complain of amalgam-related symptoms also suffer more frequently from other, unrelated complaints, such as chronic craniofacial pain, than controls.

RESINS

There are few data to indicate significant toxicity from most resin components, apart from allergic reactions (Ch. 17), though bisphenol-A-glycidyldimethacrylate (BIS-GMA) may have some oestrogenic activity *in vitro*. Bisphenol A has also recently been implicated in heart disease and diabetes, though only miniscule amounts are found in dental resin restorations, and much more is present in other items such as plastic bottles and can linings. Indeed, a recent survey by the Centers for Disease Control and Prevention (CDC) found bisphenol in the urine of 95% of people in USA.

TOOTH-WHITENING PRODUCTS

Tooth-whitening products are widely available for sale over-the-counter (OTC) or dispensed by dentists for use at home. Most release hydrogen peroxide (H_2O_2). Self-applied bleaching agents either contain or generate H_2O_2, as gel in trays, paint-on films or whitening strips. A nightguard bleach is typically used with 10% carbamide peroxide (which contains ≈3% hydrogen peroxide), OTC whitening strips contain ≈6% H_2O_2, while in-office bleach uses 25–35% hydrogen peroxide. These can potentially all produce comparable whitening but strips are slightly more effective at whitening than is a gel in a tray. In the UK, Cosmetic Product (Safety) Regulations apply to products that contain or release more than 0.1% H_2O_2.

Recently, attention has focused on dentist-prescribed home bleaching, in which the teeth and oral soft tissues can be in contact with peroxide-type agents for extended periods of time, providing a very different situation from either in-office bleaching or peroxide-containing toothpastes and mouthwashes, from both dose and time standpoints. For home oral health care products, such as mouth rinses and toothpastes, which contain low concentrations of H_2O_2 (1% or less), the daily exposure to H_2O_2 will be lower than when using self-administered bleaching agents that either contain or produce high-levels of H_2O_2 for an extended period of time. Hydrogen peroxide is a highly reactive substance that can damage oral soft tissues and hard tissues when at high concentrations and with exposures of prolonged duration. Direct exposure of skin or eyes to 30% H_2O_2 may cause severe irritation or burns, while ingestion may irritate the oesophagus and stomach, causing bleeding and sudden distension. Vesicle formation and ulceration can occur following inadvertent exposure of oral soft tissues to such concentrated solutions of H_2O_2. The much lower concentrations used in dental whitening products do not appear to produce such adverse effects, but tooth sensitivity and gingival irritation are common.

FLUORIDE

Some studies, now criticized for their analyses, had suggested associations of bladder cancer with occupational fluoride exposure and of osteosarcoma with water fluoridation. A recent systematic review confirmed the benefit of fluoride in protection against dental caries, but showed that water fluoride to a concentration of 1 ppm had no proven adverse effects on bone strength, bone mineral density, fracture incidence (either protective or deleterious), cancer incidence or mortality, or on other conditions such as Down syndrome, congenital abnormalities or stillbirths. For details, see http://www.nhmrc.gov.au/publications/synopses/_files/eh41.pdf.

DRUGS

Relatively few drugs are used in general dentistry, and the rarity of hypersensitivity reactions and lack of evidence of significant interactions of local anaesthesia (LA) with drugs (especially tricyclic or other antidepressants) must be stressed. However, stepping outside this relatively safe arena can raise the level of risk. Sedative techniques are more likely and general anaesthesia (GA) is much more likely to produce adverse reactions. Drugs used in the practice of oral medicine and surgery also may produce adverse reactions or interactions.

Children need lower doses of virtually all drugs. Older people tend to be more liable to adverse drug reactions, and the reactions tend to be more serious and last longer than in younger people. Older people are also more likely to be given drugs.

Many drug reactions could not be predicted and it is only by recording suspected adverse drug reactions to an appropriate authority (Figs 29.1 and 29.2) that serious adverse reactions of apparently safe drugs can be elicited (e.g. the cardiotoxicity of cyclo-oxygenase-2 inhibitors). Drug interactions are possible and it is also important to bear in mind that OTC and herbal preparations, foods and other substances can sometimes interact by affecting drug absorption or efficacy, or causing other interactions (Appendix Ch. 29).

DRUG ADVERSE EFFECTS

Many adverse drug reactions are probably not, at present, recognized. A full medical history should always be taken, asking specifically about adverse drug reactions. Obviously the medical status can influence the choice of drugs.

DRUG ALLERGIES

Any suggestion of previous drug reaction or allergy, and particularly any adverse reaction during anaesthesia or imaging, should be taken seriously. Patients with allergy to one drug, and probably those patients with Sjögren syndrome or HIV disease, may be particularly liable to drug allergies (Appendix Ch. 29).

DRUG-INDUCED HYPERSENSITIVITY SYNDROME (DIHS)

This may manifest with a glandular fever-like syndrome (fever, rash, cervical lymphadenopathy, raised white cell count with atypical lymphocytes, and liver dysfunction) following the use of various drugs – especially anticonvulsants such as carbamazepine and phenytoin, isoniazid and sulfonamides. Many cases are associated with the reactivation of human herpesvirus 6 (HHV-6) or other herpesviruses.

DRUG OVERDOSE

The excessive use of virtually any drug can cause harm.

ANAESTHETICS

The use of excessive amounts of LA agents can be dangerous. However, lidocaine with epinephrine/adrenaline, the most widely used drugs in dentistry, have proved to be remarkably safe in practice over very many years, but gross overdose can be dangerous. One dentist has been found guilty of manslaughter, having given 16 cartridges of lidocaine with epinephrine to an elderly patient who subsequently died.

ANALGESICS

Non-steroidal anti-inflammatory drugs (NSAIDs) should not be taken by patients taking anticoagulants, alcohol or high-dose methotrexate. They should also be avoided in older or renally impaired patients taking digoxin, and avoided over the long term in those taking other NSAIDs. It is possible, but unconfirmed, that NSAIDs should not be given to patients taking lithium. NSAIDs are probably appropriate in the short term for patients taking antihypertensives, unless they have severe congestive heart disease or renal function is compromised.

Aspirin is a safe analgesic, but readily causes platelet dysfunction, and excessive doses have led to post-extraction bleeding. It should also not be given to patients taking oral hypoglycaemics, valproic acid or carbonic anhydrase inhibitors.

Acetaminophen/paracetamol is also safe but, when given in repeated doses, can cause severe liver damage. It may be given in the short term to any patient with a healthy liver, but should

COMMITTEE ON SAFETY OF MEDICINES

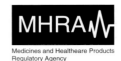

Medicines and Healthcare Products
Regulatory Agency

SUSPECTED ADVERSE DRUG REACTIONS

If you are suspicious that an adverse reaction may be related to a drug or combination of drugs please complete this Yellow Card. For reporting advice please see over. Do not be put off reporting because some details are not known.

PATIENT DETAILS   Patient Initials: _____   Sex: M / F   Weight if known (kg): _____

Age (at time of reaction): _____   Identification number (Your Practice / Hospital Ref.)*: _____

SUSPECTED DRUG(S)
Give brand name of drug and
batch number if known

	Route	Dosage	Date started	Date stopped	Prescribed for
_____	_____	_____	_____	_____	_____
_____	_____	_____	_____	_____	_____

SUSPECTED REACTION(S)
Please describe the reaction(s) and any treatment given:

Outcome

Recvered ☐
Recovering ☐
Continuing ☐

Date reaction(s) started: _____   Date reaction(s) stopped: _____   Other ☐

Do you consider the reaction to be serious?   Yes / No

If yes, please indicate why the reaction is considered to be serious (please tick all that apply):

Patient died due to reaction ☐   Involved or prolonged inpatient hospitalisation ☐

Life threatening ☐   Involved persistent or significant disability or incapacity ☐

Congenital abnormality ☐   Medically significant; please give details: _____

OTHERS DRUGS (including self-medication & herbal remedies)

Did the patient take any other drugs in the last 3 months prior to the reaction?   Yes / No

If yes, please give the following information if known:

Drug (Brand, if known)	Route	Dosage	Date started	Date stopped	Prescribed for
_____	_____	_____	_____	_____	_____
_____	_____	_____	_____	_____	_____
_____	_____	_____	_____	_____	_____
_____	_____	_____	_____	_____	_____

Additional relevant information   e.g, medical history, test results, known allergies, rechallenge (if performed), suspected drug interactions. For congenital abnormalities please state all other drugs taken during pregnancy and the last menstrual period.

REPORTER DETAILS
Name and Professional Address: _____

_____

Post code: _____   Tel No: _____
Speciality: _____
Signature: _____   Date: _____

CLINICIAN (if not the reporter)
Name and professional Address: _____

_____
Post code: _____

Tel No: _____   Speciality: _____

If you would like information about other adverse reactions associated with the suspected drug, please tick this box ☐

* This is to enable you to identify the patient in any future correspondence concerning this report

Please attach additional pages if necessary

Fig. 29.1   Form for reporting serious adverse drug reactions in the UK

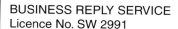

Postage will be paid by licensee

Do not affix Postage Stamps if posted in Gt. Britain, Channel Islands, N. Ireland or the Isle of Man

BUSINESS REPLY SERVICE
Licence No. SW 2991

Medicines and Healthcare products Regulatory Agency
CSM FREEPOST
London
SW8 5BR

SECOND FOLD HERE

Remember if in Doubt - Report

SUSPECTED ADVERSE DRUG REACTIONS REPORTING ADVICE

New Black triangle (▼) Druge - report ALL suspected adverse reactions
(New medicinal drugs can be indentified by the presence of a black triangle(▼)
both on the product information for the drug and BNF and MIMS)

Other Drugs - only report SERIOUS suspected adverse reactions
For instance those which are:
- Fatal
- Life threatening
- Involves or prolongs inpatient hospitalisation
- Involves persistent or signifigant disability or incapacity
- Congenital abnormality
- Medically signifigant (please exercise your judgement)

Please remember the areas of particular concern– delayed drug effects, the elderly, congenital abnormalities, children (including offlabel use of medications) and any herbal remdies

For more information contact:
- The National Yellow Card Information Service on Freephone 0800-7316789
- The MHRA website http://medicines.mhra,gov.uk
- Reporters can send suspected advers drug reaction reports by electronic Yellow Card, via the MHRA Website.
- More detailed guidelines are given in the BNF

DO NOT BE PUT OFF REPORTING BECAUSE SOME DETAILS ARE NOT KNOWN

FIRST FOLD HERE

Fig. 29.2 Form for reporting serious adverse drug reactions in UK

not be given to heavy drinkers or to persons who have recently stopped alcohol after chronic intake.

Opioids should not be given to heavy alcohol drinkers.

ANTIBIOTICS

There are potential life-threatening interactions of some antimicrobials (erythromycin, clarithromycin, metronidazole, ketoconazole and itraconazole) with a host of other drugs whose metabolism is impaired by them.

Antibiotics may also interfere with the effects of warfarin via suppression of gut bacteria that produce vitamin K. Commonly employed antibiotics may also impair the effectiveness of oral contraceptive agents, though the evidence for this is not strong (Fig. 29.3).

OTHERS

Starch glove powder can cause direct skin irritation, can interfere with wound healing and can impair implant osseo-integration and composite bonding.

Possible contraindications to the main drugs prescribable by the dental surgeon are tabulated in Appendix Ch 29.

DRUG REACTIONS

Drug doses should be reduced in children, the elderly, and those with liver or kidney dysfunction. Patients should be warned if serious adverse reactions are li kely (e.g. systemic corticosteroids), and provided with the appropriate warning card.

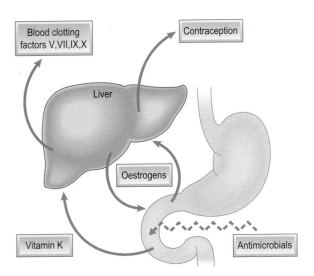

Fig. 29.3 Effects of antimicrobials on the contraceptive pill and vitamin K (hence on warfarin)

DRUG INTERACTIONS

Almost any drug may cause interactions, so no drug should be given unless there are good indications. Drug metabolism can be affected by other drugs. Polypharmacy should be avoided and only drugs with which the dentist is familiar should be used. Possible drug interactions are more likely when GA is used (Appendix Ch. 29), in older people and in patients with learning disability (Appendix Ch. 29).

Drug absorption can be impaired by other drugs; for example, iron, magnesium and aluminium in drugs can impair absorption of tetracyclines. Aluminium can impair absorption of azole antifungals. Metoclopramide enhances absorption of acetaminophen/paracetamol and aspirin.

ORAL ADVERSE EFFECTS OF DRUGS

Oral side-effects caused by drugs are relatively uncommon but may be important. Some drugs almost invariably cause oral side-effects; for example, the most common drug-induced oral disorders are dry mouth (caused by many drugs with an atropinic action), ulcers (from cytotoxic drugs and others), candidosis (usually caused by tetracyclines, ampicillin or corticosteroids), gingival swelling (usually caused by phenytoin, ciclosporin and calcium-channel blockers), and lichenoid reactions (from NSAIDs and many others). Drugs that may occasionally cause oral complications are given in Appendix Ch. 29.

Some habits, such as the use of oral snuff (smokeless tobacco), can cause gingival recession and leukoplakia, and possibly predispose to oral cancer; oral use of cocaine can cause gingival ulceration or desquamation.

Drug-related cheilitis

Cheilitis is commonly caused by contact reactions to cosmetics or foods, but drugs may be implicated (Box 29.1).

Box 29.1 Cheilitis

Drugs most commonly implicated
- Etretinate
- Isotretinoin
- Protease inhibitors
- Vitamin A
- Lip salves/lipsticks

Drug-related contact stomatitis (stomatitis venenata)

Fixed drug eruptions comprise repeated ulceration at the same site in response to a particular drug (Box 29.2). However, intraoral contact stomatitis is a dubious entity. In any such reactions, the lips or perioral skin are far more likely to be affected.

Box 29.2 Contact stomatitis

Drugs most commonly implicated
- Antibiotics
- Antiseptics
- Barbiturates
- Dentifrices
- Mouthwashes
- Phenacetin
- Sulfonamides
- Tetracyclines

Drug-related erythema multiforme

A wide range of drugs may give rise to erythema multiforme, and it may be impossible clinically to distinguish drug-induced erythema multiforme from disease due to other causes (Box 29.3).

Box 29.3 Erythema multiforme (and Stevens–Johnson syndrome and toxic epidermal necrolysis)

Drugs most commonly implicated
- Allopurinol
- Barbiturates
- Carbamazepine
- NSAIDs
- Penicillin
- Phenytoin
- Sulfonamides

Drug-related infections

Opportunistic infection secondary to cytotoxic chemotherapy can cause oral ulceration. In particular herpes simplex virus 1, varicella-zoster and cytomegalovirus give rise to oral ulceration. Less commonly ulceration may be due to Gram-negative bacterial infections.

Candidosis arises secondary to treatment with broad-spectrum antibiotics, corticosteroids (both systemic and inhaled preparations) and other immunosuppressive regimens (e.g. ciclosporin) and cytotoxic drugs (Box 29.4). More rarely, mucormycosis and aspergillosis may cause thrush-like areas in patients on long-term immunosuppressive treatment.

Human papillomavirus infection manifesting as warty-like growths may develop in patients on long-term immunosuppressive therapy. Oral hairy leukoplakia, usually affecting the dorsum and lateral borders of the tongue and floor of mouth, may be a consequence of Epstein–Barr virus infection in patients on treatment with corticosteroids (topical and systemic), ciclosporin or other long-term immunosuppressive regimens.

Box 29.4 Infections

Drugs most commonly implicated
- Broad-spectrum antimicrobials
- Corticosteroids
- Drugs causing xerostomia
- Immunosuppressives

Drug-related leukoplakia

Tobacco and alcohol use are important risk factors for leukoplakia and oral cancer. A greater frequency of lesions with epithelial dysplasia of the lips (but not oral mucosa) has also been observed in some iatrogenically immunosuppressed patients. Sanguinarine, the principal alkaloid of the bloodroot plant (*Sanguinaria canadensis*), which is used in some mouthwashes and dentifrices for its antiplaque activity, may be associated with the development of oral leukoplakia.

Drug-related lichenoid reactions

Since noticed as a side-effect of antimalarial therapy, there has been an ever-growing list of drugs that may give rise to mucocutaneous lichen planus-like eruptions (lichenoid reactions) (Box 29.5). The drugs now most commonly implicated are the NSAIDs and the angiotensin-converting enzyme (ACE) inhibitors.

Box 29.5 Lichenoid eruptions

Drugs most commonly implicated
- ACE inhibitors
- Antimalarials
- Beta-blockers
- NSAIDs

Drug-related lupus-like disorders

Systemic lupus erythematosus (SLE) may be induced by a wide variety of different drugs (Box 29.6).

Box 29.6 Lupoid reactions

Drugs most commonly implicated
- Hydralazine
- Isoniazid
- Procainamide

Drug-related malodour (halitosis)

Oral malodour may be related to treatment with isosorbide dinitrate, dimethyl sulfoxide or disulfiram, although drugs causing xerostomia can indirectly cause or aggravate this problem.

Drug-related movement disorders

Several different drug-induced movements can affect the mouth and face, particularly tardive dyskinesia (secondary to antipsychotics) and dystonias (e.g. with metoclopramide; Box 29.7). Although these disorders principally affect the face, there can be abnormal movements of the tongue, for example dystonia secondary to carbamazepine therapy.

Box 29.7 Involuntary facial movements

Drugs most commonly implicated
- L-Dopa
- Metoclopramide
- Phenothiazines

Drug-related neoplasms

Non-Hodgkin lymphoma, usually manifesting as ulceration of the gingivae, fauces or palate, or Kaposi sarcoma (see later) are rare complications of long-term immunosuppressive therapy.

Drug-related neuropathies

Facial or oral paraesthesia, hypoaesthesia or anaesthesia can be due to interferon-alpha, acetazolamide, labetalol, sultiame, vincristine and occasionally with some other agents, such as hepatitis B vaccination and some of the protease inhibitors (Box 29.8).

Box 29.8 Trigeminal paraesthesia or hypoaesthesia

Drugs most commonly implicated
- Acetazolamide
- Articaine
- Labetalol
- Protease inhibitors
- Vincristine

Drug-related pain and dysaesthesia

Captopril and lisinopril may very rarely cause a scalded-type sensation of the mouth.

Drug-related pemphigoid and other bullous disorders

Drug-induced pemphigoid may be due to drugs acting as haptens or drug-induced immunological dysfunction (Box 29.9).

Box 29.9 Pemphigoid-like reactions

Drugs most commonly implicated
- Furosemide
- Penicillamine

Drug-related pemphigus

Pemphigus-like reactions may occasionally be associated with drugs with active thiol groups in the molecule, such as penicillamine and captopril, or by rifampicin or diclofenac (Box 29.10).

Box 29.10 Pemphigus-like reactions

Drugs most commonly implicated
- Captopril
- Diclofenac
- Penicillamine
- Rifampicin

Drug-related pigmentation

Superficial transient discolouration of the dorsum of the tongue and other soft tissues and teeth, which may be of various colours (typically yellowish or brown), may be caused by some foods and beverages (coffee and tea), habits (tobacco, betel and crack cocaine use) and some drugs (iron salts, bismuth, chlorhexidine or antibiotics), especially if these also induce xerostomia (Box 29.11).

Box 29.11 Superficial mucosal pigmentation

Drugs/materials most commonly implicated
- Amalgam
- Drugs causing xerostomia
- Smoking/tobacco

Localized areas of pigmentation of the mucosa may be due to amalgam, while gingival pigmentation may be secondary to the gold or metal alloys of crowns. Heavy metal salts, used in the past, caused pigmentation, particularly of the gingival margin.

Blue, blue–grey or brown mucosal pigmentation can be an adverse effect of antimalarials, phenothiazines and phenytoin or amiodarone. Minocycline frequently causes widespread brown pigmentation of the gingivae and mucosae.

Discolouration of saliva may be caused by rifampicin and rifabutin and a few other drugs (Box 29.13).

Box 29.12 Tooth discolouration

Drugs most commonly implicated
- Chlorhexidine
- Fluorides
- Iron
- Tetracyclines

Box 29.13 Red saliva

Drugs most commonly implicated
- Clofazimine
- L-Dopa
- Rifabutin
- Rifampicin

Drug-related salivary gland pain

Salivary gland pain can be a side-effect of some drugs such as bethanidine, bretylium, clonidine, methyldopa and some cytotoxics (Box 29.14).

Drug-related sialorrhoea

Anticholinesterases are the main cause of sialorrhoea (Box 29.15).

Box 29.14 Salivary gland pain or swelling

Drugs most commonly implicated
- Antihypertensives
- Chlorhexidine
- Cytotoxics
- Iodides

Box 29.15 Sialorrhoea (hypersalivation)

Drugs most commonly implicated
- Anticholinesterases
- Clozapine

Others

Drug-related swelling

Gingival enlargement is a well-recognized oral side-effect of treatment with phenytoin, ciclosporin and the calcium-channel blockers (Box 29.16).

Box 29.16 Gingival swelling

Drugs most commonly implicated
- Amlodipine
- Basiliximab
- Ciclosporin
- Diltiazem
- Felodipine
- Lacidipine
- Nifedipine
- Oral contraceptives
- Phenytoin
- Verapamil

Drug-induced mucosal swelling predominantly affects the lips and floor of mouth (although rare isolated swelling of the uvula is possible). It is typically due to type I hypersensitivity reactions.

Many drugs, particularly penicillins, ACE inhibitors and aspirin can cause angioedema.

Drug-related taste disturbance

Drugs commonly impair taste by causing a loss of acuity (hygeusia) or distortion of function (dysgeusia) either by interfering in the chemical composition or flow of saliva or, more specifically, affecting taste receptor function or signal transduction (Box 29.17). Xerostomia also disturbs taste.

Drug-related ulceration

Oral ulceration may follow burns from the local application of aspirin or toothache preparations, potassium tablets, pancreatic supplements and other agents, such as trichloroacetic acid or hydrogen peroxide.

Mucositis and ulceration is caused by many chemotherapy regimens, particularly those involving methotrexate, 5-fluorouracil, doxorubicin, melphalan, mercaptopurine or bleomycin (Box 29.18).

Aphthous-like ulcers can be caused by NSAIDs and beta-blockers, and possibly by nicorandil and alendronate.

Box 29.17 Taste disturbance

Drugs most commonly implicated

- Antithyroids
- Aurothiomalate
- Azithromycin
- Aztreonam
- Baclofen
- Biguanides
- Calcitonin
- Captopril
- Cilazapril
- Clarithromycin
- Cytotoxic drugs
- Metronidazole
- Penicillamine
- Protease inhibitors
- Terbinafine
- Thiouracil

Box 29.18 Ulceration

Drugs most commonly implicated

- Cytotoxics
- Immunosuppressive agents
- NSAIDs (e.g. indometacin)

Drug-related xerostomia

Common habits such as tobacco smoking, alcohol use (including in mouthwashes) and use of beverages containing caffeine (coffee, some soft drinks) can cause some oral dryness.

Drugs are the most common cause of reduced salivation (Box 29.19). Those most commonly implicated in dry mouth are the tricyclic antidepressants, antipsychotics, atropinics and antihistamines. The complaint of dry mouth is therefore particularly common in patients treated for hypertensive, psychiatric or urinary problems.

Box 29.19 Xerostomia

Drugs most commonly implicated

- Alpha-receptor antagonists for treatment of urinary retention
- Anticholinergics
- Antidepressants (serotonin agonists, or noradrenaline and/or serotonin re-uptake blockers)
- Antipsychotics such as phenothiazines
- Appetite suppressants
- Atropinics
- Muscarinic receptor antagonists for treatment of overactive bladder
- Protease inhibitors

The cause for which the drug is being taken may also be important. Patients with anxiety or depression may complain of dry mouth even in the absence of drug therapy or evidence of diminished salivary flow.

Table 29.1 Some therapeutic monoclonal antibodies[a]

Monoclonal	Mechanism	Applications
Abciximab	Inhibits platelet GPIIb/ILIA	Prevent coagulation in coronary angioplasty
Adalimumab	Inhibits TNF-alpha	Rheumatoid arthritis Crohn disease
Alemtuzumab	Targets CD52 on T and B lymphocytes	B-cell leukaemia
Basiliximab	Inhibits IL-2 on T cells	Acute transplant rejection
Cetuximab	EGFR inhibitor	OSCC
Daclizumab	Inhibits IL-2 on T cells	Acute transplant kidney
Etanercept	Contains TNF receptor	Rheumatoid arthritis
Gemtuzumab	Targets leukaemia cells	Relapsed acute myeloid leukaemia
Infliximab	Inhibits TNF-alpha	Rheumatoid arthritis Crohn disease
Nimotuzumab	EGFR inhibitor	Glioma
Palivizumab	Inhibits RSV protein	RSV infections
Rituximab	Targets CD20 on B lymphocytes	Non-Hodgkin lymphoma
Trastuzumab	Targets HER2/neu (erbB2) receptor	Breast cancer

[a]See also http://en.wikipedia.org/wiki/List_of_monoclonal_antibodies. EGFR, epidermal growth factor receptor; IL-2, interleukin 2; OSCC, oral squamous cell carcinoma; RSV, respiratory syncytial virus; TNF-alpha, tumour necrosis factor-alpha.

MONOCLONAL ANTIBODIES

Monoclonal antibodies specifically bind to a substance and can serve to detect or purify that substance or act as a therapeutic medicine. When used as medications, the generic name ends in *—mab*. Monoclonal antibodies are available to treat cancer, cardiovascular disease, inflammatory diseases, transplant rejection, multiple sclerosis and viral infections (Table 29.1).

IMMUNOMODULATOR AGENTS

An immunomodulator is a substance (e.g. a drug) that has an effect on the immune response (Table 29.2). This effect can be stimulatory or suppressive. Immunostimulatory agents include, for example, vaccines and colony-stimulating factors. Immunosuppressive agents can be classified into (see Chs 16, 18 and 35):

- glucocorticosteroids
- cytostatic agents
- antibodies
- drugs acting on immunophilins
- others (e.g. interferons, TNF-binding agents, mycophenolate).

Table 29.2 Immunomodulators

Group	Mechanisms	Examples
Antimetabolites	Purine synthesis inhibitor	Azathioprine Mycophenolic acid
	Pyrimidine synthesis inhibitor	Leflunomide Teriflunomide
	Antifolate	Methotrexate
IL-1 receptor antagonists	Block IL-1	Anakinra
IL-2 inhibitors	FKBP/cyclophilin/calcineurin	Abetimus Ciclosporin Gusperimus Pimecrolimus Tacrolimus
Inhibitors of mTOR	Inhibit mTOR – a serine/threonine protein kinase that regulates cell growth, cell proliferation, cell motility, cell survival, protein synthesis and transcription	Ridaforolimus (deforolimus) Everolimus Sirolimus Temsirolimus Zotarolimus
TNF-alpha inhibitors	Inhibit TNF	Lenalidomide Thalidomide

IL-1, interleukin 1; IL-2, interleukin 2; FKBP, FK-binding protein; TNF-alpha, tumour necrosis factor alpha.

HYPERBARIC OXYGEN THERAPY (HBO)

Hyperbaric oxygen therapy is the medical use of oxygen at a level higher than atmospheric pressure. Indications, contraindications and possible adverse effects are summarised in Table 29.3

Table 29.3 Hyperbaric oxygen therapy

Possible indications	Contraindications	Possible adverse effects
Air embolism	Pneumothorax	Oxygen toxicity
Carbon monoxide poisoning	Upper respiratory infections	Barotrauma affecting sinuses, middle ear, or teeth
Crush injuries or gas gangrene	Middle ear barotrauma	Possible ocular complications
Burns	Chest surgery	
Skin flaps which are compromised	Emphysema	
Intractable soft tissue infections	Malignant disease	
Bone disorders such as osteomyelitis or osteoradionecrosis	Medication with disulfiram, doxorubicin, mafenide acetate or cisplatin	

USEFUL WEBSITES

http://www.nhmrc.gov.au
http://nccam.nih.gov/
http://aafp.org
http://bnf.org/bnf/bnf/
http://www.drugdigest.org/DD/Interaction/ChooseDrugs
http://www.dial,org.uk
http://www.dvla,gov.uk/medical.aspx
http://www.ukmi.nhs.uk
http://en.wikipedia.org/wiki/List_of_monoclonal_antibodies
http://www.fda.gov/Drugs

FURTHER READING

Bassin, E.B., Wypij, D., Davis, R.B., Mittleman, M.A., 2006. Age-specific fluoride exposure in drinking water and osteosarcoma (United States). Cancer Causes Control 17, 421–428.

Bellinger, D.C., Trachtenberg, F., Barregard, L., et al., 2006. Neuropsychological and renal effects of dental amalgam in children: a randomized clinical trial. JAMA 295, 1775–1783.

Bellinger, D.C., Trachtenberg, F., Zhang, A., Tavares, M., Daniel, D., McKinlay, S., 2008. Dental amalgam and psychosocial status: the New England Children's Amalgam Trial. J Dent Res 87, 470–474.

Bjerrum, L., Andersen, M., Petersen, G., Kragstrup, J., 2003. Exposure to potential drug interactions in primary health care. Scand J Prim Health Care 21, 153–158.

Clarkson, T.W., Magos, L., 2006. The toxicology of mercury and its chemical compounds. Crit Rev Toxicol 36, 609–662.

Cook-Mozaffari, P., 1996. Cancer and fluoridation. Community Dent Health 13 (Suppl 2), 56–62.

Corbett, C.E., El Khouri, M., Costa, A.N., et al., 2007. Health evaluation of gold miners living in a mercury-contaminated village in Serra Pelada, Pará, Brazil. Arch Environ Occup Health 62, 121–128.

DeRouen, T.A., Martin, M.D., Leroux, B.G., et al., 2006. Neurobehavioral effects of dental amalgam in children: a randomized clinical trial. JAMA 295, 1784–1792.

Diz Dios, P., Scully, C., 2002. Adverse effects of antiretroviral therapy: focus on orofacial effects. Expert Opin Drug Saf 1, 307–317.

Douglass, C.W., Joshipura, K., 2006. Caution needed in fluoride and osteosarcoma study. Cancer Causes Control 17, 481–482.

Edlich, R.F., Greene, J.A., Cochran, A.A., et al., 2007. Need for informed consent for dentists who use mercury amalgam restorative material as well as technical considerations in removal of dental amalgam restorations. J Environ Pathol Toxicol Oncol 26, 305–322.

Eilers, H., Niemann, C., 2003. Clinically important drug interactions with intravenous anaesthetics in older patients. Drugs Aging 20, 969–980.

Gelberg, K.H., Fitzgerald, E.F., Hwang, S.A., Dubrow, R., 1995. Fluoride exposure and childhood osteosarcoma: a case-control study. Am J Public Health 85, 1678–1683.

Göhring, T.N., Schicht, O.O., Imfeld, T., 2008. [Is amalgam a health hazard?] Ther Umsch 65, 103–110.

Grandjean, P., Olsen, J.H., Jensen, O.M., Juel, K., 1992. Cancer incidence and mortality in workers exposed to fluoride. J Natl Cancer Inst 84, 1903–1909.

Halbach, S., Vogt, S., Köhler, W., et al., 2008. Blood and urine mercury levels in adult amalgam patients of a randomized controlled trial: interaction of Hg species in erythrocytes. Environ Res 107, 69–78.

Hasson, H., Ismail, A.I., Neiva, G., 2006. Home-based chemically-induced whitening of teeth in adults. Cochrane Database Syst Rev (4) CD006202.

Heyer, N.J., Echeverria, D., Farin, F.M., Woods, J.S., 2008. The association between serotonin transporter gene promoter polymorphism (5-HTTLPR), self-reported symptoms, and dental mercury exposure. J Toxicol Environ Health A 71, 1318–1326.

Jones, D.W., 2004. Putting dental mercury pollution into perspective. Br Dent J 197, 175–177.

Li, Y., 2003. The safety of peroxide-containing at-home tooth whiteners. Compend Contin Educ Dent 24, 384–389.

Magos, L., Clarkson, T.W., 2006. Overview of the clinical toxicity of mercury. Ann Clin Biochem 43, 257–268.

Melchart, D., Köhler, W., Linde, K., et al., 2008. Biomonitoring of mercury in patients with complaints attributed to dental amalgam, healthy amalgam bearers, and amalgam-free subjects: a diagnostic study. Clin Toxicol (Phila) 46, 133–140.

Metz, M.J., Cochran, M.A., Matis, B.A., Gonzalez, C., Platt, J.A., Pund, M.R., 2007. Clinical evaluation of 15% carbamide peroxide on the surface microhardness and shear bond strength of human enamel. Oper Dent 32, 427–436.

Mohundro, M., Ramsey, L.A., 2003. Pharmacologic considerations in geriatric patients. Adv Nurse Pract 11, 21–22, 25–8.

Naik, S., Tredwin, C., Scully, C., 2006. Hydrogen peroxide tooth-whitening (bleaching): review of safety in relation to possible carcinogenesis. Oral Oncol 42, 668–674.

Pemberton, M.N., Oliver, R.J., Theaker, E.D., 2004. Micronazole oral gel and drug interactions. Br Dent J 196, 529–531.

Pollick, H.F., 2006. Concerns about water fluoridation, IQ, and osteosarcoma lack credible evidence. Int J Occup Environ Health 12, 91–94.

Porter, S.R., Scully, C., 2000. Adverse drug reactions in the mouth. Clin Dermatol 18, 525–532.

Ramesh, N., Vuayaraghavan, A.S., Desai, B.S., Natarajan, M., Murthy, P.B., Pillai, K.S., 2001. Low levels of p53 mutations in Indian patients with osteosarcoma and the correlation with fluoride levels in bone. J Environ Pathol Toxicol Oncol 20, 237–243.

Rode, D., 2006. Are mercury amalgam fillings safe for children? An evaluation of recent research results. Altern Ther Health Med 12, 16–17.

Scully, C., 2003. Drug effects on salivary glands; dry mouth. Oral Dis 9, 165–176.

Scully, C., Bagan, J.V., 2004. Adverse drug reactions in the orofacial region. Crit Rev Oral Biol Med 15, 221–239.

Scully, C., Field, A., Randall, C., 2008. Over-the-counter remedies for oral soreness. Periodontology 2000 48, 76–84.

Stockley, I.H. (Ed.), 2002. Stockley's drug interactions, 6th edn. Pharmaceutical Press, London.

Tredwin, C., Naik, S., Lewis, N.J., Scully, C., 2006. Hydrogen peroxide tooth-whitening (bleaching) products: review of adverse effects and safety issues. Br Dent J 200, 371–376.

Walsh, L.J., 2000. Safety issues relating to the use of hydrogen peroxide in dentistry. Austral Dent J 45, 257–269.

Yorifuji, T., Tsuda, T., Takao, S., Harada, M., 2008. Long-term exposure to methylmercury and neurologic signs in Minamata and neighboring communities. Epidemiology 19, 3–9.

Appendix 29.1   Drugs implicated in xerostomia

Alfuzosin	Duloxetine	Mirtazapine	Sibutramine
Amiloride	Ecstasy	Morphine	Sucralfate
Amitriptyline	Elliptinium	Moxonidine	Tamsulosin
Amoxapine	Ephedrine	Nabilone	Terazosin
Benzhexol	Fenfluramine	Nefopam	Thiabendazole
Benztropine	Fluoxetine	Nortriptyline	Tiapride
Biperiden	Furosemide	Olanzapine	Tiotropium
Bupropion	Guanfacine	Omeprazole	Tizanidine
Buspirone	Hyoscine	Orphenadrine	Tolterodine
Cannabis	Imipramine	Oxitropium	Tramadol
Cetirizine	Indoramine	Oxybutynin	Tranylcypromine
Chlormezanone	Interferon-alpha	Paroxetine	Trazodone
Chlorpromazine	Interleukin-2	Phenelzine	Trepium chloride
Citalopram	Ipratropium	Pipamperone	Triamterene
Clemastine	Iprindole	Pipenzolate	Trimipramine
Clomipramine	Isocarboxazid	Pirenzipine	Trospium
Clonidine	Isotretinoin	Poldine	Venlafaxine
Clozapine	Ketorolac	Procyclidine	Viloxazine
Cyclizine	Ketotifen	Propafenone	Zopiclone
Cyclobenzaprine	Lansoprazole	Propantheline	
Desipramine	L-Dopa	Propiverine	
Dexamfetamine	Lithium	Sertraline	

(Continued)

Appendix 29.1 Drugs implicated in xerostomia—cont'd

Diazepam	Lofepramine	Pseudoephedrine	
Dicyclomine	Lofexidine	Quetiapine	
Dideoxyinosine	Loratadine	Reboxetine	
Dihydrocodeine	Maprotiline	Rilmenidine	
Disopyramide	Mepenzolate	Risperidone	
Donepezil	Methyldopa	Rizatriptan	
Dosulepin	Mianserine	Selegiline	
Doxepin			

Appendix 29.2 Drugs implicated in salivary gland pain or swelling

Bethanidine	Famotidine	Naproxen	Phenytoin
Bretylium	Guanethidine	Nicardipine	Ranitidine
Cimetidine	Insulin	Nifedipine	Ritodrine
Clonidine	Interferon	Nitrofurantoin	Trimepramine
Clozapine	Isoprenaline	Oxyphenbutazone	
Deoxycycline	Methyldopa	Phenylbutazone	

Appendix 29.3 Drugs implicated in hypersalivation

Alprazolam	Guanethidine	Mefenamic acid	Tacrine
Amiodarone	Haloperidol	Mercurials	Tobramycin
Buprenorphine	Imipenem/cilastatin	Nicardipine	Triptorelin
Buspirone	Iodides	Niridazole	Venlafaxine
Clonazepam	Kanamycin	Pentoxifylline	Zaleplon
Diazoxide	Ketamine	Remoxipride	
Ethionamide	Lamotrigine	Risperidone	
Gentamicin	L-Dopa	Rivastigmine	

Appendix 29.4 Drugs implicated in discolouration of saliva

Clofazimine	L-Dopa	Rifabutin	Rifampicin

Appendix 29.5 Drugs implicated in disturbed taste

Acarbose	Celecoxib	Hyoscyamine	Perindopril
	Cholestyramine		
Acetazolamide	Choline magnesium trisalicylate	Imipenem	Phenformin
Alcohol	Cilazapril	Indometacin	Phenindione
Allopurinol	Cisplatin	Interferon-gamma	Phenylbutazone
Amiloride	Clarithromycin	Iodine	Phenytoin
Amitriptyline	Clidinium	Isotretinoin	Procaine penicillin
Amphetamines	Clofibrate	L-Dopa	Propafenone

Appendix 29.5 Drugs implicated in disturbed taste—cont'd

Amphotericin	Clomipramine	Levamisole	Propranolol
Amrinone	Cocaine	Levodopa	Propylthiouracil
Aspirin	Diazoxide	Lincomycin	Quinapril
Atorvastatin	Dicyclomine	Lisinopril	Ramipril
Auranofin	Diltiazem	Lithium	Rifabutin
Aurothiomalate	Dipyridamole	Lomefloxacin	Rivastigmine
Azathioprine	Disodium etidronate	Losartan	Selegiline
Azelastine	Enalapril	Lovastatin	Sodium lauryl sulfate
Aztreonam	Esomeprazole	Methimazole	Spironolactone
Baclofen	Ethambutol	Methotrexate	Sulfasalazine
Biguanides	Ethionamide	Methyl methacrylate	Terbinafine
Bisphosphonates	Famotidine	Methylthiouracil	Tetracycline
Bleomycin	Flunisolide	Metronidazole	Thiamazole
Bretylium	Fluoxetine	Nifedipine	Tocainide
Calcitonin	Flurazepam	Niridazole	Topiramate
Captopril	5-Fluorouracil	Nitroglycerin	Trandolapril
Carbamazepine	Fluvoxamine	Ofloxacin	Triazolam
Carbimazole	Glycopyrrolate	Omeprazole	Venlafaxine
Carboplatin	Griseofulvin	Penicillamine	Zopiclone
Ceftirizine	Hexetidine	Pentamidine	
Cephamandole	Hydrochorothiazide	Pergolide	
Chlormezanone	Hydrocortisone	Propantheline	

Appendix 29.6 Drugs implicated in oral ulceration

Adalimumab	Dideoxycytidine	Losartan	Phenylbutazone
Alendronate	Emepromium	Molgramostim	Phenytoin
Allopurinol	Flunisolide	Naproxen	Potassium chloride
Aurothiomalate	Gold	Nicorandil	Proguanil
Aztreonam	Indometacin	NSAIDs	Sertraline
Captopril	Interferons	Olanzapine	Sulindac
Carbamazepine	Interleukin-2	Pancreatin	Tacrolimus
Clarithromycin	Isoprenaline	Penicillamine	Vancomycin
Diclofenac	Ketorolac	Phenindione	

Appendix 29.7 Drugs implicated in lichenoid reactions

Allopurinol	Ethionamide	Metformin	Procainamide
Amiphenazole	Flunarizine	Methyldopa	Propranolol
Barbiturate	Gaunoclor	Metronidazole	Propylthiouracil
BCG vaccine	Gold	Niridazole	Prothionamide
Captopril	Griseofulvin	Oral contraceptives	Quinidine
Carbamazepine	Hepatitis B vaccine	Oxprenolol	Quinine
Carbimazole	Hydroxychloroquine	Para-aminosalicylate	Rifampicin

(Continued)

Appendix 29.7 Drugs implicated in lichenoid reactions—cont'd

Chloral hydrate	Interferon-alpha	Penicillamine	Rofecoxib
Chloroquine	Ketoconazole	Penicillins	Streptomycin
Chlorpropamide	Labetalol	Phenindione	Tetracycline
Cholera vaccine	Levamisole	Phenothiazines	Tocainide
Cinnarizine	Lincomycin	Phenylbutazone	Tolbutamide
Clofibrate	Lithium	Phenytoin	Triprolidine
Colchicine	Lorazepam	Piroxicam	
Dapsone	Mepacrine	Practolol	
Dipyridamole	Mercury (amalgam)	Prazosin	

Appendix 29.8 Drugs implicated in oral candidosis

Broad-spectrum antimicrobials	Corticosteroids	Drugs causing xerostomia	Immunosuppressives

Appendix 29.9 Drugs implicated in pemphigoid-like reactions

Amoxicillin	Ibuprofen	Penicillin V	Salicylic acid
Azapropazone	Isoniazid	Penicillamine	Sufasalazine
Clonidine	Mefenamic acid	Phenacetin	Sulfonamides
Furosemide	Nadolol	Practolol	

Appendix 29.10 Drugs implicated in pemphigus-like reactions

Ampicillin	Cephalexin	Oxyphenbutazone	Probenecid
Arsenic	Diclofenac	Penicillamine	Procaine penicillin
Benzylpenicillin	Gold	Phenobarbital	Rifampicin
Captopril	Interferon-beta	Phenylbutazone	
Cephadroxil	Interleukin-2	Piroxicam	

Appendix 29.11 Drugs implicated in erythema multiforme (and Stevens–Johnson syndrome and toxic epidermal necrolysis)

Acetylsalicylic acid	Digitalis	Mesterolone	Streptomycin
Allopurinol	Diltiazem	Minoxidil	Sulindac
Amlodipine	Ethambutol	Nifedipine	Sulfasalazine
Arsenic	Ethyl alcohol	Omeprazole	Tenoxicam
Atropine	Fluconazole	Oxyphenbutazone	Tetracyclines
Busulfan	Fluorouracil	Penicillin derivatives	Theophylline
Carbamazepine	Furosemide	Phenolphthalein	Tocainide
Chloral hydrate	Gold	Phenylbutazone	Tolbutamide
Chloramphenicol	Griseofulvin	Phenytoin	Trimethadione
Chlorpropamide	Hydantoin	Piroxicam	Vancomycin
Clindamycin	Hydrochlorothiazide	Progesterone	Verapamil

Appendix 29.11 Drugs implicated in erythema multiforme (and Stevens–Johnson syndrome and toxic epidermal necrolysis)—cont'd

Codeine	Indapamide	Pyrazolone derivatives	Zidovudine
Co-trimoxazole	Measles/mumps/rubella vaccine (MMR)	Quinine	
Diclofenac	Meclofenamic acid	Retinol	
Diflunisal	Mercury	Rifampicin	

Appendix 29.12 Drugs implicated in lupoid reactions

Ethosuximide	Isoniazid	Phenytoin	Sulfonamides
Gold	Methyldopa	Phenothiazines	Tetracyclines
Griseofulvin	Para-aminosalicylate	Procainamide	
Hydralazine	Penicillin	Streptomycin	

Appendix 29.13 Drugs implicated in cheilitis

Actinomycin	Ethyl alcohol	Lithium	Sulfasalazine
Atorvastatin	Etretinate	Menthol	Tetracycline
Busulfan	Gold	Methyldopa	Vitamin A
Clofazimine	Indinavir	Penicillamine	
Clomipramine	Isoniazid	Selegiline	
Cyancobalamin	Isotretinoin	Streptomycin	

Appendix 29.14 Drugs implicated in oral mucosal pigmentation

Adrenocorticotropic hormone (ACTH)	Chlorhexidine	Iron	Phenothiazines
Amodiaquine	Chloroquine	Lead	Quinacrine
Anticonvulsants	Clofazimine	Manganese	Quinidine
Arsenic	Copper	Mepacrine	Silver
Betel	Cyclophosphamide	Methyldopa	Thallium
Bismuth	Doxorubicin	Minocycline	Tin
Bromine	Gold	Oral contraceptives	Vanadium
Busulfan	Heroin	Phenolphthalein	Zidovudine

Appendix 29.15 Drugs implicated in oral mucosal pigmentation; different colours

Blue	Brown (hypermelanosis)	Black	Grey	Green
Amiodarone	Aminophenazone	Amiodiaquine	Amodiaquine	Copper
Antimalarials	Betel nut	Betel nut	Chloroquine	
Bismuth	Bismuth	Bismuth	Fluoxetine	
Mepacrine	Busulfan	Methyldopa	Hydroxychloroquinine	
Minocycline	Clofazimine	Minocycline	Lead	
Phenazopyridine	Contraceptives		Silver	
Quinidine	Cyclophosphamide		Tin/zinc	

(Continued)

Appendix 29.15   Drugs implicated in oral mucosal pigmentation; different colours—cont'd

Blue	Brown (hypermelanosis)	Black	Grey	Green
Silver	Diethylstilbestrol			
Sulfasalazine	Doxorubicin			
	Doxycycline			
	Fluorouracil			
	Heroin			
	Hormone replacement therapy			
	Ketoconazole			
	Menthol			
	Methaqualone			
	Minocycline			
	Phenolphthalein			
	Propranolol			
	Smoking			
	Zidovudine			

Appendix 29.16   Drugs implicated in gingival swelling

Drugs most commonly implicated	Drugs occasionally implicated	
Amlodipine	Basiliximab	Mephenytoin
Ciclosporin	Co-trimoxazole	Nitrendipine
Diltiazem	Erythromycin	Norethisterone + mestranol
Felodipine	Diphenoxylate	Phenobarbital
Lacidipine	Ethosuximide	Primidone
Nifedipine	Interferon-alpha	Sertraline
Oral contraceptives	Ketoconazole	Topiramate
Phenytoin	Lamotrigine	Valproate
Verapamil	Lithium	Vigabatrin

Appendix 29.17   Drugs implicated in angioedema

ACE inhibitors	Disulfite sodium	Ketoconazole	Penicillin derivatives
Asparaginase	Droperidol	Mianserin	Pyrazolone derivatives
Carbamazepine	Enalapril	Miconazole	Quinine
Clindamycin	Epoetin-alpha	Naproxen	Streptomycin
Clonidine	Ibruprofen	Nitrofurantoin	Sulfonamides
Co-trimoxazole	Indometacin	Penicillamine	Thiouracil

Appendix 29.18 Drugs implicated in trigeminal paraesthesia or hypoaesthesia

Acetazolamide	Interferon-alpha	Nitrofurantoin	Streptomycin
Amitryptiline	Isoniazid	Pentamidine	Sulfonylureas
Articaine	Labetalol	Phenytoin	Sultiame
Chlorpropamide	Mefloquine	Prilocaine	Tolbutamide
Colistin	Methysergide	Propofol	Tricyclics
Ergotamine	Monoamine oxidase inhibitors	Propranolol	Trilostane
Gonadotropin-releasing hormone analogues	Nalidixic acid	Prothionamide	Vincristine
Hydralazine	Nicotinic acid	Stilbamidine	Streptomycin

Appendix 29.19 Drugs implicated in involuntary facial movements

Carbamazepine	Methyldopa	Phenytoin
L-Dopa	Metoclopramide	Tetrabenazine
Lithium	Metirosine	Trifluoroperazine

Appendix 29.20 Drugs implicated in halitosis

Dimethyl sulfoxide (DMSO)	Disulfiram	Isorbide dinitrate

Appendix 29.21 Drugs implicated in orofacial pain

Benztropine	Penicillins	Vinca alkaloids
Biperidin	Phenothiazines	Vitamin A
Griseofulvin	Stilbamidine	
Lithium	Ticarcillin	

Appendix 29.22 Drugs implicated in tooth discolouration

Antibiotics	Fosinopril	Pentamidine	Terbinafine
Clarithromycin	Imipenem	Perindopril	Tetracyclines
Enalapril	Lisinopril	Propafenone	Trandolapril
Essential oil	Metronidazole	Quinapril	Zopiclone
Etidronate	Penicillin	Ramipril	

This chapter focuses mainly on medical issues related to ethnic and cultural groups, homeless people, immigrants, people in custodial institutions, Roma and socioeconomically deprived people.

ETHNIC AND CULTURAL GROUPS

This section tabulates some of the main aspects (Table 30.1).

Population mobility increases inexorably, leading to enormous changes in the structure of many populations across the world. This is especially evident in the developed world. For example, the proportion of the UK population born outside Europe has reached 10% overall, with regional variations from, for example, 3% in the far south-west to 30% in east London. Ongoing expansion of the European Union has produced major changes.

It is difficult to characterize all the different faiths and cultures, since differences exist according to social class, background, ethnicity, and other factors, but Table 30.2 attempts to highlight some relevant aspects.

Communication is crucial between dental professionals and patients from different faiths, cultures and countries. Professional interpreters may therefore be required.

HOMELESS PEOPLE

Homeless people, and those who live in poor accommodation, tend to have more illness, mainly due to exposure, inadequate diet, inadequate hygiene, stress, violence, accidents and exposure to communicable diseases and drug abuse. Mental health problems, including psychotic illness, depression and anxiety, alcohol addiction or injecting drug use are common. There are high rates of blood-borne and other infections, such as hepatitis B and C, and human immunodeficiency (HIV), all of which can be associated mainly with drug use and neglect of health TB is common (Ch. 15). Most report negative oral health impacts: most have caries and inflammatory periodontal disease and over half have current orofacial pain. Additional oral health

Table 30.1   Ethnic and cultural groups: languages, religions, habits and medical aspects (Adapted with permission from Scully C, Wilson N. Culturally sensitive oral health care. Quintessence, London, 2006)

Ethnic group	Main language(s)	Main religion(s)	Diet, habits and medical aspects
Albanians (Kosovars)	Albanian	Islam Christianity	Alcohol use and smoking endemic, and younger generation uses narcotics at an increasing rate
Afro-Caribbeans	English French Spanish	Christianity	Seventh Day Adventists consume no pork, tea or coffee or alcohol. Rastafarians often use marijuana, but may be vegan or eat no pork. Crack and cocaine use common in Jamaicans
Arabs	Arabic	Islam	See Table 30.
Armenians	Armenian	Christianity	–
Bangladeshi	Bengali, Urdu	Islam	Healthy diet, dislike oral medication. Females prefer female health care workers. Often smoke or use paan
Bosnian	Serbo-Croat	Islam	Healthy diet, dislike oral medication and females prefer female health care workers
Cambodian	Khmer	Buddhist	Traditional medicine may be preferred
Chinese	Cantonese	Taoism Confucianism Buddhism	Traditional Chinese medicine may be used. Doctor-shopping common. Often eat rice diet and smoke heavily May not like venepuncture
Eritreans	Tigrinya, Arabic	Christianity Islam	Coptic Christians do not consume meat or dairy products for more than half of each year
Ethiopians	Amharic	Christianity Islam	Coptic Christians do not consume meat or dairy products for more than half of each year
Ghanaian	Twi	Islam Christianity	Traditional medicine may be used
Greeks	Greek	Christianity	Healthy diet High tobacco use

Table 30.1 Ethnic and cultural groups: languages, religions, habits and medical aspects (Adapted with permission from Scully C, Wilson N. Culturally sensitive oral health care. Quintessence, London, 2006)—cont'd

Ethnic group	Main language(s)	Main religion(s)	Diet, habits and medical aspects
Gujaratis	Gujarati	Hindu	Often eat no meat, eggs or fish
Indian	Hindi, Punjabi, English	Hindu (mainly) Islam Christianity Sikhism Zoroastrianism	Traditional medicine (Ayruvedic) Often vegetarian or vegan High tobacco and betel use Rarely, vitamin B_{12} deficient from veganism
Iranian	Farsi	Islam	–
Iraqi	Arabic	Islam	–
Irish	English	Christianity	May be high alcohol intake
Japanese	Japanese	Buddhism Shintoism	Diet often of rice, raw fish and eggs
Koreans	Korean (Han-gul)	Confucianism Shamanism Taoism Buddhism	Traditional medicine commonly used. Be aware of communication styles and patterns, such as no eye contact, smiling at inopportune times represents lack of respect and intelligence
Kurds (a diverse ethnic group from Kurdistan, encompassing parts of Turkey, Iran, Iraq, Syria)	Kurdish	Islam	–
Laotians	Laotian	Buddhism	–
Latin Americans	Spanish Portuguese	Christianity	–
Liberians	English		Traditional medicine may be used
Nigerians	Four peoples/languages: Hausa, Yoruba, Ibo and Fulani	Islam Christianity	Traditional medicine may be used
Pakistanis	Punjabi	Islam	See Table 30.2
Portuguese	Portuguese	Christianity	High tobacco use
Somalis	Somali Arabic	Islam	May have qat habit
South Africans (whites)	English Afrikaans	Christianity	–
Soviet Union	Russian	Christianity	–
Sudanese	Arabic English	Islam Christianity	Traditional medicine may be used
Tamils	Tamil	Hindu	Vegetarian
Tibetans	Tibetan Chinese	Buddhism	Ayurvedic tradition
Turks	Turkish	Islam	See Table 30.2
Vietnamese	Vietnamese Cantonese	Buddhism Christianity	Vegetarian

impacts include eating, smiling, concentrating and talking. Dental anxiety status is related to dental disease experience, which impacts negatively on quality of life. Various studies have confirmed that few had dental care in the previous year.

The problems, summarized in Table 30.3, serve to perpetuate the homelessness and impede access to health care. There is a need to provide more accessible and affordable health services to homeless people.

IMMIGRANTS

Immigrants and refugees can arrive from diverse social, economic, educational, cultural, religious and ethnic backgrounds for a variety of reasons: for work, education or economic advantage, or fleeing war, political upheaval or persecution, or joining families from which they have been separated. Many arrive with inadequate resources and suffer social exclusion and inequality of health care provision. The acute phase following

Table 30.2 Main faiths/religions and their medical relevance[a] (see also Table 30.1)

Faith/religion	Main festival or religious occasion(s)	Dietary aspects	Possible main medical problems	Other comments
Buddhism	Wesak	Often vegetarian	–	–
Jehovah's Witnesses	Christmas, Easter	–	Jehovah's Witnesses firmly believe that blood has sacred meaning, and that it should not be removed from the body and stored, nor should donor blood be taken in during a transfusion. They often refuse blood transfusions and organ transplants, and human blood products like platelets (Ch.8)	Jehovah's Witness Watchtower Society biblical ban on the storage/use of animal blood, but the Watchtower Society has ruled that Hemopure, a highly purified haemoglobin solution made by Biopure Corporation from fractionated bovine (cow) blood (http://www.biopure.com) can be used by Jehovah's Witnesses (Appendix 30.1)
Hinduism	Diwali, Mahashivaratri, Ram Navami, Janmastami	Often eat no meat (particularly beef) or meat products, eggs or fish Some drink no tea, coffee or alcohol, and eat no garlic or onions	Vitamin B_{12} deficient from veganism	–
Islam (Muslim)	Ramadan, Mawlid, al-Nabi	Eat no pork, drink no alcohol. Eat only Halal meat. During Ramadan, between sunrise and sunset, eat and drink nothing (including water), and smoke nothing, unless ill, young, old or pregnant	May be non-compliant with oral medication during fasts such as Ramadan. Alcohol-free oral products should be used. Meningitis vaccination indicated at Hajj and Umra	Often cover much of the body and head/face. Right hand is considered clean, and used for eating and handshaking. Handshakes are appropriate only between men or between women. It is not acceptable for a man to shake the hand of a Shiite woman Women not permitted to be alone with a man who is not her husband or relative. At public events, women are segregated from men
Judaism	Rosh Hashanah, Yom Kippur, Pesach	Eat no pork or shellfish, and only kosher meat Fast for 25h from eve of Yom Kippur	Orthodox Jews may refuse organ transplants. Liable to Tay–Sachs disease (inherited neurological defects), Canavan disease (inherited brain disorder), Fanconi anaemia, pemphigus	No work on Sabbath (Saturday)
Sikhism	Vaisakhi, Diwali, Hola	Eat no fish or eggs, usually no beef or pork Often vegetarian	Vitamin B_{12} deficient from veganism	Invariably cover head

[a] It is impossible to generalize: always consider the individual and their wishes and needs.
The reader is referred elsewhere for detail: Scully C, Wilson N. Culturally sensitive oral healthcare. Quintessence, London, 2006.

immigration, particularly from the developing world, war zones and tropical regions, attracts most concern (Table 30.4), and is particularly when health can be neglected.

Many come from health care systems that differ from traditional Western medicine, and may involve traditional remedies. Lifestyle factors predispose some to specific diseases (e.g. areca nut use and oral submucous fibrosis). Hereditary factors are sometimes also important, as in sickle cell disease, thalassaemia and glucose-6-phosphate dehydrogenase deficiency.

Other problems may include malnutrition, intestinal parasites (*Enterobius, Trichuris, Strongyloides* and *Ascaris*), filariasis, leishmaniasis, hepatitis A, B and C, tuberculosis, low immunization rate, typhoid fever, yellow fever, malaria, trachoma, syphilis, dengue fever, HIV infection, diarrhoeal illnesses,

leprosy, hypertension, coronary disease, gastrointestinal problems, diabetes, depression, lactose intolerance, carcinomas of cervix, breast and mouth, vitamin D deficiency, alcoholism and substance abuse.

The second phase, transition, typically takes at least 5 years, with acculturation and modification of social norms, attitudes, values, behaviours and diet, bringing changes not least in the use of health care services. Most younger people become well integrated into the community.

The third phase, 10 or more years after arrival, is typified by the resettled refugee suffering a variety of chronic conditions seen at least partly as a consequence of resettlement, but many have acculturated and others continue to live and often work in their own communities, in a multicultural society.

Table 30.3 Medical problems prevalent in homeless people[a]

Assaults	Physical
	Psychological
	Sexual
Cardiovascular	Hypertension
	Peripheral vascular disease
Exposure	Hypothermia
Gastrointestinal	Vomiting and diarrhoea
Infections	Infestations (lice, fleas, scabies)
	Lower respiratory infections, such as influenza, pneumonia, tuberculosis
	Sexually transmitted infections
	Upper respiratory viral infections
	Viral hepatitis
Mental	Depression
	Schizophrenia
	Stress, anxiety, substance abuse
Nutritional	Malnutrition
Substance abuse	Alcohol
	Illegal drugs and volatile substance abuse
	Tobacco

[a] Often multiple or complex problems, over and above the problems afflicting others, and poor access to health care services.

PEOPLE IN CUSTODIAL CARE

Prisoners' general health is compromised by lifestyle behaviours such as the use of tobacco, alcohol and drugs of abuse, high sugar diets and homosexual practices. In particular, there are high levels of violence, mental illness and infectious disease, such as hepatitis virus infections and HIV. Prisoners' oral health status often includes high levels of caries and relatively low levels of both missing and filled teeth, and the oral health is poor and also poor in comparison with non-institutionalized individuals where appropriate comparisons have been made.

The main barriers to health care are cost, anxiety and access.

ROMA

Roma is the preferred term (or Romanies) for people commonly but incorrectly known as gypsies. Most Roma refer to themselves as *rom* or *rrom*. Worldwide there is an estimated population of at least 15 million Roma but many are not registered for fear of discrimination. Most Roma are from east Europe (Romania, Bosnia, Bulgaria, Kosovo and Slovakia) or America. 'New age travellers' are *not* Roma.

Roma are generally a nomadic people with an alternative lifestyle and refusal to conform, and they speak Romani – derived primarily from Sanskrit. There is not a separate Romani religion; they traditionally adopt the dominant religion of the country in which they live, and are usually Hindu, Christian, Protestant or Muslim (Sufism).

Traditional Roma place a high value on the extended family. At the top of the family is the oldest man or grandfather, and men generally have much more authority than women. Virginity is essential in unmarried women, and both women and men tend to marry young; there may even be child marriage.

Roma often suffer from unemployment, socioeconomic deprivation and discrimination, are frequently accused of petty crime, and can find barriers to education. Dietary habits include high fat and salt content in foods and a large percentage of Roma smoke and are obese. These factors can put Roma at increased risk for hypertension, diabetes, occlusive vascular disease, strokes and myocardial infarction. Crowded living conditions can lead to an increase incidence of gastrointestinal infections and respiratory infections. Nutritional deficits, hepatitis B, tuberculosis and post-traumatic stress disorder may be increased in Roma populations. Social (or societal) isolation also leads to an increase in consanguineous marriages, and thus an increased risk for birth defects.

In the health care setting, only the elder males of some groups are likely to communicate with health care personnel. Women are not permitted to interrupt men or to be alone with a man who is not her husband or relative. Washing hands after touching the lower body before touching the upper body is required. Separate soap and towels are used on the upper

Table 30.4 The phases of acculturation (Scully C, Wilson N. Culturally sensitive oral healthcare. Quintessence, London, 2006)

Phase	Possible medical and social problems	Barriers to care	Possible outcomes
Acute	Communicable illnesses (TB, HBV, HIV) and tropical diseases, malnutrition, trauma, conflict intergenerationally and with other cultures, domestic violence, gambling and substance abuse	Lack of language fluency and understanding of health care system	Linguistic and cultural isolation. Help-seeking behaviour becomes one of emergency care only
Transition	Hypertension, diabetes, psychological disorders and other post-traumatic stress	Lack of language fluency and understanding of health care system by older generation	Younger generations integrate into host health care system; continued isolation of older generations
Integration	Hypertension, coronary heart disease and diabetes are the most common disorders. Morbidity and mortality from cancers, particularly cervical, are high	Emotional difficulties as family structures break down	Intergenerational conflicts can arise, and there can be heavy alcohol consumption

HBV, hepatitis B virus; HIV, human immunodeficiency virus; TB, tuberculosis.

and lower parts of the body and they must not be allowed to mix. When a clan member must enter a hospital, family members are expected to remain with that person day and night to watch over, protect, and perform caring and curing rituals. Roma are especially fearful of any surgical procedure that requires general anaesthesia (GA) because of their belief that a person under GA undergoes a 'little death'. For the family to gather around the person recovering from GA is especially important.

SOCIOECONOMICALLY DEPRIVED PEOPLE

Socioeconomic status is considered to be a major social basis for inequalities and an important predictor of health at all ages. Socioeconomic deprivation appears to predispose to a wide range of health issues, from disease, to access to provision of and outcomes of health care. Examples are shown in Box 30.1.

Socioeconomically disadvantaged men and women have higher overall mortality rates than persons with a higher socioeconomic status. Moreover, relationships between class and mortality are consistent for almost every cause of death, with only a few exceptions, notably certain cancers. In almost all countries, the rates of death due to common causes (e.g. cardiovascular disease and cancer), causes related to smoking, causes related to alcohol use, and causes amenable to medical intervention (e.g. tuberculosis and hypertension) and poorer self-assessments of health are substantially higher in groups of lower socioeconomic status.

Socioeconomic factors also influence oral health in terms of, for example, hygiene practices, diet, gingivitis and dental caries. Attending a state school, being female and having parents with low educational attainment were identified as risk factors both for having dental caries and for having a high level of caries. Lack of oral health care may lead to periapical abscesses, and other odontogenic infections, which have caused morbidity and even mortality.

Such inequalities in health care might be reduced by improving educational opportunities, income distribution, health-related behaviour and access to health care. Policies related to preventive social, economic and behavioural interventions in areas such as poverty and income, education, unemployment, housing, transportation, the environment (including pollution) and nutrition may well have a much greater effect on reducing health disparities than would traditional medical interventions.

USEFUL WEBSITES

http://www.who.int/topis/social-environment/en
http://www.ic.nhs.uk/news-and-media/press-releases/april-2005–march-2006/health-of-ethnic-minorities
http://www.kingsfund.org.uk/health_topics/black_and.html
http://www.nrcemh.nhsscotland.com/

FURTHER READING

Acheson, D., Barkers, D., Chambers, J., Graham, H., Marmot, M., Whitehead, M., 1998. Independent inquiry into inequalities in health report. Stationery Office, London.

Allard, S.W., Tolman, R.M., Rosen, D., 2003. Proximity to service providers and service utilization among welfare recipients: the interaction of place and race. J Policy Anal Manage 22, 599–613.

Berkman, L.F., Kawachi, I., 2000. Social epidemiology. Oxford University Press, New York.

Berkman, L., Epstein, A.M., 2008. Beyond health care – socioeconomic status and health. N Engl J Med 358, 2509–2510.

Bezrucha, S., 2005. Review of: The status syndrome: how social standing affects our health and longevity. N Engl J Med 352, 1159–1160.

Bolin, K.A., 2006. Survey of community, migrant, and homeless health center dentists in Texas. Tex Dent J 123, 12–20.

British Dental Association, 2003. Dental care for homeless people. BDA, London.

Bunt, G.R. (Ed.), 2005. Faith guides for higher education. Higher Education Authority, The Centre for Philosophical and Religious Studies, Leeds.

Bussey-Jones, J., Genao, I., 2003. Impact of culture on health care. J Natl Med Assoc 95, 732–735.

Ciaranello, A.L., Molitor, F., Leamon, M., et al., 2006. Providing health care services to the formerly homeless: a quasi-experimental evaluation. J Health Care Poor Underserved 17, 441–461.

Cohen, D.A., Farley, T.A., Mason, K., 2003. Why is poverty unhealthy? Social and physical mediators. Soc Sci Med 57, 1631–1641.

Collins, J., Freeman, R., 2007. Homeless in North and West Belfast: an oral health needs assessment. Br Dent J 202, E31. [Epub ahead of print].

Conte, M., Broder, H.L., Jenkins, G., Reed, R., Janal, M.N., 2006. Oral health, related behaviors and oral health impacts among homeless adults. J Public Health Dent 66, 276–278.

Conway, D.I., McMahon, A.D., Smith, K., Taylor, J.C., McKinney, P.A., 2008. Socioeconomic factors influence selection and participation in a population-based case-control study of head and neck cancer in Scotland. J Clin Epidemiol 61, 1187–1193.

Cortellazzi, K.L., Pereira, S.M., Tagliaferro, E.P., et al., 2008. Risk indicators of gingivitis in 5-year-old Brazilian children. Oral Health Prev Dent 6, 131–137.

De Palma, P., Frithiof, L., Persson, L., Klinge, B., Halldin, J., Beijer, U., 2005. Oral health of homeless adults in Stockholm, Sweden. Acta Odontol Scand 63, 50–55.

De Palma, P., Nordenram, G., 2005. The perceptions of homeless people in Stockholm concerning oral health and consequences of dental treatment: a qualitative study. Spec Care Dent 25, 289–295.

Demakakos, P., Nazroo, J., Breeze, E., Marmot, M., 2008. Socioeconomic status and health: the role of subjective social status. Soc Sci Med 67, 330–340.

Department of Health, 2003. Strategy for modernizing dental services for prisoners in England. Department of Health, London.

Díaz-Cruz, A.A., 2006. Dental assistant apprenticeship program within the U.S. Disciplinary Barracks. Dent Assist 75, 28–29.

Box 30.1 Some health areas more prevalent in lower socioeconomic groups

- Arthritis
- Asthma
- Cancer
- Coronary heart disease, and death from first infarcts
- Height
- Obesity
- Oral health
- Mental health problems
- Physical health problems
- Psychiatric referral, admission rates and length of stay
- Surgical outcomes
- Uptake of blood pressure and medical checks

Dogan, M.C., Haytac, M.C., Ozali, O., Seydaoglu, G., Yoldas, O., Oztunc, H., 2006. The oral health status of street children in Adana, Turkey. Int Dent J 56, 92–96.

Epstein, A.M., 2004. Health care in America – still too separate, not yet equal. N Engl J Med 351, 603–605.

Fan, J., Hser, Y.I., Herbeck, D., 2006. Tooth retention, tooth loss and use of dental care among long-term narcotics abusers. Subst Abus 27, 25–32.

Gibson, G., Reifenstahl, E.F., Wehler, C.J., et al., 2008. Dental treatment improves self-rated oral health in homeless veterans – a brief communication. J Public Health Dent 68, 111–115.

Haugejorden, O., Klock, K.S., Astrøm, A.N., Skaret, E., Trovik, T.A., 2008. Socio-economic inequality in the self-reported number of natural teeth among Norwegian adults – an analytical study. Community Dent Oral Epidemiol 36, 269–278.

Heidari, E., Dickinson, C., Fiske, J., 2008. An investigation into the oral health status of male prisoners in the UK. J Disabil Oral Health 9, 3–12.

Hunter, D.J., Richards, T., 2008. Health and wealth in Europe. BMJ 336, 1390.

Irwin, A., Valentine, N., Brown, C., et al., 2006. The Commission on Social Determinants of Health: tackling the social roots of health inequities. PLoS Med 3, e106–e106.

Kahabuka, F.K., Mbawalla, H.S., 2006. Oral health knowledge and practices among Dar es Salaam institutionalized former street children aged 7–16 years. Int J Dent Hyg 4, 174–178.

Kanli, A., Kanbur, N.O., Dural, S., Derman, O., 2008. Effects of oral health behaviors and socioeconomic factors on a group of Turkish adolescents. Quintessence Int 39, e26–e32.

King, T.B., Gibson, G., 2003. Oral health needs and access to dental care of homeless adults in the United States: a review. Spec Care Dent 23, 143–147.

King, T.B., Muzzin, K.B., 2005. A national survey of dental hygienists' infection control attitudes and practices. J Dent Hyg 79 (2), 8.

Kuthy, R.A., McQuistan, M.R., Riniker, K.J., Heller, K.E., Qian, F., 2005. Students' comfort level in treating vulnerable populations and future willingness to treat: results prior to extramural participation. J Dent Educ 69, 1307–1314.

Lang, I.A., Gibbs, S.J., Steel, N., Melzer, D., 2008. Neighbourhood deprivation and dental service use: a cross-sectional analysis of older people in England. J Public Health (Oxf) 30 (4), 472–478.

Lee, J.W., 2005. Public health is a social issue. Lancet 365, 1005–1006.

London Health Commission, 2007. Health in London; looking back, looking forward. London Health Commission, London.

Lunn, H., Morris, J., Jacob, A., Grummitt, C., 2003. The oral health of a group of prison inmates. Dent Update 30, 135–138.

Luo, Y., McGrath, C., 2006. Oral health status of homeless people in Hong Kong. Spec Care Dent 26, 150–154.

Mackenbach, J.P., Stirbu, I., Roskam, A.J., et al.; European Union Working Group on Socioeconomic Inequalities in Health, 2008. Socioeconomic inequalities in health in 22 European countries. N Engl J Med 358, 2468–2481.

Mautino, K.S., 2003. Immigration and ancillary health care providers. J Immigr Health 5, 45–47.

McGinnis, J.M., Williams-Russo, P., Knickman, J.R., 2002. The case for more active policy attention to health promotion. Health Aff (Millwood) 21, 78–93.

Mello, T., Antunes, J., Waldman, E., Ramos, E., Relvas, M., Barros, H., 2008. Prevalence and severity of dental caries in schoolchildren of Porto, Portugal. Community Dent Health 25, 119–125.

Nahouraii, H., Wasserman, M., Bender, D.E., Rozier, R.G., 2008. Social support and dental utilization among children of Latina immigrants. J Health Care Poor Underserved 19, 428–441.

Namal, N., Can, G., Vehid, S., Koksal, S., Kaypmaz, A., 2008. Dental health status and risk factors for dental caries in adults in Istanbul, Turkey. East Mediterr Health J 14, 110–118.

Palinkas, L.A., Pickwell, S.M., Brandstein, K., et al., 2003. The journey to wellness: stages of refugee health promotion and disease prevention. J Immigr Health 5, 19–28.

Pikhart, H., Bobak, M., Malyutina, S., Pajak, A., Kubínová, R., Marmot, M., 2007. Obesity and education in three countries of the Central and Eastern Europe: the HAPIEE study. Cent Eur J Public Health 15, 140–142.

Raimer, B.G., Stobo, J.D., 2004. Health care delivery in the Texas prison system: the role of academic medicine. JAMA 292, 485–489.

Reifel, N., 2005. Federal role in dental public health: dental care for special populations. J Calif Dent Assoc 33, 553–557.

Sabbah, W., Tsakos, G., Chandola, T., Sheiham, A., Watt, R.G., 2007. Social gradients in oral and general health. J Dent Res 86, 992–996.

Sabbah, W., Watt, R.G., Sheiham, A., Tsakos, G., 2008. Effects of allostatic load on the social gradient in ischaemic heart disease and periodontal disease: evidence from the Third National Health and Nutrition Examination Survey. J Epidemiol Community Health 62, 415–420.

Scully, C., 2001. Oral piercing in adolescents. CPD Dentistry 2, 79–81.

Scully, C., Wilson, N., 2006. Culturally sensitive oral healthcare. Quintessence, London.

Thomas, S.J., Atkinson, C., Hughes, C., Revington, P., Ness, A.R., 2008. Is there an epidemic of admissions for surgical treatment of dental abscesses in the UK?. BMJ 336, 1219–1220.

Vallejos-Sánchez, A.A., Medina-Solís, C.E., Maupomé, G., et al., 2008. Sociobehavioral factors influencing toothbrushing frequency among schoolchildren. J Am Dent Assoc 139, 743–749.

Walsh, T., Tickle, M., Milsom, K., Buchanan, K., Zoitopoulos, L., 2008. An investigation of the nature of research into dental health in prisons: a systematic review. Br Dent J 204, 683–689, discussion 667.

Webb, E., Kuh, D., Peasey, A., et al., 2008. Childhood socioeconomic circumstances and adult height and leg length in central and eastern Europe. J Epidemiol Community Health 62, 351–357.

Wilmoth, J.M., Chen, P.C., 2003. Immigrant status, living arrangements, and depressive symptoms among middle-aged and older adults. J Gerontol B Psychol Sci Soc Sci 58, S305–S313.

Appendix 30.1   Acceptable alternatives products suitable for Jehovah's Witnesses (Adapted with permission from http://www.ajwrb.org

Blood-oxygen monitoring devices

Transcutaneous pulse oximeter
Paediatric ultra-microsampling equipment
Multiple tests per blood draw

Haematopoietic agents

Intravenous iron
Folic acid
Vitamin B$_{12}$
Vitamin C
Granulocyte colony-stimulating factor
Interleukin-11
Recombinant stem-cell factor

Operative and anaesthetic techniques

Hypotensive anaesthesia
Induced hypothermia
Mechanical occlusion of bleeding vessel

Haemostatic agents

Avitene
Gelfoam
Oxygel
Surgicel
Desmopressin (DDAVP)
Epsilon-aminocaproic acid (Amicar)
Tranexamic acid (Cyklokapron)
Vasopressin (Pitressin)
Aprotinin (Trasylol)
Vincristine (Oncovin)
Conjugated oestrogens
Vitamin K
Recombinant factor VIIa
Recombinant factor IX

Volume expanders: crystalloids

Ringer's lactate
Saline

Volume expanders: colloids

Dextran
Gelatin
Hetastarch
Pentastarch

Oxygen therapy

Hyberbaric oxygen therapy
Perfluorocarbon solutions

Surgical devices and techniques

Electrocautery
Ligature vessel

Personal decisions

Medical products and therapy

Albumin
Any drug buffered with albumin
Immune globulins
Natural clotting factors
Cryoprecipitate
Plasma protein fractions
Tissue adhesives
Natural interferons
Haemoglobin-based blood substitutes
Platelet-derived wound healing factors

Medical tests

Red or white blood cell tagging

Surgical procedures

Dialysis and heart–lung equipment
Blood salvage without blood storage

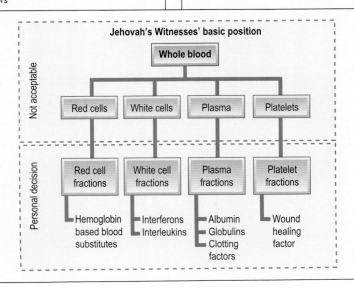

This chapter discusses the health of dental staff but some occupations, especially the construction industry, are especially dangerous, far more so than the health care professions.

HEALTH OF DENTAL STAFF

The main causes of death among dentists in Britain, USA and other industrialized countries are cardiovascular disease, cancer and suicides, as in non-dental groups of similar socioeconomic status. The standardized mortality ratio (SMR) – the ratio of observed deaths in an occupation or from any disease to the national average death rate for the same age and sex – however, is lower in dentists than in the general population. The risks in male dentists from liver cirrhosis and suicide are somewhat higher than in the general population, and dentists are also a risk group for malignant melanoma – presumably a consequence of sun exposure on vacations. Dentists, however, have a lower SMR for cancers, ischaemic heart disease, cerebrovascular disease and chronic lung diseases (bronchitis, emphysema and asthma).

Infections and physical, chemical and radiation hazards are the main occupational problems in dentistry. There are also risks from accidents and damage to eyes, hearing, mental health, the musculoskeletal system, the fetus in pregnancy, respiratory systems and the skin (Table 31.1).

In the UK, governmental concern and the defining of safe work practices and measures for implementing them by the Health and Safety at Work etc. Act (1974) and Regulations, such as the Ionizing Radiations Regulations (1988) and Control of Substances Hazardous to Health Regulations (1988), have brought the matter of occupational hazards in dentistry into sharper focus.

Table 31.1 Occupational hazards in dentistry

Infections	Bacteria	Legionellosis Syphilis Tuberculosis
	Viruses	Common cold and other respiratory viruses Hand, foot and mouth disease Hepatitis viruses Herpangina Herpesviruses HIV/AIDS and other retroviruses Human papilloma virus Parvovirus
	Prions	
Physical and chemical	Accidents and assaults	
	Burns (chemical heat/cold/radiation)	
	Chemical sterilizers	
	Disinfectants	
	Electrical accidents	
	Fires and explosions	
	Flammable or explosive agents	
	Formaldehyde	
	Inhalational anaesthetic agents	
	Mercury	
	Minerals	
	Non-anaesthetic agents	
	Poisons	
	'Sick building syndrome'	
	Solvents	
	Vibration injury	
	X-ray processing chemicals	

(Continued)

Table 31.1 Occupational hazards in dentistry—cont'd		
Radiation	Ionizing radiation	X-rays
	Non-ionizing radiation	Electromagnetic radiation Light (ultraviolet, blue, white) Lasers
	Video display units (VDUs or monitors)	
	Pacemaker cardioverter and hearing aid interference	
To specific body systems	Eyes	
	Hearing	
	Mental health	Reaction of staff to stress Adapting to stress
	Musculoskeletal complaints	
	Pregnancy	General anaesthetic agents Mercury Ionizing radiation Infectious agents
	Respiratory system	
	Skin	
Other systems	Bone marrow Brain Cardiovascular system Gastrointestinal tract Kidneys Liver	

HIV/AIDS, human immunodeficiency virus/acquired immune deficiency syndrome.

INFECTIONS (SEE ALSO CH. 21)

Overall, the major infectious hazards are respiratory and hepatitis B and C infections and, to a very much lesser extent, human immunodeficiency virus (HIV), prions and health care-associated infections (HCAI) such as meticillin-resistant *Staphylococcus aureus*, *Clostridium difficile*, *TB* and *Legionella*. Blood, serum and saliva are the sources most likely to transmit serious infection and dental instruments (and bites) are often contaminated with all these body fluids. Since there is a potential for transmission of various infections, where at all possible dental equipment should be single-use and all reusable instruments must be sterilized or at least decontaminated (Fig. 31.1). Dental staff should pay considerable attention to avoidance of needlestick (percutaneous inoculation; sharps) infections/injuries and bites.

Standard (universal) infection control must be implemented; infection control guidelines can be found at http://www.udp.org.uk/resources/bda-cross-infection.pdf.

The main points to minimize cross-infection are shown in Box 31.1.

NEEDLESTICK/OCCUPATIONAL EXPOSURE TO INFECTIONS

Exposure-prone procedures (EPPs) are defined by the UK Department of Health as those where there is a risk that injury to the worker may result in exposure of the patient's open tissues to the blood of the worker. These procedures include

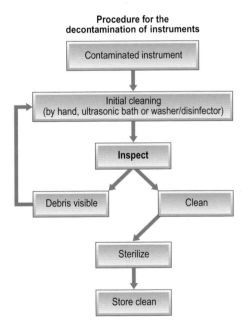

Procedure for the decontamination of instruments

Contaminated instrument → Initial cleaning (by hand, ultrasonic bath or washer/disinfector) → **Inspect** → Debris visible / Clean → Sterilize → Store clean

Fig. 31.1 Instrument decontamination

those where the worker's gloved hands may be in contact with sharp instruments, needle tips or sharp tissues (spicules of bone or teeth) inside a patient's open body cavity, wound or confined anatomical space where the hands or fingertips may not be completely visible at all times.

The majority of procedures in dentistry are defined as exposure prone, with the exception of:

- examination using a mouth mirror only
- taking extra-oral radiographs
- visual and digital examination of the head and neck
- visual and digital examination of the edentulous mouth
- taking impressions of edentulous patients
- the construction and fitting of full dentures.

However, taking impressions from dentate or partially dentate patients would be considered exposure prone, as would the fitting of partial dentures and fixed or removable orthodontic appliances, where clasps and other pieces of metal could result in injury to the dentist.

Health care workers need not refrain from performing EPPs pending follow-up of occupational exposure to an HIV-infected source. The combined risks of contracting HIV infection from the source patient and then transmitting this to another patient during an EPP are so low as to be considered negligible. However, in the event of the worker being diagnosed HIV-positive, such procedures must cease in accordance with this guidance. (From http://www.dh.gov.uk/en/Publicationsandstatistics/Publications/PublicationsPolicyAndGuidance/Browsable/DH_5368137.)

The four UK Health Departments decontamination policies are generally driven by the EU Medical Devices Directive (MDD) 93/42/EEC and the Medical Device Regulations (MDR) 2005 (Box 31.2).

British Dental Association (BDA) Advice Sheet *A12 Infection control in dentistry*, which was often used for guidance, has been superseded by a document, often referred to as 'HTM 01-05', published by the UK Department of Health in 2008 as 'Health Technical Memorandum 01-05: Decontamination in primary care dental practices' and superseded by a new edition published in April 2009. (See http://www.dh.gov.uk/en/Publicationsandstatistics/Publications/PublicationsPolicyAndGuidance/DH_089245.)

Disinfection after cleaning reduces the number of viable micro-organisms on instruments, making them safer to handle.

It is not acceptable to use chemical disinfectants to disinfect instruments (unless this is specifically recommended by the manufacturer) and therefore thermal disinfection is necessary.

Thermal disinfection can be achieved by using an automated washer–disinfector (WD). Two types of sterilizer are found in general dental practice: the *vacuum benchtop sterilizer Type B* is suitable for wrapped and unwrapped solid items, hollow items and porous loads, and as such is particularly suitable for sterilizing dental handpieces. It is the standard for use in dental practice, since wrapped items can be readily transported, remain sterile up to point of use, and can be stored for use at a later date, minimizing the risk of cross-contamination. The *Type N benchtop sterilizer* is the other type – an unwrapped instrument and utensil sterilizer suitable for solid devices that are not wrapped.

Provided that the proper irrigation and cleaning of lumens and internals of handpieces has been achieved in combination with a WD, handpieces may also be processed in a Type N sterilizer. Where remaining hollow items used in the practice are single-use, a Type N sterilizer may be the appropriate solution, although this type of technology is being increasingly overtaken by the vacuum-type sterilizer (Type B). Instruments processed in a Type N sterilizer should ideally be used directly from the sterilizer as transportation and storage of sterilized items may pose a risk of re-contamination, and should be risk assessed and controlled to minimize the risk.

Some instruments cannot be steam sterilized and must then be decontaminated according to the manufacturer's instructions. If sending instruments for repair or disposal, ensure they are decontaminated first.

Health care facilities, particularly hospitals, are also well recognized reservoirs of infection and may be responsible for a wide range of nosocomial (hospital) infections such as meticillin-resistant *Staphylococcus aureus* (MRSA), etc. (Ch. 21). *Legionella* is ubiquitous in dental unit water supplies (Ch. 15);

strategies to reduce the level of bacterial contamination in dental unit water are shown in Box 31.3.

PHYSICAL AND CHEMICAL HAZARDS

BURNS

In dentistry, an obvious but avoidable cause of heat burns is instruments just removed from the steriliser, often caused by the difficulty in gauging their temperature through the rubber gloves worn by all staff. Autoclaves and laboratory and surgery compressors can also be an explosive risk.

High-speed handpieces, provided the water-cooling is working efficiently, cannot cause burns but, if not cooled, they can overheat and burn the patient's mouth. Other possible causes of thermal burns include hot gutta percha, hot dental composition, hot wax, boiling water, steam, naked flames, flammable or explosive fluids, lasers or diathermy and even operating lights. Fluids heated in a microwave oven may be hotter than they appear, as the container remains cooler. Diathermy is a form of high-frequency electrical energy used either for local tissue warming or for cutting, which can cause burns. Accidents have resulted from metallic parts of the dental chair becoming involved in the electric current path. The localized increase in current density can then cause superficial burns of the skin. Some serious accidents of this nature have also resulted from the use of diathermy units in operating theatres, where higher powers are used and the current path is normally completed by a large area electrode, to reduce the current density, placed under the patient. The risk from such diathermy is that of superficial burning, should the current be misdirected, but any part of the body can be involved if the current density is high enough.

Burns are more likely to occur in the laboratory. Bunsen burners are often causes of burns and long hair and gloves or clothing can catch light in a Bunsen flame. Burns from the melting and casting of alloys can be more severe. Hot wax knives can cause burns.

CHEMICAL HAZARDS

Where work practices are poor, staff can be exposed to a wide range of noxious chemical substances in a dental environment including gases, vapours, liquids, fumes, dusts and solids. The UK Control of Substances Hazardous to Health (COSHH) Regulations (1988 S1 No. 1657) place specific obligations on employers and the self-employed to control hazardous substances. Such a substance is 'any natural or artificial substance whether it is in solid or liquid form or in the form of a gas or vapour (including micro-organisms) which can constitute a hazard'. In summary, there are the following requirements on employers to:

(a) assess health risks created by work involving substances hazardous to health
(b) prevent or control exposure to substances hazardous to health
(c) provide and use control measures, personal protective equipment, etc. and take all reasonable steps to ensure these are properly used or applied
(d) maintain control measures in an efficient state, and good working order and repair
(e) monitor exposure to substances hazardous to health
(f) provide suitable health surveillance where appropriate for the protection of all employees exposed to substances hazardous to health.

All employees, and so far as is reasonably possible, persons on the premises where the work is being carried out who may be exposed to substances hazardous to health must be properly informed, instructed and trained. Employees must take steps to protect themselves and others, make full use of control measures and report immediately any defect. COSHH is enforced in the same way as the Health and Safety at Work, etc. Act or any other Regulations made under it. Part IA1 of the Approved List for the Classification Packaging and Labelling of Dangerous Substances Regulations (1984; ISBN 011 8839012) lists very toxic, corrosive, harmful or irritant, substances hazardous to health.

Most of the chemicals used in dentistry are currently listed on either the European Union dangerous substances list – Annex 1 of the 67/548/EEC Directive – or are designated as sensitizers by relevant Agencies or Institutions, such as the American Conference of Governmental Industrial Hygienists (ACGIH) or the German Senate Commission of the Deutsche Forschungs Gemeinschaft (DFG).

Generally, the primary contact for the health worker is the skin and the eyes (allergic and irritative dermatitis, ocular irritative diseases) with acute effects and sensitive effects. While formaldehyde and glutaraldehyde have known systemic effects, they are toxic for inhalation as are other volatile organic compounds (VOCs). Volatile organic compounds identified in the dental environment include benzene, toluene, ethylbenzene, xylenes, methyl methacrylate and aldehydes (formaldehyde, acetaldehyde, propionaldehyde and benzaldehyde).

Occupational exposure should be minimized wherever possible and it should be a fundamental principle to reduce exposure as much as possible by safe work practices, particularly storing material in correctly labelled, appropriate, preferably unbreakable, containers; avoiding spills and splatter; avoiding contacts with eyes and skin; and washing away spilt material with running tap water (see later). Better still is to consider whether a hazardous substance can be substituted with an innocuous one.

Acids

Chemical burns are all too common. Acids such as phosphoric acid, chromic acid and trichloracetic acid can cause burns. Many stronger acids and corrosives are used in the laboratory: hydrofluoric, sulfuric and nitric acids, and caustic soda are especially dangerous. Such acids and pickling solutions must be stored safely in appropriate and clearly labelled containers and with proper safety precautions (see later).

Anaesthetic gases

Dental clinical personnel may be chronically exposed to anaesthetic gases and vapours, especially if the anaesthetic equipment is faulty, poorly maintained or used without an effective scavenging system, or if the agents are abused. Nitrous oxide and halothane have known adverse effects but there are as yet few data on any possible adverse occupational effects of isoflurane, enflurane or other agents apart from occasional asthma (see Ch. 15). However, such pollutants are inhaled and absorbed, and appear in the blood and secretions such as breast milk. Headache is common, especially where halothane is used, and there are rare confirmed cases of occupationally acquired halothane hepatitis. However, occupational exposure does not appear to give rise to neuropsychiatric disorders. Mental and neurological performance are not significantly impaired by exposure to inhalational anaesthetic agents under normal working conditions but are, not surprisingly, impaired after exposure to excessive amounts of inhalational anaesthetics – to a greater degree by nitrous oxide than by halothane.

Abuse of nitrous oxide, however, is a well-recognized hazard in medicine and dentistry and can produce neurological damage, a myeloneuropathy caused by nitrous oxide, interfering with vitamin B_{12} metabolism and subsequent DNA production, similar to that of subacute combined degeneration of the spinal cord. Nitrous oxide impairs the enzyme methionine synthetase, which normally catalyses the conversion of homocysteine to methionine. There is early sensory impairment, L'Hermitte's sign (shooting pains when the neck is flexed), leg weakness, ataxia, impotence and loss of sphincter control. Fortunately, the myeloneuropathy improves after exposure to the gas is stopped though some damage remains, especially in the central nervous system. Interference with vitamin B_{12} metabolism probably also underlies the bone marrow damage leading to megaloblastosis seen in bone marrow biopsies of dentists chronically overexposed to nitrous oxide but, surprisingly, macrocytic anaemia does not seem to result. Nitrous oxide appears to be the agent most frequently responsible for occupational exposure.

It has been suggested that dental personnel exposed to inhalational general anaesthesia (GA) may be predisposed to disorders of health and reproduction, but the evidence is not unequivocal. Male dentists have been reported to have more liver, kidney and neurological disorders than controls, while their partners have been reported to have an increased rate of spontaneous abortions. Female dentists exposed to inhalational GA agents have been reported to have an increased risk of spontaneous abortion, congenital abnormalities in children and higher rates of cancer, renal and hepatic diseases. Dental nurses chronically exposed to GA agents may suffer from similar problems and (it has been suggested) may have an increased incidence of cancer of the cervix. A recent critical review of the available evidence has indicated that none of the criteria for the demonstration of toxicity by trace concentrations of GA agents has been adequately fulfilled, and that anxieties over occupational exposure may have been unjustifiably exaggerated. The consensus of data from animal experiments at subanaesthetic concentrations has not yielded convincing evidence of toxicity. Epidemiological studies have also provided no convincing evidence of any effect of chronic exposure to anaesthetic agents on mental performance, cancer or fetal disorders such as low birthweight, stillbirth or malformation.

In contrast to anaesthetic personnel, exposure of dental staff to inhalational GA agents is usually for short periods, except where relative analgesia is frequently used. Though there is little evidence of any significant hazard from dental gases in the surgery atmosphere, the following precautions should be taken where GA or relative analgesia (inhalational sedation) is used. To reduce contamination of the surgery atmosphere by gases, relative analgesia should not be overused, the machine should be carefully used, adequate surgery ventilation should be provided and, most importantly, a scavenger system should be used. Scavenging systems reduce air pollution by inhalational GA agents but, even when used, nitrous oxide levels in dental surgeries using relative analgesia can still exceed 150 ppm. Pregnant staff, or staff likely to become pregnant, should not work in a contaminated environment unless there is an effective scavenging system.

Antiseptics

Dentists, dental staff and patients may also be exposed to chemical agents that are used as topical antiseptics in the dental practice. For example, for caries, cavities or root canals, zinc oxide is used as a pulp capping agent and a root canal antiseptic; hydrogen peroxide is used as a root canal irrigant; m-cresol, formaldehyde and glutaraldehyde as root canal antiseptics; and iodoform as a root canal filling agent. Carbol camphor, eugenol, guaiacol and thymol are endodontic medicaments used as pulp sedatives. Benzalkonium chloride, benzethonium chloride, chlorhexidine and iodine are antiseptics directly administered to the oral mucosa.

Disinfectants

Dentists and dental personnel may also be exposed to substances that generally belong to the category of disinfectants (such as hydrogen peroxide, sodium hypochlorite, chlorhexidine, formalin, etc.). Personnel may also be exposed to organic solvents and active (antibacterial) ingredients of disinfectants when they clean surfaces or instruments (with solvent-based disinfectants or water-based agents). Examples of active ingredients of the disinfectants used in dental environment are o-phenylphenol, benzoyl-p-chlorophenol and n-alkyl-n-benzyl-n,n-dimethyl-ammonium chloride and many others (Table 31.2).

Methyl methacrylate

Acrylic monomer is the most common organic solution used in dentistry; the main component is methyl methacrylate, but it may also contain other monomers such as N-butylmethacrylate, isobutylmethacrylate, laurylmethacrylate, 1,4-butanediol dimethacrylate or ethylene glycol dimethacrylate. Polymerization inhibitors, such as hydroquinone, p-methoxyphenol or butylated cresols; plasticizers such as dibutyl phthalate;

Table 31.2 Disinfectants

Acids	Alkalis	Oxidants	Inorganic halogens	Heavy metal salts
Inorganic				
Boric acid, hydrochloric acid, sulfochromic acid, tartaric acid	Calcium hydrate, potassium hydroxide, sodium carbonate, sodium hydroxide	Peroxide, potassium permanganate	Calcium chloride, chlorine derivates: chloramines, chlorate, hypochlorites, Iodine	Mercuric bichloride, mercuric ossicyanide
Alcohols	**Aldehydes/phenols**	**Mercury organic compounds**	**Chlorine/iodine organic compounds**	**Quaternary ammonium derivates**
Organic				
Ethyl alcohol, isopropyl alcohol	Chlorine cresol, chlorine xylenol, cresol Dichlorine, formaldehyde, glutaraldehyde, hexachlorophene, phenol, polyphenols Xylenol	Mercurochrome, mercuric phenyl nitrate	Chloramine, dichloramine Iodine, povidone/betadine	Benzalkonium, benzoxonium, benzetonium chloride, cetrimide

ultraviolet light absorbers such as benzophenone; and activators such as dimethyl-*p*-toluidine may also be found.

Methyl methacrylate and cyanoacrylate may be used for solvent abuse but, in the absence of abuse, there is little evidence of a serious hazard if reasonable care is taken. Chemical hepatitis due to overexposure to methyl methacrylate monomer has been rarely reported, as have methyl methacrylate and cyanoacrylate-induced occupational asthma or dermatitis. Methyl methacrylate monomer may cause transient nausea if inhaled in large quantities, possibly by central depression of gastric motor function and, *rarely*, monomer has caused dyspnoea and hypertension. It may also soften soft contact lenses.

In technicians using methylmethacrylate the monomer is absorbed through skin, even to some extent where 'protective' creams are used. Unfortunately, many gloves are permeable to monomer, and barrier creams may impede the setting of acrylic. Urine analysis shows low methacrylate levels in the morning, but clear evidence of percutaneous absorption throughout the working day. Handling of methyl methacrylate may occasionally cause transient finger and palmar paraesthesia, pain and whitening of the fingers in the cold and local neurotoxicity and an eczema-like reaction. Contact dermatitis as a result of handling methyl methacrylate monomer is also a possibility, but is surprisingly rare.

Methyl methacrylate is embryotoxic and fetotoxic to rats (as is toluene). Though there is no evidence of such a danger to humans from methyl methacrylate, this should be borne in mind as a hazard, but probably no more than a theoretical one, in the case of female dental technicians.

There is no evidence of any permanent toxic effects from methyl methacrylate monomer under conditions of normal use.

Volatile, highly flammable chemicals

Methyl methacrylate monomer and gases such as oxygen are commonly used in dentistry. These must be stored properly in a correctly labelled strong container and not used near flames, or a fire or explosion could result. Many alcohols, acetone, and solvents and thinners are toxic and may be flammable

---

Box 31.4 Especially hazardous flammable fluids that may be used in dentistry

- Acetone
- Alcohols (ethyl alcohol, methyl alcohol, isopropyl alcohol)
- Benzene[a]
- Butane
- Ethers
- Ethylene oxide[a]
- Methyl methacrylate monomer
- Propane
- Toluene
- Xylene

Acids
- Chromic
- Hydrochloric
- Hydrofluoric
- Nitric
- Phosphoric
- Sulfuric
- Trichloracetic

Alkalis
- Ammonium hydroxide
- Sodium hydroxide
- Sodium hypochlorite

Other dangerous fluids
- Carbon tetrachloride[a]
- Chloroform[a]
- Methylene chloride

[a]Possible carcinogens

(Box 31.4). Some can also cause dermatitis, damage the eyes and respiratory tract, and chronic exposure may cause renal or liver damage; some such as toluene are teratogenic.

X-ray developers

Developers for radiographs contain hydroquinone; fixatives contain acetic acid and sodium thiosulfate. These solutions may cause dermatitis, conjunctivitis or bronchitis.

They should be handled carefully and with rubber gloves, avoiding contact with the eyes (it is best to wear protective eyewear) and avoiding excessive inhalation.

'SICK BUILDING SYNDROME'

The term 'sick building syndrome' refers to vague symptoms that develop in some office workers during the working week, but abate at weekends and vacations. The cause is unclear.

RADIATION HAZARDS

Radiation hazards in dental practice are mainly from ionizing radiation, as in X-rays, but there may also be hazards from the light sources used for curing composite materials and occasionally other sources, such as lasers.

IONIZING RADIATION

Ionizing radiation is that with a wavelength shorter than 10 nm, which can be artificial (such as X-rays) or come from natural sources. Exposure can induce genetic mutations in the germinal tissues (teratogenic effect) or induce malignant tumours in other tissues (oncogenic effect). Exposure to ionizing radiation must therefore be kept to the absolute minimum. Ionizing radiation is a hazard especially to the fetus or young child, or where cells are proliferating rapidly, as in the gonads and bone marrow. Acute high-level overexposure may cause radiation sickness, gastrointestinal and haematological damage, but most occupational exposure is at a lower level and prolonged; radiosensitive, rapidly dividing cells (such as in the fetus, skin or bone marrow) are then at risk.

Additional and possibly more important radiation hazards are those from accidents (e.g. Chernobyl), nuclear explosions and from domestic radon exposure in buildings situated over uranium-bearing strata, in such areas as parts of Cornwall, Devon, Somerset and Aberdeen, but also in some areas of Cumbria, Staffordshire, the West Midlands and Mid-Glamorgan. More than 75% of the annual exposure of the UK population to ionizing radiation is from natural sources such as radon (an alpha-emitting gas); this is recognized as a hazard which might equal in magnitude that from cigarette smoking and from toxic waste.

Therapeutic radiation may also predispose later to malignant tumours and there has been concern about diagnostic radiation in this respect. Therapeutic radiation affects not only malignant tumours but also the normal tissues in the surrounding area and in the radiation beam. The risk of injury depends on the size, number and frequency of radiation fractions, volume of irradiated tissue, duration of treatment, method of radiation delivery and other factors such as concomitant chemotherapy. Long-term follow-up studies of patients who had radiation treatment have also shown significant risk for tumours to develop in the radiation field. For example, radiotherapy for Hodgkin disease may lead later to breast cancer; patients irradiated for breast carcinoma, particularly smokers may develop lung cancer.

There is an increased risk of salivary tumours in patients who have received radiation to the tonsils and nasopharynx. More worryingly, radiotherapy in the past for benign diseases of the skin (acne, tinea capitis, haemangiomas), and for tonsillitis, led to substantially increased risks of thyroid cancer, parotid, parathyroid and central nervous system (CNS) tumours. Radiation treatment for benign conditions has increased with the advent of stereotactic delivery and, in particular, single high-dose gamma-knife therapy. This is used for benign CNS tumours (e.g. vestibular schwannoma, meningioma, pituitary adenoma and haemangioblastoma). There are concerns regarding the use of radiotherapy in childhood and in tumour-predisposing syndromes. The advent of new techniques such as intensity-modulated radiation therapy (IMRT) may reduce the adverse effects of radiation on normal tissues but this is controversial. Proton therapy may offer further improvement in dose localization over photons (X-rays) and reduce the risk of second malignancies.

NON-IONIZING RADIATION

Non-ionizing radiation has many forms.

Electromagnetic (radiofrequency) radiation is emitted by a variety of sources ranging from transmitter towers to electric power lines, computer terminals, electric clocks, microwave ovens and electric blankets. The public has become concerned about possible adverse effects from electromagnetic fields emanating from power transmission lines, but the evidence indicates that there is little, if any, reliable evidence for a health risk and, in any event, there is more exposure to electromagnetic radiation from household appliances and wiring than from power lines. Moreover, *natural* electromagnetic radiation is at least 100 times as intense as those induced by power lines. There is no evidence that exposure to electromagnetic radiation at these radiofrequencies and power levels poses any other health hazard to normal persons but some individuals fitted with cardiac pacemakers could be at risk (Ch. 5).

Ultraviolet (UV) light is emitted especially by the sun and the universally recognized consequence of overexposure is sunburn, but there are hazards to the eyes mainly (cataracts) and skin (predisposition to melanoma and squamous or basal cell carcinoma). UV and other lights may be used in dentistry (Table 31.3).

UVB (wavelengths between 286 and 320 nm) is responsible for most sunburn and also snow blindness (actinic retinitis). UVA (wavelengths between 320 and 400 nm) is the most dangerous and causes chronic damage to the eye, cataracts and damage to the retina. UVA light sources in dentistry include

Table 31.3 Light hazards

Radiation	Based on	Applications
Conventional blue or white light	Light-emitting diode (LED) or tungsten quartz halogen	Bonding, composite resin sealants and restorative materials, luting agents
Plasma arc lamps	430–490 nm	Rapid cure resins
Intense pulsed light (IPL)	Xenon lamp	Aesthetic surgery

UV sources for curing of restorative resins and fissure sealants and UV plaque lights (320–365 nm) but these have largely been replaced by blue light sources. Protective eyewear should be worn to absorb the wavelengths of any light sources used.

Blue light (400–500 nm) sources were developed to overcome the dangers of UV radiation and activate diketones in dental composite materials. However, blue light is not entirely safe, since it contains high-energy photons with the potential to form reactive free radicals in the eye, and these produce peroxides that denature photoreceptors in the retina. Blue light may be up to 30 times more damaging than UV light to the retina and may possibly also predispose to cataract.

White (visible) light (400–700 nm) is much safer, but also emits minute amounts of both UV and blue light, and green light (490–600 nm), so protective eyewear that absorbs these wavelengths should still be worn.

Laser is the acronym for Light Amplification by Stimulated Emission of Radiation. In general, lasers rapidly heat and acoustically shock tissues, and all are potentially hazardous, particularly because of eye damage, burns, and the risks of fire or electric shock. *All* lasers should therefore always be used with great care and *never* shone into the eyes, in unintended directions or on to brightly plated instruments that reflect the laser. Protective eyewear must be worn.

The effect of a laser on target tissue depends on the wavelength, beam power, degree of focus, duration of exposure and distance to target, as well as the absorption by the tissue. The wavelength of the photons (radiation) is controlled by the type of laser and lasing medium. There are hundreds of different lasers in use but the main ones used in health care are the carbon dioxide (CO_2), Nd:YAG (neodymium, yttrium, aluminium, garnet), and argon-ion lasers (Table 31.4).

The CO_2 laser emits infrared light (wavelength 10.6 μm), which is invisible but absorbed by water-containing tissues. It damages tissue by heat, and can be used to cut soft and hard tissues. Because the CO_2 laser is invisible, it is used co-axially with a helium–neon laser to produce a visible red beam. CO_2 lasers are expensive and potentially very dangerous.

The Nd:YAG laser (wavelength 1.06 μm) and krypton lasers are also used clinically and have the great advantage that they can be transmitted down a fibreoptic path. The Nd:YAG (near infrared) laser is invisible and therefore used with a helium–neon laser. It is used in dentistry for cutting dentine and soft tissues and also for photocoagulation.

The argon laser produces a blue–green light of 0.5 μm wavelength and can be transmitted by fibreoptics. It is used in dentistry mainly for polymerizing some composite materials. It is also used for photocoagulation.

Soft lasers include the helium–neon (He–Ne) laser, which produces light of 0.63 μm wavelength, and the diode laser (0.90 μm wavelength), which emits light in the near infrared or visible part of the spectrum and, if restricted to only milliwatt powers, produces little if any heating or a direct photochemical effect on tissues. The beam of a soft laser penetrates directly only to a depth of about 0.8 mm and is less damaging than others but still must be used with care as there is some hazard to the retina.

Video display units (VDUs or monitors) operate in the same way as television receivers, emitting light that forms the image on the screen, but excitation of the phosphors by the electron

Table 31.4 Lasers		
Laser	**Based on**	**Applications**
Argon	488 nm	Tooth whitening Increase resin adhesion, polymerization and reduce microleakage
Argon	514.5 nm	Soft tissue surgery
Carbon dioxide	10 600 nm	Soft tissue surgery
Diode	800–830 nm	Soft tissue surgery
Diode	980 nm gallium aluminium arsenide (GaAlAs)	Bleaching
Erbium	2940 nm and 2780 nm	Hard and soft tissue procedures
Nd:YAG	1064 nm	Soft tissue surgery
Potassium titanyl phosphate (KTP)	532 nm	Aesthetic surgery

beam also causes emission of minute amounts of ultraviolet and infrared rays, and low-energy X-rays. Very low frequency (VLF) and extremely low frequency (ELF) electromagnetic radiation is also emitted but the levels are exceedingly low – often lower than from domestic appliances.

The evidence indicates that VDUs are not responsible for cataracts, reproductive disorders, fetal congenital abnormalities or facial dermatitis. Musculoskeletal disorders and stress may be induced by VDUs. There is some evidence that these can be genuine problems, and that pains and stiffness in the neck, shoulders, back and wrists, and carpal tunnel syndrome – repetitive strain injury (RSI) – are not uncommon, but this is related more to poor posture and the elimination of tasks that once required office workers to get up and move around once in a while, rather than concentrating on the VDU itself. Prolonged work at VDUs is fatiguing, particularly for those with minor visual defects, as correction for middle-distance viewing is rarely carried out adequately, and it is possible that the resulting eyestrain may lead to blurred vision, tension and headaches. This in turn can lead to depression and some of the other symptoms sometimes ascribed to working with VDUs.

A further concern has been that the flickering of the VDU display might provoke epileptic attacks but there is no good evidence.

HAZARDS TO SPECIFIC BODY SYSTEMS
EYES

Care should be taken to avoid eye infections and damage from projected particles when using the air rotor, grinding metals or cutting wire. Penetrating wounds can cause deep injuries and even loss of sight. Chemicals such as phosphoric acid, sodium hypochlorite, trichloracetic and chromic acids can also cause serious eye damage. Radiation is an eye hazard.

Blue and UV light sources with wavelengths shorter than 400–500 nm (this is mainly a UV danger) cause cumulative eye damage; the shortest wavelengths are most damaging. Protective glasses should be used to filter out all light under about 500 nm and therefore glasses with red-, orange- or yellow-coloured lenses of sufficient optical density are indicated when using blue or UV light. Ordinary dark glasses do *not* filter out these offending wavelengths; indeed, by absorbing visible light, they can cause pupil dilatation and therefore aggravate the problem.

HEARING

Loud noise (85 dB or more) can irreversibly damage the inner ear hair receptor cells of the organ of Corti in the cochlea. Ultrasonic scalers may produce slight tinnitus after prolonged use but this rarely appears to be clinically significantly either to patients or to staff. Otherwise, the overall evidence suggests that hearing is not impaired in clinical dental staff compared with age-matched controls provided modern well-maintained equipment (such as air rotors) is used.

MENTAL HEALTH

Despite the low risks in dentistry, dental staff clearly perceive that occupationally related diseases, especially stress, are common. Dentistry, even for students, appears to be somewhat stressful but perhaps less so than medicine and some other professions. Dentists and dental hygienists complain particularly of musculoskeletal discomfort and of stress; dental nurses complain mainly about allergies and respiratory infections.

Drug abuse in dentistry and medicine is increasing, and the incidence of alcohol and other drug abuse (including nitrous oxide or other inhalational anaesthetics) by doctors and dentists is probably somewhat higher than for comparable groups in the population.

MUSCULOSKELETAL COMPLAINTS

Dental professionals, probably as a result of poor working positions and possibly stress, tend to develop musculoskeletal complaints. Although there appear to be few reliable objective studies of postural and skeletal problems in dental staff, one radiograph survey in Finland showed cervical spondylosis in about 50% of dentists compared with about 20% of farmers of the same age. Dentists also had somewhat more radiographic changes in the shoulder joint, but less lumbar spondylosis.

Activities involving repetitive wrist and hand movements, especially in women, may result in oedema beneath the transverse carpal ligament at the wrist. This can lead to compression of the median nerve and subsequent pain (especially at night), paraesthesia, hypoaesthesia and weakness in the wrist and hand (carpal tunnel syndrome). Though this is a common consequence of a variety of activities and is predisposed to by, for example, pregnancy or hypothyroidism, carpal tunnel syndrome has been reported in hygienists and endodontists in particular. Symptoms and signs consistent with partial carpal tunnel syndrome have been noted in one-quarter or more of hygienists in some surveys, but the diagnosis is far less frequent. Typists may also suffer the same symptoms.

Rest and analgesics usually provide adequate relief but, occasionally, splinting or corticosteroid injections are required. Surgical decompression may be indicated for recalcitrant cases.

PREGNANCY

Hazards from exposure to anaesthetic gases, mercury, ionizing radiation and infections have caused concern among female dental staff, but most evidence suggests that there is little if any specific occupational risk to the outcome of pregnancy. Pregnant female staff may, understandably, be concerned about possible risks to their fetus from ionizing radiation but, provided the rules of radiation protection are carefully followed, even female radiography or radiology staff appear to be at no significant risk. However, non-immune or immunocompromised female staff and their fetus may be at risk from various infections, notably rubella, cytomegalovirus and varicella-zoster virus. Pre-conception immunization and universal cross-infection control procedures should obviate this risk.

RESPIRATORY SYSTEM

Aerosols are suspensions of fine particles less than 50 μm in size, most of which are smaller than 5 μm, remain airborne for 24 h or more, are dispersed widely by air currents, and may enter the lungs. They can contain micro-organisms. These, and larger particles that tend not to pass to the lungs, may also settle on the conjunctiva or nasal mucosa. Infections can damage the respiratory system; the agents of most concern owing to their high morbidity or mortality are the respiratory viruses such as avian flu, and bacterial infections such as tuberculosis and legionellosis (Ch. 15). These have been transmitted to dental staff and there is also well-documented transmission to clinical dental staff of viruses such as adenoviruses and a variety of agents including *Chlamydia trachomatis*, but these incidents are rare. Fortunately, neither hepatitis B virus nor HIV appears to be transmitted by the airborne route.

Dusts can also damage the respiratory system. Dusts can be created during various dental procedures and can constitute a hazard where work practices are poor, especially in the dental laboratory (Table 31.5).

Table 31.5 Possibly hazardous mineral dusts in dentistry	
Mineral	**Found in some**
Albite	Porcelain veneers
Andalusite	Silicate cement powders
Calcium sulfate	Gypsum products
Chrysolite	Asbestos ring liners
Cristobalite	Casting investments
Diatomite	Alginates
Labradorite	Porcelain veneers
Metals (various)	See text
Microcline	Porcelain veneers
Orthoclase	Porcelain veneers
Quartz	Casting investments
Sillimanite	Silicate cement powders
Spinelles	Cement powders

There is little evidence of occupational lung disease among clinical dental staff but the drilling of teeth and old amalgams creates dust (and mercury vapour) if there is inadequate water-cooling, and the mixing of alginate impression materials can also create dust. Alginates contain alginate salts and calcium sulfate, silica compounds and diatomaceous earth, and may contain fluorine salts, zinc oxide or barium sulfate and various filler particles. These materials may be inhaled, especially during dispensing and mixing, and produce a hazard because of either the lead content or the siliceous fibres, though objective evidence for injury from these is very slight.

In the laboratory, there are a number of possible sources of dust, from pumice to various metals. The possible consequences of such inhalation are unclear but there are reports of mild dyspnoea, respiratory infections, pneumoconioses and possibly lung cancer in dental laboratory technicians. To date, most reports of pneumoconiosis in dental technicians relate to silica dust inhalation from polishing and sandblasting using outdated equipment. Cancer may be due more to tobacco use than dust inhalation.

Chemicals can also damage the respiratory system, directly or via allergic reactions. Clinical staff have occasionally developed asthma after exposure to enflurane. Occupational asthma has been precipitated in nurses and dental technicians by methyl methacrylate and cyanoacrylates. Formaldehyde, chlorhexidine, glutaraldehyde, cobalt, nickel, beryllium and chromium are other potential causes.

Electrostatic or HEPA (high-efficiency particulate air) air filters significantly reduce aerosols containing micro-organisms or dusts. Face masks rarely filter particles smaller than 5 μm in diameter and their filtering efficiency varies from 14% to 99%. Nevertheless, face masks do filter a great deal of debris. They should preferably be changed every hour. In the laboratory, local lathe ventilation is mandatory; a plexiglass shield will reduce splatter and dust extraction is vital.

SKIN

The main skin problems in dentistry are maceration (water-logging) and dermatitis from repeated hand-washing, candidosis secondary to maceration, and infections such as herpetic whitlow and contact dermatitis. It has been suggested that as many as one-third of dental staff suffer from contact allergies.

Dermatitis can result from direct chemical irritation of the skin or, in a susceptible individual, from an allergic response (contact allergy) which is a type 4 (delayed hypersensitivity) reaction (see Table 31.6). Hand dermatitis is particularly

Table 31.6 Some skin irritants and allergens used in dentistry

Irritants	Recognized allergens	Rarely allergic
Abrasives (pumice, silica, calcium carbonate)	Epoxy resin	Acrylic monomer
Adhesives (epoxy and cyanoacrylates)	Ethylenediamine dihydrochloride	Amethocaine (tetracaine)
Amalgam	p-Chloro-m-xylenol	Balsam of Peru
Detergents	Formaldehyde	Beeswax
Essential oils (eugenol)	Lanolin	Benzalkonium chloride
Etching compounds (phosphoric acid, 38%)	Latex	Benzocaine
Germicidal solutions	Mercaptobenzothiazole (rubber gloves, rubber	Benzophenone
Resins and catalysts	bands and dams, Band-Aids)	Benzoyl peroxide
Soaps	Neomycin	Bronopol
Solvents	Nickel	Camphor (plasticizer in acrylics)
	Parabens (medications, toothpaste)	Chlorhexidine
	Potassium dichromate	Chlorocresol
	Rosin (colophony)	Chlorothymol
	Thiomersal (disinfectants)	Cinnamon oil
		Cobalt
		Eugenol
		Glutaraldehyde
		Gold
		Hexachlorophane
		Hexylresorcinol
		Hydroquinone (inhibitor for acrylic resin systems)
		N-Isopropyl-N-phenyl-p-phenylenediamine (IPPD; rubber)
		MEK peroxide (catalyst for acrylic resin systems)
		Menthol
		Methyl dichlorobenzene sulfonate
		Methyl-p-toluene sulfonate
		Methyl salicylate (toothpastes)
		Nickel
		Penicillin
		Povidone–iodine
		Procaine
		Resorcinol monobenzoate (ultraviolet inhibitor in clear plastics)
		Triethylenetetramine (catalyst for epoxy resins)
		Zirconium (polishing paste)

frequently seen in dental technicians where up to one-third may suffer; the most common causes are direct irritation and a reaction to acrylic monomer.

Clinical dental staff may develop dermatitis, mainly from repeated hand washing, or chemicals or latex gloves.

USEFUL WEBSITES

www.dh.gov.uk/en/Publicationsandstatistics/PublicationsPolicyAndGuidance/DH_097678
http://www.mhra.gov.uk/Publications/Safetyguidance/DeviceBulletins/CON014775
http://www.mhra.gov.uk/index
http://www.aafp.org/
http://www.cdc.gov/niosh/topics

FURTHER READING

American Academy of Pediatric Dentistry Clinical Affairs Committee; American Academy of Pediatric Dentistry Council on Clinical Affairs, 2005–2006. Policy on minimizing occupational health hazards associated with nitrous oxide. Pediatr Dent 27 (7 Reference Manual), 49–50.

Andersson, T., Bruze, M., Gruvberger, B., Björkner, B., 2000. In vivo testing of the protection provided by non-latex gloves against a 2-hydroxyethyl methacrylate-containing acetone-based dentin-bonding product. Acta Derm Venereol 80, 435–437.

Bennett, A.M., Fulford, M.R., Walker, J.T., et al., 2000. Microbial aerosols in general dental practice. Br Dent J 189, 664–667.

Brown, P.N., 2004. What's ailing us? Prevalence and type of long-term disabilities among an insured cohort of orthodontists. Am J Orthod Dentofacial Orthop 125, 3–7.

Bruzell Roll, E.M., Jacobsen, N., Hensten-Pettersen, A., 2004. Health hazards associated with curing light in the dental clinic. Clin Oral Investig 8, 113–117.

Evans, D.G.R., Birch, J.M., Ramsden, R.T., Sharif, S., Baser, M.E., 2006. Malignant transformation and new primary tumours after therapeutic radiation for benign disease: substantial risks in certain tumour prone syndromes. J Med Genet 43, 289–284.

Fasunloro, A., Owotade, F.J., 2004. Occupational hazards among clinical dental staff. J Contemp Dent Pract 5, 134–152.

Godwin, C.C., Batterman, S.A., Sahni, S.P., et al., 2003. Indoor environment quality in dental clinics: potential concerns from particulate matter. Am J Dent 16, 260–266.

Harrel, S., Molinari, J., 2004. Aerosols and splatter in dentistry: a brief review of the literature and infection control implications. J Am Dent Assoc 135, 429–437.

Helmis, C.G., Tzoutzas, J., Flocas, H.A., et al., 2007. Indoor air quality in a dentistry clinic. Sci Total Environ 377, 349–365.

Henderson, K.A., Matthews, I.P., 2000. Environmental monitoring of nitrous oxide during dental anaesthesia. Br Dent J 188, 617–619.

Hörsted-Bindslev, P., 2004. Amalgam toxicity – environmental and occupational hazards. J Dent 32, 359–365.

Hylander, L.D., Lindvall, A., Gahnberg, L., 2006. High mercury emissions from dental clinics despite amalgam separators. Sci Total Environ 362, 74–84.

Iyer, R., Jhingran, A., 2006. Radiation injury: imaging findings in the chest, abdomen and pelvis after therapeutic radiation. Cancer Imaging 6 (Spec No A), S131–S139.

Kedjarune, U., Kukiattrakoon, B., Yapong, B., et al., 2000. Bacterial aerosols in the dental clinic: effect of time, position and type of treatment. Int Dent J 50, 103–107.

Leggat, P.A., Kedjarune, U., Smith, D.R., 2007. Occupational health problems in modern dentistry: a review. Ind Health 45, 611–621.

Pandis, N., Pandis, B.D., Pandis, V., Eliades, T., 2007. Occupational hazards in orthodontics: a review of risks and associated pathology. Am J Orthod Dentofacial Orthop 132, 280–292.

Puriene, A., Aleksejuniene, J., Petrauskiene, J., Balciuniene, I., Janulyte, V., 2007. Occupational hazards of dental profession to psychological wellbeing. Stomatologija 9, 72–78.

Scully, C., Cawson, R.A., Griffiths, M.J., 1990. Occupational hazards to dental staff. British Dental Journal, London.

Szymanska, J., 2004. Risk of exposure to Legionella in dental practice. Ann Agric Environ Med 11, 9–12.

Szymanska, J., 2000. Work-related vision hazards in the dental office. Ann Agric Environ Med 7, 1–4.

Szymanska, J., 2000. Work-related noise hazards in the dental surgery. Ann Agric Environ Med 7, 67–70.

Szymanska, J., 2005. Microbiological risk factors in dentistry. Current status of knowledge. Ann Agric Environ Med 12, 157–163.

Tang, W.M., Chiu, K.Y., Ng, T.P., Yau, W.P., 2003. Practicing cementing technique with a toy: Play-Doh. J Arthroplasty 18, 799–800.

Toroglu, M.S., Bayramoglu, O., Yarkin, F., Tuli, A., 2003. Possibility of blood and hepatitis B contamination through aerosols generated during debonding procedures. Angle Orthod 73, 571–578.

Veronesi, L., Bonanini, M., Dall'Aglio, P., Pizzi, S., Manfiedi, M., Tanzi, M.L., 2004. Health hazard evaluation in private dental practices: a survey in a province of northen Italy. Acta Biomed 75, 50–55.

Webber, L.M., 2000. Bloodborne viruses and occupational exposure in the dental setting. SADJ 55, 494–496.

World Health Organization (WHO), 2000. Air quality guidelines for Europe. Regional Publications, European Series, No. 91, 2nd edn., WHO Regional Office for Europe, Copenhagen.

Zimmer, H., Ludwig, H., Bader, M., et al., 2002. Determination of mercury in blood, urine and saliva for the biological monitoring of an exposure from amalgam fillings in a group with self-reported adverse health effects. Int J Hyg Environ Health 205, 205–211.

CONTRACEPTION

There is a range of methods of contraception with varying degrees of effectiveness, as shown in Table 32.1. The most widely used and effective forms are the oral contraceptive pill (OCP; 'the Pill') and the male condom (this also confers protection against transmission of infections).

EFFECTIVE CONTRACEPTION

The OCP is effective, but not completely, in preventing pregnancy and provides no protection against sexually transmitted infections. Contraception is thus best achieved by planned regular use of oral contraceptives plus barrier precautions such as a male or female condom.

Oral contraceptive pill

General aspects

Oral contraceptive pills are usually mixtures of synthetic oestrogens and progestogens taken regularly every day. The mini-pill contains only a progestogen but is less effective than the combination pill and is prescribed less often. OCPs may act especially by inhibiting ovulation via action on the hypothalamic–pituitary axis; by altering the composition of uterine cervical mucus; and by impeding implantation of the ovum. Emergency contraception may prevent pregnancy when taken within 72 h of intercourse but is not reliable. The two types of synthetic oestrogen used in OCPs are ethinylestradiol and mestranol. The synthetic progesterone is progestogen. Norethindrone and levonorgestrel are other examples. Most OCP

Table 32.1 Methods of contraception

Contraceptive Methods	Efficacy (%)
Majority use	
Oral contraceptive pill (OCP) including the mini-pill	99
Male condom	98
Minority use	
Contraceptive coil (intrauterine contraceptive device)	95
Contraceptive patch	99
Contraceptive injection	99
Contraceptive implants	99
Cap or diaphragm	95
Mirena (intrauterine system)	99
Female condom	95
Withdrawal method	? (low)
Natural family planning (the rhythm method)	? (low)

side-effects are thought to be caused by the oestrogen component, which is now only 50 mg or less.

Oral contraceptive pills can have adverse effects. The major risk is the higher incidence of thromboembolic disease (thrombosis of deep veins and coronary or cerebral thrombosis), but the incidence of cardiovascular or cerebrovascular disease is normally so low in young women that these complications are still uncommon even with a four- or fivefold increase in incidence. Hypertension, diabetes, jaundice and liver tumours, usually benign, are amongst the many other disorders more frequent in those taking OCPs (Table 32.2: Ch.29). There is some evidence that long-term use of OCPs may increase the risk of cancer of the cervix and possibly of breast cancer, but they appear to lower the risk of ovarian cancer by 40–50%, and may also reduce the risk of endometrial cancer. *However, the risks from adverse effects of OCPs are low compared with the health risks associated with pregnancy.*

Table 32.2 Adverse effects of oral contraceptives

Minor	Moderate	Serious
Nausea	Intermenstrual bleeding	Thromboembolic disease[a]
Depression		Hypertension[a]
Loss of libido		Myocardial infarction[a]
Breast pain		Gallstones
Fluid retention		Liver benign tumours
Weight gain		Cancer of cervix and breast

[a]More frequent in smokers and older women.

Oral contraceptive pills are absorbed from the intestine, but their effect may be impaired by: excessive intestinal motility, as in diarrhoea; antimicrobials, such as amoxicillin, ampicillin or tetracycline, which suppress the gut flora that deconjugate bile salts, thereby interrupting the enterohepatic recycling of the oestrogen; or drugs that enhance the liver enzymes that metabolize the OCPs, such as carbamazepine. As a result these drugs may at least theoretically increase the risk of pregnancy, though the risk must be minimal (Table 32.3: Ch. 29). Women prescribed such drugs should best be advised to take additional contraceptive measures whilst taking the drug and for at least 7 days afterwards (4 weeks in the case of rifampicin).

Dental aspects

Oral contraceptives may worsen gingivitis and possibly periodontitis, may increase the risk of dry sockets and, on radiography, there may be jaw radio-opacities or altered trabecular patterns.

The predisposition to myocardial infarction, thromboembolic disease and hypertension theoretically necessitates precautions for operations under general anaesthesia (GA). However, if the patient is otherwise well, GA, in hospital of course, is not contraindicated. Despite the risk of thromboembolism, the disadvantages of discontinuing oral contraceptives before GA outweigh the advantages.

The significance of drug interactions for dental antibiotics with the OCP is probably low. OCPs can also interact with anticoagulants to disturb anticoagulant control and they can impair the effect of tricyclic antidepressants.

Condoms

Male and female latex rubber condoms are available, are relatively inexpensive, have a high success rate and virtually no side-effects and also protect against sexually transmitted infections (STIs).

Other effective contraception

- *IUCD (intrauterine contraceptive device):* originally termed the coil or loop, because the early devices were coil-shaped or loop-shaped, many now are T-shaped and contain some copper (to increase efficacy), the IUCD acts by inhibiting the movement of sperm through the uterus, altering the mucus and affecting the endometrium.
- *Contraceptive injection:* progestogens that act by inhibiting ovulation, thickening cervical mucus, inhibiting the progress of sperm and thinning the endometrium. They include *Depo-Provera (medroxyprogesterone)*, which protects against pregnancy for 12 weeks, or *Noristerat (norethisterone)*, which protects for 8 weeks.
- *Contraceptive implants:* contain etonorgestrel (Implanon), are usually inserted subcutaneously in the left arm, above the elbow, and are effective for 3 years.
- *Cap or diaphragm:* a mechanical impediment to sperm entry into the uterus.
- *Intrauterine system (Mirena):* this intrauterine system contains a reservoir of progestogen steadily released for up to 5 years.

Table 32.3 Some drugs interacting with oral contraceptives pills (OCPs) to reduce their effect and predispose to pregnancy

Significantly interfering with OCP	Slightly interfering with OCP
Anticonvulsants	Oral antibiotics
– Barbiturates	– Ampicillin
– Phenytoin	– Amoxicillin
– Carbamazepine	– Metronidazole
– Primidone	– Tetracyclines
– Dichloralphenazone	
Antibiotics	
– Rifampicin	

- *Contraceptive patch (Evra):* this lasts for 1 week, so new patches are used each week for 3 weeks, followed by a week's break – just like the OCP.

UNRELIABLE FORMS OF CONTRACEPTION

- *Withdrawal method:* coitus interruptus (Latin for 'interrupted intercourse').
- *Natural family planning (the rhythm method):* avoiding intercourse when ovulation is probable, as assessed by the calendar method, temperature method or mucus test.

SEXUALLY TRANSMITTED INFECTIONS

Sexually transmitted diseases (STDs) or infections (STIs) include bacterial, viral and fungal infections, and infestations (Table 32.4), and were formerly termed venereal diseases (VDs). Non-specific urethritis (NSU) and *Chlamydia* are probably the most common. There can be infection with more than one STI, and STIs generally increase the liability to transmission of viruses such as HIV, especially if there is mucosal or cutaneous ulceration. The group of most common serious STIs has been given the acronym SHAG (syphilis, herpes, anogenital warts and gonorrhoea).

Young people (age 16–24 years) now account for half of all STI cases, the incidence of which are virtually all increasing. In the UK in 2008, nearly half a million people attended clinics for STIs. Sexually promiscuous people can be the source of transmission to literally hundreds of others (Fig. 32.1).

Table 32.4 The most important sexually transmitted diseases and their causal agents

	Micro-organism	Diseases
Bacteria	Treponema pallidum	Syphilis
	Mycoplasma genitalium	Non-specific urethritis
	Ureaplasma urealyticum	Non-specific urethritis
	Neisseria gonorrhoeae	Gonorrhoea
	Chlamydia trachomatis	Chlamydia
		Lymphogranuloma venereum
	Haemophilus ducreyi	Chancroid
	Calymmatobacterium granulomatis	Granuloma inguinale
	Staphylococcus aureus	MRSA in MSM
Viruses	Herpes simplex virus [human (alpha) herpesvirus]	Genital herpes
	Human papillomavirus	Genital warts (condyloma acuminatum)
	Hepatitis B and probably C viruses	Hepatitis
	Human immunodeficiency virus	HIV/AIDS
Fungi	Candida	Thrush
Parasites	Phthirus pubis (crab lice)	Pubic lice
	Sarcoptes scabiei	Scabies
	Trichomonas vaginalis	Trichomoniasis

AIDS, acquired immune deficiency syndrome; HIV, human immunodeficiency virus; MRSA, meticillin-resistant *Staphylococcus aureus*; MSM, men who have sex with men.

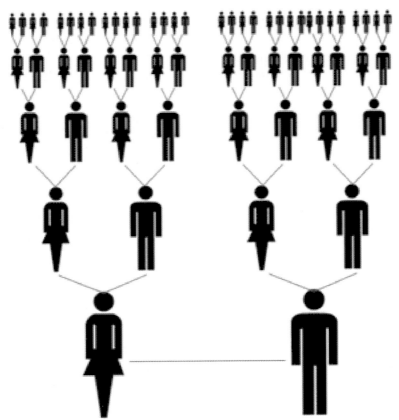

**When you have sex with someone, you are having sex
With everyone they have had sex with, and with
Everyone they have had sex with, and with
Everyone they have had sex with, and with
Everyone they have had sex with, and with
Everyone they have had sex with, and with
Everyone they have had sex with, and with
Everyone they have had sex with, and with**

Fig. 32.1 Chart demonstrating the spread of STIs to other partners (From www.positive-choice.org)

PREVENTION

Sexually transmitted diseases are not highly contagious, and are transmitted only by direct intimate contact with mucosae/body fluids. They can be caught during sex, including oral and anal sex, but not from hugging, toilet seats or sharing towels, or normal social contact. Since STIs are passed from person to person through unsafe sexual practices, the risk of infection can be reduced by avoiding casual and unprotected sexual intercourse by:

- *A*bstinence
- *B*eing monogamous
- *C*ondom use always.

A man should always use a condom during sexual intercourse, each time, from start to finish, and a woman should make sure that her partner uses one. A woman can also protect herself from STIs by using a female condom.

Although any person can be at risk of contracting STDs, members of certain groups can be at especially high risk (Box 32.1 and Fig. 32.2).

CHLAMYDIA

General aspects

Chlamydia trachomatis, the most frequently reported bacterial STI in the USA and UK, can be transmitted during vaginal, anal or oral sex. In women, it initially infects the cervix and urethra, or rectum. In men, infection is urethral, or rectal. *Chlamydia* can be found in the pharynx of women and men having oral sex with an infected partner.

Clinical features

About three-quarters of infected women and half of infected men have no symptoms. If symptoms do occur, they usually appear within 1–3 weeks after exposure. Rectal *Chlamydia* may cause pain, discharge or bleeding.

Women may develop an abnormal vaginal discharge or dysuria (burning sensation when urinating). Some have lower abdominal pain, low back pain, nausea, fever, pain during intercourse (dyspareunia), or intermenstrual bleeding (between periods). *Chlamydia* can cause pelvic inflammatory disease (PID), which can permanently damage the fallopian tubes, uterus and surrounding tissues, or cause ectopic pregnancies.

Men may have a urethral discharge or dysuria. Complications among men are rare but include epididymitis with pain, fever and, rarely, sterility.

Chlamydial infections can lead to premature delivery and babies who are born to infected mothers can get chlamydial pneumonia and conjunctivitis (pink eye). Chlamydia may cause lymphogranuloma venereum. Rarely, genital chlamydial infection in adults can cause arthritis accompanied by skin lesions and inflammation of the eye and urethra (Reiter syndrome).

General management

Azithromycin (single dose) or doxycycline (twice daily for a week) are the most commonly used treatments.

GONORRHOEA

General aspects

Gonorrhoea, caused by *Neisseria gonorrhoeae*, is less common than most other STIs, but is about 15 times more common than syphilis.

Clinical features

Gonorrhoea usually causes urethritis or proctitis in males, and urethritis, proctitis or endocervicitis in females. However, gonorrhoea in all sites is often asymptomatic, a fact that increases the chances of transmission. An important complication is urethral stenosis. In neonates of infected women, it can cause blindness.

General management

Diagnosis depends on laboratory tests including Gram-stained smears (to show the Gram-negative diplococci within leukocytes), bacterial culture and sensitivity tests. Repeated smears or culture may be required, particularly in female contacts. Serological tests are uninformative.

Penicillin is usually the drug of choice in the UK and is often given as 2 g ampicillin plus 1 g probenecid as a single oral dose. Patients hypersensitive to penicillin can be treated with co-trimoxazole. Antimicrobial resistance in *N. gonorrhoeae* occurs as plasmid-mediated resistance to penicillin and tetracycline, and

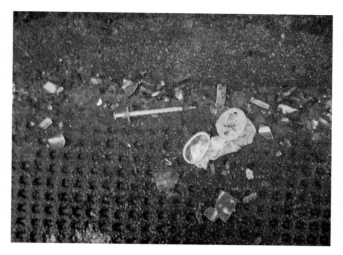

Fig. 32.2 The outfall from street prostitution; heroin syringe and condoms

chromosomally mediated resistance to penicillins, tetracyclines, spectinomycin and fluoroquinolones. The current Centers for Disease Control and Prevention (CDC)-recommended options for treating *N. gonorrhoeae* infections are the cephalosporins: ceftriaxone, available only as an injection, is the recommended treatment for all types of gonorrhoeal infection. The only oral agent recommended by CDC for treatment of uncomplicated urogenital or rectal gonorrhoea is a single dose of cefixime 400 mg.

Dental aspects

In contrast to the high incidence of urethral gonorrhoea, infection in the oropharynx seems to be uncommon, except perhaps in male homosexuals. Fellatio is probably the main cause of such infections, but it has been shown that saliva normally strongly inhibits the growth of *N. gonorrhoeae*. Though a rarity, gonococcal stomatitis may be suspected when there is acute stomatitis and/or pharyngitis without features ascribable to other oral diseases, with severe but ill-defined inflammation or painful ulceration in a young adult, and especially with a history of recent orogenital or oroanal contact. The tonsils become red and swollen with a greyish slough and there is regional lymphadenitis. However, the infection can be asymptomatic and the throat may appear normal. A throat swab should be taken in suspected cases for Gram-staining to show polymorphs containing Gram-negative diplococci and there should be confirmation by culture and identification of *N. gonorrhoeae*, since saprophytic neisseriae are common in the mouth. Penicillin is effective in 97% of oropharyngeal infections; azithromycin is an alternative.

There is no evidence that oral gonococcal infections can be transmitted by coughing and droplet infection, or by saliva to the dentist (especially if normal cross-infection control is practised). Furthermore, dental procedures on an infected patient will not produce haematogenous spread or deep infection.

NON-SPECIFIC CERVICITIS (NSC)

Fewer than half of those who have cervicitis are infected with *Chlamydia*: others have gonorrhoea, and a few have other bacterial or herpes simplex virus infection. Frequently no cause is found and it is then referred to as 'non-specific'.

NON-SPECIFIC URETHRITIS

Non-specific urethritis (NSU) is urethritis not caused by *Chlamydia* or gonorrhoea, and manifests with dysuria and stains on underwear. *Mycoplasma genitalium* or *Ureaplasma urealyticum* may be implicated. Diagnosis is from a smear showing numerous polymorphonuclear leukocytes. Treatment is doxycycline or azithromycin.

SYPHILIS

Syphilis is an STI caused by the bacterium *Treponema pallidum*, which may damage cardiovascular or nervous systems, and the fetus, and can also be fatal. The incidence of syphilis, though low, is currently rising and over 80% of cases are in men who have sex with men. In HIV infection it can be atypical and severe (lues maligna).

Other treponemal infections [*non-venereal* (endemic) treponematoses] can be acquired where poverty, overcrowding and unhygienic practices facilitate the transmission of infection (Appendix 32.1).

Primary syphilis

Over 80% of syphilis cases are in homosexual men. The incubation period is about 3 weeks (range 10–90 days).

Clinical features

Treponema pallidum causes a chancre (primary or Hunterian chancre), which begins as a small, firm, pink and typically single macule (usually on the glans penis or vulva). This changes to a papule and then ulcerates to form a painless round ulcer with a raised margin and indurated base. Primary chancres occasionally involve the lips or tongue. Untreated chancres heal in 3–8 weeks, but are highly infectious and are associated with enlarged painless regional lymph nodes.

Management of primary syphilis

Diagnosis is by microscopy of lesional exudate and serology. In oral lesions, the diagnosis can be confused by oral commensal treponemes, so, to minimize confusion, specific fluoresceinated antibodies should be used or oral lesions should be thoroughly swabbed with sterile gauze or cotton wool to remove as many contaminating oral bacteria as possible, then gently but thoroughly scraped with an instrument such as a sterile plastic spatula. The scraping is then transferred to a slide, covered with a coverslip and examined as quickly as possible by dark-ground microscopy. If the lesion is a chancre, many large but slender, regular, helical forms with a leisurely rotational movement across the field are seen. A negative test does not rule out syphilis, though this investigation is important, since serology is often negative at this stage. Biopsy may be uninformative and unlikely to be diagnostic unless specific antibodies are used.

Non-specific (reaginic) serological tests, useful for screening such, include the Venereal Disease Research Laboratory (VDRL), rapid plasma reagin (RPR) card test, automated reagin test (ART) and toluidine red-treated serum test (TRUST). Treponemal enzyme immunoassays (EIAs) are an appropriate alternative for screening but another treponemal assay such as TPHA (*Treponema pallidum* haemagglutination test) should be used for confirmation. The VDRL test appears positive towards the end of primary syphilis and remains positive in untreated secondary or tertiary syphilis, but usually becomes negative 1–2 years after treatment. It is positive in all treponematoses. False-positive results may be seen after immunizations, in autoimmune disease and in other infections (HIV, viral pneumonia, tuberculosis, malaria or leptospirosis).

Specific serological tests such as the fluorescent treponemal antibody absorbed (FTA-Abs) test, the TPHA and the treponemal immobilization (TPI) test overcome the problem of the false-positive results found in the VDRL, but still cannot differentiate syphilis from other treponematoses. The FTA-Abs is probably best reserved for specimens giving discrepant results. Specific tests become positive during primary and remain positive through untreated secondary or tertiary syphilis, as does the VDRL but, in contrast to VDRL, most of the specific tests remain positive even in treated syphilis.

Primary syphilis is treated with procaine penicillin or doxycycline or erythromycin.

Patients must be followed up clinically and serologically for 2 years and contacts traced.

Secondary syphilis

Secondary syphilis follows the primary stage after 6–8 weeks but a chancre may still be present.

Clinical features

Syphilis is the great mimic. Signs and symptoms are often non-specific, with fever, headache, malaise, a rash (characteristically symmetrically distributed coppery maculopapules on the palms) and generalized painless lymph node enlargement with unusual enlargement of the epitrochlear nodes. It is in this stage that oral lesions classically appear but these are seen in only about one-third of patients: painless ulcers (mucous patches and snailtrack ulcers), split papules and condyloma lata are typical. The mucosal lesions are highly infectious.

Management of secondary syphilis

Mucosal lesions should be examined for *T. pallidum* as described above and blood should be taken for serological examination. Treatment is as for primary syphilis (see below; Herxheimer reaction).

Tertiary syphilis

If untreated, syphilis progresses to a tertiary stage 3–10 or more years after infection in about 30% of patients. The remainder are serologically reactive and said to have latent syphilis.

Clinical features

The gumma is the main feature. It is a localized non-infectious granuloma varying in size from a pinhead to several centimetres, which breaks down to form a deep punched-out ulcer. Skin gummas heal with depressed shiny scars (tissue-paper scars). Bone gummas may affect the long bones (especially the tibia – 'sabre tibia') or skull, producing lytic lesions and periostitis with new bone formation. Mucosal gummas may destroy bone, particularly the palate, or involve the tongue. The main oral manifestation of late-stage syphilis is leukoplakia, particularly of the dorsum of tongue, which has a high potential for malignant change.

Cardiovascular syphilis (aortitis, coronary arterial stenosis or aortic aneurysms) affects about 10% of patients, as a late complication.

Neurosyphilis, sometimes with sensorineural deafness, also affects about 10%. *Meningovascular neurosyphilis* has highly variable early symptoms but late effects may be hydrocephalus or lesions of the IInd, IIIrd and VIIIth cranial nerves, and the pupils are also unequal and unresponsive to light (Argyll Robertson pupils). *Paretic neurosyphilis* begins insidiously with subtle mental disturbance going on to severe personality changes, complete dementia and widespread paralyses (general paresis of the insane; GPI). *Tabes dorsalis (locomotor ataxia)* is characterized by atrophy of lumbar posterior nerve roots and sometimes the optic nerves, and clinically characterized by sudden attacks of lightning-like pain and paraesthesiae of leg or trunk, with loss of normal pain sensation and of deep proprioceptive reflexes. These cause a peculiar tabetic gait in which the feet are slapped on to the ground as a result of loss of sense of their position, and the neuropathic joints then become disorganized (Charcot's joints).

Neurosyphilis is a rare cause of atypical trigeminal neuralgia but is now of little dental significance, though its presence should be suspected in a patient with a gumma or syphilitic leukoplakia, which typically involves the dorsum of the tongue.

Management of tertiary syphilis

The diagnosis of tertiary syphilis is confirmed by serology. Treatment is with procaine penicillin, 600 000 units daily for 3 weeks, and lifelong follow-up. Systemic corticosteroids are given at the start of antibiotic therapy to reduce the possibility of a Jarisch–Herxheimer reaction (febrile reaction often with exacerbation of the local syphilitic lesions).

Syphilis may be associated with HIV infection and then takes an atypical, accelerated course in which progress to the tertiary stage may be rapid and gummata may develop while the secondary stage is still active (lues maligna). Relapse is common despite treatment, or the response to penicillin may be poor. The antibody response is also atypical and unpredictable.

Congenital syphilis

Syphilis in the pregnant patient (after the fifth month) may result in infection of the fetus, with learning disability, deafness and blindness, and typically results in a saddle nose and Hutchinson's teeth – screwdriver-shaped incisors. Affected children are highly infectious until about 2 years of age. Penicillin is the usual treatment.

TRICHOMONIASIS

General aspects

Trichomoniasis (TV) is a common STI caused by the parasite *Trichomonas vaginalis*. Women can acquire the disease from infected men or women, but men usually contract it only from infected women. The vagina is the most common site of infection in women, and the urethra is the most common site of infection in men. Transmission is via penis-to-vagina intercourse or vulva-to-vulva contact. Rarely, it is caught by sharing towels or washcloths with an infected person.

Clinical features

Symptoms are more common in women. TV usually causes an odiferous vaginal discharge, often foamy and yellow in colour, with vulval pruritus and erythema. In males, TV is usually symptomless but may cause dysuria.

General management

Metronidazole and tinidazole are usually effective treatments.

OTHER STIs

Hepatitis (Ch. 9), herpes (Ch. 11), HIV (Ch. 20), human papillomavirus (HPV; Ch. 21), and parasites such as crab lice and scabies (Ch. 21) are discussed elsewhere.

STIs SEEN MAINLY IN PEOPLE FROM THE DEVELOPING WORLD

Chancroid

Chancroid, caused by the small Gram-negative bacterial rod, *Haemophilus ducreyi*, is a frequent cause of genital ulcers in developing countries but is uncommon in industrialized nations.

Clinical features

After an incubation period of 2–10 days, a papule or pustule erupts that erodes to form a painful deep ulcer with ragged margins. More than one-half of patients have multiple ulcers. Painful regional lymphadenopathy is common.

General management

Treatment is with azithromycin, ceftriaxone, erythromycin or ciprofloxacin.

Granuloma inguinale (donovanosis)

This is a chronic, ulcerative, granulomatous disease caused by *Calymmatobacterium granulomatis*, a Gram-negative bacillus seen in people from the Americas, Far East and Africa.

Clinical features

After an incubation period of 1–4 weeks, a papule or nodule appears usually in the inguinal or anogenital region and

Table 32.5 Possible complications from body art

Procedure	Complications		
Dental grillz	Can impair oral hygiene, cause tooth movement or surface loss		
Piercings	Pain, oedema, haemorrhage, infection	*Staphylococcus aureus* infections, osteomyelitis, toxic shock syndrome and endocarditis, *Pseudomonas aeruginosa* infection and HIV transmission, Ludwig angina, bleeding into the pharynx and airways, and acute hypotension	Oral piercings can interfere with speech and mastication, cause mucosal or gingival trauma, chipped or fractured teeth, hypersalivation, calculus accumulation, and foreign body granulomas or allergies
Tattooing	Pain, oedema, haemorrhage, infection	*Staphylococcus aureus* infections, and transmission of HBV, HCV and HIV	Foreign body granulomas or allergies, or scarring
Tongue-splitting	Pain, oedema, haemorrhage, infection		

HBV, hepatitis B virus; HCV, hepatitis C virus; HIV, human immunodeficiency virus.

progresses to a locally destructive granulomatous ulcer. Three main types of donovanosis have been described: ulcerative, exuberant and cicatricial.

General management

Direct examination of a piece of granulation tissue compressed between two slides and stained by Giemsa for the presence of Donovan bodies (clusters of bacilli lying within leukocytes) is the best diagnostic method.

Tetracycline, ampicillin or trimethoprim–sulfamethoxazole are first-line therapy.

Lymphogranuloma venereum

Lymphogranuloma venereum (LGV) or lymphogranuloma inguinale, caused by *Chlamydia trachomatis*, is seen worldwide, but is particularly common in people from Latin America, India, Indonesia and Africa.

Clinical features

Lymphogranuloma venereum primarily affects the external genitalia, the inguinal lymph nodes and lymphatics. About 10 days after exposure a small vesicle appears, and then ruptures and heals without scarring. About 1 week to 2 months later there may be swelling and tenderness of the regional lymph nodes and suppuration. Healing involves scarring, which blocks lymphatic channels causing oedema (elephantiasis).

General management

Diagnosis is by serological tests and isolation of *C. trachomatis*. A non-specific skin test (Frei test) is available. LGV is treated with sulfonamides, tetracycline, erythromycin or rifampicin.

BODY ART

Tattooing and more invasive procedures, with distortion or mutilation of body parts, have been commonplace in many cultures for centuries and often have sexual connotations. For example, facial scarification and female circumcision are common in some African cultures. In some East African groups, the uvula is removed in children in the belief that health will be improved. In some groups in developing countries such as in some Amazonian tribes and in the Surma tribe of Ethiopia, large plates are worn in the lower lip.

In the developed world, the expression of individualism through body art such as tattooing and body piercing, and the wearing of jewellery in 'unconventional' sites has become popular. Oral piercings, tongue splitting and 'dental grills' (also termed bling tooth jewellery, grillz or fronts) are increasingly seen. Grillz are generally removable and made from metal (silver, gold or platinum) with some encrusted with expensive precious stones and jewels.

Complications possible from body art are shown in Table 32.5.

USEFUL WEBSITES

http://health.nih.gov/topic/SexualHealthGeneral
http://www.dh.gov.uk/en/Publichealth/Healthimprovement/Index.htm
http://www.cdc.gov/std
http://www.hpa.org.uk

FURTHER READING

Antonio, A.G., Kelly, A., Maia, L.C., 2005. Premature loss of primary teeth associated with congenital syphilis: a case report. J Clin Pediatr Dent 29, 273–276.

Bruce, A.J., Rogers 3rd, R.S., 2004. Oral manifestations of sexually transmitted diseases. Clin Dermatol 22, 520–527.

Cliffe, S.J., Tabrizi, S., Sullivan, E.A., on behalf of the Pacific Islands Second Generation HIV Surveillance Group, 2008. Chlamydia in the Pacific region, the silent epidemic. Sex Transm Dis 35, 801–806.

Dalmau, J., Alegre, M., Roé, E., Sambeat, M., Alomar, A., 2006. Nodules on the tongue in an HIV-positive patient. Scand J Infect Dis. 38, 822–825.

Dan, M., Poch, F., Amitai, Z., Gefen, D., Shohat, T., 2006. Pharyngeal gonorrhea in female sex workers: response to a single 2-g dose of azithromycin. Sex Transm Dis 33, 512–515.

Eccleston, K., Collins, L., Higgins, S.P., 2008. Primary syphilis. Int J STD AIDS 19, 145–151.

Egglestone, S.I., Turner, A.J.L., 2000. Serological diagnosis of syphilis. Commun Dis Public Health 3, 158–162.

Gurlek, A., Alaybeyoglu, N.Y., Demir, C.Y., et al., 2005. The continuing scourge of congenital syphilis in 21st century: a case report. Int J Pediatr Otorhinolaryngol 69, 1117–1121.

Leão, J.C., Gueiros, L.A., Porter, S.R., 2006. Oral manifestations of syphilis. Clinics 61, 161–166.

Lewis, D.A., McDonald, A., Thompson, G., Bingham, J.S., 2004. The 374 clinic: an outreach sexual health clinic for young men. Sex Transm Infect 80, 480–483.

Menni, S., 2007. Acquired primary syphilis on a child's lip. Acta Derm Venereol 87, 284.

Platt, L., Rhodes, T., Judd, A., et al., 2007. Effects of sex work on the prevalence of syphilis among injection drug users in 3 Russian cities. Am J Public Health 97, 478–485.

Appendix 32.1 Non-venereal treponematoses (endemic treponematoses)

Disease	Aetiology/epidemiology	Clinical features	Management
Bejel (endemic syphilis)	Caused by *Treponema pallidum*, prevalent among nomads in the Arabian peninsula and sub-Saharan Africa	No obvious primary stage. Secondary and tertiary stages are encountered, mainly manifesting on skin and mucosae: mucous patches, angular stomatitis, rashes, pigmentary changes and tenderness of long bones may be seen. About one-third of patients develop lesions of the late or tertiary stage of the disease which are mainly gummatous. Skin lesions are usually extensive, chronic, destructive, healing with scarring and depigmentation. Gummatous destruction of the nasal septum, lips, soft palate and nasopharynx may lead to facial deformity (rhinopharyngitis mutilans)	Dark-ground microscopy and serology are needed to confirm the diagnosis. Penicillin is the drug of choice; tetracycline and erythromycin are alternatives
Pinta	Caused by *T. carateum*, almost exclusively confined to Central and South America and transmitted by either direct or indirect contact	Incubation period is usually 2–3 weeks. The primary lesion is a slowly developing subcutaneous granulomatous lesion on the trunk, leg or face usually in young adults of 15–30 years of age. Secondary lesions (pintides) are papules thata develop into plaques with scaly and centrally pigmented areas tending eventually to become depigmented and atrophic. Hyperkeratosis of the palms and soles may be seen and facial skin is extensively affected	Dark-ground microscopy and serology are needed for the diagnosis. Penicillin is the treatment of choice
Yaws (framboesia; pian; bouba)	Caused by *T. pertenue*, seen throughout Equatorial Africa, Asia, Central and South America, the South Pacific Islands and Australia, and transmitted either by contact with the early infectious lesions or via contaminated utensils or possibly insects	Incubation period is between 9 and 90 days. The primary papular stage may be of very short duration. One to three months later, painless papillomas or framboesial granulomas appear in the axilla, groin or around the body orifices. Skin lesions may spontaneously heal in about 3–6 months. Most patients then have a stage of latency which may last a lifetime, but in some, about 5 years after the primary infection, gummatous nodular ulcerative lesions may develop. Bone and cartilage lesions are frequently found, including osteitis, periostitis and dactylitis. In infected growing children 'sabre tibia' may develop. Bone involvement may result in thickening of the face on either side of the nose giving rise to a characteristic facial appearance called 'goundou'. The other type of lesion is a destructive lesion of the palate, eventually destroying parts of the nose (gangosa) and causing a 'saddle-nose' defect	Dark-field microscopy, biopsy and serology are useful. Treatment is with penicillin, erythromycin or tetracycline

SPORTS

Participation in physical activity is a huge part of everyday life, and exercise has clear benefits to both health and quality of life (Ch. 36). However, there may be risks from trauma, and sometimes from other issues such as travel, disordered eating, menstrual disturbances, and supplement use.

TRAUMA (SEE ALSO CH. 24)

Head, orofacial and other injuries are a risk in many sports; therefore the wearing of helmets, and face and mouth protection is often indicated along with other protection.

Motion sports

Head injuries and maxillofacial and dental trauma are all too common in any sport involving fast movement including any involving vehicles, roller-blading, skateboarding, snow-boarding and skiing. Helmets are mandatory and, in some instances, protection for knees and elbows and wrists is indicated.

Contact sports

Contact sports include football (soccer and rugby), boxing, martial arts (e.g. wrestling, karate and judo), gymnastics, hockey and, to a degree, there is contact in some other sports such as baseball and basketball. Injuries to the teeth and orofacial soft tissues are common, particularly in football, boxing, martial arts and hockey.

Most sports injuries affect the maxillary incisors and involve young males. In soccer and rugby, players have about a 10% chance of injury per season. Injuries may include head injury, cerebral concussion and neck injuries, which can be fatal or lead to paraplegia. Maxillofacial and dental injuries account for about 13% of the costs of all soccer injuries.

Prevention and adequate preparation are the key elements in minimizing injuries from such sports. Teaching skills such as tackling, use of appropriate equipment, safe playing areas and the wearing and utilization of properly fitted protective equipment such as helmets and mouthguards are essential. A properly fitted mouthguard may also reduce the chances of sustaining a concussion from a blow to the jaw. Mouthguards are usually made of vinyl or acrylic, and three types are available (Box 33.1).

Non-contact sports

Non-contact sports such as tennis and volleyball can also be dangerous. Custom-made protectors could offer the best protection against dental damage.

Box 33.1 Mouthguards

- Custom-made protectors – offer the best protection (vacuum custom-made and pressure laminated custom-made). Ethylene vinyl acetate (EVA) is recommended.
- Mouth-formed protectors – moulded on to the teeth ('boil and bite') and give variable protection, but are useful where orthodontic appliances are worn
- Stock protectors – cheap and easily adjusted, but less comfortable, protective or retentive

Water sports

Athletes who swim more than 6 h per week in pools chemically treated to maintain safe water quality standards, may develop tooth stains mis-termed 'swimmers calculus' and/or tooth erosion. The stains can usually be removed with professional cleaning.

Scuba divers depend on air in the form of compressed air from a tank, transmitted to the mouth by way of a regulator held in the mouth by the teeth, so that there is an airtight seal between the teeth and lips. Inability to hold the mouthpiece because of missing teeth poses a contraindication for scuba diving. Dental concerns in divers include temporomandibular joint (TMJ) and muscle pain from holding the regulator ('diver's mouth syndrome'), barotrauma and barodontalgia (from the effects of pressure changes), and the management of prostheses. Many divers experience TMJ and/or facial muscle pain or headache from the continuous jaw clenching. Mouthpieces are usually made of neoprene or silicone rubber and held in place by bite tabs that fit into the dentition at the canine and premolar area. The average dive is 30–60 min and requires constant jaw muscle effort. Extending the bite tabs to cover the molar teeth balances the weight of the regulator, and can relieve stress on the TMJ.

Barodontalgia (pain in the tooth caused by pressure changes) can arise in divers (or people in aircraft or at high altitude) if there are pulp lesions, abscesses or sinusitis. Antral pain may have a similar cause. Teeth that have been opened for endodontic treatment and temporarily sealed have been known to explode from air trapping and expansion on surfacing – mainly in deep divers using a helium–oxygen mixture. Full porcelain crowns can also shatter from relatively shallow dives of 65 feet. Raised pressure in the middle ear can occasionally cause facial palsy (baroparesis) but this typically resolves spontaneously over a few hours.

Divers cannot wear full or partial dental prostheses while diving as they may be dislodged and aspirated. To completely eliminate the possibility of dislodgement, a custom mouthpiece to obviate the chance of aspiration of the prosthesis can be made. Full arch impressions are taken with the patient holding silicone putty in the roof of the mouth until it is set, then mounted in a hinge articulator and sent to the laboratory with the silicone putty impression.

DRUG USE IN SPORTS

Sports people may wish to take drugs as medication for disease, to enhance their performance (and in doing so to gain an unfair advantage) or for 'recreational' reasons.

Anabolic steroids are available legally only by prescription, for conditions when the body produces abnormally low amounts of testosterone, such as delayed puberty and some types of impotence. They are also used to treat body wasting in, for example, patients with HIV/AIDS. Athletes (and others) may misuse anabolic (androgenic) steroids – synthetic substances related to male sex hormones – to enhance performance (and also to improve physical appearance) taken orally or injected, typically in cycles of weeks or months ('cycling'), rather than continuously.

Anabolic steroids given to adolescents may accelerate pubertal changes and cause premature skeletal maturation, halting growth. The major toxic effects include kidney and liver tumours (and jaundice), fluid retention and hypertension, increases in low-density lipoprotein (LDL) and decreases in high-density lipoprotein (HDL), severe acne, trembling, hostility and aggression, and other psychiatric effects. Gender-specific adverse effects include: for men, testicular atrophy, low sperm count, infertility, baldness, breast development and prostate cancer; and for women, facial hair growth, baldness, menstrual changes, clitoris enlargement and deepened voice. Injecting anabolic steroids is also associated with the risk of contracting or transmitting human immunodeficiency virus (HIV) or viral hepatitis.

Blood doping is the process of artificially increasing the amount of erythrocytes in an attempt to improve athletic performance. In the past this was accomplished by autologous transfusion, a practice now outlawed. Erythropoietin (EPO) stimulates erythrocyte production and equally is outlawed. It increases blood viscosity, may lead to thromboses and is one of the causes of 'sudden death syndrome' seen in occasional athletes (Table 33.1; see also www.uksport.gov.uk).

Gamma hydroxybutyrate (GHB) is also used by some bodybuilders. Drugs such as modanifil have been used to help alertness.

The International Olympic Committee permits or prohibits the use of various drugs (Table 33.2). A comprehensive list of banned substances from the World Anti-Doping Agency (WADA) is available at http://www.wada-ama.org/rtecontent/document/2006_LIST.pdf.

Some drugs are banned at all times; others are permissible when not competing but not during competition, and some are banned in some sports but not others. Banned substances can include alcohol and caffeine above a certain level. Some agents are permitted for use for certain complaints (Table 33.3). If a doctor believes that there is a good reason why a patient who is a sportsperson needs a banned substance, it is possible to issue a therapeutic use exemption (TUE) certificate.

Table 33.1 Causes of sudden death in athletes

Cardiac causes	Other causes
Anomalous origin of coronary artery	Alcohol
Aortic rupture (Marfan syndrome)	Amphetamine
Aortic stenosis	Cocaine
Coronary artery disease	Erythropoietin (EPO)
Electrical conduction system abnormalities	Head trauma
Hypertrophic cardiomyopathy	Vascular event
Myocarditis	
Obstructive cardiomyopathy	
Right ventricular dysplasia	

http://www.drfalsetti.com/faq10.html

Table 33.2 Examples of agents not permitted for use by athletes[a]

Classes not permitted	Examples not permitted
Stimulants	Amphetamine, bromantan, caffeine, cocaine, ephedrines, methyphenidate, pseudoephedrine, phenylephrine, phenylpropanolamine
Narcotics	Morphine, buprenorphine, diamorphine, pethidine, methadone
Anabolic agents	Androstenedione, clenbuterol, DHEA, methandienone, 19 nor-steroids, stanozolol, testosterone
Diuretics	Bendrofluazide, furosemide, mannitol, triamterene, hydrochlorothiazide
Peptide hormones, mimetics and analogues	Growth hormone, corticotrophin, chorionic gonadotrophin, pituitary and synthetic gonadotrophins
Blood, red cells, plasma expanders Erythropoietin (EPO)	
Corticosteroids systemically	
Beta-blockers	
Local anaesthetics, if not restricted to medically justified local injection	
Insulin	

[a]Check with governing bodies as regulations may vary, or apply under specific circumstances/conditions.
DHEA, dihydroepiandrosterone.

Table 33.3   Examples of agents permitted for use by athletes for certain complaints[a]

Complaints	Drugs permitted
Allergies	Astemizole, cetirizine, chlorphenamine, loratidine, terfenadine
Diarrhoea	Diphenoxylate, loperamide
Bacterial infections	Antibiotics (all)
Fungal infections	Amphotericin, fluconazole, nystatin, miconazole, terbinafine
Viral infections	Aciclovir, idoxuridine
Asthma	Cromoglicate, theophylline, fluticasone (under specific conditions), beclometasone, salbutamol, formoterol, terbutaline, salmeterol
Coughs and colds	Antihistamines, dextromorphan, guaiphenesin, pholcodine
Oral or ENT problems	Sprays or drops containing: betamethasone, dexamethasone, docusate, hydrocortisone, beclometasone, fluticasone, tramazoline
Eye problems	Ointments or drops containing: antazoline, betamethasone, hydrocortisone, beclometasone, chloramphenicol
Hayfever	Antihistamines
Pain and inflammation	Aspirin, acetaminophen, NSAIDs, codeine, dextropropoxyphene
Nausea ad vomiting	Cimetidine, cinnarizine, domperidone, metoclopramide, prochlorperazine

[a]Check with governing bodies as regulations may vary, or apply under specific circumstances/conditions.
ENT, ear, nose and throat; NSAIDs, non-steroidal anti-inflammatory drugs.

Smokeless tobacco

Smokeless tobacco is associated with some sports in the USA, and the public should be educated on the potentially dangerous properties of this in terms of oral keratoses and malignant change.

EATING DISORDERS

Some athletes, mainly women, in cross country, track and field, gymnastics, dancing, figure skating, volleyball and basketball may be prone to develop eating disorders (Ch. 27). Tooth erosion may be seen.

DENTAL ASPECTS

In endurance sports such as long-distance running, triathlons or cycling, athletes may consume a high amount of refined carbohydrates ('carbo-load'), as well as carbohydrate gels or drinks (sports drinks – often containing carbohydrates, electrolytes, B vitamins and an acid such as citric, malic, tartaric or phosphoric). Preventive dental care and prevention of caries and erosion is therefore important. Local anaesthesia (LA) given for dental procedures is permitted. Analgesics such as aspirin, acetaminophen and non-steroidal anti-inflammatory drugs (NSAIDs) are permitted. Opioids are banned and opiate-related analgesics are problematical: *codeine* is not on the WADA list of banned substances, and combinations such as co-codamol and co-proxamol appear acceptable. However, screening does not always differentiate adequately between the various narcotic or codeine-related compounds, so they are best avoided. Antimicrobials of all types are generally allowed. Anxiolytics may sometimes be banned. Alcohol and beta-blockers are banned in certain sports, and therefore alcohol-containing oral health care products are also best avoided. Some vitamin, herbal and nutritional supplements are banned.

Preparations used for topical oral use are generally permitted: topical corticosteroids are permitted but systemic corticosteroids are best avoided, or a TUE is required.

TRAVEL AND LEISURE

International travel is undertaken by ever-growing numbers of people for social, recreational, professional and humanitarian purposes, and can result in a variety of health risks in unfamiliar environments with variable standards of health care. Most risks can be minimized by common sense, with suitable precautions taken before, during and after travel (see UK Department of Health booklet *Health advice for travellers* (T7.1) or www.dh.gov.uk).

Travellers are more likely to be killed or injured in accidents or through violence than to be struck down by an exotic infectious disease. Assaults are common in some areas and lone travellers are particularly vulnerable. Accidents and injuries are also common in recreational waters in association with swimming, diving, sailing and other activities.

The countries to be visited and the duration of the visit are important in determining the likelihood of exposure to many problems, such as infectious agents and violence, and will influence decisions on the need for certain vaccinations or antimalarial or other medication. The behaviour of the traveller is also important: exposure to the risk of assault or accidents, or to insects, rodents or other animals, infectious agents and contaminated food and water, are often lifestyle choices. A business trip to a city in the developed world, for example, typically involves far fewer risks than a visit to remote rural areas in the tropics. For example, going outdoors in the evenings in a malaria-endemic area without precautions such as protective clothing, repellants and antimalarials is highly risky. The duration of the visit may also determine whether the traveller may be subjected to wide changes in temperature and humidity, or to other environmental factors.

FLYING

Flight phobia (fear of flying) is common, particularly since 11 September 2001. There also appears to be an increase in the use of alcohol on flights, with air rage – a form of disruptive behaviour – linked to high levels of stress and frequently precipitated by alcohol.

Dehydration is common. Cabin humidity is low, usually less than 20%, and may cause discomfort of the eyes, mouth and nose, especially in Sjögren syndrome. Fluid should be taken to prevent dehydration – non-alcoholic beverages (water and fruit juices) rather than alcohol, which contributes to dehydration.

Deep vein thrombosis (DVT; Ch. 8) can develop from prolonged immobility leading to pooling of blood, which is probably aggravated by dehydration. Most DVTs are in the calves and cause no symptoms; some cause swelling, stiffness and discomfort. They are usually reabsorbed but, occasionally, pulmonary embolism may follow with serious consequences including chest pain, dyspnoea and even death, sometimes many hours or days later. Exercise and properly fitted, graduated compression stockings specially designed for air travel may be helpful. Aspirin is often advised prophylactically for its antiplatelet activity for long-distance flights, along with ample fluids and exercise in-flight.

Jet lag – the disruption of sleep patterns and other circadian rhythms (the body's internal clock) caused by crossing multiple time zones in a short period of time – is commonplace. The adverse effects of jet lag may lead to indigestion, general malaise, insomnia, and reduced physical and mental performance. Melatonin may help resynchronize the body's internal clock.

Pain in people with ear, nose, and sinus or dental infections or after recent surgery or injury may occur where there is expansion of trapped air or gas that may be present in air-filled body cavities. This occurs especially after abdominal trauma and gastrointestinal surgery, craniofacial and ocular injuries, brain operations, and eye operations involving penetration of the eyeball. Because cabin air pressure is relatively low, the blood oxygen saturation is slightly reduced leading to mild hypoxia. Travellers with pre-existing cardiovascular or pulmonary disease or anaemia (especially sickle cell disease) are highly sensitive to hypoxia, which can be dangerous and even life-threatening.

Infections can occasionally be transmitted in aircraft as in any confined space, and influenza and tuberculosis have been transmitted between passengers on long-haul flights. Modern aircraft recirculate up to 50% of cabin air by passing it through HEPA (high-efficiency particulate air) filters, which clean recirculated cabin air, but incompletely. Viruses in particular can be recirculated. Passengers may occasionally also be infected by insects in the aircraft and there have been outbreaks of malaria in the vicinity of airports, due to the escape of transported mosquitoes ('airport malaria').

Contraindications for air travel are shown in Box 33.2.

Box 33.2 Contraindications for air travel

- Infants under 7 days old
- Women in the last 4 weeks of pregnancy (8 weeks for multiple pregnancies) and until 7 days after delivery
- People with serious medical/surgical conditions
  - Angina pectoris, recent myocardial infarction or stroke
  - Serious or acute contagious disease
  - Decompression sickness after diving
  - Raised intracranial pressure
  - Recent surgery or injury where trapped air or gas may be present
  - Severe chronic respiratory disease, breathlessness at rest or unresolved pneumothorax
  - Sickle cell disease
  - Uncontrolled hypertension of more than 200 mmHg (27 kPa) systolic pressure
  - Recent psychiatric illness

HIGH ALTITUDES

At high altitude, atmospheric pressure is lowered and the fall in oxygen pressure can lead to hypoxia as discussed above. At 1500–3500 m, exercise tolerance is impaired and ventilation is stimulated. At 3500–5500 m, there is hypoxia and altitude sickness is possible.

Rapid ascent may lead to acute hypoxia: the affected person becomes faint and may lose consciousness. Acute mountain sickness may develop after 1–6 h at high altitudes: headache is followed by anorexia, nausea and vomiting, and insomnia, fatigue, lassitude and irritability. The outcome is sometimes fatal due to the development of pulmonary and cerebral oedema.

Travellers making a rapid ascent to high altitude (>3000 m) can consider prophylactic medication (acetazolamide). Those planning to climb or trek at high altitude benefit from a period of gradual adaptation.

HOT OR HUMID CLIMATES

Exposure to hot, dry, dusty air may lead to irritation and infection of the eyes and respiratory tract, and may lead to heat exhaustion and heat stroke. Dehydration is particularly likely unless care is taken to maintain adequate fluid intake. Consumption of salt-containing food and drink helps to replenish the electrolytes in case of heat exhaustion and after excessive sweating.

Fungal skin infections (e.g. tinea) can be aggravated by heat and humidity, and a daily shower, wearing loose cotton clothing and applying talcum powder to sensitive skin areas help control their development or spread.

SUN EXPOSURE

Ultraviolet (UV) radiation from the sun includes both UVA (wavelength 315–400 nm) and UVB (280–315 nm) radiation and radiation may penetrate clear water to a depth of 1 m or more. UVB radiation is particularly intense in summer and in the 4-hour period around solar noon. Both forms of UV radiation are damaging to skin and eyes. Adverse acute effects include sunburn, particularly in light-skinned people, acute keratitis ('snow blindness') and actinic cheilitis. Long-term adverse effects can include accelerated skin ageing, skin cancers (melanoma, basal cell carcinoma and squamous carcinoma), lip cancer (squamous carcinoma), cataracts, photosensitization (to drugs such as oral contraceptives, antimalarials and antimicrobials, and to perfumes containing oil of bergamot or other citrus oils) and immune suppression, increasing the risk of infectious disease, and limiting the efficacy of vaccinations.

INFECTIONS PREVALENT IN THE DEVELOPING WORLD (APPENDIX 33.1; SEE ALSO CHs. 21, 32)

Infections are mainly acquired in the tropics, but can appear elsewhere, particularly in areas bordering the tropics and subtropics, war zones or where there are other disasters that lead to poor water and food hygiene, and the proliferation of rodents and other pests; infections are occasionally imported into developed countries (e.g. airport malaria, SARS, bird flu and swine flu).

The main infective hazards are shown in Box 33.3 but there are many others, some potentially lethal, such as dengue fever.

SEXUALLY TRANSMITTED INFECTIONS (SEE CH. 32)

INFESTATIONS (SEE CH. 21)

BLOOD-BORNE INFECTIONS

Hepatitis B and C, HIV and other agents can be transmitted by direct contact with infected blood or other body fluids, especially by inoculation. Ebola fever, Lassa fever and Marburg disease are highly contagious.

FOOD-BORNE AND WATER-BORNE HEALTH RISKS

Infections transmitted by ingesting contaminated food and water include 'travellers' diarrhoea' (caused by a wide range of viruses and bacteria), which may affect up to 80% of travellers to high-risk destinations. Food-borne infections are seen worldwide, especially from shellfish. Most diarrhoeal attacks are self-limiting, with recovery in a few days. It is important, especially for children, to avoid becoming dehydrated, so fluids (e.g. bottled, boiled or treated water, or weak tea) should be taken. If diarrhoea continues for more than 1 day, oral rehydration salt (ORS) solution should be taken. Antidiarrhoeal medicines (e.g. loperamide) are not generally recommended but may be used exceptionally. If the stools contain blood, medical help should be obtained, or a course of antibiotics may be taken (for children and pregnant women, azithromycin; other adults, ciprofloxacin).

Other hazards may include brucellosis, cholera, cryptosporidiosis, giardiasis, hepatitis A and E, legionellosis, leptospirosis, listeriosis and typhoid fever. Contaminated food may also spread worms, such as cysticercosis and echinococcosis (Ch. 21). Illness can also be caused by biological toxins found in seafood, which may be paralytic, neurotoxic or amnesic (e.g. shellfish; ciguatera toxin; scombroid or puffer fish). 'Red tides' are harmful algal blooms in water that result in production of potentially lethal neurotoxic brevetoxins, mainly domoic acid and saxitoxins. Brevetoxins cause neurotoxic shellfish poisoning (NSP). Domoic acid is a neurotoxin that causes amnesic shellfish poisoning (ASP): saxitoxin causes paralytic shellfish poisoning (PSP).

Swimming or paddling in water in the developing world may lead to schistosomiasis or other infections. Direct person-to-person contact or physical contact with contaminated surfaces in the vicinity of swimming pools and spas anywhere may spread the viruses that cause molluscum contagiosum and warts (human papillomaviruses), and fungal infections of the hair, fingernails and skin, especially tinea pedis (athlete's foot).

Contamination of spas and whirlpools can lead to infection by *Legionella*, *Pseudomonas aeruginosa* and non-tuberculous mycobacteria. Otitis externa and infections of the urinary tract, respiratory tract, wounds and cornea have also been linked to spas.

DISEASES TRANSMITTED FROM SOIL

Soil-transmitted diseases include those caused by spores, such as anthrax, tetanus and deep mycoses. Some intestinal parasites, such as ascariasis and trichuriasis, are transmitted via soil and infections may result from consumption of soil-contaminated vegetables.

ZOONOSES (DISEASES TRANSMITTED FROM ANIMALS)

A zoonosis is an infection seen in wild or domestic animals that can be transmitted to humans. Infections can be caused by bacteria, viruses, fungi, prions or parasites, which include protozoa and helminths. A partial list of animals that can carry infectious organisms that may be zoonotic is shown in Box 33.4. Rats can, for example, transmit rat-bite fever – infection by bacteria [*Streptobacillus moniliformis* (Haverhill fever) or *Spirillum minus* (sodoku)] – and a wide range of other diseases from typhus to leptospirosis.

Zoonoses include a wide range of infections (such as malaria, dengue fever, Chagas disease, rabies, brucellosis, leptospirosis and certain viral haemorrhagic fevers), which can be transmitted to humans through animal bites or from parasites such as fleas or ticks, or contact with contaminated body fluids or faeces from animals, or by consumption of foods of animal origin, particularly meat and milk products. A partial list of important zoonoses is shown in Box 33.5.

Other zoonoses might be glanders and SARS (severe acute respiratory syndrome; possibly, civet cats may spread the disease, or may catch the disease from humans).

The risk of infection can be reduced by avoiding close contact with any insects or animals – including wild, captive and domestic animals – in places where infection is likely to be present. Pets are no exception and, apart from the dangers from bites (Ch. 24), various infections can be contracted. Particular care should be taken to prevent children from approaching and handling any animals.

Box 33.4 Animals apart from humans that can transmit zoonoses

- Bats
- Birds
- Cats
- Cattle
- Chickens
- Chimpanzees
- Dogs
- Ducks
- Fish
- Fleas
- Geese
- Goats
- Horses
- Hamsters
- Insects (various)
- Monkeys
- Opossums
- Pigs
- Rabbits and hares
- Raccoons
- Rats
- Rodents
- Sheep
- Snails
- Sloths

Box 33.5 Zoonoses

- Anthrax
- Avian influenza (bird flu)
- Bolivian hemorrhagic fever
- Brucellosis
- *Borrelia* (Lyme disease and others)
- Borna virus infection
- Bovine tuberculosis
- Campylobacteriosis
- Chagas disease
- Creutzfeldt–Jakob disease (vCJD) – a transmissible spongiform encephalopathy from bovine spongiform encephalopathy or 'mad cow disease'
- Crimean–Congo haemorrhagic fever
- Cryptosporidiosis
- Cutaneous larva migrans
- Dengue fever
- Ebola
- Echinococcosis
- Hantavirus
- Hendra virus
- Henipavirus
- Korean haemorrhagic fever
- Lábrea fever
- Lassa fever
- Leishmaniasis
- Leptospirosis
- Listeriosis
- Lyme disease (see *Borrelia*)
- Lymphocytic choriomeningitis virus
- Malaria
- Marburg virus infection
- Monkey B virus
- Nipah virus
- Ocular larva migrans
- Ornithosis (psittacosis)
- Orf
- Oropouche fever
- Plague
- Q fever
- Psittacosis ('parrot fever')
- Rabies
- Rift Valley fever
- Ringworms (*Tinea canis*, mainly)
- Salmonellosis
- Sodoku
- Swine flu
- Toxoplasmosis
- Trichinosis
- Tuberculosis (badgers, cows, elephants)
- Tularemia ('rabbit fever')
- Typhus and other rickettsial diseases
- Venezuelan haemorrhagic fever
- Visceral larva migrans
- Yellow fever

FLEAS

General and clinical aspects

Fleas are parasites of humans and other animals, transmitted to those in close proximity, living mainly on the hairy parts of the body, depositing eggs that can cause an itchy rash. Rodent fleas in particular can act as vectors of life-threatening infections, such as typhus (*Rickettsia prowazeki*) (Ch. 21) and plague (*Yersinia pestis*), and have been responsible for recent outbreaks of plague in India and other areas.

General management

Improved hygiene and malathion are indicated.

LICE

General and clinical aspects

Lice infestations, which are increasing in many areas, especially in vagrants, can be of three main types:

- head lice (*Pediculosis humanis* var. capitis) infest hair and are particularly common in school children
- *Pediculosis corporis* infests the body and clothes
- *Phthirius pubis* (crab lice) infests the pubic hair area and is sexually transmitted.

Lice are transmitted by close contact or via discarded clothing and feed off the host's blood when the puncture wounds can become itchy and bleed. They can, under appropriate circumstances, also transmit disease such as typhus (*Rickettsia prowazeki*), relapsing fever (*Borrelia recurrentis*) and trench fever (*R. quintana*; Ch. 21).

General management

Treatment of lice infestation is with improved hygiene and the use of malathion and carbaryl.

TICKS

General and clinical aspects

Ticks are parasitic on various animals and may transmit various bacteria and viruses to humans (Table 33.4).

Table 33.4 Tick-borne diseases of humans

Human disease	Micro-organism	Main tick implicated	Main host	Clinical features	Treatment: remove tick and use
Babesiosis	*Babesia microti*	*Ixodes scapularis*	Mice	Malaria-like illness. Fatal in elderly or asplenia	Quinine Clindamycin Atovaquone Azithromycin
Colorado tick fever	Coltivirus	*Dermacentor andersoni* or *D. variabilis*	Deer Dog	Acute high fever	Tetracycline
Human monocyte ehrlichiosis	*Erhlichia chaffeensis*	*Amblyoma americanum*	Deer	Fever, myalgia, leuko-penia, malaise, nausea	Doxycycline
Human granulocyte ehrlichiosis	*Anaplasma phagocy-tophila*	*Ixodes scapularis*	Deer Mice	Fever, myalgia, leuko-penia, malaise, nausea	Doxycycline
Lyme disease	*Borrelia burgdorferi*	*Ixodes scapularis*	Deer	Rash, arthropathy, neuropathy	Tetracyclines, penicil-lins, cephalosporins
Powasan virus	Powasan virus	*Ixodes*	Foxes, skunks, racoons	Encephalitis	–
Relapsing fever	*Borrelia* spp.	*Ornithodorus*	Rodents	Fever	Tetracycline
Spotted fever (many dif-ferent types worldwide)	*Rickettsia rickettsiae* in USA (Rocky mountain spotted fever), other species worldwide	*Dermacentor andersoni* or *D. variabilis* in USA	Deer Dog	Fever, myalgia, rash, malaise, nausea Severe disease in G6PD deficiency	Tetracycline
Tick paralysis	No organism – tick toxin only	*Dermacentor andersoni*	Dog	Paralysis, including facial, leading to respi-ratory paralysis	–
Tularemia, or rabbit fever	*Franciscella tularensis*	*Amblyoma america-num, Dermacentor andersoni* or *D. variabilis*	Rabbit Dog	Ulcer, lymphadeno-pathy, fever	Streptomycin, genta-micin
Typhus	*Rickettsia prowazeki*				

G6PD, glucose-6-phosphate dehydrogenase.

General management

Prevention is by wearing long trousers and long-sleeved shirts in rural areas.

TRAVEL PRECAUTIONS

Since trauma is the greatest danger, travellers should always avoid areas of conflict, violence or natural disasters. Before travel it is advisable to consult: http://www.fco.gov.uk/en/travelling-and-living-overseas/travel-advice-by-country/.

Comprehensive travel and medical insurance should be obtained before travelling, checking any exclusions, and that the policy covers all intended activities.

PRECAUTIONS BEFORE TRAVELLING

Travellers should consult a travel medicine clinic or medi-cal practitioner at least 4–6 weeks before the journey, par-ticularly if vaccinations or antimalarials may be required, or if they intend to visit a developing country, especially if they intend to be in rural areas for prolonged periods (Table 33.5).

Table 33.5 Vaccines for travellers

1 Routine vaccination	Diphtheria/tetanus/pertussis (DTP) *Haemophilus influenzae* type b (Hib) Hepatitis B (HBV) Measles (MMR) Poliomyelitis (OPV or IPV)
2 Mandatory vaccination	Meningococcal meningitis (for Hajj, Umra) Yellow fever (certain countries)
3 Selective use[a]	Cholera Hepatitis A (HAV) Influenza Japanese B encephalitis Lyme disease Meningococcal meningitis Pneumococcal disease Rabies Tick-borne encephalitis Tuberculosis (BCG) Typhoid fever Yellow fever

[a]Check for country to be visited.
BCG, bacille Calmette–Guérin; IPV, inactivated poliomyelitis vaccine; OPV, oral poliomyelitis vaccine.
MMR, mumps, measter, rubella

Box 33.6 Prophylaxis against diarrhoeal disease

- Avoid cooked food kept at room temperature for several hours
- Eat only food that has been cooked thoroughly and is still hot
- Avoid uncooked food, apart from fruit and vegetables that can be peeled or shelled, and avoid fruits with damaged skins
- Avoid dishes containing raw or undercooked eggs
- Avoid food or ice cream bought from street vendors
- Boil unpasteurized (raw) milk before consumption
- Boil drinking water if its safety is doubtful. A certified, well-maintained filter and/or a disinfectant agent can also be used
- Avoid ice unless it has been made from safe water
- Avoid brushing the teeth with unsafe water. Bottled or packaged cold drinks are usually safe provided that they are sealed
- Avoid contaminated recreational water, particularly sewage-polluted sea water or fresh water in lakes and rivers, as well as water in swimming pools and spas

USEFUL WEBSITES

http://www.fco.gov.uk/en/travelling-and-living-overseas/
http://www.pponline.co.uk/
http://www.basem.co.uk/
http://www.sportsmedicine.com/
http://www.traveldoctor.co.uk
http://www.emedicine.com/sports/index.shtml
http://www.ncdc.gov/travel/
http://www.who.int/CSR/don/en
http://www.travax.nhs.uk
http://www.uksport.gov.uk

Infants and young children, pregnant women, older people, the disabled and those who have pre-existing health problems may need special precautions.

WHILE TRAVELLING

Avoiding contact with disease-producing organisms is best achieved by: avoiding their habitat (e.g. swamps, jungles); avoiding contact with animals; using barrier precautions (e.g. wearing long sleeves and trousers); avoiding insect bites (e.g. using insect repellants); avoiding exposure to animal excreta; and maintaining high levels of food, water and personal hygiene. Avoid food that could be contaminated; this is best achieved by drinking and using bottled water, and by eating freshly cooked meat or fish. Use of chlorine and other disinfectants controls most viruses and bacteria in water; however, parasites such as *Giardia* and *Cryptosporidium* are highly resistant to routine disinfection, but they are inactivated by ozone or eliminated by filtration. Antimicrobial prophylaxis against diarrhoeal disease is not recommended; precautions are shown in Box 33.6.

Avoid direct contact with blood and body fluids by avoiding the use of potentially contaminated needles and syringes for injection or any other medical or cosmetic procedure that penetrates the skin (including acupuncture, body piercing and tattooing), and by avoiding transfusion of unsafe blood.

ON RETURNING FROM TRAVELLING

On return, travellers should have a medical examination: if they suffer from a chronic disease, such as cardiovascular disease, diabetes mellitus or chronic respiratory disease; if they experience illness, particularly fever, persistent diarrhoea, vomiting, jaundice, urinary disorders, skin disease or genital infection; if they consider they have been exposed to a serious infectious disease; or if they have spent more than 3 months in a developing country.

PETS

Bites, scratches and infections are discussed above and in Chs. 21 and 24.

FURTHER READING

Antoun, J.S., Lee, K.H., 2008. Sports-related maxillofacial fractures over an 11-year period. J Oral Maxillofac Surg 66, 504–508.

Barnett, F., 2003. Prevention of sports-related dental trauma: the role of mouthguards. Pract Proced Aesthet Dent 15, 391–394.

Brewer, P.A., Barry, M., 2002. Survey of web-based health care information for prospective cruise line passengers. J Travel Med 9, 194–197.

Cossar, J.H., Wilson, E., Kennedy, D.H., Walker, E., 2003. A comparison of travel related ID admissions in Glasgow: (1985; 1998/99). Scott Med J 48, 49–51.

Foster, M., Readman, P., 2009. Sports dentistry – what's it all about. Dent Update 36, 135–144.

Gassner, R., Tuli, T., Hachl, O., Rudisch, A., Ulmer, H., 2003. Craniomaxillofacial trauma: a 10 year review of 9,543 cases with 21,067 injuries. J Craniomaxillofac Surg 31, 51–61.

Horvath, L.L., Murray, C.K., DuPont, H.L., 2003. Travel health information at commercial travel websites. J Travel Med 10, 272–278.

Kirkpatrick, B.D., Alston, W.K., 2003. Current immunizations for travel. Curr Opin Infect Dis 16, 369–374.

Kolars, J.C., 2002. Rules of the road: a consumer's guide for travelers seeking health care in foreign lands. J Travel Med 9, 198–201.

Lang, B., Pohl, Y., Filippi, A., 2002. Knowledge and prevention of dental trauma in team handball in Switzerland and Germany. Dent Traumatol 18, 329–334.

Lee, K.H., Steenberg, L.J., 2008. Equine-related facial fractures. Int J Oral Maxillofac Surg 37, 999–1002.

Lo Re 3rd, V., Gluckman, S.J., 2003. Fever in the returned traveler. Am Fam Physician 68, 1343–1350.

Macpherson, A., Spinks, A., 2008. Bicycle helmet legislation for the uptake of helmet use and prevention of head injuries. Cochrane Database Syst Rev 3, CD005401.

McInnes, R.J., Williamson, L.M., Morrison, A., 2002. Unintentional injury during foreign travel: a review. J Travel Med 9, 297–307.

McIntosh, A.S., Janda, D., 2003. Evaluation of cricket helmet performance and comparison with baseball and ice hockey helmets. Br J Sports Med 37, 325–330.

Muller-Bolla, M., Lupi-Pegurier, L., Pedeutour, P., Bolla, M., 2003. Orofacial trauma and rugby in France: epidemiological survey. Dent Traumatol 19, 183–192.

Newsome, P.R.H., Tran, D.C., Cooke, M.S., 2001. The role of the mouthguard in the prevention of sports-related dental injuries; a review. Int J Paediat Dent 11, 396–404.

Papakosta, V., Koumoura, F., Mourouzis, C., 2008. Maxillofacial injuries sustained during soccer: incidence, severity and risk factors. Dent Traumatol 24, 193–196.

Solomon, T., 2003. Exotic and emerging viral encephalitides. Curr Opin Neurol 16, 411–418.

Spira, A.M., 2003. Assessment of travellers who return home ill. Lancet 361, 1459–1469.

Spira, A.M., 2003. Preparing the traveller. Lancet 361, 1368–1381.

Zazryn, T.R., Finch, C.F., McCrory, P.A., 2003. 16 year study of injuries to professional boxers in the state of Victoria, Australia. Br J Sports Med 37, 321–324.

Appendix 33.1 Infections prevalent in the developing world (see also Appendix 21.4)

Disease	Micro-organism or parasite	Infection via	Consequence	Areas of greatest risk	Prevention
Anthrax	*Bacillus anthracis*	Contact with contaminated products from, or soil infected by, animals (mainly cattle, goats, sheep)	Untreated infections may spread to regional lymph nodes and bloodstream, and may be fatal	Central Asia and worldwide	Avoid direct contact with soil and products of animal origin (e.g. souvenirs from animal skins). Vaccine available for people at high risk
Arboviruses	Many different arboviruses	Transmitted to humans by arthropods, mostly mosquitoes, sandflies or ticks	Fever, with rashes arthralgias, lymphadenopathy, CNS involvement or haemorrhagic features	Worldwide, especially Latin America, the southern USA, South-East Asia and Africa	Avoid insect bites (wear protective clothing and use insect repellants), and use prophylactic measures such as vaccination
Brucellosis	*Brucella* species	From cattle (*Brucella abortus*), dogs (*B. canis*), pigs (*B. suis*), or sheep and goats (*B. melitensis*), by direct contact with animals or unpasteurized (raw) milk or cheese	Continuous or intermittent fever and malaise	Worldwide, mainly in developing countries and around the Mediterranean	Avoid unpasteurized milk and milk products and direct contact with animals, particularly cattle, goats and sheep
Cholera	*Vibrio cholerae* bacteria, serogroups 01 and 0139	Ingestion of food or water contaminated directly or indirectly by faeces or vomit of infected persons	An acute enteric disease varying in severity	Developing countries, particularly in Africa and Asia, and to lesser extent in central and south America	Oral cholera vaccines. All care should be taken to avoid consumption of potentially contaminated food, drink and drinking water
Dengue	Dengue virus – a flavivirus	*Aedes aegypti* mosquito, which bites during day. There is no direct person-to-person transmission. Monkeys act as a reservoir host in South-East Asia and West Africa.	Dengue fever – an acute febrile illness, macular skin rash and muscle pains ('breakbone fever') Dengue haemorrhagic fever Dengue shock syndrome	Tropical and subtropical regions of Central and South America, and South and South-East Asia, and Africa below 600 m	Avoid mosquito bites
Diphtheria	Ch. 21				
Encephalitis viruses	Togaviridae or flaviviruses	Mosquito bites	Aseptic meningitis or encephalitis	Worldwide	Avoid bites of mosquitoes
Filariasis	Nematodes (roundworms) of family Filarioidea	Lymphatic filariasis transmitted through bite of mosquitoes. Onchocerciasis transmitted through bite of blackflies	Lymphatic filariasis and onchocerciasis (river blindness)	Lymphatic filariasis throughout sub-Saharan Africa and South-East Asia. Onchocerciasis in West and Central Africa, Central and South America	Avoid bites of mosquitoes and/or blackflies
Giardiasis	Protozoan parasite *Giardia lamblia*	Ingestion of *Giardia* cysts in water (unfiltered drinking and recreational waters) contaminated by faeces of humans or animals	Anorexia, chronic diarrhoea, abdominal cramps, bloating, frequent loose greasy stools, fatigue and weight loss	Worldwide	Avoid ingesting any potentially contaminated (i.e. unfiltered) drinking water or recreational water
Haemophilus meningitis	*Haemophilus influenzae* type b (Hib) bacteria	Direct contact with infected person	Meningitis in infants and young children; may also cause epiglottitis, osteomyelitis, pneumonia, sepsis and septic arthritis	Worldwide where vaccination against Hib is not practised	Vaccination against Hib

Haemorrhagic fevers, Crimean–Congo haemorrhagic fever (CCHF), dengue, Ebola and Marburg haemorrhagic fevers, Lassa fever, Rift Valley fever (RVF) and yellow fever	Most haemorrhagic fevers, including dengue and yellow fever, caused by flaviviruses; Ebola and Marburg caused by filoviruses, CCHF by bunyaviruses, Lassa fever by arenavirus, RVF by phlebovirus	Most viruses transmitted by mosquitoes. Ebola or Marburg viruses acquired by direct contact with body fluids of infected patients. CCHF transmitted by ticks. Lassa fever virus carried by rodents and transmitted by excreta, either as aerosol or direct contact. RVF acquired either by mosquito bite or direct contact with blood or tissues of infected animals	Sudden onset of fever, malaise, headache and myalgia followed by pharyngitis, vomiting, diarrhoea, rash and haemorrhages. Fatal in over 50%	Tropics and subtropical regions. Ebola and Marburg haemorrhagic fevers and Lassa fever in sub-Saharan Africa. CCHF in steppe regions of central Asia and Central Europe, as well as in tropical and southern Africa. RVF in Africa and Saudi Arabia. Other viral haemorrhagic fevers in Central and South America	Avoid mosquitoes, ticks and rodents
Hantavirus diseases – haemorrhagic fever with renal syndrome (HFRS) and hantavirus pulmonary syndrome (HPS)	Hantaviruses – family bunyaviruses. HPS caused by Sin Nombre virus (SNV)	Direct contact with the faeces, saliva or urine of infected rodents such as deer, mice or by inhalation of the virus	Vascular endothelium is damaged, leading to vascular permeability, hypotension, haemorrhages and shock. Impaired renal function with oliguria characterizes HFRS; fatal in up to 15%. Respiratory distress due to pulmonary oedema in HPS; fatal in up to 50%	Worldwide	Avoid exposure to rodents and their excreta
Hepatitis viruses	Ch. 9				
Human immunodeficiency virus (HIV)	Ch. 20				
Influenza	Ch. 15				
Japanese encephalitis	Japanese encephalitis (JE) virus – a flavivirus	Various mosquitoes of the genus *Culex*. Infects pigs and wild birds as well as humans	Fever, headache or aseptic meningitis. Severe cases rapid onset with headache, high fever and meningeal signs. May be neurological sequelae. Approximately 50% of severe cases are fatal	Asia, especially monsoon areas of South-East Asia	Vaccination. Avoid mosquito bites
Legionellosis	Ch. 15				
Leishmaniasis	Ch. 21				
Leptospirosis	Spirochaetes of the genus *Leptospira*	Contact between the skin or mucosae and water, wet soil or vegetation contaminated by urine of animals, notably rats	Sudden onset of fever, headache, myalgia, chills, conjunctival suffusion and rash. May progress to meningitis, haemolytic anaemia, jaundice, haemorrhages and hepatorenal failure	Worldwide. Most common in tropics	Avoid contact with rodents and swimming or wading in contaminated waters, including canals, ponds, rivers, streams and swamps
Listeriosis	*Listeria monocytogenes*	*Listeria* multiplies readily in refrigerated foods that have been contaminated, unpasteurized milk, soft cheeses, vegetables and prepared meat products	Meningoencephalitis and/or septicaemia in adults and newborn infants. In pregnant women, causes fever and abortion. Newborn infants, pregnant women, the elderly and immunocompromised individuals are particularly susceptible. In others, the disease may be limited to a mild acute febrile episode. In pregnancy, transmission to fetus may lead to stillbirth, septicaemia or meningitis	Worldwide	Avoid unpasteurized milk and milk products

(Continued)

Appendix 33.1 Infections prevalent in the developing world—cont'd

Disease	Micro-organism or parasite	Infection via	Consequence	Areas of greatest risk	Prevention
Lyme borreliosis	Ch. 21				
Malaria	*Vivax, ovale, malariae* or *falciparum*	Various mosquitoes	Signs of severe malaria include loss of consciousness, fever, jaundice, anaemia, renal impairment, pulmonary oedema, circulatory collapse	Developing world	Avoid mosquito bites. Take malaria prophylaxis
Meningococcal disease	*Neisseria meningitidis*	Humans	Meningitis	Saudi Arabia during Hadj	Vaccination is indicated
Paratyphoid fever	*Salmonella cholerae-suis* or *Salmonella enteritidis*	Similar to typhoid, but less severe			
Plague	*Yersinia pestis*	Fleas from rats to other animals and to humans. Direct person-to-person transmission only in the case of pneumonic plague, when respiratory droplets may transfer the infection from the patient to close contacts	Bubonic plague results from the bite of infected fleas. Lymphadenitis develops in the draining lymph nodes, with the regional nodes swelling and suppurating – characteristic buboes. Untreated, 50–60% of cases of bubonic plague are fatal. Septicaemic plague may develop from bubonic plague or occur in the absence of lymphadenitis. Dissemination of the infection in the bloodstream results in meningitis, endotoxic shock and disseminated intravascular coagulation. Pneumonic plague results from second-ary infection of lungs following dissemination from other sites producing severe pneumonia. Direct infection of others may result. Untreated septicae-mic and pneumonic plague are invariably fatal	Central, eastern and southern Africa, South America, western North America and Asia	Avoid contact with rodents dead or alive
Poliomyelitis	Ch. 13				
Q fever	*Coxiella burnetii*	Excreta or milk of cattle, sheep and goats	Fever, headache, malaise, myalgia, sore throat, chills, sweats, cough, nausea, vomiting, diarrhoea, abdominal pain and chest pain	Worldwide	Avoid contact with excreta or unpasteurized milk
Rabies	Rhabdovirus of genus *Lyssavirus*	Bite of an infected animal such as a dog, fox or bat	Acute encephalomyelitis, which is almost invariably fatal. Initial signs include sense of apprehension, headache, fever, malaise and sensory changes around bite site. Excitability, hallucinations and aerophobia common, followed in some cases by fear of water (hydrophobia) due to spasms of swallowing muscles, progressing to delirium, convulsions and death	Worldwide, especially in develop-ing countries	Avoid contact with both wild and domestic animals, includ-ing dogs and cats. Vaccination
Schistosomiasis (bilharziasis)	Parasitic blood flukes (trematodes), of which the most important are *Schistosoma mansoni, S. japonicum* and *S. haematobium*	Infection occurs in fresh water containing larval forms (cercariae) of schistosomes, which develop in snails infected as a result of excretion of eggs in human urine or faeces. The free-swimming larvae enter the skin of individuals swimming or wading in water	*S. mansoni* and *S. japonicum* cause hepatic and intestinal signs. *S. haematobium* causes urinary dysfunction	*S. mansoni* in sub-Saharan Africa, the Arabian peninsula, Brazil, Suriname and Venezuela. *S. japonicum* in China, Indonesia and Philippines (not Japan). *S. haematobium* in sub-Saharan Africa and eastern Mediterranean areas	Avoid swimming or wading in fresh water in endemic areas

Disease	Organism	Transmission	Clinical features	Distribution	Prevention
Tick-borne encephalitis (spring–summer encephalitis)	Tick-borne encephalitis (TBE) virus – a flavivirus	Bite of infected ticks	Influenza-like illness, with a second phase of fever in 10% of cases. Encephalitis develops during the second phase and may result in paralysis or death	Below 1000 m in Eastern Europe, particularly Austria, Baltic States, Czech Republic, Hungary and Russian Federation	Avoid bites by ticks by wearing long trousers and closed footwear when hiking or camping in endemic areas
Trypanosomiasis African trypanosomiasis (sleeping sickness)	Protozoan parasites Trypanosoma brucei (T. b.) gambiense and T. b. rhodesiense	Bite of infected tsetse flies	T. b. gambiense causes chronic illness after a prolonged incubation period of weeks or months. T. b. rhodesiense causes a more acute illness, with onset a few days or weeks after the infected bite; often, a striking inoculation chancre. Initial signs include headache, insomnia, enlarged lymph nodes, anaemia and rash. In late stages, there is loss of weight and involvement of CNS. Without treatment, it is invariably fatal	T. b. gambiense present in foci in tropical countries of western and Central Africa T. b. rhodesiense in East Africa, extending south as far as Botswana	Avoid contact with tsetse flies since bites are difficult to avoid because tsetse flies bite during the day, can penetrate clothing and are not repelled by insect repellents
Trypanosomiasis American trypanosomiasis (Chagas disease)	Protozoan parasite Trypanosoma cruzi	Blood-sucking triatomine bugs ('kissing bugs'). Also by transfusion if blood from infected donor	Chronic illness, progressive myocardial damage leading to cardiac arrhythmias and dilatation, and mega-oesophagus and megacolon	Mexico, Central and South America (to central Argentina and Chile)	Avoid exposure to blood-sucking bugs. Use bednets in houses and camps
Tuberculosis	Ch. 15				
Typhoid fever	Salmonella typhi	Contaminated water or food	Fever, rash, splenomegaly and leukopenia, and intestinal bleeding or perforation	Worldwide, especially North and West Africa, South Asia and Peru	Vaccination. Avoid contaminated water or food
Typhus fever (epidemic louse-borne typhus)	Rickettsia prowazekii	Human body louse	Sudden fever, headache, chills, prostration, coughing and muscular pain. After 5–6 days, a macular skin eruption (dark spots) on the upper trunk and then rest of the body except face, palms or soles. Case fatality rate up to 40%	Colder (i.e. mountainous) regions of Central and East Africa, Central and South America and Asia. In recent years, most outbreaks have taken place in Burundi; Ethiopia and Rwanda	Avoid infestation by body lice
West Nile fever	West Nile virus	Bite of an infected mosquito, and can infect people, horses, many types of birds and some other animals	Rarely, severe sometimes fatal encephalitis	Africa, USA	Avoid mosquito bites
Yellow fever	Yellow fever virus – an arbovirus of the flavivirus genus	Bite of Aedes aegypti mosquitoes Yellow fever virus infects humans and monkeys	Acute illness characterized initially by fever, chills, headache, muscular pain, anorexia, nausea and/or vomiting, with bradycardia. About 15% progress to second phase, with fever resurgence, jaundice, abdominal pain, vomiting and haemorrhages. 50% die after 10–14 days	Tropical areas of Africa and Central and South America below 2500m	Vaccination. Avoid mosquito bites during the day as well as at night

CNS, central nervous system.

INTRODUCTION

GENERAL ASPECTS

Substance or chemical dependence or abuse (drug misuse) covers misuse of a range of mind-altering substances. Addiction or dependence are significant problems worldwide, and these substances affect health, social interactions, work and study, and can result in financial difficulties and problems with the law. In some countries, use or possession may result in serious punishments – even execution.

Substance abuse is increasingly common in many parts of the world: In the USA, the highest rates of illicit drug use are, in males, in entertainment, food preparation and service, cleaning services and construction; and in females, in workers involved in food preparation, social workers, and the legal professions, including lawyers and legal assistants. Abuse of alcohol is highest among construction workers, car mechanics, food preparation workers, light truck drivers and labourers. Unmarried workers or those having three or more jobs in the previous 5 years report about twice the rate of illicit drug and heavy alcohol use as married workers or those who had two or fewer jobs.

The lowest rates of illicit drug use are in workers in occupations that require public trust, such as police officers, teachers and child care workers. One USA study of medical personnel, however, found over half had tried marijuana or cocaine recreationally, or opioids or tranquillizers for self-treatment. More than a half of UK dental students in 2003 had used cannabis and over one-third admitted other illicit drug use. Alcohol abuse is also relatively common among doctors and dentists. Clinicians in the UK with such issues can receive support from the Practitioner Health Programme initiated by NCAS (National Clinical Assessment Service; http://www.php.nhs.uk/).

The 2007/08 British Crime Survey and an annual survey of school pupils in England 2007 and 2008 showed a number of trends relating to drug use (Box 34.1). In 2008, 1 in 20 of people aged 15–16 in UK had used cocaine.

Drug abuse causes central nervous system (CNS) effects, which produce changes in the mind, behaviour, thoughts and mood, levels of awareness or perceptions and sensations. It is defined as self-administration without any medical indication and despite adverse medical and social consequences, and in a manner that deviates from the cultural norm and is harmful.

Drugs of misuse may be obtained legally from a doctor or chemist, or may be illicitly obtained, and may be taken orally, inhaled or injected into the skin, muscle or a vein. Drugs abused include stimulants (uppers), depressants (hypnotic/sedatives/downers), hallucinogens (psychedelics), analgesics and anabolic steroids (Table 34.1).

The drugs most commonly abused include alcohol, amphetamine/amfetamines, barbiturates, benzodiazepines, cannabis, cocaine, ecstasy, methaqualone, nicotine and opium alkaloids. New agents are appearing frequently, often in an attempt to circumnavigate the law and often under a variety of names; for example, benzylpiperazine (BZP; A2, legal E, legal XTC, legal high, Jax, London Underground, Pep twisted or Pep love) appeared recently as an alternative to ecstasy but almost inevitably it caused serious adverse effects (see http://www.deadiversion.usdoj.gov/drugs_concern/index.html).

Substance *dependence* is present when at least three of the conditions listed in Box 34.2 apply.

Club drugs are those used by teenagers and young adults who are part of a nightclub, bar, trance or rave scene – night-long dances, often held in warehouses (Table 34.2). Club drugs in high doses can cause a sharp rise in body temperature (malignant hyperthermia) leading to muscle breakdown and kidney and cardiovascular system failure (see http://www.whitehousedrugpolicy.gov/streetterms/Default.asp).

Date rape drugs such as gamma-hydroxybutyric acid (GHB), Rohypnol and ketamine are CNS depressants used because they are often colourless, tasteless and odourless, and can be added to beverages and ingested unknowingly by the victim, with the intention of causing loss of inhibitions and memory. They can readily cause unconsciousness.

Use of some of these drugs is illegal and being found in possession of these or, particularly, if there is any intention of dealing (supplying), there can be criminal charges (Table 34.3). Illegal drugs are classified in the UK under the Misuse of Drugs Act 1971 into three classes: A, B and C, depending on how dangerous they are to health, a classification which can only be changed and added to by the Home Secretary.

COMPLICATIONS ASSOCIATED WITH CHEMICAL DEPENDENCE

The drugs used mimic brain neurotransmitters but, in contrast to natural neurotransmitters (which are released at the right location, at the correct time and are quickly removed), abused drugs end up at the wrong location, are removed slowly and can produce adverse effects..

There may be intense drug dependence (or psychological addiction) and severe psychological or physical effects (physical addiction) if a drug of abuse is stopped (withdrawal syndrome). Drug use may also lead to health and social problems, with serious mental, physical and legal sequelae (Fig. 34.1).

Box 34.1 Drug use in 2007 / 2008

- A general downward trend in drug use since 2001 among 11–15-year-olds
- One third had smoked tobacco
- One half had drunk alcohol
- Cannabis use among this age group had continued to fall since 2001
- Most young people did not feel that drug use is acceptable behaviour within their age group
- Use of solvents and glues was reportedly increased

Table 34.1 Main groups of substances abused

	Stimulants (uppers)	Depressants (hypnotic/ sedatives /downers)	Hallucinogens (psychedelics)	Analgesics	Anabolic steroids
Actions	Speed brain activity	Slow brain activity	Distort brain activity	Decrease pain	Promote growth and muscle
Examples	Amphetamine/ amfetamine, caffeine, cocaine, crack, dextroamphetamine/ amfetamine, diethylpropion, methylphenidate, nicotine, phenmetrazine, tobacco	*Anxiolytics:* alprazolam, benzodiazepines, chlorazepate, meprobamate *Barbiturate Ethanol (alcohol) Inhalants:* amyl nitrite, butyl nitrite, enflurane, ether, halothane, isoflurane, nitrous oxide, petrol, solvents (various)	Lysergic acid diethylamide (LSD), mescaline (peyote), methyl-dimethoxy amphetamine/amfetamine (STP; DOM), methylene dioxyamphetamine (MDA), 3,4-methylenedioxy-methamphetamine (MDMA; ecstasy), phencyclidine (PCP), psilocybin *Cannabinoids:* marijuana	*Opioids:* codeine, fentanyl, heroin, hydrocodone, lomotil, meperidine, methyl-phenyl-tetrahydropyridine (MPTP), morphine, oxycodone, propoxyphene	Nandrolone (Deca-Durabolin), Sustanon 250, Dianabol, Anavar, stanozolol
Main CNS and adverse effects	Exhilaration, energy, reduced appetite, weight loss, alertness; rapid or irregular heart beat; raised heart rate, blood pressure, metabolism	Feeling of well-being; lowered inhibitions; slowed pulse and breathing; lowered blood pressure; poor concentration, confusion, fatigue; impaired coordination, memory, judgement; respiratory depression and arrest	Altered states of perception and feeling; nausea, psychoses, persisting perception disorder (flashbacks)	Pain relief, euphoria, drowsiness, nausea, confusion, constipation, sedation, respiratory depression and arrest, unconsciousness, coma	No intoxication effects

CNS, central nervous system.

Box 34.2 Features suggesting substance dependence

- Some of the symptoms of the disturbance must have persisted for at least 1 month or have recurred repeatedly over a longer period of time
- Substances are often taken in larger amounts or over longer period than intended
- Persistent desire or one or more unsuccessful efforts to cut down or control substance use
- Excessive time is spent in activities to obtain the substance (e.g. theft), taking the substance (e.g. chain smoking) or recovering from its effects
- Important social, occupational or recreational activities are given up or reduced because of substance misuse
- There is continued substance use despite knowledge of having persistent or recurrent social, psychological or physical problems caused by use of the substance
- Growing tolerance – greatly increased amounts of the substance (> 500% increase) are needed to achieve the desired effect, or greatly diminished effect with continued use of the same amount
- Characteristic withdrawal symptoms
- Substances often taken to relieve or avoid withdrawal symptoms

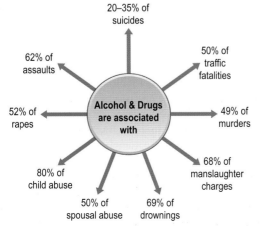

Fig. 34.1 Outcomes from substance abuse

Intravenous use and mixing drugs (polydrug use) are particularly hazardous; those who misuse drugs also not uncommonly misuse several substances, including alcohol and tobacco, and may neglect their health – general and oral. Drugs bought on the street are also not necessarily pure, and are frequently adulterated, often with unknown ingredients that may be dangerous in their own right, complicating the whole picture of drug misuse.

Heroin and cocaine are especially dangerous. Tobacco and alcohol also cause significant harm, but cannabis appears to be less harmful in general.

CLINICAL FEATURES

Signs and symptoms that may indicate drug addiction include behavioural and social features as well as health aspects (Table 34.4).

681

Table 34.2 Current popular club drugs

Street name	Constituents	Effects	Comments
Cat	Methcathinone	Produces a cocaine-like high with hallucinations similar to mescaline	Analogue of methamphetamine
China white	Beta-hydroxy methylfentanyl	6000 times the potency of natural heroin. Responsible for many narcotic overdose deaths	Analogue of fentanyl
Double stack or PMA	Paramethoxyamphetamine	Does not produce the pleasurable MDMA effects, so users take more drug. Dramatic rise in body temperature in excess of 109°F. Death from hyperthermia	Analogue of methamphetamine
DXM	Dextromethorphan	Hallucinations and a heavy 'stoned' feeling in users but no desirable ecstasy effects	Often passed off as ecstasy. Found in OTC cold remedies
Ecstasy	MDMA	Resembles methamphetamine, but also produces mild hallucinations and a feeling of emotional closeness to other people	The most sought-after club drug
Eve	3,4-Methylenedioxy-ethamphetamine (MDE)	Does *not* produce the ecstasy feeling of emotional closeness	Analogue of ecstasy
GBL (gamma-butyrolactone and 1,4-butanediol)	Gamma-butyrolactone and 1,4-butanediol. Together they convert to GHB	Taken alone, or especially when mixed, or with alcohol, produces stupor, vomiting and coma	Related to GHB. Sold over the internet to avoid laws against GHB
GHB, super-G, liquid G, liquid ecstasy	Gamma-hydroxybutyric acid	Taken alone, or especially when mixed with alcohol, produces a stupor, vomiting and coma	A clear, odourless liquid with a slight salty taste. Originally thought to be a human growth hormone, it was abused by body builders until banned in 1991 by FDA
Ice	Methamphetamine	Produces a 10-h high	A smokable form of recrystallized methamphetamine similar to crack
Nexus or 2C-B	4-Bromo-2,5-dimethoxyphenethylamine	Produces strong, ecstasy-like feelings of closeness and sexual enhancement	Phenylethylamine analogue of powerful hallucinatory drug DOB (4-bromo-2,5-dimethoxyamphetamine)
Rohypnol	Flunitrazepam	Mixed with alcohol, as a 'date rape' drug	Analogue of diazepam but ten times as powerful
Special K	Ketamine	Produces hallucinations and stupor and is highly addictive	Analogue of phencyclidine (PCP)
YABA	Methamphetamine	Produces a 10-h high	Ultrapure form of methamphetamine often combined with caffeine

FDA, US Food and Drug Administration; MDMA, 3,4-methylenedioxy-methamphetamine; OTC, over the counter.

There can be serious medical and behavioural consequences affecting both the user (and any fetus) and others in the community from the use or misuse of drugs. Drug misuse is particularly troublesome to the community because of the amount of crime committed to obtain money to buy the drugs. Assaults, theft and prostitution are often used to fund the drug habit. Maxillofacial injuries and sexually transmitted and other infectious diseases are thus common consequences. Intravenous injection is frequently used for misuse of drugs, often with filthy injection technique, sharing of needles or syringes (with the risk of blood-borne infections) and even use of water from a lavatory pan to dissolve the drug. Infective endocarditis and consequent cardiac lesions may be a consequence of infected injections. Venous thromboses are common, making intravenous injection difficult. Viral hepatitis (particularly B, C, D and others), chronic liver disease, human immunodeficiency virus (HIV) and other blood-borne agents are common consequences of intravenous drug abuse or drug 'snorting'.

Care should be taken with any patient who has subjective symptoms with no objective evidence of the disorder; makes a self-diagnosis and requests a specific drug, especially a psychoactive agent; appears to have a dramatic but unexpected complaint such as trigeminal neuralgia requiring potent analgesics; firmly rejects treatments that exclude psychoactive drugs; has no interest in the diagnosis or investigations, or refuses a second opinion.

Recognition of abuse in a health care worker may include, in addition to the above, patient and staff complaints about deteriorating attitude and behaviour, worsening personal and professional isolation, excessive amounts of time spent near a drug supply, heavy 'wastage' of drugs, sloppy record-keeping, suspect ledger entries and drug shortages; inappropriate prescriptions or insistence on personal administration of injected narcotics to patients.

Table 34.3 Main drug classes and penalties for possession and supply

	UK MISUSE OF DRUGS ACT CLASS		
	A	**B**	**C**
Danger to health	Considered most dangerous	Considered dangerous	Considered least harmful
Drugs	Cocaine (including crack; nicknamed charlie, coke, snow) Dicanol Heroin (nicknamed smack, H, gear, scag, brown) LSD (lysergic acid diethylamide; nicknamed acid, trips, blotters, tabs) Magic mushrooms (nicknamed liberties, shrooms) MDMA (3,4-methylenedioxy-methamphetamine/ amfetamine; nicknamed ecstasy, E, pills, XTC, disco biscuits, Mitsubishis, Rolexs, dolphins) Mescalin Methylamphetamine (crystal meth) Methadone Morphine Opium PCP (phencyclidine; nicknamed angel dust) Pethadine Poppy straw Psilocybin STP (amphetamine/amfetamine; nicknamed serenity, tranquillity and peace)	Amphetamine/amfetamine (an ingredient of ecstasy; nicknamed speed, whizz, dexies) Barbiturates Cannabis, cannabis resin and cannabinol (marijuana, grass, pot, weed) Codeine (in concentrations above 2.5%) DF118 (dihydrocodeine) Ritalin	Anabolic steroids (nicknamed roids) Benzodiazepines including valium and Rohypnol (nicknamed roofies and sometimes referred to as date-rape drugs) GHB (gamma-hydroxybutrate; nicknamed liquid ecstasy and sometimes referred to as date-rape drugs) Ketamine (nicknamed special K, vitamin K, green) Methaqualone
Maximum penalties: – Possession	7 years in prison and/or a fine	5 years in prison and/or a fine	2 years in prison and/or a fine
– Supply	Life in prison and/or a fine	14 years in prison and/or a fine	5 years in prison and/or a fine

Table 34.4 Features possibly suggesting drug misuse

Presentation	Features	Behaviour	Social history
Specifically requests drugs of misuse No fixed abode	Progressive deterioration in personal appearance and hygiene, deterioration of handwriting, alcohol on the breath, nicotine on fingers, the smell of marijuana, tremors, avoidance of eye contact, constricted or dilated pupils, a history of liver disease, wearing long sleeves when inappropriate Puncture marks, scars or pigmentation over veins Jaundice	Personality change – mood swings, anxiety, depression, lack of impulse control, suicidal thoughts or gestures, and deteriorating interpersonal relations with rare admittance or acceptance of blame for errors or oversights. Unusually elated, drowsy or restless	Frequent changes of health carers Family disruption Frequent changes in or loss of employment Self-discharge from health care History of offences to obtain money Work absenteeism, frequent disappearances from work, improbable excuses and frequent or long trips to the lavatory or stockroom where drugs are kept Unreliability in keeping appointments, meeting deadlines and work performance

GENERAL MANAGEMENT

Common management difficulties are behavioural problems including irregular health care, poor attendance and compliance, effects of trauma and hazards of cross-infection with hepatitis viruses, HIV and, increasingly, tuberculosis (TB). Drug misusers who collapse, become hyperthermic, drowsy or panicky may well need emergency care (Table 34.5).

Many drugs of abuse can alter behaviour or interact with drugs used for medical or dental purposes (Ch. 29). A further major problem with chemically dependent patients is their poor compliance – the failure to follow directions either during or after health care procedures. There may also be the possibility of communicable diseases: the lifestyle of some drug addicts is often such that sexually transmitted, TB or other serious infections can be a complication, and there is the frequent risk of maxillofacial and other injuries during assaults or fights.

There can therefore be substantial difficulties in interactions between health care workers and drug users. However, it is unethical to withhold treatment from any patient on the basis of a moral judgement that the patient's activities or lifestyle might have contributed to the condition for which treatment was being sought.

MAIN GROUPS OF DRUGS ABUSED

(See http://www.talktofrank.com/home_html.aspx.)

Patterns of drug misuse change rapidly, depending on fashion and cultural factors, availability and cost. Alcohol, tobacco, solvents, cannabis and ecstasy have been popular for many years but, apart from these, heroin is still the main drug of misuse followed closely by methadone and cocaine (Table 34.6).

Table 34.5 Emergency care of drug users

Patient problem	Possible causal drugs	STEP		
		1	2	3
Consciousness lost	Alcohol, heroin, tranquillizers, solvent abuse, ecstasy	Place in recovery position. Call ambulance	Cardiopulmonary resuscitation	
Dehydrated and hot	Ecstasy, speed	Reassure and calm person. Give non-alcoholic drinks (1 pint per hour). Move to cool area. Remove hot clothing	Call ambulance	Cardiopulmonary resuscitation
Drowsy	Heroin, tranquillizers, solvent abuse	Reassure	Place in recovery position. Avoid coffee	Call ambulance
Panicky	Ecstasy, LSD, magic mushrooms, speed	Reassure and calm the person	Keep in quiet area, accompanied	Call ambulance

Table 34.6 Common drugs of misuse and the possible consequences

Drug type	Risks from misuse	Examples	Intravenous use and possible consequent blood-borne virus infection transmission, or endocarditis, or septicaemia
Stimulants	Behavioural disturbances and psychoses	Amphetamine/amfetamines Cocaine Crack cocaine MDMA (ecstasy)	+ + – +
Sedatives	Fatal overdose Seizures on withdrawal	Alcohol Barbiturates Benzodiazepines	– + +
Opioids	Respiratory arrest in overdose	Buprenorphine Dipipanone Heroin Methadone	+ + + +

MDMA, 3,4-methylenedioxy-methamphetamine.

STIMULANTS

Stimulants are derivatives of epinephrine or are similar substances that cause excitement and euphoria (a 'high'), which may last several hours. Withdrawal symptoms of restlessness, agitation, sleeplessness and depression may follow. Heavy use of strong stimulants for weeks may cause paranoia and auditory hallucinations – effects which may not be reversible without medication (Table 34.7).

HERBAL PREPARATIONS

Stimulants used in various cultures include betel, caffeine, cocaine, kava, khat, kratom, marijuana, salvia and tobacco (Table 34.8).

Common herbal sources of psychedelics include *psilocybe* mushrooms, various *ayahuasca* preparations (prepared from *Banisteriopsis* spp. of vine from Amazonia), *peyote* (from a cactus in south-west USA), *San Pedro cactus* (from a cactus in Peru, Bolivia, Chile, Ecuador), and seeds of *morning glory* (from the *Convolvulus* family) and *Hawaiian baby woodrose* (a vine from India, the Caribbean, Hawaii and Africa).

INHALANTS

Inhalants are volatile chemical vapours that produce psychoactive effects. Many are available over the counter, including solvents (paint thinners, gasoline, glues), gases (butane, propane, aerosol propellants, nitrous oxide), nitrites (isoamyl, isobutyl, cyclohexyl – used to enhance sexual arousal) and sprays (e.g. deodorants; Table 34.9). 'Laughing gas', 'poppers', 'snappers' and 'whippets' are commonly used terms.

Inhalant misuse is increasingly common in children and young adults, and has led to many deaths. Sniffing inhalants produces psychotomimetic effects somewhere between those of alcohol and general anaesthesia (GA), in that initially users may feel slightly stimulated; with successive inhalations, they may feel less inhibited and less in control. Users may appear drunk and giggling with slurred speech and unsteadiness. Adverse effects include headache, nausea or vomiting, wheezing, unconsciousness, cramps, weight loss, muscle weakness, depression, memory impairment, damage to cardiovascular and nervous systems, and unconsciousness.

Sniffing highly concentrated chemicals such as fluorocarbons and butane-type gases can directly induce liver damage, neurological damage, delusions, hypoxia, arrhythmias and sometimes sudden death. High concentrations of inhalants also cause death from suffocation by displacing oxygen in the lungs and then in the CNS so that breathing ceases. Deliberately inhaling from an attached paper or plastic bag or in a closed area greatly increases the chances of suffocation. Users can also choke on their own vomit.

Table 34.7 Common stimulants

Main stimulant groups	Chemical names	Street names (see Appendix)	Comments
Adrenaline derivatives	Ephedrine and pseudo-ephedrine Phentermine Amphetamine/amfetamine	Bennies, black beauties, crosses, hearts, LA turnaround, speed, truck drivers, uppers	Raised heart rate, blood pressure, metabolism; feelings of exhilaration, energy, increased mental alertness, rapid or irregular heart beat, reduced appetite, weight loss, heart failure rapid breathing Hallucinations/tremor, loss of coordination; irritability, anxiousness, restlessness, delirium, panic, paranoia, impulsive behaviour, aggressiveness, tolerance, addiction
Caffeine		Found in tea and coffee, cola and a number of energy drinks	Energy, increased mental alertness/rapid or irregular heart beat
Cocaine	Cocaine hydrochloride	Blow, bump, C, candy, charlie, coke, crack, flake, rock, snow, toot, white	Raised temperature, chest pain, respiratory failure, nausea, abdominal pain, strokes, seizures, headaches, malnutrition
MDMA	Methylenedioxy-methamphetamine	DOB, DOM, MDA; adam, clarity, ecstasy, eve, lover's speed, peace, STP, X, XTC	Mild hallucinogenic effects, increased tactile sensitivity, empathic feelings, hyperthermia, impaired memory and learning
Methamphetamine		Chalk, crank, crystal, fire, glass, go fast, ice, meth, speed	Aggression, violence, psychotic behaviour, memory loss, cardiac and neurological damage, impaired memory and learning, tolerance, addiction
Methylphenidate		Ritalin; JIF, MPH, R-ball, skippy, the smart drug, vitamin R	Increase or decrease in blood pressure, psychotic episodes, digestive problems, loss of appetite, weight loss
Nicotine		Bidis, chew, cigars, cigarettes, smokeless tobacco, snuff, spit tobacco	Tolerance, addiction, additional effects attributable to tobacco exposure – adverse pregnancy outcomes, chronic lung disease, cardiovascular disease, stroke, cancer

Chronic solvent misuse can impair memory and concentration, and a few cases of permanent damage to the brain, liver or kidneys have been reported. Respiratory damage, anaemia, lead poisoning and cranial nerve palsies can follow chronic misuse of petrol/gasoline. A syndrome of learning disability hypotonia, scaphocephaly and high malar bones has also been reported in children of mothers who inhaled petrol during pregnancy (fetal gasoline/petrol syndrome). Specific chemicals may also have additional adverse effects (Table 34.10). Signs of solvent misuse include slurred speech, euphoria, anorexia and a circumoral (glue sniffers') rash. Jaundice may be seen and the pulse may be irregular.

DEPRESSANTS

Sedatives (including alcohol) depress the nervous system, causing drowsiness, loss of concentration, judgement and memory, disorientation and, in severe cases, unconsciousness (Table 34.11).

HALLUCINOGENS

Hallucinogenic drugs cause sensory distortions, including mood changes, feelings of disassociation, auditory and visual disturbances, and changes to taste or smell. Hallucinations are quite dangerous, as sufferers may represent extreme danger either to themselves or to others (Table 34.12).

ANABOLIC STEROIDS (SEE CH. 33)

ALPHABET OF DRUGS OF MISUSE

Appendix 34.1 gives street names for many drugs of abuse.

ALCOHOL

Alcohol (ethanol) is the most common drug of abuse, and consumption is rising throughout the world. Alcohol accounts for about as much of the burden of world disease as tobacco and hypertension, and is exceeded only by the burdens caused by malnutrition and unsafe sex (Fig. 34.2). Alcohol in drinks is generally measured in units (Table 34.13): one alcohol unit (AU) equates to 10–12 ml of pure ethanol, contained in a standard bottle or a can of regular beer, a glass of dinner wine (125 ml), a small glass (30 ml) of spirits and a measure (60 ml) of aperitif. Moderate alcohol use is defined as 1 AU daily for women and 2 for men. A safe maximum daily alcohol consumption is generally regarded as 3 units for a man, 2 for a woman. Alcohol misuse, defined as a daily intake in excess of 5 units, is the most common form of drug misuse. The World Health Organization estimates that there are almost 80 million people worldwide with diagnosable alcohol misuse disorders. Over 25% of the UK

Table 34.8 Stimulants used in various cultures

Stimulant	Sources	Comments
Betel	See text	
Caffeine	See text	
Cocaine	See text	
Kava	Kava (ava, intoxicating pepper, kawa kawa, kew, sakau, tonga, yangona) from *Piper methysticum* (intoxicating pepper), a shrub native to South Pacific Islands, including Hawaii. The term kava also refers to the non-fermented, psychoactive beverage prepared from the rootstock. Kava-containing dietary supplements are marketed for the treatment of anxiety and insomnia	Pacific Island societies have long used kava beverages for social, ceremonial and medical purposes. The pharmacologically active compounds are kava-lactones. Effects include euphoria, muscle relaxation, sedation and analgesia. High doses can have transient CNS depressant effects (e.g. sedation and muscle weakness). Individuals may experience a numb or tingling of the mouth upon drinking kava due to its local anaesthetic activity. Liver damage (hepatitis and cirrhosis) and failure have been associated with commercial extracts of kava. Kava inhibits CYP450 enzymes and has potential for drug interactions
Khat	Khat (qat, kat, chat, miraa, quaadka), the leaves of *Catha edulis*, a shrub native to East Africa and the Arabian Peninsula, widely used as a recreational drug by indigenous people from those areas and the Middle East	Khat has amphetamine-like effects from cathinone and cathine. Cathinone (alpha-aminopriopiophenone), the principal active stimulant, is structurally similar to D-amphetamine and almost as potent as a CNS stimulant. Cathine (D-norpseudoephedrine) is about ten times less potent than cathinone as a CNS stimulant
Kratom	Kratom (*Mitragyna speciosa* Korth; thang, kakuam, thom, ketum, biak) – a tree indigenous to Thailand, Malaysia and Myanmar	Used as an herbal drug. Mitragynine (9-methoxy-corynantheidine) is the primary active alkaloid and has opioid-like activity
Marijuana	See text	
Salvia	*Salvia divinorum* (Maria Pastora, sage of the seers, diviner's sage, salvia, Sally-D, magic mint) – a perennial herb native to the Sierra Mazateca region of Oaxaca, Mexico	Salvinorin A (divinorin A) is believed to be the ingredient responsible for hallucinogenic effects
Tobacco	See text	

CYP450, cytochrome P450.

Table 34.9 Inhalants: solvents and gases

Solvents		Gases		
Industrial or household solvents	Art or office supply solvents	Butane and propane in household or commercial products	Aerosol propellants	Anaesthetics
Paint thinners or solvents, degreasers (dry-cleaning fluids), petrol (gasoline) and glues	Correction fluids, felt-tip-marker fluid, and electronic contact cleaners	Whipping cream aerosols or dispensers (whippets) and refrigerant gases	Spray paints, hair or deodorant sprays, and fabric protector sprays	Nitrous oxide, halothane, ether and chloroform

Table 34.10 Adverse effects from inhalants

Chemical	Found in	Effects
Benzene	Gasoline/petrol	Bone marrow damage
Chlorinated hydrocarbons	Correction fluids, dry-cleaning fluids	Liver and kidney damage
Hexane	Glues, gasoline/petrol	Peripheral neuropathies or limb spasms
Methylene chloride	Varnish removers, paint thinners	Blood oxygen depletion
Nitrites	'Poppers', 'bold' and 'rush'	Blood oxygen depletion
Nitrous oxide	Whipping cream, gas cylinders	Peripheral neuropathies or limb spasms
Toluene	Paint sprays, glues, dewaxers	Liver, kidney and CNS damage, hearing loss
Trichloroethylene	Cleaning fluids, correction fluids	Hearing loss

CNS, central nervous system.

Table 34.11 Main depressants

Main groups	Chemical names	Street name(s) (see Appendix)	Comments
Alcohol	Ethanol	Booze	Reduced pain and anxiety; feeling of well-being; lowered inhibitions; slowed pulse and breathing; lowered blood pressure; poor concentration, confusion, fatigue; impaired coordination, memory, judgement; respiratory depression and arrest, addiction
Barbiturates	Amytal, nembutal, seconal, phenobarbital	Barbs, reds, red birds, phennies, tooies, yellows, yellow jackets	Sedation, drowsiness, depression, unusual excitement, fever, irritability, poor judgement, slurred speech, dizziness
Benzodiazepines	Various	Ativan, Halcion, Librium, Valium, Xanax; candy, downers, sleeping pills, tranks	Sedation, drowsiness, dizziness
	Flunitrazepam	Rohypnol; forget-me pill, Mexican valium, R2, Roche, roofies, roofinol, rope, rophies	Visual and gastrointestinal disturbances, urinary retention, memory loss for the time under the drug's effects
GHB	Gamma-hydroxybutyrate	G, Georgia home boy, grievous bodily harm, liquid ecstasy	Drowsiness, nausea/vomiting, headache, loss of consciousness, loss of reflexes, seizures, coma, death
Methaqualone	Methaqualone	Mandrax, quaaludes	Euphoria, depression, poor reflexes, slurred speech, coma

Table 34.12 Main hallucinogens

Main hallucinogen groups	Chemical names	Street names (see Appendix)	Comments
Ketamine	Ketamine	Ketalar SV; cat, K, Special K, vitamin K	Altered states of perception and feeling; nausea, temporary blindness, aggression, chronic mental disorders, persisting perception disorder (flashbacks) plus, at high doses, delirium, depression, respiratory depression and arrest
LSD	Lysergic acid diethylamide	Acid, blotter, boomers, cubes, microdot, yellow sunshines	Increased body temperature, heart rate, blood pressure; loss of appetite, sleeplessness, numbness, weakness, tremors
MDMA	Methylenedioxy-methamphetamine	Ecstasy	Increased body temperature, heart rate, blood pressure; loss of appetite, sleeplessness, numbness, weakness, tremors
Mescaline	Trimethoxy-phenethylamine	Buttons, cactus, mesc, peyote	Increased body temperature, heart rate, blood pressure; loss of appetite, sleeplessness, numbness, weakness, tremors
PCP and analogues	Phenylcyclidine	Phencyclidine; angel dust, boat, hog, love boat, peace pill	Possible decrease in blood pressure and heart rate, panic, aggression, violence, loss of appetite, depression
Psilocybin	Psilocybin	Magic mushroom, purple passion, shrooms	Nervousness, paranoia
THC compounds (tetrahydrocannabinoids; cannabis)	Marijuana	Hashish, boom, chronic, gangster, hash, hash oil, hemp, blunt, dope, ganja, grass, herb, joints, Mary Jane, pot, reefer, sinsemilla, skunk, weed	Euphoria, slowed thinking and reaction time, confusion, impaired balance and coordination, cough, frequent respiratory infections; impaired memory and learning; increased heart rate, anxiety; panic attacks; tolerance, addiction

population appear to drink to excess (44% of men in Scotland also drink to excess). There appears to be a genetic predilection to alcoholism.

The term 'alcohol' as used in medicine and by the lay public typically applies to ethanol (CH_3CH_2OH), which is produced by yeast fermentation of carbohydrates, such as in fruit and starch. Fermentation is incomplete in beer and complete in wine, with resulting alcohol contents between 3–8% and 7–18% by volume, respectively. Spirits (e.g. whisky, brandy and vodka) are produced by distillation of fermented products, and are 30% or greater alcohol by volume.

A cocktail is a mixed drink usually containing one or more alcoholic beverages, flavourings and one or more fruit juices, sauces, honey, milk, cream or spices, etc. A subgroup of cocktails are pre-mixed and bottled cocktails, generally known as alcopops, RTDs (ready to drink), or FABs (flavoured alcoholic beverages), usually made from vodka, beer, whisky or rum to reach an alcohol concentration of 4–7% by volume, and are sweet and fruit flavoured because they are mixed with cola, lemonade, ginger ale, etc.

Most ethanol, which is rapidly absorbed through the gastric and duodenal mucosa, is metabolized by the liver, with a small fraction also metabolized by oral and other mucosae of the upper digestive tract. Alcohol dehydrogenase catalyses ethanol oxidation to acetaldehyde, which is oxidized into non-toxic acetate by aldehyde dehydrogenase. In turn, acetate is oxidized into fatty acids, carbon dioxide and water. Ethanol blocks nitrosamine metabolism in the liver, thus allowing it to circulate to

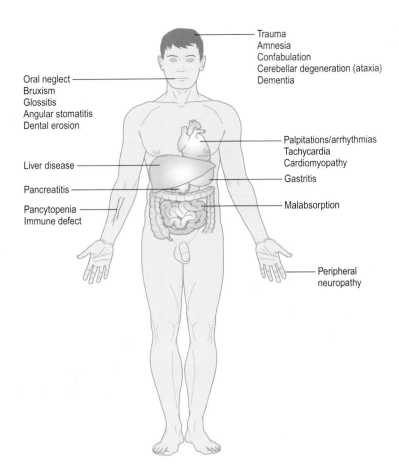

Trauma
Amnesia
Confabulation
Cerebellar degeneration (ataxia)
Dementia

Oral neglect
Bruxism
Glossitis
Angular stomatitis
Dental erosion

Palpitations/arrhythmias
Tachycardia
Cardiomyopathy

Liver disease

Gastritis

Pancreatitis

Pancytopenia
Immune defect

Malabsorption

Peripheral
neuropathy

Fig. 34.2 Alcoholism

Table 34.13	Alcohol in various alcoholic beverages		
Beverage	**Strength of alcohol**	**Amount**	**Units of alcohol**
Beer, cider, lager	3.5%	Half-pint	1
	3.5%	Pint	2
	Export strength 5%	Pint	2.5–3
	8%	Pint	4.5
Alcopop	5%	330 ml	1.7
Wine	10%	One glass	1
	10%	750 ml	7.5
	12%	750 ml	9
	Fortified (e.g. sherry) 15–20%	700 ml	16
Spirits	40%	One measure	1
	40%	700 ml	32

Clinical features

Alcohol is a CNS depressant and can have a range of mental effects (Box 34.3). The acute effects are mainly on judgement, concentration and coordination, and alcohol-influenced individuals may become aggressive and fail to comply with instructions. Effects are dose-related, eventually interfering with cerebellar function, causing ataxia and motor incoordination and ultimately unconsciousness (Table 34.14). After a large alcoholic binge, suppression of the cough reflex can result in inhalation of vomit and death.

Harmful use is when alcohol is causing physical and/or mental damage. Dependence is a strong overpowering desire to use alcohol, despite obvious harmful consequences. The probability of developing alcoholism is greater in several groups, especially those to whom alcohol is freely available (Table 34.15).

Box 34.3 Mental effects of alcohol

- Acute intoxication
- Harmful use
- Dependence syndrome
- Withdrawal state
- Psychotic disorder
- Amnesic syndrome

other organs, such as the kidneys and oesophagus, where it can be activated into carcinogens. Alcoholic beverages also contain polyphenols – plant secondary metabolites, which play an important protective role via their potent antioxidant activity. Resveratol in red wine is one example. In contrast, since the diet of alcoholics is often deficient, B-vitamin deficiencies may be found.

Table 34.14 Acute effects of alcohol

BLOOD ALCOHOL LEVEL IN MG/DL					
< 100	100–200	200–300	300–400	400–500	> 500
Dry and decent	Delighted and devilish	Delinquent and disgusting	Dizzy and delirious	Dazed and dejected	Dead drunk

Table 34.15 Alcoholism

Risk factors	Suggestive findings	Outcomes
Armed forces Bachelors over 40 Bored housewives Commercial travellers Doctors Entertainers Publicans and other workers in the drinks industry	Absenteeism Accidents Assaults Cirrhosis Family history of alcoholism Frequent job changes Gamma-glutamyl transpeptidase raised Macrocytosis Marital disharmony Medical history Social history Violence	Brain damage and epilepsy Cancers Fetal alcohol syndrome Gastrointestinal disease: gastritis and peptic ulcer Heart disease: cardiomyopathy Inadequate diet leading to immune defects, peripheral polyneuropathies and organic brain disorders Impaired haemostasis Impaired wound healing Infections, especially pneumonia and tuberculosis Injuries (including maxillofacial), from accidents or assaults Liver disease: alcoholic hepatitis and cirrhosis Muscle disease: myopathy Nutritional defects Pancreatic disease; pancreatitis

Alcohol misuse (alcoholism) is consumption of alcohol to such a degree as to cause deterioration in social behaviour, or physical illness, and the development of dependence, from which withdrawal is difficult or causes adverse effects.

Alcohol interferes with CNS function and is causally related to more than 60 different medical conditions; some, such as suicide, homicide and different forms of accidents (e.g. falls, poisoning, accidents caused by flames or by motor vehicles) are acute consequences of alcohol use. Alcohol is an important, if not the main, causal factor in over 25% of road traffic accidents and also in many other accidents or assaults. Acute alcoholic hepatitis may follow binge-drinking; cirrhosis commonly results from chronic alcoholism. Alcohol contributes to the spread of sexually transmitted diseases (including HIV), to impaired wound-healing and predisposition to respiratory infections, especially pneumonia and tuberculosis.

Late signs or symptoms of chronic excessive alcohol drinking include palpitations and tachycardia, cardiomyopathy, liver disease, chronic pancreatitis, malnutrition, peripheral neuropathy, amnesia and confabulation (in Wernicke and Korsakoff CNS syndromes). Cerebellar degeneration with ataxia, dementia, haemorrhagic stroke and various forms of cancer are consequences of chronic alcohol use (Table 34.16).

A diet poor in fruits and vegetables is typical of heavy drinkers and can cause nutritional defects leading to immune defects and peripheral polyneuropathies (burning hands and feet), pellagra, amblyopia (visual defects) and organic brain disorders (Wernicke encephalopathy and Korsakoff psychosis).

Alcoholics are predisposed to infections, especially pneumonia and tuberculosis, and alcohol use also contributes to the spread of sexually transmitted infections, including HIV.

Alcohol is now the most common teratogen apart from smoking, and drinking during pregnancy has a detrimental effect on

Table 34.16 Effects of chronic alcohol use

	Possible effects	Biochemical changes
Cardiac	Cardiomyopathy, hypertension, arrhythmias	–
CNS	Intoxication, dependency, dementia Wernicke–Korsakoff syndrome	Raised blood alcohol Decreased thiamine levels
Gastric	Gastritis, ulceration, carcinoma	–
Haematological	Pancytopenia Folate deficiency Thiamine deficiency Immune defect	Macrocytosis, anaemia Thrombocytopenia, leukopenia Reduced blood clotting factors: II, VII. IX, X
Hepatic	Hepatitis, fatty liver (steatosis), cirrhosis, liver cancer	Raised gamma-glutamyl transpeptidase, CDT, liver enzymes, bilirubin
Intestinal	Glucose and vitamins malabsorption	Reduced folate, thiamine and vitamins B_{12}, A, D, E and K
Musculoskeletal	Myopathy, gout	–
Oesophageal	GORD, Mallory–Weiss syndrome, carcinoma	–
Pancreatic	Pancreatitis	Raised serum amylase
Reproductive	Impotence, dysmenorrhoea, low birthweight babies, fetal alcohol syndrome	–

CDT, carbohydrate deficient transferrin; GORD, gastro-oesophageal reflux disease.

fetal development. It can lead to spontaneous abortion or the fetal alcohol syndrome (FAS), the prevalence of which is similar to that of Down syndrome. FAS affects growth, the CNS and orofacial features. Most affected children are of short stature; microcephaly is common and is associated with a low IQ, difficulties in eating and speech, and muscular incoordination. The FAS patient is irritable as an infant, hyperactive as a child and highly unsociable as an adult. Facial features include hypoplastic maxillae, a low nasal bridge, an indistinct philtrum with a hypoplastic upper lip, and other features, including small teeth with dysplastic enamel.

The mortality rate in alcoholism is significantly raised and over 15 years may be about 300% above the norm. Diseases that can be caused or aggravated by alcohol include injuries, including maxillofacial, from accidents or assaults.

Whereas the health risks of heavy alcohol consumption and alcohol abuse are well known, there are studies indicating beneficial effects of lower intake levels, for conditions such as diabetes mellitus and cardiovascular diseases.

Alcohol should only be drunk in moderation, with meals, and when consumption cannot put others at risk. Alcohol should not be consumed by: children; women trying to conceive or already pregnant; anyone about to drive a motor vehicle, fly a plane or take on any other skilled activity; health care workers about to treat patients; and anyone taking prescription or over-the-counter medicines.

General management

Findings that suggest alcoholism may be present in the social or medical history (Table 34.17) or by discovery of used bottles at home, at work or elsewhere. Recognition of the alcoholic is notoriously difficult and the history is often

Table 34.17 Findings suggesting alcoholism	
Social history	**Medical history**
Absenteeism	Accidents
Assaults	Cirrhosis
Violence	Macrocytosis
Frequent job changes	Folate deficiency or raised CDT or gamma-glutamyl transpeptidase
Marital disharmony	Family history of alcoholism

hopelessly unreliable. Signs or symptoms of chronic excessive alcohol intake include: slurred speech; smell of alcohol on the breath; signs of self-neglect (whether of the mouth or shabbiness of clothes); an evasive, truculent, over-boisterous or facetious manner; indigestion (particularly heartburn); anxiety (often with insomnia); or tremor of the hands. Later signs or symptoms of chronic excessive alcohol drinking include palpitations and tachycardia, cardiomyopathy and signs of malnutrition.

The CAGE questionnaire may be helpful and a positive response to any of the following questions suggests a diagnosis of alcoholism.

- Have you ever felt the need to **C**ut down on drink?
- Have you ever felt **A**nnoyed by criticism of your drinking?
- Have you ever felt **G**uilty about drinking?
- Do you drink a morning **E**ye opener?

Two or more affirmative answers indicate probable alcoholism. A five-shot questionnaire if producing scores over 5 suggests alcoholism (Table 34.18).

Laboratory investigations that may be diagnostically helpful include macrocytosis on blood examination, raised levels of alcohol, gamma-glutamyl transpeptidase (gamma-GT or GGT) and other hepatic enzymes, levels above 1.3% of carbohydrate-deficient transferrin isoforms (%CDT), and folate deficiency of no obvious cause.

Alcohol can interact with other drugs, sometimes inducing the cytochrome P450 enzyme system to accelerate their metabolism, in others depressing their metabolism. Warfarin, paracetamol/acetaminophen and benzodiazepines may be affected.

Treatment of alcoholism is by drinking in a less damaging way and accepting help to deal with the crises and the physical, behavioural and social damage that result; or learning to abstain from alcohol. Admission to manage rehabilitation and ensure abstinence, nutrition replacement of thiamine and folate, and drugs to reduce dependence (naltrexone, acamprosate or chlormethiazole) or to cause unpleasant side-effects if alcohol is taken (disulfiram) may help.

If the alcohol supply is reduced or cut off, or if blood alcohol levels fall sharply, the abstinence or withdrawal syndrome (AWS) may appear with morning 'shakes', typically trembling of the hands, but possibly involving the whole body. Morning nausea and vomiting are sometimes called 'toothbrush heaves'. Other withdrawal symptoms are diarrhoea, sweating, rapid pulse and raised blood pressure, confusion, agitation, fits, illusions, misperceptions, hallucinations or delusions. The full-blown syndrome is called 'delirium tremens' or 'DTs'. The whole withdrawal syndrome lasts about a week and requires medical supervision and use of benzodiazepines or chlormethiazole.

Dental aspects

Many alcoholics present no dental management problems, though there may be issues related to informed consent if the person is inebriated, but challenges may also include erratic attendance for dental treatment and aggressive behaviour. Alcoholics are best given an early morning appointment, when they are least likely to be under the influence of alcohol.

The main relevant medical complications are that cirrhosis delays the metabolism of many drugs and may cause a bleeding tendency. Chronic alcoholism may also depress the bone marrow to cause anaemia and thrombocytopenia. Other problems may include cardiomyopathy, poly-substance misuse, smoking and drug interactions.

General anaesthesia is best avoided, especially if patients have pre-medicated themselves with alcohol, and increased the risk of vomiting and inhalation of vomit. Alcoholics are especially prone to aspiration lung abscess. Alcoholic heart disease is also a contraindication.

Sedatives (including benzodiazepines and antihistamines) or hypnotics generally have an additive effect with alcohol,

Table 34.18 Five-shot questionnaire for detecting alcoholism

	SCORES				
	0	0.5	1.0	1.5	2.0
How often do you have a drink containing alcohol?	Never	< monthly	2–4 times/month	2–3 times/week	≥ 4 times/week
How many drinks containing alcohol do you have on a typical day when you are drinking?	1 or 2	3 or 4	5 or 6	7 or 8	10 or more
Have people annoyed you by criticizing your drinking?	No		Yes		
Have you ever felt bad or guilty about drinking?	No		Yes		
Have you ever had a drink first thing in the morning to steady your nerves or get rid of a hangover?	No		Yes		

although these interactions are not entirely predictable. Heavy drinkers, however, become tolerant not only of alcohol but also of other sedatives. Alcoholics are also notoriously resistant to GA. Once liver disease develops, the position is reversed: drug metabolism is then impaired (Ch. 9) and drugs have a disproportionately greater effect.

Aspirin and non-steroidal anti-inflammatory drugs (NSAIDs) should be avoided: they are more likely in the alcoholic patient to cause gastric erosions and precipitate bleeding. Opioids may enhance sedation. The hepatotoxic effects of acetaminophen are enhanced, though it is probably the safest analgesic.

Alcohol-containing preparations, such as some mouthwashes, should be avoided in patients given metronidazole within the last 48 h. Metronidazole inhibits the liver breakdown of acetaldehyde, which accumulates to cause widespread vasodilatation, nausea, vomiting, sweating, headache and palpitations similar to the Antabuse reaction. The effects of penicillins and erythromycin may be reduced by alcohol.

Wound healing may also be impaired in the severely chronic alcoholic and, in the USA, alcoholism may be a common factor in patients with osteomyelitis following jaw fractures. The most common oral effect of alcoholism is neglect, leading to advanced caries and periodontal disease, and there is sometimes tooth surface loss from caries, dental erosion from regurgitation and/or attrition from bruxism.

Alcohol may be a cause of leukoplakia and oral cancer. There may be folate deficiency or other anaemia causing glossitis and sometimes angular stomatitis or recurrent aphthae. A rare manifestation is bilateral painless swelling of the parotids or other major salivary glands (sialosis).

Other orofacial features include a smell of alcohol on the breath, telangiectases and possibly rhinophyma ('grog blossom').

AMPHETAMINE/AMFETAMINES

Amphetamine/amfetamines stimulate alpha- and beta-adrenergic receptors in the CNS and peripheral nervous system, and essentially have similar effects to cocaine. They are used for euphoriant effect, to stave off fatigue in order to continue work or for slimming. Amphetamine/amfetamines are usually taken orally but can also be injected, snorted or smoked (ice; crystal).

Amphetamine/amfetamines raise the blood pressure (BP) and sometimes temperature, and cause sleeplessness and anorexia.

Acute amphetamine/amfetamine toxicity causes dry mouth, dilated pupils, tachycardia, aggression, talkativeness, tachypnoea and hallucinations, leading to seizures, hyperpyrexia, arrhythmias and collapse. High doses can cause mood swings and psychoses – including hallucinations and paranoia – and can cause respiratory failure and death. Chronic amphetamine/amfetamine toxicity causes restlessness, hyperactivity, loss of appetite and weight, tremor, repetitive movements, picking at the face and extremities, and bruxism, and there can be xerostomia and increased caries incidence.

Amphetamine/amfetamines have no true withdrawal syndrome and, in this respect, addiction is quite different from opioid or barbiturate dependence. Unfortunately, psychoses can persist after the drug has been stopped. Addicts may be remarkably resistant to GA and, if taking drugs intravenously, may have many of the infective problems of opioid addicts. If GA is required, intravenous barbiturates may induce convulsions, respiratory distress or coma, and should be avoided. Opioids are also contraindicated. Amphetamine/amfetamines enhance the sympathomimetic effects of epinephrine and thus vasoconstrictors are best avoided, since hypertension and cardiotoxicity can result. Monoamine oxidase inhibitors are contraindicated.

BARBITURATES

Barbiturates are depressant drugs used mainly to treat anxiety, tension and sleep disorders. They cause sedation, and depress respiration and heart rate, as well as impairing thought processes and memory and causing incoordination and ataxia. With chronic use, addicts begin to think slowly, have increasing emotional lability, concentration and judgement are increasingly impaired, and the barbiturate addict becomes irritable and shows signs of self-neglect.

Although tolerance to barbiturates develops, the lethal dose remains the same, with only a small gap between relatively safe and lethal levels. Barbiturates are often used to adulterate more expensive drugs such as heroin and are responsible for many of the fatal overdoses. Accidental overdose is a relatively common cause of death from respiratory failure and CNS depression, especially if alcohol is also taken. There is no antidote to overdose; artificial ventilation is used until respiratory function recovers.

Two main types of barbiturate addict are recognized and either may also misuse other drugs. Middle-aged women, often living alone, taking large quantities of barbiturates orally and living in a dream world, form the largest group; chronic toxicity such as rashes and ataxia often develop. Young addicts, who take barbiturates ('sleepers') for immediate effect by injection, are at risk of complications from filthy injection technique, including multiple abscesses, gangrene, hepatitis, HIV infection, infective endocarditis or occasionally tetanus.

Should barbiturates be withdrawn, the addict initially improves and any ataxia disappears but, within 12–16 h, a dangerous withdrawal syndrome can develop. Nausea, anxiety, tremor, insomnia, tachycardia, weakness and postural hypotension are followed by abdominal pain. After 36–48 h, in heavy users, there may be loss of consciousness, often fits and sometimes death. The syndrome has a slower onset in those who have been using long-acting barbiturates.

Dental management may be complicated by barbiturates enhancing the sedative effects of some drugs, or inducing liver drug-metabolizing enzymes and causing resistance to anaesthetics. Other problems may include hepatitis B and C, HIV infection and sexually transmitted disease, epilepsy, maxillofacial injuries and tetanus.

Oral complications of barbiturate misuse are rare. A bullous mucosal reaction has been reported but manifestations such as atypical facial pain, related to the underlying condition for which the drug was prescribed, are more common.

BENZODIAZEPINES

Benzodiazepines are prescribed to treat anxiety, acute stress reactions and panic attacks. Memory loss is a major feature. Psychological dependence on benzodiazepines is common but the effects are considerably less severe than with most other sedatives. Physical dependence can develop fairly quickly – sometimes within 1 month.

Withdrawal symptoms are frequently delayed in onset compared with the barbiturates but may last 8–10 days. Typical effects include insomnia, anxiety, loss of appetite, tremor, perspiration and perceptual disturbances, and occasionally fits or psychoses. The anxiety, tremor and insomnia that follow the drug's withdrawal are incorrectly attributed to the return of the original anxiety state.

Sudden withdrawal, particularly of short-acting benzodiazepines, is dangerous since it can cause confusion, fits, toxic psychosis or a condition resembling delirium tremens.

BETEL

Betel quid or paan chewing is widely used and claimed to produce a sense of well-being, euphoria, warm sensation of the body, sweating, salivation, palpitation, heightened alertness and increased capacity to work. Betel quid is a mixture of areca (betel) nut and slaked lime, to which tobacco can be added, all wrapped in betel leaf. Arecoline (methyl-1-methyl-1,2,5, 6-tetrahydropyridine-3-carboxylate) is the primary active ingredient of areca nut responsible for the CNS stimulant effects, which are comparable to those of nicotine (which has a similar chemical structure). Arecoline is an agonist of acetylcholine

muscarinic M_1, M_2 and M_3 receptors, which causes associated pupillary constriction, bronchial constriction, etc. Plasma noradrenaline and adrenaline also rise during betel quid chewing. The specific quid components vary between communities and individuals where it is used, having a major social and cultural role in communities throughout and from the Indian subcontinent, South-East Asia and locations in the western Pacific. Betel use is well recognized by tooth staining (Fig. 34.3) and can have a number of health consequences (Table 34.19), especially submucous fibrosis.

Oral submucous fibrosis (OSMF), though not regarded as a connective tissue disease, has pathological changes closely similar to those of scleroderma. It is a chronic disease that is almost entirely confined to Asians, related to the use of areca nut in gutkha or pan masala, or in other chewables (kharra, chewable tobacco). OSMF causes severe and often disabling fibrosis of the oral tissues, and is characterized by fibrous bands that form beneath the oral mucosa and progressively contract so that mouth-opening is increasingly severely limited. As many as 10% of OSMF patients develop oral carcinoma. Intralesional corticosteroids and regular stretching of the oral soft tissues with an interdental screw may delay fixation in the closed position. Failing this, operative treatment may become necessary.

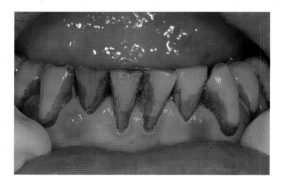

Fig. 34.3 Betel staining

Table 34.19 Possible adverse health effects from betel chewing	
Health effect	**Examples**
Cancer and potentially malignant conditions	Hepatocellular cancer Oesophageal cancer Oral cancer Oral submucous fibrosis Pancreatic cancer
Cardiovascular and diabetes	Hypertension Metabolic syndrome
Adverse birth outcomes	Lower birthweight Lower male to female sex ratio Reduced birth length
Others	Contact dermatitis Chronic kidney disease Liver cirrhosis Periodontitis Urinary calculi (related to use of calcium hydroxide 'chuna' in the betel quid)

CAFFEINE

Caffeine is an alkaloid stimulant widely used in many cultures. Found in over 60 plants, it is most commonly derived from coffee or tea plants. Other sources include kola, cacao, guarana and yerba mate. Chocolate contains a small amount. Caffeine is called guaranine when found in *guarana*, mateine when found in *mate* and *theine* when found in *tea*. There is far more caffeine in coffees than in teas. Significant amounts of caffeine are also added to some soft drinks and 'energy' drinks (e.g. Red Bull, Relentless, Cocaine; the amount of caffeine has to be stated on the label where it contains > 150 mg caffeine/L). Some of these 'energy drinks' are banned in some countries.

Caffeine is psychoactive and diuretic, competitively inhibiting adenosine, leading to a rise in brain dopamine, serotonin and catecholamines. Caffeine metabolites include theobromine (which increases the blood flow to the brain and muscles), theophylline (which relaxes bronchioles and increases heart rate and efficiency) and paraxanthine (which increases lipolysis, releasing glycerol and fatty acids for use as a muscle energy source). Coffee and tea also contain other xanthine alkaloids, for example cardiac stimulants theophylline and theobromine (tea only) and other substances such as polyphenols, which can insolubly complex with caffeine and alter its activity.

Caffeine tolerance develops very quickly, especially among heavy coffee and energy drink consumers, and when caffeine use is stopped the falling serotonin levels can cause anxiety, irritability, inability to concentrate and diminished motivation or depression. Excess caffeine can lead to caffeine intoxication, caffeine-induced anxiety disorder or caffeine-induced sleep disorder.

Studies suggesting caffeine intake is associated with a risk of miscarriage or a reduced risk of developing Parkinsonism or cardiovascular disease are inconclusive. Some Latter-day Saints (Mormons), Christian Scientists and Gaudiya Vaishnava Hindus do not consume caffeine.

COCAINE

Cocaine hydrochloride, derived from the plant *Erythroxylon coca,* is one of the most widely abused drugs. It is powerfully addictive: having once tried cocaine, individuals may not be able to control the extent to which they will continue to use it. Cocaine is widely used worldwide, and in all levels of society. 'Crack' is the street name given to cocaine processed with ammonia or sodium bicarbonate (baking soda) and water, and heated to remove the hydrochloride (producing a crackling sound) to a free base for smoking.

Cocaine is often snorted – inhaled through the nose, where it is rapidly absorbed into the bloodstream – giving a 'high' lasting 15–30 min. It may also be used by injecting, or smoking – extremely high doses reach the brain quickly and bring an intense immediate high, which can last 5–10 min.

Cocaine has profound and almost immediate CNS effects, potentiating catecholamines and interfering with dopamine reabsorption. Euphoric effects appear in less than 5 min and include hyperstimulation and diminished fatigue and appetite. Cocaine causes feelings of well-being and heightened mental activity: the cocaine addict is garrulous, witty and the life and soul of the party – aptly described as a 'sexed-up extrovert with dilated pupils'. High doses of cocaine and/or prolonged use can trigger paranoia, visual hallucinations (snowlights) and tactile hallucinations. The latter are typically of insects crawling over the skin (formication, 'cocaine bugs').

Physical effects of cocaine also mimic those of catecholamines, and include dilated pupils, constricted peripheral blood vessels, and raised temperature, pulse rate and BP. Toxic reactions include angina, coronary spasm, ventricular arrhythmias, myocardial infarction, cerebrovascular accidents, convulsions and respiratory depression. Cocaine-related deaths are often a result of cardiac arrest, cerebrovascular accidents or seizures followed by respiratory arrest.

As a constituent of Brompton cocktail (cocaine, heroin or morphine, and alcohol), cocaine is also sometimes used to make terminal disease more tolerable. However, when people choose to mix cocaine and alcohol, they are also compounding the dangers, since the liver combines them, manufacturing cocaethylene, which intensifies the euphoric effects, and increases the risk of sudden death. Use of cocaine plus heroin intravenously ('speedballing') is also highly dangerous.

Prolonged cocaine snorting can result in ischaemic necrosis with ulceration of the nasal mucous membrane and nasal septum collapse, ulceration of the palate, and to sphenoidal sinusitis. It occasionally leads to brain abscess.

On stopping cocaine, symptoms proceed through a crash phase of depression and craving for sleep, a withdrawal phase of lack of energy, and then an extinction phase of recurrence of craving evoked by various external stimuli but of lesser intensity. Depression, fatigue bradycardia and psychoses may be seen. Behavioural interventions, particularly cognitive behavioural therapy, can be effective in reducing cocaine misuse.

Behavioural problems or drug interactions may interfere with dental treatment. Injected cocaine brings the risk from the same blood-borne infections as in other addicts.

It is important to avoid epinephrine-containing LA in persons using cocaine until at least 2 h have elapsed, because of enhanced sympathomimetic action and subsequent arrhythmias, acute hypertension or cardiac failure. Therefore, it is best not to give dental treatment until 6 h after the last dose of cocaine has been taken. When GA is needed, isoflurane and sevoflurane are preferred to halothane, which may induce arrhythmias. Ketamine and suxamethonium are also best avoided.

Oral use of cocaine temporarily numbs the lips and tongue, and can cause gingival erosions. The main oral effects of cocaine addiction may be a dry mouth and bruxism or dental erosion. Caries and periodontal disease, especially acute necrotizing gingivitis, are more frequent. Cocaine may precipitate cluster headaches. Children born to cocaine-using mothers are more prone to have ankyloglossia.

DIPIPANONE

Dipipanone is less sedating than morphine and is sometimes abused in tablet form and in combination with an anti-emetic (Diconal).

DEXTROPROPOXYPHENE

Co-proxamole (because of the dextropropoxyphene, a weak opioid) is also abused.

ECSTASY (3,4-METHYLENEDIOXY-METHAMPHETAMINE; MDMA)

Ecstasy is a synthetic, psychoactive amphetamine-like drug with sympathomimetic activity, and both stimulant and hallucinogenic properties. Like other amphetamines, it produces euphoria and appetite suppression, but is more potently hallucinogenic.

Ecstasy is usually taken orally, giving effects after 20–60 min. Unfortunately, the tablets may contain other amphetamine derivatives, caffeine, ketamine or salicyclic acid, or ecstasy may be used along with cannabis, alcohol, amphetamine/amfetamine or cocaine (increasing the hazards of use).

Adverse effects from ecstasy include neurological effects (e.g. ataxia and seizures), psychiatric sequelae (e.g. agitation or paranoia), cardiovascular effects (e.g. tachycardia, arrhythmias or infarction) as well as renal or hepatic failure or other effects – but these are unrelated to the dose. Ecstasy causes brain injury, affecting dopamine-containing neurons that use serotonin to communicate with other neurons. The serotonin system plays a direct role in regulating mood, aggression, sexual activity, sleep and sensitivity to pain. Ecstasy users face risks similar to those caused by cocaine and amphetamine/amfetamines – psychological difficulties, including confusion, depression, sleep problems, drug craving, severe anxiety and paranoia – during and sometimes weeks after taking it, and physical symptoms such as muscle tension, involuntary teeth-clenching, nausea, blurred vision, rapid eye movement, faintness, and chills or sweating.

Ecstasy can cause a sharp rise in body temperature (malignant hyperthermia) leading to muscle breakdown, and kidney and cardiovascular system failure.

Ecstasy has been widely used in 'raves' and users need to take water or non-alcoholic drinks frequently and in large amounts to avoid potentially fatal hyperthermia ('chill-out'). Deaths are rare but usually caused by high temperatures, raised heart rate and BP and myocardial infarcts, hyponatraemia or asthma. At special risk are people with circulatory or heart disease. People who develop a rash resembling acne after using ecstasy may be risking severe side-effects, including liver damage, if they continue to use the drug. After long-term use, tolerance develops but there is no physical dependence or withdrawal symptoms.

Teeth-clenching and bruxism appear to be common; temporomandibular joint dysfunction, dry mouth, attrition, erosion, mucosal burns or ulceration, circumoral paraesthesiae and periodontitis have been reported. Ecstasy can interact with adrenaline, tricyclic or selective serotonin reuptake inhibitor (SSRI) antidepressants.

GHB (GAMMA-HYDROXYBUTYRATE)

GHB is abused for euphoric, sedative and anabolic (bodybuilding) effects. GHB and two of its precursors, gamma-butyrolactone (GBL) and 1,4-butanediol (BD), have been involved in poisonings, overdoses, date rapes and deaths. Coma and seizures can follow misuse of GHB and, when combined with methamphetamine, there appears to be an increased risk of seizure. Combining use with other drugs such as alcohol can result in nausea, difficulty in breathing and unconsciousness.

GHB may also produce withdrawal effects, including insomnia, anxiety, tremors and sweating.

HEROIN (SEE OPIATES AND OPIOIDS)

KETAMINE

Ketamine is a GA agent related to phencyclidine (PCP), which can cause a dream-like state and hallucinations, and has been used as a date-rape drug. Ketamine effects come on and recede faster than those of LSD but include aggression (as with PCP) and temporary blindness, and the drug can cause delirium, amnesia, impaired motor function, hypertension, depression and potentially fatal respiratory problems.

LSD (LYSERGIC ACID DIETHYLAMIDE)

LSD (acid) is a major hallucinogen manufactured from lysergic acid, found in ergot, a fungus that grows on rye and other grains. Within 30–90 min of taking LSD orally, it produces several different emotions at once or swinging rapidly from one to another (a 'trip'). Synaesthesia, the overflow from one sense to another when, for example, colours are heard, is common. These effects can last up to 12 h and, even up to months after a 'trip', many LSD users experience flashbacks – recurrence of certain aspects of a person's experience – without the user having taken the drug again.

There is often lability of mood, panic ('bad trip') and delusions of magical powers, such as being able to fly. If taken in a large enough dose, LSD causes delusions, visual hallucinations and paranoia. The sense of time and self becomes distorted. LSD intoxication can cause severe, terrifying thoughts and feelings, and despair, and fatal accidents have been precipitated. Taking LSD is especially risky because each tablet can contain very different amounts of drug from as little as 25 µg to as much as 250 µg – enough to cause serious side-effects.

The physical effects from LSD are similar to those of catecholamines and include: dilated pupils; raised body temperature, heart rate and BP; sweating; loss of appetite; sleeplessness; dry mouth; and tremors. The effects of LSD are unpredictable but prolonged, often to about 12 h, depending on the amount taken, and the user's personality, mood and expectations, and the surroundings in which the drug is used. LSD is not considered an addictive drug since it does not produce the compulsive drug-seeking type of behaviour as shown by users of cocaine, amphetamine/amfetamine, heroin, alcohol and nicotine. Most users of LSD voluntarily limit or stop its use over time.

MARIJUANA (CANNABIS)

Marijuana is the most commonly abused illicit drug aside from alcohol in the developed world, and is used religiously in Rastafarianism. A dry, shredded, green/brown mix of flowers, stems, seeds and leaves of the hemp plant *Cannabis sativa* or *Cannabis indica*, it usually is smoked as a cigarette (joint, nail) or in a pipe (bong). It also is smoked in blunts – cigars that have been emptied of tobacco and refilled with marijuana – often in combination with another drug. Use also might include mixing marijuana in food or brewing it as a tea. As a more concentrated, resinous form it is called hashish and, as a sticky black liquid, hash oil.

The main active chemical in marijuana is THC (delta-9-tetrahydrocannabinol), which binds to receptors in parts of the brain that influence pleasure, memory, thought, concentration, sensory and time perception, and coordinated movement. The marijuana currently used is many times more potent than that used in the 1950s.

The short-term adverse effects of marijuana use can include difficulties with memory and learning, distorted perception, difficulty in thinking and problem-solving, and loss of coordination. Critical skills related to attention, memory and learning are significantly impaired: students who smoke marijuana obtain lower examination grades and are less likely to graduate compared with non-smoking peers. Depression, anxiety and personality disturbances are all associated with marijuana use. Schizophrenia may be triggered in susceptible people.

Marijuana affects BP and heart rate, and lowers the oxygen-carrying capacity of the blood. Smoking marijuana may more than quadruple the risk of myocardial infarction in the first hour, and frequently leads to respiratory illnesses such as infections, daily cough and sputum production, and obstructed airways.

Marijuana smoke contains 50–70% more carcinogenic hydrocarbons than tobacco smoke and THC impairs immune function. Marijuana has been implicated in lung and oral cancer, as well as some other malignant disease, but the evidence is equivocal and could be related to concurrent tobacco use.

Babies born to women who used marijuana during pregnancies display abnormal responses to visual stimuli, tremulousness and a high-pitched cry, features that may indicate neurological maldevelopment. Later there may be behavioural problems and poor performance on tasks of visual perception, language comprehension, sustained attention and memory.

No medications are currently available for treating marijuana misuse.

There are no specific aspects of addiction that influence dental management in most patients, but there is a tendency to a dry mouth and increased cravings for certain foods ('the munchies'), xerostomia, increased carriage of *Candida*, and oral white lesions.

METHAMPHETAMINE

Methamphetamine is an addictive stimulant with stronger CNS effects than amphetamine/amfetamine, releasing high levels of dopamine, which enhance mood and body movement. Unlike amphetamine/amfetamine, users of methamphetamine may become addicted quickly, and use it with increasing frequency and in increasing doses. Methamphetamine is also neurotoxic, damaging brain cells that contain dopamine and serotonin and, over time, lowering levels of dopamine, which can result in parkinsonism. Methamphetamine also raises heart rate and

BP and can cause cardiovascular collapse, strokes, hyperthermia and convulsions, which can be fatal. 'Meth mouth' is the term given to the neglect and poor oral hygiene seen in methamphetamine users.

METHYLPHENIDATE (RITALIN)

Methylphenidate is a CNS stimulant often prescribed for children with attention-deficit hyperactivity disorder (ADHD). It has effects similar to, but more potent than, caffeine but less potent than amphetamine/amfetamines. It may amplify dopamine release, thereby improving attention and focus. Some individuals misuse it for stimulant effects: appetite suppression, euphoria, wakefulness and enhanced focus/attentiveness.

NICOTINE AND TOBACCO

Tobacco is one of the most common lifestyle habits worldwide. Derived from plants of the genus *Nicotiniana*, it releases the stimulant nicotine, one of the most heavily used and highly addictive drugs. Nicotine binds to a CNS receptor and, like cocaine, heroin and marijuana, raises the level of dopamine as well as opioids and glucose, and activates the nucleus accumbens. The type of nicotine cholinergic receptor and the enzyme CYP2A6 influence the chances of addiction. Nicotine also causes a discharge of adrenaline from the adrenals, which stimulates the CNS, and other endocrine glands, and a sudden release of glucose. Stimulation is followed by depression and fatigue, leading the abuser to seek more nicotine. Addiction to nicotine results in withdrawal symptoms, if a person tries to stop smoking, with excessive anger, hostility and aggression.

Tobacco is frequently smoked in cigarettes but there are several other forms used in different cultures (Table 34.20).

Table 34.20 Main types of tobacco smoking in different cultures

Africa	Arab countries	South Asia	Western countries
Cigarettes	Cigarettes, hookah (shisha – water pipe)	Cigarettes, bidi (cheerot), chuta (reverse smoking) kreteks, hookah	Cigarettes, cigars, pipe

Nicotine is absorbed readily from tobacco smoke in the lungs, acting in seconds on the brain but affecting the body for up to 30 min. Tobacco smoking is a major hazard to health, since the smoke also contains a dozen gases (mainly carbon monoxide) and tar, which varies from about 15 mg for a regular cigarette to 7 mg in a low-tar cigarette. About 4000 compounds, including around 40 known carcinogens, such as nitrosamines and aromatic amines, are present, and promote many diseases including cancers (Table 34.21 and Fig. 34.4). There is also now suspicion that nicotine itself may also be carcinogenic.

Cigarette smoking is particularly linked to cancers of the lung, oesophagus, mouth and bladder, and increases the risk of cardiovascular disease, chronic obstructive pulmonary disease, hypertension and stroke – and is a leading cause of death. If women smokers also take oral contraceptives, they are more prone to cardiovascular and cerebrovascular diseases than are other smokers; this is especially true for women older than 30.

Table 34.21   Diseases associated with cigarette smoking

System	Diseases
Cardiovascular	Ischaemic heart disease Peripheral vascular disease Buerger disease
Respiratory	Sinusitis Chronic obstructive pulmonary disease
Carcinomas	Oropharyngeal and oral Bronchus Bladder Breast Colorectal Larynx Pancreas
Fetus	Higher prevalence of abortion Low birthweight Higher risk of perinatal and sudden infant deaths
Gastrointestinal	Periodontal disease Peptic ulcer
Central nervous system	Alcoholism Cerebrovascular disease Dementia

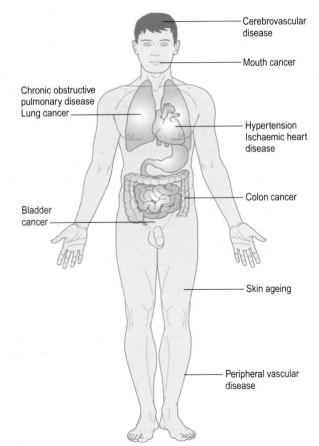

Fig. 34.4   Health effects of tobacco use

Women who smoke generally have an earlier menopause. Pregnant women who smoke cigarettes run a greater risk of having stillborn or premature infants or infants with low birthweight, and the children have a raised risk for developing conduct disorders. Second-hand smoke (passive smoking) causes lung cancer in adults and greatly increases the risk of respiratory illnesses in children and sudden infant death.

Tobacco smoking may be recognized from the odour, or staining of fingers, teeth and even lips (Fig. 34.5), but a smoking history should be taken (Table 34.22).

Smoking cessation should be a gradual process, because withdrawal symptoms are less severe in those who quit gradually than in those who quit quickly. Rates of relapse are highest in the first few weeks and months, and diminish considerably after 3 months. There are five crucial steps in advising people to stop smoking, known as the 'five As':

- ask
- assess
- advise
- assist
- arrange.

Ask

It is very important that every patient who is seen by a health professional has the status of their tobacco use noted on clinic records and the information kept as up to date as possible. Such

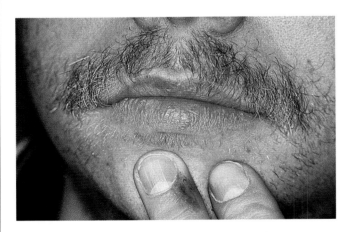

Fig. 34.5   Tar staining on lips and fingers in a tobacco smoker

Table 34.22   Smoking history

Questions	SMOKER		
	Current	Former	Never
What smoked?			
How many per day?			
Age starting?			
How many years?			
Quit attempt?			
Quit success?			
Exposed to passive smoke?			

a record should cover whether the patient is a smoker and, if so, the frequency of smoking and how long they have smoked. If the patient uses other forms of tobacco, this should be noted.

Assess

The health professional should inquire whether the patient is keen to quit, but ideally should cover more detailed information on whether he or she has ever tried to give up in the past. Any aids used in smoking cessation in the past should be noted. By collecting this sort of information, it is possible to help patients identify the best means of quitting.

Advise

Every smoker must be told of the value that stopping smoking will have for them and of the dangers that exist in continuing. Particularly if a risk lesion, such as a white or red patch of the oral mucosa, was found, it is important to discuss the sequelae of continuing smoking and give plain, precise and personalized advice to them. Other reasons for quitting (e.g. the benefits for preventing heart disease) should be included in the overall advice. Pharmacological treatments combined with psychological treatment results in some of the highest long-term abstinence rates, so the advice, where appropriate, should include directions to use nicotine replacement therapy (NRT). There is little difference in effect between the different types of NRT (Table 34.23).

Bupropion is as effective as NRT, but can cause dry mouth, headache and gastrointestinal symptoms, and is contraindicated in pregnancy, people who have seizures, the under-18s people with eating disorders, people with a CNS tumour, people on epileptogenic medications and the very old. Varenicline has a better efficacy and fewer adverse effects than bupropion, but it may cause some nausea, depression and interfere with driving.

Assist

Other clinic staff should be encouraged to help any smoker who wishes to stop. Setting a date for quitting and arranging to remind a smoker through reception staff may be helpful. In the UK, the patient could be provided with the telephone number to call the NHS smoking helpline or to visit an appropriate website. Useful leaflets should be available in the surgery for distribution.

Arrange

Arranging a follow-up is important, preferably within 1 week of quitting. Heavy smokers may also be referred to local smoking cessation services and helplines. This is important since studies show that people are twice as likely to quit successfully with intensive counselling.

Fortunately, smoking is increasingly being banned in public places in many countries.

Smokeless tobacco

Tobacco use in other forms is also deleterious to health (Table 34.24); nicotine is also absorbed readily when tobacco is chewed.

Difficulties in dental management of smokers may include associated disorders such as chronic obstructive pulmonary disease, ischaemic heart disease, alcoholism or peptic ulcer. Smokers metabolize some other drugs more rapidly and require, for example, higher doses of benzodiazepines than non-smokers.

Smoking may cause mucosal keratinization and pigmentary incompetence, and is linked to oral cancer. Smoker keratosis, in which there is diffuse hyperkeratosis of the palate, is typically caused by pipe smoking, is benign and rapidly reversible even after years of pipe smoking. Oral snuff dipping and chewing tobacco predispose to leukoplakia and oral cancer. Up to 46% of regular users develop leukoplakia. Currently there is particular concern over the mucosal reactions and the carcinogenic potential of smokeless tobacco by children and adolescents, which is widespread, especially in the USA. Smoking also predisposes to periodontal disease, particularly necrotizing gingivitis, to implant failure, to dry socket, to candidosis and to xerostomia. Cigarette smoking is the most common cause of extrinsic staining of teeth.

Stopping smoking reduces the risk of oral cancer so that, by 5 years, it is down to that of a non-smoker. However, stopping smoking is not merely difficult but may bring other problems. Aggravation or the onset of recurrent aphthae is noted by some, while others take to eating sweets as a substitute for smoking and may then have more caries activity, or put on weight. Use of nicotine-containing chewing gum may reduce the risk of aphthae but may cause hypersalivation. Bupropion may cause dry mouth.

NITRITES

Aliphatic nitrites, including amyl, butyl and cyclohexyl nitrite (used as 'poppers' to enhance sexual activity) may be inhaled. They are dangerous if ingested.

NITROUS OXIDE

Nitrous oxide induces impaired consciousness with a sense of dissociation and often of exhilaration (laughing gas). Addiction to nitrous oxide is an occupational hazard of anaesthetists

Table 34.23 Nicotine replacement therapies (NRTs)		
Type of NRT	**Delivery system**	**Possible adverse effects**
Chewing gum	Gum is chewed gently to release nicotine	Jaw ache Gastric irritation Unsuitable for denture wearers
Inhalor/inhalator	Puff steadily for about 20 min/h	–
Lozenges	Suck until dissolution	–
Nasal spray	1–2 doses per hour for 2 months	Irritation of nasal mucosa
Sublingual tablets	4 mg hourly for 3 months	–
Transdermal patches	Worn during waking hours	Local skin irritation

and others who have access, such as dental surgeons. Cases of nitrous oxide misuse have been reported in the USA among dental and medical students who stole large hospital cylinders. The reason that it has not become a widely abused drug is simply the practical problem of carrying such heavy cylinders around.

Chronic misuse of nitrous oxide can lead to interference with vitamin B_{12} metabolism and neuropathy. Vague neurological symptoms have also been reported by dental staff working in environments contaminated by nitrous oxide.

Other GA agents that may be misused include halothane (liver damage can result; Ch. 9), methoxyflurane (fluorosis, hypertension and renal damage can result) and ketamine. Ether and chloroform were widely abused in the past but now rarely so, as other agents are more readily available.

OPIATES AND OPIOIDS

General aspects

Opiate analgesics (derived from the opium poppy) can produce pain relief and euphoria, but also drowsiness/respiratory depression and arrest, nausea, confusion, constipation, sedation, unconsciousness, coma, tolerance and addiction (Table 34.25).

Opiates – morphine and heroin (diacetylmorphine) – are narcotics derived from the opium poppy. These, and synthetic compounds (opioids) such as methadone, dipipanone, dihydrocodeine and pethidine, are widely used potent analgesics that act by mimicking the natural brain peptides enkephalins and endorphins. Misuse is widespread, mainly in urban areas, particularly new towns and major cities amongst adolescents and young adults. Opiates can be abused orally, sometimes smoked, sniffed or injected subcutaneously (skin popping), but the maximum effect is obtained by intravenous injection. Many addicts also misuse alcohol, cocaine or other drugs. Misuse leads to tolerance at an early stage and dependence after some months.

Heroin is highly addictive and differs from morphine mainly in the difficulty in overcoming addiction; indeed, heroin is probably the most addictive drug known. Heroin users will do almost anything to fund their addiction, which is why heroin use is often associated with antisocial and criminal behaviour, such as burglary. Heroin can be sniffed, smoked from a tin-foil ('chasing the dragon') or injected.

Clinical features

The short-term effects of heroin misuse appear soon after a single dose with a surge of euphoria ('rush') accompanied by a warm flushing of the skin, a dry mouth and heavy extremities – probably due to histamine release – which can last up to 4 h. Mental functioning then becomes clouded due to the depression of the CNS and the heroin user goes into an alternately wakeful and drowsy state ('on the nod'). The addict is said to be 'a depressed introvert with constricted pupils'. Loss of weight, emaciation, pupil constriction, lack of concentration, poor work performance, irritability, a desire to be left alone, absences from home or self-neglect may be indicators. Constipation, respiratory depression, orthostatic hypotension, infections, neglect of general health and hygiene, and poor diet are common. However, early signs of misuse can be difficult or impossible to detect, but may be suspected if needle marks are seen, syringes found or medical complications develop. Needle marks or venous thromboses, particularly in the forearms and legs, are common, but addicts are remarkably adept at finding veins that escape casual inspection, such as lingual or penile veins.

Table 34.24 Non-smoking tobacco use in different cultures

Africa	Arab countries	South Asia	Western countries
Toombak	Shama/shammaah Nass/naswar Zarda	Pan (paan; betel quid) ingredients can be used alone (e.g. mishri, zarda and kiwan) Khaini Gutkah Oral cleaning products (e.g. gudakha) Bajar and creamy snuff	Chewing tobacco (plug, loose leaf and twist) Snuff Snuss

---

Table 34.25 Main opiate and opioid analgesics that are abused

Chemical names	Street names	Comments
Codeine	Captain Cody, Cody, schoolboy; (with glutethimide) doors and fours, loads, pancakes and syrup	Less analgesia, sedation and respiratory depression than morphine
Fentanyl	Apache, China girl, China white, dance fever, friend, goodfella, jackpot, murder 8, TNT, tango and cash	100 times more potent analgesic than morphine
Heroin (diacetylmorphine)	Rock, harry, brown sugar, dope, H, horse, junk, skag, skunk, smack, white horse	Staggering gait, constipation, miosis
Methadone	The done	
Opium	Laudanum, paregoric; big O, black stuff, block, gum, hop	

Syringes and needles are often reused or shared by others; therefore, infective complications such as hepatitis B, C and D, HIV, septicaemia and pneumonia are common. Acute right-sided staphylococcal endocarditis, from injection of skin bacteria, can be rapidly fatal or leave substantial cardiac damage. Sexually transmitted infections are also widespread. Heroin is also a respiratory depressant and its use predisposes also to pneumonia, lung abscesses and fibrosis. Heroin misuse is associated with other serious health disorders, including spontaneous abortion. Long-term effects include collapsed veins, infective endocarditis, abscesses and cellulitis. The mortality rate among opioid addicts is 2–6% per annum; deaths are usually from overdose, suicide, assaults and HIV/AIDS.

'Street' heroin contains only about 10% heroin – most is filler such as lactose, flour, fruit sugars or powdered milk, that do not readily dissolve and result in infection or infarction in lungs, liver, kidneys or brain, and can cause thromboses, abscesses and gangrene. Drugs such as ecstasy may also have been added.

With regular heroin use, tolerance develops so that, as progressively higher doses are taken over time, physical dependence and addiction develop. With physical dependence, the body has adapted to the presence of the drug, and withdrawal symptoms result if the drug is reduced or stopped. Most deaths from heroin are from overdose.

General management

Opiate withdrawal is unpleasant but not usually dangerous. Early features include lacrimation, rhinorrhoea, sweating and persistent yawning. After about 12 h, a phase develops of restless tossing sleep (yen) with pupil dilatation, tremor, gooseflesh ('cold turkey'), anorexia, nausea, vomiting, muscle spasms with kicking movements ('kicking the habit'), orgasms, diarrhoea and abdominal pains. Pulse rate and blood pressure also rise. Once the main features have subsided, there may be weakness and insomnia for weeks or months. Sudden withdrawal in heavily dependent users who are in poor health is occasionally fatal.

Medical supervision and opioid agonists such as methadone (a synthetic medication taken orally as a syrup that blocks the effects of heroin for about 24 h), buprenorphine, naltrexone or LAAM (synthetics that can block heroin effects for up to 72 h) are used.

Dental aspects

Dental treatment for narcotic addicts can often be given without fear of complications. In the established addict, non-narcotic analgesics may be ineffective in controlling dental pain, so that large doses of opioids may have to be given. However, opioids should not be given or prescribed without first seeking expert advice and their only indication in dentistry is for severe post-operative pain. Pentazocine, being a narcotic antagonist, should not be used for such patients as it may precipitate a withdrawal syndrome. Many addicts tolerate pain poorly and complain that LA is insufficient for operative procedures. Opioids may enhance the sedation of conscious sedation agents and GA. Methadone can affect the P450 drug metabolism system.

General anaesthesia requires admission to hospital. Nausea and vomiting are common if the narcotics are stopped pre-operatively. Those under treatment for addiction have a period of several weeks during which they are particularly hypersensitive to pain and stress. In such patients, opioids must be avoided. Although the withdrawal syndrome subsides within about a week, the addict is, for a few weeks thereafter, intolerant of stress and pain. The respiratory response to carbon dioxide is depressed and GA may then be hazardous.

Simulation of pain is a common manoeuvre to obtain analgesics. Prescription pads may be stolen or drug cabinets raided. Dental drugs that may attract the opiate addict include pethidine, codeine, pentazocine and dextropropoxyphene (in co-proxamol). Other management aspects include behavioural disturbances and withdrawal symptoms, cardiac lesions, maxillofacial injuries, hepatitis or chronic liver disease, infective endocarditis, sexually transmitted diseases, including HIV infection, venous thromboses – making intravenous injection difficult – tetanus, and drug interactions.

There are no specific oral effects of opiate dependence but there is often oral neglect, advanced periodontal disease and caries. Diet and sometimes the medications predispose to caries either by containing sugar and/or causing xerostomia. Opiate addicts tend also to adopt a cariogenic diet. Caries is often left untreated by the patient who, because of the opioid, may be undisturbed by the pain.

Adverse effects relevant to dentistry include impaired ability to metabolize drugs, hypertension, arrhythmias, hypercoagulability and disturbed behaviour, such as aggression, irritability, paranoia, headache and psychoses. In relation to the use of GA, gastrointestinal inflammation may predispose to vomiting, and there may be scoline sensitivity. Low plasma cortisol levels might be an indication for a corticosteroid cover before operation. Bleeding tendency or drug intolerance may influence dental care.

Lofexidine and methadone can cause xerostomia. Sugar-free preparations should be used but they are acidic and may predispose to tooth erosion. Preventive oral health care is indicated.

PARAMETHOXYAMPHETAMINE

Paramethoxyamphetamine (PMA) is an MDMA (ecstasy)-like substance that has been involved in the deaths of some people who mistakenly thought they were taking MDMA. Deaths were mainly due to complications from hyperthermia.

PCP (PHENCYCLIDINE; ANGEL DUST)

PCP was developed as an intravenous anaesthetic but discontinued because patients often became agitated, delusional and irrational. PCP has a reputation for causing unpleasant psychological effects, users often becoming violent or suicidal, and a danger to themselves and to others. Many people therefore, after using the drug once, will not knowingly use it again.

PCP is addictive and snorted, smoked or eaten. Low to moderate doses of PCP cause a slight rise in breathing rate, a pronounced rise in BP and pulse rate, flushing and profuse sweating. Generalized numbness of the extremities and muscular incoordination also may occur.

High doses of PCP cause a fall in BP, pulse rate and respiration, which may be accompanied by nausea, vomiting, blurred vision, flicking up and down of the eyes, drooling, loss of balance, and dizziness, and sometimes a syndrome closely resembling schizophrenia and manic depressive psychosis. It can also cause seizures, illusions and hallucinations, coma and death. Speech is often sparse and garbled.

Long-term PCP use can cause memory loss, difficulties with speech and thinking, depression and weight loss. PCP may cause facial grimacing and flushing, hypersalivation and jaw clenching.

PENTAZOCINE

Pentazocine, despite its dysphoric effects, is also used as a drug of dependence, particularly amongst medical and paramedical personnel in the USA. Pentazocine tablets together with an antihistamine (Ts and blues) have been used intravenously as an alternative to the more expensive heroin.

ROHYPNOL (FLUNITRAZEPAM)

Rohypnol is a benzodiazepine that has been used by perpetrators to commit rapes, especially when mixed with alcohol, as it can incapacitate victims and prevent them from resisting sexual assault; since it causes 'anterograde amnesia', individuals may not remember such events. Rohypnol may be lethal when mixed with alcohol and/or other depressants.

USEFUL WEBSITES

http://www.nida.nih.gov/Drugpages/html
http://www.whitehousedrugpolicy.gov/streetterms
http://www.emedicinehealth.com/drug_dependence_and_abuse/article_em.htm
http://www.ic.nhs.uk.statistics-and-data-collections/health-and-lifestyles-related-surveys/smoking-drinking-and-druk-use-among young people in england/drug-use-smoking-among-young-people-in-england-2008-full-report

---

FURTHER READING

Akhter, R., Hassan, N.M., Aida, J., Takinami, S., Morita, M., 2008. Relationship between betel quid additives and established periodontitis among Bangladeshi subjects. J Clin Periodontol 35, 9–15.

Allen, S.E., Singh, S., Robertson, W.G., 2006. The increased risk of urinary stone disease in betel quid chewers. Urol Res 34, 239–243.

Araujo, M.W., Dermen, K., Connors, G., Ciancio, S., 2004. Oral and dental health among inpatients in treatment for alcohol use disorders: a pilot study. J Int Acad Periodontol 6, 125–130.

Autti-Rämö, I., Fagerlund, A., Ervalahti, N., Loimu, L., Korkman, M., Hoyme, H.E., 2006. Fetal alcohol spectrum disorders in Finland: clinical delineation of 77 older children and adolescents. Am J Med Genet A 140, 137–143.

Avon, S.L., 2004. Oral mucosal lesions associated with use of quid. J Can Dent Assoc 70, 244–248.

Babor, T.F., Higgins-Biddle, J.C., Saunders, J.B., Monteiro, M.G., 2001. AUDIT – The alcohol use disorders identification test guidelines for use in primary care, 2nd edn. World Health Organization, Geneva.

Brand, H.S., Dun, S.N., Nieuw Amerongen, A.V., 2008. Ecstasy (MDMA) and oral health. Br Dent J 204, 77–81.

Brazier, W.J., Dhariwal, D.K., Patton, D.W., Bishop, K., 2003. Ecstasy related periodontitis and mucosal ulceration – a case report. Br Dent J 194, 197–199.

Calhoun, F., Attilia, M.L., Spagnolo, P.A., Rotondo, C., Mancinelli, R., Ceccanti, M., 2006. National Institute on Alcohol Abuse and Alcoholism and the study of fetal alcohol spectrum disorders. The International Consortium. Ann Ist Super Sanitá 42, 4–7.

Carda, C., Carranza, M., Arriaga, A., Díaz, A., Peydró, A., Gomez de Ferraris, M.E., 2005. Structural differences between alcoholic and diabetic parotid sialosis. Med Oral Patol Cir Bucal 10, 309–314.

Carda, C., Gomez de Ferraris, M.E., Arriaga, A., Carranza, M., Peydró, A., 2004. Alcoholic parotid sialosis: a structural and ultrastructural study. Med Oral 9, 24–32.

Carpenter, J.M., Syms, M.J., Sniezek, J.C., 2005. Oral carcinoma associated with betel nut chewing in the Pacific: an impending crisis? Pac Health Dialog 12, 158–162.

Carranza, M., Ferraris, M.E., Galizzi, M., 2005. Structural and morphometrical study in glandular parenchyma from alcoholic sialosis. J Oral Pathol Med 34, 374–379.

Carretero Pelaez, M.A., Esparza Gomez, G.C., Figuero Ruiz, E., Cerero Lapiedra, R., 2004. Alcohol-containing mouthwashes and oral cancer. Critical analysis of literature. Med Oral 9, 120–123.

Chaloupka, F.J., Grossman, M., Saffer, H., 2002. The effect of price on alcohol-consumption and alcohol-related problems. Alcohol Res Health 26, 22–34.

Chen, C.C., Li, T.C., Chang, P.C., et al., 2008. Association among cigarette smoking, metabolic syndrome, and its individual components: the metabolic syndrome study in Taiwan. Metabolism 57, 544–548.

Chikte, U.M., Naidoo, S., Kolze, T.J., Grobler, S.R., 2005. Patterns of tooth surface loss among winemakers. South Afr Dent J 60, 370–374.

Chuajedong, P., Kedjarune-Leggat, U., Kertpon, V., Chongsuvivatwong, V., Benjakul, P., 2002. Associated factors of tooth wear in southern Thailand. J Oral Rehabil 29, 997–1002.

Chung, F.M., Chang, D.M., Chen, M.P., et al., 2006. Areca nut chewing is associated with metabolic syndrome: role of tumor necrosis factor-alpha, leptin, and white blood cell count in betel nut chewing-related metabolic derangements. Diabetes Care 29, 1714.

Cole, P., Rodu, B., Mathisen, A., 2003. Alcohol-containing mouthwash and oropharyngeal cancer: a review of the epidemiology. J Am Dent Assoc 134, 1079–1087.

Corrao, G., Rubbiati, I., Bagnardi, V., Zambon, A., Poikolainen, K., 2000. Alcohol and coronary heart disease: a meta-analysis. Addiction 95, 1505–1523.

Enberg, N., Wolf, J., Ainamo, A., Alho, H., Heinälä, P., Lenander-Lumikari, M., 2001. Dental diseases and loss of teeth in a group of Finnish alcoholics: a radiological study. Acta Odontol Scand 59, 341–347.

Ezzati, M., Lopez, A.D., Rodgers, A., van der Hoorn, S., Murray, C.J.L.; Comparative Risk Assessment Collaborating Group, 2002. Selected major risk factors and global and regional burden of disease. Lancet 360, 1347–1360.

Fasanmade, A., Kwok, E., Newman, L., 2007. Oral squamous cell carcinoma associated with khat chewing. Oral Surg Oral Med Oral Pathol Oral Radiol Endod 104, e53–e55.

Ferlay, J., Bray, F., Pisani, P., Parking, D.M. (Eds), 2001. Gobocan 2000 Cancer incidence, mortality and prevalence worldwide. International Agency for Research on Cancer, Lyons.

Ferraris, M.E., Carranza, M., Arriaga, A., 2000. A structural and immunocytochemical study of palatine and labial salivary glands from chronic alcoholics. Acta Odontol Latinoam 13, 113–121.

Foxcroft, D.R., Ireland, D., Lister-Sharp, D.J., Lowe, G., Breen, R., 2003. Longer-term primary prevention for alcohol misuse in young people: a systematic review. Addiction 98, 397–411.

Furr, A.M., Schweinfurth, J.M., May, W.L., 2006. Factors associated with long-term complications after repair of mandibular fractures. Laryngoscope 116, 427–430.

Gallivan, K.H., Reiter, D., 2001. Acute alcohol withdrawal and free flap mandibular reconstruction outcomes. Arch Facial Plast Surg 3, 264–266.

García-Algar, O., Vall, O., Alameda, F., et al., 2005. Prenatal exposure to arecoline (areca nut alkaloid) and birth outcomes. Arch Dis Child Fetal Neonatal Ed 90, F276–F277.

Goodisson, D., MacFarlane, M., Snape, L., Darwish, B., 2004. Head injury and associated maxillofacial injuries. N Z Med J 117 U1045.

Graham, C.H., Meechan, J.G., 2005. Dental management of patients taking methadone. Dental Update 32, 477–485.

Guh, J.Y., Chen, H.C., Tsai, J.F., Chuang, L.Y., 2007. Betel-quid use is associated with heart disease in women. Am J Clin Nutr 85, 1229–1235.

Hashibe, M., Straif, K., Tashkin, D.P., Morganstern, H., Greenland, S., Zhang, Z.F., 2005. Epidemiologic review of marijuana use and cancer risk. Alcohol 35, 265–275.

Hornecker, E., Muuss, T., Ehrenreich, H., Mausberg, R.F., 2003. A pilot study on the oral conditions of severely alcohol addicted persons. J Contemp Dent Pract 4, 51–59.

Hoyme, H.E., May, P.A., Kalberg, W.O., et al., 2005. A practical clinical approach to diagnosis of fetal alcohol spectrum disorders: clarification of the 1996 institute of medicine criteria. Pediatrics 115, 39–47.

Hsiao, T.J., Liao, H.W., Hsieh, P.S., Wong, R.H., 2007. Risk of betel quid chewing on the development of liver cirrhosis: a community-based case-control study. Ann Epidemiol 17 (6), 479–485.

Hsu, S.D., Singh, B.B., Lewis, J.B., 2002. Chemoprevention of oral cancer by green tea. Gen Dent 50, 140–146.

IARC Working Group on the Evaluation of Carcinogenic Risks to Humans, 2004. Betel-quid and areca-nut chewing and some areca-nut derived nitrosamines. IARC Monogr Eval Carcinog Risks Hum 85, 1–334.

Jang, Y.C., Kim, Y.J., Lee, J.W., et al., 2006. Face burns caused by flambé drinks. J Burn Care Res 27, 93–96.

Jones, L., Lekkas, D., Hunt, D., McIntyre, J., Rafir, W., 2002. Studies on dental erosion: an in vivo-in vitro model of endogenous dental erosion – its application to testing protection by fluoride gel application. Aust Dent J 47, 304–308.

Kamisawa, T., Tu, Y., Egawa, N., Sakaki, N., Inokuma, S., Kamata, N., 2003. Salivary gland involvement in chronic pancreatitis of various etiologies. Am J Gastroenterol 98, 323–326.

Kastin, B., Mandel, L., 2000. Alcoholic sialosis. N Y State Dent J 66, 22–24.

Kwasnicki, A., Longman, L., Wilkinson, G., 2008. The significance of alcohol misuse in the dental patient. Dent Update 35, 7–20.

Lin, C.F., Shiau, T.J., Ko, Y.C., Chen, P.H., Wang, J.D., 2008. Prevalence and determinants of biochemical dysfunction of the liver in Atayal Aboriginal community of Taiwan: is betel nut chewing a risk factor?. BMC Gastroenterol 8, 13.

Llewellyn, C.D., Johnson, N.W., Warnakulasuriya, K.A.A.S., 2001. Risk factors for squamous cell carcinoma of the oral cavity in young people – a comprehensive literature review. Oral Oncol 37, 401–418.

Lugasi, A., Hovari, J., 2003. Antioxidant properties of commercial alcoholic and nonalcoholic beverages. Nahrung 47, 79–86.

Lussi, A., Jaeggi, T., Zero, D., 2004. The role of diet in the aetiology of dental erosion. Caries Res 38 (Suppl 1), 34–44.

Mack, F., Mundt, T., Mojon, P., et al., 2003. Study of health in Pomerania (SHIP): relationship among socioeconomic and general health factors and dental status among elderly adults in Pomerania. Quintessence Int 34, 772–778.

Mandel, L., 2005. Dental erosion due to wine consumption. JADA 136, 71–75.

Mandic, R., Teymoortash, A., Kann, P.H., Werner, J.A., 2005. Sialadenosis of the major salivary glands in a patient with central diabetes insipidus – implications of aquaporin water channels in the pathomechanism of sialadenosis. Exp Clin Endocrinol Diabetes 113, 205–207.

McGrath, C., Chan, B., 2005. Oral health sensations associated with illicit drug abuse. Br Dent J 198, 159–162.

Meurman, J.H., Vesterinen, M., 2000. Wine, alcohol, and oral health, with special emphasis on dental erosion. Quintessence Int 31, 729–733.

Molin, S., Plewig, G., 2007. [Betel quid chewing: traditional habit with side effects.]. MMW Fortschr Med 149, 46–47.

Mutsvangwa, T., Douglas, T.S., 2007. Morphometric analysis of facial landmark data to characterize the facial phenotype associated with fetal alcohol syndrome. J Anat 210, 209–220.

Naidoo, S., Chikte, U., Laubscher, R., Lombard, C., 2005. Fetal alcohol syndrome: anthropometric and oral health status. J Contemp Dent Pract 6, 101–115.

Naidoo, S., Harris, A., Swanevelder, S., Lombard, C., 2006. Foetal alcohol syndrome: a cephalometric analysis of patients and controls. Eur J Orthod 28, 254–261.

Naidoo, S., Norval, G., Swanevelder, S., Lombard, C., 2006. Foetal alcohol syndrome: a dental and skeletal age analysis of patients and controls. Eur J Orthod 28, 247–253.

Nathwani, N.S., Gallagher, J.E., 2008. Methadone: dental risks and preventive action. Dent Update 35, 542–544, 547–8.

Petti, S., Scully, C., 2005. The role of the dental team in preventing and diagnosing cancer: 5. Alcohol and the role of the dentist in alcohol cessation. Dent Update 32, 454–462.

Rafeek, R.N., Marchan, S., Eder, A., Smith, W.A., 2006. Tooth surface loss in adult subjects attending a university dental clinic in Trinidad. Int J Dent 56, 181–186.

Reece, A.S., 2007. Dentition of addiction in Queensland: poor dental status and major contributing drugs. Aust Dent J 52, 144–149.

Rehm, J., Room, R., Graham, K., Monteiro, M., Gmel, G., Sempos, C.T., 2003. The relationship of average volume of alcohol consumption and patterns of drinking to burden of disease – an overview. Addiction 98, 1209–1228.

Room, R., Babor, T., Rehm, J., 2005. Alcohol and public health. Lancet 365, 519–530.

Sandler, N.A., 2001. Patients who misuse drugs. Oral Surg 91, 12–14.

Sant'Anna, L.B., Tosello, D.O., 2006. Fetal alcohol syndrome and developing craniofacial and dental structures – a review. Orthod Craniofac Res 9, 172–185.

Schreiber, A., 2001. Alcoholism. Oral Surg 92, 127–131.

Scully, C., 2007. Cannabis; adverse effects from an oromucosal spray. Br Dent J 203, 336–337.

Scully, C., 2009. Aspect of Human Disease 34. Alcoholism Dental Update 36, 317.

Scully, C., Bagán, J.V., 2004. Adverse drug reaction in the orofacial region. Critical Reviews in Oral Biology and Medicine 15, 221–239.

Scully, C., Bagan, J.V., Eveson, J.W., Barnard, N., Turner, 2008. Sialosis: 35 cases of persistent parotid swelling from two countries. Br J Oral Maxillofac Surg 46, 468–472.

Shepherd, J.P., Sutherland, I., Newcombe, R.G., 2006. Relations between alcohol, violence and victimization in adolescence. J Adolesc 29, 539–553.

Shults, R.A., Elder, R.W., Sleet, D.A., et al., and the Task Force on Community Preventive Services, 2001. Reviews of evidence regarding interventions to reduce alcohol-impaired driving. Am J Prev Med 21, 66–88.

Signoretto, C., Burlacchini, G., Bianchi, F., Cavalleri, G., Canepari, P., 2006. Differences in microbiological composition of saliva and dental plaque in subjects with different drinking habitus. New Microbiol 29, 293–302.

Simpura, J., Karlsson, T., 2001. Trends in drinking patterns among adult population in 15 European countries, 1950 to 2000: a review. Nordic Stud Alcohol Drugs 18, 31–53.

Smith, A.J., Hodgson, R.J., Bridgeman, K., Shepherd, J.P., 2003. A randomized controlled trial of a brief intervention after alcohol-related facial injury. Addiction 98, 43–52.

Smullen, J., Koutsou, G.-A., Foster, H.A., Zumbé, A., Storey, D.M., 2007. The antibacterial activity of plant extracts containing polyphenols against Streptococcus mutans. Caries Res 41, 342–349.

Tilakaratne, W.M., Klinikowski, M.F., Saku, T., Peters, T.J., Warnakulasuriya, S., 2006. Oral submucous fibrosis: review on aetiology and pathogenesis. Oral Oncol 42, 561–568.

Tredwin , C., Scully, C., Bagan, J.V., 2005. Drug-induced dental disorders. Adverse Drug Reaction Bulletin 232, 891–894.

Tredwin , C., Scully, C., Bagan, J.V., 2005. Drug-induced disorders of teeth. Journal of Dental Research 84, 596–602.

Tsai, J.F., Chuang, L.Y., Jeng, J.E., et al., 2001. Betel quid chewing as a risk factor for hepatocellular carcinoma: a case-control study. Br J Cancer 84, 709–713.

Tsai, J.F., Jeng, J.E., Chuang, L.Y., et al., 2004. Habitual betel quid chewing and risk for hepatocellular carcinoma complicating cirrhosis. Medicine (Baltimore) 83, 176–187.

Underwood, B., Fox, K., 2001. A survey of alcohol and drug use among UK based dental undergraduates. BDJ Launchpad 8, 26–29.

Versteeg, P.A., Slot, D.E., van der Velden, U., van der Weijden, G.A., 2008. Effect of cannabis usage on the oral environment: a review. Int J Dent Hyg 6, 315–320.

Warburton, A.L., Shepherd, J.P., 2002. Alcohol-related violence and the role of oral and maxillofacial surgeons in multi-agency prevention. Int J Oral Maxillofac Surg 31, 657–663.

Warburton, A.L., Shepherd, J.P., 2006. Tackling alcohol related violence in city centres: effect of emergency medicine and police intervention. Emerg Med J 23, 12–17.

Weinfeld, A.B., Davison, S.P., Mason, A.C., Manders, E.K., Russavage, J.M., 2000. Management of alcohol withdrawal in microvascular head and neck reconstruction. J Reconstr Microsurg 16, 201–206.

World Health Organization (WHO), 2004. Department of Mental Health and Substance Abuse. Global status report on alcohol 2004. WHO, Geneva.

World Health Organization (WHO), 2002. World Health Report 2002: reducing risks, promoting healthy life. WHO, Geneva.

Yang, M.S., Lee, C.H., Chang, S.J., et al., 2008. The effect of maternal betel quid exposure during pregnancy on adverse birth outcomes among aborigines in Taiwan. Drug Alcohol Depend 95, 134–139.

Young, W.G., 2005. Tooth wear: diet analysis and advice. Int Dent J 55, 68–72.

Zero, D.T., Lussi, A., 2006. Behavioral factors. Monogr Oral Sci 20, 100–105.

Zero, D.T., Lussi, A., 2005. Erosion – chemical and biological factors of importance to the dental practitioner. Int Dent J 55 (4 Suppl 1), 285–290.

Appendix 34.1 Some street names and other terms for drugs of misuse

Street names	Drug
Acapulco gold	Cannabis
Acid	LSD
Angel dust/mist	Phencyclidine
Animal tranquillizer	Phencyclidine
Base	Cocaine
Beans	Amphetamine/amfetamine
Bennies	Amphetamine/amfetamine
Bhang[a]	Cannabis
Billy	Amphetamine/amfetamine
Biscuits	Ecstasy
Black tar	Heroin
Blanco	Heroin
Blow	Cannabis
Blue angel/devil/heaven	Amylobarbital
Bolivian	Cocaine
Booze	Alcohol
C	Cocaine
Cadillac	Cocaine
Candy	Barbiturates
Charas	Cannabis
Charlies	Cocaine
Chip	Heroin
Christmas trees	Barbiturates
Coke	Cocaine
Co-pilot	Methamphetamine
Crack	Cocaine free base
Crystal	Methamphetamine
Crystal joints	Phencyclidine
Cubes	LSD
Dagga[a]	Cannabis
Dennis the Menace	Ecstasy
Dexies	Dexamphetamine/amfetamine
Disco (disco biscuit)	Ecstasy
Doe	Methamphetamine
Dope	Heroin
Dot	LSD

Street names	Drug
Downers	Barbiturates
Drinamyl	Amphetamine/amfetamines
E	Ecstasy
Ecstasy	Methylenedeoxy-methamphetamine
Edwards	Ecstasy
Elephant	Phencyclidine
Freebase	Cocaine
Ganga[a]	Cannabis
GHB	Gamma-hydroxybutyrate
Girl	Cocaine
Gold dust	Cocaine
Goofballs	Barbiturates
Goon	Phencyclidine
Grass	Cannabis
Gunk	Morphine
H	Heroin
Hash (hashish[a])	Cannabis
Hocus	Morphine
Hog	Phencyclidine
Horse	Heroin
Horse tranquillizer	Phencyclidine
Ice	Methamphetamine
Jack up	Amylobarbital
Jellies	Tranquillizers
Junk	Cocaine
K (Special K)	Ketamine
KJ	Phencyclidine
Lady	Cocaine
Lilly	Secobarbital
Love drug/dove	Methamphetamine or ecstasy
Ludes	Methaqualone
(Marihuana)[a] marijuana	Cannabis
Mesc	Mescaline
Microdot	LSD
Mist	Phencyclidine
Monkey	Morphine
Mushroom	Psilocybin
Nebbies	Pentobarbital

Street names	Drug
Panama gold	Cannabis
Paris	Methaqualone
PCP	Phencyclidine
Peace pills	Phencyclidine
Peaches	Amphetamine/amfetamine
Pink	Morphine
Poppers	Amylnitrite
Pot	Cannabis
Purple haze	LSD
Purple hearts	Dexamphetamine/amfetamine and amylobarbital
Quads	Methaqualone
Red devils	Secobarbital
Reefer	Cannabis
Rhubarb and custard	Ecstasy
Rock	Cocaine
Rocket fuel	Phencyclidine
Scuffle	Phencyclidine
Sensi	Cannabis
Shit	Heroin
Silly putty	Psilocybin
Skunk	Cannabis

Street names	Drug
Smack	Heroin
Snow	Cocaine
Soapers	Methaqualone
Soma	Phencyclidine
Speed	Amphetamine/amfetamine (intravenously)
Speedball	Opioids and amphetamine/amfetamine (or cocaine and heroin)
Spliff	Cannabis
Strawberry	LSD
Sulfate	Amphetamine/amfetamine
T	Phencyclidine
TCP	Thiencylcyclophexyl piperidine
Tea	Cannabis
Tic tac	Phencyclidine
Ts and blues	Pentazocine and tripelennamine
Vitamins	Ecstasy
Wash	Cocaine
Weed	Cannabis
White lightning	LSD
Yellow jackets	Pentobarbital

aCorrect name in country of origin.

TRANSPLANTATION AND TISSUE REGENERATION

TRANSPLANTS

Transplantation of organs and tissues has developed rapidly alongside the enormous advances in understanding of immunology, and the development of improved immunosuppressive therapy and medical and surgical technology. The organs and tissues currently transplanted are shown in Table 35.1.

INDICATIONS

Transplants are generally indicated in patients with untreatable end-stage disease, substantial limitation of daily activities and limited life expectancy. Transplantation is often the only effective treatment for end-stage disease and is frequently a life-saving procedure. Best results are in ambulatory patients with rehabilitation potential, with no other significant medical diseases, with a satisfactory psychosocial profile and emotional support system, and acceptable nutritional status. Organ donation is thus important. Transplantation may be refused by some Jehovah's Witnesses and orthodox Jews.

TYPES OF TRANSPLANT

Autologous transplantation

Autologous transplants (*autografts*) refer to cells that are collected from an individual and given back to that same individual (e.g. veins used for coronary artery bypass, and skin grafts) or blood. Autografts are the most common type of transplant used in patients with lymphoproliferative disease: stem cells are obtained from the patient before chemotherapy, frozen (stored if necessary), and then re-infused after chemotherapy (Fig. 35.1).

Allogeneic transplantation

Allogeneic transplants (allografts) refers to cells that come from another individual who may be a relative or not, but the donor's blood must be closely matched to the recipient's, which is more likely when the donor is a sibling. Isografts are allografts in which organs or tissues are transplanted from a donor to a genetically identical recipient (e.g. an identical twin). Most human tissue and organ transplants are allografts and most are not so closely matched, which means that the recipient needs to be immunosuppressed with drugs to prevent transplant rejection.

SOURCES OF ORGANS

Transplants can be from live or dead ('cadaveric') donors, or from donors who are living but 'brain dead' – a state defined by an irreversible cessation of all brain and brainstem function, determined by clinical criteria by two separate examinations

Table 35.1 Transplantation		
	Source	**Type**
Thoracic organs	Heart	Deceased donor only
	Lung	Deceased donor and living donor
	Heart/lung	Deceased donor and domino transplant
Abdominal organs	Kidney	Deceased donor and living donor
	Liver	Deceased donor and living donor
	Pancreas	Deceased donor only
	Small intestine	Deceased donor and living donor
Tissues, cells, fluids	Blood transfusion/blood parts transfusion	Living donor and autograft
	Blood vessels	Autograft and deceased donor
	Bone	Deceased donor, living donor and autograft
	Bone marrow/adult stem cell	Living donor and autograft
	Cornea	Deceased donor only
	Face replant	Autograft
	Face transplant (rare)	Deceased donor only
	Hand	Deceased donor only
	Heart valve	Deceased donor, living donor and xenograft (porcine/bovine)
	Penis	Deceased donor only
	Pancreas islet cells	Deceased donor and living donor
	Skin	Deceased donor, living donor and autograft
	Trachea	Autograft

performed 24 h apart or by ancillary studies to assess brain activities. An absence of drugs, hypothermia or metabolic derangements must be confirmed. Brain death criteria are shown in Box 35.1.

OUTCOMES

The transplantation survival rate has doubled over the past decade; renal transplant recipients, for example, now survive on average for about 35 years. Success rates vary for the different

Box 35.1 Criteria of brain death

- Known cause of condition
- Temperature higher than 95°F
- No drug intoxication or neuromuscular blocking agent
- No significant metabolic derangement
- No gag, cough or corneal reflexes
- Absence of dull-eye reflex
- Pupils fixed and dilated
- No spontaneous respirations or movements
- Negative results on apnoea test
- Isoelectric electroencephalogram (EEG)
- Computed tomographic evidence of brain herniation
- Negative results on cerebral blood flow studies (i.e. brain scan or intracranial angiography)

types of organ transplanted and can approach 90% at 1 year, the major barrier being immunological rejection of the transplant. Except for transplants between identical twins, all transplant donors and recipients are immunologically incompatible. The host cells try to destroy or reject the transplanted organ and rejection episodes may be mild or severe but, with time, can lead to graft failure or patient death. The other main cause of graft rejection is patients' failure to continue to take their immunosuppressive drugs.

Immunological evaluation primarily serves to try to avoid transplant rejection. ABO blood group determination is used to establish whether the patient is a potential target of recipient circulating preformed cytotoxic anti-ABO antibody. Transplantation across incompatible blood groups may result in a humorally mediated hyperacute rejection. Tissue typing of transplant recipients and donors determines the HLA class I and class II loci. The degree of incompatibility between the donor and recipient is defined by the number of antigens that are mismatched at each of the HLA loci. The degree of humoral sensitization to HLA antigens is determined: sensitization happens when the recipient has received multiple blood transfusions from a previous organ transplant or during pregnancy. Transplantation of an organ into a recipient sensitized against donor class I HLA antigens puts the recipient at high risk of hyperacute antibody-mediated rejection. Cross-matching is an *in vitro* assay to determine whether a potential transplant recipient has preformed anti-HLA class I antibodies against those of the organ donor. A negative cross-match must be obtained before accepting an organ for transplantation.

PREVENTION OF REJECTION

Following transplantation, all patients are placed on immunosuppressive drugs for life, prevent a T-cell alloimmune rejection. The goals are to achieve the highest rates of patient and graft survival, but also to minimize drug toxicity, infection and malignancy. The current high graft survival rate is due to effective steroid-sparing immunosuppression using azathioprine, ciclosporin, OKT3 monoclonal antibodies, daclizumab, basiliximab, mycophenolate mofetil, tacrolimus, sirolimus and interleukin (IL)-2 receptor blockers. No consensus exists as to the single best immunosuppressive protocol, and each transplant programme uses slightly different combinations of agents.

Induction immunotherapy after transplantation uses polyclonal antisera, mouse monoclonals and so-called humanized monoclonals and has increased since the introduction of IL-2 receptor-blocking antibodies (daclizumab and basiliximab). It consists of a short course of intensive treatment to lower significantly and almost abolish circulating lymphoid cells critical to the rejection response. Induction agents are given less often if the graft functions immediately, as in recipients of living kidney donors, especially HLA-ID grafts.

Maintenance immunosuppression is usually based on a calcineurin inhibitor (e.g. ciclosporin, tacrolimus or sirolimus) and/or corticosteroids, sometimes combined with corticosteroid-sparing agents, such as newer antimetabolites (e.g. mycophenolate mofetil), or antiproliferative agents, such as rapamycin (Table 35.2).

A number of drugs can interfere with immunosuppressive agents (Tables 35.3, 29.1 and 29.2).

COMPLICATIONS OF TRANSPLANTATION

The usual causes of early death of patients who survive transplant surgery are infection, multiorgan failure and acute allograft rejection.

Immunosuppressive therapy is designed to suppress T-lymphocyte function, and leads to immunoincompetence and liability to infections especially with mycobacteria, fungi and viruses. Such infections may spread rapidly, may be opportunistic and may be clinically silent or atypical. Transplant recipients have an increased risk of some malignant neoplasms, including melanoma, basal cell carcinoma, Kaposi sarcoma, lymphomas and squamous cell carcinomas of the skin and lip, and carcinoma of the cervix, external genitalia and perineum. Several of these tumours have a viral aetiology.

Transplant patients may also develop recurrent organ disease, and have an increased risk of coronary heart disease (10–20 times more prevalent). Haematopoietic stem cell transplantation may be complicated by graft-versus-host disease (GVHD).

INFECTIONS

Transplant patients are at risk from a range of infections (Table 35.4), though the infections experienced also depend on the environment and, to some extent, other treatments. Antifungal and antiviral prophylaxis may be appropriate. Infections may spread rapidly, may be opportunistic and may be clinically silent or atypical. Even mild infections are a serious threat in immunosuppressed patients and, as an adjunct to anti-infective therapy, immunosuppression may need to be reduced or even stopped temporarily by the responsible physician.

Bacterial sepsis is the most common cause of deaths during the first post-operative months. Bacterial infections are better

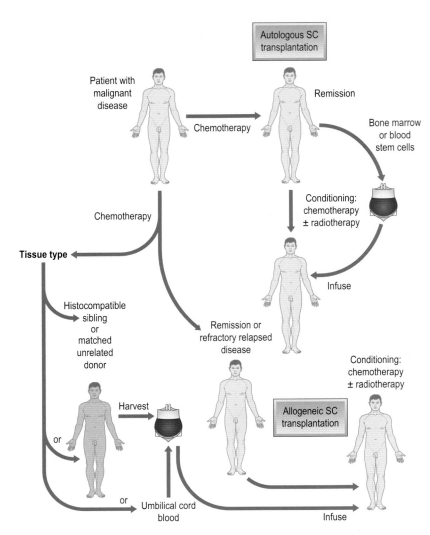

Fig. 35.1 Stem cell (SC) transplantation for lymphoproliferative disease

tolerated with ciclosporin than with azathioprine but still must be treated aggressively. *Legionella* infections are more common in immunosuppressed patients, and often cause dyspnoea and hypoxaemia before the chest radiograph shows a significant infiltrate. A patient who develops such symptoms or a pulmonary infiltrate of unknown aetiology must be treated early with erythromycin.

Viral infections account for substantial morbidity and mortality. Herpes simplex (HSV) infections are common and usually treated with a 10–14-day course of aciclovir or famciclovir. Varicella-zoster virus (VZV) infections may appear, especially herpes zoster. Cytomegalovirus (CMV) infection is one of the other most common infections, and usually appears 3 weeks or more after transplantation, presenting with fever, leukopenia and malaise. The CMV status of the donor must therefore be recorded in the recipient's records, and the CMV titre must be ordered as part of the pre-transplant evaluation so the results are available immediately after transplantation. A tissue diagnosis of CMV should be sought, either by the histological findings or by biopsy cultures. Patients with systemic CMV infections are treated with ganciclovir.

Fungi can cause severe local or even systematically invasive infections in transplant patients. Candidal species are most common and infections in sputum, blood, urine, bile or drains are an indication for systemic antifungal therapy. As a general rule, if *Candida* grows from two or more sites, even if not from blood (e.g. urine, wound), the patient should be treated and managed as having systemic candidosis. Intravenous amphotericin, or fluconazole intravenously or orally, is usually used. *Aspergillus niger, flavus* or *fumigatus* infections may infect the lungs, upper respiratory tract, skin, soft tissues and central nervous system (CNS). Aspergillosis most commonly causes a diffuse pneumonia with patchy infiltrates and, whenever aspergillosis is a possible diagnosis, amphotericin treatment should be initiated; a long course of systemic therapy is indicated if infection is confirmed. Development of a brain abscess is insidious and cure has been rare.

Cryptococcus neoformans infections may cause pulmonary, CNS and disseminated cutaneous disease in immunosuppressed patients, diagnosed by cerebrospinal fluid (CSF) examination (lumbar puncture), staining with traditional India ink stains and testing for CSF cryptococcal antigen. Amphotericin treatment systemically is indicated.

Table 35.2 Immunosuppressive agents commonly used in transplantation

Drug	Mode of action	Main adverse effects	Main drug interactions with
Azathioprine	Metabolized by thiopurine methyl transferase (TPMT) to the active mercaptopurine, which reduces DNA synthesis and inhibits lymphocyte division	Myelosuppression Leucopenia Thrombocytopenia Low TPMT increases risk of myelosuppression Hepatotoxicity	Allopurinol, cytostatic drugs, muscle relaxants, warfarin
Basiliximab	Antibody against CD25 T cells	Hypersensitivity reactions	–
Ciclosporin	Highly lipid-soluble and metabolized in the liver by cytochrome P450 (CYP3A4). Ciclosporin binds to cyclophilins (cytosolic receptors) and inhibits calcineurin. Ciclosporin prevents dephosphorylation of NFAT (nuclear translocation of nuclear factor of activated T cells), and thus blocks interleukin-2 (IL-2)	Neurotoxicity, hypertension, tremulousness, hypertrichosis, gingival swelling, hepatotoxicity, nephrotoxicity with hyperkalemia and/or renal tubular acidosis. No bone marrow effect	Carbamazepine, phenytoin, isoniazid, rifampin, phenobarbital and other drugs that induce CYP3A4 may lower ciclosporin levels. Drugs that inhibit CYP3A4 may raise ciclosporin levels Table 35.3 Acute renal failure, rhabdomyolysis, myositis and myalgias when taken concurrently with statin
Corticosteroids	May reduce inflammation by reversing increased capillary permeability and suppressing polymorphonuclear neutrophilic leukocytes (PMNs)	Hypertension, diabetes, osteoporosis and fractures, hip necrosis, cataracts, acne and obesity	–
Daclizumab	Antibody against IL-2 receptors	Hypersensitivity reactions	–
Mycophenolate mofetil	Inhibits inosine monophosphate dehydrogenase to impair cytotoxic T cells	Bone marrow suppression	Aciclovir, antacids, ganciclovir, cholestyramine
Rapamycin	Cytotoxic	Cytopenias and hyperlipidaemia	
Sirolimus	A non-calcineurin inhibitor. Inhibits lymphocyte proliferation and impairs cytotoxic T cells	Hyperlipidaemia	Table 35.3
Tacrolimus	A calcineurin inhibitor macrolide antibiotic similar to ciclosporin. Inhibits IL-2, interferon-gamma and IL-3 production; transferrin and IL-2 receptor expression; mixed lymphocyte reactions; and cytotoxic T-cell generation through an immunophilin protein – the FK-binding protein (FKBP) which inhibits nuclear translocation of nuclear factor of activated T cells (NFAT). Tacrolimus is metabolized by the same P450 system as ciclosporin	Hyperglycaemia, neurotoxicity and nephrotoxicity Cardiomyopathy if given with ciclosporin to children	Aciclovir, antacids, azathioprine, cholestyramine, probenecid Table 35.3

Mucor and *Rhizopus* infections (phycomycoses) are rarely encountered, but can cause destructive CNS or soft tissue infections. Treatment includes local excision and a long course of systemic amphotericin. *Pneumocystis* infections are common in immunosuppressed patients. A patient who develops a pulmonary infiltrate of unknown aetiology must be treated early with co-trimoxazole for *Pneumocystis* infections, which, as with *Legionella*, commonly cause dyspnoea and hypoxaemia before the chest radiographs show any significant infiltrate.

POST-TRANSPLANT MALIGNANCIES

Transplant recipients are at risk of some malignant neoplasms (but not the most common cancers), as a consequence of immunosuppression. There may be a recurrence of pre-existing cancers in recipients, donor-transmitted neoplasms or *de novo* malignancies. These malignancies are often virally induced: carcinoma of the skin, lip and cervix, may be associated with human papillomavirus (HPV); Kaposi sarcoma is associated with human herpesvirus-8 (HHV-8); and lymphomas and post-transplant lymphoproliferative disease may be associated with Epstein–Barr virus (EBV).

Skin cancer, including squamous cell carcinoma, basal cell carcinoma and melanoma, is up to 20 times more frequent in transplant recipients than in the general population and tends to be aggressive. Transplant recipients should therefore avoid sun exposure and undergo routine skin evaluations, with aggressive management of any lesions.

Kaposi sarcoma may affect the skin, oropharynx, lungs, or other viscera. Treatment involves lowering immunosuppression and then often chemotherapy or radiotherapy.

Some malignancies are seen more frequently in certain subpopulations, according to pre-existing risk factors or behaviours, such as oropharyngeal and lung cancer in those who smoke, or colon cancer in patients with pre-existing inflammatory bowel disease. Directed screening in these patients is desirable, by regular oropharyngeal examinations, chest radiographs and colonoscopies.

Table 35.3   Drug use in transplanted patients that may change blood levels of immunosuppressants, and affect treatment or health

	Drugs that may change blood levels of immunosuppressants			Drugs that increase nephrotoxicity	Drugs that increase hepatotoxicity
	Ciclosporin	Tacrolimus	Sirolimus		
Raise levels	Amphotericin Clarithromycin Erythromycin Grapefruit juice Ketoconazole Norfloxacin	Clarithromycin Diltiazem Erythromycin Fluconazole Grapefruit juice Itraconazole Ketoconazole Miconazole Nelfinavir Nifedipine NSAIDs Omeprazole Quinupristin Ritonavir Telithromycin	Ciclosporin Diltiazem Grapefruit juice Itraconazole Ketoconazole Miconazole Telithromycin Voriconazole	Amphotericin Clarithromycin Diclofenac Erythromycin Indometacin NSAIDs Sulfamethoxazole Vancomycin	Aminoglycosides Co-trimoxazole Erythromycin Halothane Quinolones Tetracyclines
Lower levels	Carbamazepine Phenytoin Sulfamethoxazole	Rifampicin	Rifampicin		

NSAIDs, non-steroidal anti-inflammatory drugs.

Post-transplant lymphoproliferative disorders

General aspects

Post-transplant lymphoproliferative disorders (PTLDs) are a heterogeneous group of B-cell proliferations, associated with EBV infection (from either virus reactivation or primary post-transplant infection) which range from B-cell hyperplasia to malignant immunoblastic lymphoma. All PTLDs, irrespective of histology, are potentially, and frequently, fatal.

Post-transplant lymphoproliferative disorders are relatively uncommon after solid organ and allogeneic bone marrow transplantation (generally about 2%), but about ten times higher if the patient receives mismatched T cell-depleted bone marrow or anti-T-cell monoclonal antibodies for GVHD. The more intense the immunosuppression, the higher the incidence of PTLD, and the earlier it appears. In cardiac transplantation, the incidence ranges from 4.9% to 13%, reflecting the greater immunosuppression used. PTLDs typically develop within 1 year of transplantation but they may appear from 1 month to 14 years post-transplantation.

Clinical features

Clinical presentation is very variable, from aggressive disease with diffuse involvement starting early in the post-transplantation period and with polyclonal lesions developing over days or weeks, to localized lesions that are indolent and slow-growing over months. Whether PTLD is localized or disseminated, the tumours are progressive and mortality rates may be as high as 60–100%.

Fever, weight loss, an infectious mononucleosis-like syndrome (anorexia, lethargy, sore throat, lymphadenopathy), gastrointestinal symptoms (diarrhoea, abdominal pain), pulmonary

Table 35.4   Main possible post-transplantation infections

Infection	Month post-transplantation		
	1	2	> 2
Fungal	Candidosis	Candidosis Deep mycoses	Candidosis Deep mycoses
Viral	Hepatitis Herpesviruses	Hepatitis Herpesviruses	Hepatitis Herpesviruses
Bacterial	Wound Urinary tract Pneumonia	Wound Urinary tract Tuberculosis Pneumonia	Tuberculosis Pneumonia

symptoms (dyspnoea) and CNS or neurological symptoms are common. The most common sites involved are lymph nodes (59%), liver (31%), lung (29%), kidney (25%), bone marrow (25%), small intestine (22%), spleen (21%), CNS (19%), large bowel (14%), tonsils (10%) and salivary glands (4%).

General management

Post-transplant lymphoproliferative disorder is diagnosed by having a high index of suspicion in a patient who has recently undergone transplantation and presents with unexplained fever, weight loss, lymphadenopathy, hepatosplenomegaly and positive histopathology, and EBV-DNA, RNA or viral protein on biopsy.

Treatment is by reduction or withdrawal of immunosuppression, plus ganciclovir for EBV. Since lowering immunosuppression carries the risk of allograft dysfunction or loss, additional treatment modalities are indicated: rituximab, an anti-CD20 monoclonal antibody, whose response rates approach 65%; interferon-alpha, a pro-inflammatory and antiviral agent; intravenous immunoglobulin; immunoglobulin and cytotoxic T lymphocytes; surgical excision; localized radiation or combination chemotherapy.

T-cell PTLD not associated with EBV infection tends to affect extranodal sites.

HAEMOPOIETIC STEM CELL TRANSPLANTATION

GENERAL ASPECTS

Haemopoietic stem cell transplantation (HSCT) is increasingly used in the treatment of haematological conditions, neoplasms and some genetic defects (Table 35.5). HSCT involves stem cells not only of myeloid, erythroid and megakaryocyte origins, but also lymphoid and macrophage. The cells are either autologous or allogeneic and obtained from bone marrow (bone marrow transplantation; BMT), peripheral blood, or from banked cryopreserved umbilical cord or fetal liver blood. Most transplants are made between HLA-identical siblings, though other family members, or matched volunteers, may be used.

GENERAL MANAGEMENT

Patients must first be profoundly immunosuppressed to reduce the chances of graft rejection by 'conditioning', often by using cyclophosphamide, plus total body irradiation (TBI) or busulfan ('reduced intensity conditioning'). All such regimens are toxic but those using reduced intensity conditioning have lower morbidity and mortality.

The donor bone marrow is then mixed with heparin and infused intravenously in order to colonize the recipient's marrow and, over the next 2–4 weeks, it starts to produce blood cells. Throughout this period and for the following 3 months, the patient is usually provided with an indwelling catheter to facilitate therapy and intravenous feeding. Recipients must also be treated with methotrexate, corticosteroids, ciclosporin, intravenous immunoglobulins, tacrolimus, sirolimus or alemtuzumab (anti-CD52 lymphocytes) for 6 months or more to prevent or ameliorate GVHD (graft versus host disease). Patients must also be isolated and protected from infections and may require transfusions of granulocytes, platelets or red cells, granulocyte colony-stimulating factors and antimicrobials since they are severely immunoincompetent until the donor marrow is fully functioning.

DENTAL ASPECTS

Oral mucositis is the most common symptom and distressing complication of HSCT, seen in 30–50% of patients and particularly problematic after TBI. Mucositis may also be a predictor of gastrointestinal toxicity and may predict the onset of hepatic veno-occlusive disease. Mucositis is also an important driver of health care costs: patients developing mucositis use more antibiotics and analgesics, have more days of fever, and stay in the hospital longer. Other oral complications include infections (which usually develop within the first month of the transplant), sinusitis, parotitis, pain or bleeding. Ciclosporin may induce gingival swelling, and this and other immunosuppressants have resulted in lip and occasionally oral carcinomas, Kaposi sarcoma or lymphomas. GVHD presents with lichenoid reactions or xerostomia.

A meticulous pre-transplant oral assessment is required and dental treatment undertaken with particular attention to establishing optimal oral hygiene and eradicating sources of potential infection. Dental treatment should be completed before transplant and elective dental care is best deferred for 6 months after transplant. If surgical treatment is needed during that period, antibiotic prophylaxis is probably warranted. Consideration must also be given to the implications of immunosuppressive therapy, bleeding tendencies, infection and veno-occlusive liver disease.

Local anaesthetic is satisfactory. Conscious sedation can be given if needed. General anaesthesia must always be given in hospital.

GRAFT-VERSUS-HOST DISEASE

GENERAL ASPECTS

Graft-versus-host disease is a serious complication of transplantation, seen mainly after HSCT, but can occasionally follow solid organ transplants, especially liver and small bowel transplantation. Allogeneic T lymphocytes recognize host major histocompatibility complex (MHC) antigens (HLA mainly) and, even in HLA-identical individuals, may recognize minor non-MHC histocompatibility antigens (mHag). Such activated T cells secrete cytokines [IL-2, interferon-gamma (IFN-gamma) and tumour necrosis factor-alpha (TNF-alpha)] causing a 'cytokine storm', exaggerated by the release of bacterial

Table 35.5 Main indications for haemopoietic stem cell transplant (HSCT)

Indications	Examples
Lymphoproliferative disease	Leukaemias Lymphomas Myelomatosis
Solid tumours	Breast cancers Colon cancers Ewing sarcoma Germinal cell tumours Gliomas Lung cancers Melanomas Ovarian carcinomas Renal carcinomas Sarcomas
Non-malignant diseases	Aplastic anaemia Autoimmune diseases Fanconi syndrome Immunodeficiencies Inborn errors of metabolism Thalassaemia

lipopolysaccharides from the gastrointestinal tract damaged by TBI. GVHD affects a number of tissues, including mucosae, and may be acute or chronic.

Acute GVHD affects the skin, liver and gut with a distinctive syndrome of fever, dermatitis, hepatitis and enteritis within 100 days of HSCT. The overall grade of acute GVHD predicts outcome, with the highest rates of mortality in those with severe (grade IV) GVHD. Response to treatment also predicts outcome in grades II–IV GVHD. Patients with no response or with progression have a mortality rate as high as 75% compared with 20–25% in those with a complete response.

Chronic GVHD also affects skin, liver and gut, but is a more diverse syndrome and develops after day 100. Chronic GVHD may be an extension of acute GVHD, but may also start *de novo* or it may emerge after a quiescent interval. The immunopathogenesis of chronic GVHD is, in part, Th2 lymphocyte-mediated, resulting in a syndrome of immunodeficiency and autoimmunity. Chronic GVHD mortality rates are higher in patients with extensive disease, progressive-type onset, thrombocytopenia and HLA-non-identical marrow donors. The overall HSCT survival rate is 42%, but patients with progressive chronic GVHD have only a 10% survival rate.

CLINICAL FEATURES

Acute GVHD may initially cause a pruritic or painful red to violaceous rash, typically first on the palms and soles, cheeks, neck, ears and upper trunk, but sometimes progressing to cover the whole body. Liver involvement causes asymptomatic rises in serum bilirubin, alanine aminotransferase (ALT), aspartate aminotransferase (AST) and alkaline phosphatase (similar to cholestatic jaundice). Gastrointestinal involvement affects the distal small bowel and colon, causing diarrhoea, bleeding, cramping pain and ileus. Other findings include a greater risk of infectious and non-infectious pneumonia, and sterile effusions, haemorrhagic cystitis, thrombocytopenia, anaemia and haemolytic–uraemic syndrome (HUS; thrombotic microangiopathy).

Chronic GVHD resembles systemic progressive sclerosis, systemic lupus erythematosus, lichen planus, Sjögren syndrome, eosinophilic fasciitis, rheumatoid arthritis and primary biliary cirrhosis. It can lead to skin and mucosal lichenoid lesions or sclerodermatous thickening, sometimes causing contractures and limitation of joint mobility. Oral effects mimic Sjögren syndrome (Ch. 18) with xerostomia and decreases in salivary immunoglobulin A and antioxidants. Ocular manifestations include symptoms of burning, irritation, photophobia and pain from lack of tears. Oral and gastrointestinal manifestations include dryness, dysphagia and increasing pain.

Pulmonary manifestations include obstructive lung disease with wheezing, dyspnoea and chronic cough unresponsive to bronchodilators. Neuromuscular manifestations include weakness, neuropathic pain and muscle cramps, and sometimes myasthenia gravis or polymyositis.

GENERAL MANAGEMENT

There are no strategies known specifically to prevent GVHD but several systemic agents such as corticosteroids, cyclophosphamide, azathioprine, methotrexate, ciclosporin, tacrolimus and mycophenolate mofetil may be beneficial; strategies under investigation include sirolimus, thalidomide, clofazimine, pentostatin, hydroxychloroquine, photopheresis therapy, anti-TNF and rituximab. Most patients undergoing HSCT are given systemic prophylaxis for GVHD with ciclosporin or tacrolimus in combination with methotrexate and/or prednisolone.

Acute GVHD is treated with intravenous methotrexate for up to 14 days. Subsequent dose-tapering or switching to an oral agent is continued over several weeks to months. *Chronic GVHD* is treated with oral prednisolone alone or in combination with ciclosporin. If the response is positive, it is continued, tapering off over 6–9 months.

DENTAL ASPECTS

Oral aspects may be encountered in addition to those discussed above in relation to HSCT. Oral GVHD may be associated with mucositis, hyposalivation, higher caries risk, altered taste, candidosis, herpes infections, lichenoid lesions, progressive systemic sclerosis-like changes, oral pain and oral cancer.

Other transplant complications may include various adverse drug effects, such as adrenal suppression, drug-induced gingival swelling, which is dose related and thus more common in those on higher doses of ciclosporin (i.e. heart, liver and lung transplant patients), arterial hypertension (an adverse effect of immunosuppressives) and diabetes mellitus (caused by some immunosuppressive medications such as corticosteroids).

Before HSCT

There should be a full oral and dental evaluation, and careful attention to oral and dental disease, bearing in mind that after transplantation the patient will be chronically immunosuppressed and at high risk from infection. A full oral health care programme should be instituted, and oral hygiene and preventive care must be maintained at a high standard throughout and following transplantation.

Immediately post-HSCT

After transplantation, elective dental care is best deferred for at least 3 months, to avoid unnecessary complications. Infection is most likely at this time – the period of intense immunosuppression. During the immediate post-transplant and chronic rejection phases, only emergency dental care is recommended and should be undertaken in a hospital. Any invasive dental treatment should only be carried out after consultation with the responsible physician and with due consideration to the liability to infection, bleeding tendency related to anticoagulation, risk of adrenal crisis in relation to steroid therapy and impaired drug metabolism; this applies probably for at least 2 years post-transplantation. Dental treatment guidelines include attention to prevent infection – use of antiseptic mouthwashes (chlorhexidine gluconate) – before treatment. Antibiotic prophylaxis is indicated for invasive dental procedures, particularly if provided within 6 months post-transplantation. In addition, steroid cover may be indicated. Macrolide antibiotics and azole antifungal drugs should be avoided because they may alter serum levels and increase the toxicity of some immunosuppressive drugs. Pre-existing illnesses of transplant candidates often need to be considered as they can influence oral health care.

General anaesthesia should be avoided, but, if essential, must only be given in hospital with appropriate expertise and facilities.

Drugs should be used with caution; aspirin and NSAIDs should be avoided since they potentiate the nephrotoxicity of ciclosporin and tacrolimus, may cause a bleeding tendency, and exacerbate peptic ulcer if the patient is on corticosteroids. Sedatives and acetaminophen are also best avoided. Several drugs, especially erythromycin and azole antifungals, may affect ciclosporin levels (Table 35.3). There may also be a greater risk from nephrotoxicity with co-trimoxazole, aminoglycosides and quinolones.

Patients may need steroid supplementation and cover during dental treatment (Ch. 6), probably for at least 2 years post-transplantation. Viral hepatitis B and C infections may be present, especially in older patients who have received blood transfusions before blood was routinely screened. Oral infections, such as HSV, VZV, CMV or EBV, to which the immunosuppressed patient is prone, are discussed in Ch. 20. Oral HSV and VZV infections can be prevented, deferred or ameliorated by prophylactic low-dose oral aciclovir.

Spontaneous bacterial peritonitis and endarteritis are possible peri- and post-transplantation, particularly after liver transplantation, and may necessitate antimicrobial prophylaxis; however, there is no evidence that, after the first 3 months following transplantation, there is any routine need for antimicrobial cover for dental interventions. Some patients carry enterococci in plaque. Rarely oral or dental infections may spread, with serious complications such as cavernous sinus thrombosis or metastatic infections, and oral bacteria are an important source of bacteraemias.

Oral candidosis may be persistent or mixed bacterial plaques may develop on the oral mucosa. Oral candidosis can usually be managed with topical nystatin, amphotericin or miconazole (Fig. 35.2). Mixed bacterial oral mucosal plaques may respond to the appropriate antibiotic, to trypsinization and possibly to an aqueous chlorhexidine mouthwash.

Routine cancer surveillance is mandatory to assure rapid diagnosis and treatment of any malignancy, since patients on immunosuppressive treatment after organ transplantation have a greatly raised incidence of malignant disease, particularly lymphomas and, to a lesser extent, skin, cervical and lip cancer. In other patients, hairy leukoplakia, leukoplakia or Kaposi sarcoma (Fig. 35.3) may be seen. This may especially be the case in those with a history of tobacco or alcohol use – often the case in adults needing liver transplants.

Drugs used in transplant patients, such as ciclosporin, nifedipine and basiliximab, may induce gingival swelling.

TRANSPLANTATION AND TISSUE ENGINEERING OF CRANIOFACIAL STRUCTURES

Craniofacial tissue replantation or transplantation to treat congenital anomalies, trauma and diseases is in its infancy. Tissue engineering also promises the regeneration or *de novo* formation

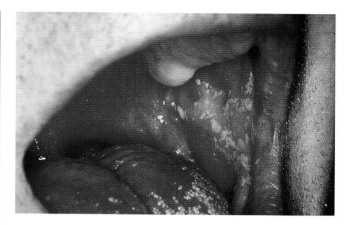

Fig. 35.2 Thrush

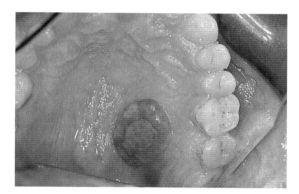

Fig. 35.3 Kaposi sarcoma in a renal transplant patient with diabetic nephrosclerosis

of dental, oral and craniofacial structures. Most craniofacial structures are derivatives of mesenchymal cells, and mesenchymal stem cells have been isolated from the dental pulp, deciduous teeth and periodontium. Several craniofacial structures, such as calvarial bone, the mandibular condyle and subcutaneous adipose tissue, have been engineered from mesenchymal stem cells, growth factor and/or gene therapy approaches.

TRANSPLANTATION OF TEETH

Autotransplantation of teeth is useful, has many indications in dentistry and has been used for decades. Transplanted teeth may, however, develop replacement resorption or ankylosis. Cryopreservation of teeth creates new possibilities (e.g. when autotransplantation is needed, but the recipient site is too small and orthodontic treatment is needed to gain space for the transplant).

The molecular control of key processes in tooth development such as initiation, morphogenesis and cytodifferentiation is being increasingly better understood and already bioengineered tooth tissues can be regenerated at the site of previously lost teeth.

TRANSPLANTATION OF SALIVARY GLANDS

Transplantation of the major salivary glands has been used successfully to provide substitute lubrication in severely dry eyes, significantly improving Schirmer's test, tear break-up time, rose Bengal staining and symptoms. Long-term graft survival is around 70%. However, the surgery is fairly complex and, in over one-third of eyes with a viable graft, salivary epiphora results, which is independent of gustatory stimuli. Since the salivary tear film is substantially hypo-osmolar, microcystic epithelial oedema can result and subsequent corneal transplantation remains unsuccessful.

Transplantation of minor salivary glands is a promising new treatment option as the procedure is simple with minimal surgical risks, the grafts remain viable in over 90% and they seem to be capable of sustaining a basal secretion for up to at least 36 months. Prospective controlled studies have to be performed to establish the long-term survival of the glands and to characterize the salivary tear film and its impact on the eye.

Salivary gland regeneration and gene transfer to salivary glands are currently experimental only.

TRANSPLANTATION OF JAWS

There is potential for regeneration within the bony tissues of the craniofacial region, and guided tissue regeneration and distraction osteogenesis (Ch. 16) are already in widespread use.

In Germany in 2004, a patient who lost his mandible in radical cancer surgery had a functional jawbone created using a combination of computer-aided design and bone stem cells. Three-dimensional computed tomography (CT) scanning and computer-aided design techniques were used to create a titanium mesh cage to replace the jaw defect, that was filled with bone mineral blocks and infiltrated with recombinant human bone morphogenetic protein (BMP) and liquid bone marrow containing stem cells from the patient's marrow. This transplant was implanted into the latissimus dorsi muscle and, 7 weeks later, transplanted as a bone–muscle free flap to repair the mandibular defect. *In-vivo* skeletal scintigraphy showed bone remodelling and mineralization inside the transplant both before and after transplantation. CT provided evidence of new bone formation. Post-operatively, the patient's mastication and aesthetics improved.

TRANSPLANTATION OF FACE

The first account of a procedure to replace all or part of a person's face was in the second century BC when an Indian surgeon, Sushruta, used autografted skin in rhinoplasty. The world's first full-face *replant* operation was in 1994, also in India, on 9-year-old Sandeep Kaur, whose face was ripped off when her hair was caught in a thresher. In 1997 a similar operation was reported from Australia.

The world's first partial face *transplant* operation was in France in 2005 and by July 2009, 7 face transplants had been carried out across the world. In the first, a triangle of facial tissue from the central face of a brain-dead woman was grafted on to a 38-year-old woman whose nose, lips, chin and adjacent cheeks had been amputated. Bone-marrow graft and immunosuppression with thymoglobulin, tacrolimus, mycophenolate mofetil and prednisone were used. The drugs were well tolerated, and there were no surgical complications. Mild rejection appeared at day 20 and was treated with prednisone. Rejection episodes

on days 18 and 214 were similarly reversed. Anatomical and psychological integration and recovery of sensation were good. Sensitivity to light touch, heat and cold had returned to normal by 6 months. Motor recovery and labial contact allowing complete mouth closure was achieved by 10 months. At 18 months, the patient was satisfied with the functional and aesthetic results.

Further cases have subsequently been reported in China (2006 and 2008), in 2008, another in France and in 2009 two in USA and two in France (one of whom died from cardiac arrest).

USEFUL WEBSITES

http://health.nih.gov/organtransplantation.html
http://www.nhlbi.nih.gov
http://kidney.niddk.nih.gov/kudiseases/pubs/transplant/
http://digestive.niddk.nih.gov/ddiseases/pubs/livertransplant/
http://www.cancer.gov/cancertopics/factsheet/therapy/bone-marrow-transplant

FURTHER READING

Al-Sarheed, M., Angeletou, A., Ashley, P.F., Lucas, V.S., Whitehead, B., Roberts, G.J., 2000. An investigation of the oral status and reported oral care of children with heart and heart–lung transplants. Int J Paediatr Dent 10, 298–305.

Buxton, P.G., Cobourne, M.T., 2007. Regenerative approaches in the craniofacial region: manipulating cellular progenitors for oro-facial repair. Oral Dis 13, 452–460.

da Fonseca, M.A., Hongs C., 2008. An overview of chronic oral graft-vs-host disease following pediatric hematopoietic stem cell transplantation. Pediatr Dent 30, 98–104.

Devauchelle, B., Badet, L., Lengelé, B., et al., 2006. First human face allograft: early report. Lancet 368, 203–209.

Duailibi, S.E., Duailibi, M.T., Zhang, W., Asrican, R., Vacanti, J.P., Yelick, P.C., 2008. Bioengineered dental tissues grown in the rat jaw. J Dent Res 87, 745–750.

Dubernard, J.-M., Devauchelle, B., 2008. Face transplantation. Lancet 372, 603–604.

Dubernard, J.M., Lengelé, B., Morelon, E., et al., 2007. Outcomes 18 months after the first human partial face transplantation. N Engl J Med 357, 2451–2460.

Fernandez de Preliasco, M.V., Viera, M.J., Sebelli, P., Rodriguez Rilo, L., Sanchez, G.A., 2002. Compliance with medical and dental treatments in child and adolescent renal transplant patients. Acta Odontol Latinoam 15, 21–27.

Filipovich, A.H., 2008. Diagnosis and manifestations of chronic graft-versus-host disease. Best Pract Res Clin Haematol 21, 251–257.

Geerling, G., Raus, P., Murube, J., 2008. Minor salivary gland transplantation. Dev Ophthalmol 41, 243–254.

Geerling, G., Sieg, P., 2008. Transplantation of the major salivary glands. Dev Ophthalmol 41, 255–268.

Guggenheimer, J., Eghtesad, B., Stock, D., 2003. Dental management of the (solid) organ transplant patient. Oral Surg Oral Med Oral Pathol Oral Radiol Endod 95, 383–389.

Guo, S., Han, Y., Zhang, X., et al., 2008. Human facial allotransplantation: a 2-year follow-up study. Lancet 372, 631–638.

Hsi, E.D., Singleton, T.P., Swinnen, L., Dunphy, C.H., Alkan, S., 2000. Mucosa-associated lymphoid tissue-type lymphomas occurring in post-transplantation patients. Am J Surg Pathol 24, 100–106.

Ikeda, E., Tsuji, T., 2008. Growing bioengineered teeth from single cells: potential for dental regenerative medicine. Expert Opin Biol Ther 8, 735–744.

Ivanovski, S., Gronthos, S., Shi, S., Bartold, P.M., 2006. Stem cells in the periodontal ligament. Oral Dis 12, 358–363.

Kagami, H., Wang, S., Hai, B., 2008. Restoring the function of salivary glands. Oral Dis 14, 15–24.

Lantieri, L., Meningaud, J.P., Grimbert, P., et al., 2008. Repair of the lower and middle parts of the face by composite tissue allotransplantation in a patient with massive plexiform neurofibroma: a 1-year follow-up study. Lancet 372, 639–645.

Lew, J., Smith, J.A., 2007. Mucosal graft-vs-host disease. Oral Dis 13, 519–529.

Mao, J.J., Giannobile, W.V., Helms, J.A., et al., 2006. Craniofacial tissue engineering by stem cells. J Dent Res 85, 966–979.

Maria, O.M., Khosravi, R., Mezey, E., Tran, S.D., 2007. Cells from bone marrow that evolve into oral tissues and their clinical applications. Oral Dis 13, 11–16.

McLoon, L.K., Thorstenson, K.M., Solomon, A., Lewis, M.P., 2007. Myogenic precursor cells in craniofacial muscles. Oral Dis 13, 134–140.

Meyer, U., Kleinheinz, J., Handschel, J., Kruse-Losler, B., Weingart, D., Joos, U., 2000. Oral findings in three different groups of immunocompromised patients. J Oral Pathol Med 29, 153–158.

Niederhagen, B., Wolff, M., Appel, T., von Lindern, J.J., Berge, S., 2003. Location and sanitation of dental foci in liver transplantation. Transpl Int 16, 173–178.

Sartaj, R., Sharpe, P., 2006. Biological tooth replacement. J Anat 209, 503–509.

Scully, C., Diz Dios, P., Kumar, N., 2007. Special care in dentistry. handbook of oral healthcare – Churchill Livingstone Elsevier, Edinburgh.

Sloan, A.J., Smith, A.J., 2007. Stem cells and the dental pulp: potential roles in dentine regeneration and repair. Oral Dis 13, 151–157.

Temmerman, L., De Pauw, G.A., Beele, H., Dermaut, L.R., 2006. Tooth transplantation and cryopreservation: state of the art. Am J Orthod Dentofacial Orthop 129, 691–695.

Warnke, P.H., Springer, I.N., Wiltfang, J., et al., 2004. Growth and transplantation of a custom vascularised bone graft in a man. Lancet 364, 766–770.

Warnke, P.H., 2006. Repair of a human face by allotransplantation. Lancet 368, 181–183.

Warnke, P.H., Wiltfang, J., Springer, I., et al., 2006. Man as living bioreactor: fate of an exogenously prepared customized tissue-engineered mandible. Biomaterials 27, 3163–3167.

Westbrook, S.D., Paunovich, E.D., Freytes, C.O., 2003. Adult hemopoietic stem cell transplantation. J Am Dent Assoc 134, 1224–1231.

Yelick, P.C., Vacanti, J.P., 2006. Bioengineered teeth from tooth bud cells. Dent Clin North Am 50, 191–203.

Zollner-Schwetz, I., Auner, H.W., Paulitsch, A., et al., 2008. Oral and intestinal Candida colonization in patients undergoing hematopoietic stem-cell transplantation. J Infect Dis 198, 150–153.

SECTION E

APPENDIX

The causes of disease are genetic (inherited) or acquired, which can be environmental (from trauma, infection, chemical or irradiation) or due to lifestyle (e.g. lack of exercise, poor diet, habits – tobacco, alcohol, drugs, betel and other habits). Many diseases result from an interaction of several of these factors.

GENERAL HEALTH PROMOTION

Since disease arises from interactions of genetic, environmental and lifestyle factors, it may be prevented by avoiding or minimizing these factors. Already the effects of genetic diseases like haemophilia can be minimized by providing the missing protein (blood clotting factor VIII) and, in the future, genetic manipulation may be more widely possible. Disease can be more readily prevented by avoiding certain environmental and lifestyle factors, or minimizing themas – summarized in Table 36.1 and Fig. 36.1. Lifestyle choices are crucial. Lifestyle refers to how

Table 36.1	Prevention of disease		
Environmental		**Lifestyle**	
Trauma	Avoid alcohol use, accidents, aggression and dangerous environments, activities and sports	Exercise	Take regular daily exercise for 30 min minimum
Infection	Avoid needlestick injuries and use latex protection (condoms, gloves, rubber dam) Be vaccinated	Diet	Eat a balanced diet with five portions of fruit/vegetables daily, minimise sugar and avoid food fads
Chemical	Label and take care with toxic agents	Substance dependence	Abstain if possible from use of tobacco; alcohol; recreational drugs, betel
Irradiation	Minimize exposure (to sun, X-rays, lasers, damaging lights, etc.) and use safety measures such as protective eyewear and screens		

individuals live their life and how they handle problems and interpersonal relations – 'the unique way in which individuals try to realise their fictional final goal and meet or avoid the three main tasks of life: work, community, love' (Adler). Apart from a lifestyle designed to improve or maintain good health by avoid my contracting infections including sexually transmitted infections (Ch. 32), the three most important measures are to

take regular exercise, eat a healthy diet, and avoid substance dependence and other deleterious habits.

EXERCISE

Physical inactivity often occurs together with an unhealthy diet, contributing to obesity, diabetes, heart disease and cancer. In contrast, when exercise is combined with a proper diet, weight can be controlled and obesity – a major risk factor for many diseases – prevented.

There are real health benefits from exercise, from protecting against cardiac disease (hypertension, atheroma and coronary artery disease) to reducing the chances of cancer and Alzheimer disease. In addition, exercise can: increase stamina; improve brain function; reduce stress (by releasing endorphins), depression and anxiety; control weight, and build and maintain healthy bones, muscles and joints; reduce the risk of developing diabetes; and reduce the risk of developing or dying from some of the leading causes – myocardial infarct, stroke, and cancer.

To achieve health benefits, at the very least enough regular moderately intense physical activity to burn an extra 200 calories daily is needed. At a minimum, this means about 30 minutes of activity daily – such as a brisk walk.

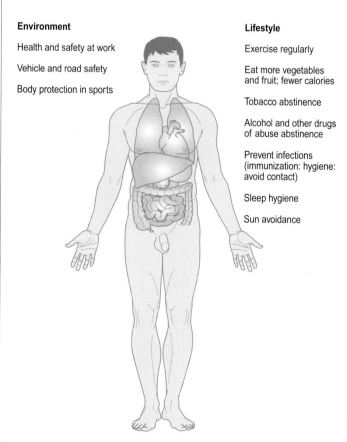

Environment

Health and safety at work

Vehicle and road safety

Body protection in sports

Lifestyle

Exercise regularly

Eat more vegetables and fruit; fewer calories

Tobacco abstinence

Alcohol and other drugs of abuse abstinence

Prevent infections (immunization: hygiene: avoid contact)

Sleep hygiene

Sun avoidance

Fig. 36.1 Health promotion

There are at least ten scientifically proven reasons for taking regular exercise, as follows.

1 *Exercise helps minimize obesity.* Exercise, by burning calories, helps minimize obesity (Ch. 27). Men who are obese are more likely than non-obese men to die from cancer of the colon, rectum or prostate; obese women are more likely to die from cancer of the gallbladder, breast, uterus, cervix or ovaries. Other health problems from obesity include diabetes, ischaemic heart disease (IHD), hypertension, stroke, gallbladder disease; liver disease; osteoarthritis; gout; sleep apnoea; menstrual irregularities and infertility in women; and psychosocial effects.

2 *Exercise helps increase levels of HDL or 'good' cholesterol.* Levels of high-density lipoproteins (HDL) when low, and low-density lipoproteins (LDL) when high, predict a risk for IHD. Exercise helps increase HDL and lower LDL levels and, by strengthening the heart and lowering blood pressure, protects against atheroma, myocardial infarcts and strokes (Ch. 5).

3 *Exercise helps lower high blood pressure.* Hypertension can be reduced by exercise. Blood pressure levels predict the risk for coronary heart disease and stroke. Physical activity also reduces obesity, which is associated with hypertension (Ch. 5).

4 *Exercise helps promote healthy blood sugar levels.* High blood sugar levels in diabetes, a risk factor for coronary heart disease, can be lowered by exercise (Ch.6).

5 *Exercise helps improve the metabolic syndrome.* The metabolic syndrome (syndrome X or insulin resistance syndrome) is a cluster of abdominal obesity (excess body fat around the waist), insulin resistance (causing high blood sugar) and increased blood pressure, which increases the risk for diabetes, heart disease and stroke (Ch. 23). Having just one of these factors contributes to the risk of serious disease and, in combination, the risk is even greater. Exercise improves these factors.

6 *Exercise helps build muscle strength.* Exercise, by building or preserving muscle mass and strength, and improving the ability to use calories, helps reduce body fat. By increasing muscle strength and endurance, and improving flexibility and posture, regular exercise also helps prevent back pain. Exercise helps build muscle but this benefit fades if exercise stops for any reason, so *regular* exercise is needed.

7 *Exercise helps promote bone density.* Regular exercise from a young age can increase bone density and help avoid or minimize osteoporosis (Ch. 16).

8 *Exercise helps improve mobility.* People who exercise regularly have been shown to be more mobile and independent compared with those having a sedentary lifestyle (Ch. 25).

9 *Exercise helps the immune system.* Exercise helps the immune system combat infections. The mechanism is unclear, but it is known that exercise increases the numbers of circulating leukocytes – and these are defensive against infections. In contrast, when exercise is performed without food intake, and is too continuous, prolonged, or of high intensity (as in athletes), immune function can be depressed.

10 *Exercise helps improve mood.* People who exercise regularly have been shown to be generally happier and less liable to depression compared with those having a sedentary lifestyle (Ch. 10).

DIET

The key to a healthy diet is eating the right amount of food for the activity undertaken *and* eating a range of foods to ensure a balanced diet is achieved. This includes: fruit and vegetables; wholegrain bread, pasta and rice; some protein-rich foods such as meat, fish, eggs and lentils; and some dairy foods; but is low in fat (especially saturated fat), salt and sugar. Generous amounts of vegetables and fruit daily appear to protect against cancers of stomach, colon and lung, and possibly against cancers of the mouth, larynx, cervix, bladder and breast. Carbohydrates as wholegrain unrefined products may help protect against colon cancer, diverticulitis and caries. A high-fibre diet may also offer some protection against hypertension and IHD. Minimizing the intake of saturated fats (especially those from dairy sources) and partially halogenated vegetable fats may lower the risk of IHD and some cancers.

The *Dietary Guidelines for Americans* nicely describes a healthy diet as one that:

- emphasizes a variety of fruits, vegetables, whole grains, and fat-free or low-fat milk and milk products
- includes lean meats, poultry, fish, beans, eggs and nuts
- is low in saturated fats, trans-fats, cholesterol, salt (sodium) and added sugars
- stays within daily calorie needs.

See http://www.healthierus.gov/dietaryguidelines and US Department of Agriculture's food guidance system (My Pyramid; http://www.mypyramid.gov).

Ready meals, convenience foods and takeaways are often high in added salt, sugar or fat, and should only be eaten in moderation.

CALORIES

A calorie is the amount of energy required to heat 1 g of water through 1°C; however, because this is a small energy quantity, it more common to use the kilocalorie or Calorie – equivalent to 1000 calories. Energy is usually expressed either in kilojoules or in kilocalories. These two units – joules and calories – are directly related. To convert one to the other, the number of calories multiplied by 4.186 gives the number of joules; or the number of kilocalories multiplied by 4.186 gives the number of kilojoules.

ELEMENTS (MINERALS) AND TRACE ELEMENTS

Iron (Fe) is an important component of haemoglobin. Sodium (Na), potassium (K), calcium (Ca), and phosphorus (P) are needed in large quantities to take part in physiological reactions such as nerve impulse transmission or to form bones and teeth. Trace elements vital to good health include iodine (I), which is necessary for thyroxine, and fluorine (F), which helps to protect against caries.

VITAMINS (CH. 27)

SUBSTANCE DEPENDENCE

Substance dependence is defined as self-administration without any medical indication and despite adverse medical and social consequences, and in a manner that deviates from the cultural norm and is harmful. This applies to tobacco, alcohol and a range of drugs of abuse (Ch. 34).

TOBACCO (SEE CH. 34)

Nicotine is absorbed readily from tobacco smoke in the lungs, is one of the most heavily used addictive drugs, and is highly addictive. Cigarette smoking is a major hazard to health and promotes many diseases (Box 36.1).

Smoking cessation should be gradual, because withdrawal is less severe in those who quit gradually. Aids include nicotine chewing gum or patches, or drugs.

Box 36.1 Health problems from tobacco

- Cigarette smoking is particularly linked to atherosclerotic heart disease, cancers of the lung, oesophagus, mouth and bladder, and chronic obstructive pulmonary disease
- Carbon monoxide in the smoke increases the risk of cardiovascular disease
- Tobacco use is a major cause of stroke and leading cause of death
- Smokers metabolize some other drugs more rapidly and require, for example, higher doses of benzodiazepines than non-smokers
- Women who smoke generally have an earlier menopause. If women smokers also take oral contraceptives, they are more prone to cardiovascular and cerebrovascular diseases than are other smokers; this is especially true for women older than 30
- Pregnant women who smoke cigarettes run a greater risk of having stillborn or premature infants or infants with a low birthweight
- Children of women who smoked while pregnant have a raised risk for developing conduct disorders
- Second-hand smoke (passive smoking) causes lung cancer in adults and greatly increases the risk of respiratory illnesses in children and sudden infant death
- Tobacco use can also damage oral health and cause:
  - Oral cancer
  - Keratosis
  - Periodontal disease, particularly necrotizing gingivitis
  - Implant failure
  - Dry socket
  - Candidosis
  - Dry mouth (xerostomia)
  - Halitosis
  - Staining of teeth

ALCOHOL (SEE CH. 34)

Alcohol is damaging to health and high in calories, so cutting down can help control weight. Women can drink up to 2–3 units of alcohol a day and men up to 3–4 units a day without significant risk to their health. A unit is half a pint of standard strength beer, lager or cider, or a pub measure of spirit. A glass of wine is about 2 units and alcopops are about 1.5 units.

DRUG ABUSE (SEE CH. 34)

Use of illegal drugs can cause dry mouth, dilated pupils, tachycardia, aggression, talkativeness, tachypnoea and hallucinations, leading to hyperpyrexia, seizures, arrhythmias and collapse. High doses can cause mood swings and psychoses, including hallucinations and paranoia, and can cause respiratory failure and death. Intravenous use of illegal drugs can easily lead to life-threatening infections including hepatitis and HIV/AIDS.

USEFUL WEBSITES

http://health.nih.gov/category/WellnessLifestyle
http://phpartners.org/hpro.html
http://www.dh.gov.uk/en/Publichealth/Healthimprovement/Healthyliving/index.htm
http://www.patient.co.uk/showdoc/16/
http://www.equip.nhs.uk/topics/Healthtopics/healthyliving.aspx

---

EPONYMOUS AND ACRONYMOUS DISEASES AND SIGNS

This chapter includes synopses of many relevant conditions; if a specific condition is not located here, please see index, as it may be elsewhere in the book. For eponymous medical signs, see also http://en.wikipedia.org/wiki/List_of_eponymous_medical_signs.

Abrikossof tumour. Granular cell tumour.

Adamantiades syndrome. Behçet syndrome.

Addison disease. Autoimmune hypoadrenocorticism (Ch. 6).

Adie's (Holmes–Adie) pupil. A benign condition in which one pupil is dilated and reacts only very slowly to light or convergence.

Albers–Schonberg disease. Osteopetrosis.

Albright syndrome (McCune–Albright syndrome). Polyostotic fibrous dysplasia with skin pigmentation and an endocrine abnormality (usually precocious puberty in girls) (Ch. 16).

Allgrove syndrome. Autosomal recessive condition due to chromosome 12 mutation. Achalasia of cardia, adrenal insufficiency, alacrima (triple A syndrome) plus xerostomia.

Alstrom syndrome. Congenital nerve deafness and retinitis pigmentosa.

Apert syndrome. Craniofacial synostosis with craniosynostosis, facial dysmorphology, hands and feet defects, and learning disability.

Argyll Robinson pupils. Small, irregular, unequal pupils which fail to react to light but react to accommodation. Caused by neurosyphilis and other diseases.

Arnold–Chiari syndrome. A congenital malformation in which the brainstem and the cerebellum are longer than normal and protrude into the spinal cord.

Ascher syndrome. Congenital double lip with blepharoclasia and thyroid goitre.

Avellis syndrome. Unilateral paralysis of the larynx and palate.

Battle's sign. Bruising over the mastoid bone, a sign of basilar skull fracture.

Becker syndrome. Severe muscular dystrophy resulting in progressive weakness of limb and breathing muscles almost exclusively in boys.

Beckwith–Wiedemann syndrome. Congenital gigantism, omphalocele or umbilical hernia.

Beeson's signs. Myalgia, facial oedema and fever in trichinosis.

Behçet syndrome. The triad of oral aphthous ulcers, genital ulceration and uveitis.

Bell palsy. A common lower motor neuron facial palsy, caused by inflammation in the stylomastoid canal (Ch. 13).

Bence Jones protein. Overproduction of gamma-globulins in myelomatosis, particularly of immunoglobulin light chains that spill over into the urine (Bence Jones proteinuria) (Ch. 8).

Berardinelli–Seip syndrome. An autosomal recessive form of generalized lipodystrophy.

Biemond syndrome. Congenital obesity and hypogonadism.

Binder syndrome. Congenital maxillonasal dysplasia, and absent or hypoplastic frontal sinuses.

Blackfan–Diamond syndrome. Congenital red cell aplasia.

Block–Sulzberger disease (incontinentia pigmenti). Congenital hyperpigmented skin lesions, skeletal defects, learning disability and hypodontia.

Bloom syndrome. Congenital telangiectasia, depigmentation, short stature and susceptibility to oral carcinoma.

Boeck syndrome. Sarcoidosis (Ch. 15).

Book syndrome. Autosomal dominant disorder of palm and sole hyperhidrosis, hypodontia and premature whitening of hair.

Bourneville disease (epiloia, tuberous sclerosis). Autosomal dominant phakomatosis including fibromas at the nail bases (subungual fibromas), hamartomas in the brain, kidneys and heart, and nodules in the nasolabial folds (adenoma sebaceum) (Ch. 13).

Bruton syndrome. Sex-linked agammaglobulinaemia, cervical lymph node enlargement, oral ulceration, recurrent sinusitis and absent tonsils.

Burkitt lymphoma. (Ch. 8).

Byar–Jurkiewicz syndrome. Gingival fibromatosis, hypertrichosis, giant fibroadenomas of the breast and kyphosis.

Cannon disease. Congenital white sponge naevus.

Carabelli cusp. Congenital additional palatal cusp on upper molars.

Carney syndrome. Autosomal dominant multisystem tumorous disorder of myxomas and lentigos.

Carpenter syndrome. Autosomal recessive acrocephalopolysyndactyly type II.

Castleman disease (angiolymphoid hyperplasia). Nodal lymphoproliferation that may progress to a malignant vascular tumour or lymphoma. Sometimes associated with paraneoplastic pemphigus.

CATCH22. **C**ardiac abnormality, **A**bnormal facies, **T**-cell deficit (due to thymic hypoplasia), **C**left palate, and **H**ypocalcaemia (due to hypoparathyroidism). A chromosome **22** defect (Di George syndrome).

Chediak–Higashi syndrome. Congenital immune defect in which neutrophils have large inclusions.

Christmas disease. Deficiency of blood clotting factor IX (Ch. 8).

Chvostek sign. Tapping the skin over the facial nerve elicits involuntary twitching of the upper lip or ipsilateral side of face – seen in hypoparathyroidism (Ch. 6).

Clutton joints. Syphilitic neuropathic joints.

Cockayne syndrome. Premature ageing, dwarfism, deafness and neuropathy.

Coffin–Lawry syndrome. Congenital osteocartilaginous anomalies and learning disability.

Coffin–Siris syndrome. Congenital defective neutrophil function, susceptibility to infection and skin pigmentation.

Costen syndrome. Outmoded term relating to patients with facial pain, otalgia and possible occlusal abnormalities.

Cowden syndrome. Congenital multiple hamartoma syndrome, with oral papillomatosis and risk of breast and thyroid cancer.

Coxsackie virus. Named after Coxsackie in New York State. Coxsackie viruses can cause herpangina, hand, foot and mouth disease, and other illnesses.

CREST syndrome. **C**alcinosis, **R**aynaud disease, **O**esophageal involvement, **S**clerodactyly and **T**elangiectasia (see Scleroderma) (Ch. 18).

Crohn disease. Chronic inflammatory idiopathic granulomatous disorder of the ileum or any part of the gastrointestinal tract, including the mouth (Ch. 7).

Cronkhite–Canada syndrome. Hypogeusia is the dominant initial symptom, followed by diarrhoea and ectodermal changes (alopecia, nail dystrophy, and skin and buccal melanotic hyperpigmentation).

Cross syndrome. Athetosis, learning disability, gingival fibromatosis and hypopigmentation.

Crouzon syndrome. Autosomal dominant premature fusion of cranial sutures, mid-face hypoplasia and proptosis.

Curry–Jones syndrome. Unilateral coronal synostosis and microphthalmia, plagiocephaly, craniofacial asymmetry, iris coloboma, broad thumbs, hand syndactyly, foot polydactyly, erosive skin lesions, gastrointestinal abnormalities and developmental delay.

Cushing syndrome. Moon face with buffalo hump, hirsutism and hypertension due to an ACTH-producing pituitary adenoma (Ch. 6).

Danon disease. Rare genetic condition causing muscular dystrophy, cardiomyopathy and learning problems.

Darier disease (Darier–White disease). Autosomal dominant skin disorder with follicular hyperkeratosis, and sometimes white oral papules.

Destombes–Rosai–Dorfman syndrome. Rosai–Dorfman syndrome (see below).

DiGeorge syndrome. Congenital immunodeficiency with hypoplasia of thymus and parathyroids, characteristic facies with down-slanting palpebral fissures and ocular and nasal anomalies, and cardiac, thyroid and parathyroid defects due to a third and fourth branchial arch defect related to a chromsome 22 anomaly (CATCH 22 syndrome – see above) (Ch. 20).

Down syndrome (trisomy 21). Chromosomal anomaly causing learning disability, short stature, brachycephaly, mid-face retrusion and upward sloping palpebral fissures (mongoloid slant) (Ch. 28).

Duhring disease. Dermatitis herpetiformis.

Duncan disease. Rare sex-linked lymphoproliferative syndrome, characterized by severe Epstein–Barr virus mononucleosis, immunoblastic sarcoma or lymphoma.

Eagle syndrome. Elongated styloid process associated with dysphagia and pain on chewing, and on turning the head towards the affected side.

ECHO viruses. **E**nteric **C**ytopathogenic **H**uman **O**rphan viruses.

Ehlers–Danlos syndrome. Congenital disorders of collagen characterized by joint hyperflexibility, hyperextensible skin, bleeding and bruising, and mitral incompetence (Ch. 16).

Ellis–van Creveld syndrome (chondroectodermal dysplasia). Congenital polydactyly, dwarfism, ectodermal dysplasia; hypodontia and hypoplastic teeth; multiple fraenae.

Epstein–Barr virus. Herpesvirus implicated in infectious mononucleosis, hairy leukoplakia, nasopharyngeal carcinoma and some lymphomas.

Epstein pearls. Small cysts due to persistence of epithelial rests in the alveolar ridge.

Fabry disease (angiokeratoma corporis diffusum universale). X-linked recessive error of glycosphingolipid metabolism with skin angiokeratomas, hypertension, fever, renal disease and risk of myocardial infarction.

Fallot tetralogy. Combination of ventricular septal defect (VSD) and pulmonary stenosis, with aorta 'overriding' (sitting 'astride') the VSD and with right ventricular hypertrophy.

Fanconi anaemia. Rare autosomal recessive syndrome of congenital anaemia, congenital skeletal defects (e.g. abnormal radii), hyperpigmentation and pancytopenia; associated with abnormal susceptibility to oral or other head and neck carcinomas and leukaemia at an early age (Ch. 8).

Felty syndrome. Rheumatoid arthritis and neutropenia.

Fitzgerald–Gardner syndrome. Gardner syndrome (see below).

Fordyce disease (Fordyce spots). Congenital ectopic sebaceous glands seen mainly in the buccal mucosa or lips.

Freeman–Sheldon syndrome. Rare form of multiple congenital contracture syndrome (arthrogryposis).

Frey syndrome. Skin gustatory sweating and flushing after trauma to skin over a salivary gland, due to crossover of sympathetic and parasympathetic innervation to the gland and skin.

Friedreich ataxia. Inherited progressive central nervous system damage causing features ranging from muscle weakness and speech problems to heart disease. Usually an autosomal recessive trait, leading to degeneration of many tracts of the spinal cord extending up to the brainstem, and thus severe ataxia, loss of reflexes and secondary deformities. Degenerative heart disease with arrhythmias may be associated. Treatment is symptomatic.

Froehlich syndrome. Congenital obesity, hypogonadism, and risk of learning disability and open bite.

Gardner syndrome. Autosomal dominant syndrome of intestinal polyposis, bony abnormalities, soft tissue tumours, multiple osteomas, fibromas and pigmented lesions of fundus of eye.

Garre osteomyelitis. Proliferative periostitis.

Gasserian ganglion. Trigeminal ganglion.

Gilles de la Tourette syndrome. In this familial early-onset syndrome, seen mainly in males, chronic motor tics involving the head and neck especially are associated with compulsive vocal tics and sometimes swearing (coprolalia). Tongue-thrusting and lip-smacking are common and sometimes regarded as lewd (copropraxia). Many of those affected have obsessive–compulsive tendencies or have attention-deficit hyperactivity, but intelligence is usually normal. Temporomandibular or other oral pain may result and self-mutilation, such as tongue- and lip-biting, may be associated. The dopamine receptor blocker haloperidol is usually effective and suggests that there is overactivity in the basal ganglia. Pimozide and/or clonidine may also be used. Drugs used to treat the syndrome may cause xerostomia or tardive dyskinesia. Interactions of these drugs with general anaesthetic agents, other CNS depressants and atropine means that dental treatment for such patients is best carried out under local analgesia.

Glossopharyngeal neuralgia. Severe pain in the posterior tongue, fauces, pharynx and sometimes beneath the angle of the mandible.

Goldenhar syndrome. Variant of congenital hemifacial microsomia, with microtia (small ears), macrostomia, agenesis of mandibular ramus and condyle, vertebral abnormalities, and epibulbar dermoids.

Goltz syndrome (focal dermal hypoplasia). X-linked disorder with multiple mesenchymal defects, skin lesions, and oral warts and dental defects.

Gorham disease. Rare osteolysis without sex, race or age predilection, affecting bones. Jaw is the main location; histology mostly shows haemangioma-like proliferation.

Gorlin–Goltz syndrome (Gorlin syndrome; multiple basal cell naevi syndrome). Autosomal dominant trait, with multiple basal cell carcinomas, odontogenic keratocysts, vertebral and rib anomalies.

Graves disease. Hyperthyroidism with ophthalmopathy and exophthalmos (Ch. 6).

Grinspan syndrome. Lichen planus, diabetes and hypertension (probably actually due to lichenoid reactions to antihypertensive and antidiabetic drugs).

Guillain–Barré syndrome. Acute infective polyneuritis; facial palsy may be seen.

Hailey–Hailey disease. Autosomal dominant benign familial pemphigus presenting in second or third decade with skin and oral blisters and vegetations.

Hajdu–Cheney syndrome. Ulcerating lesions on the palms of the hands and soles of the feet; with softening and destruction of bones (acro-osteolysis).

Hallerman–Streiff syndrome. Congenital cranial anomalies, micro-ophthalmia, cataracts, mandibular hypoplasia and abnormal temporomandibular joint.

Hand–Schuller–Christian disease. Langerhans histiocytosis causing skull lesions, exophthalmos and diabetes insipidus (Ch. 8).

Hansen disease. Leprosy.

Heck disease. Focal epithelial hyperplasia. Caused by HPV 13 or 32, seen especially in various ethnic groups such as American native Indians and Inuits.

Heefordt syndrome (uveoparotid fever). Sarcoidosis associated with lacrimal and salivary swelling, uveitis, fever and sometimes facial palsy (Ch. 15).

Henoch–Schonlein purpura. Allergic purpura, typically following streptococcal infection.

Hermansky–Pudlak syndrome. Congenital albinism and bleeding tendency.

Hirschsprung disease. Congenital aganglionic megacolon.

Hodgkin disease. Nearly one-half of all lymphomas are Hodgkin disease, which can affect any age group, particularly males in middle age (Ch. 8).

Horner syndrome. Usually unilateral miosis (pupil constriction); ptosis (drooping of the upper eyelid); loss of sweating of the ipsilateral face; enophthalmos (retruded eyeball). Caused by interruption of sympathetic nerve fibres peripherally (e.g. as a result of trauma to the neck, or lung cancer infiltrating the superior cervical sympathetic ganglion) (Ch. 13).

Horton cephalgia. Migrainous neuralgia.

Hunter syndrome. A mucopolysaccharidosis.

Hunterian chancre. Syphilitic primary chancre.

Hurler syndrome (Hurler–Scheie syndrome). Congenital mucopolysaccharidosis causing growth failure, learning disability, large head, frontal bossing, hypertelorism, coarse facial features (gargoylism) and mandibular radiolucencies (Ch. 23).

Hutchinson–Gilford syndrome (progeria). See Werner syndrome.

Hutchinson teeth. Screwdriver-shaped incisor teeth in congenital syphilis.

Hutchinson triad. Hutchinson's teeth, interstitial keratitis and deafness.

Immerslund–Grasbeck syndrome. Congenital vitamin B_{12} deficiency.

Jackson–Lawler syndrome. A type of pachyonychia in congenital syphilis with no oral leukoplakia, but neonatal teeth and early loss of secondary teeth.

Jadassohn–Lewandosky syndrome. Pachyonychia congenita.

Jones syndrome. See Curry–Jones syndrome.

Kaposi sarcoma. Malignant neoplasm of endothelial cells caused by human herpesvirus 8 seen mainly in AIDS, immunosuppressed patients, elderly Jews and those of Mediterranean or Middle Eastern origin (Ch. 20).

Kartagener syndrome. Congenital dextrocardia, immunodeficiency and sinusitis.

Kawasaki disease (mucocutaneous lymph node syndrome). Idiopathic disorder with fever, lymphadenopathy, desquamation of hand and feet, cheilitis and cardiac lesions.

Kearns–Sayre syndrome. A mitochondrial cardiomyopathy.

Kikuchi–Fujimoto disease. A self-limiting lymphadenopathy that can be confused histologically and clinically with lymphoma or systemic lupus erythematosus.

Kimura disease. A chronic inflammatory disorder, mostly in males, causing a painless, slowly enlarging, soft-tissue mass, lymphadenopathy and peripheral eosinophilia.

Kindler syndrome. Autosomal recessive skin disorder with blistering, photosensitivity, progressive poikiloderma and diffuse cutaneous atrophy.

Klinefelter syndrome. A chromosomal abnormality affecting men and causing hypogonadism.

Klippel–Feil anomalad. Congenital association of cervical vertebrae fusion with short neck, low-lying posterior hairline, syringomyelia and other neurological anomalies, and sometimes unilateral renal agenesis and cardiac anomalies.

Koplik spots. Small white spots on the buccal mucosa in measles prodrome.

Kveim test. Outdated skin test for sarcoidosis using antigen from the lymph nodes or spleen of human sarcoidosis patients, injected intracutaneously.

Laband syndrome (Zimmerman–Laband syndrome). Hereditary gingival fibromatosis with skeletal anomalies and large digits.

Langerhans cell histiocytoses (histiocytosis X). Rare tumours arising from dendritic intraepithelial antigen-presenting cells (Langerhans cells) (Ch. 8).

Larsen syndrome. Autosomal recessive condition, consisting of cleft palate, flattened facies, multiple congenital dislocations and deformities of feet.

Laugier–Hunziker–Baran syndrome. A rare, acquired, benign hyperpigmentation of the lips, oral mucosa and nails.

Laurence–Moon–Biedl syndrome. Congenital retinitis pigmentosa, obesity, polydactyly, learning disability and blindness.

Leigh disease. A progressive neurodegenerative disorder related to respiratory chain deficiency.

Lesch–Nyhan syndrome. Congenital defect of purine metabolism causing learning disability, choreoathetoid cerebral palsy and self-multilation.

Letterer–Siwe disease. Rapidly progressive disseminated form of Langerhans histiocytosis, often fatal because of pancytopenia and multisystem disease (Ch. 8).

Lewar disease. Pulse granuloma.

Löfgren syndrome. Acute benign form of sarcoidosis, with erythema nodosum and bilateral hilar lymphadenopathy (Ch. 15).

Lowe syndrome (cerebrohepatorenal syndrome). Congenital hypotonia and flexion contractures.

Ludwig angina. Infection of sublingual and submandibular fascial spaces.

Lyme disease. *Borrelia burgdorferii* infection from deer ticks, causing rashes, fever, arthopathy and facial palsy. First recognised in Lyme, Connecticut, USA.

Madelung disease. Benign symmetrical lipomatosis.

Maffucci syndrome. Multiple enchondromas, haemangiomas (often in the tongue) and risk of malignant chondrosarcomas.

MAGIC syndrome. Mouth And Genital ulcers and Interstitial Chondritis – a variant of the Behçet syndrome.

Mallory–Weiss syndrome. Mucosal gastric tear near the oesophageal/stomach junction causing bleeding.

Mantoux test. Skin test for delayed-type hypersensitivity reaction to bacillus Calmette–Guérin (BCG; for tuberculosis).

Maroteaux–Lamy syndrome. A mucopolysaccharidosis.

Marcus Gunn syndrome. Jaw-winking syndrome (eyelid winks during chewing), with ptosis.

Marfan syndrome. Autosomal dominant condition in which patient is tall, thin and has arachnodactyly (long, thin, spider-like hands) (Ch. 16).

Marie–Sainton syndrome. Cleidocranial dysplasia.

Meig syndrome. Ascites, pleural effusion and benign ovarian tumour.

Melkersson–Rosenthal syndrome. Facial swelling similar to that in Crohn disease or orofacial granulomatosis, with facial palsy and fissured tongue.

Mendelson syndrome. Inhalation of gastric contents causing pulmonary oedema.

Ménière disease. Labyrinthine dysfunction with vertigo, tinnitus and sensorineural hearing loss, with nausea and sometimes nystagmus. Betahistine and cinnarizine have been promoted as specific treatments but phenothiazines, prochlorperazine or thiethylperazine may be required.

Miescher cheilitis. Oligosymptomatic orofacial granulomatosis or Crohn disease affecting the lip alone.

Migrainous neuralgia (cluster headaches; histamine cephalgia; Sluder headaches). Pain in the head and face, defined by the International Headache Society as unilateral, excruciatingly severe attacks of pain in the ocular, frontal and temporal areas, recurring in separate bouts with daily or almost daily attacks for weeks or months, usually with ipsilateral lacrimation, conjunctival injection, photophobia and nasal stuffiness and/or rhinorrhoea.

Mikulicz disease. Salivary gland and lacrimal gland swelling often related to Sjögren syndrome.

Mikulicz syndrome. Salivary gland and lacrimal gland swelling related to malignant disease.

Mikulicz ulcer. Minor aphthous ulceration.

Miller syndrome. Autosomal recessive post-axial acrofacial dysostosis.

Moebius syndrome. Congenital anomaly involving multiple cranial nerves, mainly the abducens (VI) and facial (VII), often associated with limb anomalies.

Moon molars. Hypoplastic molars from congenital syphilis.

Morquio syndrome. A mucopolysaccharidosis (Ch. 23).

Munchausen syndrome. The fabrication of stories by the patient, aimed at the patient receiving operative intervention (Ch. 10).

Murray–Puretic–Drescher syndrome (juvenile hyaline fibromatosis). Autosomal recessive disease characterized by large cutaneous nodules, especially around the head and neck, joint contractures, gingival swelling and osteolytic lesions.

Nager syndrome. Acrofacial dysostosis.

Nelson syndrome. Hyperpigmentation caused by ACTH overproduction in response to adrenalectomy – used for breast cancer (Ch. 6).

Neumann bipolar aphthosis. The association of recurrent aphthae with genital ulceration; this is probably emerging Behçet syndrome.

Nikolsky sign. Blistering, or the extension of a blister, on gentle pressure (seen in pemphigus and pemphigoid) (Ch. 11).

Noonan syndrome. Congenital short stature and webbed neck, sometimes with cardiac anomalies, pulmonary stenosis and cherubism.

Ollier syndrome. Multiple enchondromas.

Osler–Rendu–Weber disease (hereditary haemorrhagic telangiectasia; HHT). Autosomal dominant disorder where telangiectases are present orally and periorally and in the nose, gastrointestinal tract and occasionally on the palms (Ch. 8).

Paget disease. Disease of bone (Ch. 16).

Papillon–Lefevre syndrome. Congenital defect in cathepsin C, causing palmoplantar hyperkeratosis, juvenile periodontitis, which affects both dentitions, and immunodeficiency.

Parrot nodes. Frontal bossing in congenital syphilis.

Parry–Romberg syndrome. Hemifacial atrophy.

Patterson–Brown-Kelly syndrome (Plummer–Vinson syndrome). Dysphagia (due to a post-cricoid candida web), microcytic hypochromic anaemia, koilonychia and angular cheilitis (secondary to the anaemia) (Ch. 8).

Paul–Bunnell test (Paul–Bunnell–Davidsohn). Serological test for heterophile antibodies in infectious mononucleosis (glandular fever).

Peutz–Jegher syndrome. Autosomal dominant condition of circumoral melanosis and intestinal polyposis.

Pfeiffer syndrome. Craniosynostosis.

Pierre Robin sequence. Congenital micrognathia, cleft palate and glossoptosis.

Pindborg tumour. Calcifying epithelial odontogenic tumour.

Plummer–Vinson syndrome. See Patterson–Kelly-Brown syndrome.

Popischill–Feyrter aphthae. Palatal ulceration in neonates.

Prader–Willi syndrome. Congenital obesity, hypogonadism, learning disability, diabetes and dental defects.

Quincke oedema. Angioedema.

Ramon syndrome. Cherubism, arthritis, epilepsy, gingival fibromatosis and learning disability.

Ramsay–Hunt syndrome. Lower motor neuron facial palsy with vesicles in ipsilateral pharynx, external auditory canal, and face – due to herpes zoster of the geniculate ganglion of the VIIth nerve.

Rapp–Hodgkin syndrome. Ectodermal dysplasia, kinky hair, cleft lip/palate, popliteal pterygium and ectrodactyly.

Raynaud syndrome. Vascular spasm in response to cooling, seen in the digits in connective tissue disorders (Ch. 18).

Reiter disease. Association of arthritis, urethritis and balanitis, and conjunctivitis, found mainly in men with sexually transmitted disease and HLA-B27.

Rett syndrome. Congenital bruxism and hand-wringing, often with learning disability.

Reye syndrome. Rare serious illness affecting brain and liver, in children after viral infection and treated with aspirin.

Reynolds syndrome. A rare autoimmune disease, consisting of the combination of primary biliary cirrhosis and progressive systemic sclerosis.

Rieger syndrome. Congenital ocular anomalies, iridal hypoplasia, glaucoma, maxillary hypoplasia and dental hypoplasia with oligodontia and microdontia.

Riley–Day syndrome. Inherited familial dysautonomia, seen particularly in Ashkenazi Jews. Sympathetic dysfunction, enlarged salivary glands, sialorrhoea and self-mutilation.

Robinow syndrome. Fetal facies syndrome, a rare autosomal syndrome of short stature, characteristic facial dysmorphism, genital hypoplasia and mesomelic brachymelia.

Romberg syndrome (Parry-Romberg syndrome hemifacial atrophy). Progressive atrophy of half the face, associated with contralateral Jacksonian epilepsy and trigeminal neuralgia.

Rosai–Dorfman syndrome (sinus histiocytosis with massive lymphadenopathy or Destombes–Rosai–Dorfman syndrome). A benign histiocytic proliferative disorder that primarily affects lymph nodes.

Rothmund–Thomson syndrome. Congenital poikiloderma, hypogonadism, dwarfism, cataracts and microdontia.

Rubinstein–Taybi syndrome (broad thumb–great toe syndrome). Short stature, small head, prominent beaked nose, down-slanting eyes, developmental delay, broad, sometimes angulated thumbs and first toes. Undescended testes occur in males. Other variable features include congenital heart disease, kidney abnormalities, eye and hearing problems.

Rud syndrome. Recessive disorder marked by ichthyosis, hypogonadism, learning disability, epilepsy and dwarfism.

Rutherfurd syndrome. Corneal dystrophy, gingival fibromatosis and delayed tooth eruption.

Ruvalcaba–Myrhe–Smith syndrome. Congenital macrocephaly, learning disability, intestinal polyps, pigmented macules on penis, tongue polyps.

Sabin–Feldmann test. Serological test for toxoplasmosis.

Saethre–Chotzen syndrome. Autosomal dominant craniosynostosis with cleft palate and other disturbances of the facial skeleton and extremities.

Sanfilippo syndrome. A mucopolysaccharidosis.

SAPHO syndrome. Synovitis, Acne, Pustulosis, Hyperostosis and Osteitis.

Scheie syndrome. A mucopolysaccharidosis (Ch. 23).

Schmidt syndrome. Congenital hypoadrenocorticism, hypoparathyroidism, diabetes and malabsorption, with candidosis.

Seckel syndrome. Congenital microcephaly, learning disability, zygomatic and mandibular hypoplasia.

Shprintzen syndrome. Velocardiofacial syndrome.

Shwachman–Diamond syndrome. Rare disorder affecting the pancreas, bone marrow – with neutropenia and thrombocytopenia – and skeletal defects.

Sipple syndrome. Multiple endocrine neoplasia (MEN) type 3 (MEN 3; sometimes called 2b) affecting several endocrine glands with multiple mucosal neuromas, phaeochromocytoma and medullary thyroid carcinoma (Ch. 6).

Sjögren syndrome. Xerostomia and keratoconjunctivitis sicca (i.e. dry mouth and dry eyes) (Ch. 18).

Sjögren–Larsson syndrome. Congenital ichthyosis, learning disability, cerebral palsy and indifference to pain.

Sluder syndrome. Migrainous neuralgia.

Sly syndrome. A mucopolysaccharidosis.

Smith–Lemli–Opitz syndrome. Congenital short stature, learning disability, syndactyly, urogenital and maxillary anomalies.

SSS syndrome (silent sinus syndrome). A rare entity of unilateral enophthalmos and hypoglobus secondary to thinning of the maxillary sinus roof in the absence of sinonasal inflammatory disease.

Stevens–Johnson syndrome. Severe erythema multiforme (Ch. 11).

Stickler syndrome. Collagenopathy affecting collagens II and IX, causing a distinctive facial appearance, eye abnormalities, hearing loss and joint problems.

Still disease. Juvenile rheumatoid arthritis.

Sturge–Weber syndrome (encephalotrigeminal angiomatosis). Congenital hamartomatous angioma of upper face (naevus flammeus), oral mucosa and underlying bone (with hemihypertrophy of bone and accelerated eruption of associated teeth), extending intracranially to cause convulsions, and contralateral hemiplegia and intracerebral calcifications, and sometimes learning disability.

Sutton's ulcers. Major aphthae.

Sweet syndrome. Acute neutrophilic dermatosis; red mucosal lesions and aphthae.

Takayasu disease. Pulseless aorta and large arteries.

Thibierge–Weissenbach syndrome. The CREST syndrome – scleroderma with calcinosis and ischaemia.

Treacher Collins syndrome (mandibulofacial dysostosis). Autosomal dominant defect in first branchial arch with downward-sloping (antimongoloid slant) palpebral fissures, hypoplastic malar, mandibular retrognathia, deformed pinnas, hypoplastic sinuses, colobomas in outer third of the eye, middle and inner ear hypoplasia (deafness).

Trotter syndrome. Acquired unilateral deafness, pain in mandibular (third) division of trigeminal nerve, ipsilateral palatal immobility, and trismus due to invasion of nasopharynx and trigeminal nerve, by a malignant tumour. Pterygopalatine fossa syndrome is a similar condition where first and second divisions of trigeminal nerve are affected.

Turner teeth. Hypoplastic tooth due to damage to the developing tooth germ.

Tzanck cells. Abnormal squamous cells in pemphigus or herpetic infections

Urbach–Wiethe disease. Lipoid proteinosis.

Van der Woude syndrome. Cleft lip or palate with lip pits and hypodontia.

Vincent disease (acute ulcerative gingivitis). Non-contagious anaerobic infection with overwhelming proliferation of *Borrelia*

vincentii and fusiform bacteria. Predisposing factors include smoking, viral respiratory infections and immune defects such as in HIV/AIDS.

von Hippel–Lindau disease. Autosomal dominant condition with café-au-lait spots, retinal angiomatosis, CNS haemangioblastomas, phaeochromocytomas, pancreatic neuroendocrine tumours and renal cancer.

Von Recklinghausen disease. Multiple neurofibromas with skin pigmentation, skeletal abnormalities and central nervous system involvement (Ch. 13).

Von Willebrand disease. Common bleeding disorder caused by defective blood clotting factor VIII and platelet dysfunction (Ch. 8).

Waardenburg syndrome. Congenital heterochromia iridis (differently coloured eyes), deafness and white forelock, with prognathism.

Waldeyer ring. Lymphoid tissue surrounding the entrance to the oropharynx (tonsils and adenoids).

Warthin tumour. A benign salivary gland neoplasm – adenolymphoma or papillary cystadenoma lymphomatosum.

Wegener granulomatosis. Idiopathic disseminated malignant granulomatous disorder which may affect lungs, kidneys and mouth, sometimes related to *Staphylococcus aureus* (Ch. 8).

Weil disease. Leptospirosis.

Werner syndrome. Congenital alopecia, dwarfism, senility, early atherosclerosis, delayed tooth eruption and mandibular hypoplasia.

Whipple disease. A bacterial infection with *Tropheryma whippelii*, which affects primarily middle-aged white men.

Williams syndrome. Genetic disorder of cognitive impairment (usually mild learning disability), unique personality characteristics, distinctive ('elfin') facial features, and cardiovascular disease (elastin arteriopathy).

Wilson disease. Hepatolenticular degeneration.

Wiskott–Aldrich syndrome. X-linked recessive immunodeficiency with thrombocytopenia, eczema, infections and lymphoreticular malignancies (Ch. 20).

Witkop disease. Hereditary benign intraepithelial dyskeratosis – seen mainly in parts of the USA.

Yersiniosis. Infection with *Yersinia pseudotuberculosis*.

Zimmerman–Laband syndrome. See Laband syndrome.

Zinsser–Engman–Cole syndrome. Rare syndrome of skin pigmentation, oral leukoplakia, nail dystrophy, pancytopenia and predisposition to malignancy.

Zollinger–Ellison syndrome. Comprises intractable peptic ulcers, high gastric acidity and gastrin-secreting, non-beta islet cell tumours (nesidioblastomas), usually of the pancreas, but sometimes duodenum (Ch. 7).

USEFUL WEBSITES

http://www.all-acronyms.com/cat/7

FURTHER READING

Scully, C., Langdon, J., Evans, J. 2009. Marathon of eponyms: 1 Albers–Schonberg disease (osteopetrosis). Oral Dis 15, 246–247.

Scully, C., Langdon, J., Evans, J. 2009. Marathon of eponyms: 2 Bell palsy (idiopathic facial palsy). Oral Dis 15, 307–308.

Scully, C., Langdon, J., Evans, J. 2009. Marathon of eponyms: 3 Crouzon syndrome. Oral Dis 15, 367–368.

Scully, C., Langdon, J., Evans, J. 2009. Marathon of eponyms: 4 Down syndrome. Oral Dis 15, 434–436.

Scully, C., Langdon, J., Evans, J. 2009. Marathon of eponyms: 5 Ehlers–Danlos syndrome. Oral Dis 15, 517–518.

Scully, C., Langdon, J., Evans, J. 2009. Marathon of eponyms: 6 Frey syndrome (gustatory sweating). Oral Dis 15, 608–609.

Scully, C., Langdon, J., Evans, J. Marathon of eponyms: 7 Gorlin syndrome. Oral Dis (in press).

Scully, C., Langdon, J., Evans, J. Marathon of eponyms: 8 Hodgkin disease or lymphoma. Oral Dis (in press).

Scully, C., Langdon, J., Evans, J. Marathon of eponyms: 9 Immerslund–Grasbeck syndrome. Oral Dis (in press).

Scully, C., Langdon, J., Evans, J. Marathon of eponyms: 10 Jadassohn–Lewandosky syndrome. Oral Dis (in press).

Scully, C., Langdon, J., Evans, J. Marathon of eponyms: 11 Kaposi sarcoma. Oral Dis (in press).

Scully, C., Langdon, J., Evans, J. Marathon of eponyms: 12 Ludwig angina. Oral Dis (in press).

Scully, C., Langdon, J., Evans, J. Marathon of eponyms: 13 Melkersson–Rosenthal syndrome. Oral Dis (in press).

Scully, C., Langdon, J., Evans, J. Marathon of eponyms: 14 Noonan syndrome. Oral Dis (in press).

Scully, C., Langdon, J., Evans, J. Marathon of eponyms: 15 Osler–Rendu–Weber disease. Oral Dis (in press).

Scully, C., Langdon, J., Evans, J. Marathon of eponyms: 16 Paget disease of bone. Oral Dis (in press).

Scully, C., Langdon, J., Evans, J. Marathon of eponyms: 17 Quinke oedema. Oral Dis (in press).

Scully, C., Langdon, J., Evans, J. Marathon of eponyms: 18 Robin sequence. Oral Dis (in press).

Scully, C., Langdon, J., Evans, J. Marathon of eponyms: 19 Sjögren syndrome. Oral Dis (in press).

Scully, C., Langdon, J., Evans, J. Marathon of eponyms: 20 Treacher Collins syndrome. Oral Dis (in press).

Scully, C., Langdon, J., Evans, J. Marathon of eponyms: 21 Urbach–Wiethe disease. Oral Dis (in press).

Scully, C., Langdon, J., Evans, J. Marathon of eponyms: 22 Virchow node. Oral Dis (in press).

Scully, C., Langdon, J., Evans, J. Marathon of eponyms: 23 Wegener granulomatosis. Oral Dis (in press).

Scully, C., Langdon, J., Evans, J. Marathon of eponyms: 24 Xmas (Christmas) disease. Oral Dis (in press).

Scully, C., Langdon, J., Evans, J. Marathon of eponyms: 25 Yersiniosis. Oral Dis (in press).

Scully, C., Langdon, J., Evans, J. Marathon of eponyms: 26 Zinsser–Cole–Engman syndrome. Oral Dis (in press).

INDEX